CW01072747

Reflectance Confocal Microscopy for Skin Diseases

Rainer Hofmann-Wellenhof
Giovanni Pellacani • Josep Malvehy
Hans Peter Soyer
(Editors)

Reflectance Confocal Microscopy for Skin Diseases

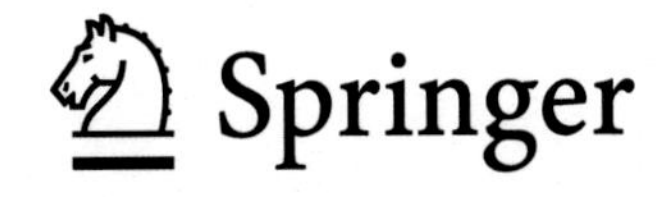

Editors
Dr. Rainer Hofmann-Wellenhof
Department of Dermatology and Venerology
Medical University of Graz
Graz
Austria

Prof. Joseph Malvehy
Department of Dermatology, Melanoma Unit
Hospital Clinic of Barcelona
Barcelona
Spain

Prof. Giovanni Pellacani
Department of Dermatology and Venereology
University of Modena and Reggio Emilia
Modena
Italy

Dr. Hans Peter Soyer
Dermatology Research Centre
The University of Queensland
School of Medicine
Princess Alexandra Hospital
Brisbane, Queensland
Australia

ISBN 978-3-642-21996-2 e-ISBN 978-3-642-21997-9
DOI 10.1007/978-3-642-21997-9
Springer Heidelberg Dordrecht London New York

Library of Congress Control Number: 2011944200

Printed on acid-free paper

Springer is part of Springer Science+Business Media (www.springer.com)

Preface

We, a group of close friends and colleagues from Austria, Spain, Italy and Australia, share an enthusiasm and passion for the macro and micro morphology of the many faces of inflammatory and neoplastic skin conditions. We have each been involved in undergraduate and postgraduate teaching as well as continuing professional development in this arena for many years. Specifically, we are excited not only by dermatopathology and dermoscopy, but in the last few years we have embraced reflectance confocal microscopy (RCM), a technique we believe will lead to a paradigmal change in the way diagnosis and monitoring in dermatology will be conducted in the future. As such, it seems logical that we were keen to elaborate a new text and atlas on this fascinating in vivo, cutaneous, black and white pathology. One of the biggest stumbling blocks for us to initially overcome in this endeavour was the fact that an excellent text and atlas on the subject in debate already exists. The book entitled "Reflectance Confocal Microscopy of Cutaneous Tumors: An Atlas with Clinical, Dermoscopic and Histological Correlations" by Salvador Gonzalez, Melissa Gill and Allan C. Halpern, Taylor and Francis Group, London (UK), 2007 is a masterpiece in its own right and one might even think that the writing and publication of a second text and atlas on RCM would simply be superfluous. We believe, however, that a novel technology like confocal microscopy will benefit from the production of additional reference books to enable a more detailed understanding of the most important concepts that cannot be easily interpreted from scientific publications in peer review journals. Reference books should complement each other and further enrich the body of teaching material required to facilitate dissemination of one area of expertise among the wider medical community.

To make a long story short, we have discussed this topic at length and worked hard to present you the SECOND text atlas on RCM providing updated concepts and new approaches in this imaging technique. We sought to have a format that reproduced the real-life confocal examination, employing wide mosaics for the general overview of the architecture and moving in a step-wise fashion towards high resolution where evaluation of cytological details is possible. For an easier use of the book in the daily practice, numerous cases have been outlined for various clinical situations, with explicit figure legends and intuitive schematics.

The unique format of the book provides:

1. Hundreds of high quality figures that reproduce the process of real imaging and reading in confocal microscopy from dermoscopy to the architectural overview and specific cellular observations
2. Inclusion of high resolution images of wide vivablocks to explore tumour architecture with precise correlation of the most relevant cellular findings presented in detailed windows
3. Inclusion of hundreds of drawings and schematics of the tumour criteria identified in confocal reflectance microscopy to facilitate reader comprehension
4. New concepts and knowledge arising from recent research in the field of confocal microscopy

We enjoyed writing this book together with the various authors of the different chapters and wish to thank them all for a great collaborative effort. We trust that our book will further help to promote in vivo cutaneous pathology to the medical community. We look forward to finding our book located beside RCM devices in both the real and virtual bookshelves of colleagues embracing this exciting new dimension of cutaneous morphology.

Graz, Austria — Rainer Hofmann-Wellenhof
Modena, Italy — Giovanni Pellacani
Barcelona, Spain — Josep Malvehy
Brisbane, Queensland, Australia — Hans Peter Soyer

Contents

Part I

Confocal Reflectance Microscopy: The Essentials

The Confocal Story

1

Elisabeth M.T. Wurm and Hans Peter Soyer

Dermatologic diagnosis is primarily based on interpretation of morphological information by visual inspection, confirmed by histopathological diagnosis if necessary. The challenge is to establish a correct diagnosis and to identify all malignant lesions while minimizing unnecessary surgical procedures. In this context, several non-invasive imaging modalities have emerged in recent years that are aimed at increasing accuracy of in vivo diagnosis. Of those, reflectance confocal microscopy has shown the most promising results. In vivo reflectance confocal microscopy produces horizontal images of the skin at a cellular resolution from the surface to the upper dermis. It enables to visualize tissue in its physiological state avoiding retraction bias due to fixation, staining and sectioning procedures that are a prerequisite to conventional light histopathology. Moreover, RCM enables observation of changes over time.

The principle of confocal scanning microscopy relies on single-point illumination and a pinhole in an optically conjugate plane (hence the name confocal) in front of the detector to eliminate out-of-focus signal and on scans of a given specimen point by point (see Chap. 2). The confocal scanning microscope was invented originally by Marvin Minsky in 1955, but was only published as a patent and went unrecognized by a broader public for decades [1]. It was not until the 1990s that confocal microscopy experienced a revival spurred by technological advancements that have helped to decrease the size of the microscope from a spacious machine filling a whole laboratory room down to handheld device that provides mobility to be applied on the bedside [2, 3] (Fig. 1.1). The interest in the use of reflectance confocal microscopy for imaging of human skin – and thus the number of related publications – has risen sharply in recent years. A search of MEDLINE (search phrases: reflectance confocal microscopy & skin) in 2000 would have displayed ten publications on RCM. By November 2010 that number has grown to more than 150 publications displayed.

Confocal laser scanning microscopy (CLSM) may be used either in reflectance mode (RCM) or fluorescence mode (FLSM). In the latter, imaging relies on endogenous and exogenous fluorophores. Fluorescent dyes are used as exogenous sources of contrast. A laser beam is used to excite the fluorophores. The company OptiScan Ltd. (Melbourne, Australia) developed a fluorescence confocal microscope for imaging of human skin. A small handheld scanner with an optical fiber is used to illuminate the tissue and to detect fluorescence signals. A single image of 250 × 250 μm can be obtained at different depths (z-stack) but it does not provide imaging of a bigger horizontal field of view (xy-mosaic).

Preliminary projects in skin imaging have not led to a breakthrough in clinical use probably due to limited imaging depth and the necessity to inject exogenous flourophores [4]. The applicability of FLSM for diagnose and therapeutic monitoring of non-invasive therapy of non-melanoma skin cancer (NMSC) have been described, however [5]. A combination of dual-mode reflectance and fluorescence mode has been reported to hold potential in detecting melanoma progression in animal models [6], and devices that combine both modes for use in humans have been recently developed.

Reflectance mode relies on inherent variations in refractive indices of skin structures [7]. In 1967, a tandem scanning reflected light microscope was developed by the group of Petran and Hadravsky [8], commonly using a mercury lamp as a light source [7]. It was first used for imaging of excised tissue and later in the late 1980s on organs in living animals, such as imaging of cat's eyes [9] and kidneys in rats [10]. Features of human skin in vivo were presented in the early 1990s [11, 12]. In 1995, Rajadhyaksha et al. [7] described features of human skin using a confocal microscope with laser beams at different wavelengths in the visible and near-infrared band (400–900 nm). In RCM, resolution is inversely related to the wavelength of the illumination source; therefore, commercial

E.M.T. Wurm • H.P. Soyer (✉)
Dermatology Research Centre, The University of Queensland, Princess Alexandra Hospital, School of Medicine
Brisbane, Queensland, Australia
e-mail: e.wurm@uq.edu.au, lissy.wurm@gmail.com; p.soyer@uq.edu.au

R. Hofmann-Wellenhof et al. (eds.), *Reflectance Confocal Microscopy for Skin Diseases*,
DOI 10.1007/978-3-642-21997-9_1, © Springer-Verlag Berlin Heidelberg 2012

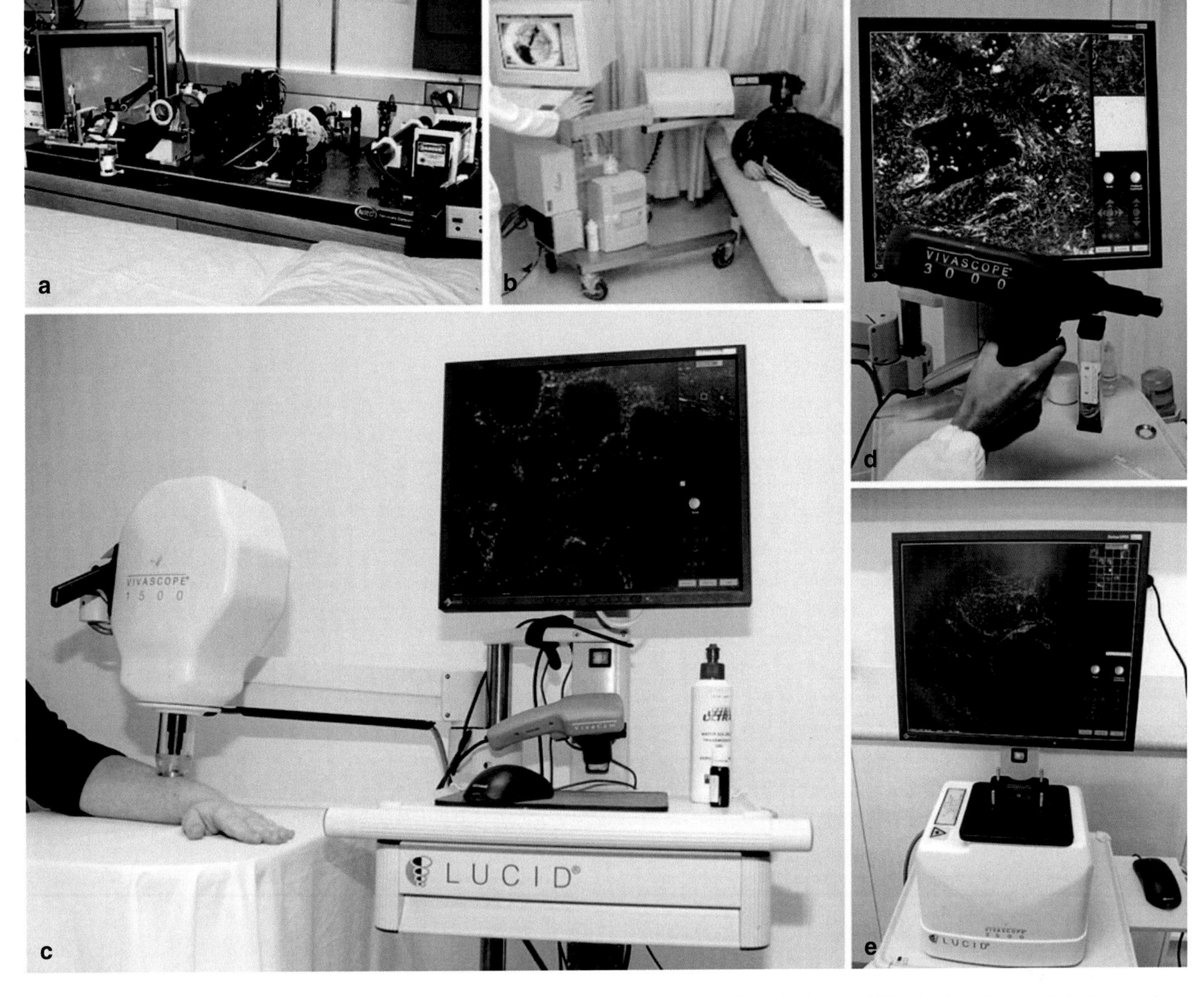

Fig. 1.1 Technical advancements have helped to decrease the size of laser scanning confocal microscopes from spacious machines down to a movable device allowing for clinical imaging at the bedside. (**a**) First confocal microscope for in vivo imaging, Wellman Labs, Dermatology Department, MGH, Harvard Medical School in 1995. (**b**) VivaScope 1000, Dermatology Department, Graz, Austria, in 2005. (**c**) VivaScope 1500, Dermatology Department, Brisbane, Australia, in 2008. (**d**) VivaScope 3000 handheld device, Dermatology Department, Modena, Italy, in 2010. (**e**) VivaScope 2000 for ex vivo imaging My-Lab, Brisbane, Australia, in 2010

confocal microscopes nowadays use laser beams in the near-infrared band [3]. In 1997, the company Lucid Inc. (Rochester, NY, USA) introduced the VivaScope 1000 with a laser source at 830 nm wavelength and a power of less than 30 mW that causes no tissue damage. Basic images had a size of 128 μm by 260 μm, allowing imaging over a square of 1.5 mm by 1.5 mm [13]. The first generation confocal microscope had a bulky configuration impeding convenient attachment to certain anatomical areas. Imaging was very time consuming. In the year 2000, the VivaScope 1500, the to date most widely used confocal microscope for imaging of human skin, was commercialized. This device is considerably smaller, more flexible and movable as opposed to its stationary predecessor. It enables real-time viewing of 500×500 μm basic confocal images. A field of up to 8×8 mm can be scanned and viewed as a mosaic of basic images stitched by software (see Chap. 3). Furthermore, this device is the first to have an integrated dermoscopic camera, underlining the importance of RCM as a natural link between dermoscopy and histopathology. By using the dermoscopic image as a gross map to navigate to a region of interest which can be viewed in real time with the RCM, a correlation between dermoscopy and confocal images is provided. Further developments are the VivaScope 3000, a handheld confocal microscope for imaging of difficult to access areas, and the ex vivo VivaScope 2500 designed for imaging of excised tissue, especially in Mohs surgery as well as Vivascope 1500 Multilaser, which combines FLSM and RCM modes.

Melanin and melanosomes are strong source of contrast that appear bright in the images [7]. This has led to a focus of confocal research in melanocytic lesions. Morphology of naevi and melanoma have been first described in detail in 2001 [14, 15], as well as the potential of the technique to detect clinically amelanotic melanoma [16]. Various diagnostic algorithms for melanoma diagnosis have been recently proposed [17–20]. Other fields of confocal research include non-melanocytic lesions and inflammatory skin diseases. Furthermore, RCM offers a unique tool to assess dynamic changes and to monitor lesions over time. As lesions often expand over what can be perceived with the naked eye, RCM can help to detect the true surgical margins preoperatively. All these applications will be addressed in this book.

As in every morphologic discipline the interpretation and thus description of structures is subjective and may depend on the socio-cultural background of the observer. In such a "young" discipline as RCM, this has led to a variation of terms used for similar features that may confound the novice. In order to overcome this, a consensus for standard RCM terminology has been published in 2007 [21] and tested for reproducibility [22]. Moreover, an international confocal microscopy working group has been founded, aiming at supporting education and collaborative research in this field. There is a learning curve to mastering diagnosis with reflectance confocal microscopy. Besides the work in the reader's hands, to date only one book about reflectance confocal microscopy of cutaneous tumors has been published [23]. To gain diagnostic confidence, a novice has to have viewed and evaluated a considerable amount of lesions which, in a real clinical setting, would require a considerable amount of time. In order to overcome this, the Skin Confocal Microscopy training platform has been created [24]. Features of this website comprise a tutorial displaying and explaining the most common features of benign and malignant skin lesions and a training platform to review single features and to diagnose lesions in a reproduced clinical setting. Although the future cannot be predicted, we are confident that morphologic evaluation is irreplaceable in dermatologic diagnosis and RCM is predestined to enhance diagnosis and move it closer to the bedside. Based on the fast-paced developments in the field of biophotonics, we foresee a future with more powerful and user-friendly confocal devices. The confocal story has just begun.

References

1. Minsky M (1988) Memoir on inventing the confocal scanning microscope. Scanning 10:128–138
2. Psaty EL, Halpern AC (2009) Current and emerging technologies in melanoma diagnosis: the state of the art. Clin Dermatol 27:35–45
3. Gonzalez S (2009) Confocal reflectance microscopy in dermatology: promise and reality of non-invasive diagnosis and monitoring. Actas Dermosifiliogr 100(Suppl 2):59–69
4. Swindle LD, Thomas SG, Freeman M, Delaney PM (2003) View of normal human skin in vivo as observed using fluorescent fiber-optic confocal microscopic imaging. J Invest Dermatol 121:706–712
5. Astner S, Dietterle S, Otberg N et al (2008) Clinical applicability of in vivo fluorescence confocal microscopy for noninvasive diagnosis and therapeutic monitoring of nonmelanoma skin cancer. J Biomed Opt 13:014003
6. Li Y, Gonzalez S, Terwey TH et al (2005) Dual mode reflectance and fluorescence confocal laser scanning microscopy for in vivo imaging melanoma progression in murine skin. J Invest Dermatol 125:798–804
7. Rajadhyaksha M, Grossman M, Esterowitz D et al (1995) In vivo confocal scanning laser microscopy of human skin: melanin provides strong contrast. J Invest Dermatol 104:946–952
8. Egger MD, Petran M (1967) New reflected-light microscope for viewing unstained brain and ganglion cells. Science 157:305–307
9. Cavanagh HD, Jester JV, Essepian J et al (1990) Confocal microscopy of the living eye. CLAO J 16:65–73
10. Andrews PM, Petroll WM, Cavanagh HD, Jester JV (1991) Tandem scanning confocal microscopy (TSCM) of normal and ischemic living kidneys. Am J Anat 191:95–102
11. Corcuff P, Leveque JL (1993) In vivo vision of the human skin with the tandem scanning microscope. Dermatology 186:50–54
12. Corcuff P, Bertrand C, Leveque JL (1993) Morphometry of human epidermis in vivo by real-time confocal microscopy. Arch Dermatol Res 285:475–481
13. Sauermann K, Clemann S, Jaspers S et al (2002) Age related changes of human skin investigated with histometric measurements by confocal laser scanning microscopy in vivo. Skin Res Technol 8:52–56
14. Busam KJ, Charles C, Lee G, Halpern AC (2001) Morphologic features of melanocytes, pigmented keratinocytes, and melanophages by in vivo confocal scanning laser microscopy. Mod Pathol 14:862–868
15. Langley RG, Rajadhyaksha M, Dwyer PJ et al (2001) Confocal scanning laser microscopy of benign and malignant melanocytic skin lesions in vivo. J Am Acad Dermatol 45:365–376
16. Busam KJ, Hester K, Charles C et al (2001) Detection of clinically amelanotic malignant melanoma and assessment of its margins by in vivo confocal scanning laser microscopy. Arch Dermatol 137:923–929
17. Pellacani G, Cesinaro AM, Seidenari S (2005) Reflectance-mode confocal microscopy of pigmented skin lesions—improvement in melanoma diagnostic specificity. J Am Acad Dermatol 53:979–985
18. Guitera P, Pellacani G, Crotty KA et al (2010) The impact of in vivo reflectance confocal microscopy on the diagnostic accuracy of lentigo maligna and equivocal pigmented and nonpigmented macules of the face. J Invest Dermatol 130(8):2080–2091
19. Gerger A, Wiltgen M, Langsenlehner U et al (2008) Diagnostic image analysis of malignant melanoma in in vivo confocal laser-scanning microscopy: a preliminary study. Skin Res Technol 14:359–363
20. Segura S, Puig S, Carrera C et al (2009) Development of a two-step method for the diagnosis of melanoma by reflectance confocal microscopy. J Am Acad Dermatol 61:216–229
21. Scope A, Benvenuto-Andrade C, Agero AL et al (2007) In vivo reflectance confocal microscopy imaging of melanocytic skin lesions: consensus terminology glossary and illustrative images. J Am Acad Dermatol 57:644–658
22. Pellacani G, Vinceti M, Bassoli S et al (2009) Reflectance confocal microscopy and features of melanocytic lesions: an internet-based study of the reproducibility of terminology. Arch Dermatol 145:1137–1143
23. Gonzales S, Gill M, Halpern A (eds) (2008) Reflectance confocal microscopy of cutaneous tumors. Thomson Publishing Services, Hampshire
24. Skin Confocal Microscopy. http://www.skinconfocalmicroscopy.org/. Accessed 15 May 2010

2 How Reflectance Confocal Microscopy Works

Isabel Kolm and Ralph P. Braun

2.1 Introduction

Because melanoma in advanced stages is still incurable, early detection is indispensable to reduce mortality. Therefore, several in vivo noninvasive diagnostic techniques, such as dermoscopy and digital epiluminescence, high-frequency ultrasonography, optical coherence tomography and reflectance confocal microscopy, have been developed during the last decades. The purpose of all this noninvasive technologies is to help the clinician in real- time diagnostics of melanoma suspicious lesions at an earlier, curable stage, while avoiding unnecessary scars from surgical biopsies of benign lesions. All of them provide additional information to the clinical inspection, and all of these techniques enable preservation of the tissue and the possibility of storage of the images to follow skin lesions over time.

However, among these techniques, reflectance confocal microscopy (RCM) is the only one that enables the en-face (horizontal plane) visualization of the skin with a resolution at the cellular level (0.5–1.0 μm in the lateral dimension and 4–5 μm in the axial ones) and therefore may provide an alternative to histopathology.

The general principles of RCM were already described by Marvin Minsky in 1957, but it took several decades until the technology improved for the imaging of human skin. The first description of RCM for the imaging of human skin in vivo was given in 1995 by Rajadhyaksha and colleagues.

2.2 Technical Principles of RCM

The device uses a diode laser as a source of monochromatic and coherent light, which penetrates into the skin and illuminates a small point inside the tissue. The light is reflected, goes through a small pinhole and forms an image in the detector. This small pinhole does not allow the reflected light (reflectance) to reach the detector from another tissue point. Therefore, only reflected light from the focal region (confocal) is detected; that is where the term confocal is derived. Light from out-of-focus planes is rejected at the pinhole. Here lies the essential difference to conventional microscopy, where the entire light enters the detector where it is transmitted to a computer and displayed on a monitor. By stepwise movement of the object table, a two-dimensional picture representing parallel sections of the skin is obtained. Figure 2.1 shows a schematic illustration of a reflectance confocal microscope.

The contrast in RCM images relies on the differences in the reflectivity of the tissue, which is depending on chemical and molecular structures. Due to these variations of the refractive index, only a certain portion of the light is reflected. Structures with a higher refractive index appear bright in RCM. Melanin and melanosomes are the strongest natural sources of contrast resulting white in RCM.

The deeper a skin section is the more laser power is needed to penetrate the skin. The commercially used RCM Vivascope 1500 uses a laser diode with a near-infrared wavelength of 830 nm. Laser power of 830 nm causes no damage to tissue, but limits the imaging depth to 200–300 μm which corresponds to the papillary dermis, depending from the skin site. Higher laser power would provide an increased signal and contrast but would be hazardous for the skin or the eyes.

2.3 Practical Aspects

The examination of a lesion by means of RCM is relatively easy, fast and a painless procedure for the patient. As the skin is not affected by material processing, the occurrence of artifacts is minimized.

A polymer or glass window is attached to a metal ring and fixed to the skin with a special adhesive tape to reduce skin movement. Before, a small amount of immersion oil is applied to the skin which optically couples the window to the

I. Kolm • R.P. Braun (✉)
Department of Dermatology, University Hospital Zurich, Zurich, Switzerland
e-mail: isabel.kolm@usz.ch; ralph.braun@usz.ch

R. Hofmann-Wellenhof et al. (eds.), *Reflectance Confocal Microscopy for Skin Diseases*,
DOI 10.1007/978-3-642-21997-9_2, © Springer-Verlag Berlin Heidelberg 2012

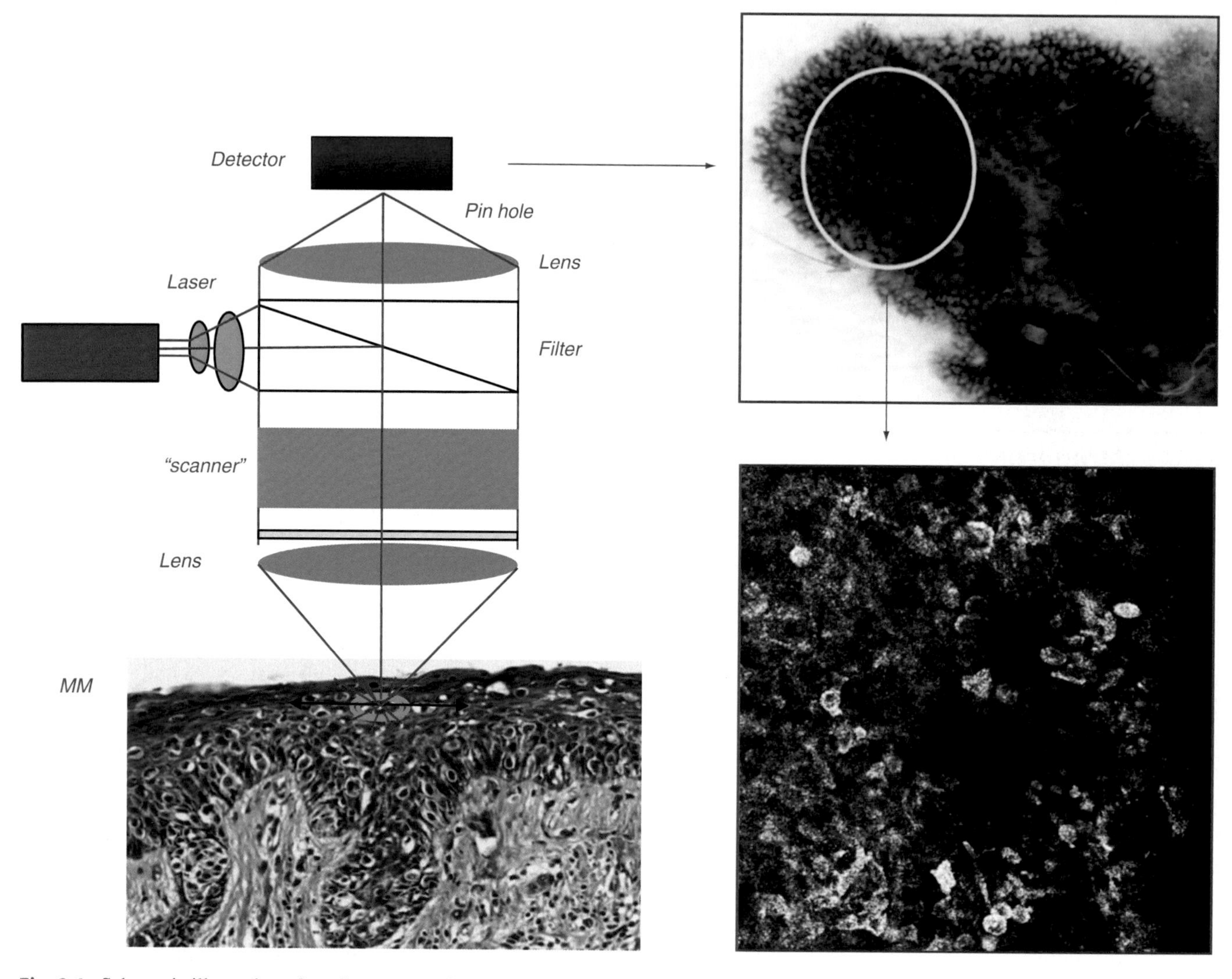

Fig. 2.1 Schematic illustration of a reflectance confocal microscope

sample. Afterwards, inside the ring an immersion liquid (water or water-based gel) is placed. The water-based immersion mediums have refractive indices close to that of the epidermis (1.34), thus reducing the spherical aberration of the beam passing through air and therefore allowing sufficient imaging through the epidermis and into the dermis. The ring is then magnetically connected to the objective lens housing to stabilize the site of imaging.

As mentioned before, RCM images are obtained horizontally from the lesion. Each single image displays a 500 μm × 500 μm large field-of-view on the screen. RCM allows the scanning of the entire area of the lesion up to 8 m × 8 mm; an automated stepper can generate a mosaic grid of contiguous horizontal images. This two-dimensional composite mosaic is called *VivaBlock* (Fig. 2.2). Additionally, an automated vertical sequence of images, each 500 μm field-of-view, can be captured in depth, providing a three-dimensional view of certain area. This is called a *VivaStack* (Fig. 2.3). The distance between each section and the section depth can be adjusted. Another useful function is the possibility to record a video at 15–25 frames per second (adjustable) to document dynamic events such as blood flow, or migration of leucocytes.

For easier correlation of the macroscopic image and the confocal image, a digital macro camera (Vivacam; Lucid Inc) is linked to the RCM. This camera produces a 5 megapixel dermoscopic image of a 10 mm field of interest enabling direct viewing of the dermoscopic structures on the RCM monitor. It is possible to navigate within the dermoscopic image and to specify areas for the subsequent RCM viewing and therefore allows choosing the interesting areas in (larger) lesions and better asses the borders of a lesion which can be very helpful for surgical planning.

2.4 Future Aspects

New developments in RCM show the potential for detection of tumors directly in surgical excisions without further processing of the tissue; for example, detection of the margin in skin excisions from Moh's surgery.

Fig. 2.2 VivaBlock. 5 mm × 5 mm area composed by 100 single images stitched together. A single image displays a 500 μm × 500 μm large field-of-view (*red square*)

Because RCM images do not visually resemble conventional stained pathology sections, intensive training for the clinician is required. But with further advances in the technology and multi-modal forms of contrast (e.g., fluorescence staining) and automated diagnostic aids, RCM is expected to become easier to use and therefore become the ideal tool for "bedside" diagnosis and an indispensable guide prior to surgical procedures.

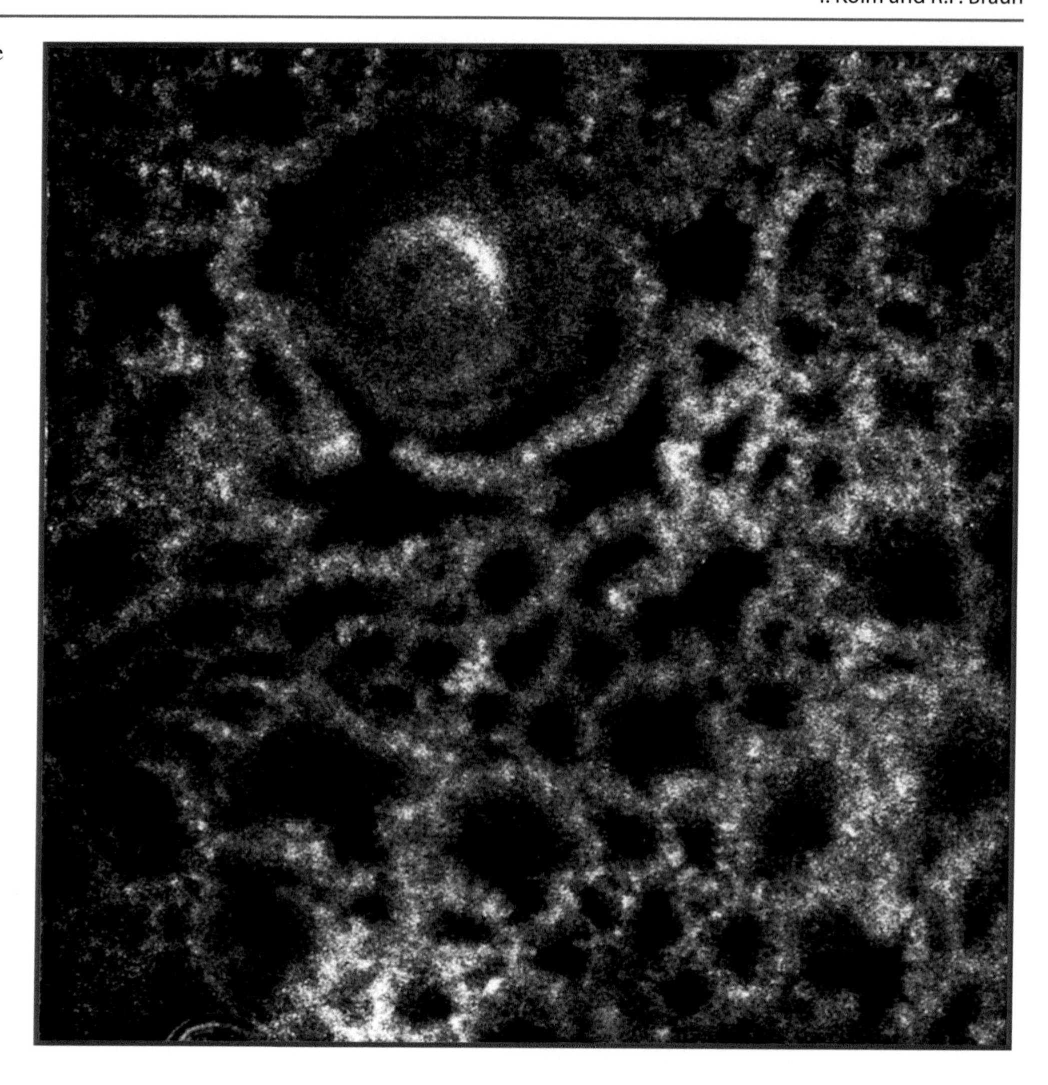

Fig. 2.3 VivaStack. A sequence of single images, captured in depth, providing a three-dimensional impression of a certain area

References

1. Esmaeili A, Scope A, Halpern AC, Marghoob AA (2008) Imaging techniques for the in vivo diagnosis of melanoma. Semin Cutan Med Surg 27:2–10
2. Minsky M (1957) Microscopy apparatus. US Patent 3,013,467
3. Rajadhyaksha M, Grossman M, Esterowitz D, Webb RH, Anderson RR (1995) In vivo confocal scanning laser microscopy of human skin: melanin provides strong contrast. J Invest Dermatol 104:946–952
4. Gareau DS, Patel YG, Rajadhyaksha M (2008) Basic principles of reflectance confocal microscopy. In: Gonzalez S, Gill M, Halpern AC (eds) Reflectance confocal microscopy of cutaneous tumors. An atlas with clinical, dermoscopic and histological correlations. Informa UK Ltd, London, pp 1–6
5. Rajadhyaksha M, Gonzalez S, Zavislan JM, Anderson RR, Webb RH (1999) In vivo confocal scanning laser microscopy of human skin, II: advances in instrumentation and comparison with histology. J Invest Dermatol 113:293–303
6. González S (2009) Confocal reflectance microscopy in dermatology: promise and reality of non-invasive diagnosis and monitoring. Actas Dermosifiliogr 100(Suppl 2):59–69
7. Gareau DS, Patel YG, Li Y, Aranda I, Halpern AC, Nehal KS, Rajadhyaksha M (2009) Confocal mosaicing microscopy in skin excisions: a demonstration of rapid surgical pathology. J Microsc 233(1):149–159
8. Calzavara-Pinton P, Longo C, Venturini M, Sala R, Pellacani G (2008) Reflectance confocal microscopy for in vivo skin imaging. Photochem Photobiol 84(6):1421–1430

A Hands-on Guide to Confocal Imaging

3

Elisabeth M.T. Wurm, Isabel Kolm, and Verena Ahlgrimm-Siess

3.1 Image Acquisition

Once the VivaScope® is started, the microscope probe can be positioned. Patient preparation before imaging a given skin lesion with the VivaScope® 1500 comprises of the following (Fig. 3.1): (i) Oil (e.g., crodamol oil) or water-based gel is used as immersion media between the skin and a subsequently applied polymer window (see below). In the majority of cases, a small drop of oil is applied to the skin (the refractive index of oil = 1.50 comes close to that of the stratum corneum = 1.55); ultrasound gel is occasionally used to fill gaps in nodular skin lesions. (ii) To minimize motion artefacts, a metal tissue ring with a disposable polymer window is attached to the skin with medical-grade adhesive. The skin lesion (or the area of interest in larger lesions) should be positioned in the centre of the tissue ring. (iii) Before confocal imaging, a dermoscopic image is captured through the tissue ring with a dedicated camera attached to the confocal microscope (VivaCam®). The dermoscopic image can be viewed simultaneously with confocal imaging and may serve as a gross map to guide RCM imaging of subregions of the lesion. To ensure a precise correlation between the dermoscopic picture and the subsequent RCM mosaic images, the housing of both the RCM probe and the VivaCam® are labelled with a direction mark (arrow). The arrows on the RCM and the VivaCam® housings should be aligned with the direction mark on the tissue ring during imaging. (iv) A small amount of water-based immersion medium (e.g., ultrasound gel; refractive index = 1.3) is applied to the adhesive ring. (v) The RCM probe is then coupled magnetically to the adaptor ring. RCM images can be now viewed on the computer screen. (vi) During real-time imaging, basic confocal images (500 × 500 μm) are displayed on the screen (Fig. 3.2). The Vivascan program enables horizontal and vertical navigation through the skin. In addition, sequential horizontal (block) (Fig. 3.3) and vertical imaging (stack) or a combination of both (cube) (Fig. 3.4) can be done by an automated stepper (see below). Short movie files may be acquired to record dynamic skin processes (e.g., blood flow). (vii) After imaging, remnants of ultrasound gel should be removed from the microscope probe with a cleansing swab.

E.M.T. Wurm
Dermatology Research Centre, The University of Queensland School of Medicine, Princess Alexandra Hospital, Brisbane, QLD, Australia
e-mail: e.wurm@uq.edu.au, lissy.wurm@gmail.com

I. Kolm
Department of Dermatology, University Hospital Zurich, Zurich, Switzerland
e-mail: isabel.kolm@usz.ch

V. Ahlgrimm-Siess (✉)
Department of Dermatology and Venerology, Medical University of Graz, Graz, Austria
e-mail: v.ahlgrimm-siess@salk.at

3.2 How to Optimize Imaging Conditions

In order to optimize imaging, it is crucial to find an appropriate patient position that allows a good microscope access to the concerning anatomical area. Since one imaging session will take approximately 5–10 min, it is advisable to find a position that is also comfortable for the patient to avoid immediate changes in the imaging depth due to body movement. The easiest way to image lesions on the scalp, lower trunk and legs is usually to have the patient lie down on the examination bed. However, breath excursions of the lower back tend to be less severe in a seated position. Lesions on the arms and upper trunk can be easily imaged with the patient sitting in an upright position and with the lower arms lying flat on an examination table. Nevertheless, imaging settings will also depend upon the equipment of a given examination room.

Before applying the tissue ring to the skin, the microscope head should be tentatively placed above the concerning skin lesion to find the best imaging position. Since hair will negatively influence imaging, it is recommended to shave abundant body hair (if the patient consents) prior to attaching the tissue ring.

R. Hofmann-Wellenhof et al. (eds.), *Reflectance Confocal Microscopy for Skin Diseases*,
DOI 10.1007/978-3-642-21997-9_3,

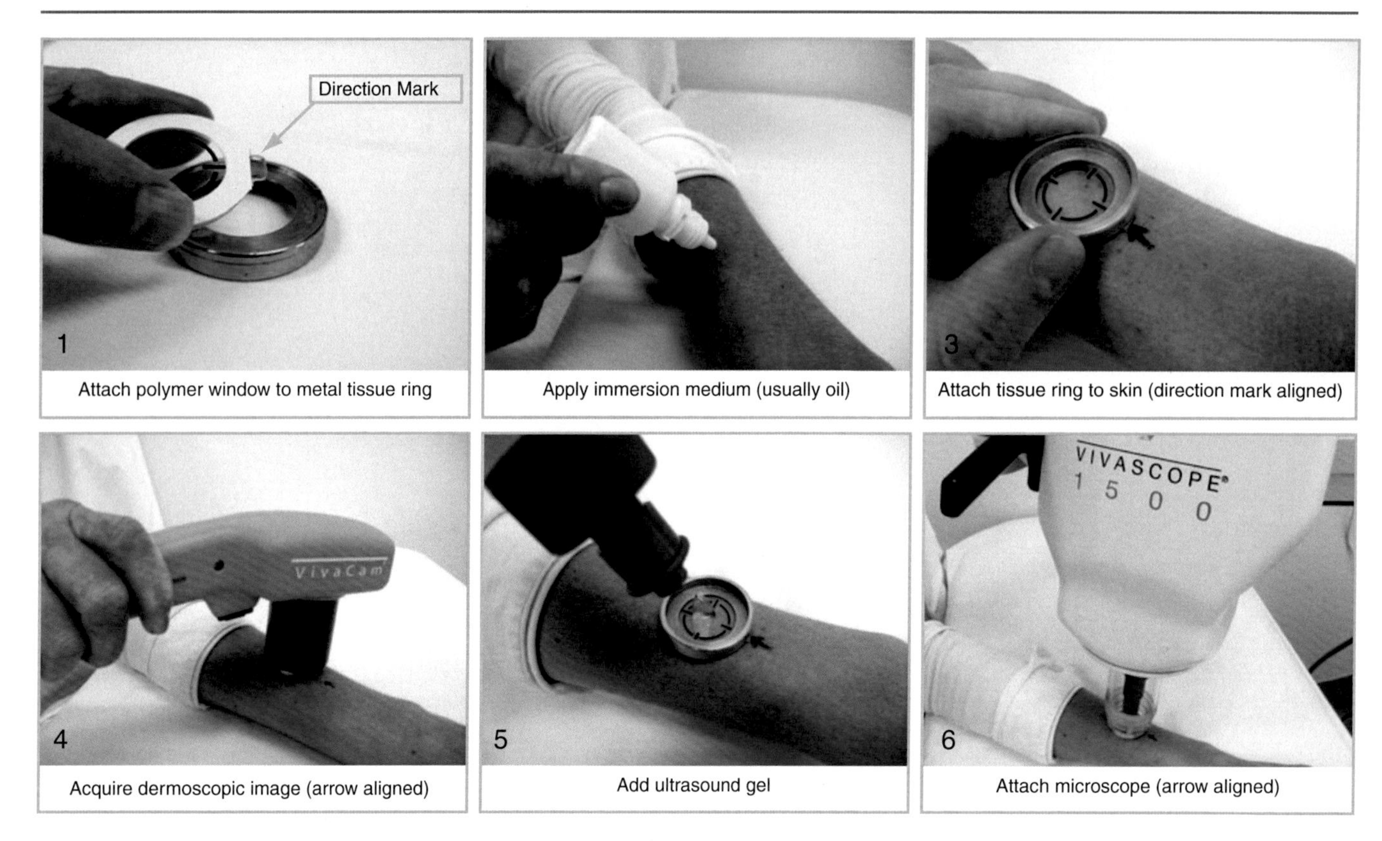

Fig. 3.1 Imaging preparation. Images 1–6 illustrate the most important steps to image acquisition with the VivaScope® 1500

Another challenge that might require examiner's creativity is imaging lesions on uneven anatomical areas, such as the nose, cheeks and fingers or of uneven and raised lesions. Extra double-sided adhesive, fixed in an overlapping position, can help to secure the position of the tissue ring on uneven body sites but decreases the aperture for imaging. A handheld substitute (VivaScope® 3000), if available, facilitates access to these body sites. On raised lesions, extra material (e.g., pre-cut foam wound dressing) placed between the polymer window and an additional adhesive ring can help to fix the tissue ring in an elevated position.

3.3 Basics of Image Interpretation

The VivaScope® 1500 provides basic images with a 500 × 500 μm horizontal field of view (*x*, *y*) at a preselected imaging depth (*z*). This basic image can be viewed in real time on the computer screen (Fig. 3.2) and can be captured as a still image, which requires about 1 MB storage space (Figs. 3.5).

A stack is a sequence of basic images captured at the same horizontal position (*x*, *y*) but at different imaging depths (*z*) ("Optical biopsy", Fig. 3.4). Stack protocols defining the variation in depth between the basic images (*z*-change) and the maximum imaging depth can be configured individually (e.g., 5 μm steps to 120 μm). Of note, the zero depth ($z=0$) needs to be set manually in each skin lesion before imaging; zero depth should be set when the strikingly bright reflection of the skin surface gets dimmer at the centre of the image, correlating to the level of the cornified layer. Defining a consistent zero depth may be hindered in elevated lesions and lesions with an uneven surface. Furthermore, when choosing a protocol for the *z*-stack, it should be considered that imaging depth is limited to approximately 150–200 μm, usually correlating to the upper dermis. Below this depth, images will be blurred and will not provide additional information.

A block ("mosaic") is a high-resolution composite of up to 256 basic images taken sequentially in the horizontal plane by an automated stepper and stitched together by a dedicated software (Fig. 3.3). A block provides a larger field of view at a preselected imaging depth. The size of the mosaics can be selected manually, ranging from 1 × 1 mm to 8 × 8 mm (equalling 2 × 2 to 16 × 16 basic images). When choosing the appropriate mosaic size for a respective skin lesion, one should consider that mosaics are always centred in the middle of the microscope ring. The evaluation of blocks is usually first

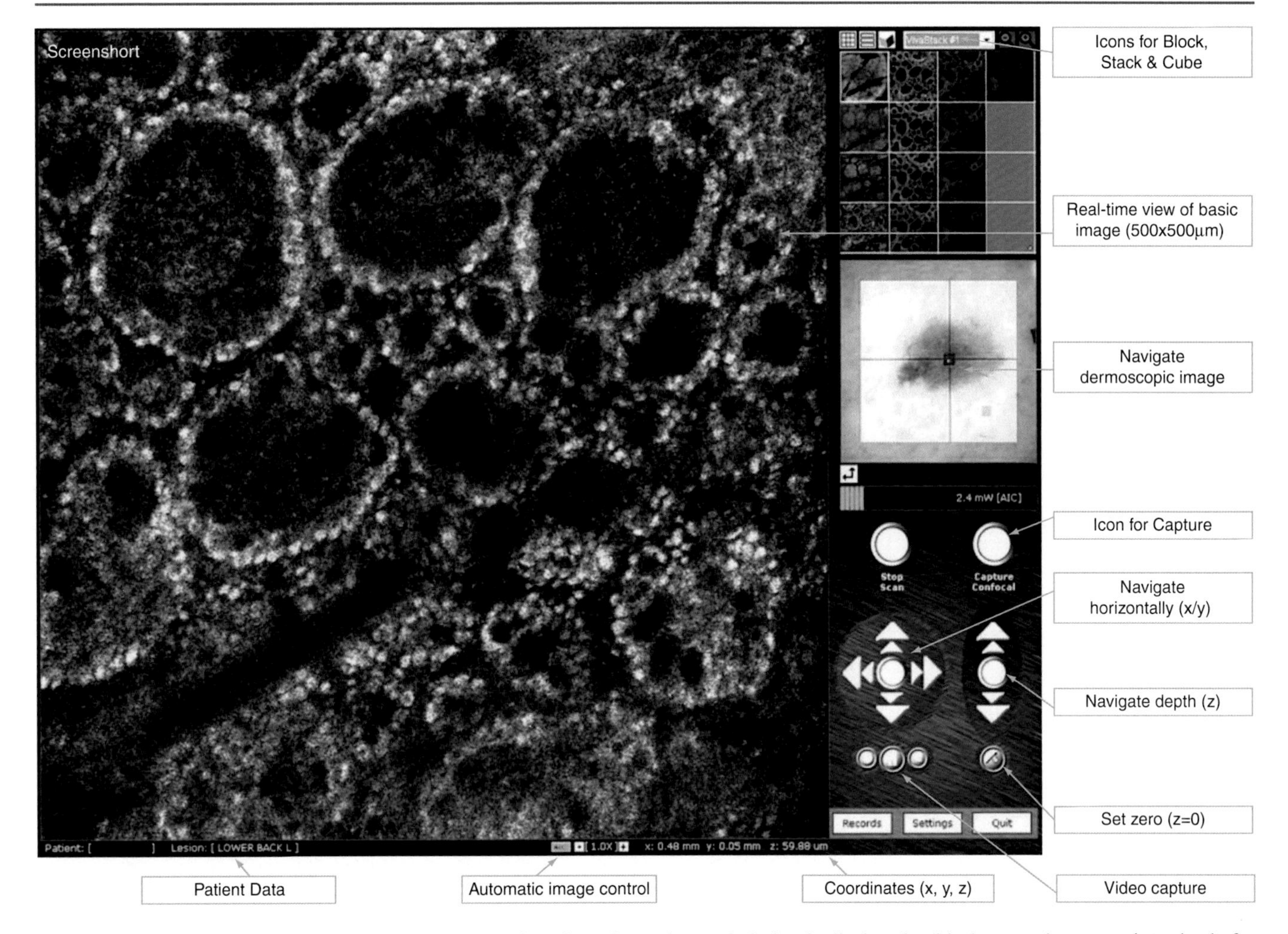

Fig. 3.2 Image acquisition. A screenshot taken during imaging of a melanocytic lesion is displayed, with the most important icons/tools for imaging labelled. (Applies to VivaScope® 1500)

done at "low magnification" (full size image) to assess the overall lesion architecture and then at "higher magnification" by zooming in to areas of interest. In addition, RCM mosaics may also serve as gross maps guiding real-time imaging. A sequence of blocks taken at preselected imaging depths by an automated stepper is called cube (Fig. 3.4). Short videos may be acquired as AVI files to document real-time imaging (e.g., blood flow through vessels).

3.3.1 Imaging Protocol

In order to facilitate image interpretation and storage, we suggest applying the following imaging protocol, especially when imaging melanocytic skin lesions (Fig. 3.6): (i) Reference mark ($z=0$) should be set in the corneal layer (see above). (ii) Acquisition of mosaics at granular/spinous layer (approximate $z=30$ µm), DEJ ($z=60$–90 µm) and upper dermis ($z=90$–120 µm) is recommended. (iii) Four adjacent stacks should be taken in the lesion centre; another two (or more) stacks in areas of special interest.

3.3.2 Confounders of Image Interpretation

Some of the most striking sources of contrast in RCM imaging, such as hair and skin folds, may not provide any relevant information but confound the novice. Due to the spherical aberration of the microscope, a bright ring appears as "flare" when entering the skin surface and disappears when going deeper into the skin. In contrast to skin folds, hairs appear usually bright, but may produce dark "shadows" at deeper skin levels. Hair follicles, skin folds and scales tend to trap air bubbles which usually appear as sharply demarcated, round to oval bright areas or as dark roundish structures with bright outlines (Fig. 3.7).

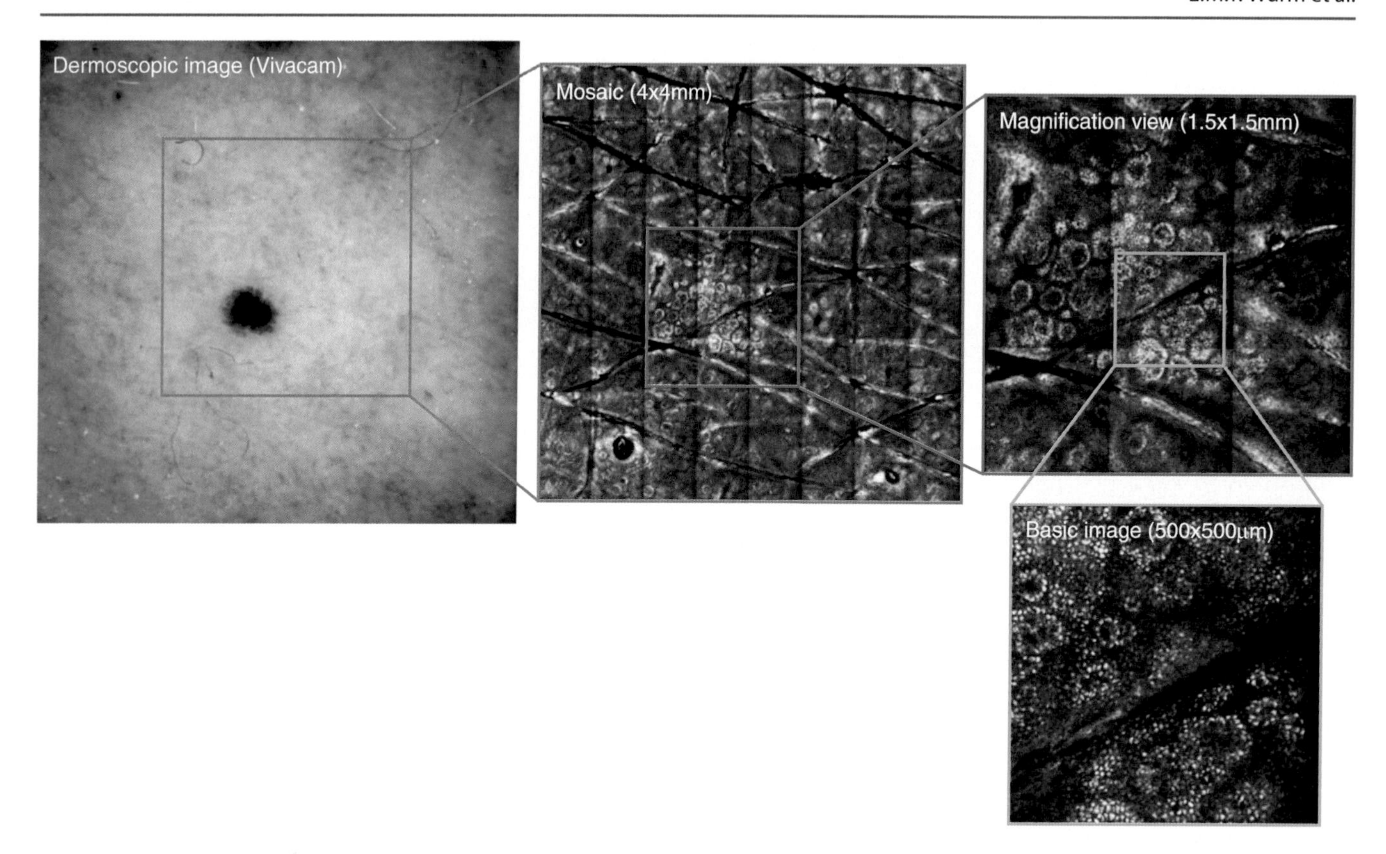

Fig. 3.3 Block/mosaic. A block is a composite mosaic of 500 × 500 µm basic images providing a larger field of view at a preselected imaging depth. The size of the mosaic is adjustable between 1 × 1 mm and 8 × 8 mm equaling 2 × 2 to 16 × 16 basic images. Like in conventional microscopy, the viewer will then zoom in to areas of interest. (Applies to VivaScope® 1500)

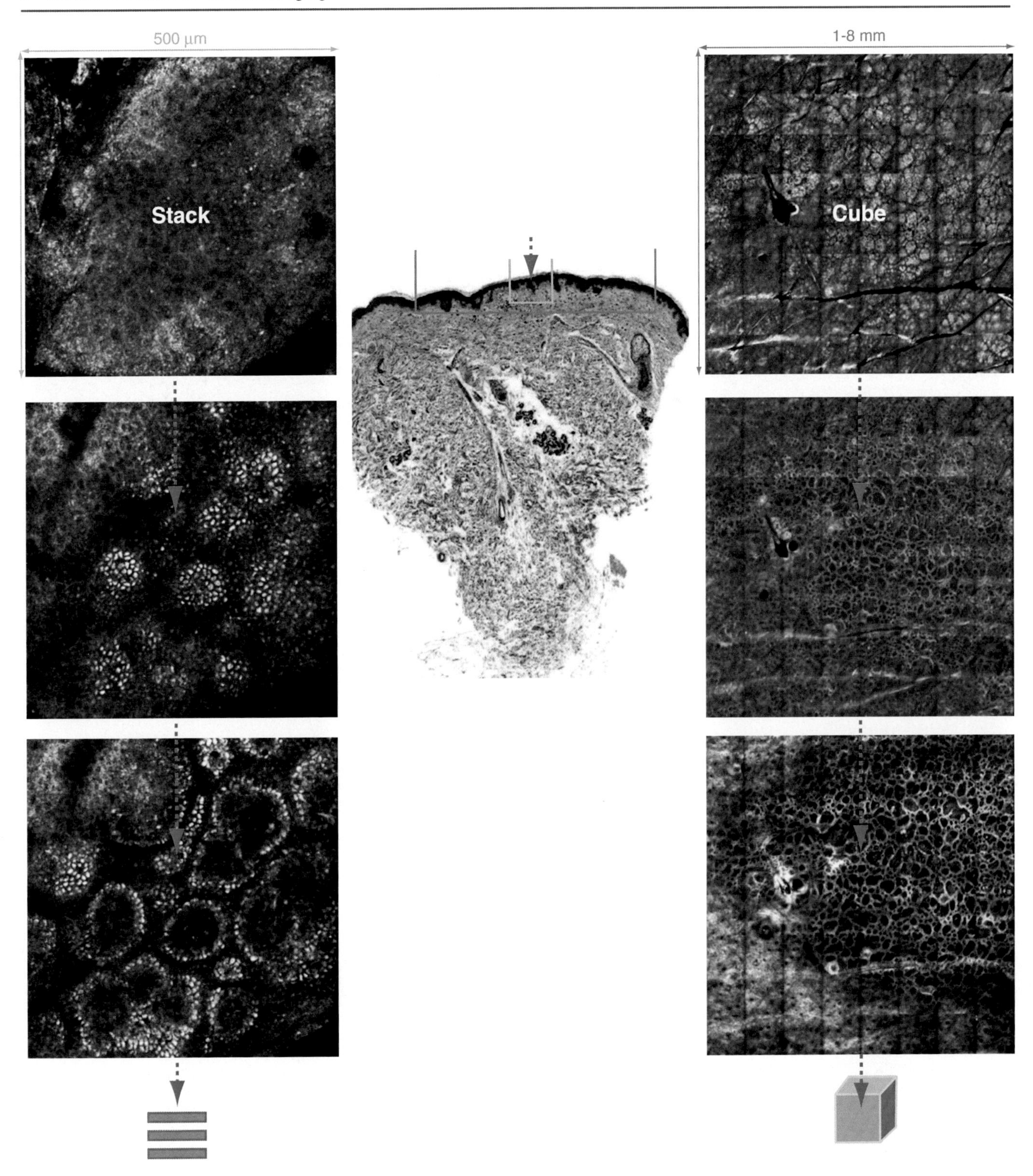

Fig. 3.4 Stack & cube. A stack is a sequence of basic images captured at the same horizontal position (*x*, *y*) but at different depths (*z*). The variation in depth between the images (*z*-change) and maximum depth is manually adjustable. A cube is a stack of mosaics. The size of the mosaics as well as the *z*-change is adjustable. (Applies to VivaScope® 1500)

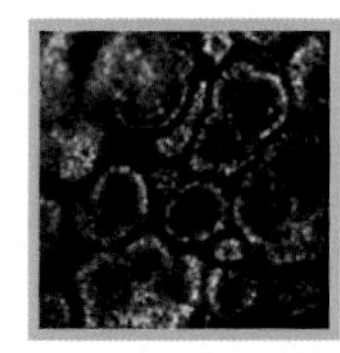

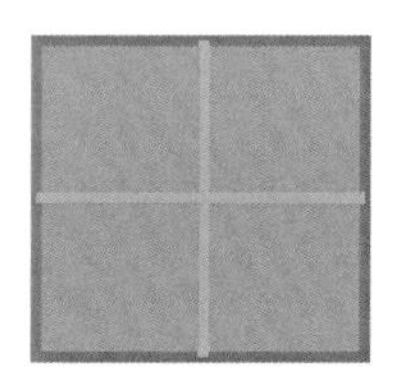

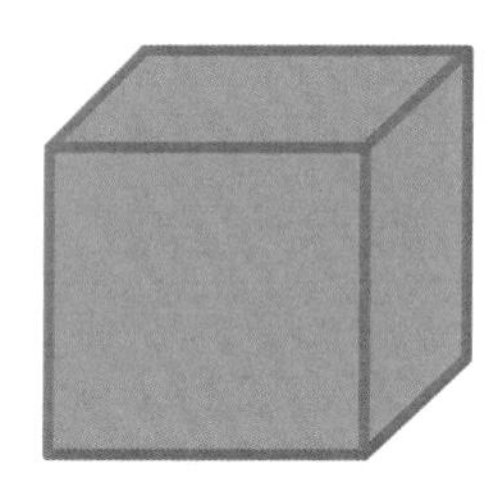

Fig. 3.5 Time expenditure & storage space. Approximate imaging time (*t*) required for image acquisition and storage space for individual imaging procedures. Of note, the time for preparation of patient and microscope is not included and will require approximately additional 5 min. (Applies to VivaScope® 1500)

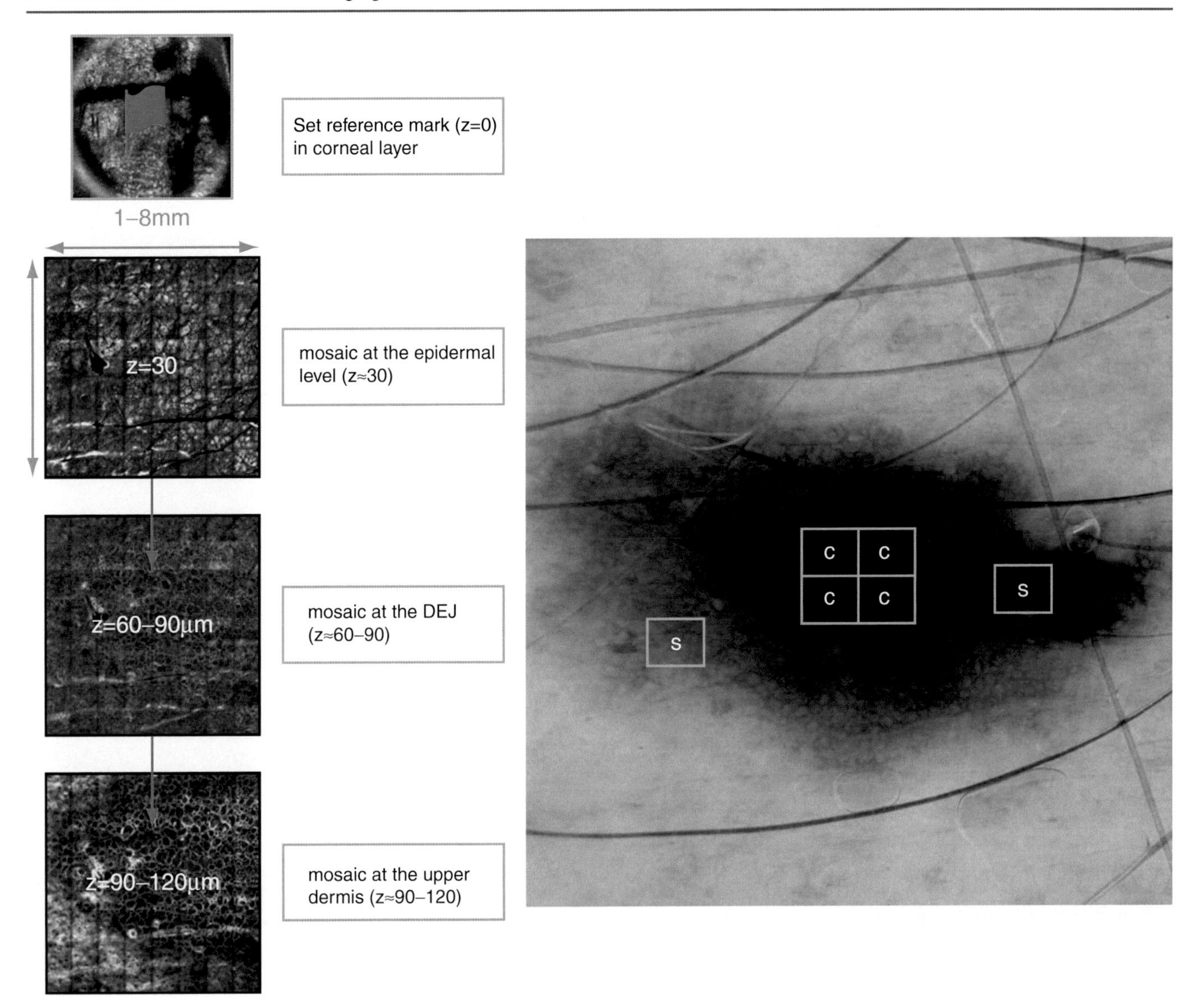

Fig. 3.6 Recommended imaging protocol for melanocytic lesions. After setting the referencing mark to zero, three mosaics (4×4 to 8×8 mm) should be acquired at the epidermal level ($z \approx 30$ μm), DEJ ($z \approx 60$–90 μm), and upper dermis ($z \approx 90$–120 μm), respectively. Four central stacks (c) and two or more stacks (s) in selected significant areas (e.g., 5 μm z-change to 100 μm depth) should be acquired. Estimated time required: 10–15 min. (Applies to VivaScope® 1500)

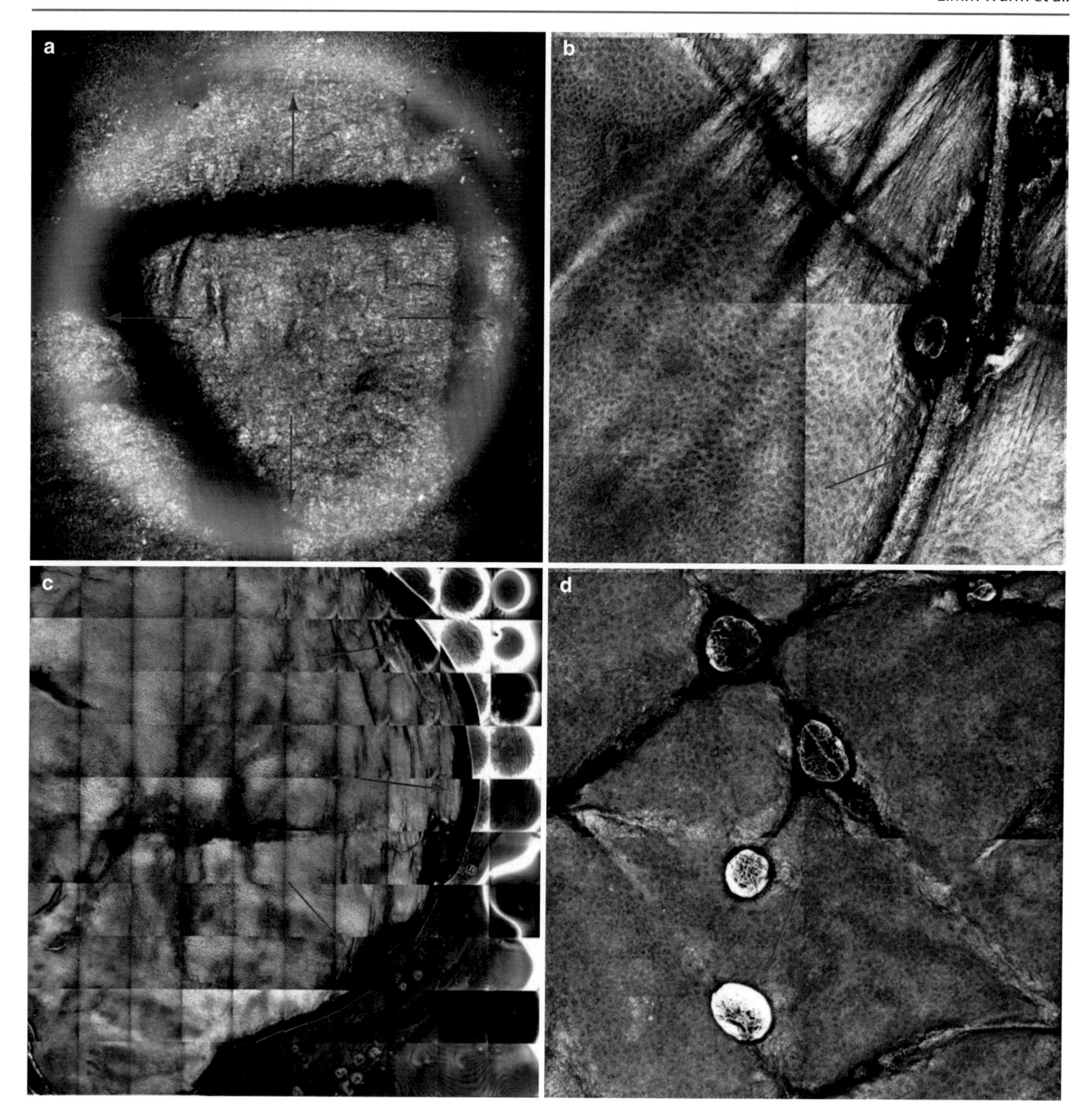

Fig. 3.7 Common confounders of image interpretation. (**a**) *Skin surface* (basic image, 500×500 μm): Due to spherical aberration, a bright ring ("flare") is visualized at the skin surface (→). (**b**) *Body hair* (mosaic view, 1×1 mm): The *lines* in this image (→) at the level of the epidermis correspond to hair shafts. In deeper levels, hair often produce confounding dark "shadows". (**c**) *Elevated lesion* (mosaic view, 5×5 mm): The outlines (→) of this elevated lesion are clearly visible. Bright and dark artefacts are seen in the surrounding area of noncontact. (**d**) *Air bubbles* (mosaic view, 1×1 mm): Air trapped in the immersion oil, often observed in skin folds and around hair follicles, appear as striking bright or dark roundish structures with bright outlines (→) and can confound the novice

Core Messages

- The microscope probe and dermoscopic camera of the VivaScope® 1500 are coupled magnetically to an adhesive tissue ring attached to the skin to enable precise image correlation and to minimize motion artefacts.
- Basic RCM images (500 × 500 μm) are displayed on the screen during real-time navigation through the skin.
- Sequential vertical imaging by an automated stepper enables an optical biopsy (stack). Automated sequential imaging in the horizontal plane provides a mosaic (block) with a larger field of view (1×1 mm to 8×8 mm). Sequential vertical imaging of mosaics is called cube.
- An imaging protocol should be followed to facilitate image interpretation.
- To optimize imaging it is crucial to find an appropriate patient position. Extra material can help to secure the position of the tissue ring on uneven body sites/raised lesions.
- Some of the most striking sources of contrast in RCM imaging (hair, skin folds, air bubbles) may confound image interpretation.

Part II

Normal Skin

4 Epidermis, Dermis and Epidermal Appendages

Susana Puig, Cristina Carrera, Gabriel Salerni, and Joanne Rocha-Portela

4.1 Epidermal Layers

4.1.1 Stratum Corneum (Fig. 4.1 and 4.2)

The stratum corneum is the top layer of the intact epidermis. This layer produces the first bright confocal image [1]. The stratum corneum is located 0–15 μm from the skin surface and appears as a highly refractive surface surrounded by visible skin folds [2, 3]. It is the greater bright image compared with other epidermal layers because of back-scattered light caused by difference in the refractive indexes at the interface between the microscope immersion medium (water or gel) and the skin (stratum corneum) [3–5]. The corneocytes are large, polygonal-shaped anucleated, each with 10–30 μm of dimension [2, 6]. Skin folds (dermatoglyphs) appear as non-refractile or dark linear furrows between groups of keratonocytes [2]. Within these groups, the corneocytes appear as bright polygonal structures with dark outlines [6].

4.1.2 Stratum Granulosum (Fig. 4.3.1 and 4.3.2)

The stratum granulosum is located 15–20 μm below the skin surface [6]. This is the first layer of viable epidermis with large and sparsely located nuclei [5]. In confocal images, granular cells are polygonal keratinocytes with 25–35 μm of dimension [6]. Within the cytoplasm, there is 0.5–1.0 μm bright grainy structure due to organelles and keratohyalin granules [1, 6]. The cytoplasm appears bright and granular like a ring surrounding the round to oval dark central nuclei [1, 2, 6]. The keratinocytes have well-demarcated outlines that form a grid that resembles a honeycombed pattern [3, 4].

S. Puig (✉) • C. Carrera • G. Salerni • J. Rocha-Portela
Melanoma Unit, Department of Dermatology, Hospital Clinic, IDIBAPS, CIBERER, Barcelona, Spain
e-mail: susipuig@gmail.com

4.1.3 Stratum Spinosum (Fig. 4.4.1 and 4.4.2)

Further penetration from superficial to deeper epidermal layers showed the nuclei becoming small with increased number density [5]. These are the upper and lower spinous layers, extending 20–100 μm below the skin surface [2, 5, 6]. In confocal images, a spinous keratinocyte is smaller cell of size 15–25 μm, polygonal in shape, with dark oval-round central nuclei surrounded by refractive white thin cytoplasm [4, 6, 7]. The keratinocytes show regular demarcation of the cells and are arranged in a honeycomb pattern [2, 3].

4.1.4 Stratum Basalis (Fig. 4.5.1 and 4.5.2)

Below the spinous layers, at an average depth of 50–100 μm below the skin surface, there is a single layer of basal cells at the dermo-epidermal junction [6]. Basal cells are uniform in size and shape, smaller in size, about 7–12 μm and are higher refractive than spinous keratinocytes because of the melanin caps forming bright disks on top of the nuclei [4, 5]. Melanin and melanosomes are strong sources of contrast for reflectance confocal microscopy of the epidermis [3, 5]. Melanocytes and pigmented keratinocytes appear as solitary bright, round or oval structures in the basal layer because of the high refractive index of melanin [1, 3]. In normal skin, it is difficult to distinguish between melanocytes and pigmented keratinocytes, since melanocytes rarely show branching outlines that may correspond to their dendrites [4]. In skin phototypes II–IV, the basal keratinocytes are arranged as clusters of round cells with refractive cytoplasm forming a cobblestone pattern in the upper confocal sections basal layer (suprapapillary plates) [2, 3, 6]. In skin phototype I, basal keratinocytes show low refractility and are difficult to elucidate [2]. Upon deeper imaging through basal layer in anatomic sites with rete ridges, basal cells and melanocytes appear as round or oval rings of bright cells surrounding dark dermal papillae ("edged papillae") [2, 4].

R. Hofmann-Wellenhof et al. (eds.), *Reflectance Confocal Microscopy for Skin Diseases*,
DOI 10.1007/978-3-642-21997-9_4, © Springer-Verlag Berlin Heidelberg 2012

4.1.5 Dermal-Epidermal Junction (DEJ) (Fig. 4.6.1 and 4.6.2)

At the undulating DEJ, the dermis forms upward finger-like projections into the epidermis called dermal papillae [2]. Confocal sections deeper through the papillae at the DEJ show dark round to oval areas corresponding to dermal papillae, centered by dermal capillary loops with individual blood cells, circumscribed by basal keratinocytes on circular loci [4, 5]. This arrangement corresponds to an "edged papillae" that is defined as the papillae presenting a demarcated rim of bright basal cells [3]. These rims increased in size until the neighboring rim touched each other tangentially, indicating that the base of the finger-like projections had been reached [2, 5]. Observation of blood flow in the dermal papillae during real-time examination may further facilitate recognition of the DEJ [3].

4.2 Dermal Layers (Fig. 4.7.1 and 4.7.2)

In confocal images below the DEJ, at average depths of 100–150 μm, it is possible to visualize the blood flow in the capillary loops within each papillae that is usually darker than the epidermis; individual circulating blood cells are best seen during real-time imaging [6]. Blood vessels appear as dark tubular or canalicular structures containing a mixture of weakly refractile and brightly refractile cells [2]. From their relative shapes, sizes, and number densities, the cells were identified as erythrocytes (6–9 μm diameter), leukocytes (6–30 μm) and platelets (2–5 μm) [6]. At average depths of 100–350 μm below the skin surface, a network of fibers and bundles can be seen within the papillary dermis (100–150 μm below the skin surface) and superficial reticular dermis (>150 μm below the skin surface) [2, 6]. These are the varying amounts of refractile collagen fibers. Collagen appears as bright elongated fibrillar structures with no cellular component, no visible nucleus, and no visible movement, distributed side by side throughout the dermis arranged in a reticulated network (fibers diameter of 1–5 μm) or as bright bundles (diameter of 5–25 μm) [2, 3, 6, 7]. Collagen fibers surround the blood vessels and are usually distributed as coils or rings in papillary dermis and parallel bundles gathered into large fascicles in reticular dermis [2, 3].

Among the dermis cells population, melanophages are easily recognized because they are rich in melanin and their solitary distribution around papillary dermal capillaries [1, 4]. They are irregularly shaped, plump-bright cells, with ill-defined borders, no visible nucleus and larger than melanocytes [1, 3].

4.3 Epidermal Appendages

Only superficial segment of the skin appendages can be identified with in vivo RCM.

4.3.1 Hair Follicle

The infundibular portion appears as an ostium often containing a hair shaft and a central lumen [3]. Follicle is characterized by cells of different sizes in an ordered pattern consistent with cellular differentiation: from small, ovoid or polygonal basal cells to larger, flatter surface cells [2, 3].

4.3.2 Hair Shaft (Fig. 4.2)

Hair shaft appears as a cylindrical or tubular long structure that has uniform high refractivity with no cellular pattern centrally, although some elliptical elongated cells may be seen at the circumference. Usually it is seen emanating from a hair follicle ostium [3].

4.3.3 Eccrine Sweat Ducts

Eccrine sweat ducts appear as bright, oval to round centrally hollow structures that spiral through the epidermis and dermis. It has a smaller diameter than hair follicle, is less straight and does not contain a central hair shaft [2].

4.3.4 Apocrine Sweat Ducts

Apocrine ducts are generally not seen because they usually insert into the follicular infundibulum just above the insertion point of the sebaceous duct and only found in groin and axila. When visualized, they are straight not coiled, resembling a follicle without a hair shaft [2].

4.3.5 Sebaceous Gland

Sebaceous glands are found in highest concentration on the face and can be visualized especially in the context of a sebaceous hyperplasia. The sebaceous acinar cells are highly refractile and have a morular appearance. Each sebocyte has a central, round, dark nucleus surrounded by a well-defined rim of a bright multi-lobular cytoplasm [2].

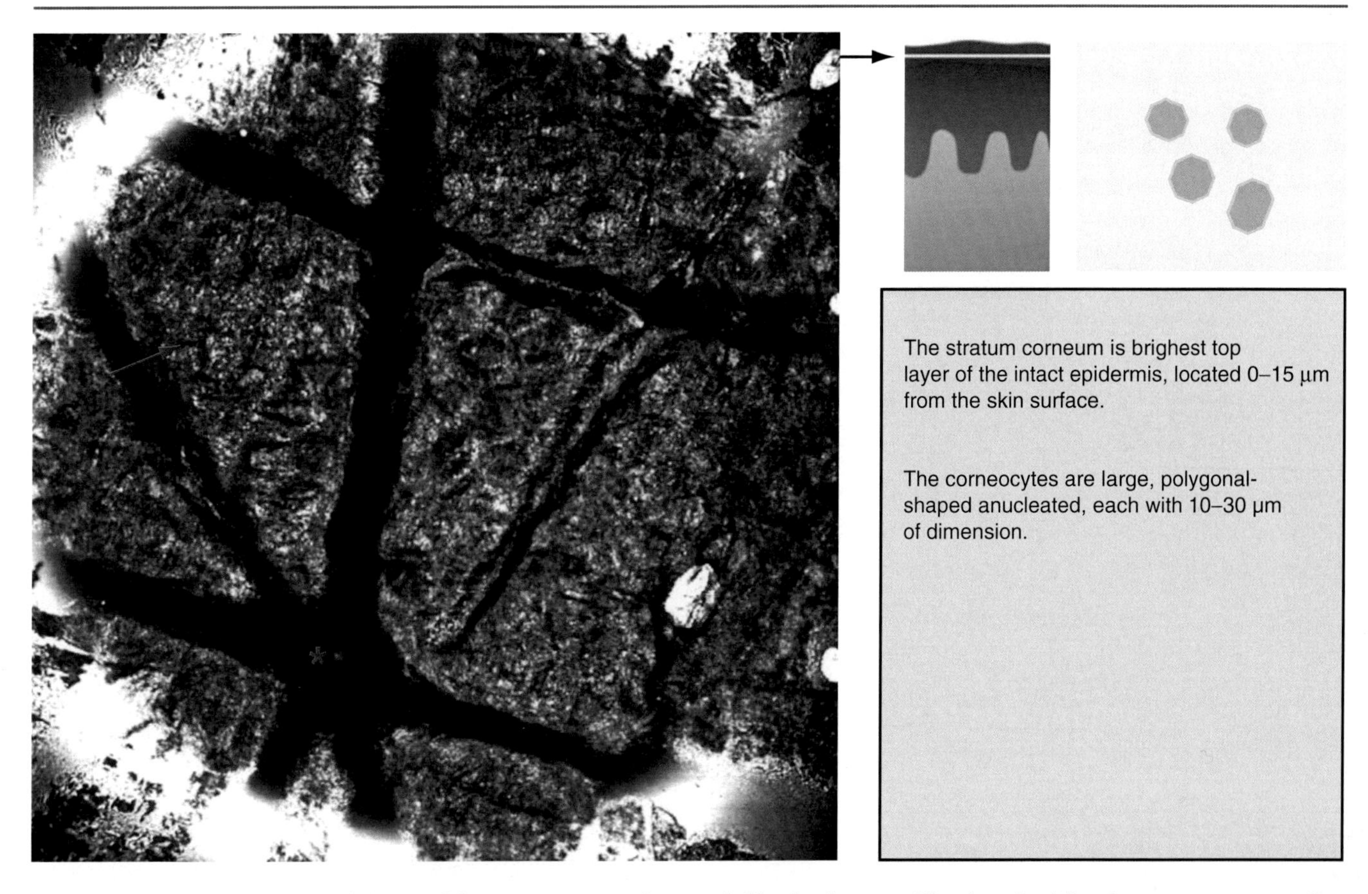

Fig. 4.1 Basic RCM image (0.5 × 0.5 mm) of the stratum corneum in normal skin of a phototype III patient. *Dark lineal structures* corresponding to skin marks (*) and large non-nucleated keratinocyte (→)

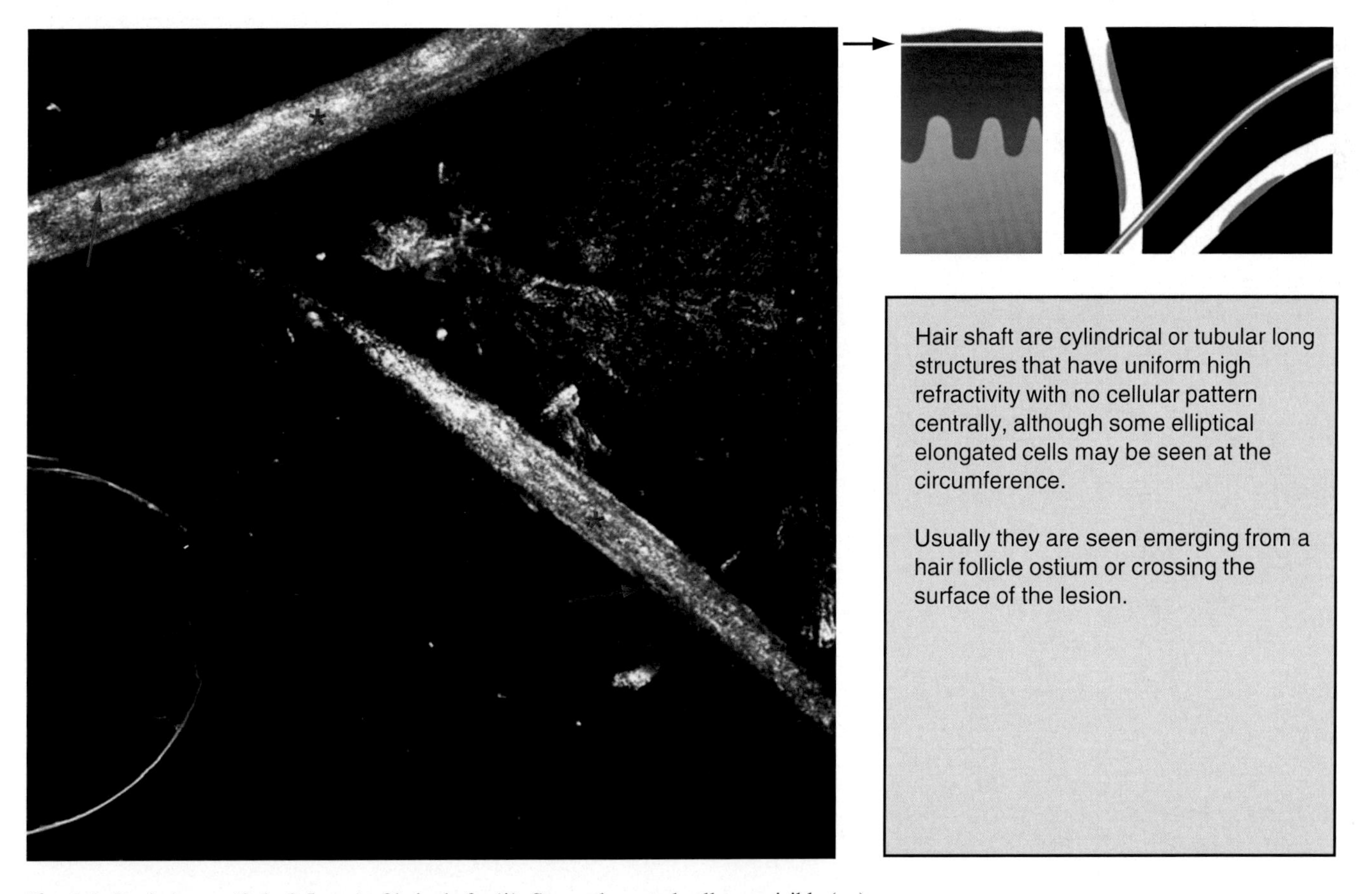

Fig. 4.2 Basic image (0.5 × 0.5 mm) of hair shafts (*). Some elongated cells are visible (→)

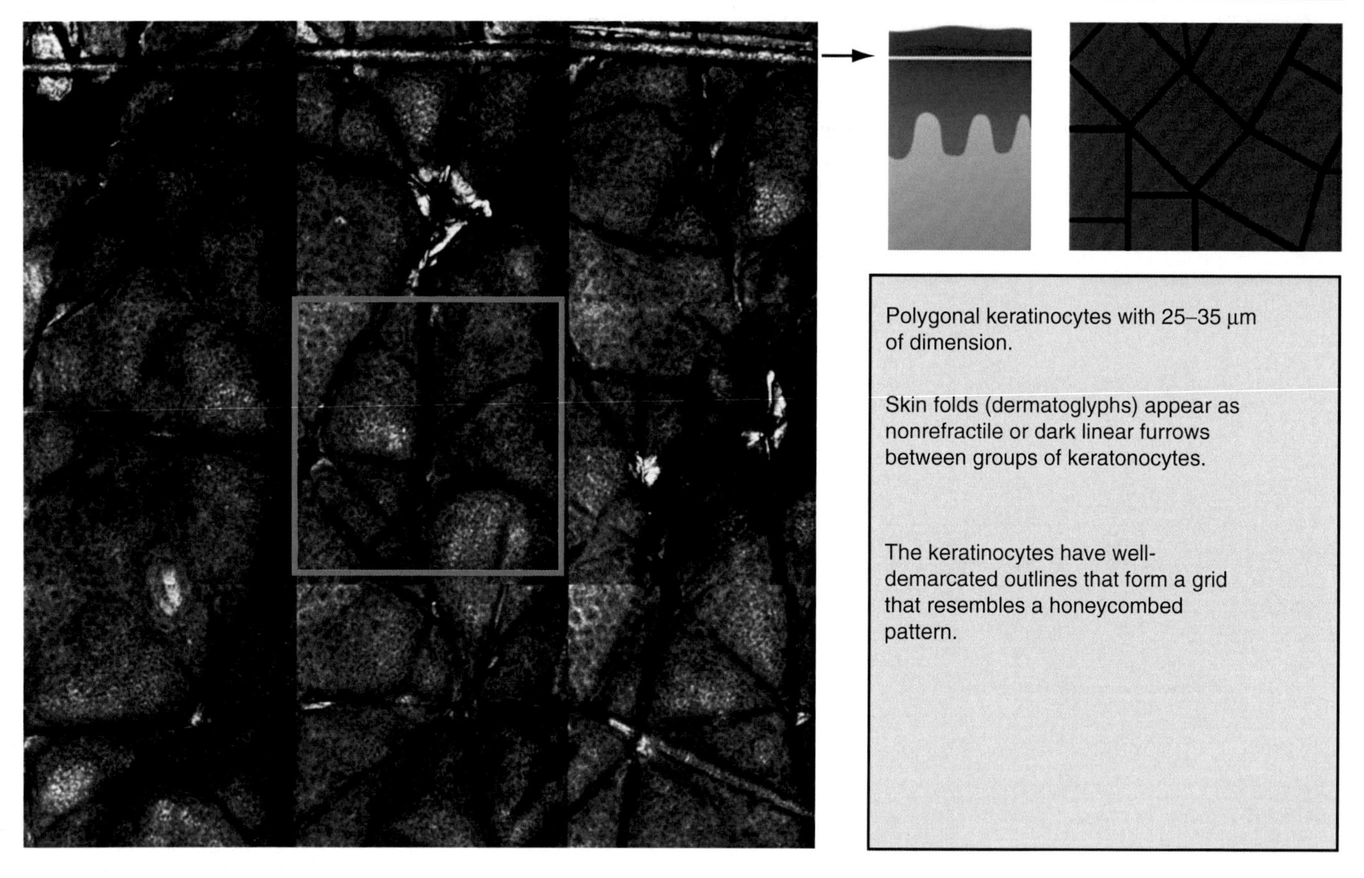

Fig. 4.3.1 RCM mosaic (1.5 × 1.5 mm) stratum granulosum in normal skin of a phototype II patient

Within the cytoplasm, there is 0.5–1.0 μm bright grainy structure due to organelles and keratohyalin granules.
The cytoplasm appears bright and granular like a ring surrounding the round to oval dark central nuclei.

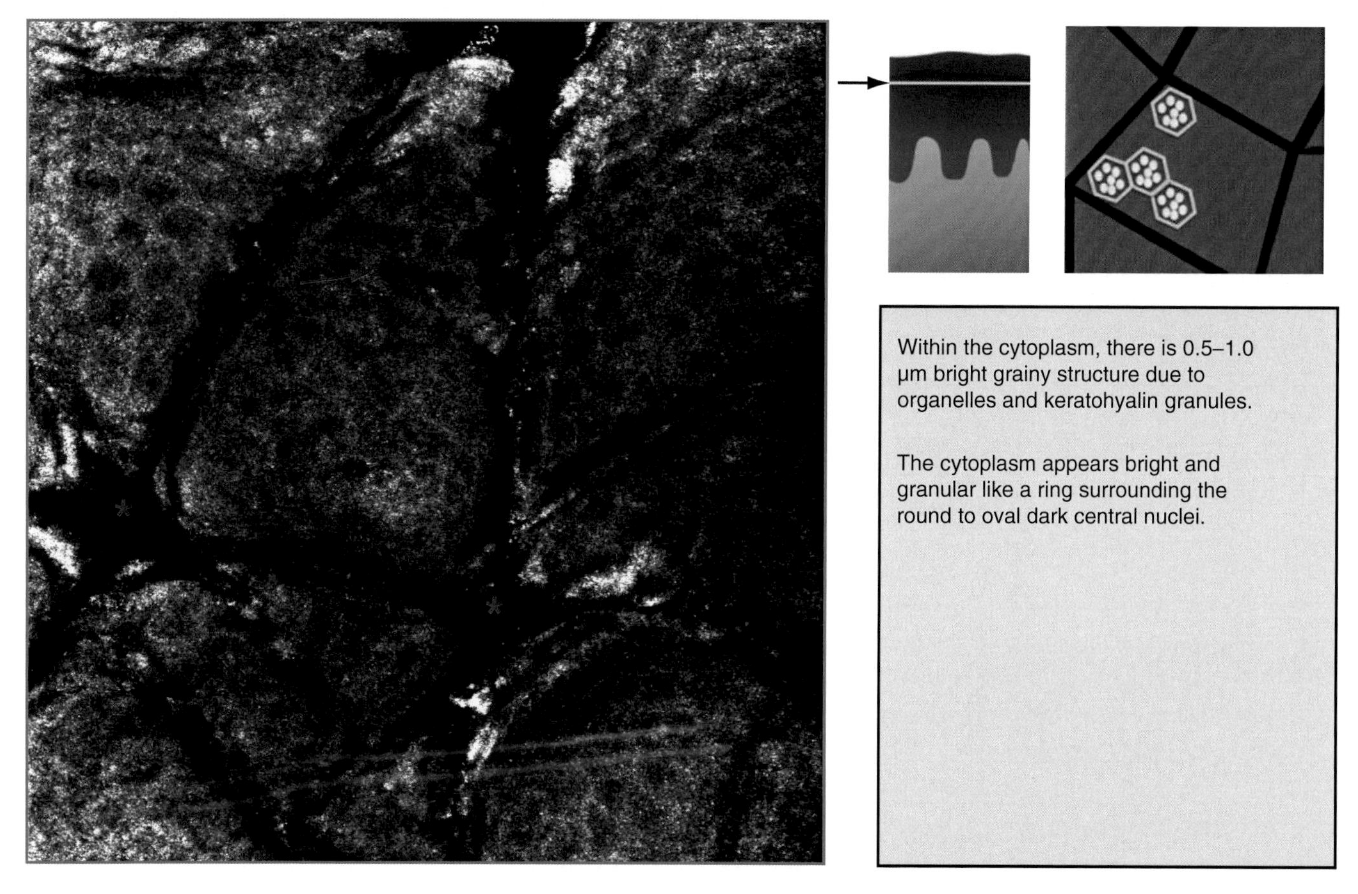

Fig. 4.3.2 Basic image (0.5 × 0.5 mm) skin folds (*) large keratinocyte with dark nucleous and granular cytoplasm (→)

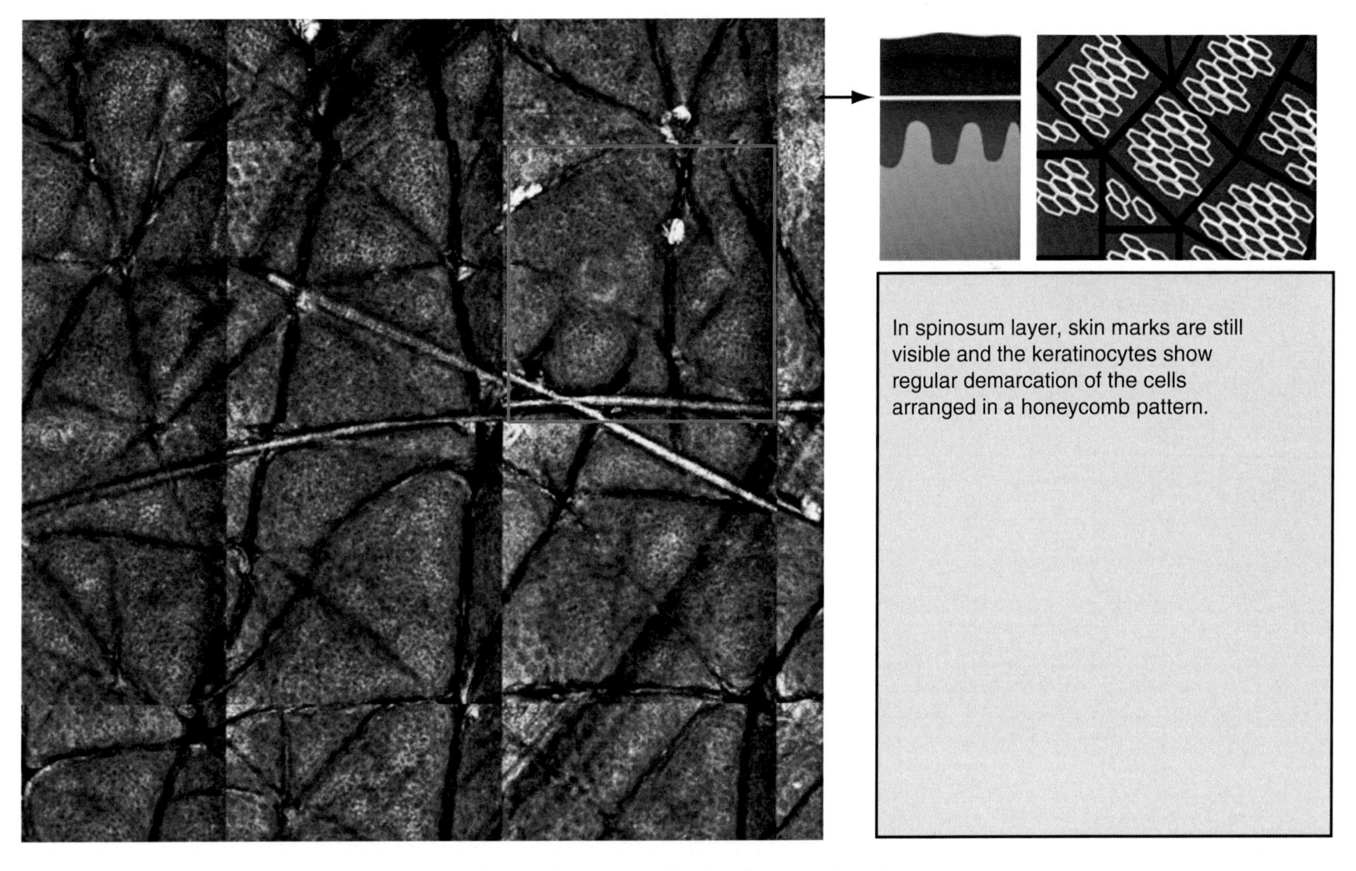

Fig. 4.4.1 RCM mosaic (1.5 × 1.5 mm) stratum spinosum in normal skin of a phototype II patient

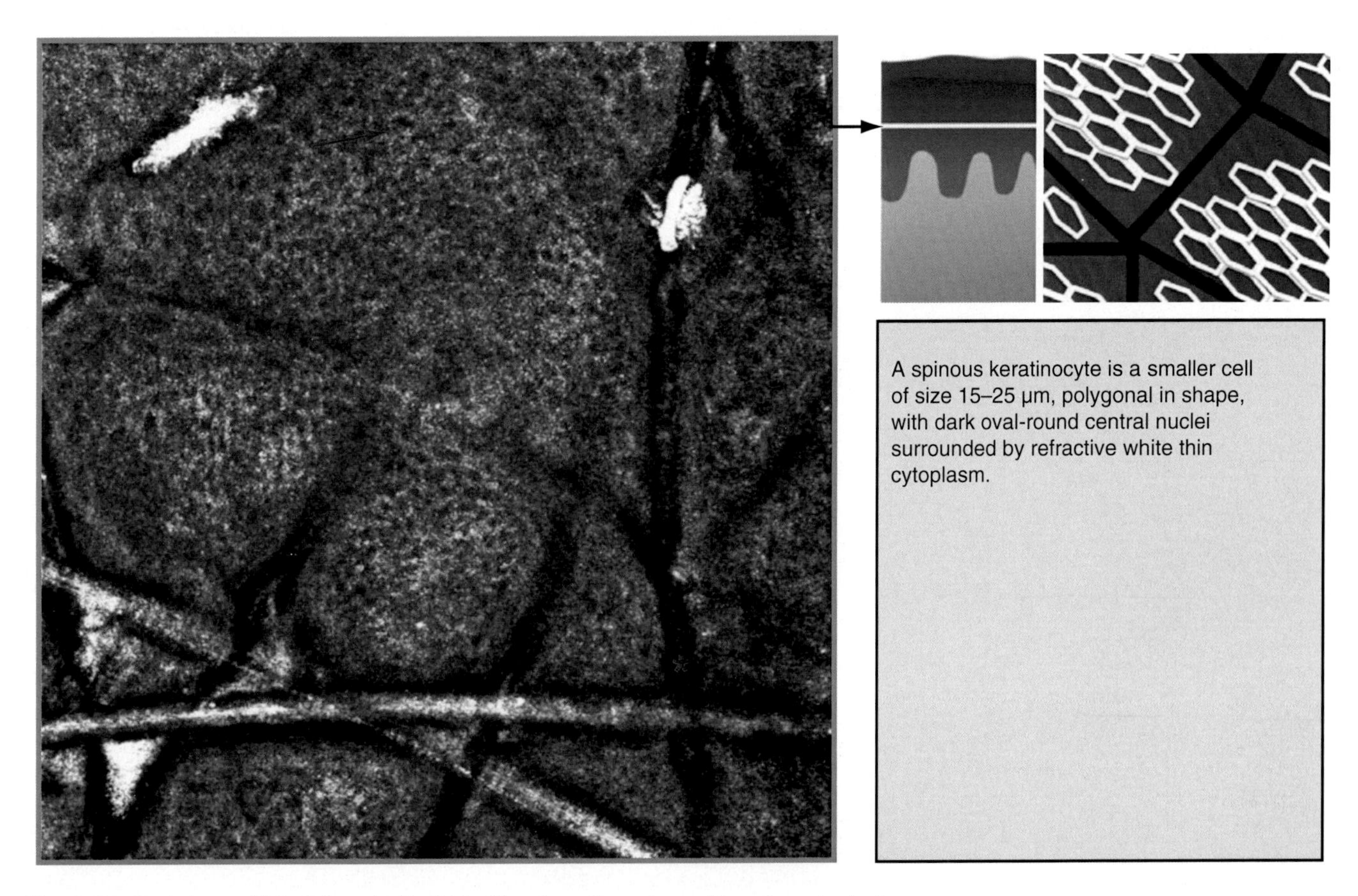

Fig. 4.4.2 Basic image (0.5 × 0.5 mm) skin folds (*) and smaller polygonal keratinocytes (→)

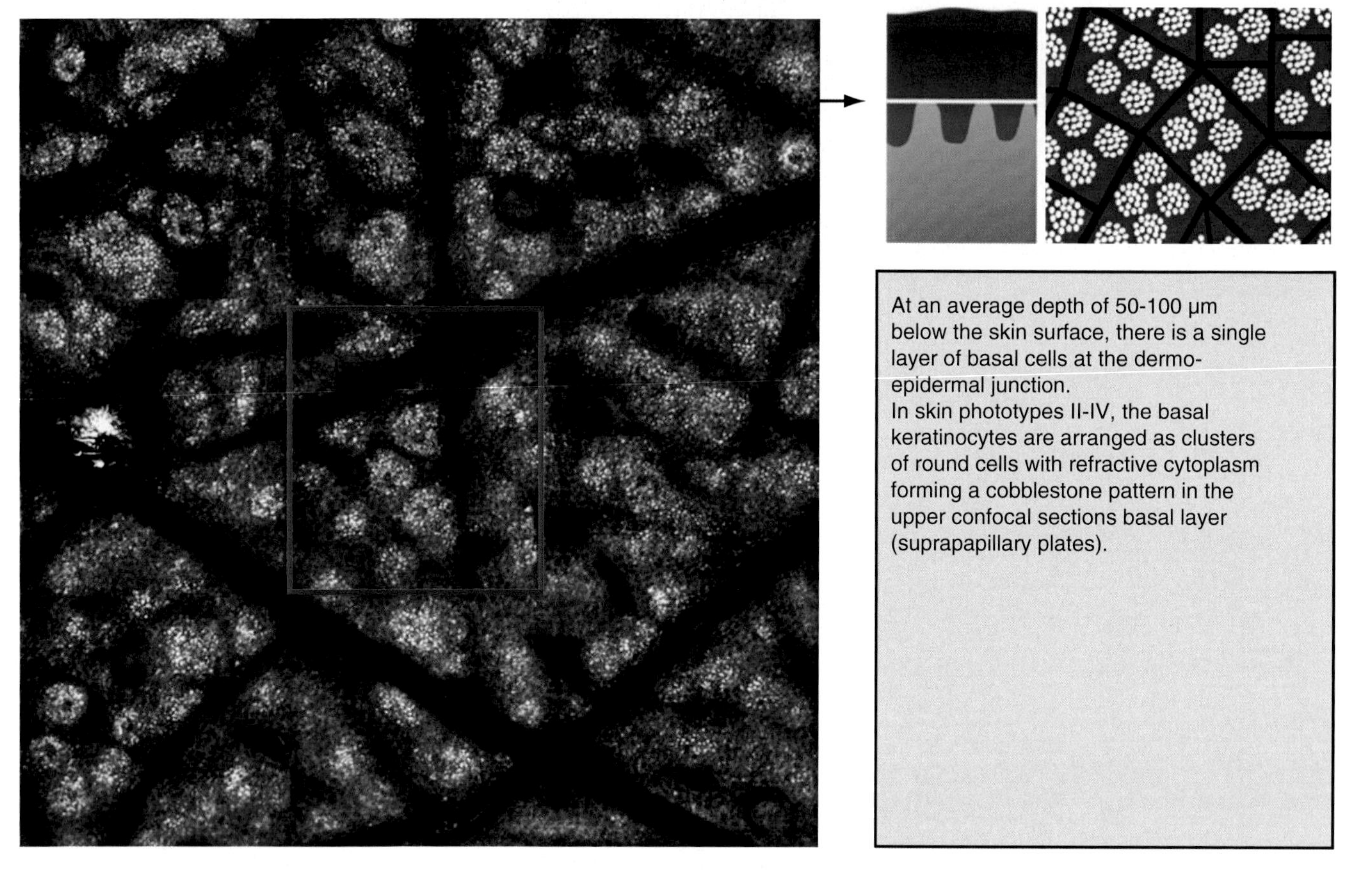

Fig. 4.5.1 RCM mosaic (1.5 × 1.5 mm) at the basal layer of normal skin in a patient phototype V

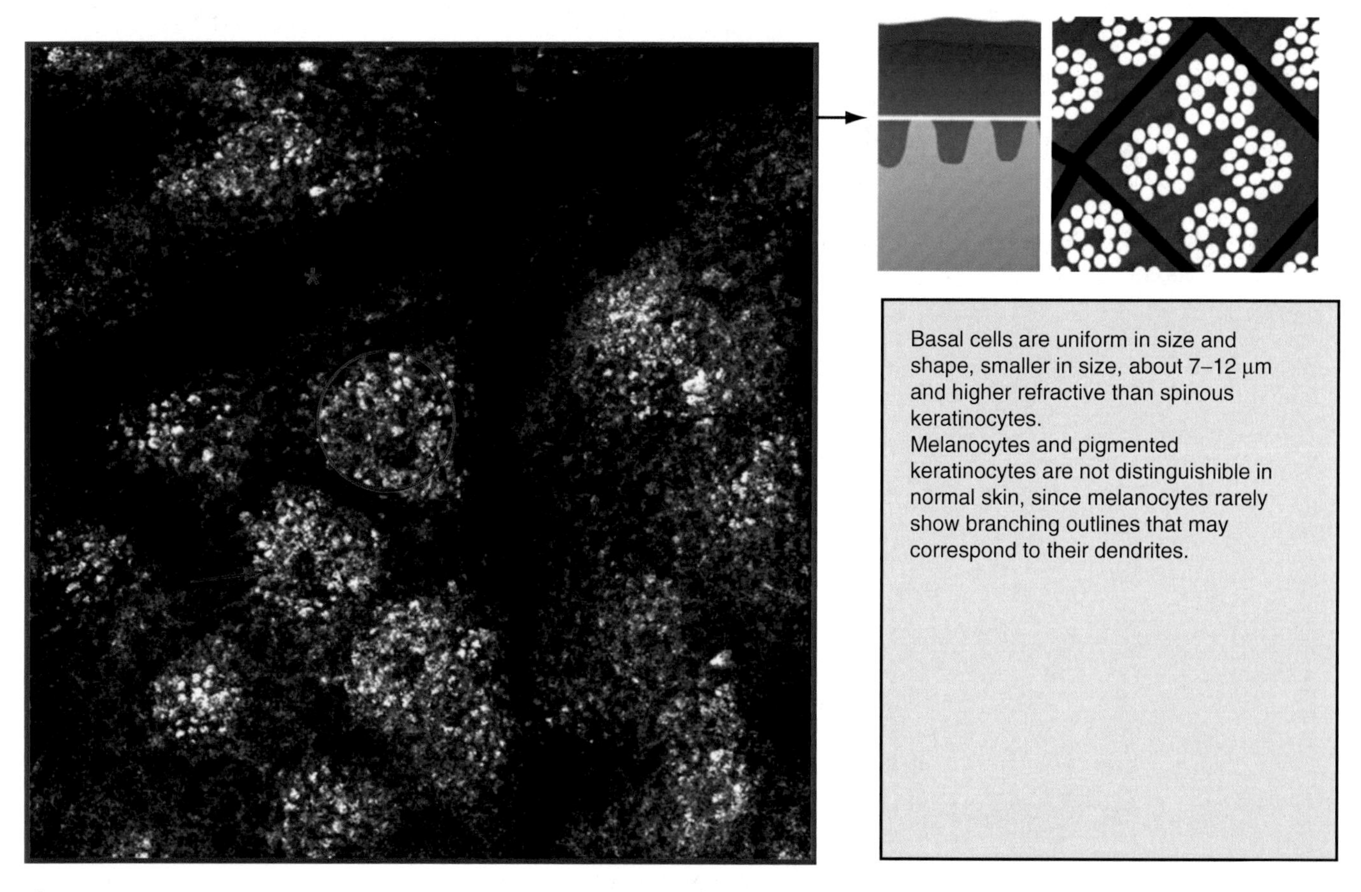

Fig. 4.5.2 Basic image (0.5 × 0.5 mm) skin folds (*) small refractile basal cells (→) in the suprapapillary plates (O)

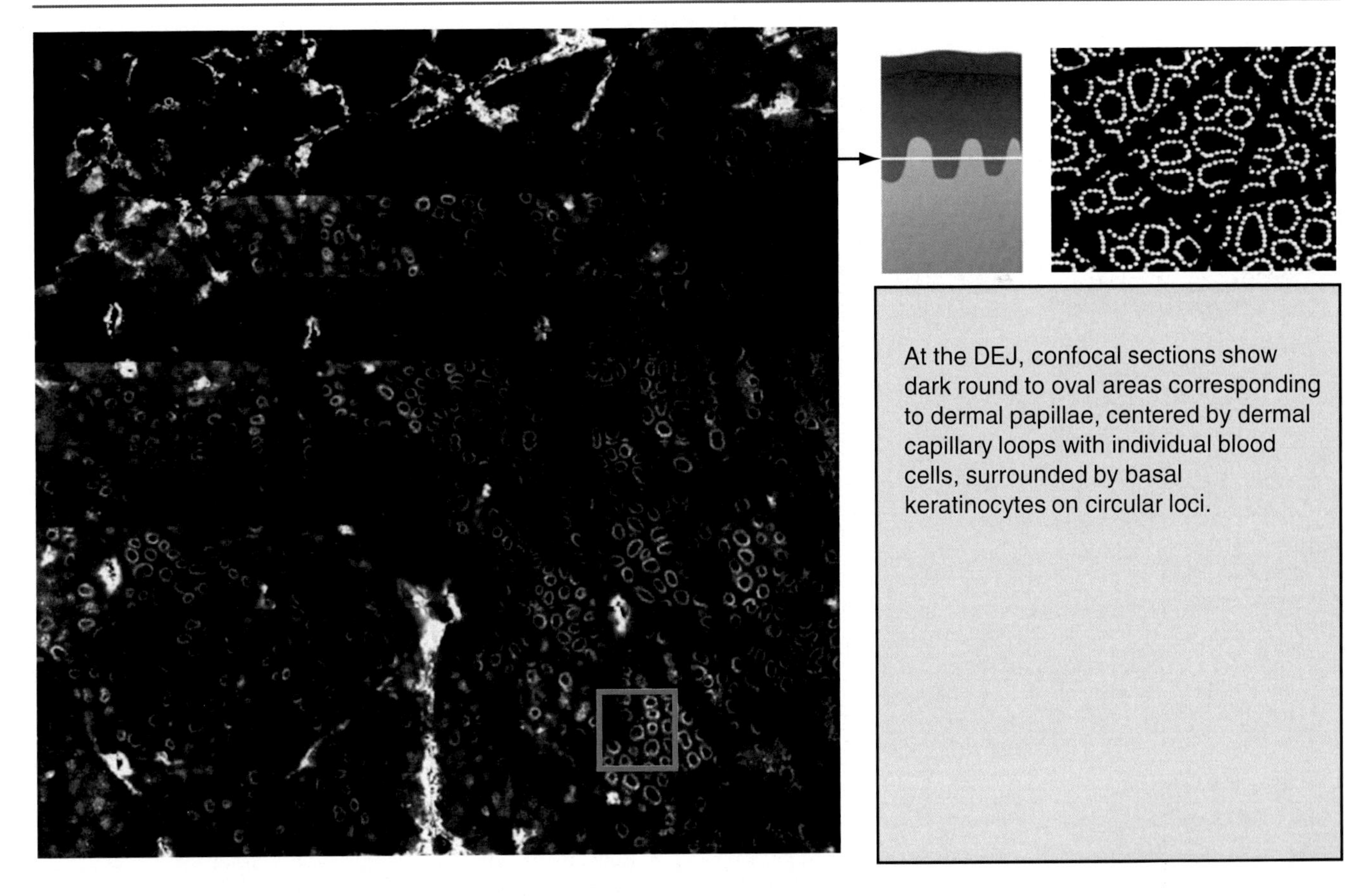

Fig. 4.6.1 RCM mosaic (1.5 × 1.5 mm) at the DEJ of normal skin in a patient phototype V

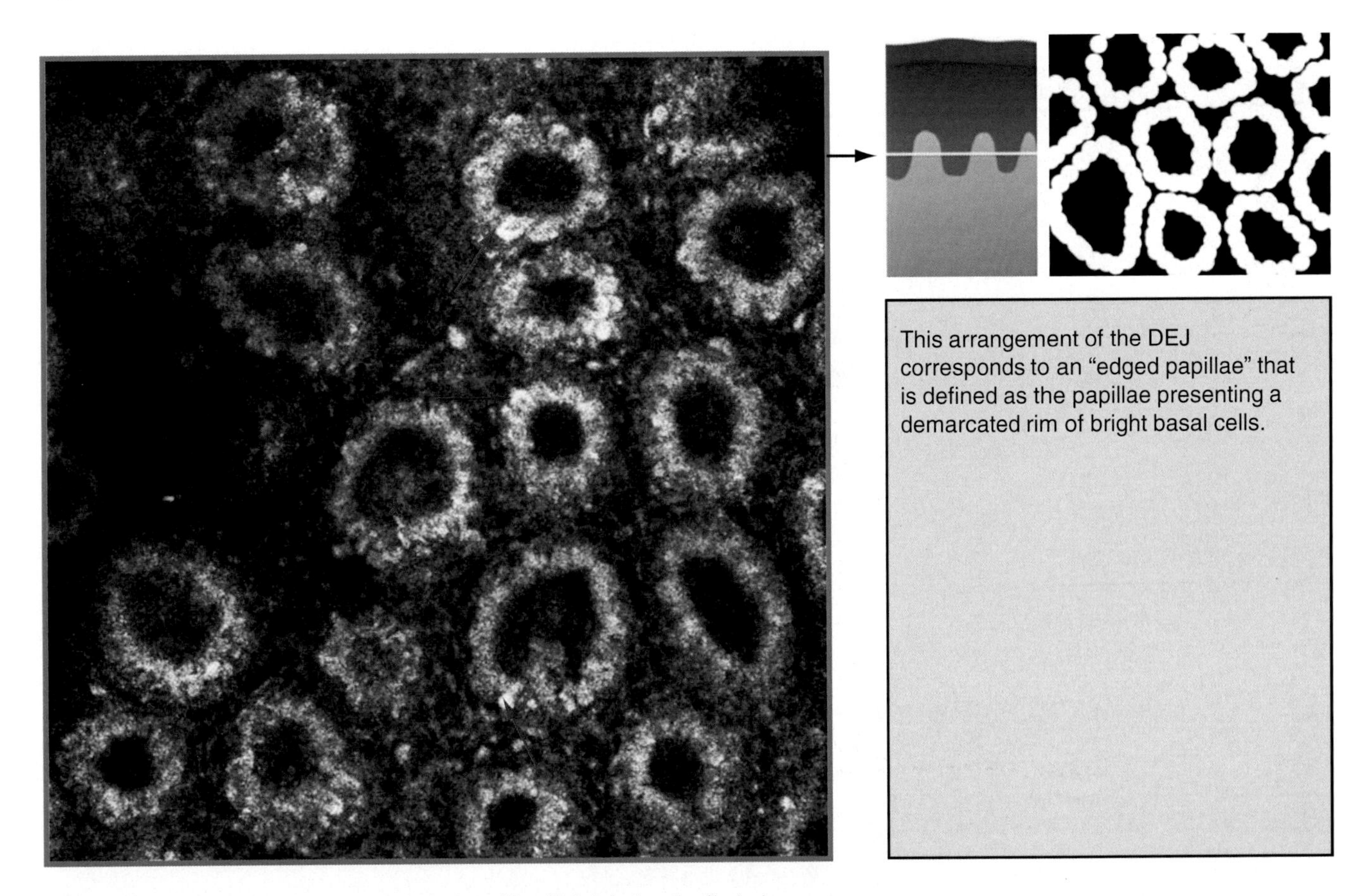

Fig. 4.6.2 Basic image (0.5 × 0.5 mm) dermal papillae (*) bright basal cells (→)

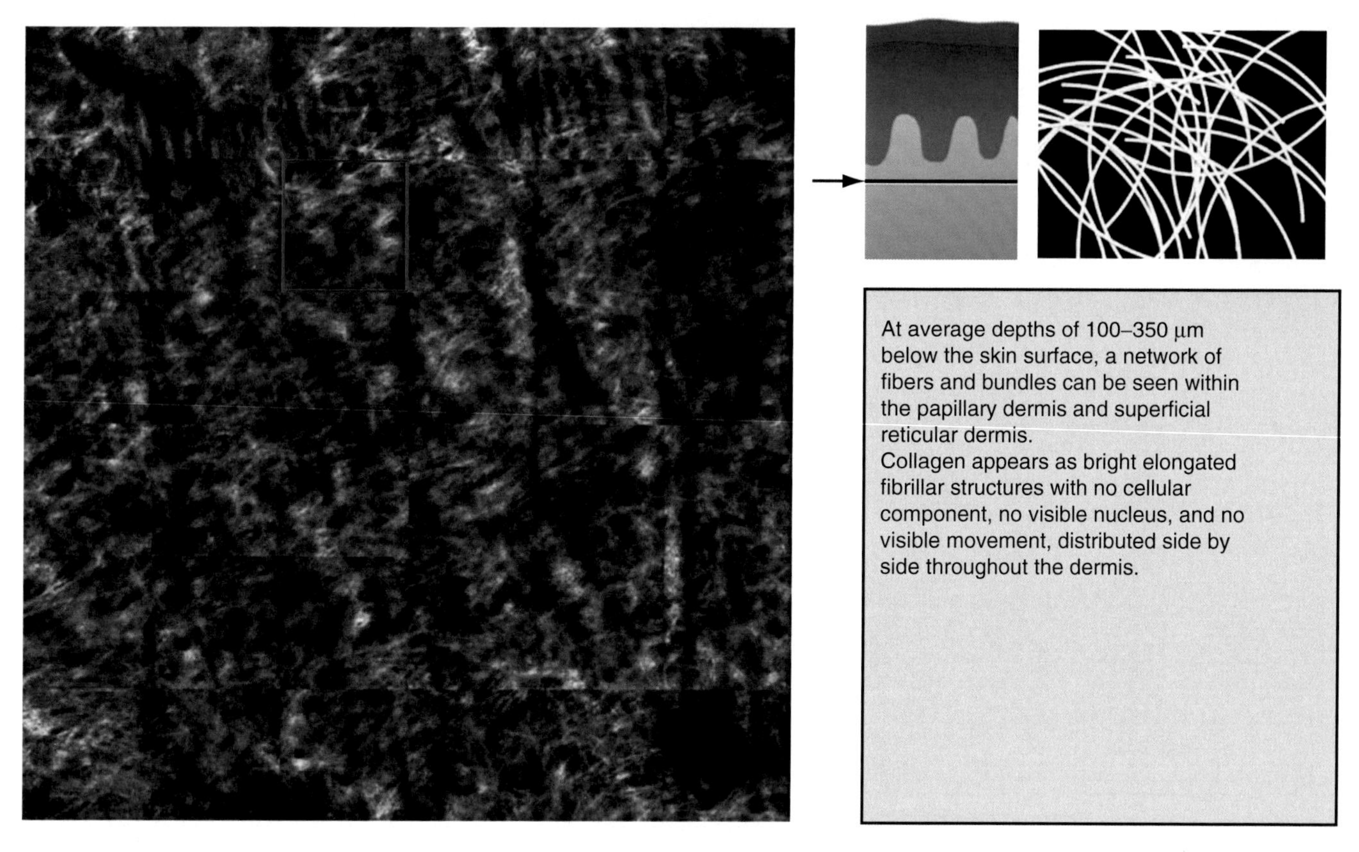

Fig. 4.7.1 RCM mosaic (1.5 × 1.5 mm) from the face of a phototype III patient

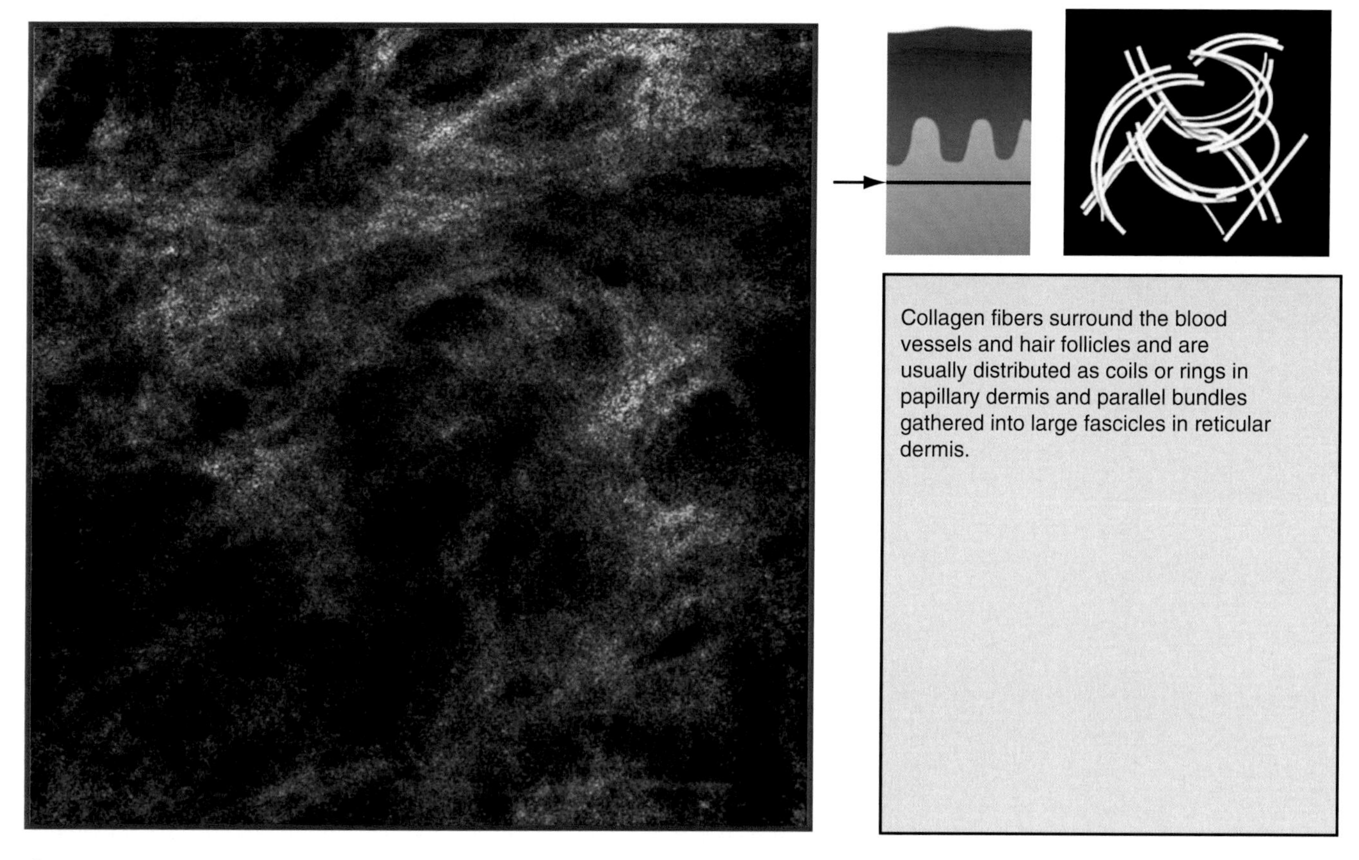

Fig. 4.7.2 Basic image (0.5 × 0.5 mm) showing widespread reticulated collagen fibers (→)

References

1. Busam KJ, Charles C, Lee G, Halpern AC (2001) Morphologic features of melanocytes, pigmented keratinocytes, and melanophages by in vivo confocal scanning laser microscopy. Mod Pathol 14:862–868
2. González S, Gill M, Halpern AC (2008) Normal skin. Reflectance confocal microscopy of cutaneous tumors: an atlas with clinical, dermoscopic and histological correlations, pp 7–13. ISBN: 9780415451048
3. Scope A, Benvenuto-Andrade C, Agero AL, Malvehy J, Puig S, Rajadhyaksha M, Busam KJ, Marra DE, Torres A, Propperova I, Langley RG, Marghoob AA, Pellacani G, Seidenari S, Halpern AC, Gonzalez S (2007) In vivo reflectance confocal microscopy imaging of melanocytic skin lesions: consensus terminology glossary and illustrative images. J Am Acad Dermatol 57:644–658
4. Calzavara-Pinton P, Longo C, Venturini M, Sala R, Pellacani G (2008) Reflectance confocal microscopy for in vivo skin imaging. Photochem Photobiol 84:1421–1430
5. Rajadhyaksha M, Grossman M, Esterowitz D, Webb RH, Anderson RR (1995) In vivo confocal scanning laser microscopy of human skin: melanin provides strong contrast. J Invest Dermatol 104: 946–952
6. Rajadhyaksha M, González S, Zavislan JM, Anderson RR, Webb RH (1999) In vivo confocal scanning laser microscopy of human skin II: advances in instrumentation and comparison with histology. J Invest Dermatol 113:293–303
7. Huzaira M, Rius F, Rajadhyaksha M, Anderson RR, González S (2001 Jun) Topographic variations in normal skin, as viewed by in vivo reflectance confocal microscopy. J Invest Dermatol 116: 846–852

5 Acral Volar Skin, Facial Skin and Mucous Membrane

Susana Puig, Cristina Carrera, Louise Lovato, and Myrna Hanke-Martinez

5.1 Acral Volar Skin

Palms and soles are areas infrequently explored with RCM, because of the peculiar characteristics of volar skin, with the thicker epidermis of the human anatomy and the limited power of RCM penetration that in these sites is not able to reach dermo-epidermal junction [1–4]. The specific characteristics of volar skin are the thickness of the epidermis, the presence of high number of eccrine glands and ducts, the absence of hair follicle units and the specific distribution of the skin marks and the eccrine ducts. The *stratum corneum*, *stratum granulosum* and *stratum spinosum* are thicker in acral sites compared with other body sites. In the images of the RCM, we can see the correlation of the ridges, conformed by groups of keratinocytes separated by dermatoglyphics, which appear as non-refractive furrow. The eccrine ducts openings are roundish bright structures with a dark center regularly distributed in the middle of the ridges of the skin marks.

5.2 Face

The skin of the face is also different from all other regions of the human body [1–3, 5, 6]. Interpapillary processes do not exist or are minimal, in part, due to frequent sun exposure and the actinic damage resulting. Facial skin has numerous pilosebaceous follicles containing small hair. Dermoscopy of melanocytic lesions of the face shows pseudonetwork, which represents the follicular openings interrupting the homogeneous pigmentation on the face.

In healthy skin types I and II, due to the little melanin in the basal layer, the images of RCM are low refractive and dermal-epidermal junction (DEJ) becomes very subtle being much less noticeable in a sun-damaged skin.

In a sun-exposed skin, the stratum corneum, the most superficial level, appears more refractive and thicker; in contrast, the granular layer becomes thinner, with an increase in the number of keratinocytes, displaying small diameter and some degree of cellular atypia in the squamous layer. The dermal papillae are more numerous, smaller and less unevenly distributed. Skin capillaries are in greater quantity and with smaller diameter. In the dermis, thick reticular refractive structures can be observed, which correspond to fragmented and distorts collagen fibers due to chronic sun exposure and the resulting solar elastosis. The immune response is also increased in this area and in inflammatory conditions there is an increase in the number of dendritic cells, such as Langerhans cells (LC). LC differentiation from dendritic melanocytes can be difficult in the evaluation of lentigo maligna melanoma.

5.3 Mucosa

Most cases of malignancy in oral mucosa and anogenital are relatively advanced at diagnosis. Early detection and appropriate treatment significantly increases survival. However, the initial lesions can often be indistinguishable from benign conditions based only on clinical examination.

Reflectance confocal microscopy can be used for the detection of precancerous lesions, dysplasia and cancer, but also in benign inflammatory conditions [7]. The limitation of confocal in vivo microscopy is the depth of penetration and therefore its inability to assess the deeper layers. In consequence, verrucous lesions with extreme hyperkeratosis not allow sufficient penetration of light to visualize the entire lesion. The correlation between images of RCM and histopathology in oral and anogenital mucosa was consistent in several previous studies. Some devices use optic fiber to perform confocal imaging in mucosa [7] but the images shown in this

S. Puig (✉) • C. Carrera • L. Lovato • M. Hanke-Martinez
Melanoma Unit, Department of Dermatology, Hospital Clinic, IDIBAPS, CIBERER, Barcelona, Spain
e-mail: susipuig@gmail.com

R. Hofmann-Wellenhof et al. (eds.), *Reflectance Confocal Microscopy for Skin Diseases*,
DOI 10.1007/978-3-642-21997-9_5, © Springer-Verlag Berlin Heidelberg 2012

chapter were obtained with the Vivascope 1500 (Lucid Corp.) in the mucosa of the inner part of the lip.

The structures that can be observed with RCM at the cellular and subcellular level in the oral mucosa (lip and tongue papillae) were previously described: the boundaries of cells and nuclei, intracellular organelles in the surface layer of the epithelium, extracellular matrix on the blade, blood flow and blood cells. In the images of the surface, epithelial cells have become larger and flatter compared with the cells of the deeper layers, which appear more spherical. With the exception of the hard palate and the dorsum of the tongue, the mucous membrane of the mouth do not produce keratin and consequently it possesses neither a granular nor a horny layer. The images obtained of the tongue are affected and limited by the surface keratinization and decreased contrast in the deeper layers. In contrast, not keratinized images in lip mucosa showed better resolution in the deeper layers. The superficial layer shows large ill-demarcated cells with prominent nucleus, then suprabasal layers show large hyporefractive (because the glycogen content) well-demarcated (because desmosomes) cells with small nucleus. Deep layers show roundish small ill-demarcated cells. In dermis, refractivity is more homogeneous with thin fibers and well-circumscribed vessels. In cancerous lesions in RCM, several features can be observed: pleomorphic cells, different densities and altered nuclear morphology that differs between confocal images of mucosal neoplastic lesions and mucosal benign lesions.

Other features that can be identified in confocal images of the oral mucosa are areas of inflammation, fibrosis, muscle fibers and salivary glands. Areas of inflammation appear dark in confocal images of the oral cavity.

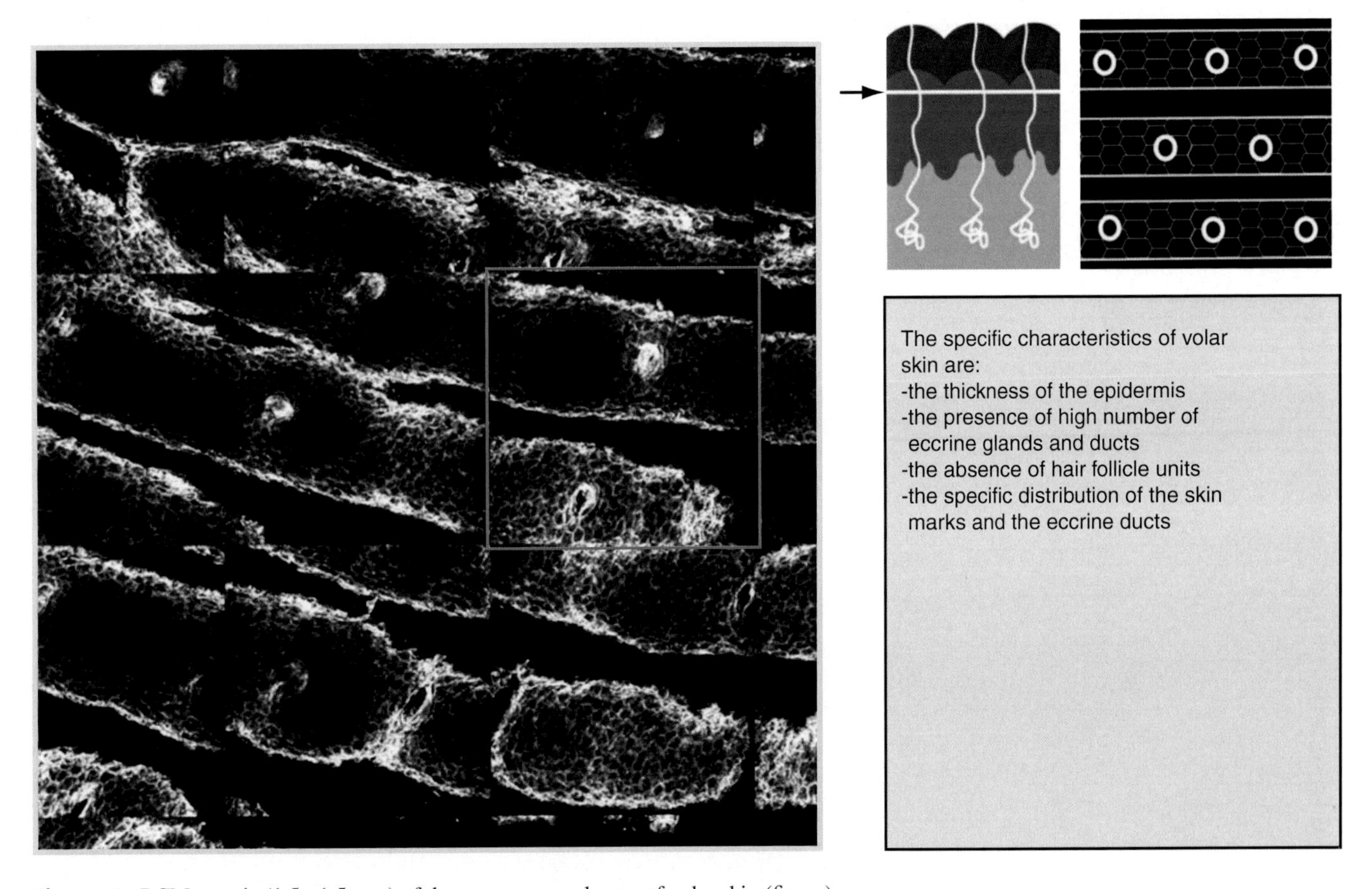

Fig. 5.1.1 RCM mosaic (1.5 × 1.5 mm) of the stratum granulosum of volar skin (finger)

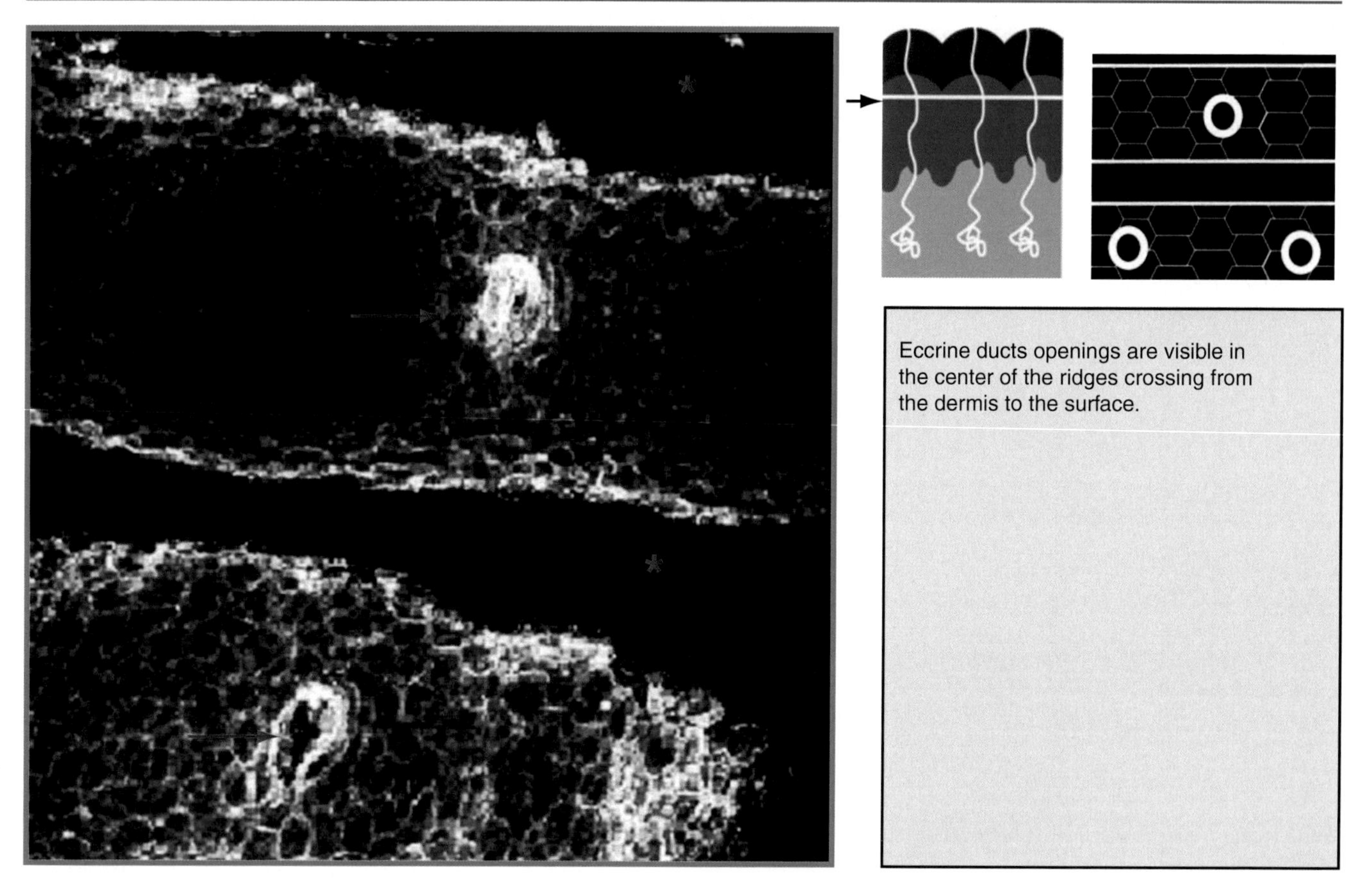

Fig. 5.1.2 Basic image (0.5×0.5 mm). The honeycomb pattern is interrupted by the presence of the furrows of the skin marks (*) in black and the presence of the acrosiringium openings (→) bright roundish structures with central dark area

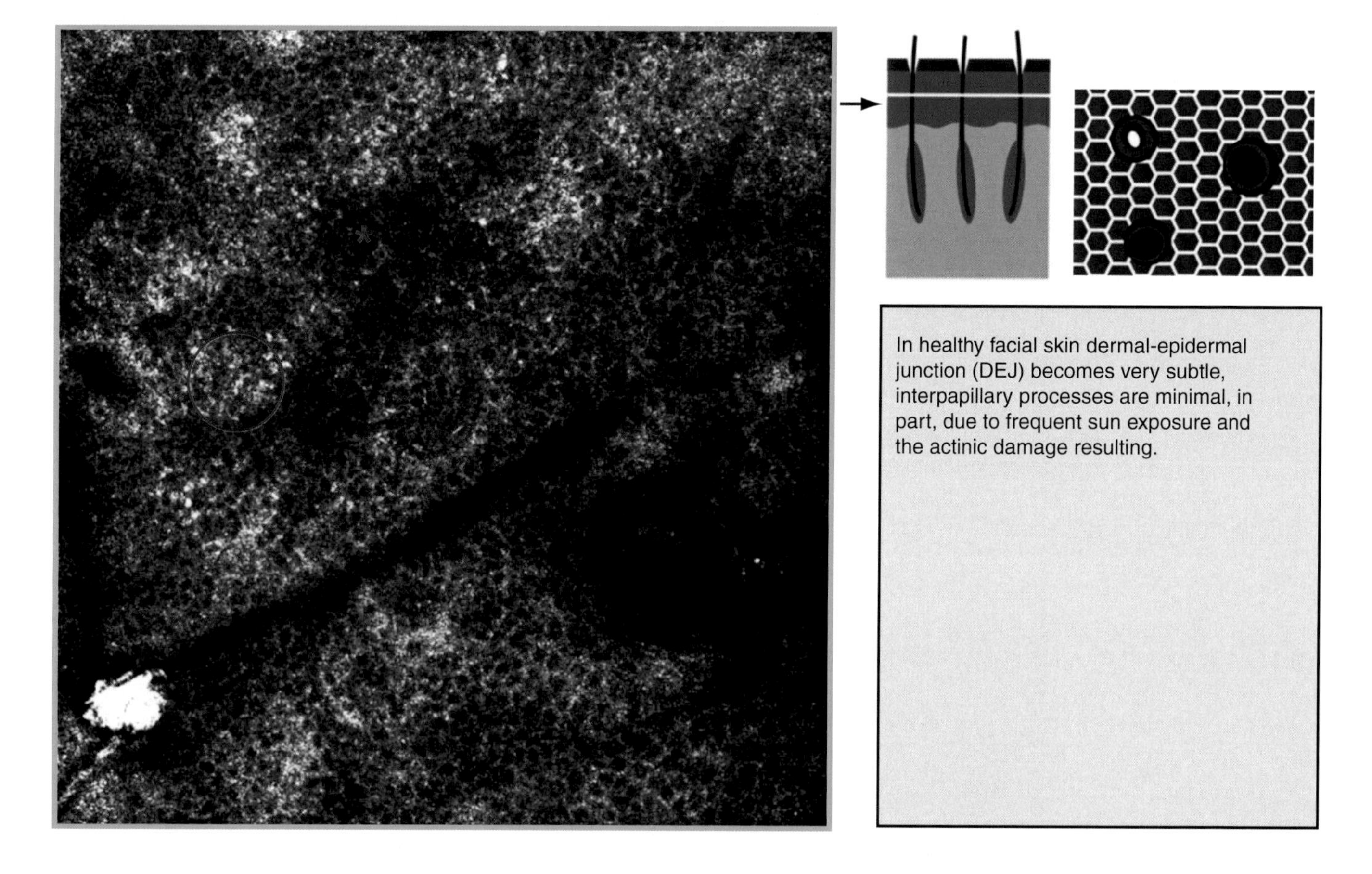

Fig. 5.2.1 Basic RCM image (0.5×0.5 mm) at the basal and suprabasal layer on the face. Interpapillary processes are minimal and dermal papilla is difficult to be identified. Hyporefractile areas are the top of the dermal papillae (*) and areas with small bright cells are keratinocytes in the basal layer (O)

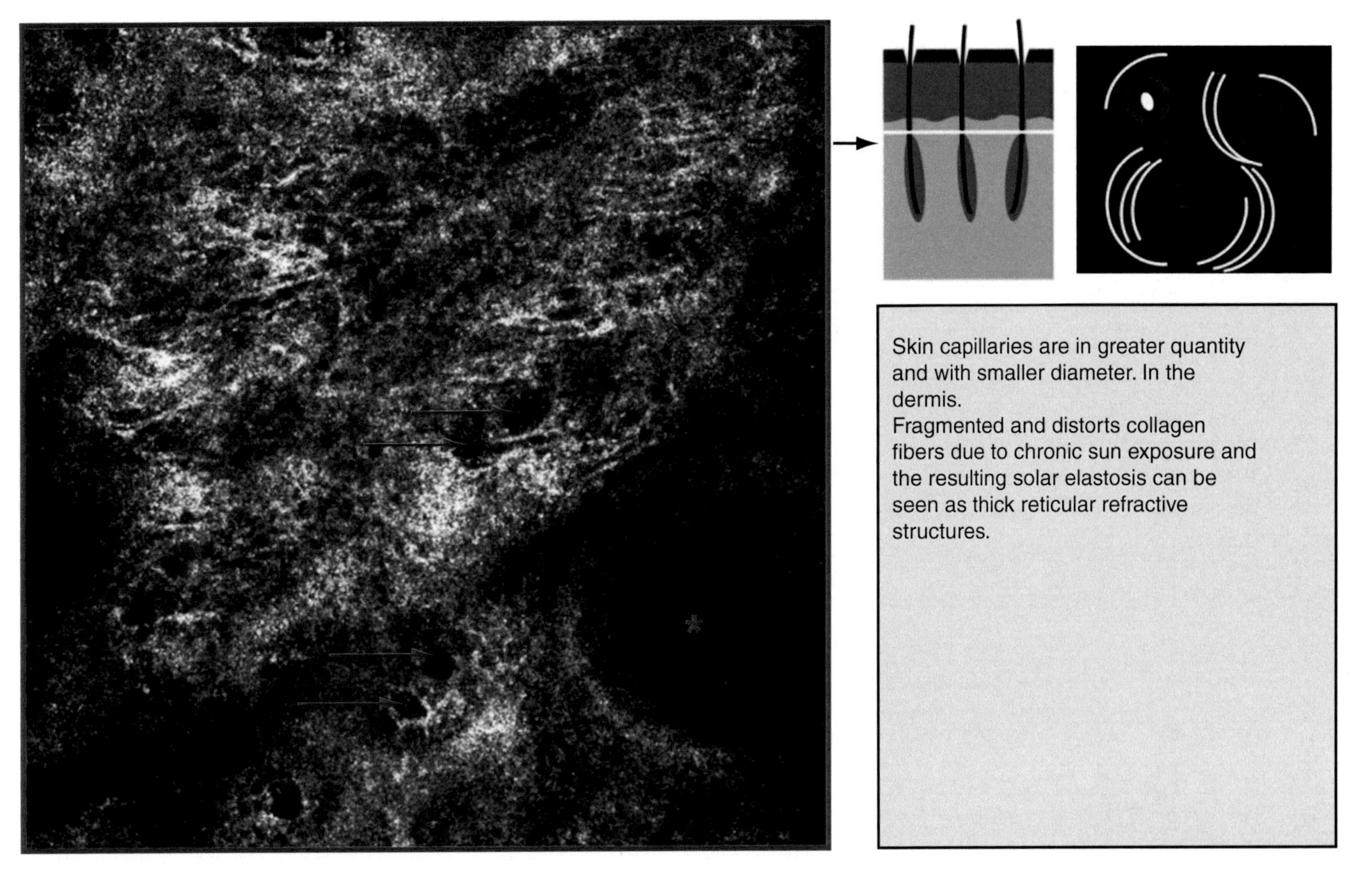

Fig. 5.2.2 Basic image (0.5 × 0.5 mm) at the papillary dermis in facial skin. Hair follicles are prominent (*) but dermal papillae are not easy visible. Small capillaries are frequently seen (→)

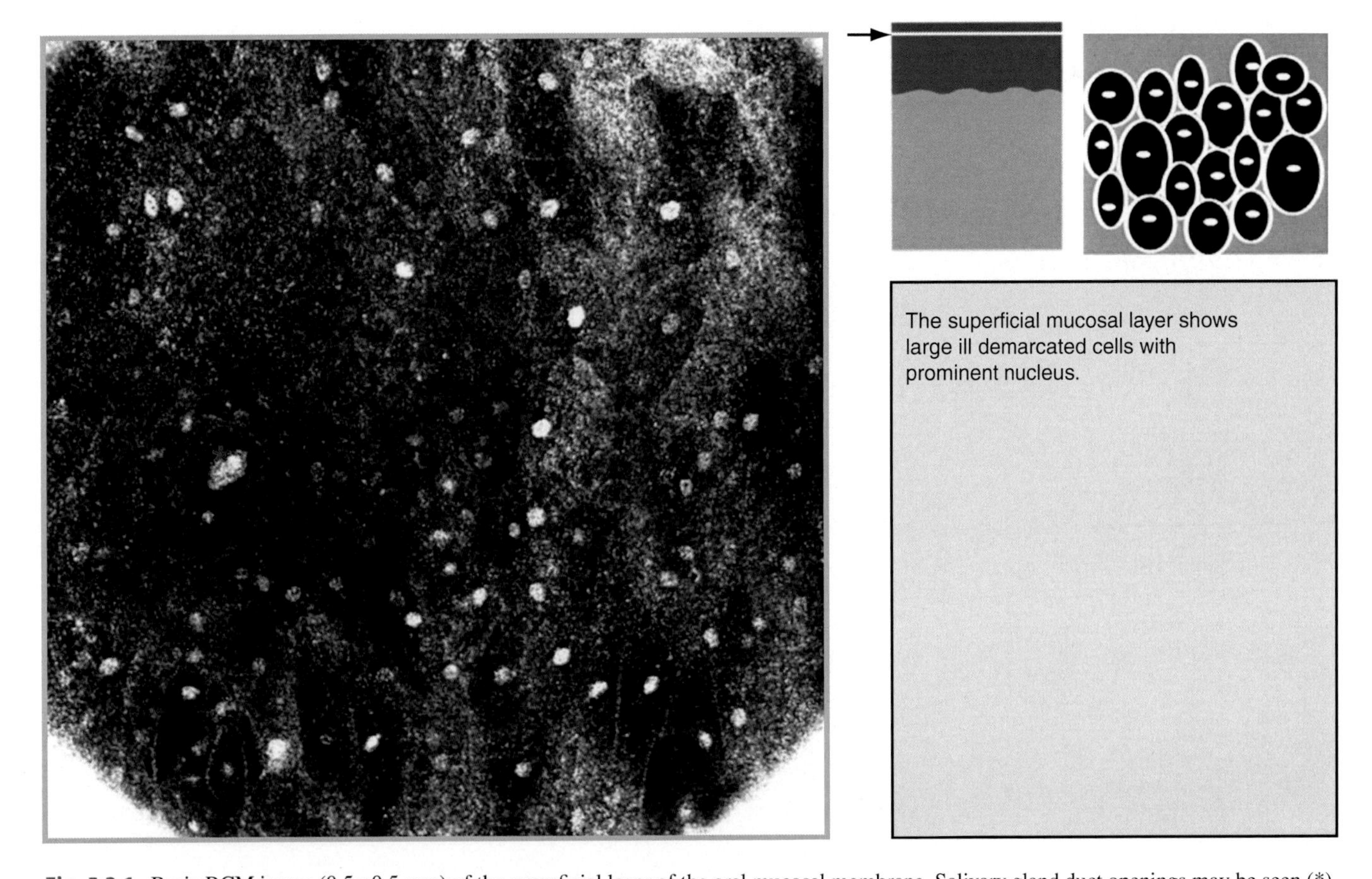

Fig. 5.3.1 Basic RCM image (0.5 × 0.5 mm) of the superficial layer of the oral mucosal membrane. Salivary gland duct openings may be seen (*)

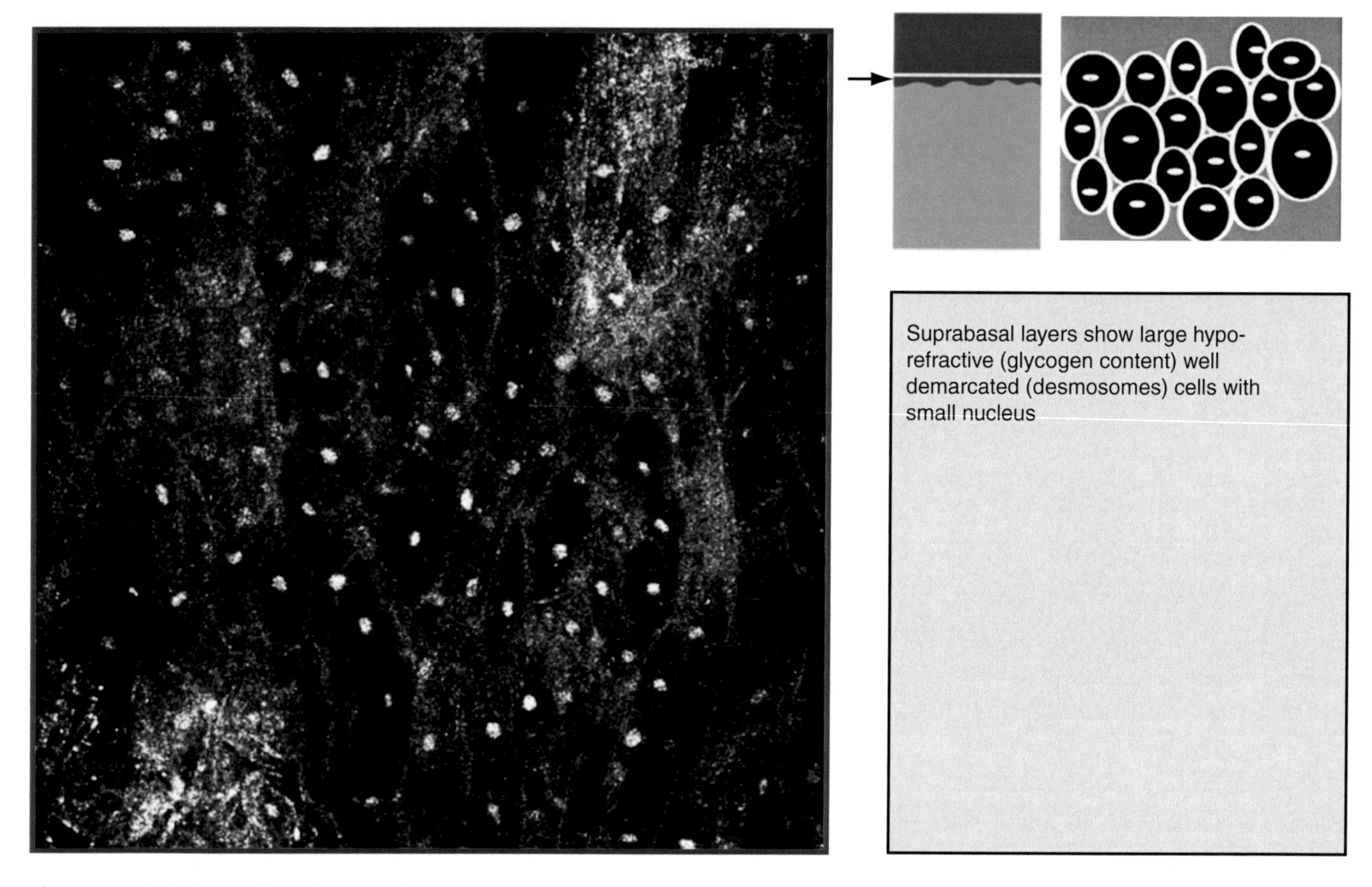

Fig. 5.3.2 Basic image (0.5 × 0.5 mm) of suprabasal layers in oral mucosae

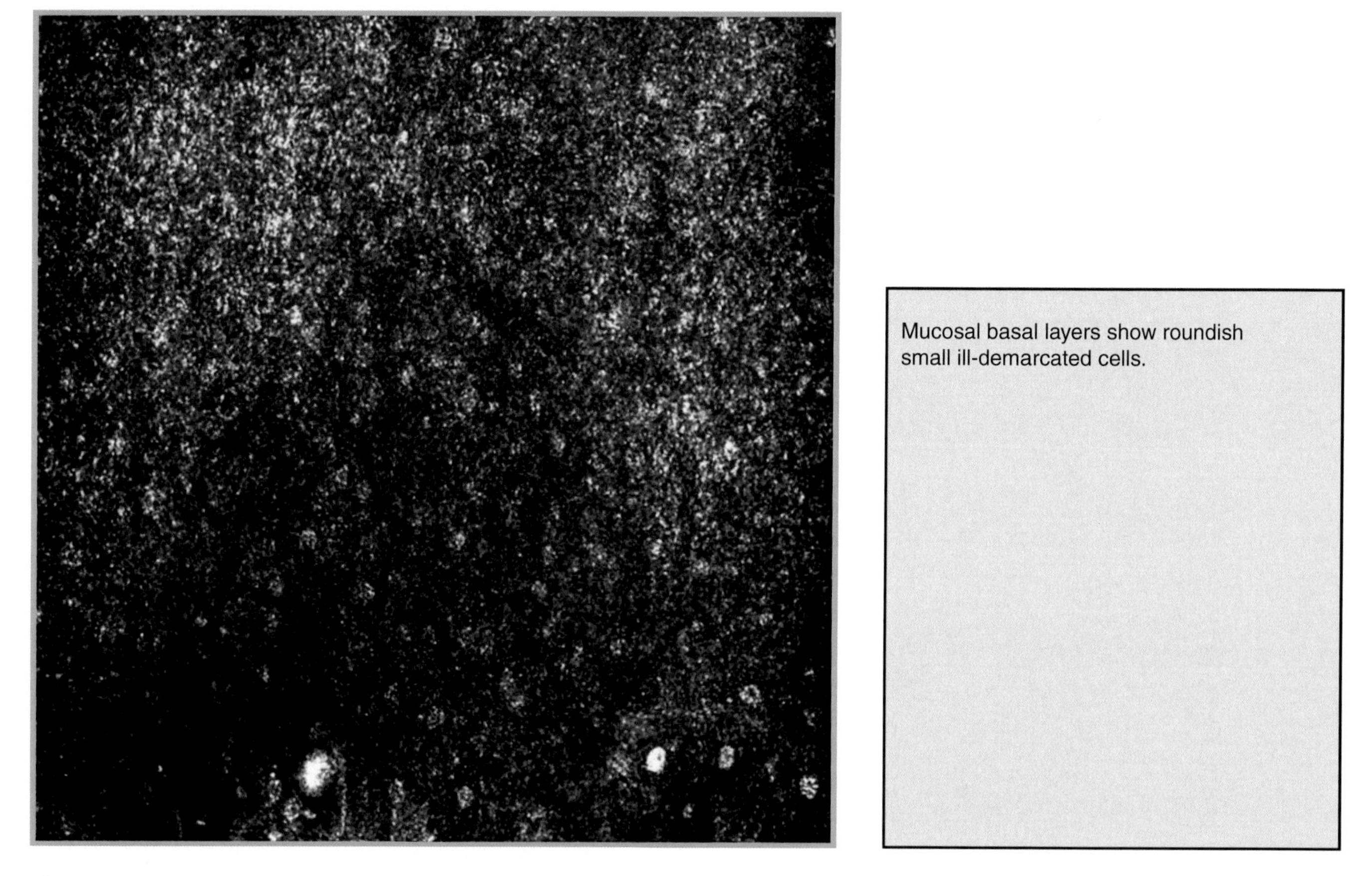

Fig. 5.3.3 Basic RCM image (0.5 × 0.5 mm) at the basal layer of oral mucosa

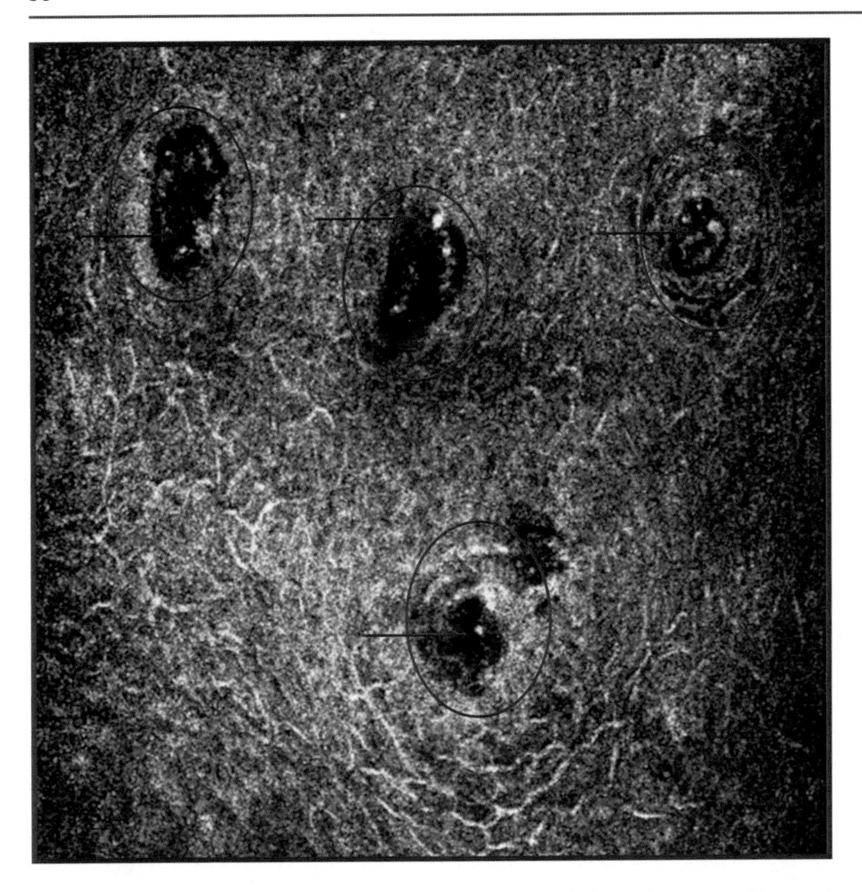

Dermal papilla are simetrically distributed with a prominent central vessel.

Fig. 5.3.4 Basic image (0.5×0.5 mm) of dermal papilla (O) in oral mucosa with prominent central curved vessels and leucocytes visible (→)

References

1. Huzaira M, Rius F, Rajadhyaksha M, Anderson RR, González S (2001) Topographic variations in normal skin, as viewed by in vivo reflectance confocal microscopy. J Invest Dermatol 116(6):846–852
2. González S, Gill M, Halpern AC (2008) Normal skin. Reflectance confocal microscopy of cutaneous tumors: an atlas with clinical, dermoscopic and histological correlations, pp 7–13. ISBN: 9780415451048
3. Robertson K, Rees JL (2010) Variation in epidermal morphology in human skin at different body sites as measured by reflectance confocal microscopy. Acta Derm Venereol 90(4):368–373
4. Kolm I, Kamarashev J, Kerl K, Hafner J, Läuchli S, French LE, Braun RP (2010) Acral melanoma with network pattern: a dermoscopy-reflectance confocal microscopy and histopathology correlation. Dermatol Surg 36(5):701–703, Epub 2010 Apr 1
5. Ahlgrimm-Siess V, Massone C, Scope A, Fink-Puches R, Richtig E, Wolf IH, Koller S, Gerger A, Smolle J, Hofmann-Wellenhof R (2009) Reflectance confocal microscopy of facial lentigo maligna and lentigo maligna melanoma: a preliminary study. Br J Dermatol 161(6):1307–1316
6. Guitera P, Pellacani G, Crotty KA, Scolyer RA, Li LX, Bassoli S, Vinceti M, Rabinovitz H, Longo C, Menzies SW (2010) The impact of in vivo reflectance confocal microscopy on the diagnostic accuracy of lentigo maligna and equivocal pigmented and nonpigmented macules of the face. J Invest Dermatol 130(8): 2080–2091
7. White WM, Rajadhyaksha M, Gonzalez S, Fabian RL, Anderson RR (1999) Noninvasive imaging of human oral mucosa in vivo by confocal reflectance microscopy. Laryngoscope 109(10):1709–1717

Part III

Melanocytic Lesions

6 Semeiology and Pattern Analysis in Melanocytic Lesions

Barbara Ferrari, Hans Peter Soyer, Alice Casari, and Giovanni Pellacani

Melanocytic lesion exploration is conducted by the examination of mosaics and/or series of consecutive high-resolution images from the surface to the dermis up to the loss of resolution (approximately up to 200 μm). Mosaics are usually acquired at three levels (superficial layers, dermal-epidermal junction, upper dermis) for the evaluation of general epidermal pattern, frequencies and distribution of pagetoid cells, regularity of the DEJ architecture, presence and distribution of nests, and structures within the papillary dermis. High-resolution images are employed for the evaluation of cyto-architectural aspects.

The spread of reflectance confocal microscopy (RCM) has rendered the development of a common language in order to analyze the lesions in univocal way. The progressively developed terminology has been summarized and tested for its reproducibility, although new definitions and improvements are still coming out from literature [1–9].

In this chapter, the main patterns subdivided for layers (epidermal layer, dermoepidermal junction and upper dermis) are described.

6.1 Superficial Epidermal Layers

6.1.1 General Aspects

Stratum spinosum and granulosum are usually constituted by large (10–20 μm) polygonal cells with dark nuclei and bright cytoplasm and cell borders giving rise to a honeycombed pattern (Fig. 6.1). In some melanocytic lesions, superficial layers consisted of small polygonal cells with refractive cytoplasm separated by a less refractive border, giving rise to a cobblestone pattern (Fig. 6.2). Honeycombed pattern with bright enlarged and broadened intercellular spaces is termed *broadened honeycombed.* The term *irregular-shaped keratinocytes* defines irregularity in size and shape of the keratinocytes (Fig. 6.3).

Sometimes melanomas present a disarray of the normal architecture of the superficial layers, characterized by unevenly distributed bright granular particles and cells, irregular in shape and size, in the absence of honeycombed or cobblestone pattern (*disarranged pattern*) (Fig. 6.4).

6.1.2 Presence and Aspects of Pagetoid Cells

The presence of large cells with bright cytoplasm and dark eccentric nucleus in superficial layers is suggestive of *pagetoid spread.* Whereas the observation of a great amount of large pleomorphic cells spreading upwards in pagetoid fashion is strictly correlated to melanoma diagnosis, few atypical cells within superficial layers can be occasionally seen in benign lesions, too.

Pagetoid cells are considered when large nucleated cells, twice the size of basal keratinocytes, with a dark nucleus and bright cytoplasm, are observable within superficial layers.

Roundish pagetoid cells, corresponding to large bright cells with well outlined border and dark nucleus within the epidermis, represent the most common finding for melanoma diagnosis (Fig. 6.5). A small percentage of Clark nevi, as well as some Spitz/Reed nevi, shows pagetoid cells, usually few and localized in the center of the lesion.

Dendritic pagetoid cells are large cells with bright cytoplasm and dark nucleus with clearly visible dendrites connected to the cell. Both the shape of the cell and the thickness, length and branching of dendrites vary consistently (Fig. 6.6). They have a lower diagnostic significance as they are sometimes observed in benign melanocytic lesions and in nonmelanocytic ones. They can represent either melanocytes spreading upward in a pagetoid fashion or Langerhans cells. Dendritic cells with a small sometimes triangular cytoplasm located in the subcorneal layer

B. Ferrari (✉) • A. Casari • G. Pellacani
Department of Dermatology and Venereology,
University of Modena and Reggio Emilia, Modena, Italy
e-mail: ferrari.barbara1@gmail.com

H.P. Soyer
Dermatology Research Centre, The University of Queensland,
Princess Alexandra Hospital School of Medicine, Brisbane,
Queensland, Australia
e-mail: p.soyer@uq.edu.au

R. Hofmann-Wellenhof et al. (eds.), *Reflectance Confocal Microscopy for Skin Diseases*,
DOI 10.1007/978-3-642-21997-9_6, © Springer-Verlag Berlin Heidelberg 2012

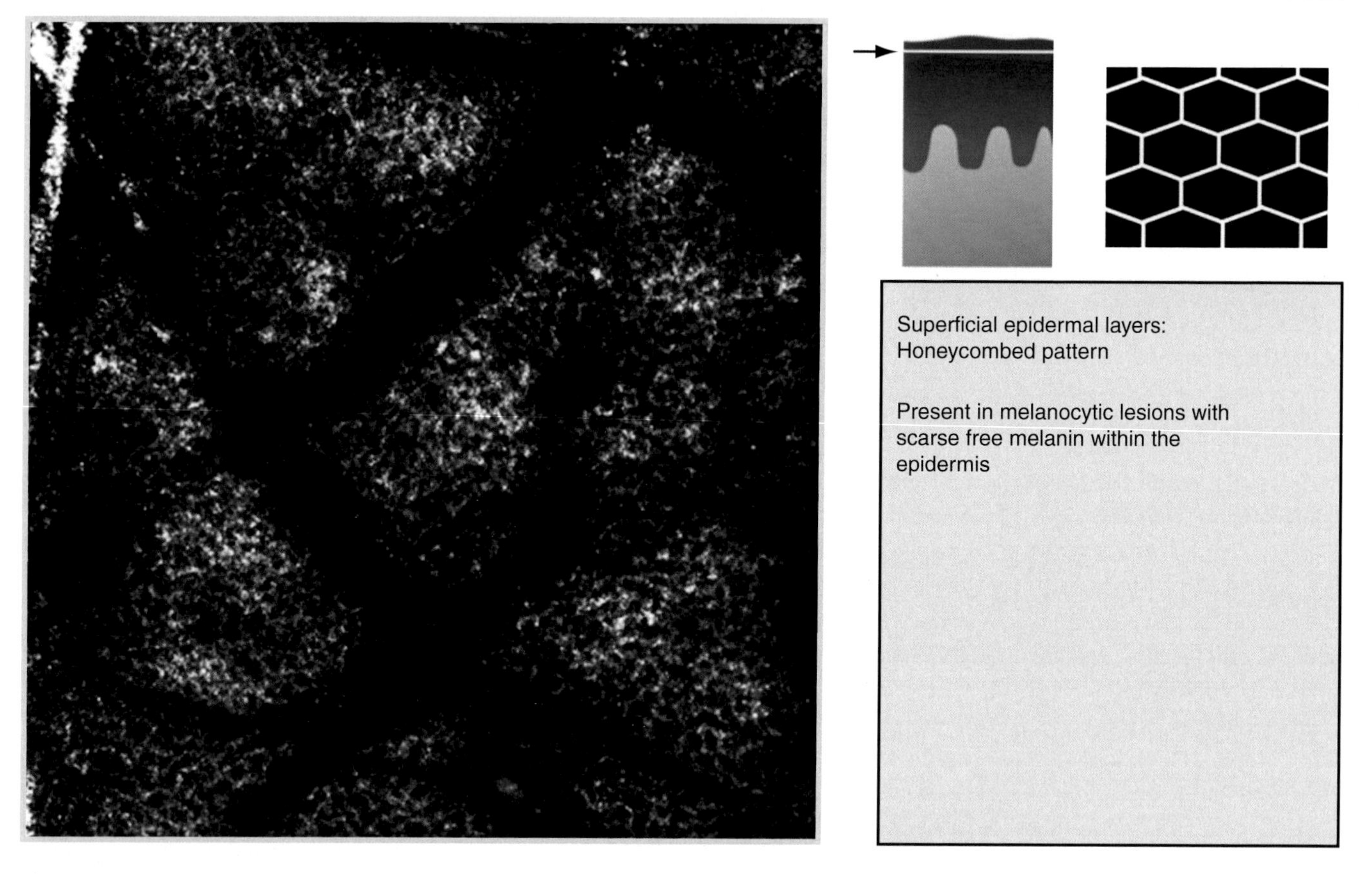

Fig. 6.1 Basic image (0.5 × 0.5 mm). Superficial epidermal layers (granulosum-spinosum): honeycombed pattern: polygonal cells with dark nuclei and bright cytoplasm and cell borders

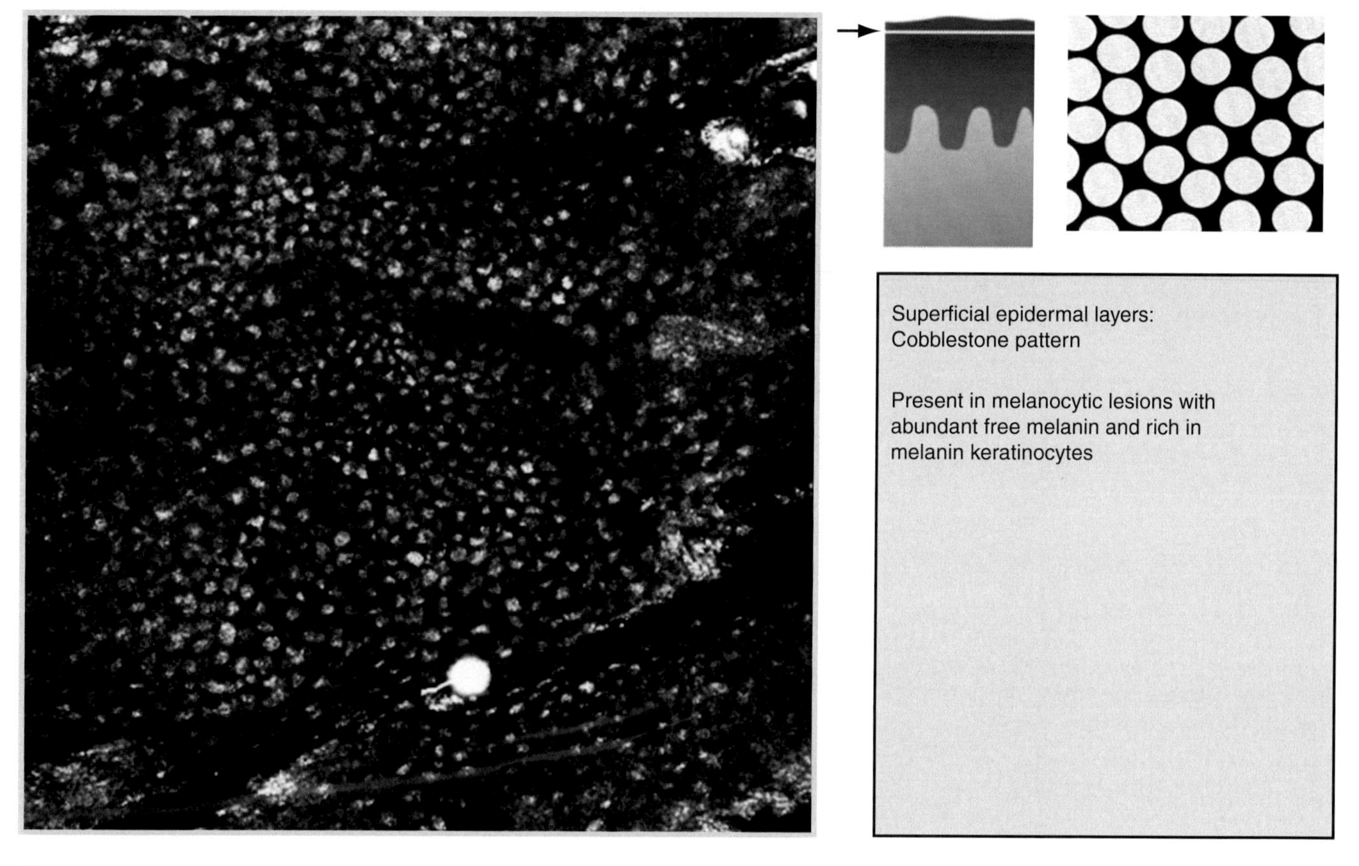

Fig. 6.2 Basic image (0.5 × 0.5 mm). Superficial epidermal layers (granulosum-spinosum: cobblestone pattern: small polygonal cells with refractive cytoplasm separated by a less refractive border

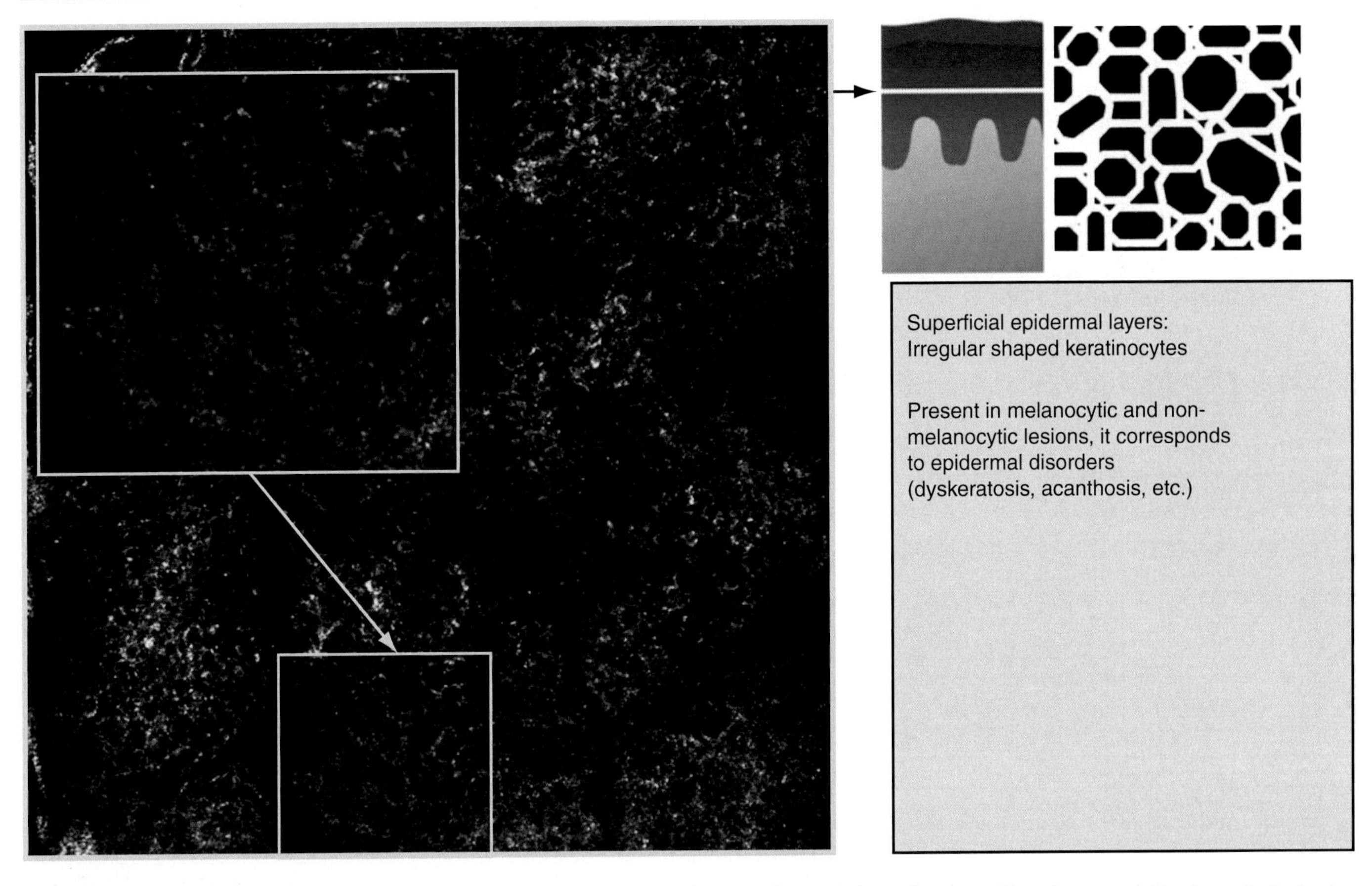

Fig. 6.3 Basic image (0.5 × 0.5 mm). Superficial epidermal layers (granulosum-spinosum): irregular-shaped keratinocytes define irregularity in size and shape of the keratinocytes

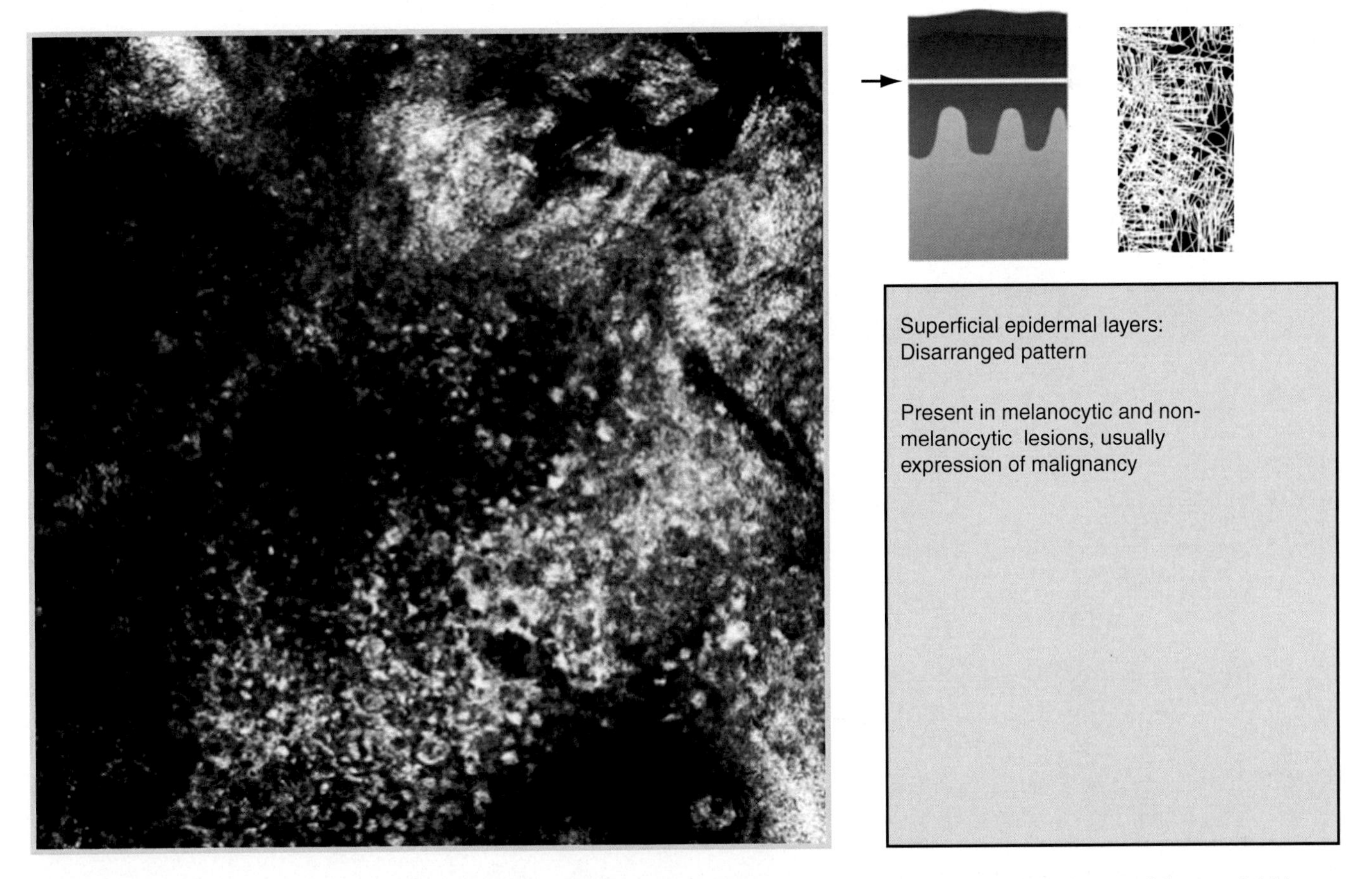

Fig. 6.4 Basic image (0.5 × 0.5 mm). Superficial epidermal layers (granulosum-spinosum): disarray of the normal architecture of the superficial layers, characterized by unevenly distributed bright granular particles and cells, irregular in shape and size, in the absence of honeycombed or cobblestone pattern

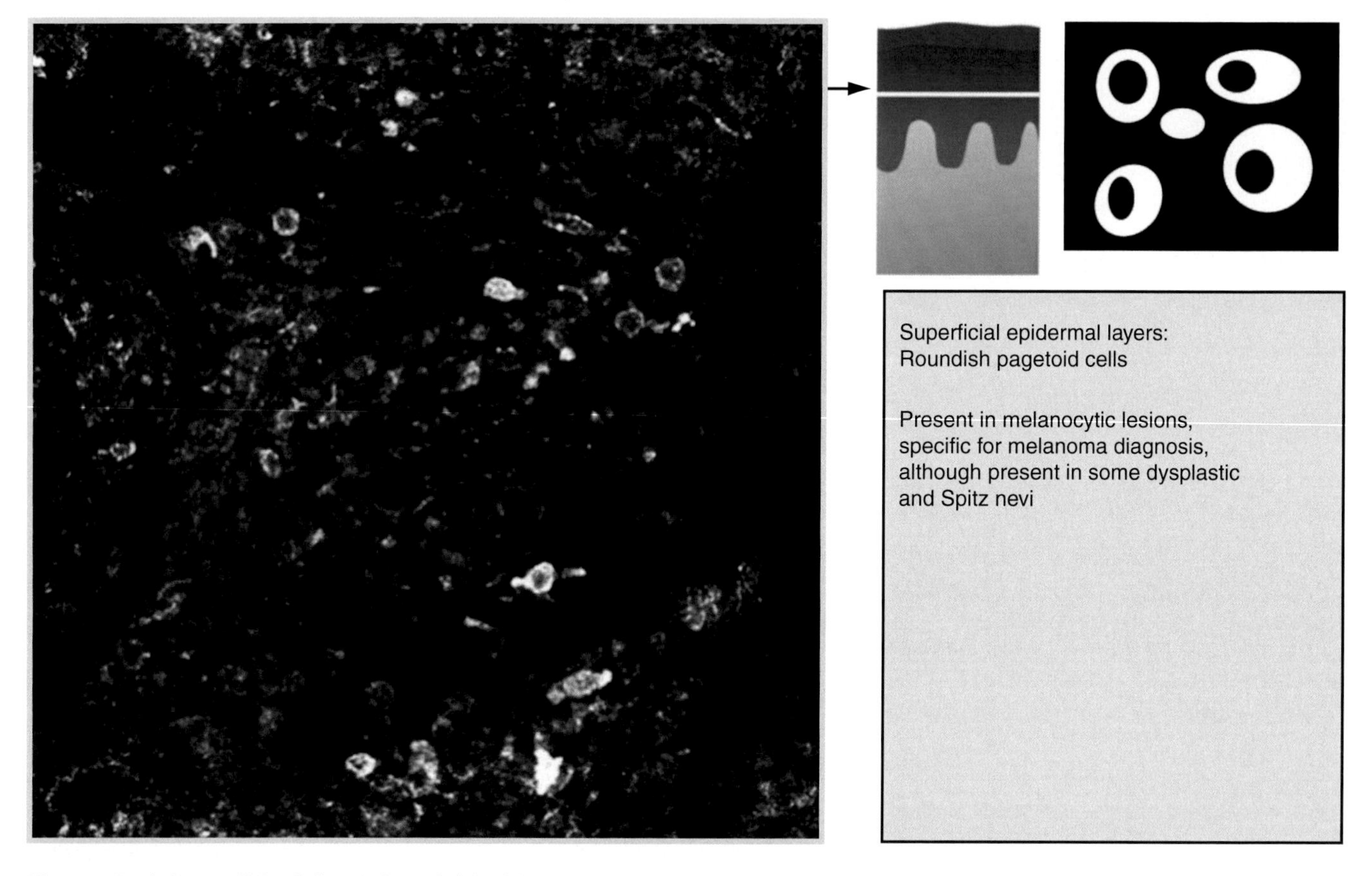

Fig. 6.5 Basic image (0.5 × 0.5 mm). Superficial epidermal layers (granulosum-spinosum): roundish pagetoid cells. Large bright cells with well outlined border and dark nucleus within the epidermis

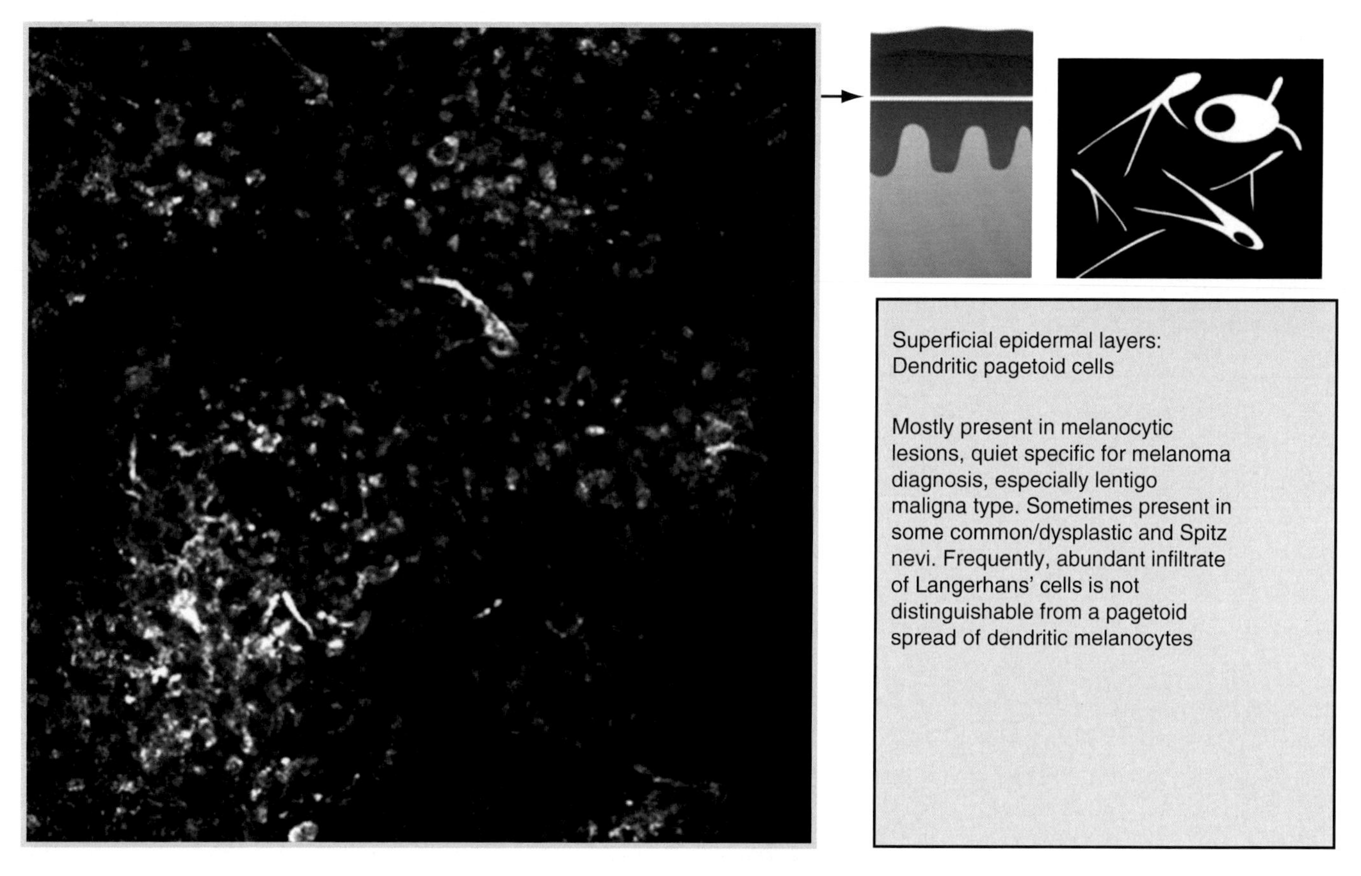

Fig. 6.6 Basic image (0.5 × 0.5 mm). Superficial epidermal layers (granulosum-spinosum): dendritic pagetoid cells. Large cells with bright cytoplasm and dark nucleus with clearly visible dendrites connected to the cell. Both the shape of the cell and the thickness, length and branching of dendrites vary consistently

are consistent with Langerhans cells. In contrast, cells with a large cell body and short and thick dendrites located in the spinous/granular layers are likely to be melanocytes. However, in some instances, as is the case in H&E pathology, the differentiation between the two dendritic cell types is impossible. Within melanomas, the lentigo maligna type is frequently characterized by the presence of numerous dendritic cells, which are found predominantly adjacent and within hair follicles.

Independent of the type of pagetoid cell, the following aspects need to be considered.

"Pleomorphism" is the variability of pagetoid cell morphology, characterized by the presence of both roundish and dendritic cells, and/or the presence of cells with bizarre shapes.

Density is classified into three different levels, considering the number of cells detectable in a square millimeter. Low density corresponds to less than 5 cells per square millimeter, moderate to 5–10 cells per square millimeter, and high to more than 10 cells per square millimeter.

Concerning the distribution, it is defined "localized" when pagetoid spread is present and concentrated in a limited portion of the lesion, "sparse" when it is possible to observe different foci of pagetoid infiltration, and "widespread" when pagetoid cells are scattered throughout the whole lesion area. A widespread distribution of the pagetoid spread is consistently associated with melanoma diagnosis, whereas atypical nevi and Spitz nevi may show few localized pagetoid cells.

6.2 Dermal–Epidermal Junction and Upper Dermis

By means of RCM, basal cells appear at a depth of approximately 50–100 μm below the stratum corneum. Going in depth, dermal papillae correspond to dark round to oval areas circumscribed by refractive cells, corresponding to melanocytes and melanin-rich keratinocytes.

6.3 Architecture

Examining skin lesions, the overall architecture is evaluated on "Mosaics" acquired at the DEJ, corresponding to a montage of full resolution individual images at a given depth "stitched" together to create a collage image with an area up to 8 × 8 mm.

At scanning magnification the general architecture of the lesion is described. One or more of the following patterns can be present:

Ringed pattern: numerous densely packed bright rings corresponding to papillae surrounded by a rim of small bright cells sharply contrasting with the dark background. The interpapillary spaces are thin. Figure 6.7 shows an example of this pattern.

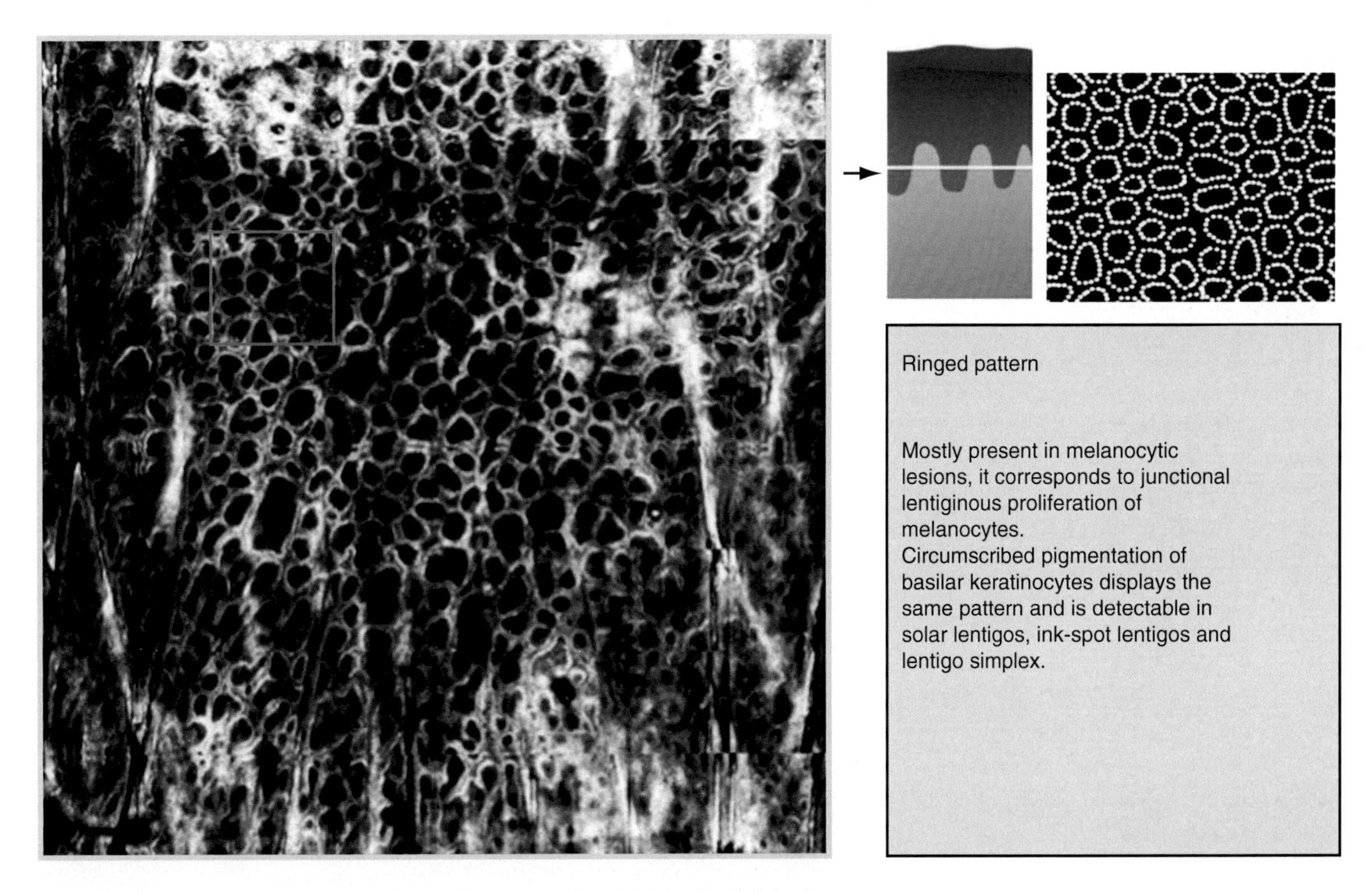

Fig. 6.7 RCM mosaic (4 × 4 mm): ringed pattern: numerous densely packed bright rings

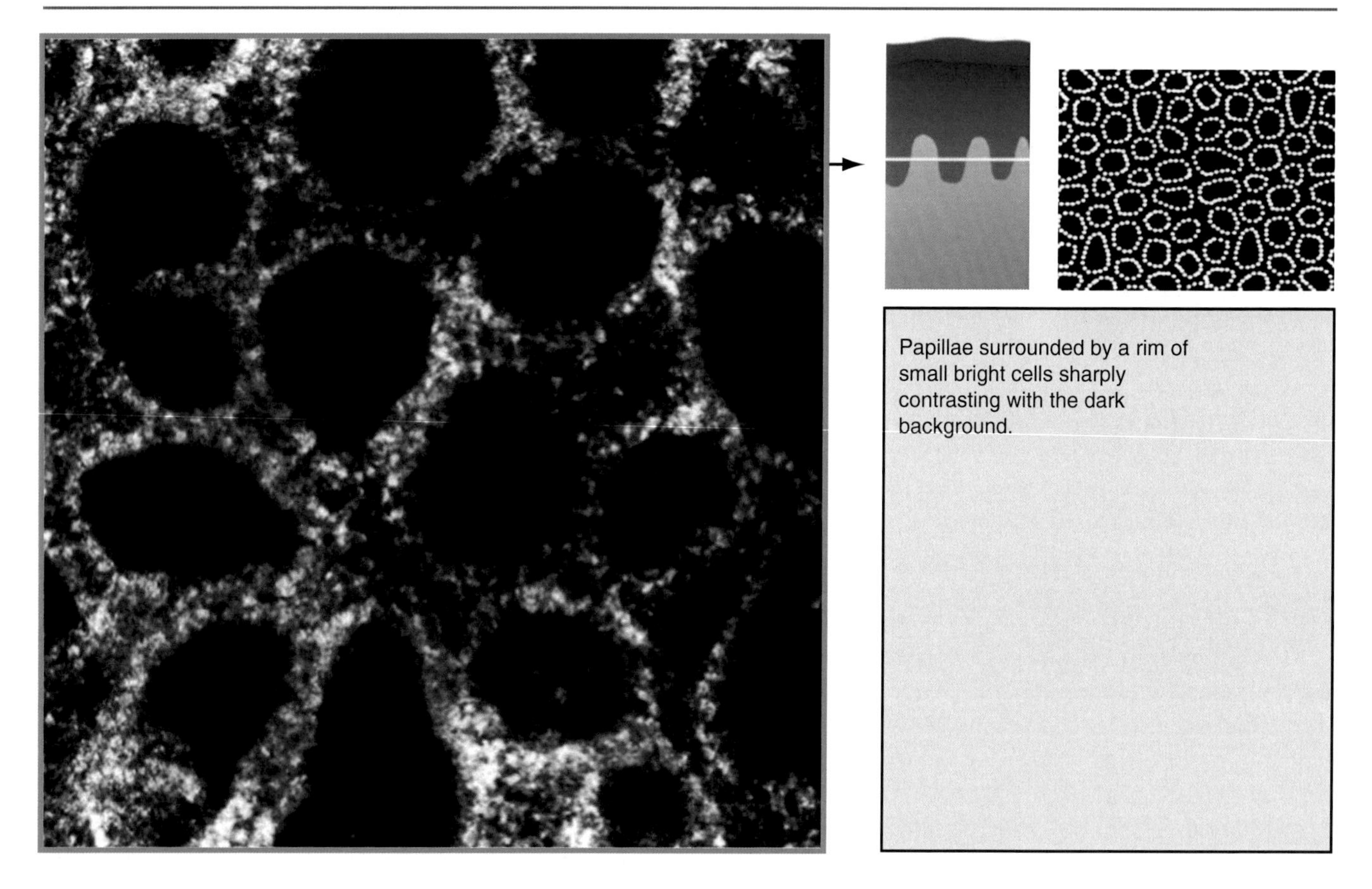

Fig. 6.7.1 Basic image (0.5 × 0.5 mm). In the detail there are papillae surrounded by a rim of small bright cells sharply contrasting with the dark background. The interpapillary spaces are thin

Meshwork pattern: a distinctive mesh characterized by small dark holes surrounded by clearly thickened interpapillary spaces. Dermal papillae usually appear smaller than in ringed pattern and are not outlined by rings. In melanocytic lesions junctional thickenings are constituted by junctional nests. Figure 6.8 shows an example of this pattern.

Clod pattern: numerous densely packed clods, constituted by clusters of melanocytes usually within dermal papillae. Figure 6.9 shows an example of this pattern.

Non-specific pattern: non-uniform architecture, non-corresponding to any of the above described patterns. It could be constituted by unevenly distributed dermal papillae, irregular in size and shape, usually without a demarcated rim of bright cells. Sometimes papillae are not visible. Figure 6.10 shows an example of this pattern.

6.4 Papillary Contour Features

After defining the overall pattern(s), characteristic descriptors of dermal–epidermal junction are taken into account, particularly focusing on the definition of the outlines of dermal papillae contours.

Edged papillae correspond to dermal papillae with clearly outlined contours. In melanocytic lesions, usually an edged papilla is either circumscribed by a rim of refractive cells, appearing as a bright ring sharply contrasting with the dark background, or by junctional nests constituted by compact melanocytic aggregates with sharp borders. Figures 6.11 and 6.12 show examples of this pattern.

Non-edged papillae are reported for the observation of dermal papillae without a demarcated contour. They are usually surrounded by single cells or by non-discrete aggregates, not forming a complete clear outline. Figure 6.13 shows an example of this pattern, whereas Fig. 6.14 shows an area presenting both edged and non-edged papillae.

The papillary architecture can be obscured by numerous cells or by non-homogeneously bright and dark areas giving rise to the disappearance of the normal papillary contour (non-visible papillae).

6.5 Aggregates

6.5.1 Junctional Nests

Junctional nests are oval compact cellular aggregates, bulging within the dermal papillae or enlarging the interpapillary spaces, formed by clustered cells, directly in connection with the basal cell layer. Usually, homogeneous compact aggregates with no atypical cells characterize

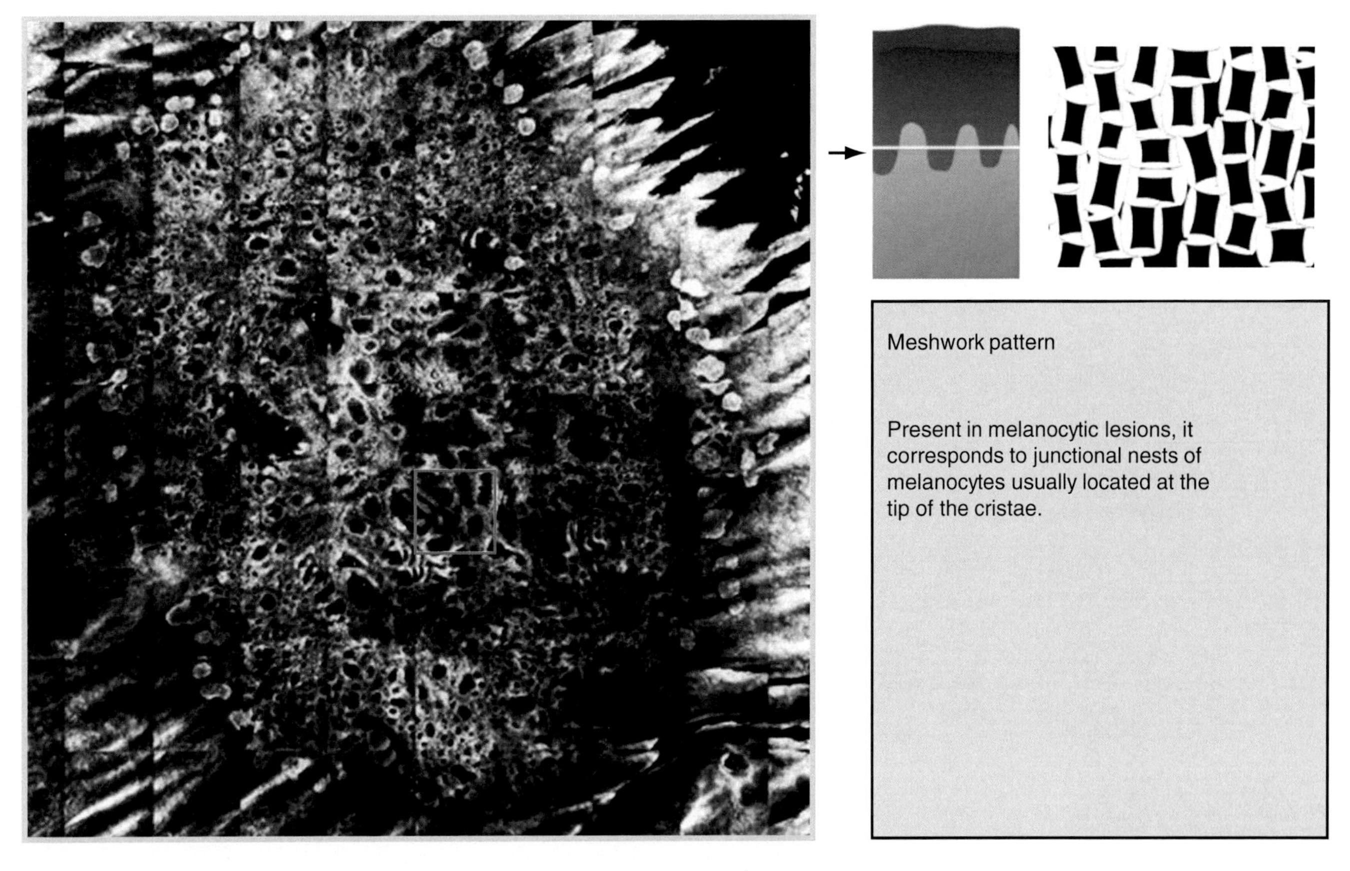

Fig. 6.8 RCM mosaic (4.5 × 4.5 mm): meshwork pattern: a net-like structure with large meshes

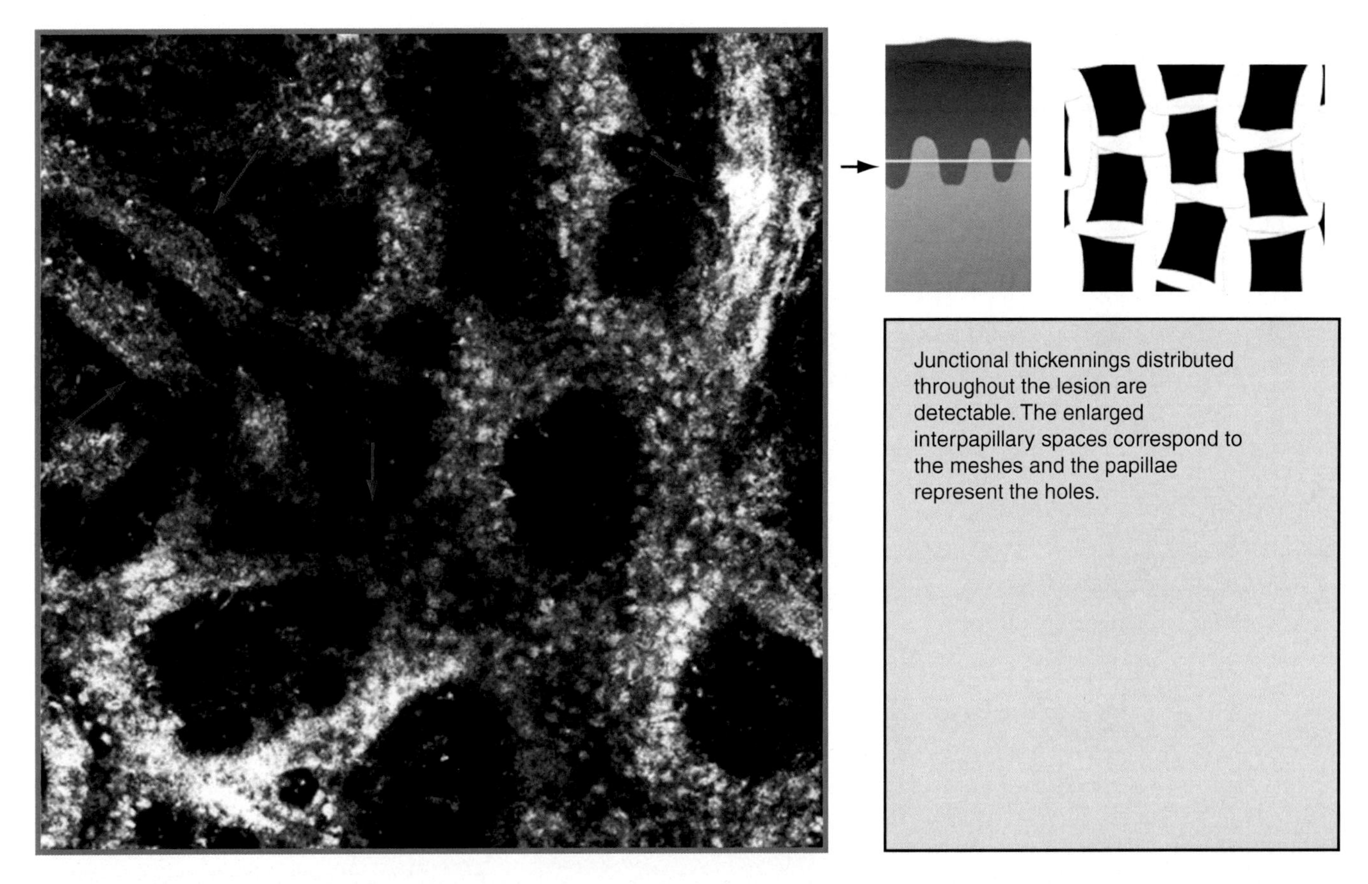

Fig. 6.8.1 Basic image (0.5 × 0.5 mm). In the detail there are junctional nests enlarging the interpapillary spaces (junctional thickenings) (→). Papilla contours are clearly outlined (edged papillae)

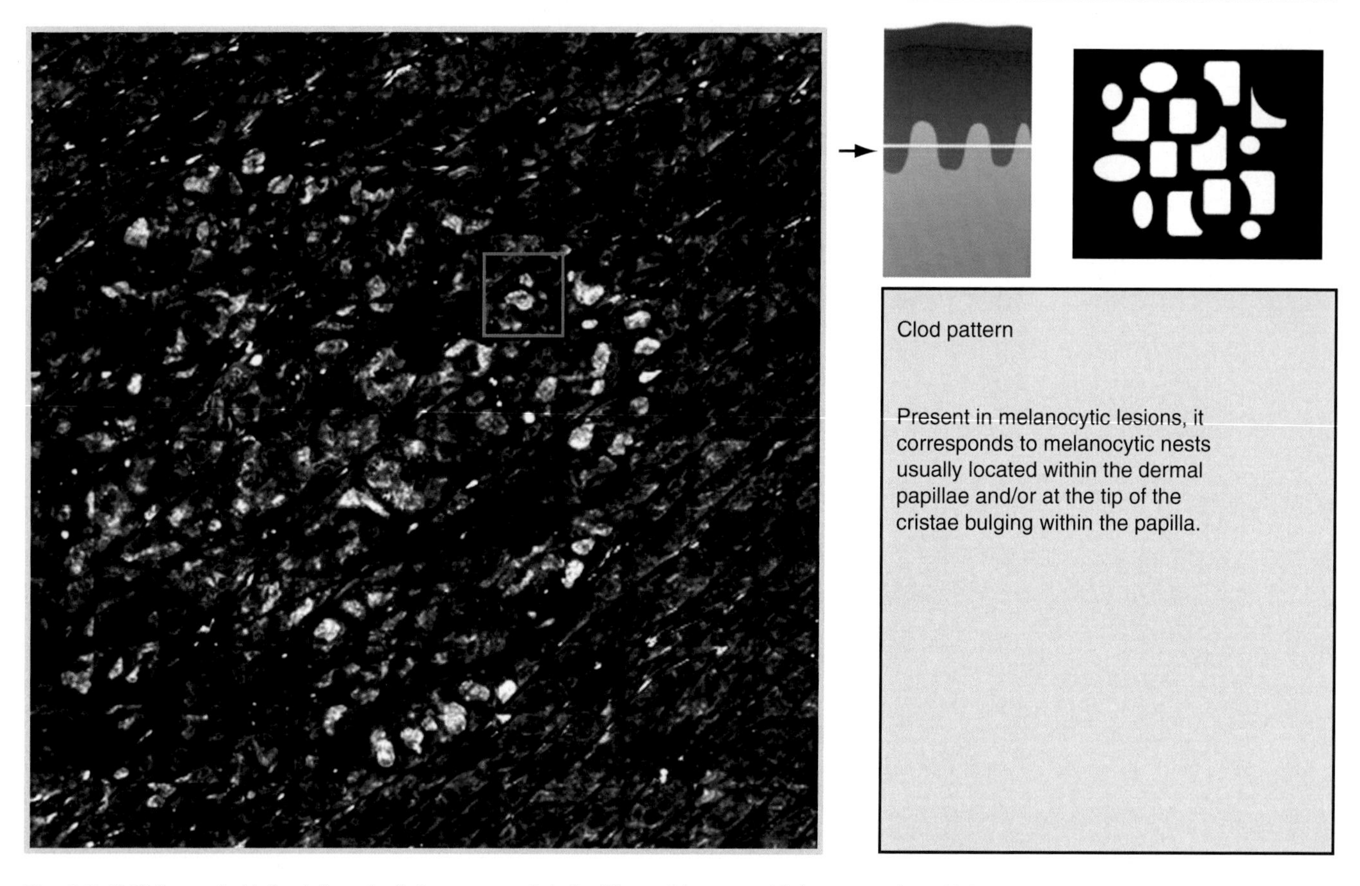

Fig. 6.9 RCM mosaic (4.5 × 4.5 mm): clod pattern: a globular-like architecture with large round-ovoidal structures

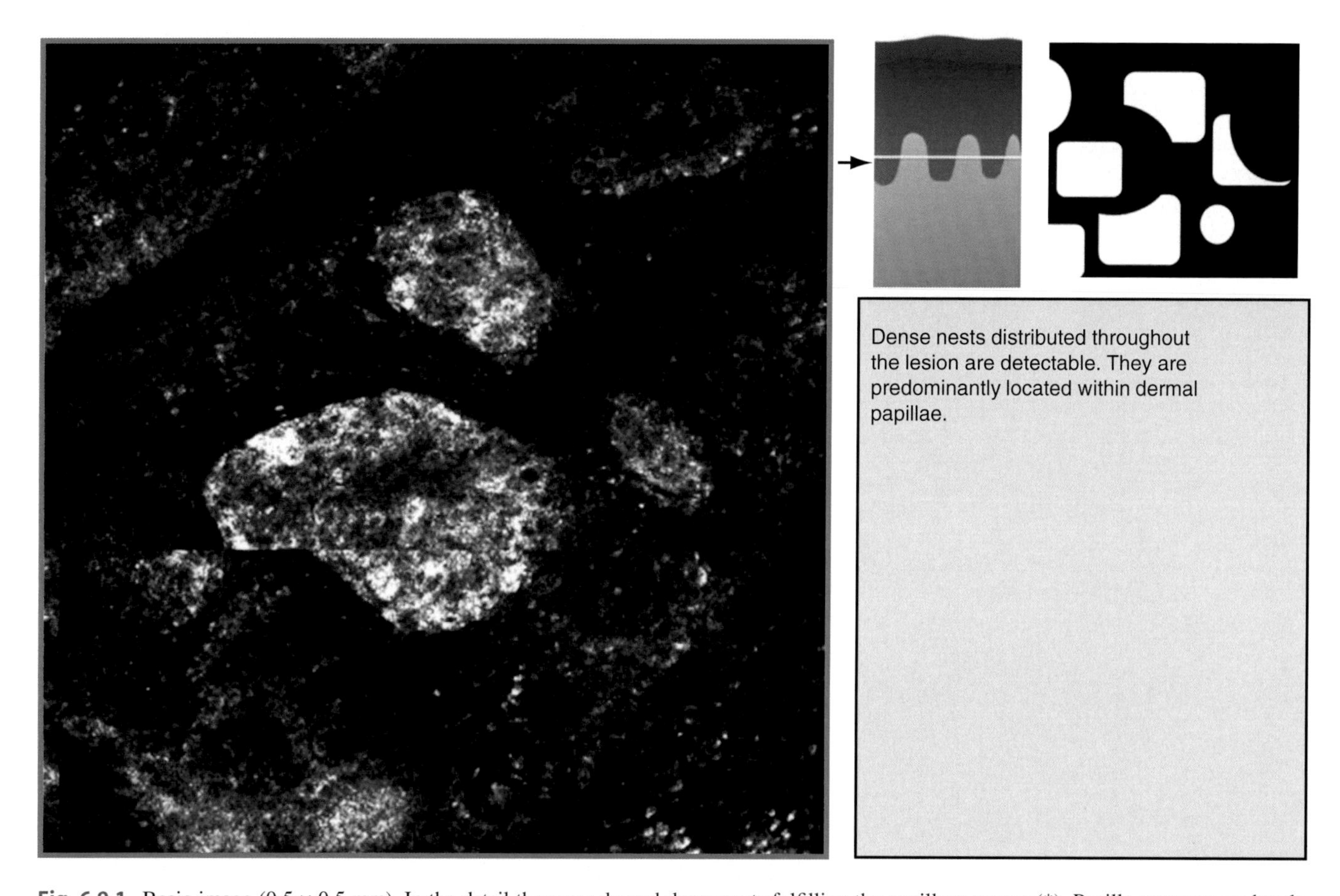

Fig. 6.9.1 Basic image (0.5 × 0.5 mm). In the detail there are dermal dense nests fulfilling the papillary spaces (*). Papilla contours are barely detectable

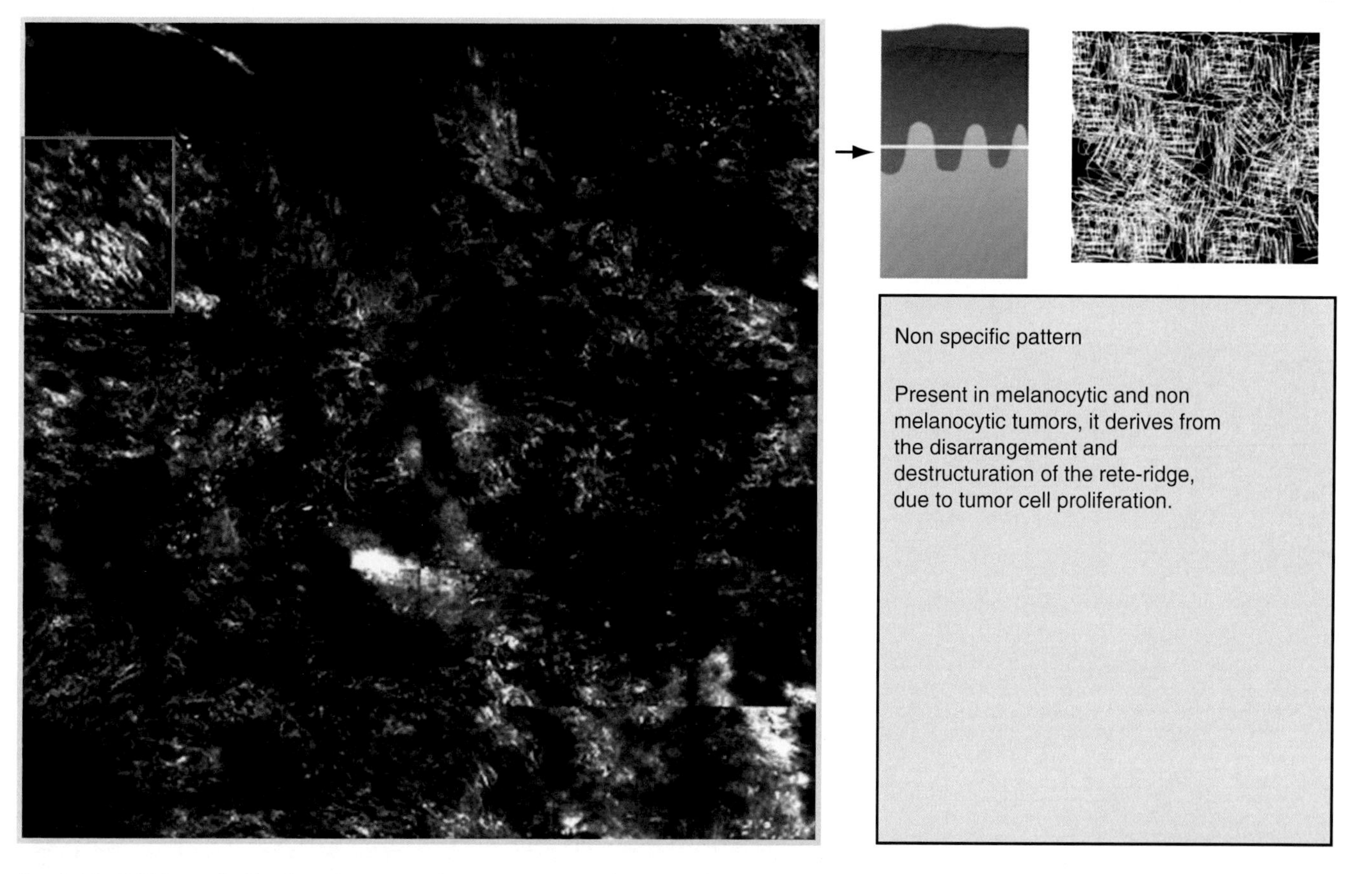

Fig. 6.10 RCM mosaic (3 × 3 mm): non-specific pattern: non-uniform architecture, by not structured unevenly reflecting areas, with a few visible dermal papillae, irregular in size and shape

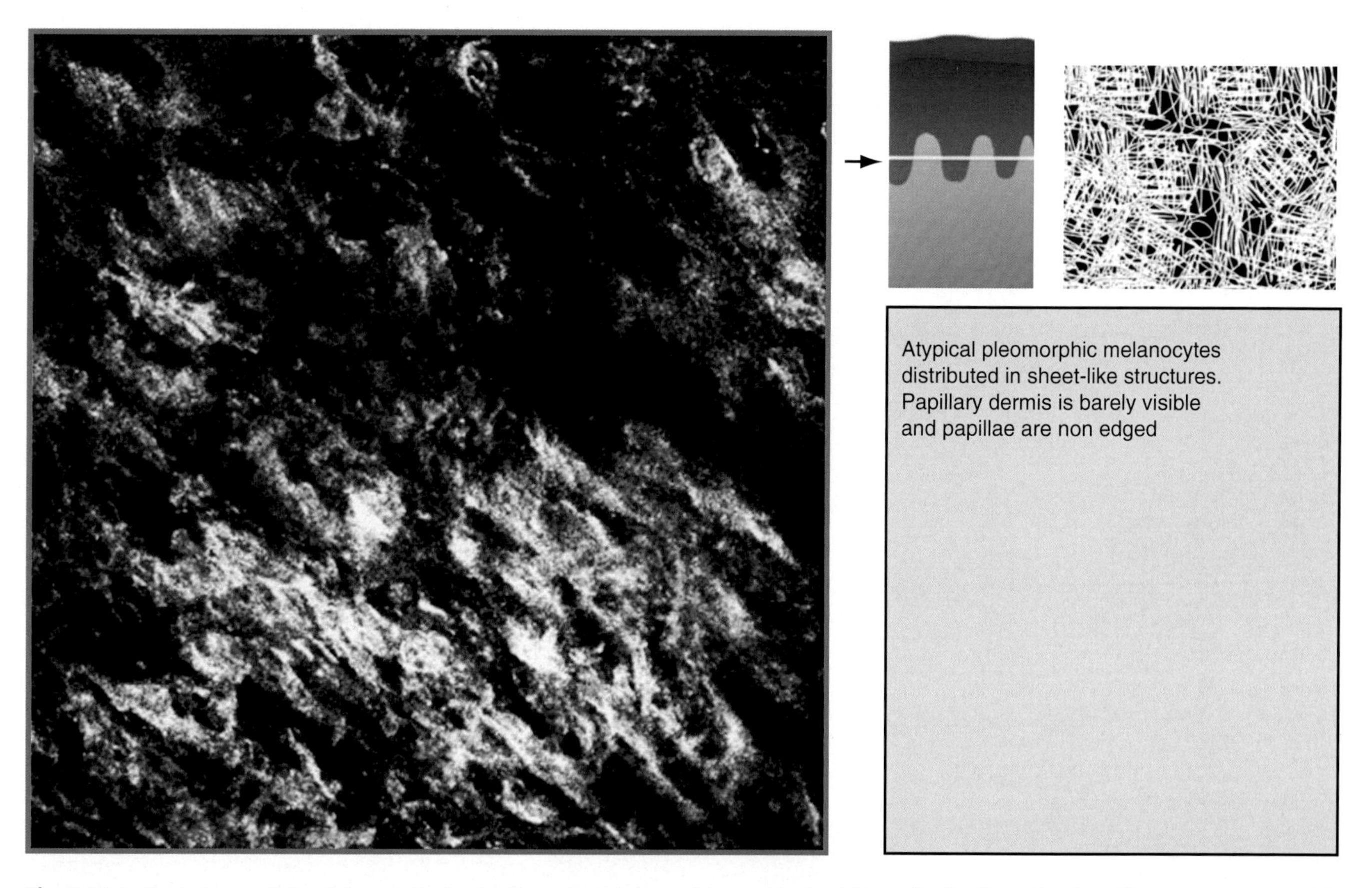

Fig. 6.10.1 Basic image (0.5 × 0.5 mm). In the detail atypical pleomorphic, mostly dendritic, cells distributed in sheet-like patter are detectable at the DEJ

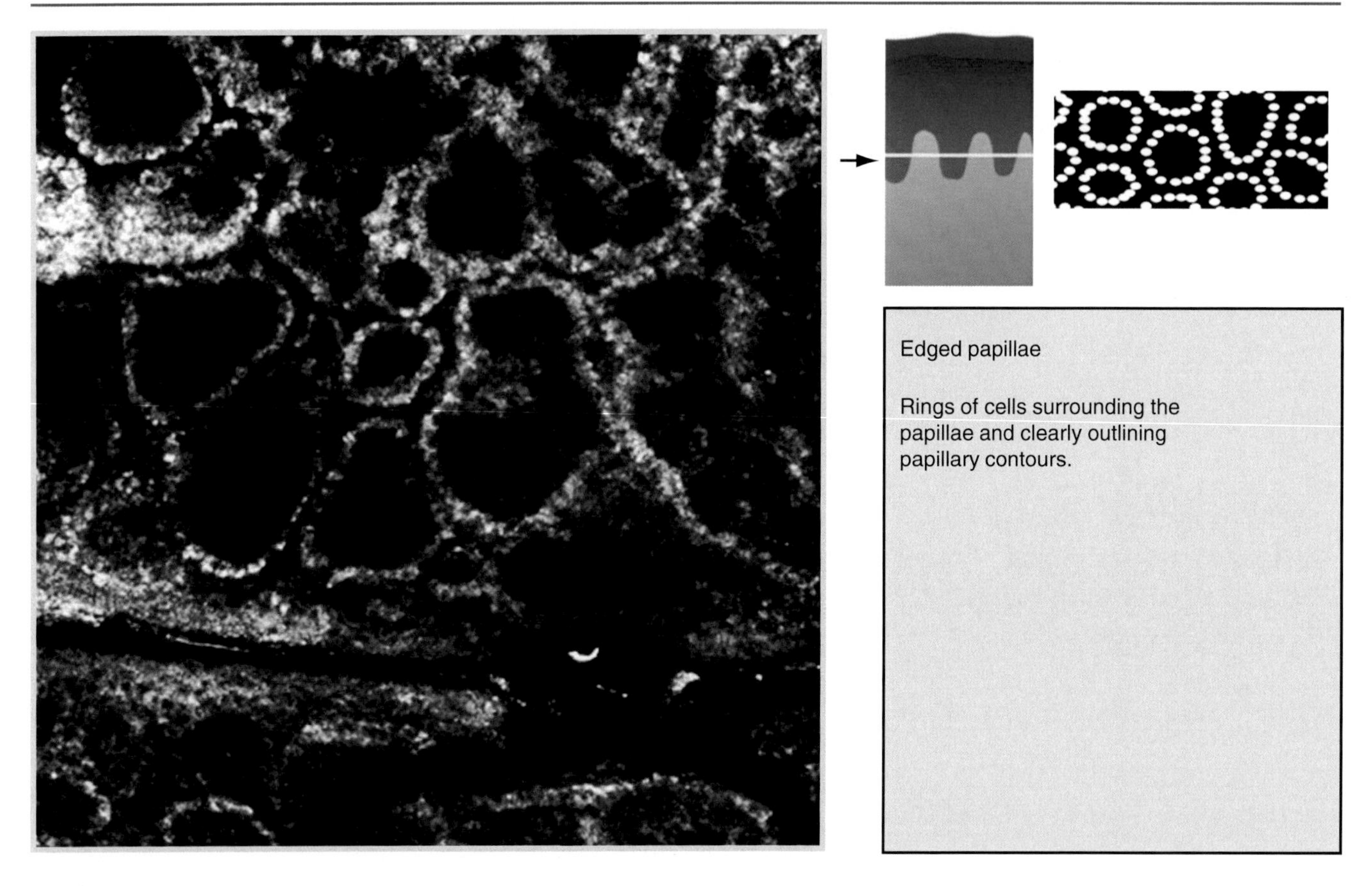

Fig. 6.11 Basic image (0.5 × 0.5 mm). Edged papillae in a ringed pattern. They correspond to dermal papillae with clearly outlined contours. In this picture, dermal papillae are circumscribed by a rim of refractive cells, appearing as a bright rings sharply contrasting with the dark background

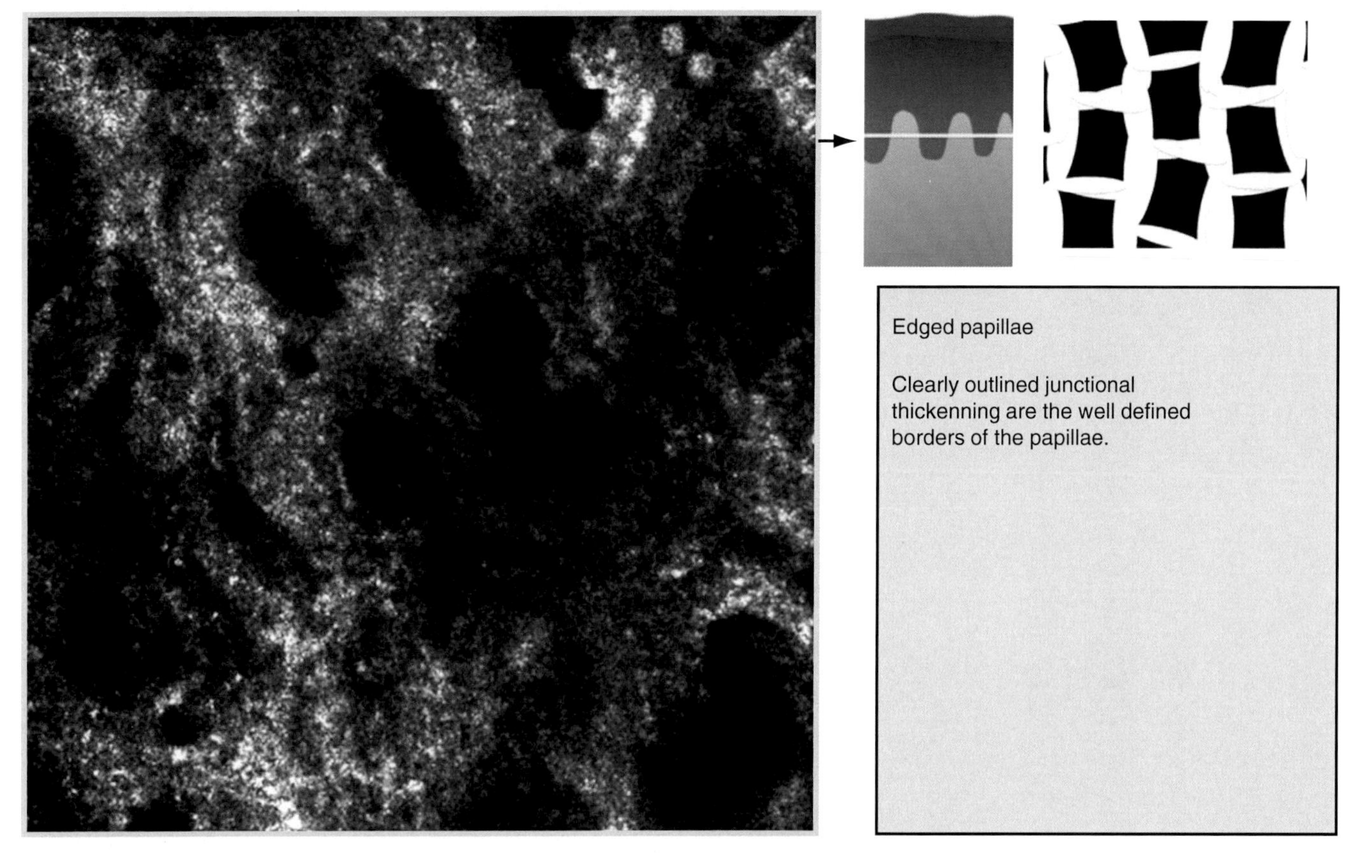

Fig. 6.12 Basic image (0.5 × 0.5 mm). Edged papillae in a meshwork pattern. They correspond to dermal papillae with clearly outlined contours. In this picture, dermal papillae are circumscribed by compact melanocytic aggregates with sharp borders

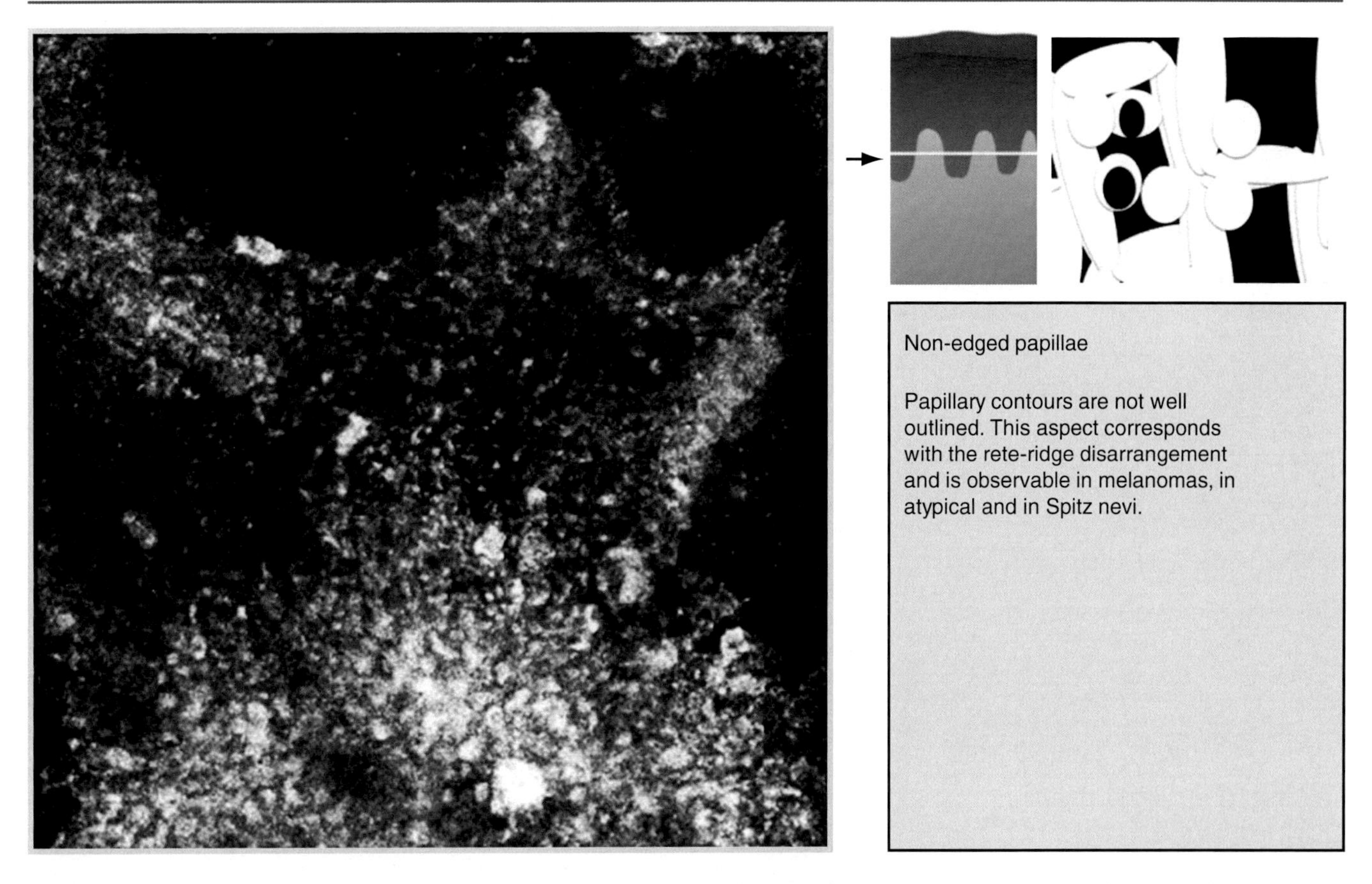

Fig. 6.13 Basic image (0.5 × 0.5 mm). Non-edged papillae. They correspond to dermal papillae without a demarcated contour. They are usually surrounded by single cells or by non discrete aggregates, not forming a complete clear outline

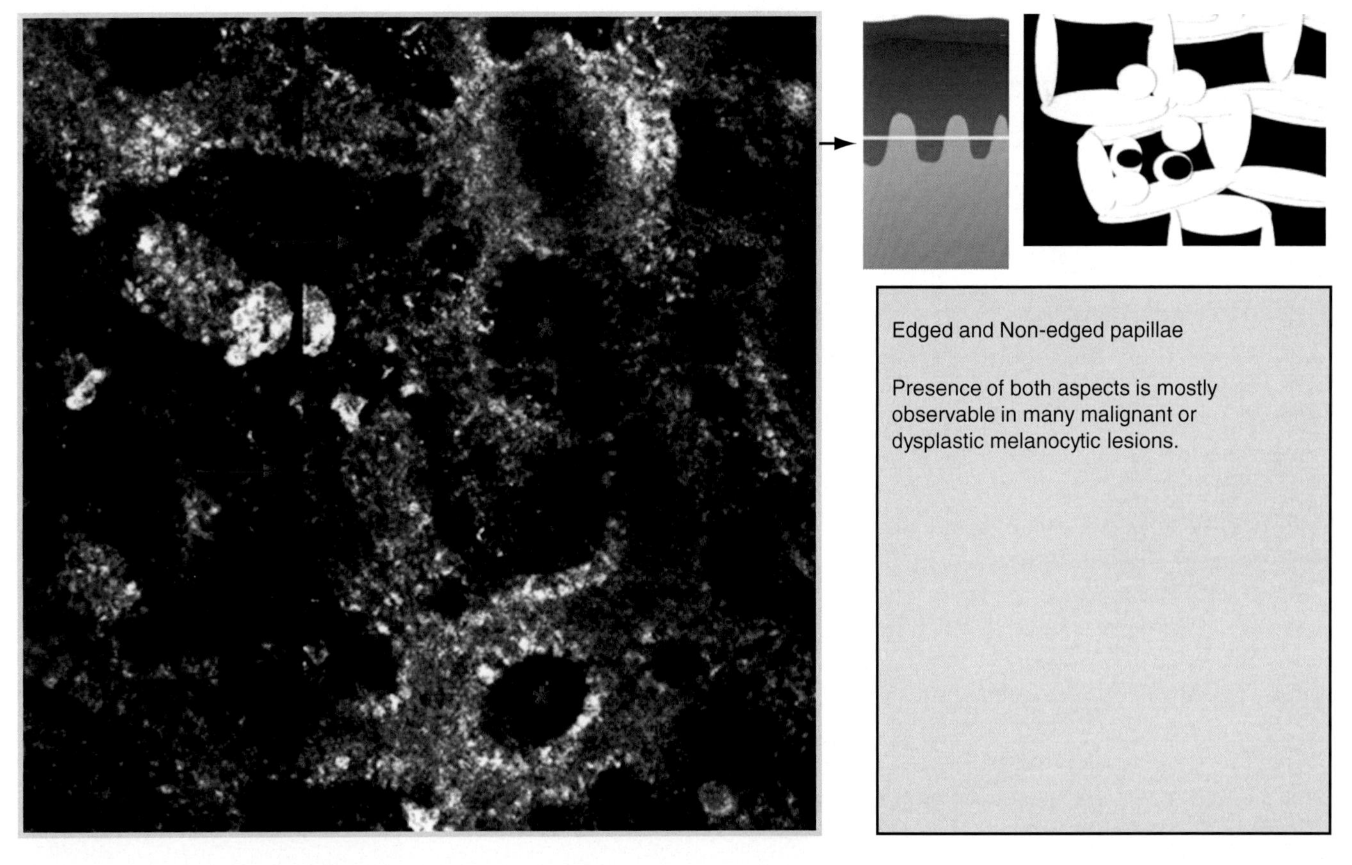

Fig. 6.14 Basic image (0.5 × 0.5 mm). Edged and non-edged papillae. In the same lesions both aspect could coexist, showing an area characterized by edged papillae (*) and another one with non-edged (→)

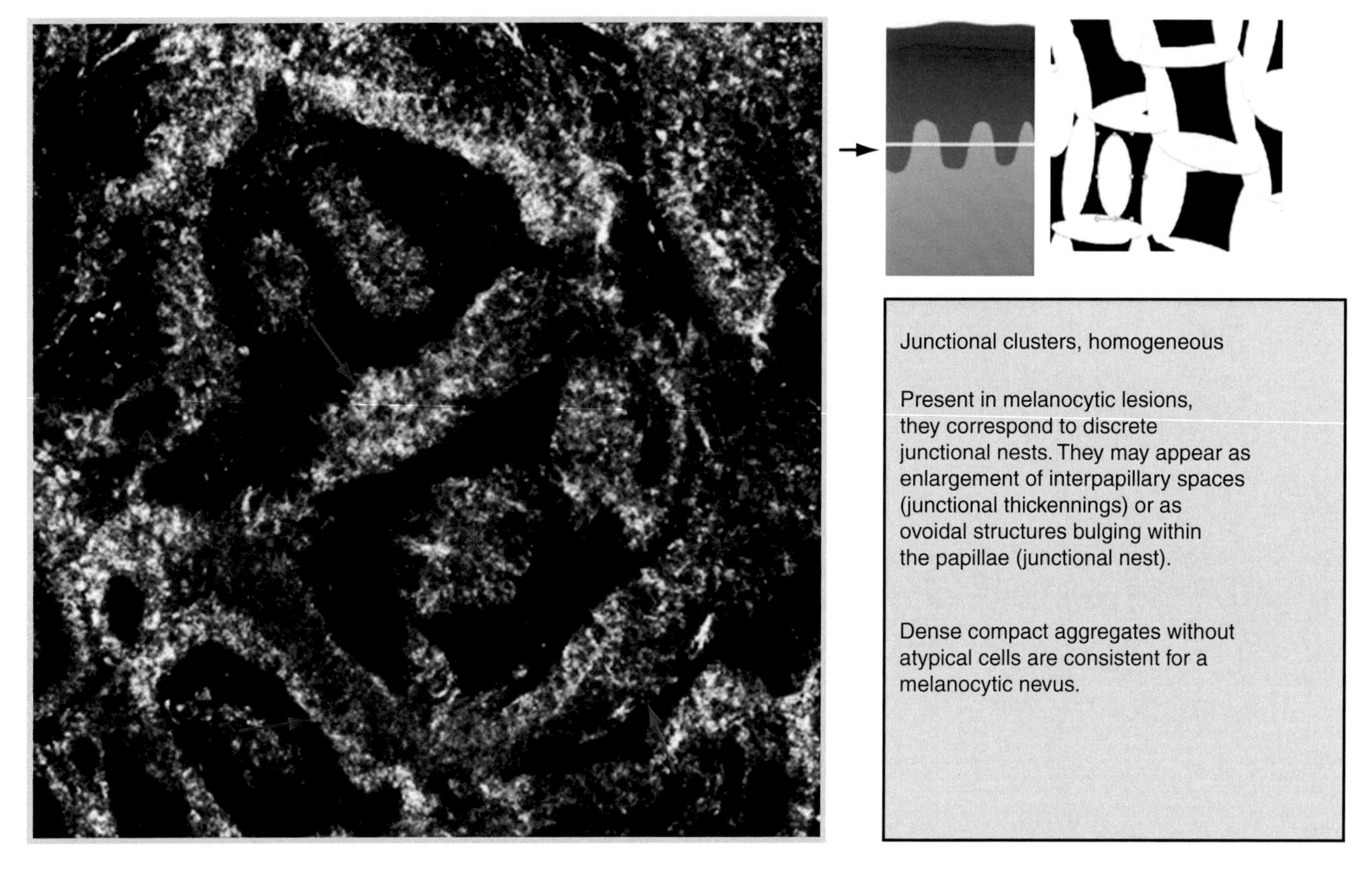

Fig. 6.15 Basic image (0.5 × 0.5 mm). Junctional nests, regular homogeneous: oval compact cellular aggregates, bulging within the dermal papillae (*), or enlarging the inter-papillary spaces (→), directly in connection with the basal cell layer. In this picture they are regular, with well defined contours clearly outlining the borders of the papillae (edged papillae), and without atypical cells

melanocytic nevi, whereas atypical nevi and melanomas may show irregular, non-homogeneous aggregates of atypical cells [5]. Figures 6.15 and 6.16 show few examples of this pattern.

6.5.2 Dermal Nests

They correspond to clusters of refractive cells forming oval to roundish structures in the papillary dermis, corresponding to melanocytic nests. Figures 6.17–6.20 show few examples of these patterns.

According to their aspect, dermal nests show up in three different main morphologies:

Dense Nests correspond to compact aggregates with sharp margin and similar cells in morphology and refractivity [6] (Fig. 6.17).

Dense & Sparse Nests (dishomogeneous clusters) correspond to nondiscrete aggregates. The margins may be sharp or undefined, and usually cells not tightly aggregated within the nest are detectable. Large dense and sparse nests with large roundish monomorphic cells are characteristic of the dermal component in congenital nevi and dermal nevi (Fig. 6.18), whereas nests variable in size composed by loose aggregates of pleomorphic cells are usually observed in melanoma (Fig. 6.19).

Cerebriform clusters: cerebriform clusters correspond to cellular clusters consisting of confluent amorphous aggregates of low reflecting cells exhibiting granular cytoplasm without evident nuclei and ill-defined borders, being the aggregates brain-like in appearance, showing a fine hyporeflective "fissure" like appearance (Fig. 6.20). Although their observation is unfrequent, cerebriform nests are specific for invasive melanomas, and they are usually located within the nodular component of the tumor.

6.5.3 Cells in Sheet-Like Structures

They correspond to cells located in the transition of the epidermis and dermis, not aggregated into clusters but closely associated and distributed on the same plane. Dermal papillae are not distinguishable due to the loss of the normal rete-ridge pattern. These cells are usually exhibiting a hyper-refractive cytoplasm and are pleomorphic.

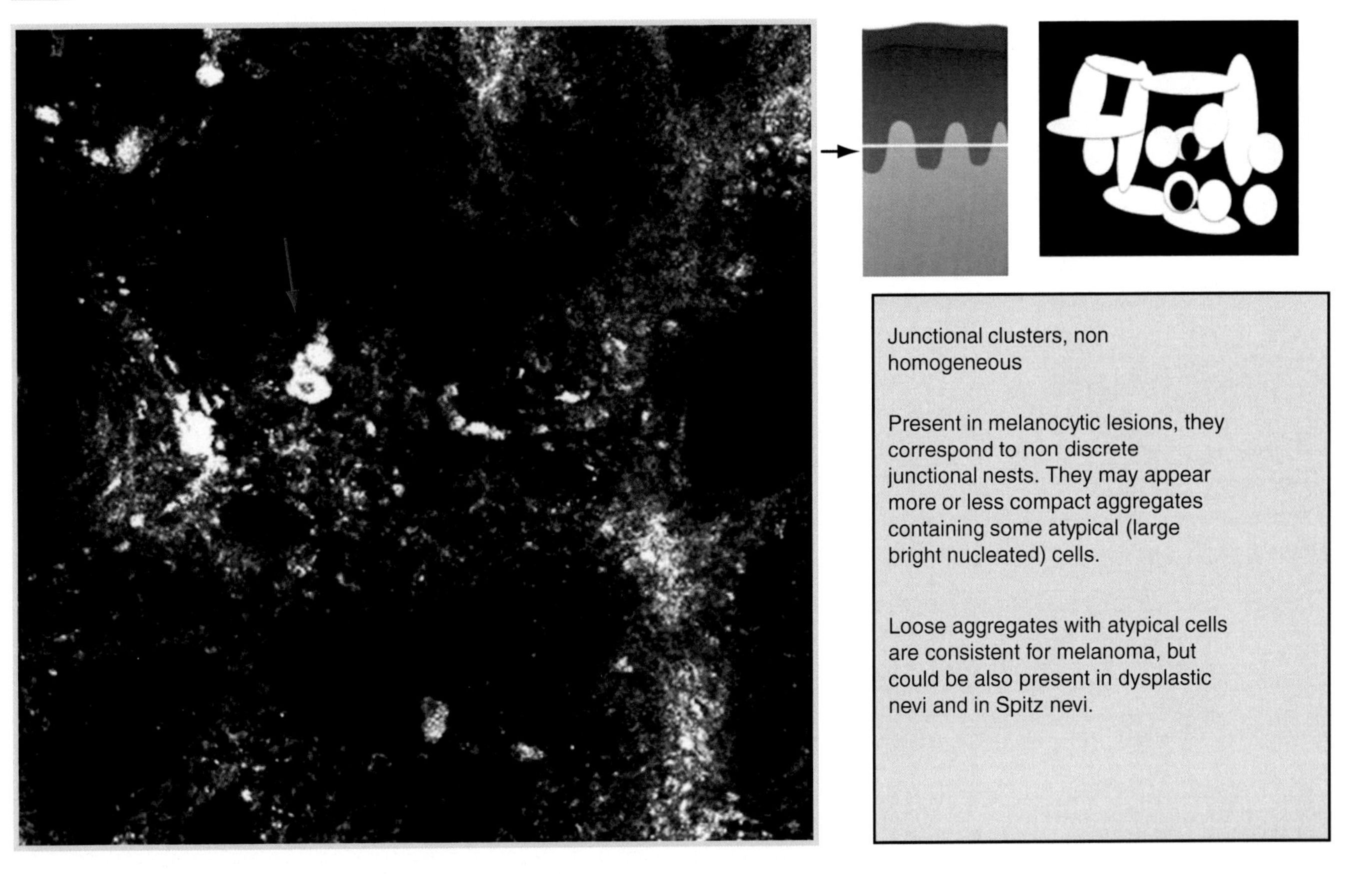

Fig. 6.16 Basic image (0.5 × 0.5 mm). Junctional nest, non homogeneous: oval lose cellular aggregates, irregularly enlarging the inter-papillary space (→), showing some atypical melanocytes. Nest contours are not clearly outlined making the papillary contours not well defined (non-edged papillae)

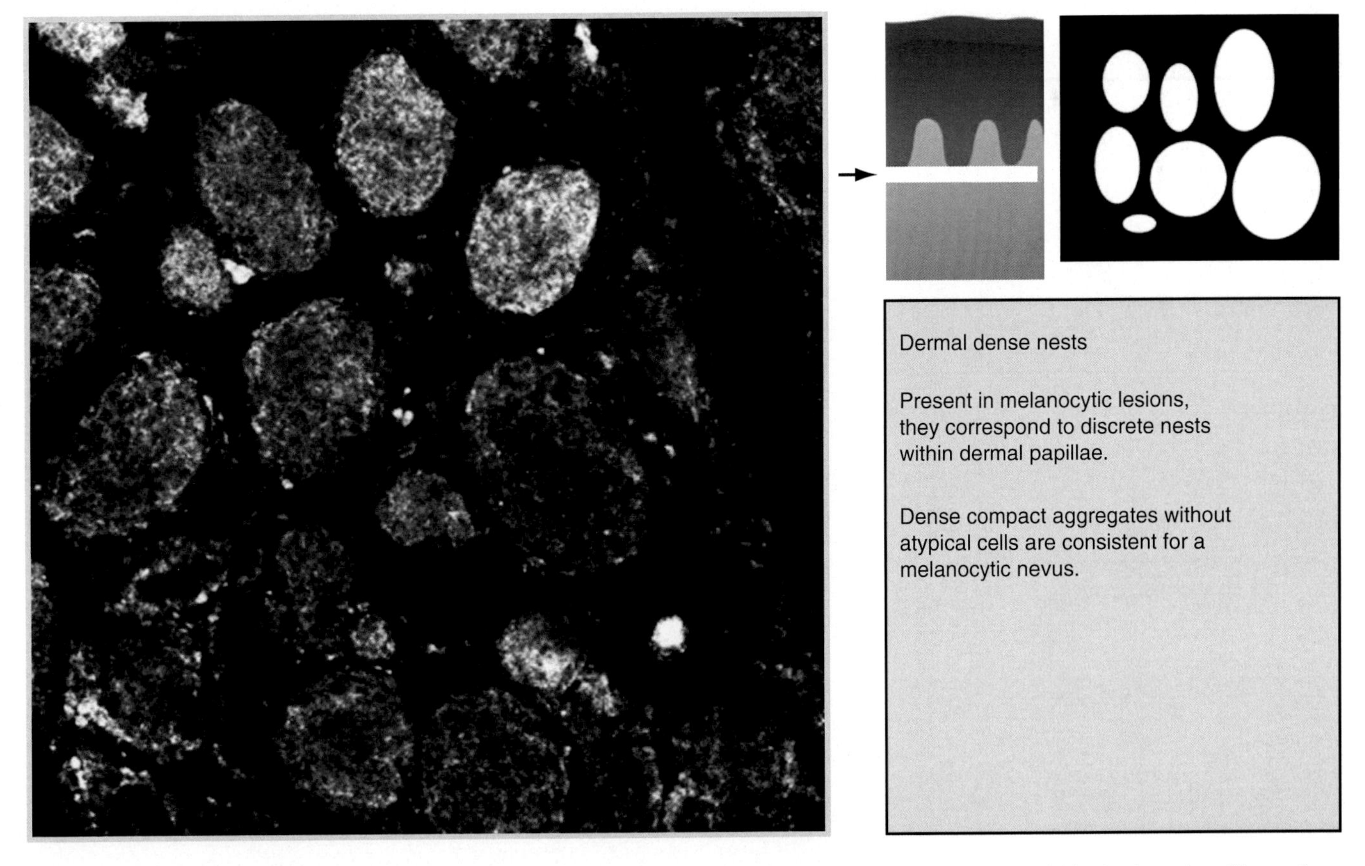

Fig. 6.17 Basic image (0.5 × 0.5 mm). Dermal dense nests, regular homogeneous: oval compact aggregates, within the dermal papillae and not connected with the epidermis

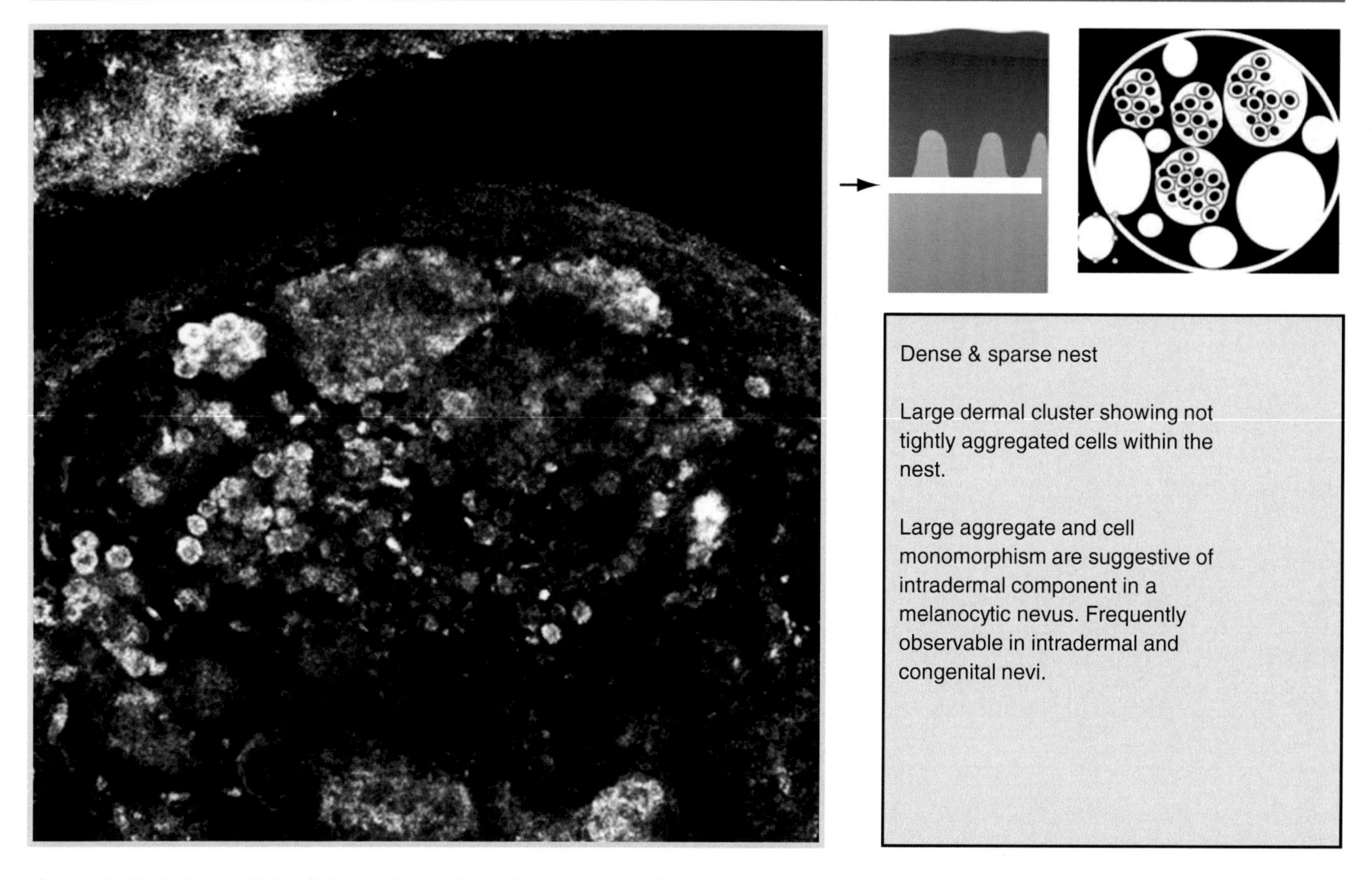

Fig. 6.18 Basic image (0.5 × 0.5 mm). Large dense & sparse nest: it is constituted by a large aggregate of roundish monomorphic cells fulfilling the dermal papilla

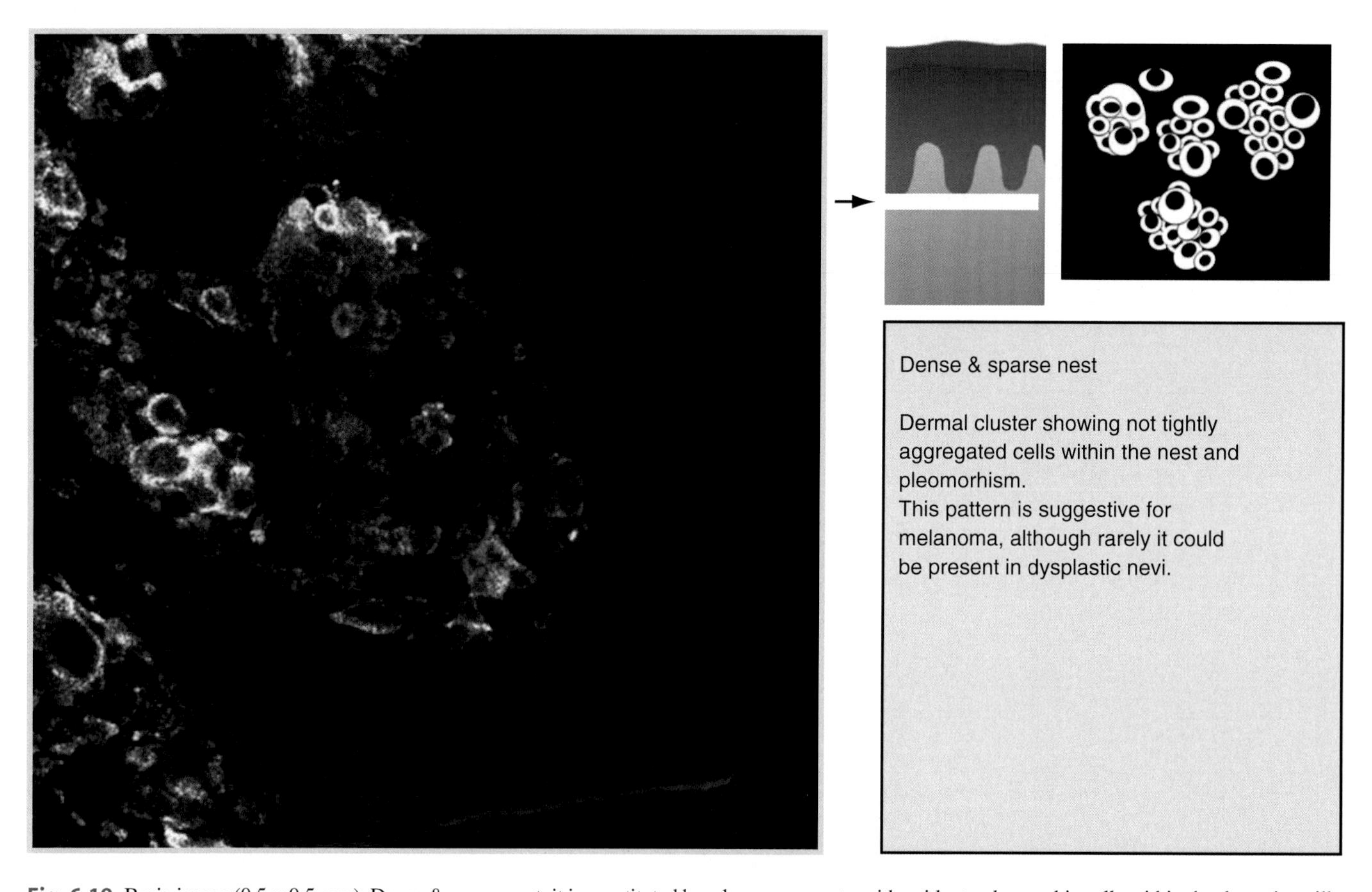

Fig. 6.19 Basic image (0.5 × 0.5 mm). Dense & sparse nest: it is constituted by a loose aggregate with evident polymorphic cells within the dermal papilla

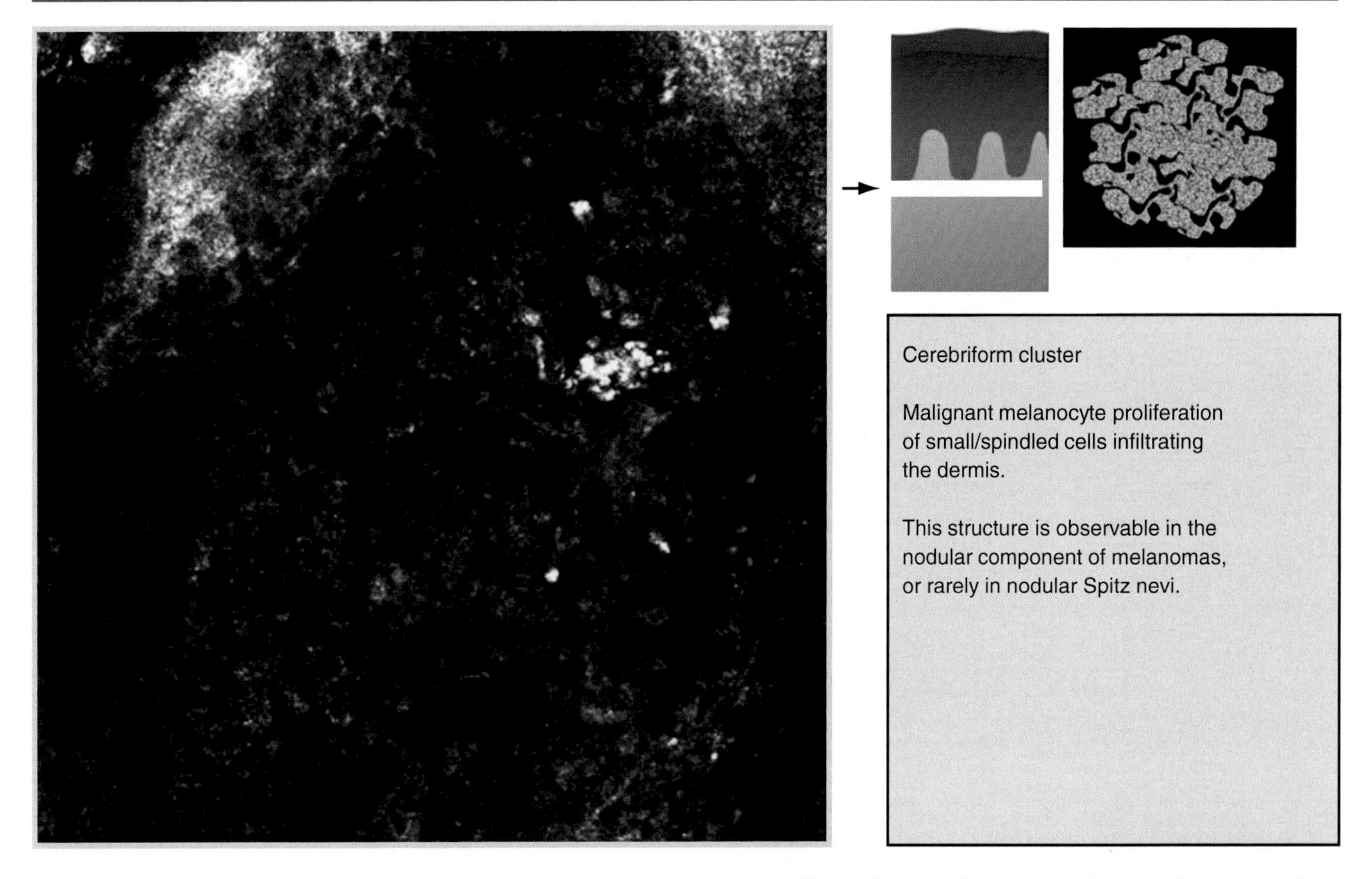

Fig. 6.20 Basic image (0.5 × 0.5 mm). Cerebriform nest: amorphous aggregates of low reflecting cells with granular low reflecting cytoplasm without evident nuclei and ill-defined borders separated by fine hyporeflective "fissure"

6.6 Cytology

Normal single melanocytes are not distinguishable from pigmented keratinocytes. On the contrary, large cells showing a bright cytoplasm with clearly outlined borders and sharply contrasted dark nucleus inside, roundish to oval in shapes, sometimes presenting dendritic-like structures, located at the dermal–epidermal junction, are defined "atypical cells" and they frequently account for atypical melanocytes.

Atypical cells are usually observed in melanocytic lesions. Rarely present in common nevi, they are frequently observed in melanomas. Few atypical cells with no marked pleomorphism are also present in atypical/dysplastic nevi. It is possible to detect atypical cells within epithelial tumor proliferation such as pigmented basal cell carcinoma or in pigmented actinic keratosis and Bowen's disease, due to the activation of melanocytes within the tumor masses.

The *aspect* is evaluated, according to the predominant cell shape, as "roundish-polygonal" or "dendritic-spindled". Pleomorphism is estimated on the variability of atypical cell morphology, and it is characterized by the presence of both roundish and dendritic cells, and/or the presence of cells with bizarre shapes. Figures 6.21 and 6.22 show an example of this pattern.

Numerosity is quantified per square millimeter, considering an average of less than 5 cells, 5 to 10 cells or more than 10, respectively.

Distribution is classified as localized, sparse or widespread, similarly to pagetoid cells distribution. Moreover for atypical cells at the DEJ, the organization is taken into account.

Atypical cells may appear as individual or aggregation of cells. At least for atypical cells within junctional or dermal nests have to be detected to consider an aggregate of atypical cells [7].

Atypical cells infiltrating dermal papillae are considered when nucleated cells round or oval in shape with well-demarcated refractive cytoplasm and prominent dark nucleus are detected.

6.7 Stroma Reaction

6.7.1 Plump Bright Cells/Small Bright Particles in Papillae

Plump bright cells are described as plump irregularly shaped bright cells with ill-defined borders and usually no visible nucleus. Bright spots and small bright particles are small

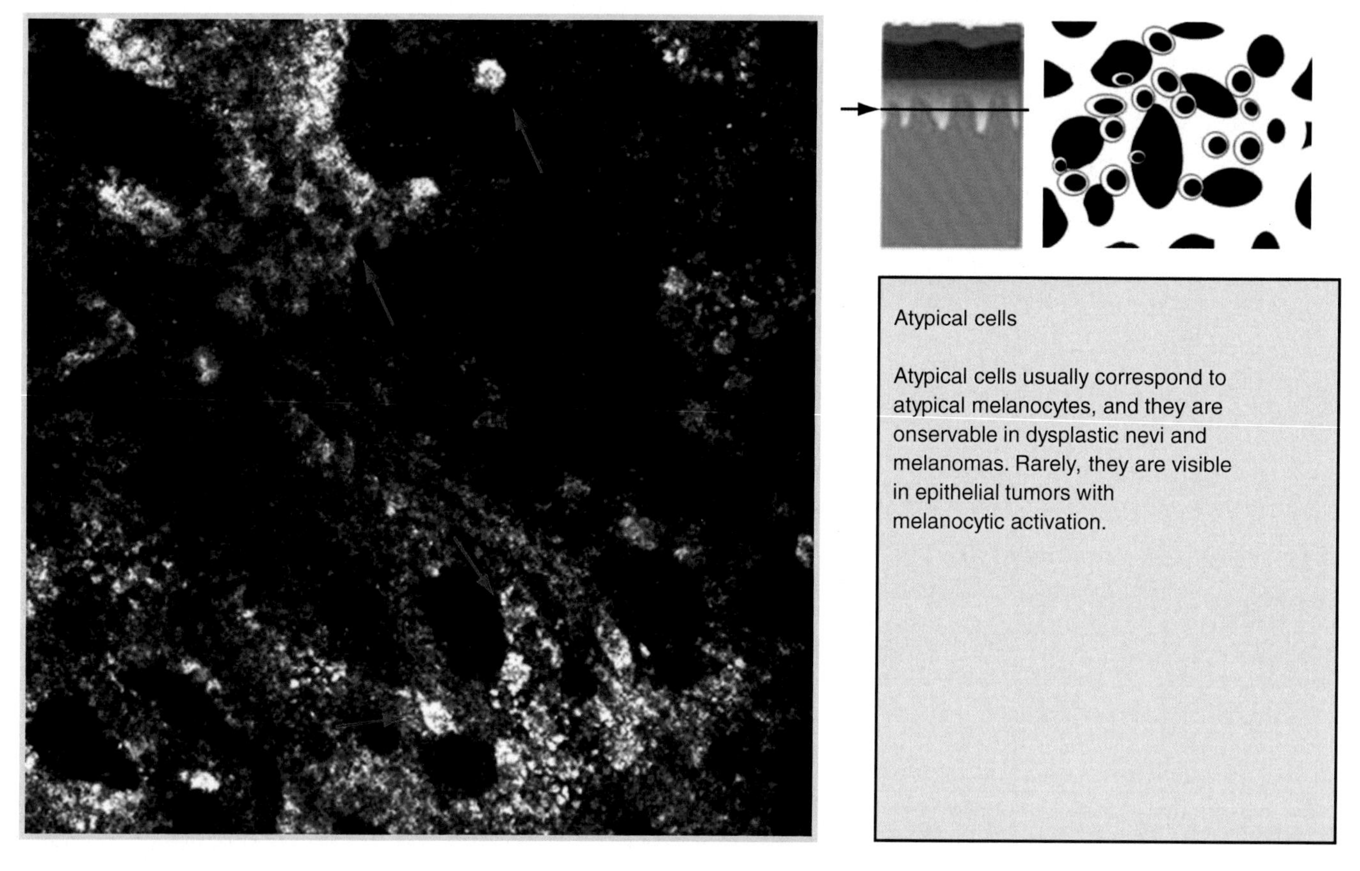

Fig. 6.21 Basic image (0.5 × 0.5 mm). Atypical cells (→). The picture shows some large cells with a bright cytoplasm, outlined borders and dark nucleus. They are in single units at the junction, within junctional clusters and infiltrating the papilla. Cells are monomorphic

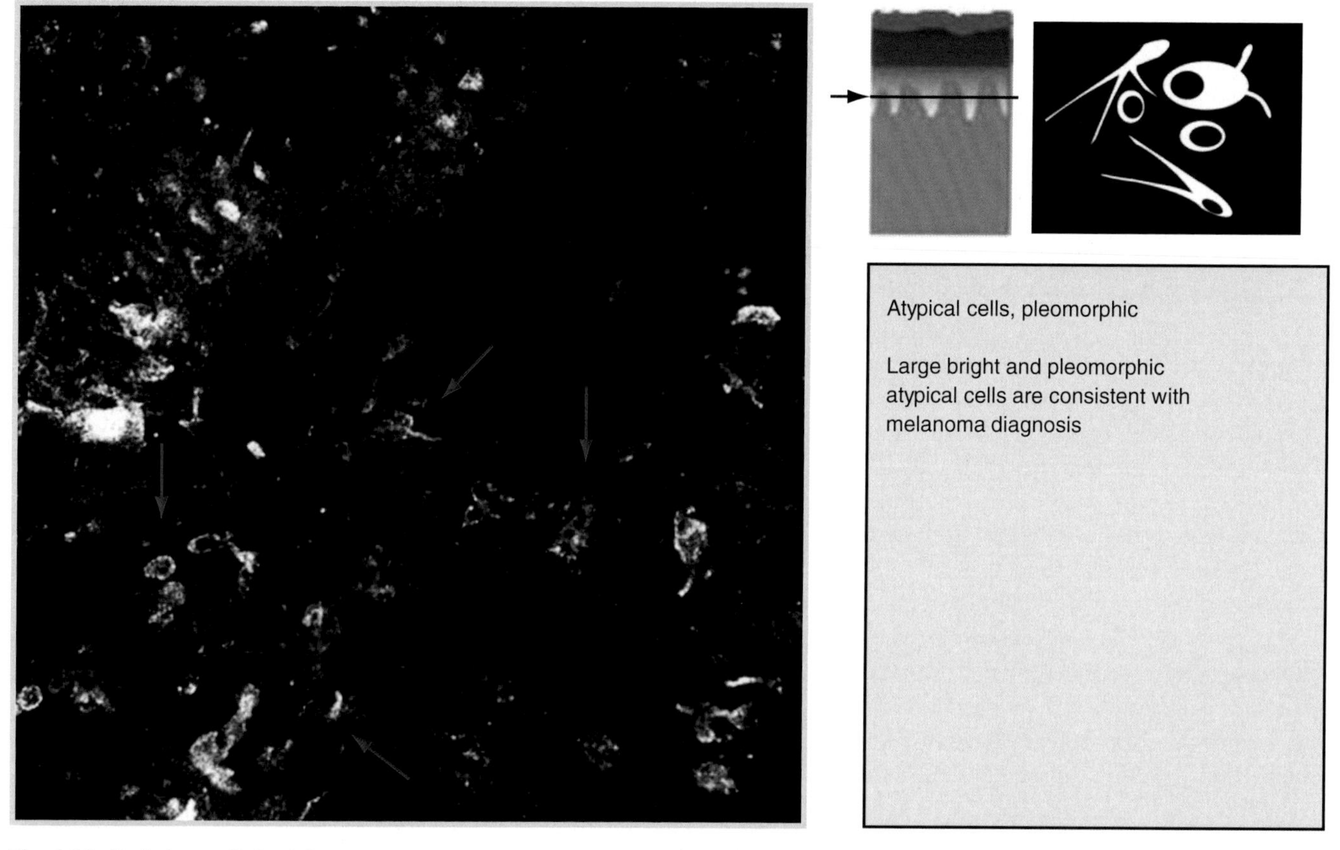

Fig. 6.22 Basic image (0.5 × 0.5 mm). Atypical cells (→). The picture displays both roundish, dendritic cells, and bizarre shape cells, defining a pleomorphic aspect

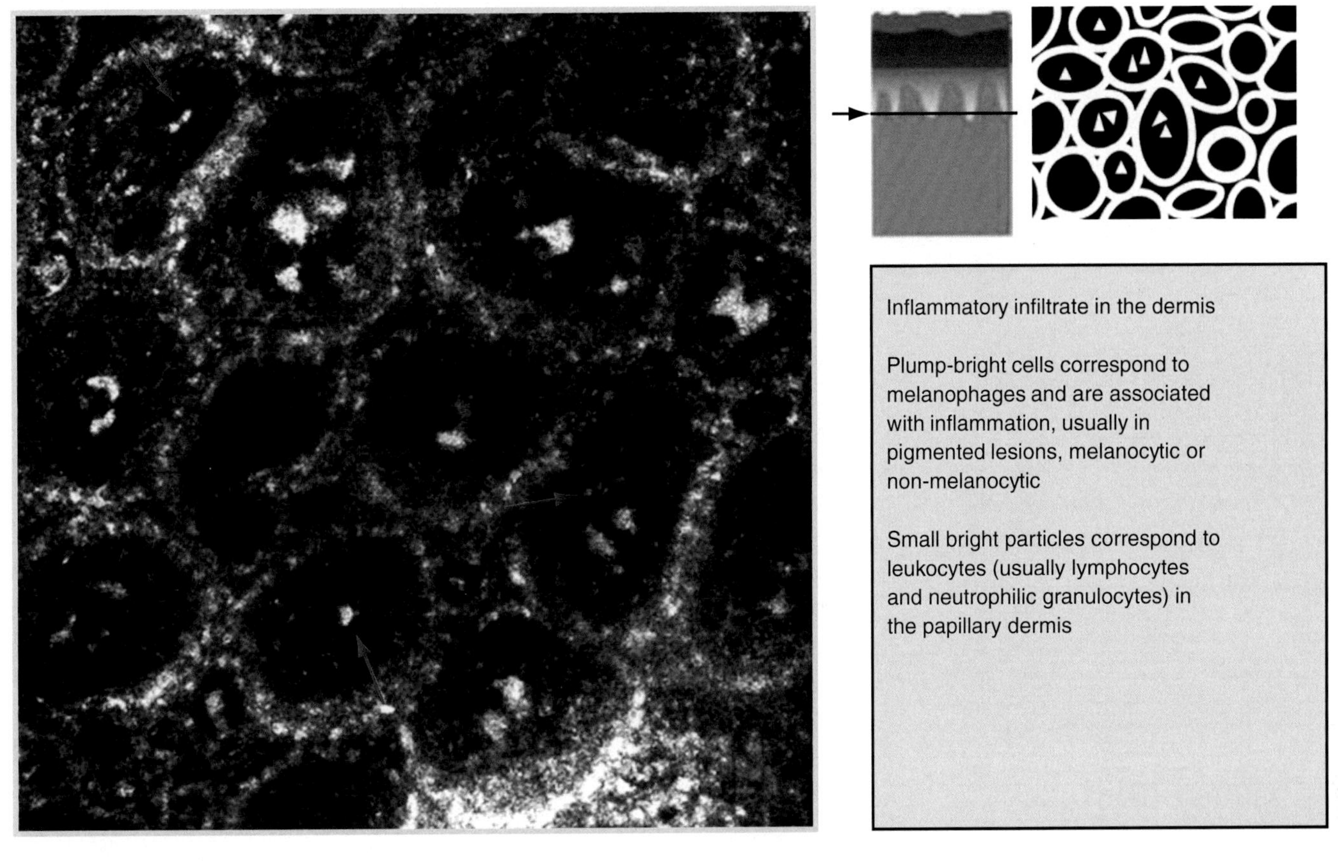

Fig. 6.23 Basic image (0.5 × 0.5 mm). Small bright particles and plump bright cells: plump irregularly shaped bright cells with ill-defined borders (*). Bright spots and small bright particles are small cells with very bright hyper-reflecting cytoplasm (→)

cells with very bright hyper-reflecting cytoplasm, sometimes visible nuclei, corresponding to leukocyte infiltration. Figure 6.23 shows an example of this pattern.

6.7.2 Coarse Collagen Structures

Collagen appears as amorphous fibrillary material which aspect could be reticulated, forming coarse web-like structures in the dermis, or in boundles, gathered into large fasciae. Figure 6.24 shows an example of coarse reticulated pattern.

6.7.3 Vessels

In the upper dermis it is possible to identify vessels. The blood flow within the vessels is clearly detectable during in vivo imaging, also in normal skin, whereas on still images only elongated and/or enlarged vessels can be evaluated. Vessels are better evaluated during live imaging or with movies.

Coarse collagen fibers
Collagen fibers are packed together forming a coarse web-like architecture. In melanocytic lesions it usually corresponds to fibroplasia. This pattern is sometimes observable in sun-damaged skin.

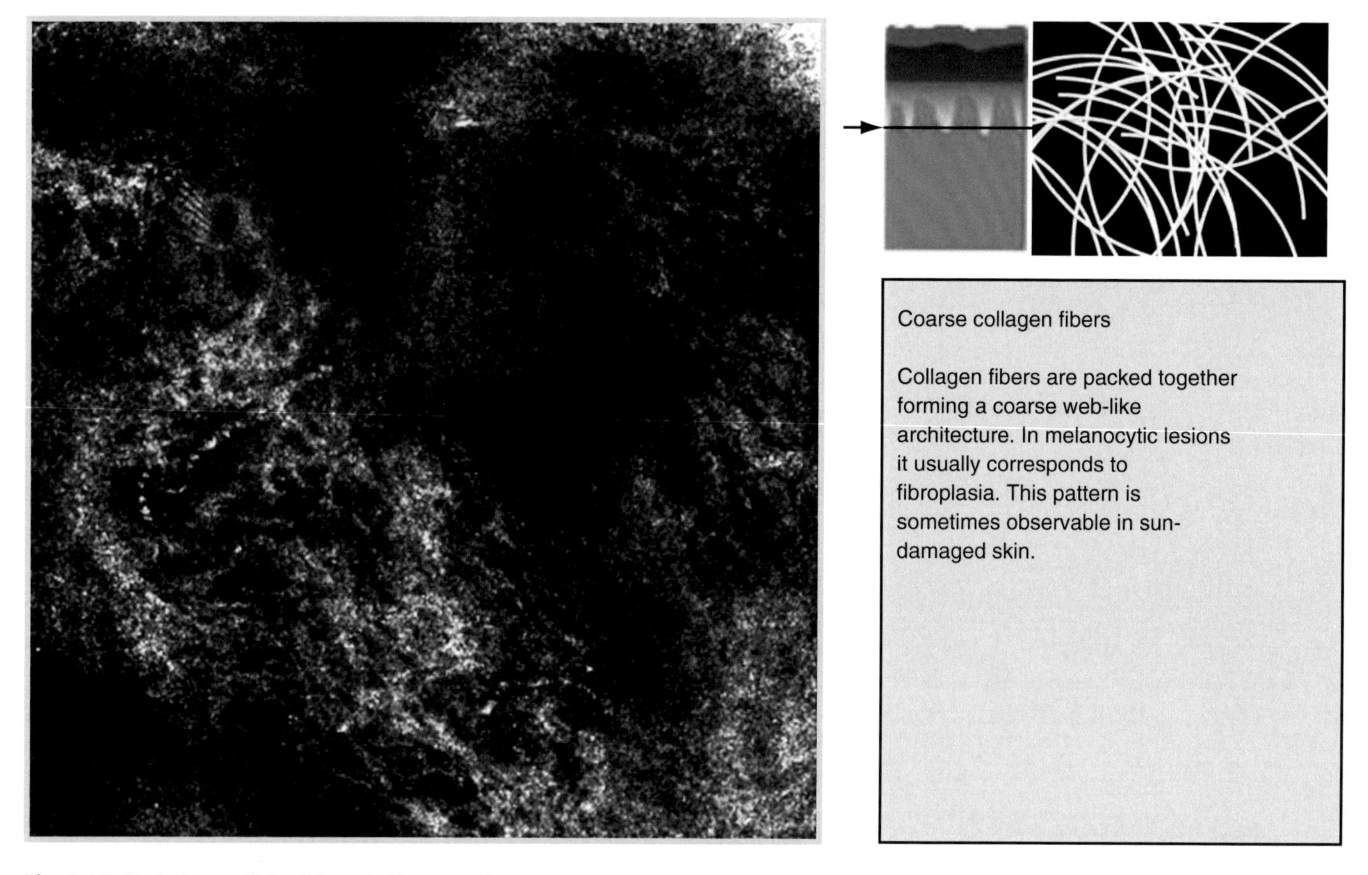

Fig. 6.24 Basic image (0.5 × 0.5 mm). Coarse collagen structures: it appear as an amorphous fibrillary material with a reticulated distribution

References

1. Busam KJ, Charles C, Lee G, Halpern AC (2001) Morphological features of melanocytes, pigmented keratinocytes, and melanophages by in vivo confocal scanning laser microscopy. Mod Pathol 14:862–868
2. Langley RGB, Rajadhyaksha M, Dweyer PJ, Sober AJ, Flotte TJ, Andersson RR (2001) Confocal scanning laser microscopy of benign and malignant melanocytic skin lesions in vivo. J Am Acad Dermatol 45:365–376
3. Pellacani G, Cesinaro AM, Seidenari S (2005) Reflectance-mode confocal microscopy for the in vivo characterization of pagetoid melanocytosis in melanomas and nevi. J Invest Dermatol 125:532–537
4. Pellacani G, Cesinaro AM, Longo C, Grana C, Seidenari S (2005) Microscopic in vivo description of cellular architecture of dermoscopic pigment network in nevi and melanomas. Arch Dermatol 141:147–154
5. Pellacani G, Cesinaro AM, Seidenari S (2005) In vivo assessment of melanocytic nests in nevi and melanomas by reflectance confocal microscopy. Mod Pathol 18:469–474
6. Pellacani G, Cesinaro AM, Seidenari S (2005) Reflectance-mode confocal microscopy of pigmented skin lesions–improvement in melanoma diagnostic specificity. J Am Acad Dermatol 53:979–985
7. Pellacani G, Scope A, Ferrari B, Pupelli G, Bassoli S, Longo C, Cesinaro AM, Argenziano G, Hofmann-Wellenhof R, Malvehy J, Marghoob AA, Puig S, Seidenari S, Soyer HP, Zalaudek I (2009) New insights into nevogenesis: in vivo characterization and follow-up of melanocytic nevi by reflectance confocal microscopy. J Am Acad Dermatol 61:1001–1013
8. Scope A, Benvenuto-Andrade C, Agero AL, Malvehy J, Puig S, Rajadhyaksha M et al (2007) In vivo reflectance confocal microscopy imaging of melanocytic skin lesions: consensus terminology glossary and illustrative images. J Am Acad Dermatol 57: 644–658
9. Pellacani G, Vinceti M, Bassoli S, Braun R, Gonzalez S, Guitera P, Longo C, Marghoob AA, Menzies SW, Puig S, Scope A, Seidenari S, Malvehy J (2009) Reflectance confocal microscopy and features of melanocytic lesions: an internet-based study of the reproducibility of terminology. Arch Dermatol 145(10):1137–1143

Dermoscopic and Histopathologic Correlations

7

Gaia Pupelli, Leonardo Veneziano, Caterina Longo,
Gisele Gargantini Rezze, Hans Peter Soyer,
and Giovanni Pellacani

Dermoscopy is a widely diffused technique that offers the possibility to analyze subsurface structures not otherwise visible by naked eye. It has been proved that dermoscopy is an essential clinical tool in the hands of experts for diagnostic definition of melanocytic and non-melanocytic skin lesions, while improving diagnostic accuracy [1]. In addition to dermoscopy, reflectance-mode confocal microscopy (RCM) holds the great advantage to explore histological details of skin tissue, in vivo and in real time. Similarly to dermoscopy RCM produces images corresponding to horizontal section of the skin from the epidermis surface to the papillary dermis but offering a cellular level resolution, similarly to histopathology. Thus, it seems to be the natural link between dermoscopy and histopathology.

In this chapter, we aimed to describe the confocal and histopathologic substrates of the most relevant dermoscopic features in melanocytic lesions. The histologic counterpart for confocal and dermoscopy is presented showing both classical vertical section and transversal ones [2]. The possibility to understand and recognize in vivo the histologic substrates of the dermoscopic relevant features renders the RCM a supportive powerful tool in daily clinical practice for skin care management.

G. Pupelli (✉) • C. Longo • G. Pellacani
Department of Dermatology and Venereology,
University of Modena and Reggio Emilia, Modena, Italy
e-mail: pupelli.gaia@gmail.com; pellacani.giovanni@unimore.it

L. Veneziano
Department of Dermatologym, Ospedale Bellaria Maggiore,
Bologna, Italy

G.G. Rezze
Departamento de Oncologia Cutânea, Hospital A.C. Camargo,
São Paulo SP, Brazil

H.P. Soyer
Dermatology Research Centre, The University of Queensland,
Princess Alexandra Hospital School of Medicine, Brisbane,
Queensland, Australia

7.1 Dermoscopic and Confocal Correlations with Histology

7.1.1 Pigment Network

According to the Consensus Net Meeting on dermoscopy, the pigment network is defined as typical or atypical [3].

Typical Network shows on RCM analysis one of two distinct RCM patterns: a ringed pattern, with a rim of bright cells revealing predominantly edged papillae, or a meshwork pattern, characterized by junctional thickenings [4].

The size and shape of the dermal papillae exactly correspond to the ones of the network holes. In the "ringed pattern" (Fig. 7.1) the network lines are correlated to two paired portions of adjacent rings, resulting at high-magnification dermoscopy in the bi-layer structure of the network grid [5]. Routine histology reveals elongated rete-ridges with an increased number of melanocytes in the basal layer and pigmented basal keratinocytes corresponding to a lentiginous pattern.

On the other hand, pigment network with an underlying "meshwork pattern" is characterized by a predominance of junctional thickenings, corresponding to enlargements of interpapillary spaces formed by compact aggregated cells. This pattern shows on histopathology nested junctional pattern with predominantly small, non-confluent, discrete nests at the tips of the rete ridges. These nests clearly predominated over single melanocytes (Fig. 7.2).

The *atypical pigment network*, on dermoscopy, corresponds to irregular and dishomogeneous dermal papillae distribution and presence of irregular aggregates or sheets of cells in the interpapillary spaces at the RCM. Frequently these papillae do not have a demarcated rim of bright cells, but are separated by loosely enlarged inter-papillary spaces. This space consists of reflecting cells or structures coinciding with the irregular network grids. In horizontal histologic sections,

R. Hofmann-Wellenhof et al. (eds.), *Reflectance Confocal Microscopy for Skin Diseases*,
DOI 10.1007/978-3-642-21997-9_7, © Springer-Verlag Berlin Heidelberg 2012

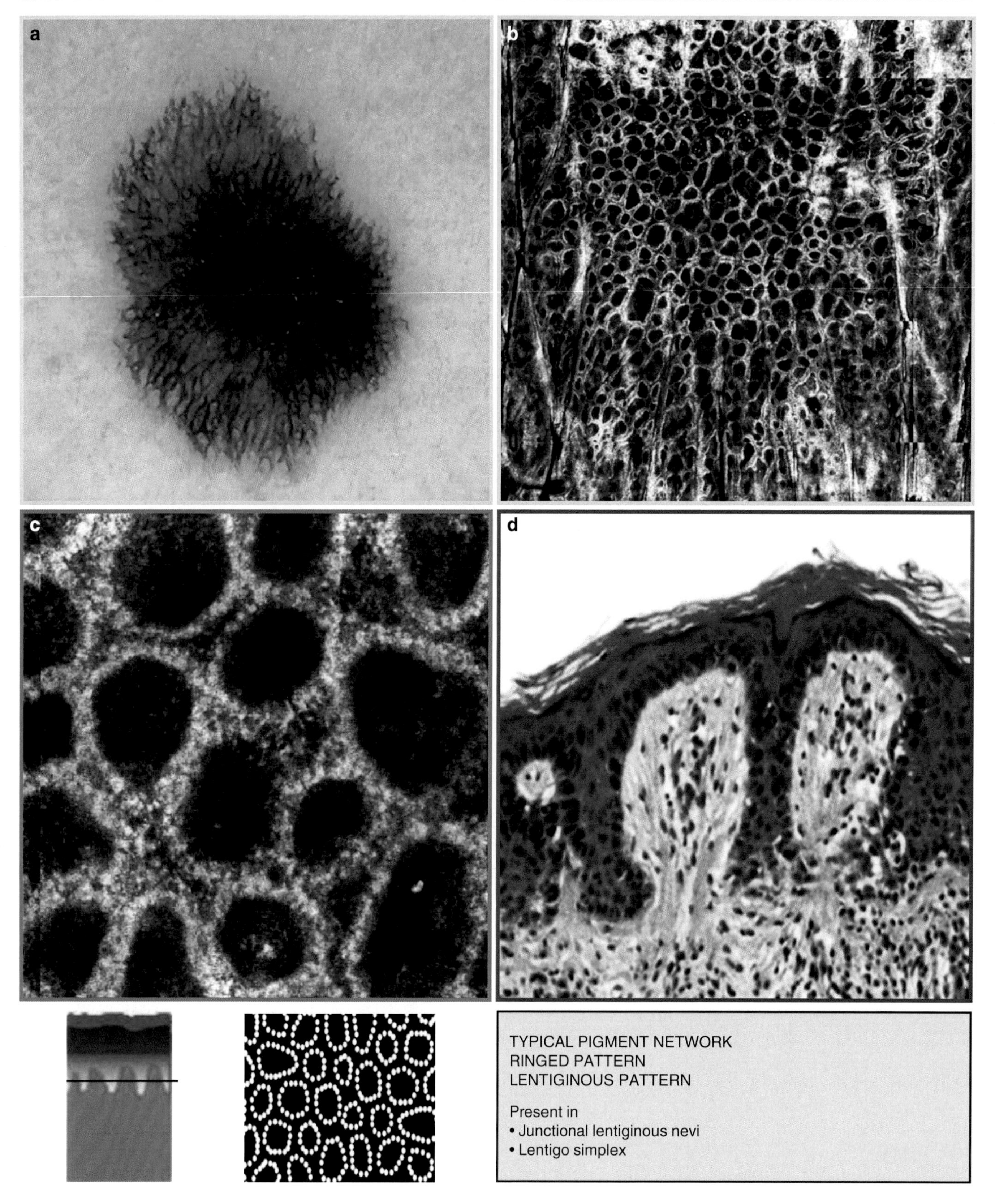

Fig. 7.1 Typical pigment network. (**a**) Dermoscopy showing a lesion characterized by pigment network. (**b**) Mosaic at DEJ (4×4 mm) displaying a ringed pattern. (**c**) Basic image at DEJ (0.5 × 0.5 mm) showing rings constituted by single monomorphous polygonal bright cells. (**d**) Corresponding histopathology showing a lentiginous pattern with elongated papillae and single melanocyte proliferation at the DEJ

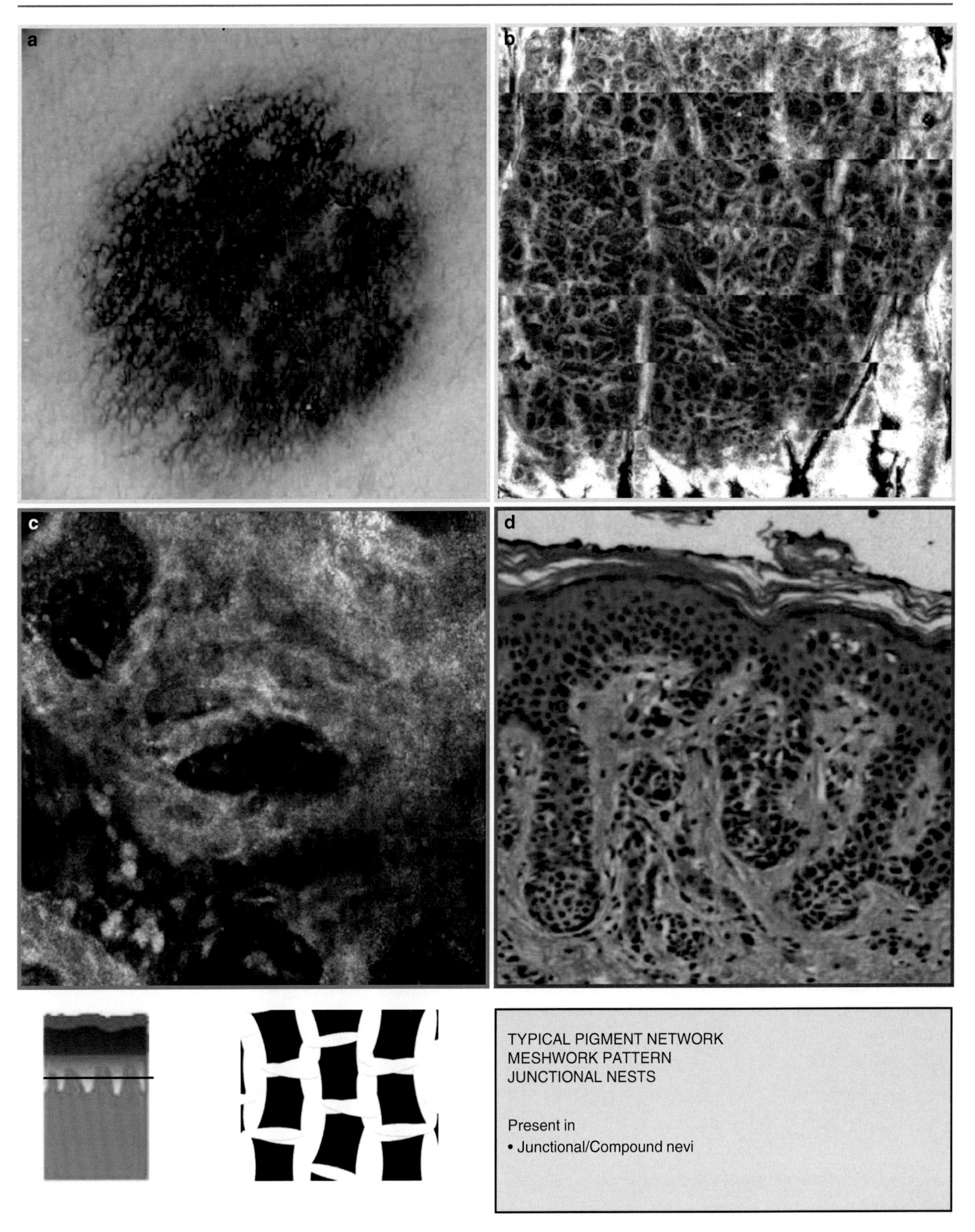

Fig. 7.2 Typical pigment network. (**a**) Dermoscopy showing a lesion characterized by pigment network. (**b**) Mosaic at DEJ (4 × 4 mm) displaying a meshwork pattern. (**c**) Basic image at DEJ (0.5 × 0.5 mm) showing enlarged interpapillary spaces with junctional thickenings. (**d**) Corresponding histopathology showing junctional nests at the tip of the cristae

an exact correspondence with confocal is visible, resulting in a disarranged network architecture with irregular enlarged meshes constituted by aggregates of atypical cells corresponding to dishomogeneous junctional nests at RCM. Traditional histopathologic examination reveals a disarrangement of the rete-ridge sometimes presenting irregular and confluent nests at the dermal–epidermal junction (Fig. 7.3).

7.1.2 Pigment Globules

7.1.2.1 Regular Pigment Globules

Brown globules at dermoscopy have an exact correspondence in shape with the dense melanocytic clusters upon RCM, appearing as compact aggregates with sharp margin of large polygonal cells similar in morphology and reflectivity (Fig. 7.4) [5]. Histopathology shows discrete melanocytic nests, composed by typical and monomorphous cells, located at dermal–epidermal junction and within papillary dermis [6].

The large polygonal structures forming the dermoscopic cobblestone pattern, typical of dermal nevi, appear upon RCM as large aggregates of clustered cells, enlarging dermal papillae and not showing connection with basal cell layer. Some large roundish nucleated cells loosely aggregated are sometimes visible in the upper portion of the cluster. Going in depth clusters assume a more compact and homogeneous aspect with no evident cell contours. Upon histologic examination nevus cells are orderly disposed as cords and nests of cells decreasing in size with depth, and separated by thin fibers.

7.1.2.2 Irregular Pigment Globules

Globules, irregular in size, shape, pigmentation and/or distribution, are frequent findings in melanomas and Spitz/Reed nevi. On RCM, they show up as irregularly shaped clusters, frequently showing loosely aggregated cell ("dense and sparse" type). Sometimes, mostly in melanomas, non-homogeneous in size and reflectivity cells are clustered together forming nondiscrete nests. Upon histology atypical globules correspond to more or less compact aggregates of pleomorphic melanocytes, variable in size and shape, predominantly distributed at the dermal–epidermal junction and in the papillary dermis (Fig. 7.5).

7.1.3 Pigment Dots

Although referred to be suggestive of malignancy, pigment dots are often detected in benign lesions. RCM offers the possibility to distinguish their nature. In fact, in benign lesions black dots correspond to ovoid homogeneously bright structures on RCM and to free melanin clumps or heavily pigmented keratinocytes within the stratum corneum, on histology. On the other hand, pigment dots generated by single melanocytes or small aggregates spreading upward in a pagetoid fashion are clearly distinguishable by RCM, showing round cells with bright cytoplasm, well-defined contours and dark nucleus, easily detectable within the epidermal contest, and almost constantly corresponding to pagetoid cells upon histopathology (Fig. 7.6).

7.1.4 Peripheral Structures

Radial streamings detected with dermoscopy appear upon RCM as a parallel series of elongated "junctional thickening-like" structures or of lines of inter-papillary basal cells projected towards the periphery, corresponding at histology to thin elongated nests or parallel oriented epidermal cristae at the periphery of the lesion [7].

On the other hand, *peripheral globules* do not differ from brown globules, corresponding to dense or dense and sparse cell clusters peripherally located upon RCM, exactly fitting in shape with dermoscopy.

At RCM *Pseudopods* show up as globular-like structures, similar to dense nests located immediately below the basal layer and characterized by sharp borders facing the outside front, but connected at the lesion core by a sheet of not closely aggregated cells. Upon histology, a well-defined nest, located at the tip of the enlarged and parallel oriented cristae, is usually observable.

7.1.5 Diffuse Pigmentation

Areas of dark brown diffuse pigmentation are generated by the abundant content of melanin within the keratinocytes and correspond to a bright cobblestone pattern on RCM. Whereas in dermoscopy the dark pigment hampers to explore the underlying structures, with confocal microscopy is still possible to examine the cyto-architectural aspects at the DEJ, helping in the diagnosis of heavily pigmented lesions.

7.1.6 Blue Hue

The *blue color* in dermoscopy derives from the presence of pigment located in the dermis. According to the location and distribution of the pigment, it is possible to distinguish different patterns within the generally called *blue areas* [8].

An homogeneous and symmetric slate-blue pigmentation with shading-off borders is typical for the blue nevus and it is generated by spindled melanocytes intermingled within collagen fibers usually located in the reticular dermis. Due to the too deep location, confocal microscopy usually is not able to detect the pigmented structures, showing the

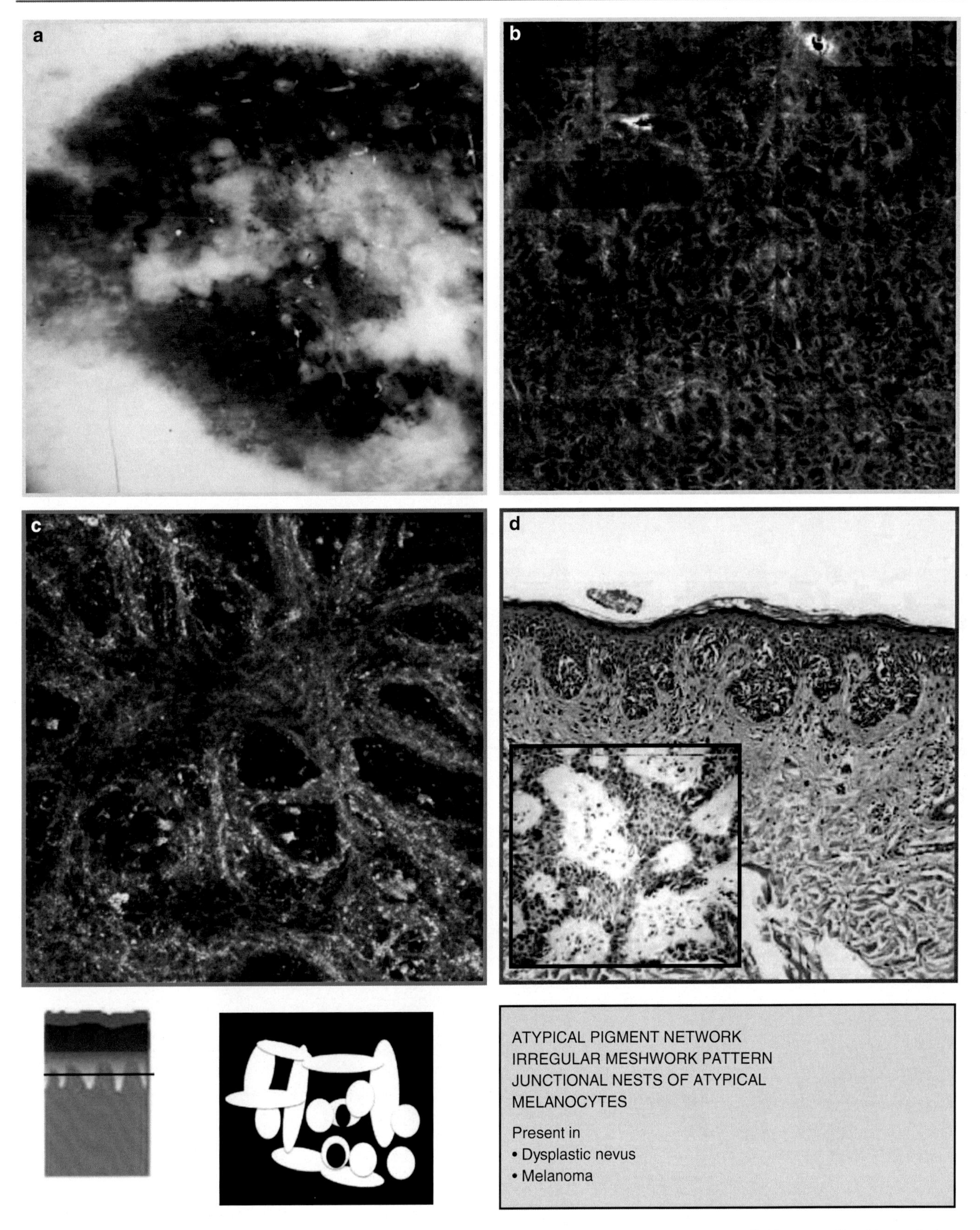

Fig. 7.3 Atypical pigment network. (**a**) Dermoscopy showing a melanoma characterized by atypical pigment network. (**b**) Mosaic at DEJ (4×4 mm) displaying an irregular meshwork architecture. (**c**) Basic image at DEJ (0.5×0.5 mm) showing enlarged interpapillary spaces with junctional thickenings and loosely aggregated cells. Atypical cells are also detectable within the nests. (**d**) Corresponding histopathology showing atypical cells in single units and aggregated in nests at the DEJ. Rete-ridge is irregular but still preserved. In the inset corresponding transversal sectioning is shown

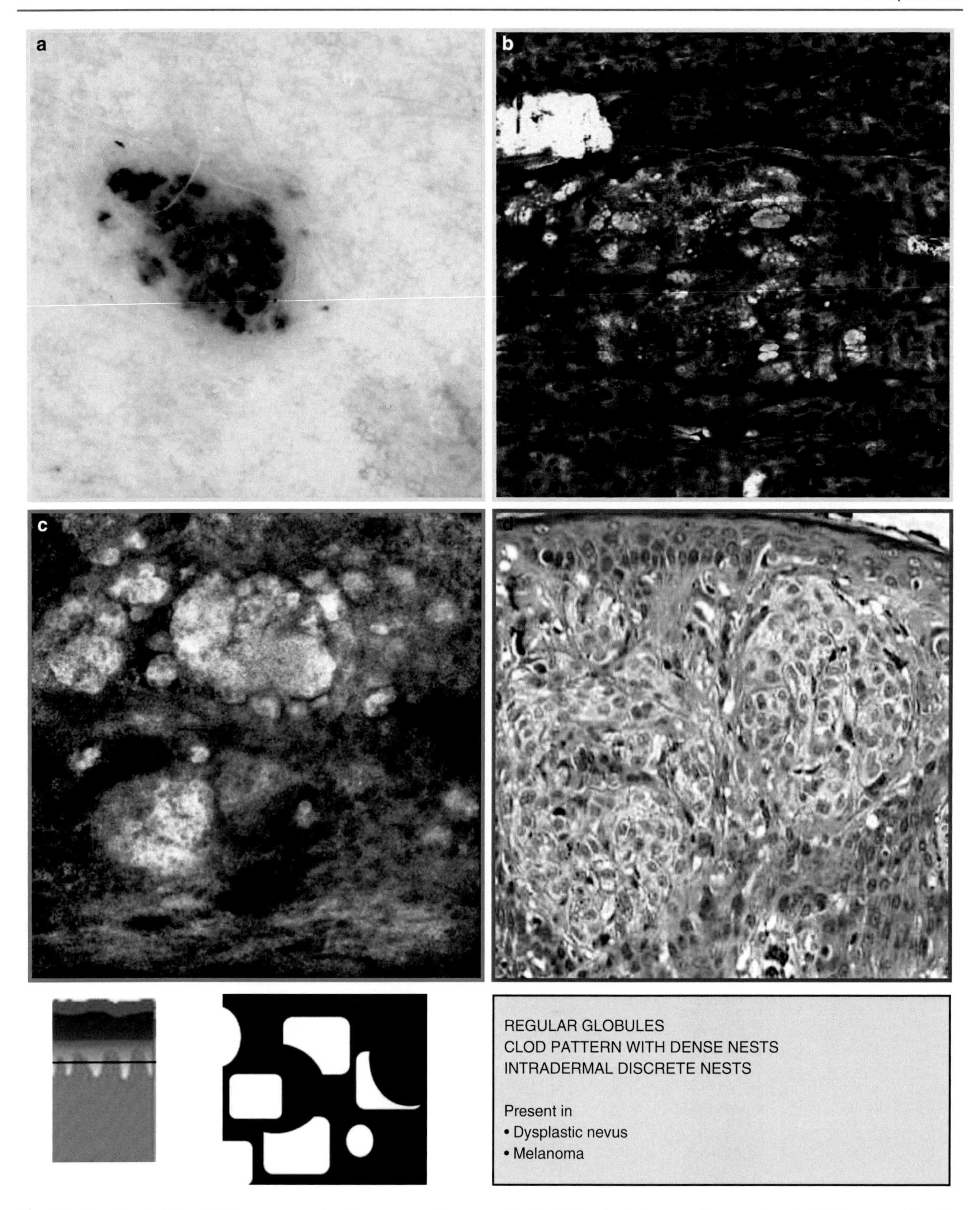

Fig. 7.4 Regular globules. (**a**) Dermoscopy showing a nevus characterized by regular nests. (**b**) Mosaic at DEJ (3.5 × 3.5 mm) displaying a clod pattern. (**c**) Basic image at DEJ (0.5 × 0.5 mm) showing aggregates of cells clustered into dense and compact nests. (**d**) Corresponding histopathology showing discrete melanocytic nests in upper dermis and in proximity of DEJ

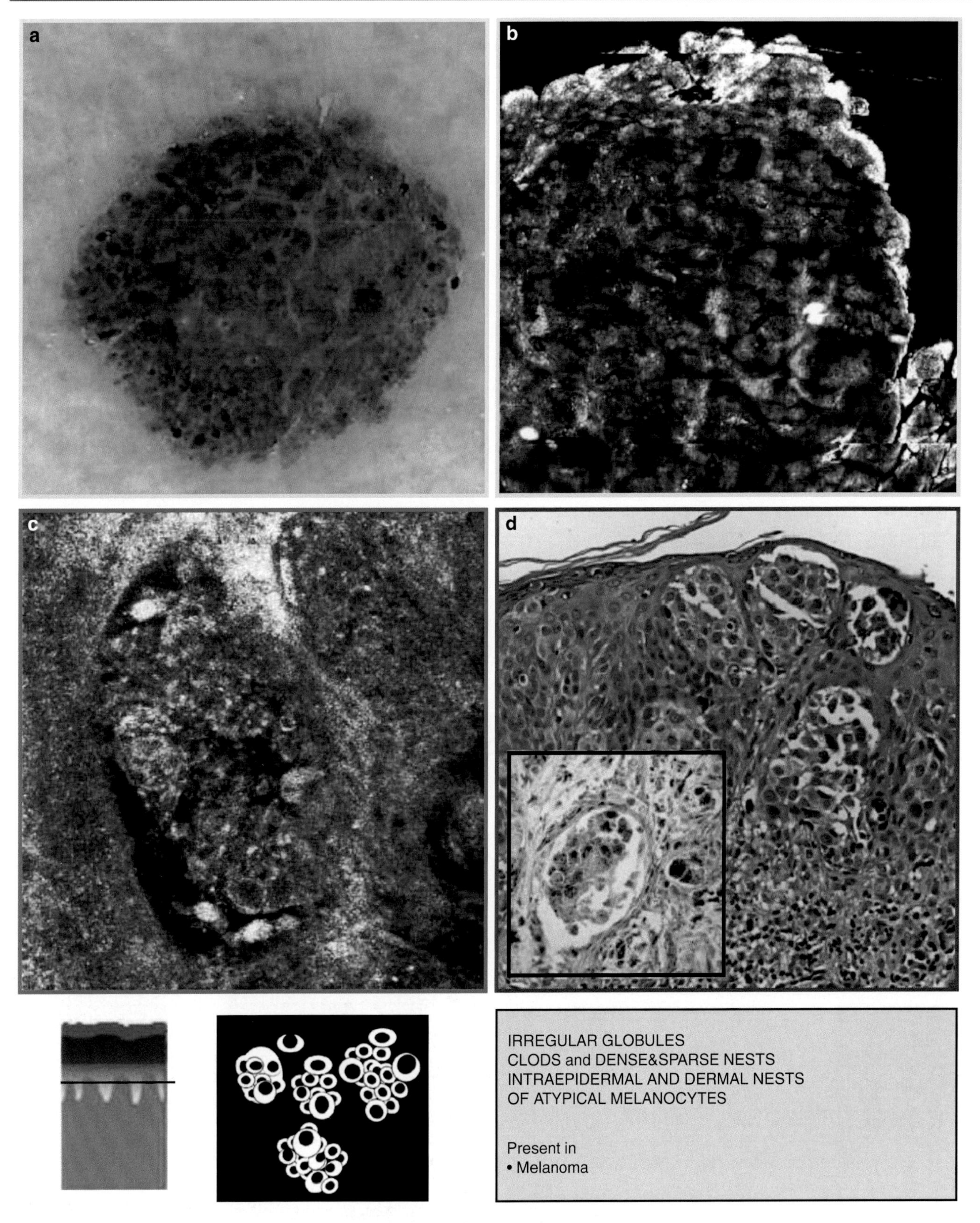

Fig. 7.5 Irregular globules. (**a**) Dermoscopy showing a melanoma characterized by irregular globules in a cobbleston arrangement. (**b**) Mosaic at DEJ (4×4 mm) displaying a clod pattern. (**c**) Basic image at DEJ (0.5 × 0.5 mm) showing dense and sparse nest constituted by atypical and pleomorphic cells. (**d**) Corresponding histopathology showing atypical cells corresponding to malignant melanocytes mostly aggregated in nests within the epidermis, at the DEJ and in the upper dermis. In the inset transversal section shows the exact correspondence with the confocal finding

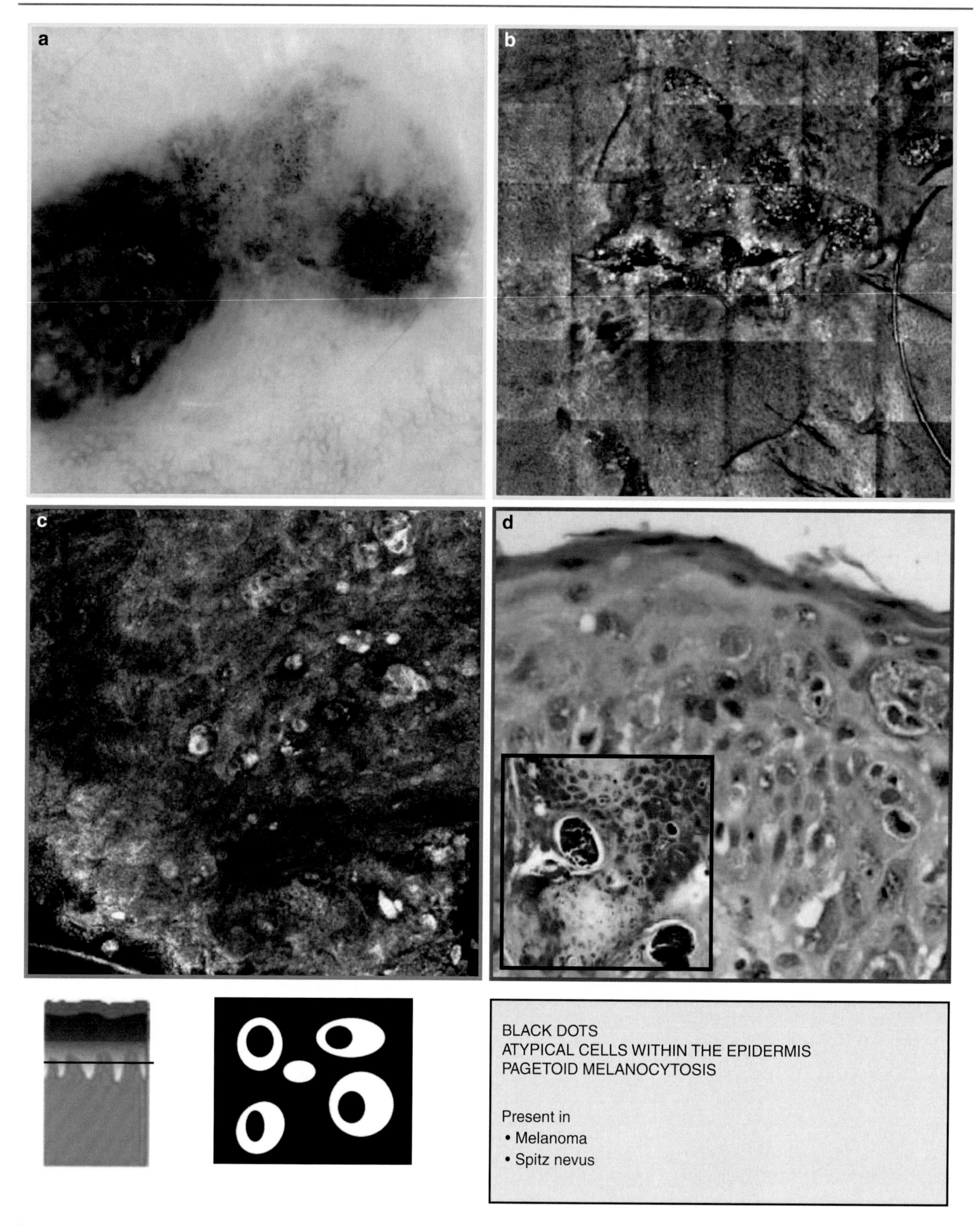

Fig. 7.6 Black dots. (**a**) Dermoscopy showing a melanoma characterized by a pigmented nodule with a peripheral area showing irregularly distributed black dots. (**b**) Mosaic at granulosum/spinosum layer (3×3 mm) displaying irregular honeycombed pattern and areas of disarrangement with numerous bright particles. (**c**) Basic image at granulosum/spinosum layer (0.5 × 0.5 mm) showing atypical polymorphic cells spreading upward in a pagetoid fashion in single units and small aggregates. (**d**) Histopathology shows atypical cells within the epidermis corresponding to pagetoid melanocytosis. In the inset transversal section showing cells and small aggregates within the epidermis

noncharacteristic normal epidermis and superficial dermis covering the pigmented lesion.

Blue areas can be arranged in blotches, mostly when the pigment is accumulated within the papillary dermis, or could merge into diffused blue areas sometimes underlying remnants of pigment structures. When they take origin from accumulation of melanophages in the dermis, as usually happen in inflamed nevi, more or less extensive clusters of plump bright cells are detectable by RCM (Fig. 7.7). In case of melanomas with a striking proliferation of malignant melanocytes in the dermis, usually along with an abundant melanophages infiltrate, both plump bright cells and bright nucleated cells, in single units or in clusters, can be identified in the papillary dermis by means of RCM, helping in the diagnosis.

The presence of a groud-glass whitish hue overlying an homogeneous background blue pigmentation give rise to the so-called *blue-white veil*, which is considered a specific clue for thick melanoma diagnosis. However, distinction between a "blue area" and a "blue-white veil" is sometimes difficult, leading to a low interobserver reproducibility. Upon RCM it is generally associated with epidermal and dermal alterations. The epidermis is usually thickened and shows different degrees of disarrangement, frequently bearing atypical melanocytes corresponding to pagetoid infiltration. In the dermis dishomogeneous nests and/or cerebriform clusters, along with numerous nonaggregated cells infiltrating dermal papillae, corresponding to collection of plump bright and atypical nucleated cells, are also usually observable. Upon histopathology, the blue-white veil finds the same confocal substrates, resulting into epidermal alterations, including orthokeratosis and hyperkeratosis, and dermal proliferation of atypical melanocytes with tendency to infiltrate the dermis along with an abundant inflammatory infiltrate.

7.1.7 Regression

Regression is defined as white scar-like or light pink well-circumscribed zones sometimes showing blue pepper-like granules, corresponding to a clinically flat part of the lesion. Regression areas are often observed in melanomas, although rarely present in benign lesions too [9]. Upon RCM, regression generally corresponds to thinned epidermis with a honeycombed pattern, only rarely with few pagetoid cells. Most of the time, the dermal–epidermal boundary is imperceptible, passing directly from the honeycombed epidermal layers to the dermis without the appearance of the reflective basal cells and papillary contours. The dermis consists of a coarse network of ill-defined collagen bundles or, less frequently, of fibrillar collagen oriented towards the same direction. Small bright reflecting spots and plump bright cells, intermingled with collagen bundles, are usually observable in correspondence of the peppering, consistent for inflammatory infiltrate. Few nucleated cells with bright cytoplasm and well-defined borders, suggestive of malignant melanocytes infiltrating the dermis, although consistent for melanoma diagnosis, can be rarely detected. Histology shows a thin, atrophic, devoid of melanin, epidermis, covering areas of fibroplasia with inflammatory infiltrate, consisting of leucocytes and few melanophages (Fig. 7.8). Also upon histology, malignant cells are seldom observed within the regression area.

7.2 Conclusion

Confocal microscopy, enabling the visualization of the cyto-architectural substrates of dermoscopy features, is helpful in the interpretation of difficult melanocytic lesions, enabling the distinction between melanomas and nevi showing similar dermoscopic features. As shown in this chapter, confocal microscopy gives rise to aspects exactly corresponding to histopathologic structures, especially when transversal sections are taken. Interpretation of the confocal figures have to consider the horizontal plane of sectioning and have to take into account the impossibility to explore structures located deeper than 200 μm, suggesting to interpret with caution lesions mostly or univocally characterized by a deep dermal component. An adequate level of knowledge of dermoscopy and histopathology is recommended in order to guarantee a good interpretation of confocal images finalized to an accurate diagnosis of melanoma.

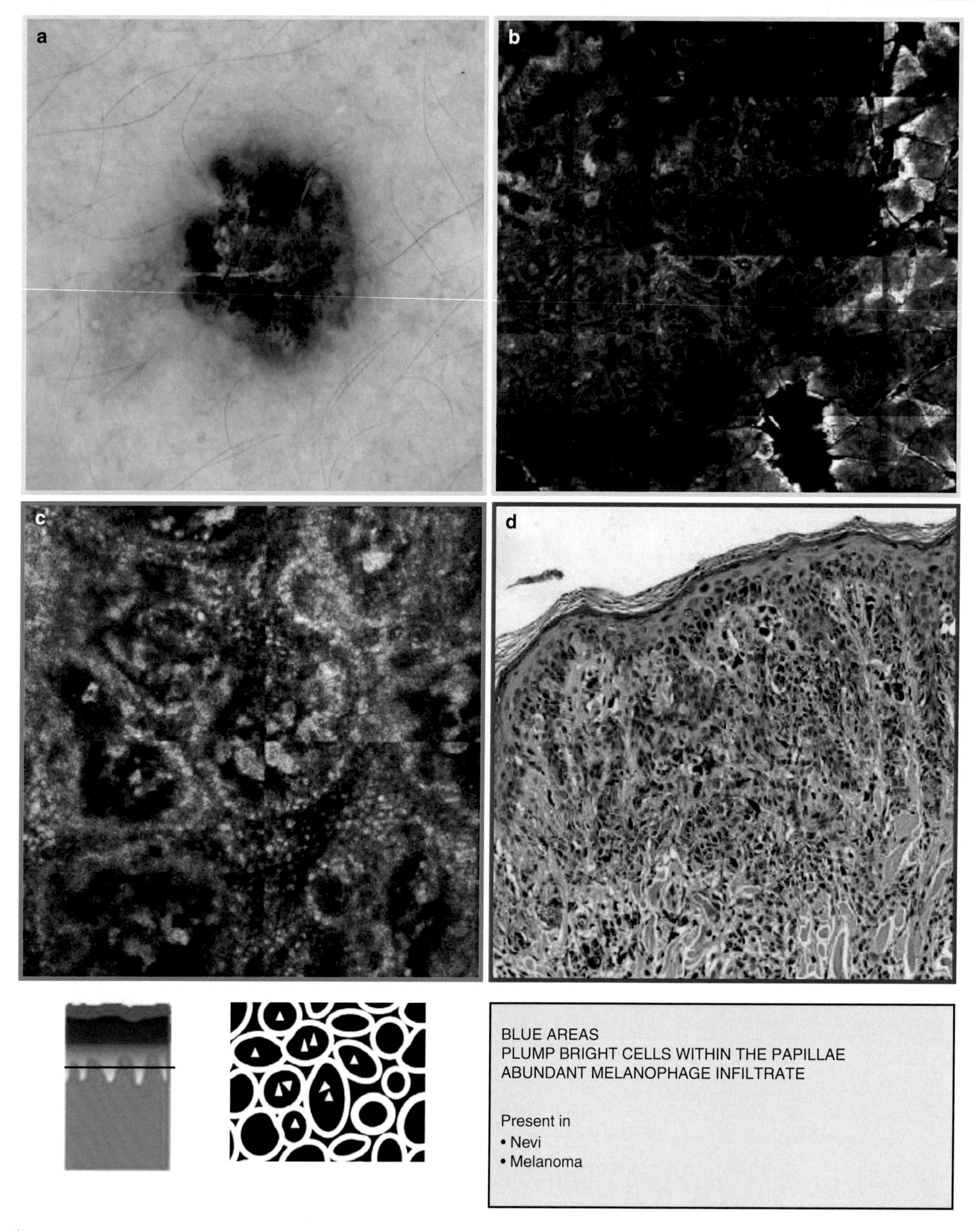

Fig. 7.7 Blue areas. (**a**) Dermoscopy showing a nevus characterized by a homogeneous blue area. (**b**) Mosaic at DEJ (3×3 mm) showing meshwork and small nests with bright structures within the papillae. (**c**) Basic image at DEJ (0.5 × 0.5 mm) showing numerous clumps of plump bright cells intermingled with small melanocytic nests. (**d**) Corresponding histopathology showing clumps of melanophages in the dermis and melanocytic nests

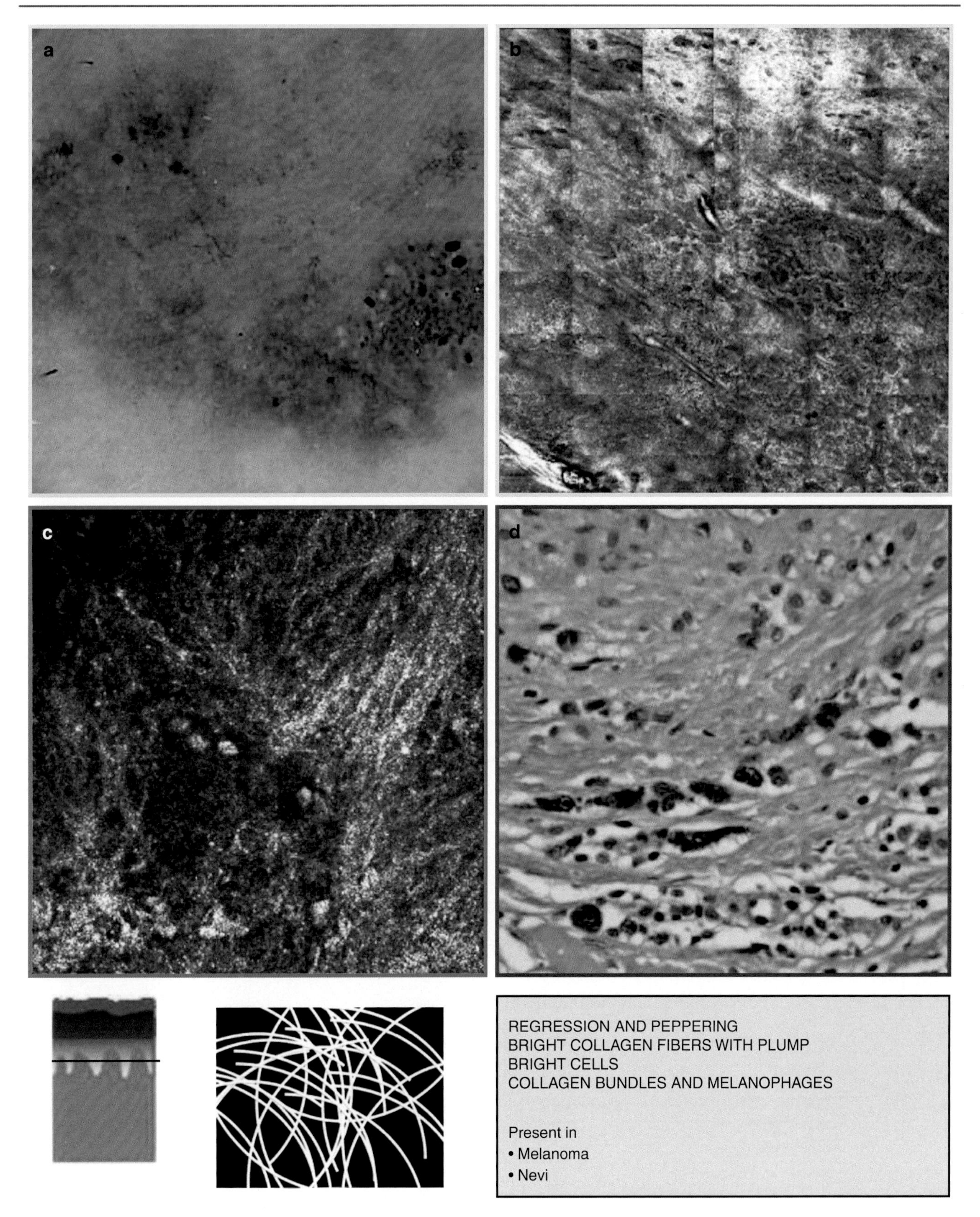

Fig. 7.8 Regression. (**a**) Dermoscopy showing a melanoma characterized by a wide area of regression (scar-like area with peppering). (**b**) Mosaic at DEJ-upper dermis (3×3 mm) showing diffuse brightness with a nonspecific architecture. (**c**) Basic image in the upper dermis (0.5 × 0.5 mm) showing bright filaments and plump bright cells. (**d**) Corresponding histopathology showing melanophages within coarse and compact bundles of collagen

References

1. Kittler H, Pehamberger H, Wolff K, Binder M (2002) Diagnostic accuracy of dermoscopy. Lancet Oncol 3:159–165
2. Pellacani G, Longo C, Malvehy J, Puig S, Carrera C, Segura S, Bassoli S, Seidenari S (2008) In vivo confocal microscopic and histopathologic correlations of dermoscopic features in 202 melanocytic lesions. Arch Dermatol 144(12):1597–1608
3. Argenziano G, Soyer HP, Chimenti S, Talamini R, Corona R, Sera F, Binder M, Cerroni L, De Rosa G, Ferrara G, Hofmann-Wellenhof R, Landthaler M, Menzies SW, Pehamberger H, Piccolo D, Rabinovitz HS, Schiffner R, Staibano S, Stolz W, Bartenjev I, Blum A, Braun R, Cabo H, Carli P, De Giorgi V, Fleming MG, Grichnik JM, Grin CM, Halpern AC, Johr R, Katz B, Kenet RO, Kittler H, Kreusch J, Malvehy J, Mazzocchetti G, Oliviero M, Ozdemir F, Peris K, Perotti R, Perusquia A, Pizzichetta MA, Puig S, Rao B, Rubegni P, Saida T, Scalvenzi M, Seidenari S, Stanganelli I, Tanaka M, Westerhoff K, Wolf IH, Braun-Falco O, Kerl H, Nishikawa T, Wolff K, Kopf AW (2003) Dermoscopy of pigmented skin lesions: results of a consensus meeting via the Internet. J Am Acad Dermatol 48(5):679–693
4. Pellacani G, Cesinaro AM, Longo C, Grana C, Seidenari S (2005) Microscopic in vivo description of cellular architecture of dermoscopic pigment network in nevi and melanomas. Arch Dermatol 141(2):147–154
5. Pellacani G, Cesinaro AM, Seidenari S (2005) In vivo assessment of melanocytic nests in nevi and melanomas by reflectance confocal microscopy. Mod Pathol 18(4):469–474
6. Yadav S, Vossaert KA, Kopf AW, Silverman M, Grin-Jorgensen C (1993) Histopathologic correlates of structures seen on dermoscopy (epiluminescence microscopy). Am J Dermatopathol 15: 297–305
7. Scope A, Gill M, Benveuto-Andrade C, Halpern AC, Gonzalez S, Marghoob AA (2007) Correlation of dermoscopy with in vivo reflectance confocal microscopy of streaks in melanocytic lesions. Arch Dermatol 143(6):727–734
8. Pellacani G, Bassoli S, Longo C, Cesinaro AM, Seidenari S (2007) Diving into the blue: in vivo microscopic characterization of the dermoscopic blue hue. J Am Acad Dermatol 57(1): 96–104
9. Pellacani G, Guitera P, Longo C, Avramidis M, Seidenari S, Menzies S (2007) The impact of in vivo reflectance confocal microscopy for the diagnostic accuracy of melanoma and equivocal melanocytic lesions. J Invest Dermatol 127:2759–2765

Part IV

Melanocytic Lesions: Nevi

Common Nevi

8

Sara Bassoli, Verena Ahlgrimm-Siess, Alice Casari,
and Giovanni Pellacani

Common, non-dysplastic nevi include a wide group of benign melanocytic lesions histologically characterized by an increased number and proliferation of typical melanocytes, in single cells or in aggregates. Cytology is usually monomorphous, characterized by small melanocytes which tend to assume a more epithelioid configuration. In this chapter, the main confocal features of clear-cut benign nevi are presented, focusing on their histological presentation, and dermoscopy correlates.

In particular, it is easier to differentiate these lesions according to their clinical presentation and histopathologic characteristic, responsible of their confocal presentations [1–3] (Table 8.1).

8.1 Flat Lesions Characterized by a Predominant Junctional Component

These lesions are characterized almost exclusively by a junctional component. In dermoscopy they are more frequently characterized by pigment network and/or homogeneous pigmentation. Globules are rarely detectable, although a few cases, predominantly corresponding to small new arising lesions in children, may show a globular pattern.

Confocal microscopy presents two main patterns, frequently singularly pattern sometimes in combination, corresponding to a ringed and/or a meshwork architecture.

S. Bassoli (✉) • A. Casari • G. Pellacani
Department of Dermatology and Venereology,
University of Modena and Reggio Emilia, Modena, Italy
e-mail: sarabassoli79@gmail.com

V. Ahlgrimm-Siess
Department of Dermatology, Medical University of Graz,
Graz, Austria

Lesions characterized by *ringed architecture* (Fig. 8.1) show well demarcated rims of bright cells surrounding the dermal papillae throughout the entire lesion. The cells surrounding the papillae are small polygonal monomorphous bright structures, where pigmented basal cell keratinocytes are indistinguishable from melanocytes. Interpapillary junctional thickenings or clusters are rarely observable. Epidermis presents a regular architecture, most frequently with a cobblestone pattern, and pagetoid cells are nonusually visible, with the exception of few sporadic dendritic cells mostly corresponding to Langerhans cells. Dermal papillae are usually dark, and it is sometimes possible to recognize the capillary vessels within a texture if tiny reticulated collagen fibers. Small bright particles are sometimes visible within the papillae in coincidence of inflammation at histopathology. Dermoscopy is characterized by a regular pigment network, sometimes with homogeneous diffuse pigmentation in the central portion. A predominance of single melanocytes over nests along with a lentiginous pattern, with preserved rete-ridge, is usually observable in histopathologic sections.

On the other hand, lesions characterized by a *meshwork pattern* (Fig. 8.2) are constituted by the predominant presence of junctional nests. Junctional nests appear as fusiform widening of the interpapillary spaces, or as roundish structures bulging within the papilla. Junctional nests are usually compact, with clearly outlined borders, constituted by a dense aggregate of monomorphous cell population, and no atypical cells are detectable within or outside the nests. Papillary contour are usually clearly outlined (edged papillae). Sometimes inflammatory infiltrate (bright particles and plump bright cells) could be present within the papillae. In dermoscopy these lesions are characterized by pigment network and/or diffuse pigmentation. Pigment globules could be sometimes visible, especially in association with large roundish nests bulging into the papillae. Rarely, a globular dermoscopic pattern is detected in these lesions, due to the predominance of large globules bulging from the DEJ contours throughout the entire lesion.

R. Hofmann-Wellenhof et al. (eds.), *Reflectance Confocal Microscopy for Skin Diseases*,
DOI 10.1007/978-3-642-21997-9_8, © Springer-Verlag Berlin Heidelberg 2012

Table 8.1 Summary of the different types of melanocytic nevi, showing histological features correlating to RCM and dermoscopy aspects

Histology	Main RCM features	Dermatoscopy
Junctional nevus – single melanocytes at the DEJ, elongated papillae, lentiginous pattern	Ringed pattern	Reticular pattern
Junctional nevus – small junctional nests, located at the tips of the ridges	Meshwork with junctional thickenings	Reticular/homogeneous pattern
Compound nevus, superficial type – nests at the junction and in the papillary dermis	Meshwork with thickenings/junctional nests + dermal nests	Reticular, homogeneous and/or globular pattern
Compound nevus deep type – Nests at the junction and in the papillary and reticular dermis	Meshwork with thickenings/junctional nests + prominent clod patterns	Complex/multicomponent pattern
Dermal nevus – compactly aggregated melanocytic nests in the dermis	Expanding dense or dense and sparse polygonal clusters	Cobblestone pattern

Junctional nests correspond in histology to the presence of discrete melanocytic nests, regularly distributed along the tips of the cristae.

In confocal, the distinction among junctional and dermal nests is sometimes impossible, because the morphologic differences are very subtle. Normally, junctional nests appear connected to the junction, while the dermal ones are disconnected and located within the dermal papillae, but these features are not always clearly visible. In these cases, it will not be possible to state with certainty if the lesion is a junctional nevus or a compound nevus with a superficial dermal component.

Fig. 8.1 RCM mosaic (5 × 5 mm) at the level of the dermal–epidermal junction, including the most part of the nevus, shows a very symmetric and regular architecture. At this magnification, a predominantly ringed pattern is recognizable, although some thickenings are visible in the lower portion of the mosaic

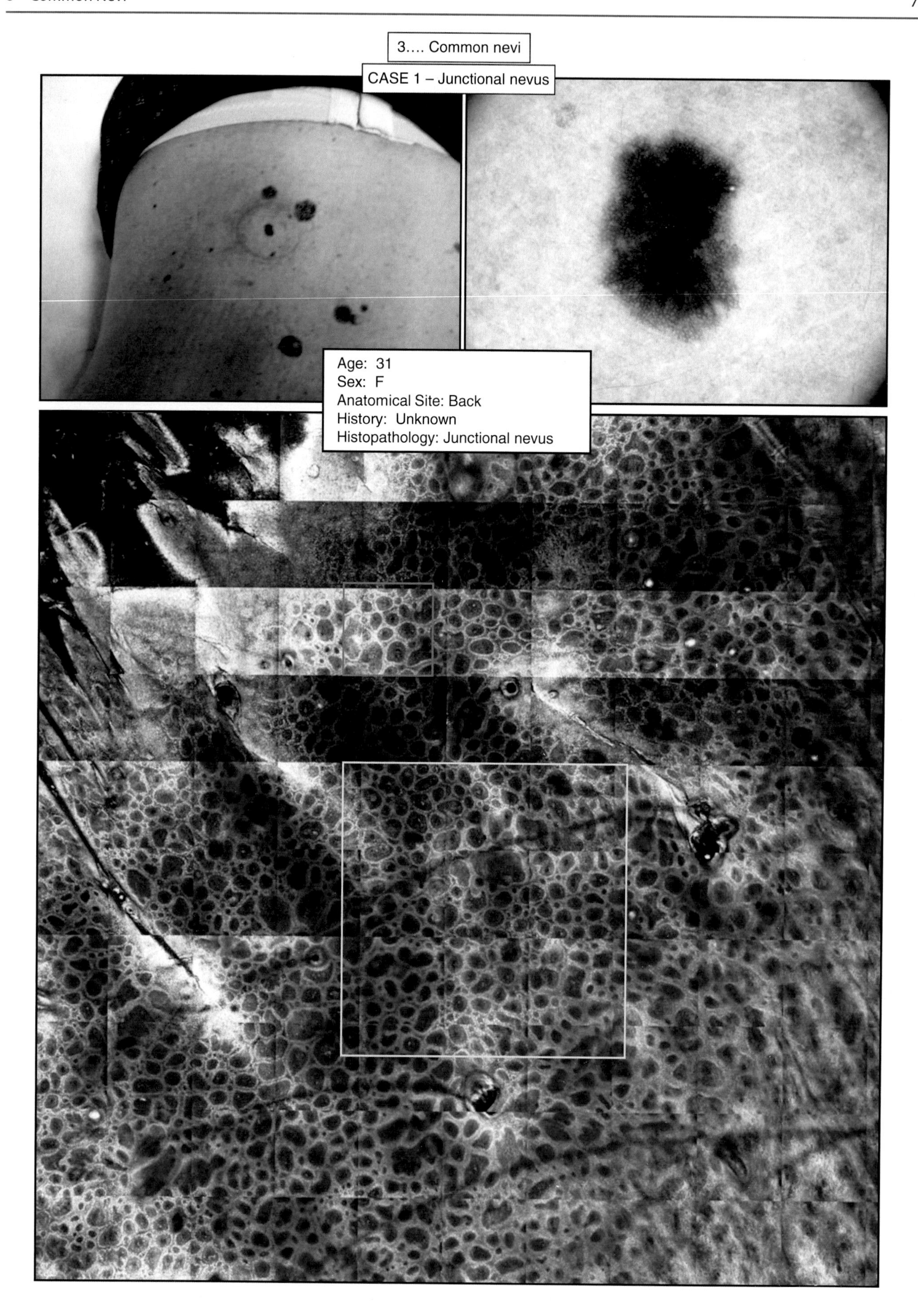
3.... Common nevi
CASE 1 – Junctional nevus
Age: 31
Sex: F
Anatomical Site: Back
History: Unknown
Histopathology: Junctional nevus

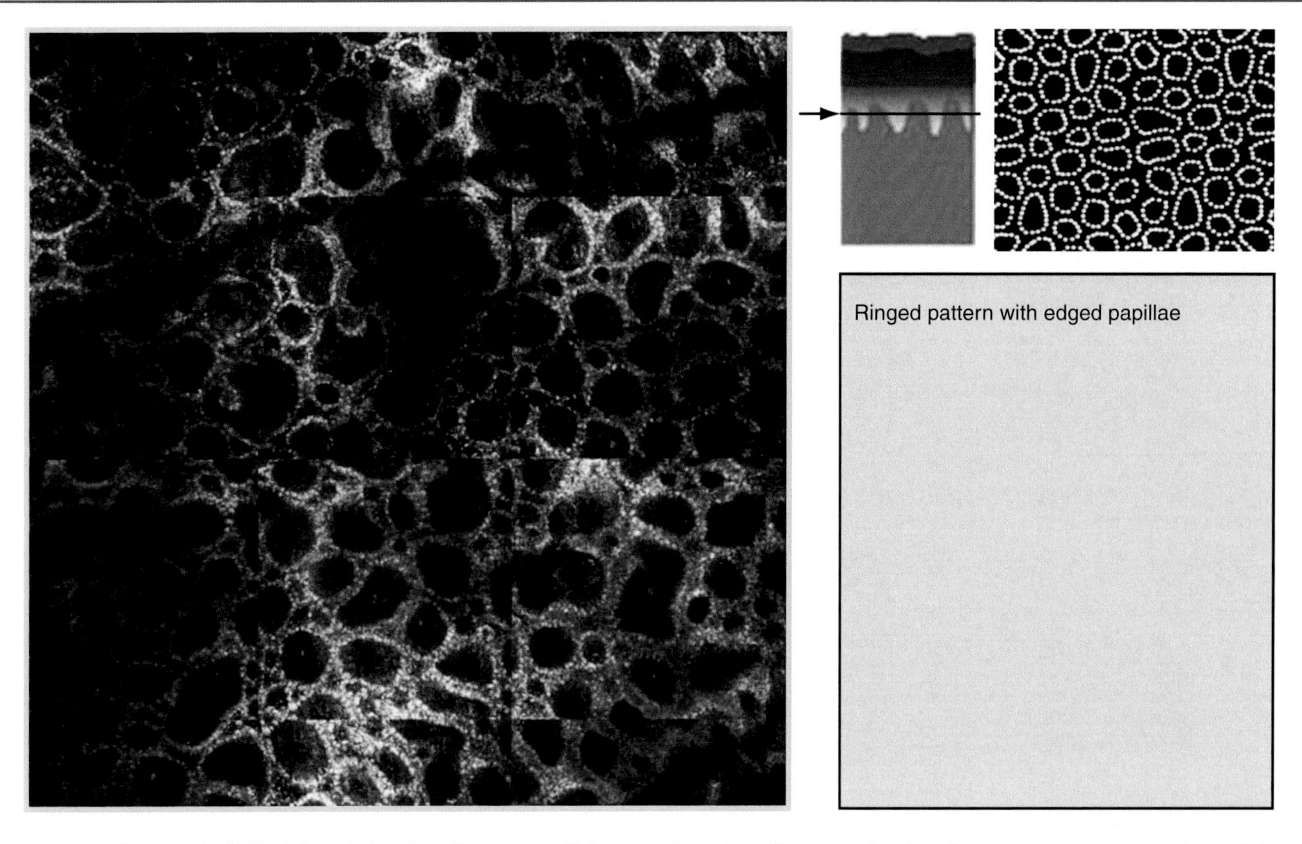

Fig. 8.1.1 RCM mosaic (1.5 × 1.5 mm) showing a better area of ringed pattern, with regular, edged papillae. Papillae are very similar to each other, and surrounded by a rim of bright, small, typical cells. Within the dermal papillae, some bright cells are present, corresponding to inflammatory infiltrate (melanophages, leukocytes)

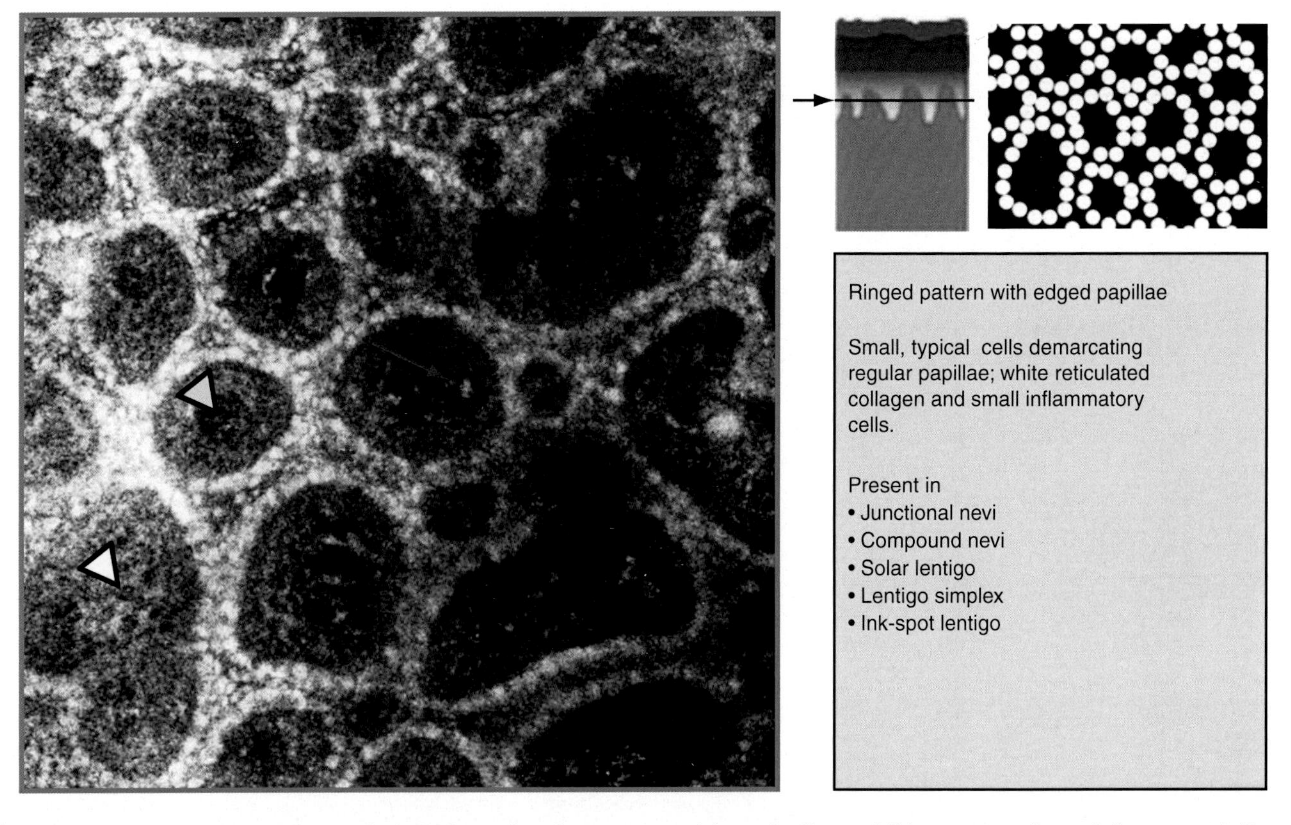

Fig. 8.1.2 Basic image (0.5 × 0.5 mm) nicely depicts a ringed pattern with regular, edged papillae: each papilla is surrounded and very well demarcated by a rim of small, bright cells (*). Within the dark hole representing the horizontal section of a dermal papilla, small bright particles and cells are visible, corresponding to inflammatory infiltrate (→); furthermore, a slight reticulated material filling the papillae is seen, corresponding to collagen (*white arrowhead*), in some cases centered by a small vessel (*yellow arrowhead*)

CASE 2 – Junctional nevus-globular type
Age: 36
Sex: M
Anatomical Site: Right forearm
History: Recent growth
Histopathology: Junctional nevus with prevalence of nests

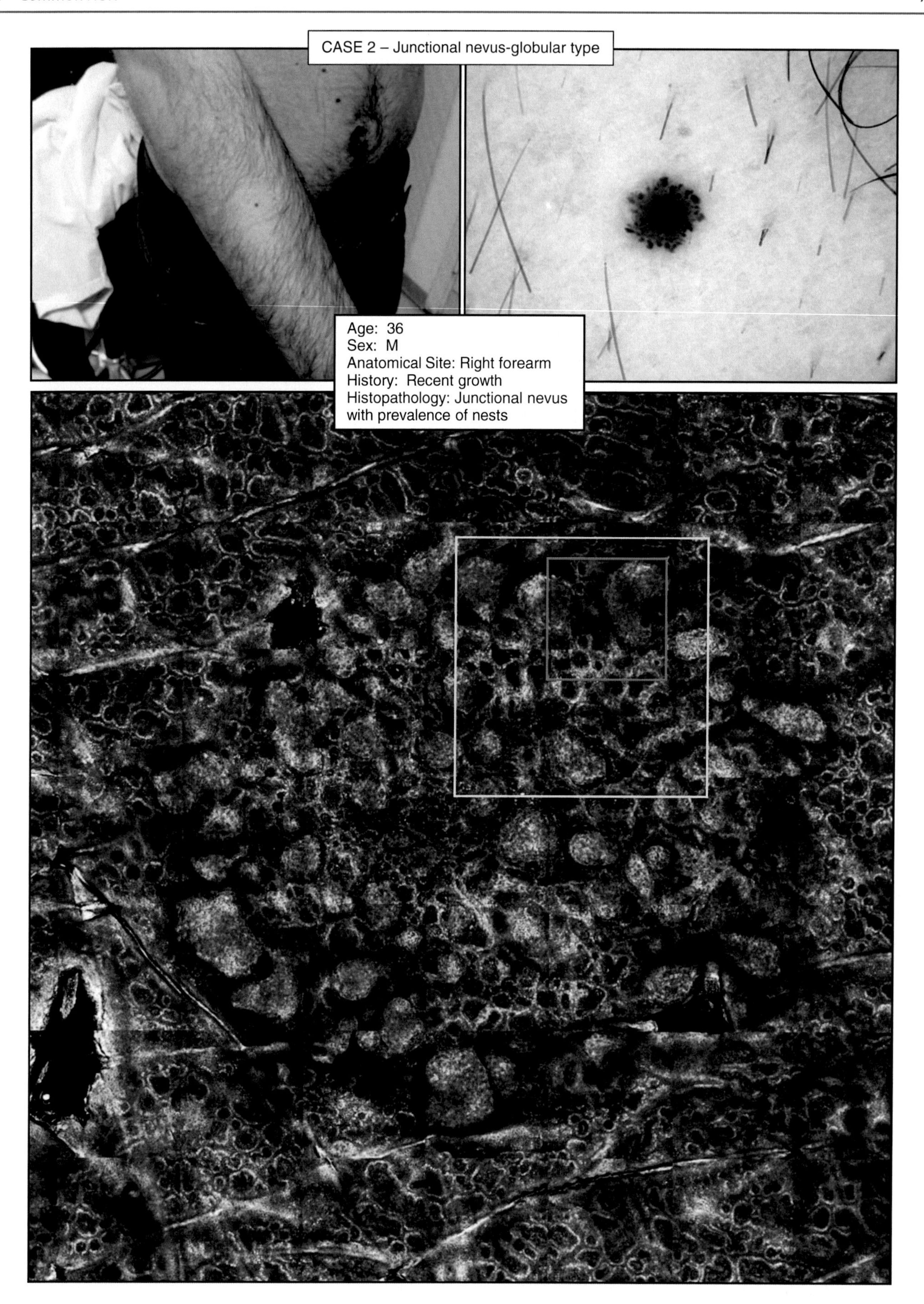

Fig. 8.2 RCM mosaic (3.5 × 3.5 mm) at the dermal–epidermal junction shows a nice correspondence with dermoscopy, revealing dense junctional nests, both at the periphery, where they are connected to the junction, and within the dermal papillae. In the center of the lesion, a meshwork pattern is observable, with edged papillae and a slight thickening of the interpapillary spaces. Globally, the lesions appears very symmetric and regular in architecture

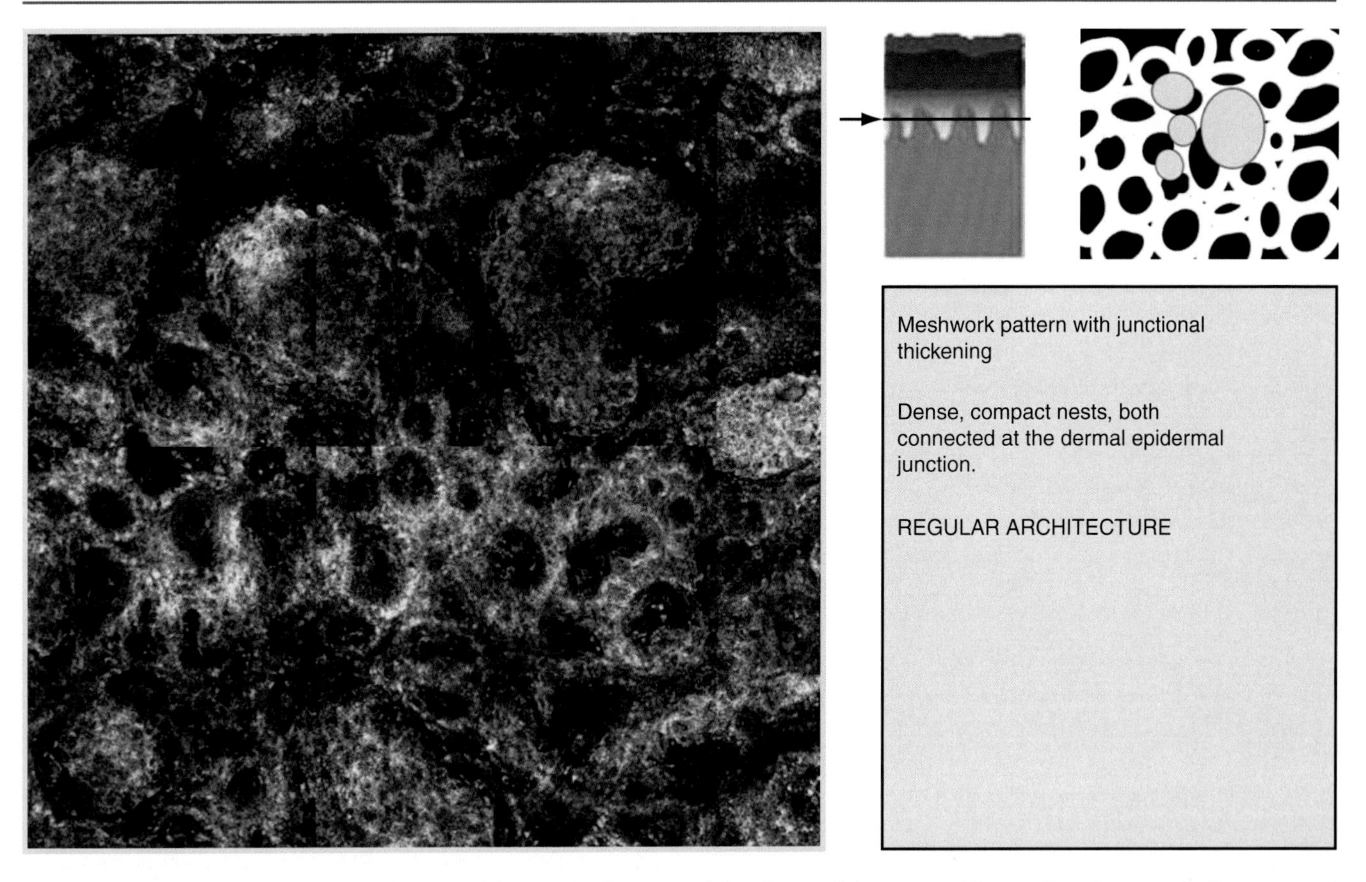

Fig. 8.2.1 RCM mosaic (1 × 1 mm): this part of the mosaic shows a peripheral area of the nevus, with a meshwork pattern in the center and junctional nests at the periphery. The nests are dense, compact and regular

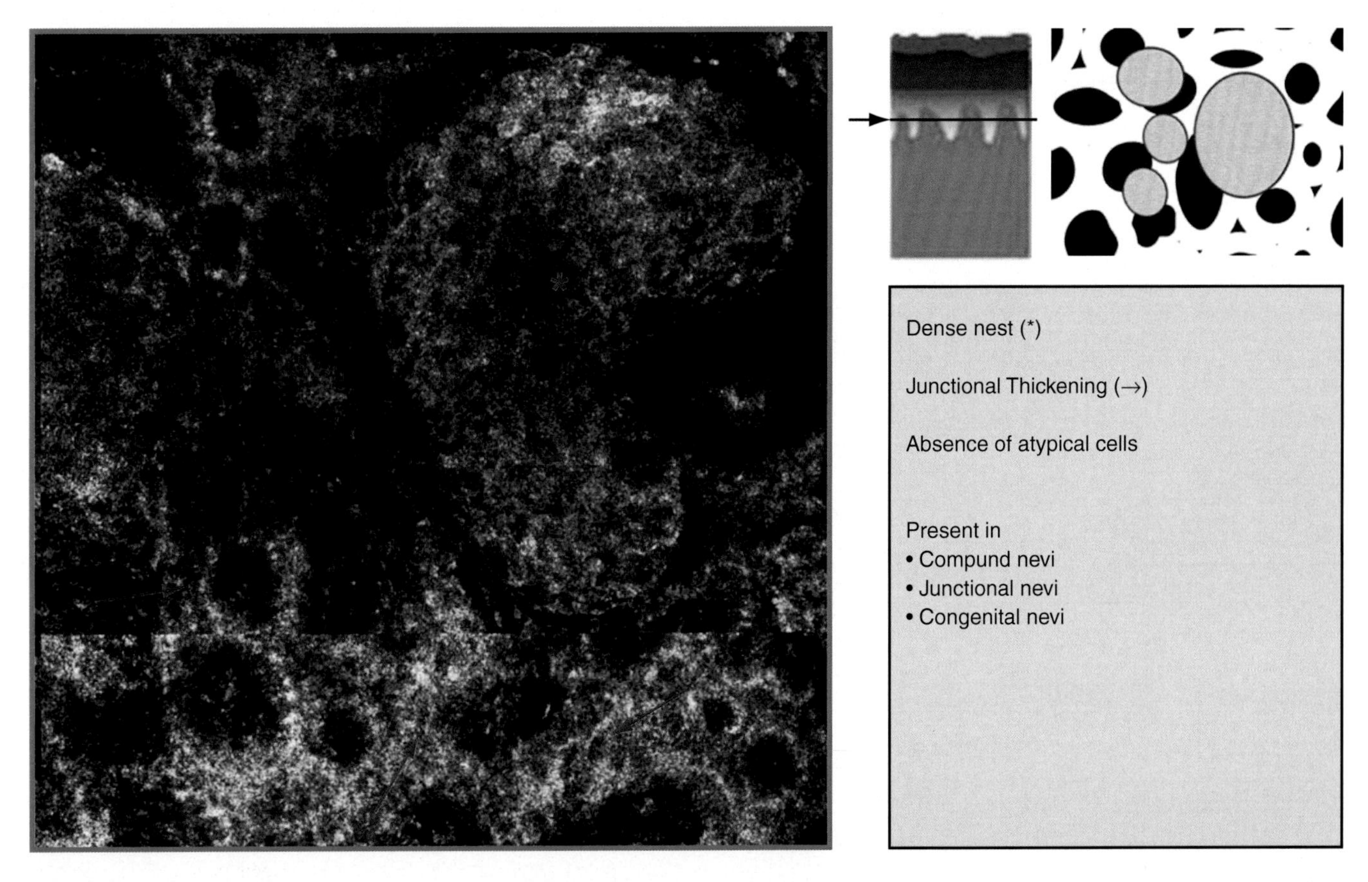

Fig. 8.2.2 Basic image (0.5 × 0.5 mm) showing a compact, regular nest with typical cells (*) that appears partially connected to the junction. Beside the nests, a meshwork pattern is seen, with a regular thickening of the interpapillary spaces (→)

8.2 Flat-Palpable and Palpable-Nodular Lesions Characterized by Junctional and Dermal Component

These lesions correspond to compound nevi in histopathology. Dermoscopy is usually variable, showing reticular, homogeneous, complex (globular + reticular or globular + homogeneous) or multicomponent pattern.

Junctional component in confocal microscopy does not differ from the one observable in the above described groups, although a *meshwork* pattern is present in the majority of cases.

Dermal component is usually characterized by aggregates of melanocytes within dermal papillae. Two main aspects are usually observable according with the dermal involvement. Lesions characterized by a superficial dermal component display dense compact nests visible within the dermal papillae and distinguishable from junctional nests only when a neat separation between the nest and the epidermis is clearly detectable throughout its entire perimeter. In histopathology these lesions are characterized by melanocytic nests at the DEJ, mostly located at the tip of the cristae, and by discrete dermal nests usually located in the papillary dermis and mostly in the center of the lesion (Fig. 8.3).

When dermal dense nests are numerous and large, a *clod* pattern is usually detectable, mostly in the center of the lesion, associated with a meshwork and/or ringed pattern more evident at the periphery. In case of massive involvement of the superficial and deep dermis, large aggregates widening the dermal papillae are visible, and the contours of the papillae show up as barely visible rings surrounding the melanocytic aggregate (Fig. 8.4). These aggregates can be described as dense & sparse nests, showing large round nucleated, but monomorphous, cells on the upper part of the nests, corresponding to the upper portion of dermal melanocytic cords and nests.

"Enlarging nevi", characterized in dermoscopy by a rim of peripheral globules, usually belong to this category, and show a predominant meshwork pattern with bulging junctional nests at the periphery, and dermal dense nests mostly located in the center of the lesion.

8.3 Palpable-Nodular Lesions Characterized Intradermal Component

These lesions correspond to intradermal nevi in histopathology. Upon dermoscopy these lesions are characterized by a cobblestone pattern or by homogeneous pigmentation.

Upon confocal microscopy, a *clod* pattern is detectable at low magnification (Fig. 8.5). The examination of the upper layers in these nevi reveals a regular epidermis, with a honeycomb pattern, while at the junctional level barely visible rings can be observed. The dermal papillae are enlarged and usually filled in by a large aggregate of melanocytes. Dermal nests could be dense, but more frequently dense & sparse, with a monomorphous melanocytic cell population evident on the upper portion of the nests similarly to the ones detectable in compound nevi with a deep dermal component. In these lesions, the vascular component can also be prominent. Vessels can be dilated, running between and within the dermal nests. In histology, intradermal melanocytes are aggregated in cord-like structures showing small melanocytes, sometimes with neuroid aspect, in the deeper portion, progressively enlarging toward the surface (Table 8.1).

In conclusion, the confocal features of benign melanocytic nevi, characterized by architectural regularity, typical confocal features and lack of melanoma characteristic aspects, such as pagetoid infiltration and atypical melanocytes at the DEJ, allow in most cases an easy and confident diagnosis.

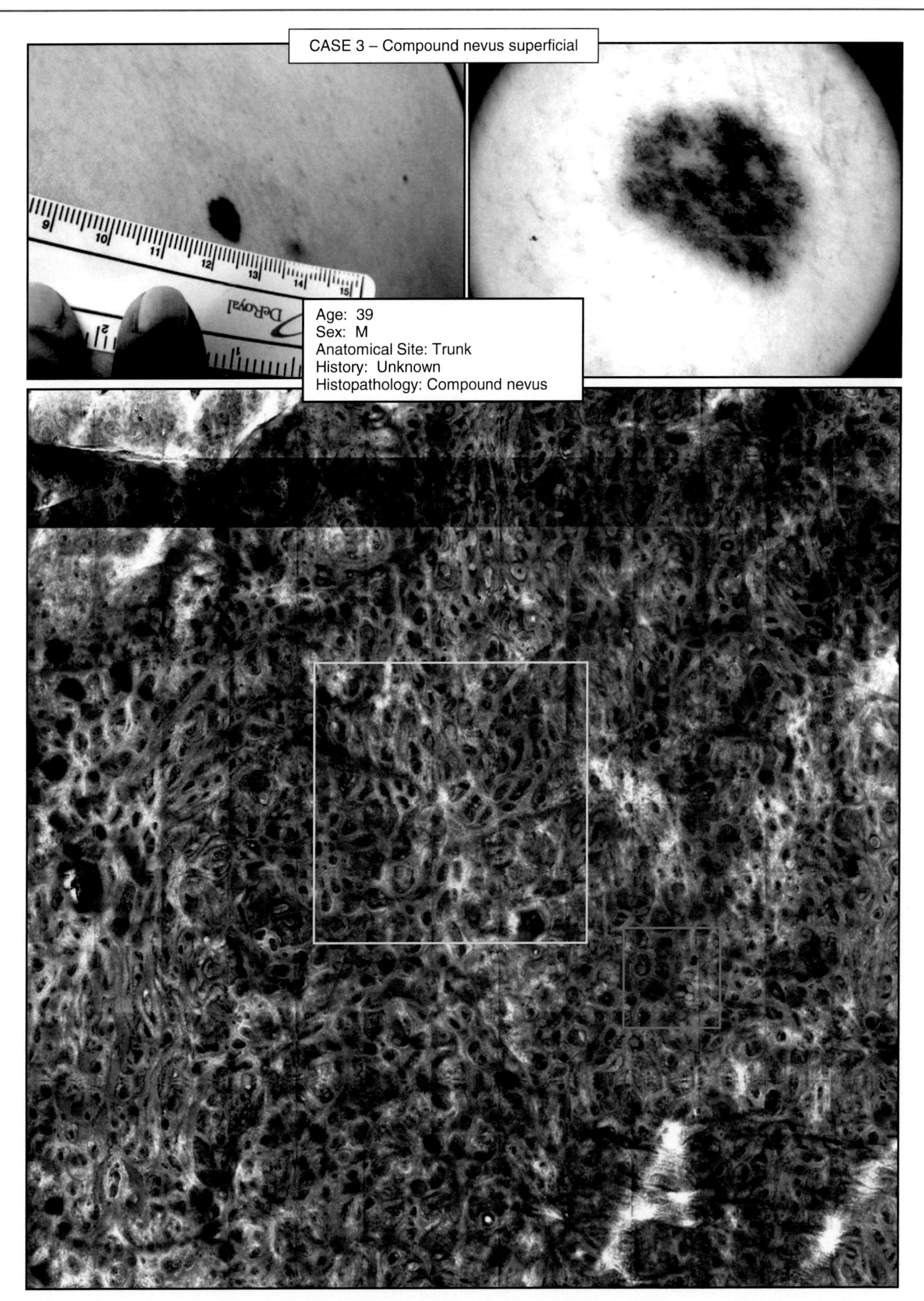

Fig. 8.3 RCM mosaic (6.5 × 6.5 mm) at the junctional–upper dermal level shows a meshwork pattern, with some small nests within the dermal papillae. The overall architecture is very regular, with edged and nonedged papillae visible but no atypical cells

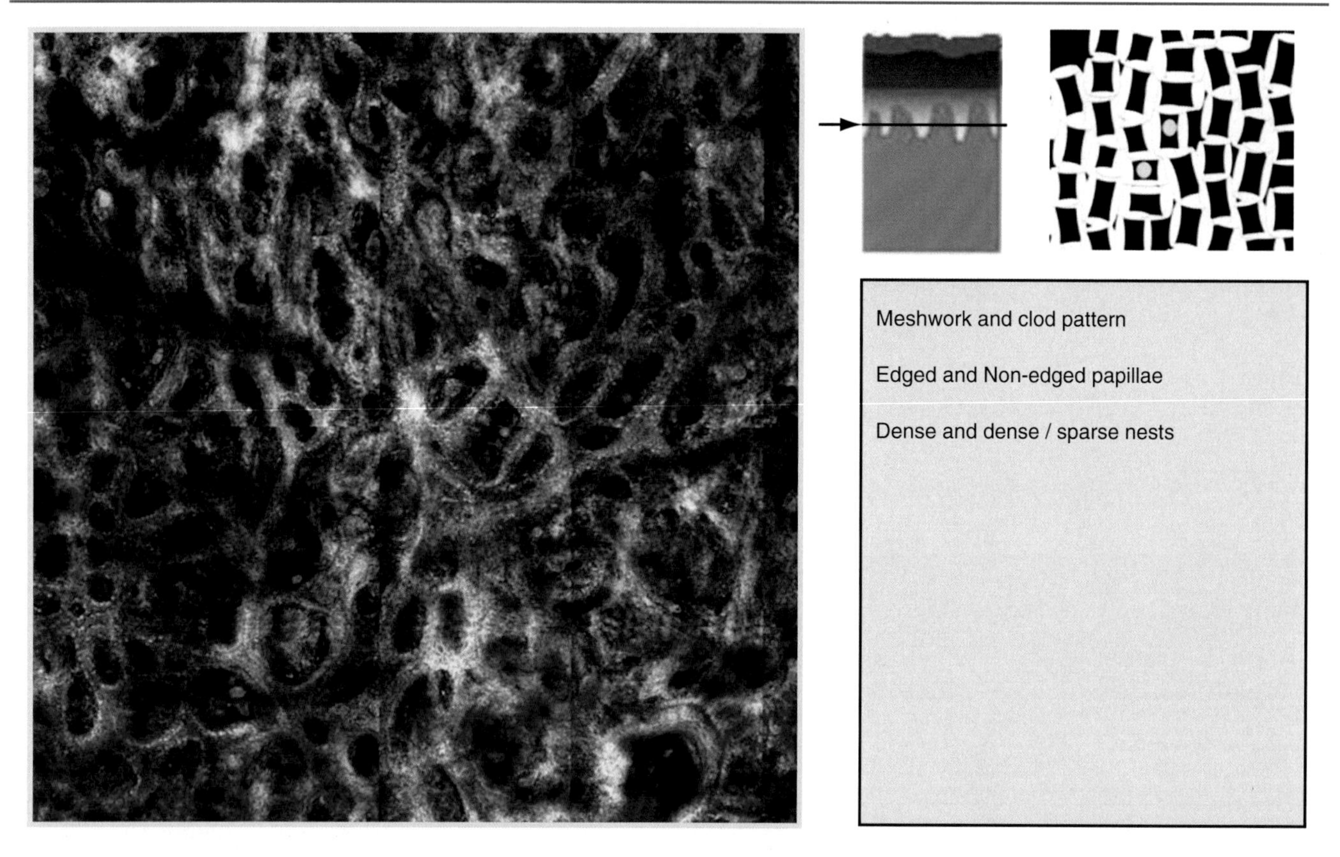

Fig. 8.3.1 RCM mosaic (2 × 2 mm) in a portion of the nevus with meshwork pattern, junctional clusters and thickenings. Also dense and dense/ sparse dermal nests are visible. The junctional clusters surround edged and nonedged papillae

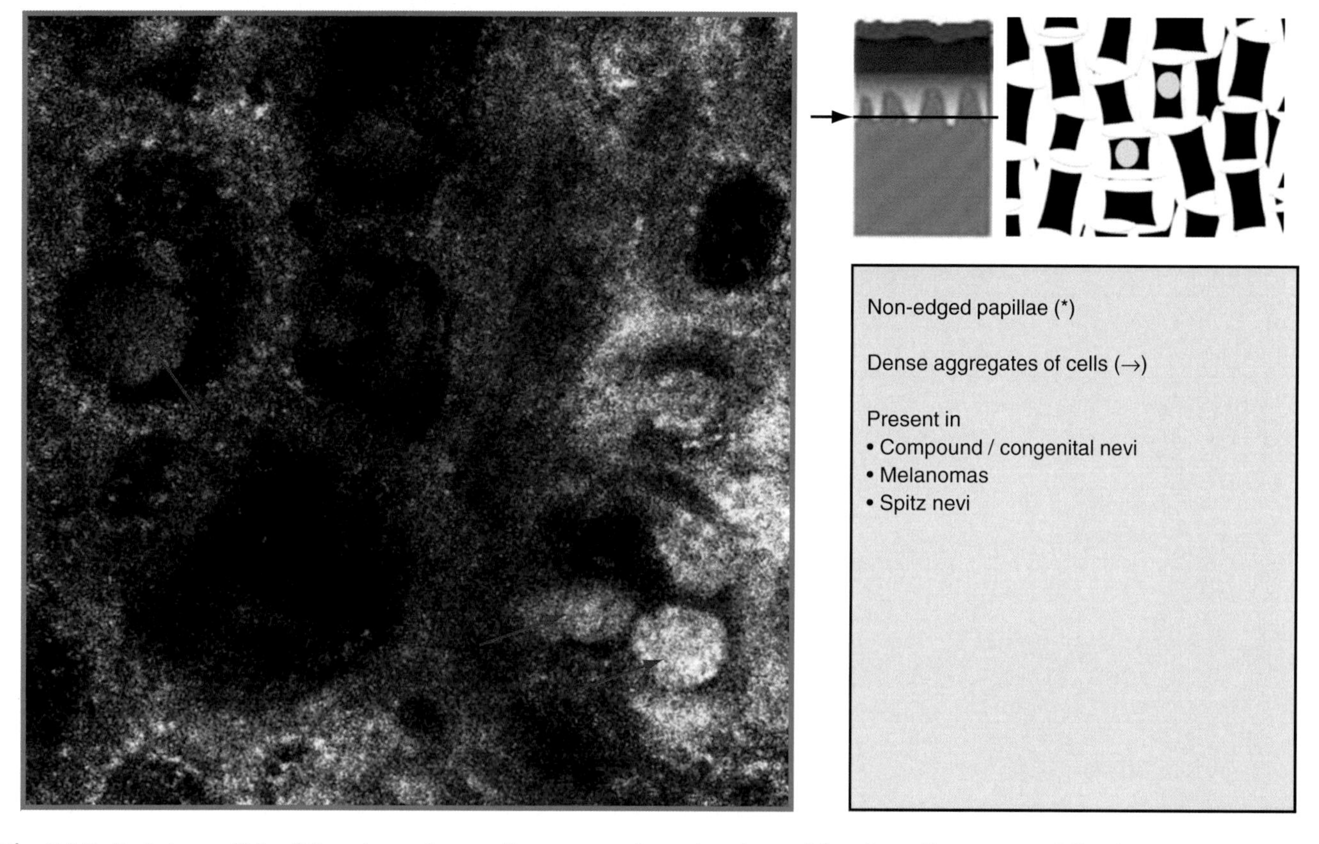

Fig. 8.3.2 Basic image (0.5 × 0.5 mm) revealing small aggregates of cells can be both dense or dense and sparse, with different grades of brightness (→). The junctional clusters surround nonedged papillae (*) and can be suspicious for malignancy, especially when associated to other suggestive confocal features. The absence of pagetoid infiltration and of architectural atypia at the DEJ leads to a diagnosis of benign nevus

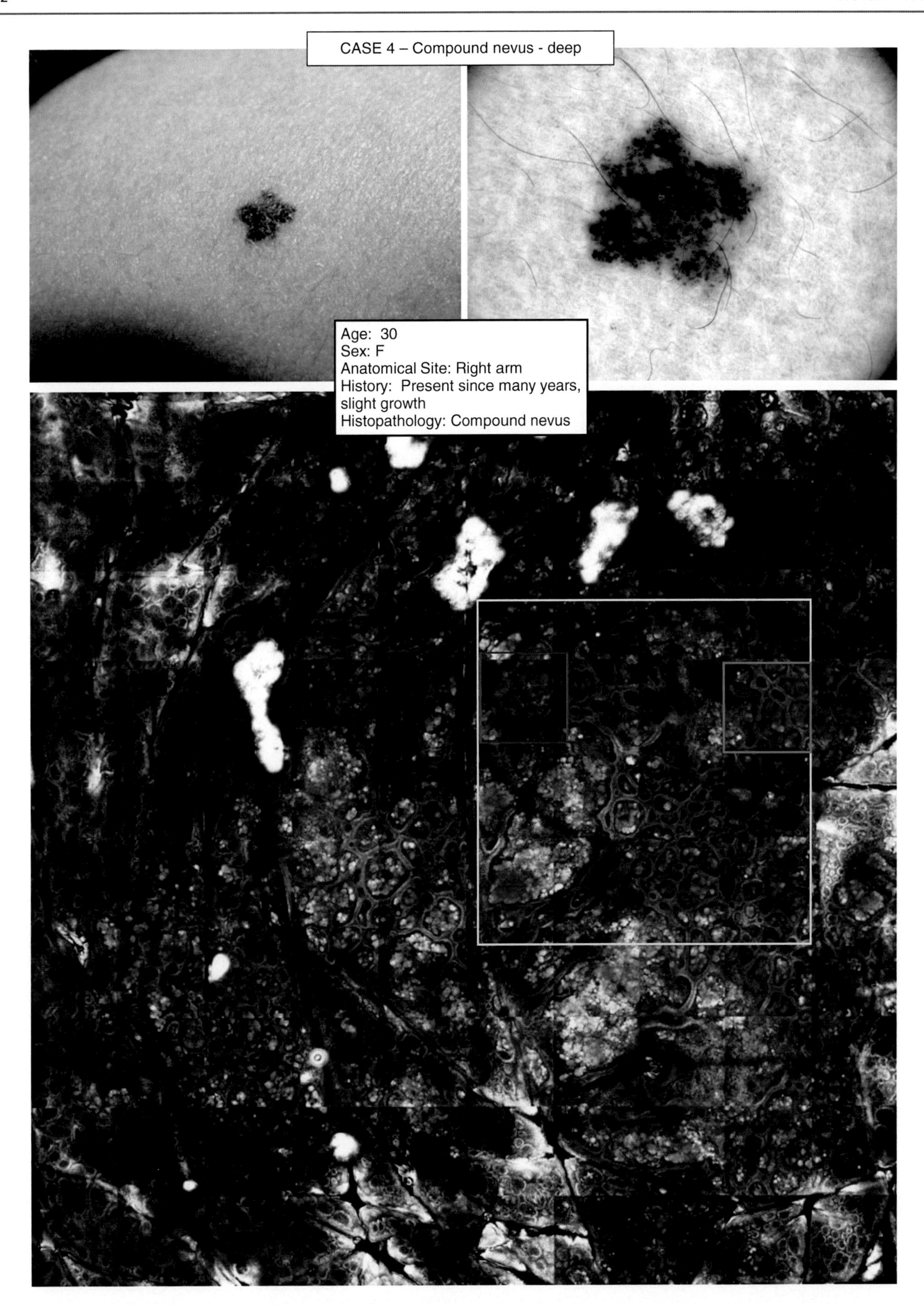

Fig. 8.4 RCM mosaic (5 × 5 mm) shows the most significant features at the level of dermal-epidermal junction/upper dermis; within regular, edged papillae, dense and sparse nests are visible, giving rise to a clod pattern associated to a ringed one. The overall appearance is of a very regular nevus with expanding nests within the papillary dermis

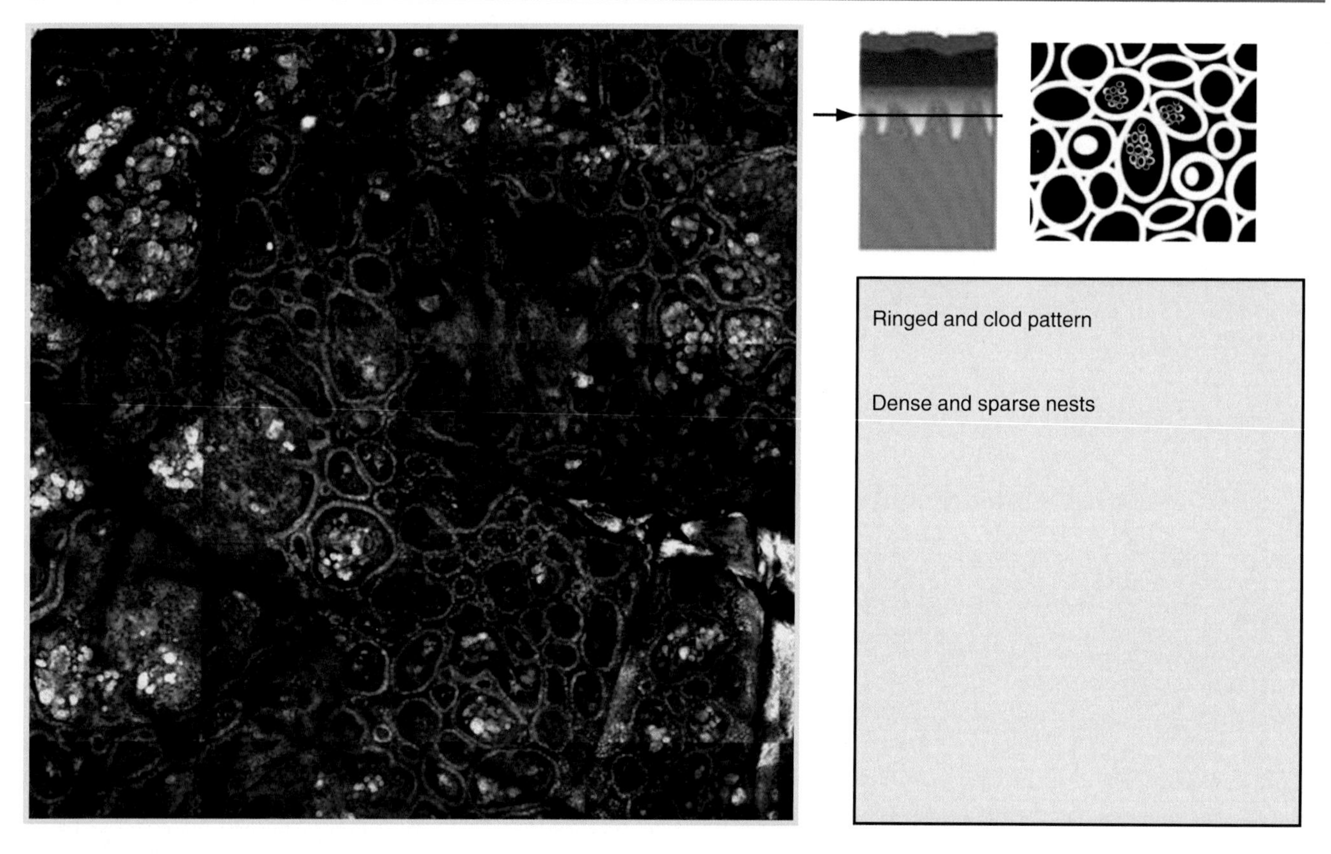

Fig. 8.4.1 RCM mosaic (2 × 2 mm) reveals a mixed pattern (ringed and clod) with dense and sparse nests within regular, edged papillae. The structure of the nests is composed by cells with variable grades of brightness, depending on a different amount of melanin in the melanocytes and to their level of depth in the dermis

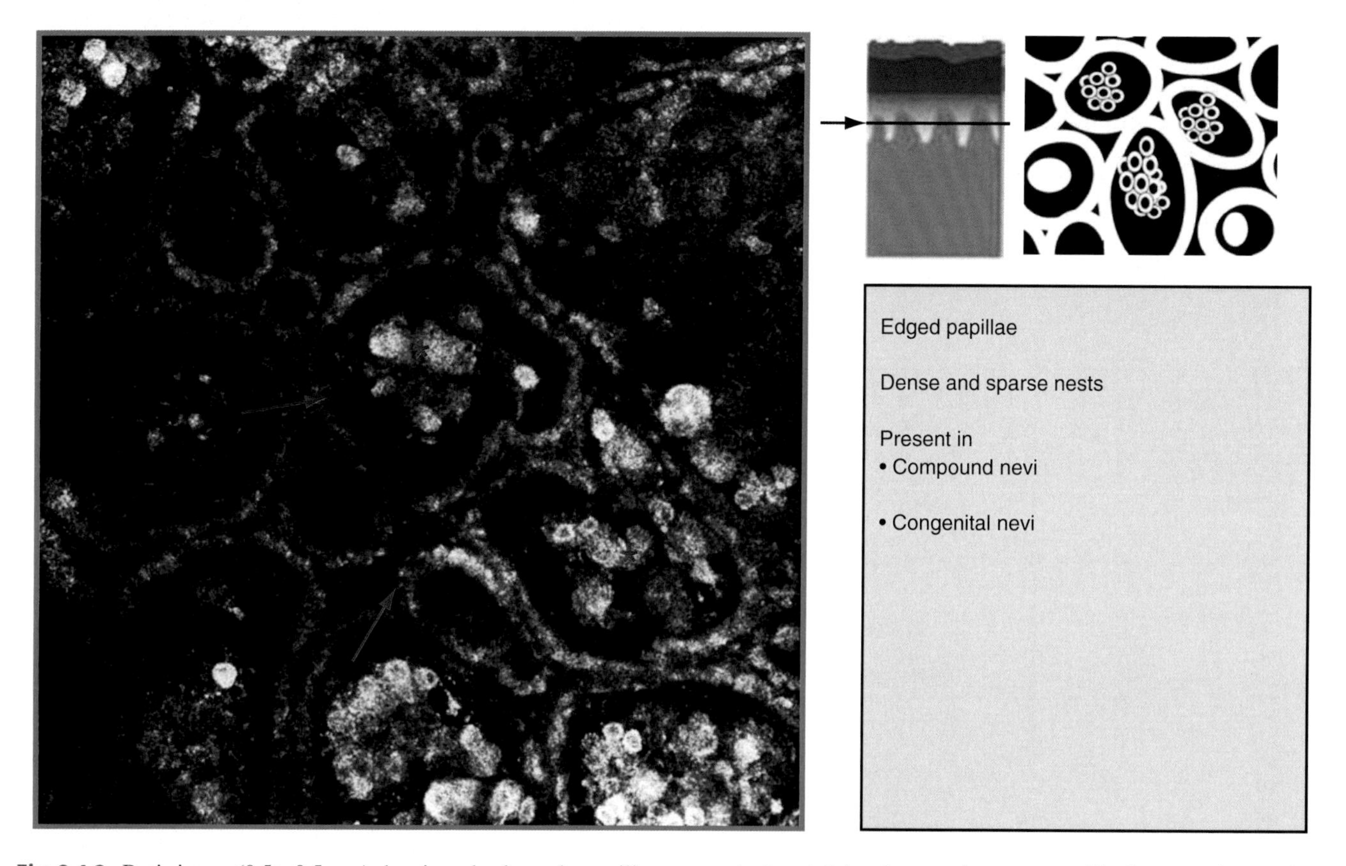

Fig. 8.4.2 Basic image (0.5 × 0.5 mm) showing edged, regular papillary spaces (→) containing dense and sparse nests (*): these are characterized by partially dischoese cells, some brighter than the others

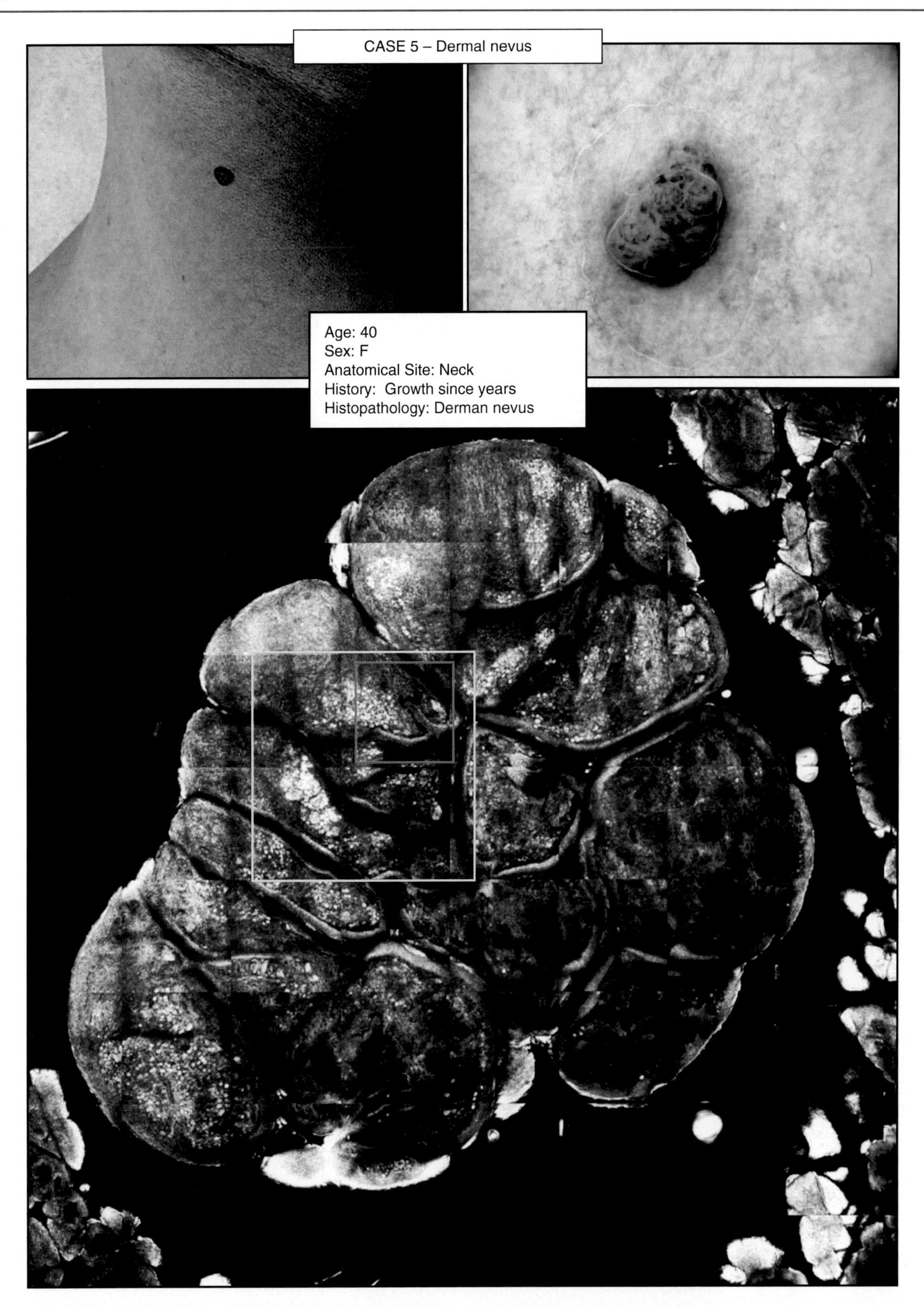

Fig. 8.5 RCM mosaic (4 × 4 mm) taken at the dermal–epidermal junction/upper dermis showing a papillomatous architecture, with fissures among the large nevus nests. The clod pattern is characteristic, with many bright cells visible throughout the all lesion. No atypical cells are seen, then the lesion is immediately classified as benign

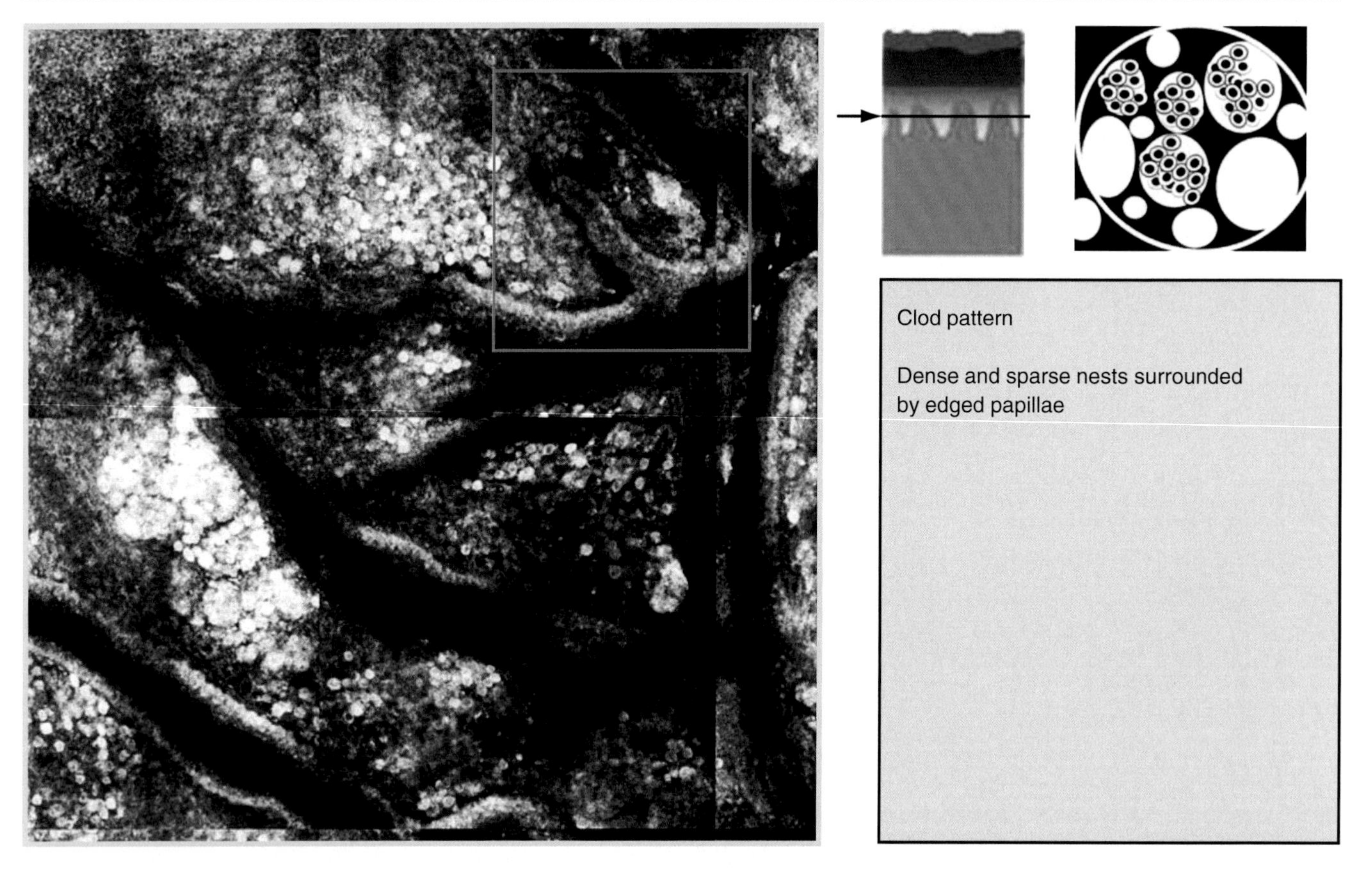

Fig. 8.5.1 RCM mosaic (2 × 2 mm) showing large, dense and sparse nests embedded in edged regular papillae; the nests are separated by a deep invagination, corresponding to the papillomatous profile of the dermal nevus

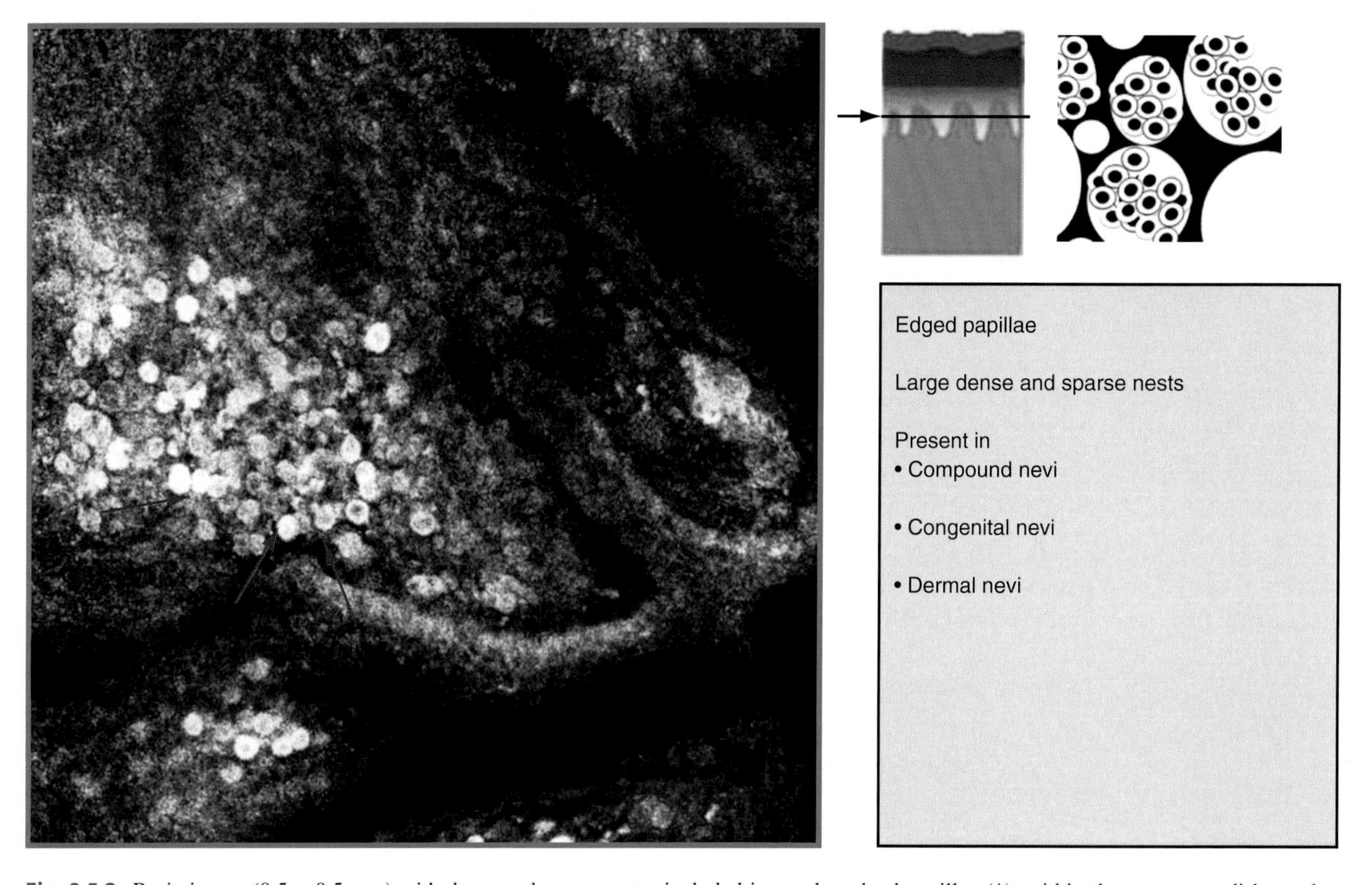

Fig. 8.5.2 Basic image (0.5 × 0.5 mm) with dense and sparse nests, included in regular edged papillae (*); within the nests, roundish regular homogeneous cells are visible, with different degrees of brightness between each others (→)

Core Messages

- Common nevi are characterized by regular architecture and absence of atypia, making their diagnosis easy with RCM.
- Junctional component is usually characterized by ringed pattern, mostly in case of lentiginous proliferation, and by meshwork pattern correlated with junctional nests.
- Dermal component is usually constituted by dense nests in case of superficial dermis involvement and by large dense & sparse nests with monomorphous melanocytes in case of deep dermal involvement.

References

1. Pellacani G, Longo C, Malvehy J et al (2008) In vivo confocal microscopic and histopathologic correlations of dermoscopic features in 202 melanocytic lesions. Arch Dermatol 144:1597–1608
2. Ahlgrimm-Siess V, Massone C, Koller S, Fink-Puches R, Richtig E, Wolf I et al (2008) In vivo confocal scanning laser microscopy of common naevi with globular, homogeneous and reticular pattern in dermoscopy. Br J Dermatol 158:1000–1007
3. Pellacani G, Scope A, Ferrari B et al (2009) New insights into nevogenesis: in vivo characterization and follow-up of melanocytic nevi by reflectance confocal microscopy. J Am Acad Dermatol 61:1001–1013

9 Atypical/Dysplastic Nevi

Giovanni Pellacani, Francesca Farnetani,
Giuseppe Argenziano, Iris Zalaudek,
Caterina Longo, and Melissa Gill

Atypical nevi, also referred as dysplastic nevi, are characterized by intermediate aspects in between to common nevi and melanomas. From a clinical point of view, they usually show up as larger and more irregular and nonhomogeneously pigmented lesions than common nevi. In dermatopathology, they are classically characterized by lentiginous melanocytic hyperplasia, epithelioid melanocytic atypia, lamellar fibroplasias and perivascular lymphocytic infiltrate [1]. From these observations a pathogenetic model for stepwise development of a MM from a nevus has been proposed. However, this model remains controversial due to nonclear and reproducible clinical definition of dysplastic nevus, limitations in recognition of early melanoma and dysplastic nevus, and weak correlation between histologic dysplasia and clinical atypia [2].

In order to make dysplasia grading more objective and reproducible, a scoring system was proposed and validated by Shea and coworkers [3]. Shea's grading takes into account the evaluation of selected architectural and cytological parameters that have to be binary evaluated as present or absent, each parameter scoring 1 point. Concerning the architectural disorders, six parameters are considered: junctional component nested at both edges, good overall symmetry, more than 50% of nests cohesive, absent or focal single-cell proliferation were negative parameters, scored 1 point in case of "absence", and prominent or at edge suprabasal spread, confluence of over the 50% of the proliferation were "positive" parameters, scored 1 point in case of "presence". A total score ranging between 0 and 1 corresponds to absent/mild architectural dysplasia; between 2 and 3 to moderate one; between 4 and 6 to severe one. As regards cytologic atypia, four parameters are considered: round or oval, and euchromatic nuclei was a negative parameter (scored 1 point in case of "absence"), whereas nuclei larger in size than basal keratinocytic nuclei, prominent nucleoli, melanocytic cell diameter over the twice of basal keratinocyte nucleus were positive features, scored 1 point in case of "presence". A total score ranging between 0 and 1 corresponds to absent/mild cytological dysplasia; 2 to moderate one; between 3 and 4 to severe one.

In vivo reflectance confocal microscopy (RCM) opens a new window in the diagnosis and definition of skin tumors. Its cellular-level resolution and horizontal sectioning resulted in excellent correlation with histopathology and dermoscopy as well. The possibility to identify specific RCM correlates for histopathologic features characterizing dysplastic nevi and to obtain a reliable in vivo grading of melanocytic dysplasia has relevant implications for clinical practice [4]. In fact, this could permit to better identify which lesion has to be necessarily excised because of the presence of equivocal histopathologic features, saving unnecessary surgery.

9.1 Correlation Between Shea's Grading Features and RCM Parameters

9.1.1 Architecture

Junctional component nested at both edges, good overall symmetry, and suprabasal spread prominent or present at edge were directly correlated with the rim of peripheral nests, architectural symmetry, widespread roundish pagetoid

G. Pellacani (✉) • F. Farnetani
Department of Dermatology and Venereology,
University of Modena and Reggio Emilia, Modena, Italy
e-mail: pellacani.giovanni@unimore.it

G. Argenziano • I. Zalaudek
Department of Dermatology, Arcispedale S Maria Nuova,
Reggio Emilia, Italy

C. Longo
Department of Dermatology, Arcispedale S Maria Nuova,
Reggio Emilia, Italy

M. Gill
Skin Medical Research and Diagnostics, P.L.L.C,
New York, NY, USA

R. Hofmann-Wellenhof et al. (eds.), *Reflectance Confocal Microscopy for Skin Diseases*,
DOI 10.1007/978-3-642-21997-9_9, © Springer-Verlag Berlin Heidelberg 2012

cells at RCM, respectively, and more than 50% of nests cohesive inversely correlated with junctional nests with cell dishomogeneity. Confluence of over the 50% of the proliferation was correlated with junctional nests irregular in size and shape, as well as absent or focal single-cell proliferation was inversely correlated with a diffused ringed architecture. Grading of architectural dysplasia according with Shea resulted highly correlated with the one obtained combining correlated RCM descriptors.

9.1.2 Cytology

Concerning cytologic atypia parameters, all but presence of prominent nucleoli were correlated with presence of atypical cells at RCM. In fact, in confocal microscopy the nucleus is a dark, nonreflecting area within the cell, and chromatin or nucleolus cannot be detected in it. Moreover, the size of nuclei is not easy to be quantified, since it depends on the sectioning level and the contrast given by the surrounding cytoplasm, obtaining a clear nucleus outline only in cells with stark bright and abundant cytoplasm. Overall cytological atypia grading was correlated with RCM atypia grading.

9.2 Confocal Aspects of Dysplastic Nevi

As well as in clinical, dermoscopy and histopathologic evaluation, atypical/dysplastic nevi show intermediate features between common (non-dysplastic) nevi and melanomas [4]. Different degrees of atypia can be detected.

9.2.1 Mild Atypical/Dysplastic Nevi

These lesions are usually characterized by a ringed architecture, corresponding to a lentiginous proliferation, in some cases widespread throughout the lesion, in other cases present only at the periphery, usually combined with a central meshwork architecture. Presence of clods and areas with nonspecific architecture is rare and presenting a limited extent. General symmetry of the architecture is preserved in the majority of cases, whereas the border contours are usually poorly defined, due to the frequent presence of a ringed pattern shading off at the periphery of the lesion, strongly correlating with the shouldering phenomenon in histopathology.

Few sporadic pagetoid cells could be detected in a third of cases, usually located in the center of the lesion, within a regular or slightly irregular epidermal architecture.

Papillae contour are mostly edged, and when non-edged papillae are observable, they rarely extend over the 10% of the lesion surface.

The identification of some large nucleated cells at DEJ is quiet common, although this population is usually characterized by few mono-morphic polygonal to roundish cells, resulting in a mild limited cell atypia upon confocal examination, and typically located in the center of the lesion.

Junctional nests are almost constantly present. They are usually compact dense aggregates, with no or few large cells detectable within. Sometimes they present an elongated shape or short interconnection, corresponding to nest fusion and bridging at histopathology. Dermal nests are rarely present and usually correspond to few dense compact aggregates.

Stroma reaction, corresponding to inflammatory infiltrates constituted by bright particles and plump bright cells and by coarse collagen fibers, is clearly detectable in less than the half of cases. Figure 9.1 presents the typical confocal features of a mild dysplastic nevus.

9.2.2 Moderate to Severe Atypical/Dysplastic Nevi

Moderately and severely dysplastic nevi show asymmetry with similar frequency as melanomas. Concerning the general pattern, moderate to severe dysplastic nevi frequently are characterized by a ringed pattern, mostly at the periphery, in association with a meshwork pattern, usually located in the center of the lesion, in a large proportion of cases. Clods are present in few cases. A non-specific pattern, present in one-third of this population, is more frequently observed in severely dysplastic nevi.

Concerning the epidermis, almost half of the lesions showed an irregular pattern, but with honeycombed or cobblestone architecture detectable in almost all cases. Moderate to severe dysplastic nevi displayed large nucleated cells in a pagetoid fashion in less than half of the cases, with a predominance of roundish cells and with an ascending trend from moderate to severe dysplastic nevi.

At the dermal–epidermal junction, papillae are clearly detectable in almost all cases, the majority showing clearly outlined contours (edged papillae), but some cases presenting also a significant extent of papillae with poorly outlined contours (non-edged papillae). Atypical junctional cells are frequently observed, mostly characterized by roundish cells. Only a small proportion of cases, almost all corresponding to severe dysplastic nevi, is characterized by a striking cytological pleomorphism, showing both roundish and dendritic cells. Anyway, characteristic for dysplastic nevus is the concentration of the atypical cells in the center of the lesion.

Almost all cases show junctional nests. They are frequently irregular in size and shape, and with short interconnections. Nest constituted by non-homogeneous cellularity are present in almost all the severe dysplastic nevi and in less than half of the moderate dysplastic ones.

Dermal nests, present in over half of the cases, are predominantly dense and compact and usually extended over less than 10% of the lesion area.

Within the papillary dermis, coarse reticulated collagen fibers and plump bright cells and/or bright particles, corresponding to an inflammatory infiltrate, are clearly visible in approximately half of the cases. Figure 9.2 corresponds to a moderate dysplastic nevus, whereas Fig. 9.3 presents a severe dysplastic nevus.

To sum up, a good correspondence between histopathologic and confocal dysplasia is detectable. Different degrees can be estimated in confocal microscopy, mostly basing on the extent and the pleomorphism of atypical cells, and the extent and cell dishomogeneity of irregular in size and shape junctional nests, frequently showing an elongated shape and/or short interconnection. Dysplastic nevi frequently display a prominent inflammatory infiltrate. Sometimes it is also possible to observe collagen alteration, resulting in coarse collagen boundles forming a gross network-like structure, although characteristic aspects correlated with the different type of histologic fibroplasias are not discernable.

Applying diagnostic confocal algorithms for melanocytic lesions, these lesions frequently result in a high scoring. So, for diagnostic purposes, the location of cytological and architectural atypia in the center of the lesion, and the absence of a striking cell pleomorphism have to be considered as characteristic for mild to moderate dysplastic nevi. On the other hand, severe dysplastic nevi usually present extensive disarrangement of the architecture, with marked and abundant cytological atypia that make these lesions almost undistinguishable from melanoma.

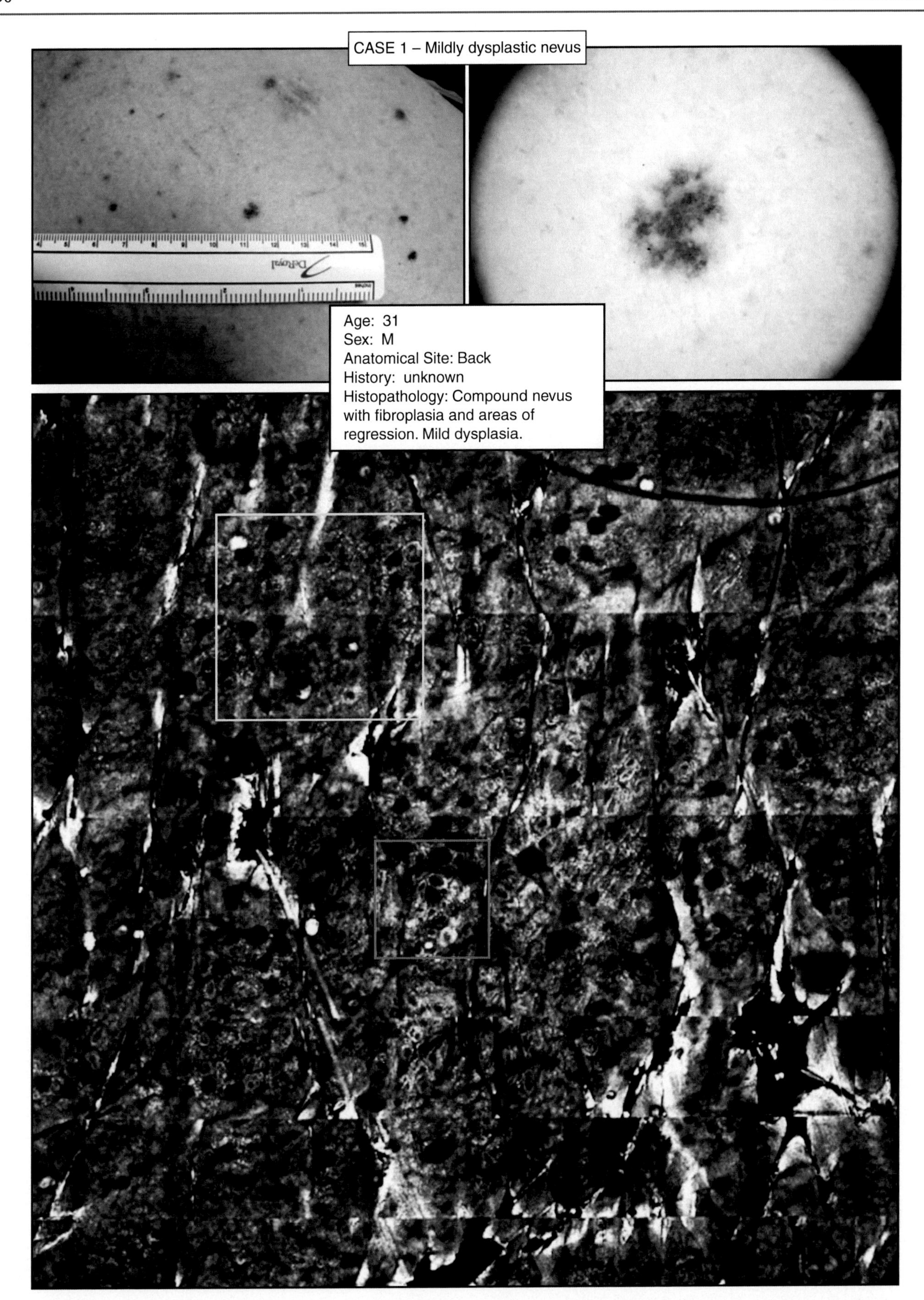

Fig. 9.1 RCM mosaic (4 × 4 mm) acquired at the suprabasal/epidermal–junctional level, showing a ringed and meshwork pattern in a slightly asymmetrical overall architecture. Also milia-like cysts and comedo-like openings are visible throughout the lesion, whereas atypical cells are lacking. The ringed and meshwork pattern fade off at the border of the lesion

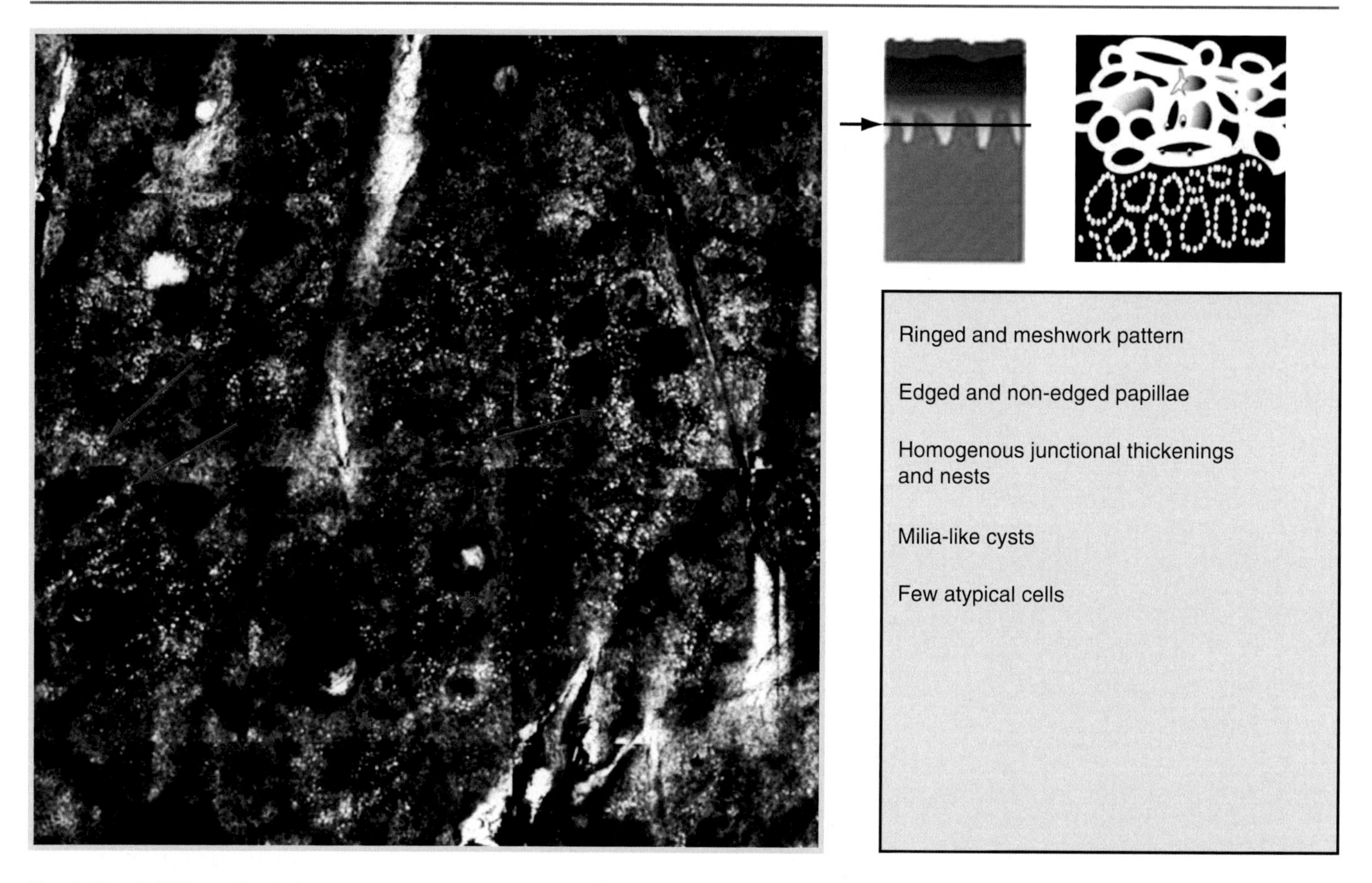

Fig. 9.1.1 RCM mosaic (1.5 × 1.5 mm) with bright and small cells, surrounding nonedged papillae and forming homogeneous junctional thickenings and nests. Some atypical cells are focally present around the papillae (→). The bright homogeneous structures surrounded by a round dark halo correspond to a milia-like cysts (*)

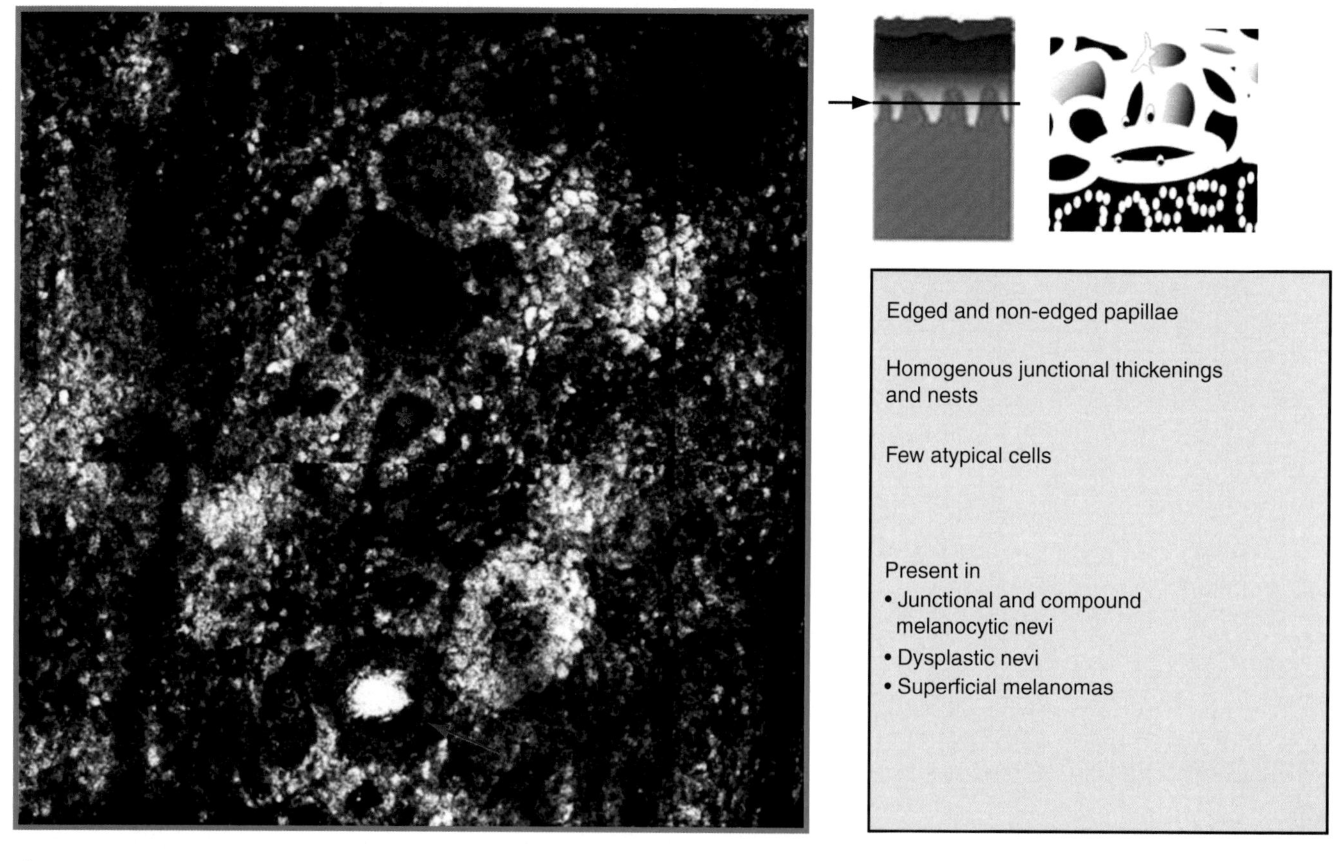

Fig. 9.1.2 Basic image (0.5 × 0.5 mm) showing mostly edged papillae (*). *Arrow* shows the milia-like cyst aspect (→)

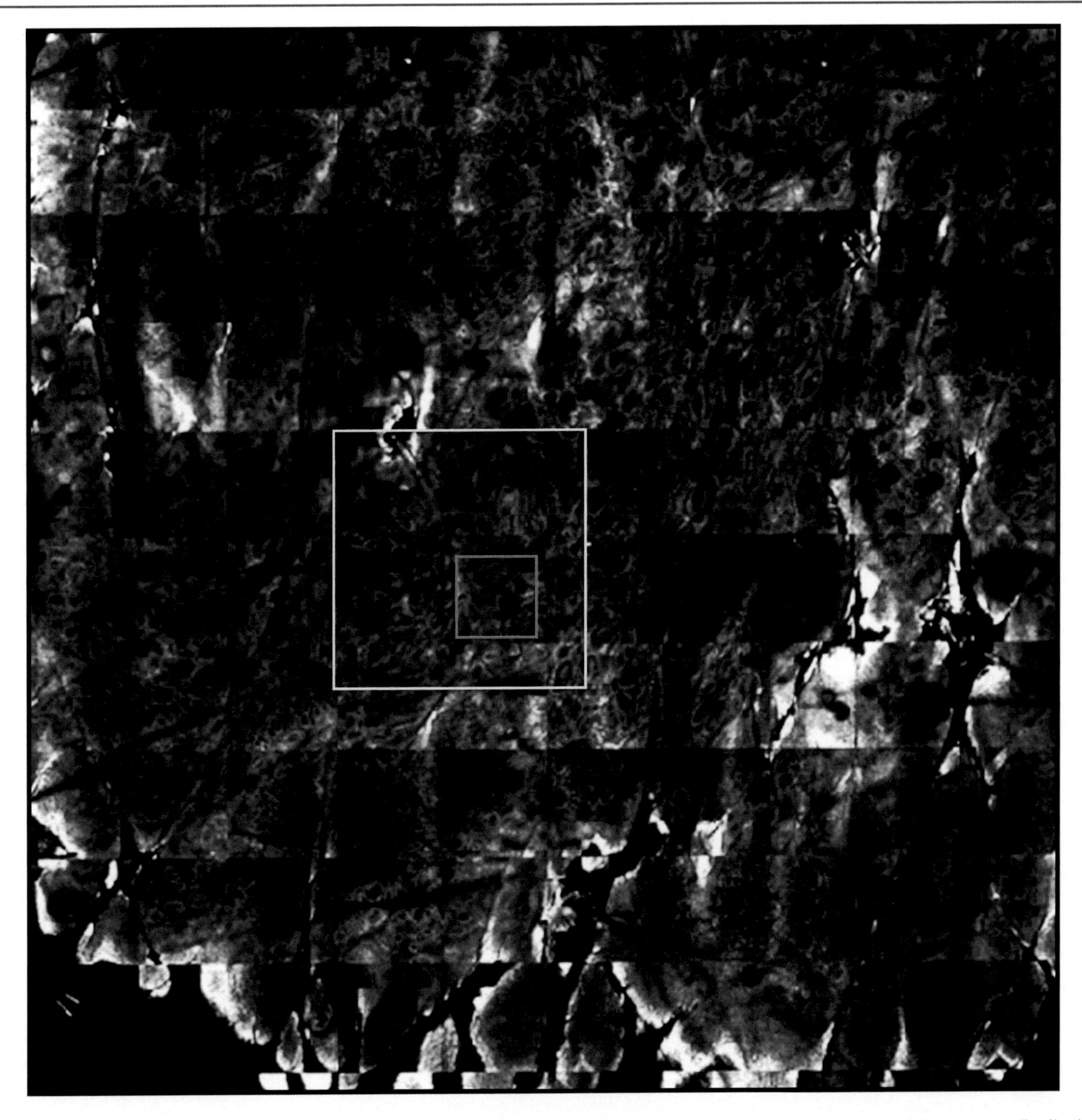

Fig. 9.1.3 RCM mosaic (4 × 4 mm) acquired at junctional level, showing a meshwork pattern. The picture displays a slightly uneven distribution of the meshes. Some rings are visible mostly at the periphery. Lesion contours are not clearly detectable

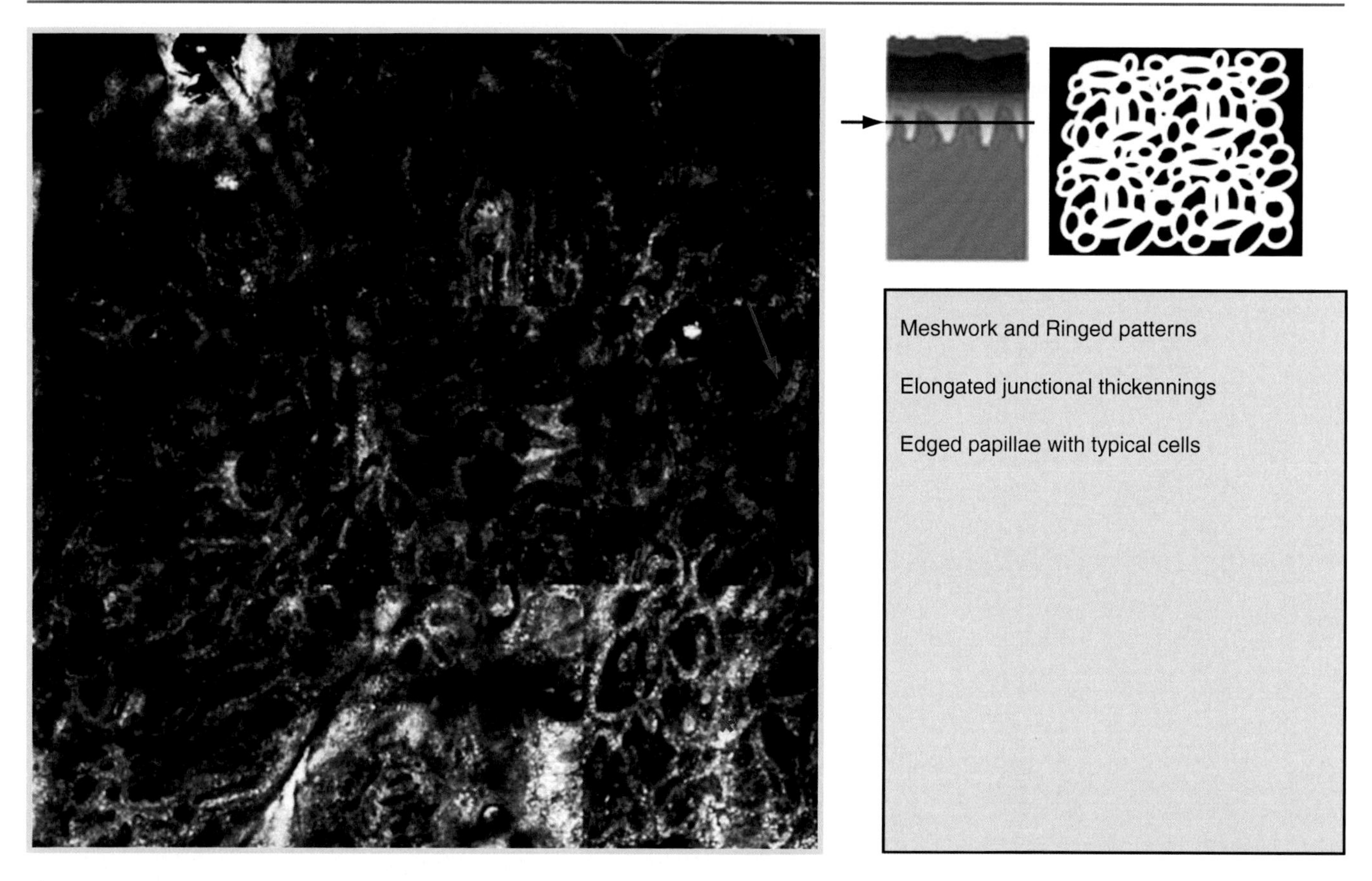

Fig. 9.1.4 RCM mosaic (1.5 × 1.5 mm) shows details of the architecture. Junctional clusters enlarging interpapillary spaces are visible. Some junctional thickenings are elongated (→). Papillae have irregular shapes but they are surrounded by rings of small polygonal bright cells

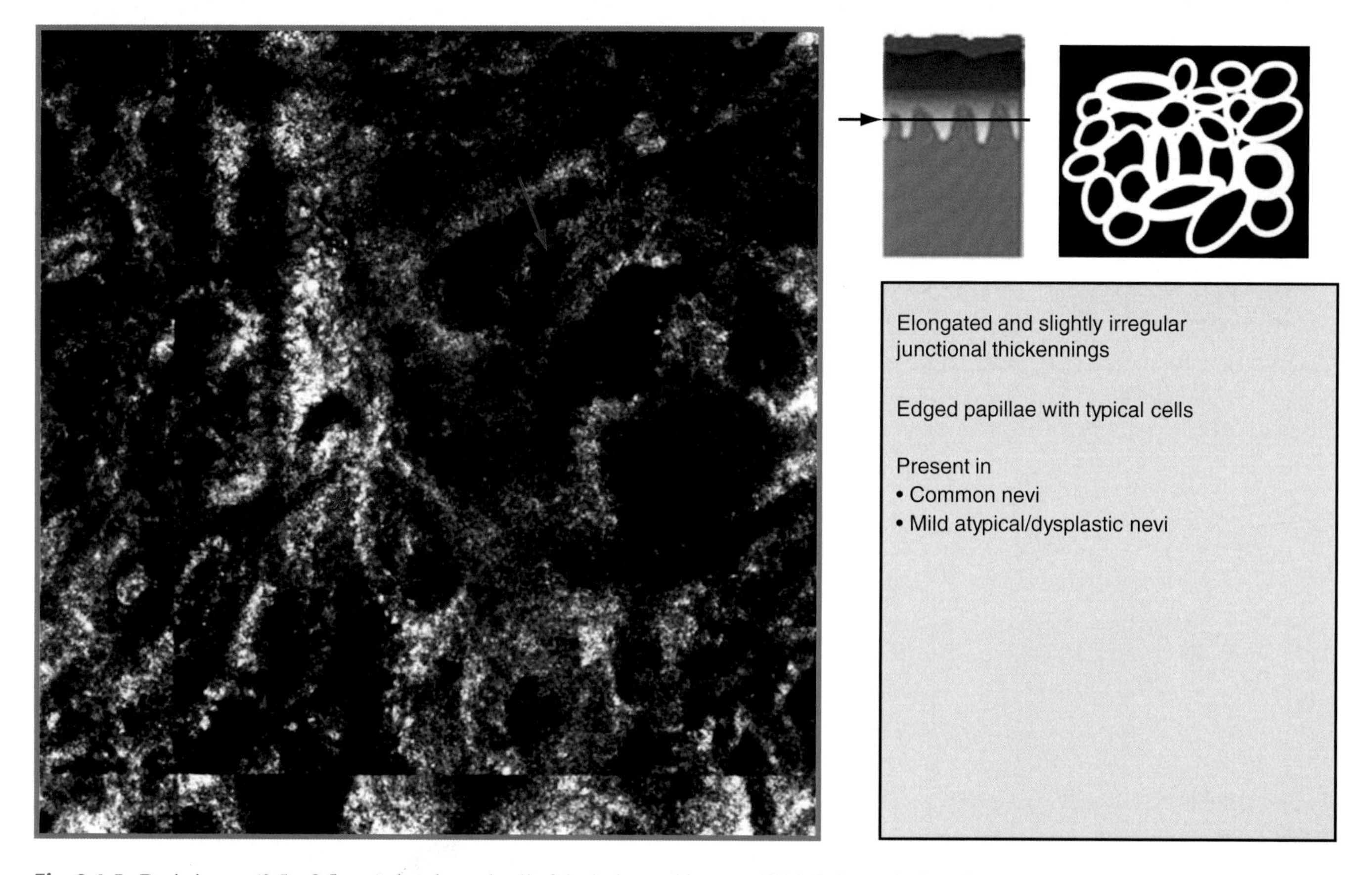

Fig. 9.1.5 Basic image (0.5 × 0.5 mm) showing a detail of the lesion architecture. Slightly irregular junctional thickenings (→) and rings of typical small cells are present (*). No atypical cells are visible

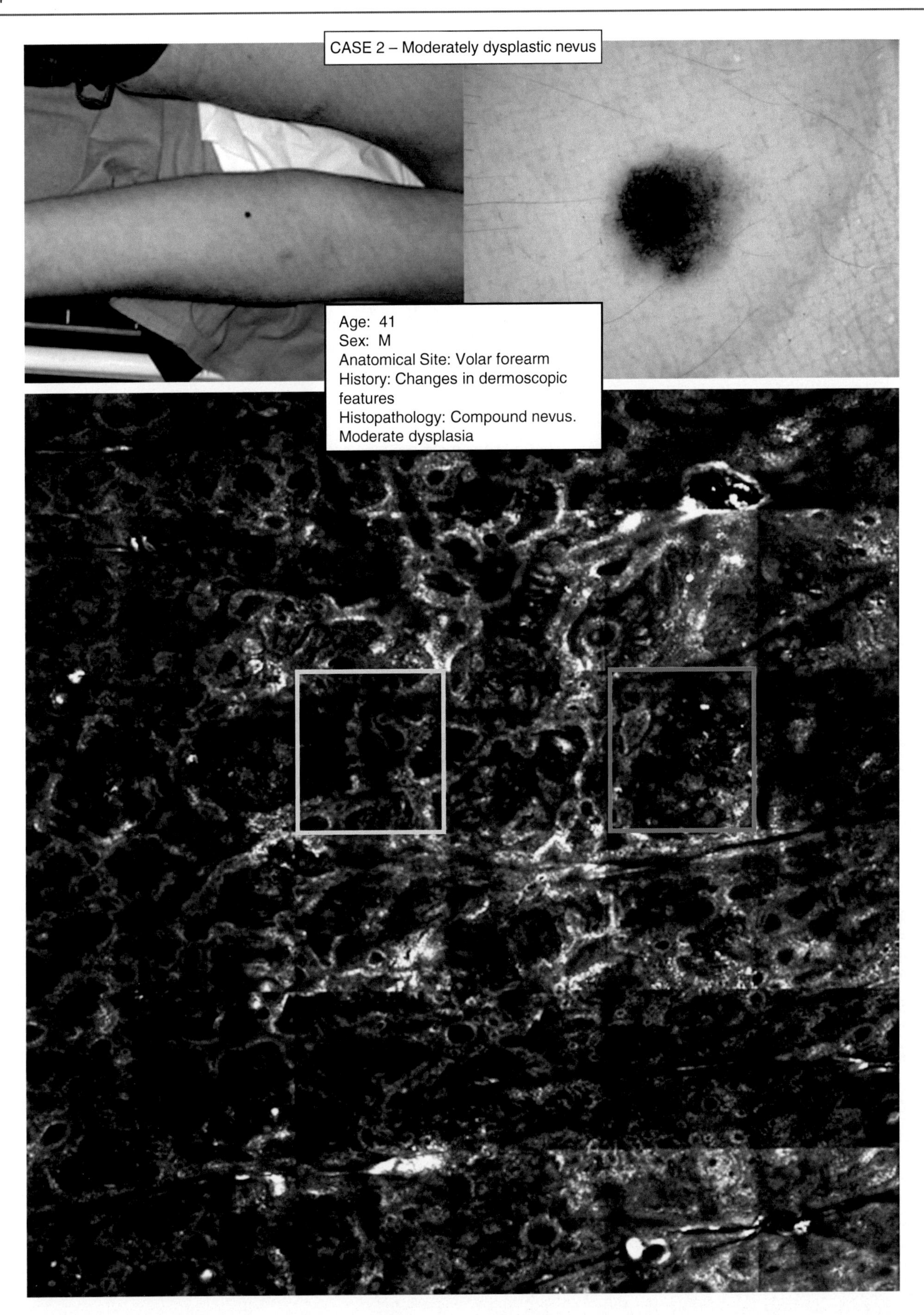

Fig. 9.2 RCM mosaic (4 × 4 mm) depicts the global architecture of the lesion, with meshwork pattern and a Evident asymmetry. The thickenings and junctional nests are dishomogeneous for brightness and distribution, and show numerous roundish atypical cells in the junctional layer, mostly located in the center of the lesion. The holes within the meshes are strongly different to each others in size and shape. The structural disorder is mostly concentrated in the center of the lesions. The borders are quiet detectable though they are blurring off

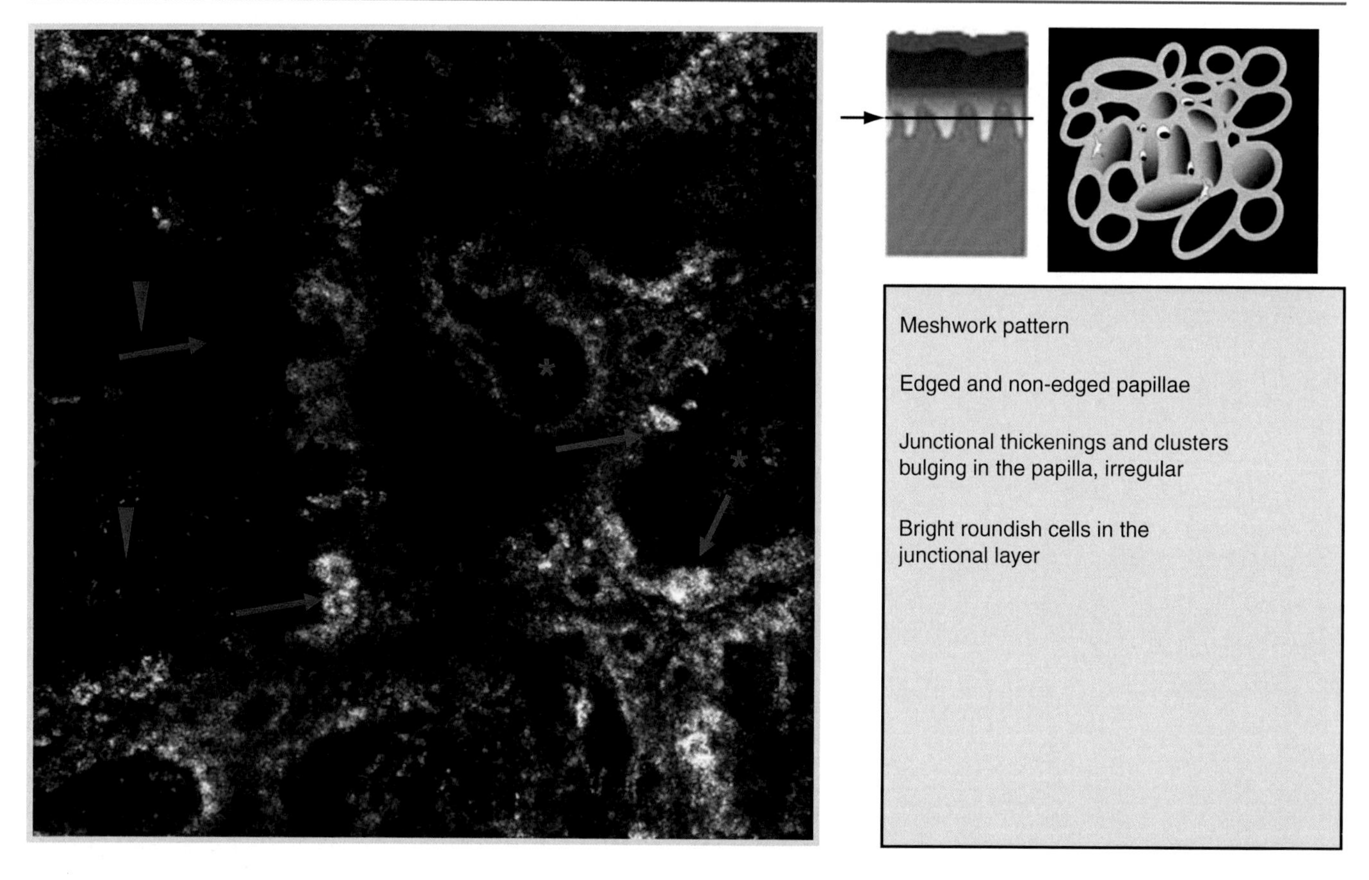

Fig. 9.2.1 Basic image (0.5 × 0.5 mm) with edged (*) and non-edged papillae (▲), different in size and shape. Irregular junctional thickenings and nests, with atypical cells visible inside, are present (→)

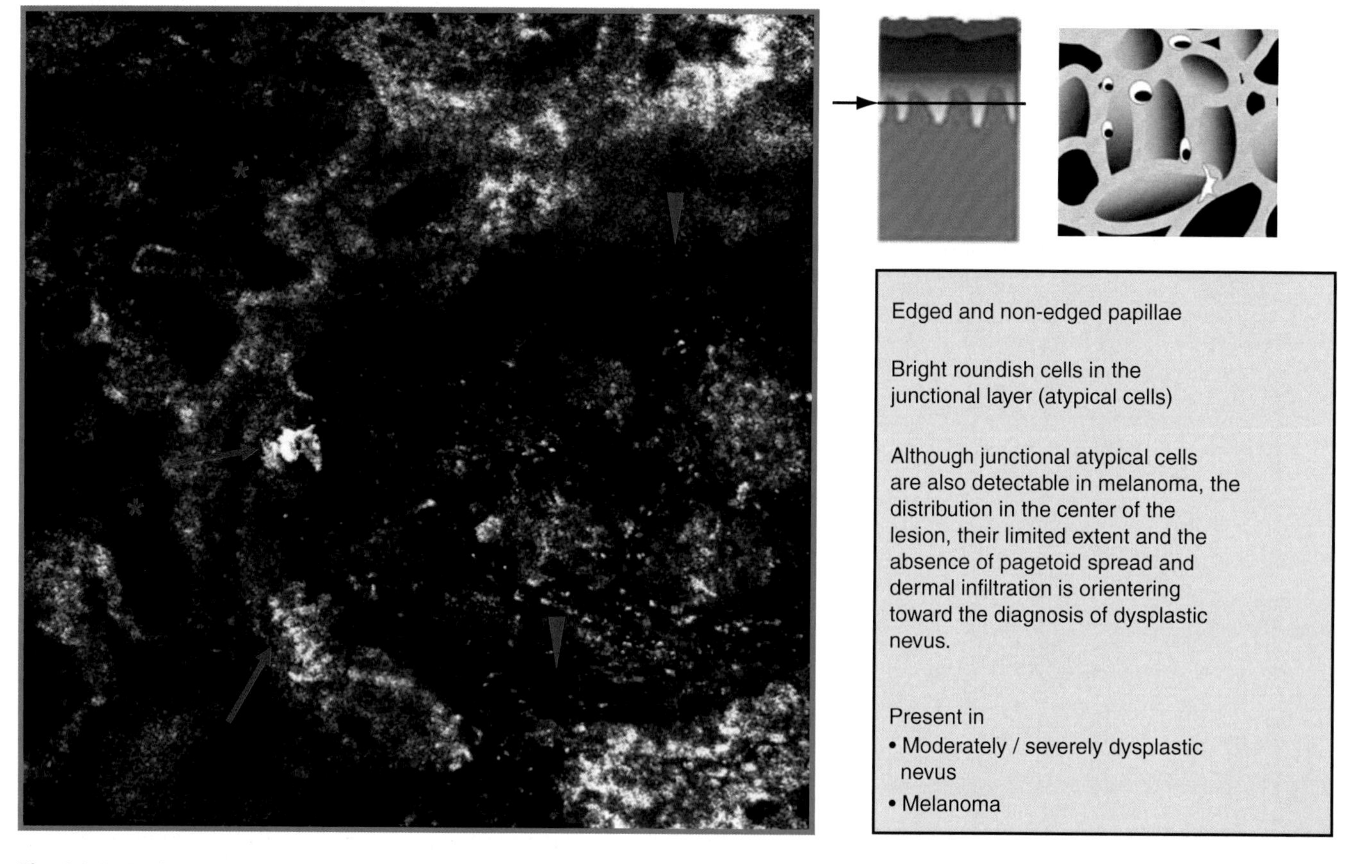

Fig. 9.2.2 Basic image (0.5 × 0.5 mm) with edged papillae (*) and non-edged papillae (▲). Large bright nucleated cells, corresponding to atypical melanocytes are clearly detectable in the junctional layer (→). The cyto-architectural features of atypia are suggestive of a dysplastic lesion

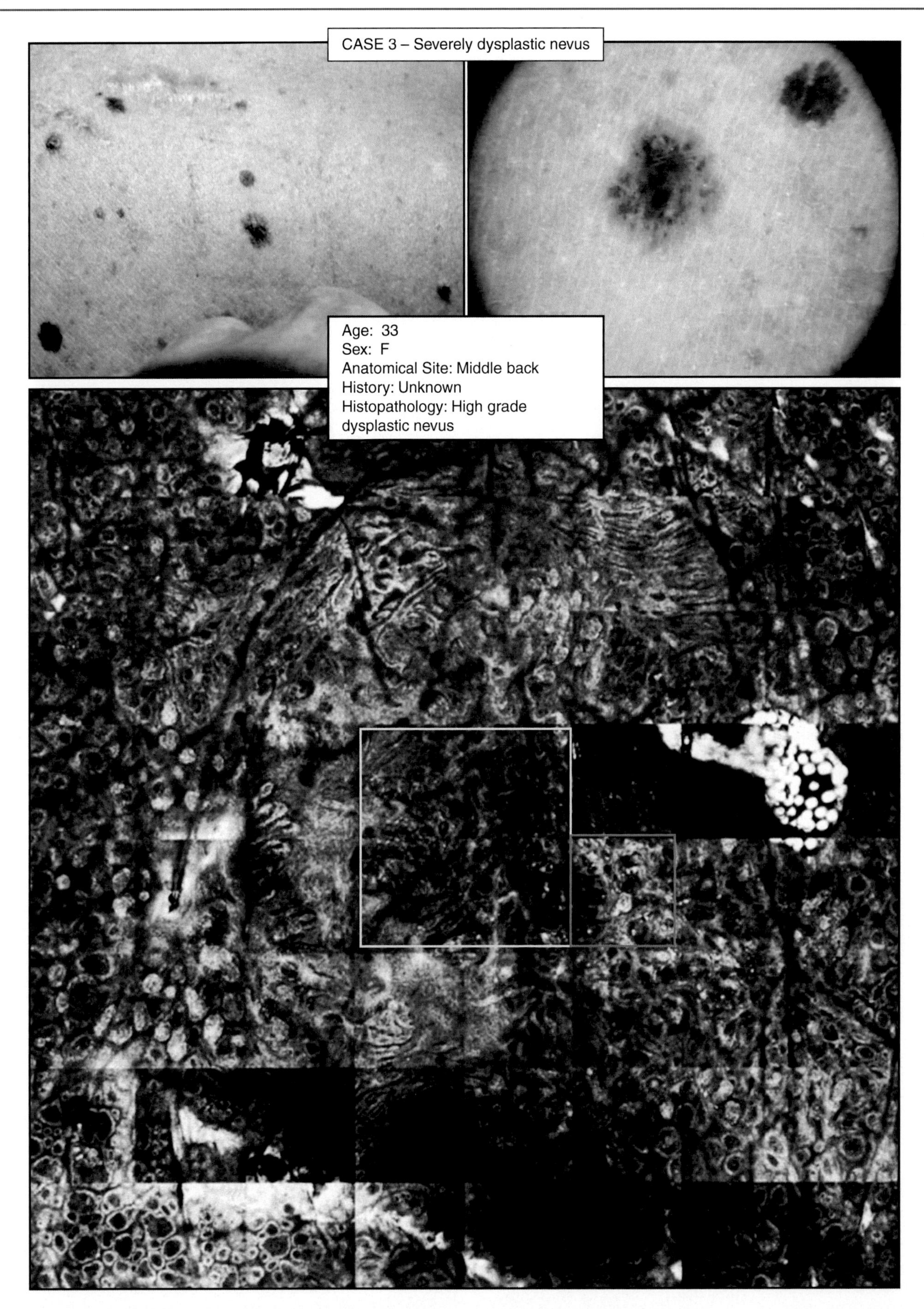

Fig. 9.3 RCM mosaic (4 × 4 mm) of a very asymmetrical lesion, with a mixed pattern (meshwork, ringed and clod). In the center of the lesion, a dishomogeneous meshwork pattern is present, with junctional nests, irregular in size and shape. At the periphery, there are junctional and dermal nests (clods), dense and sparse, and a ringed structures shading off at the periphery, corresponding to the so-called "shoulder phenomenon". In a portion of the lesion, a nonspecific pattern is visible

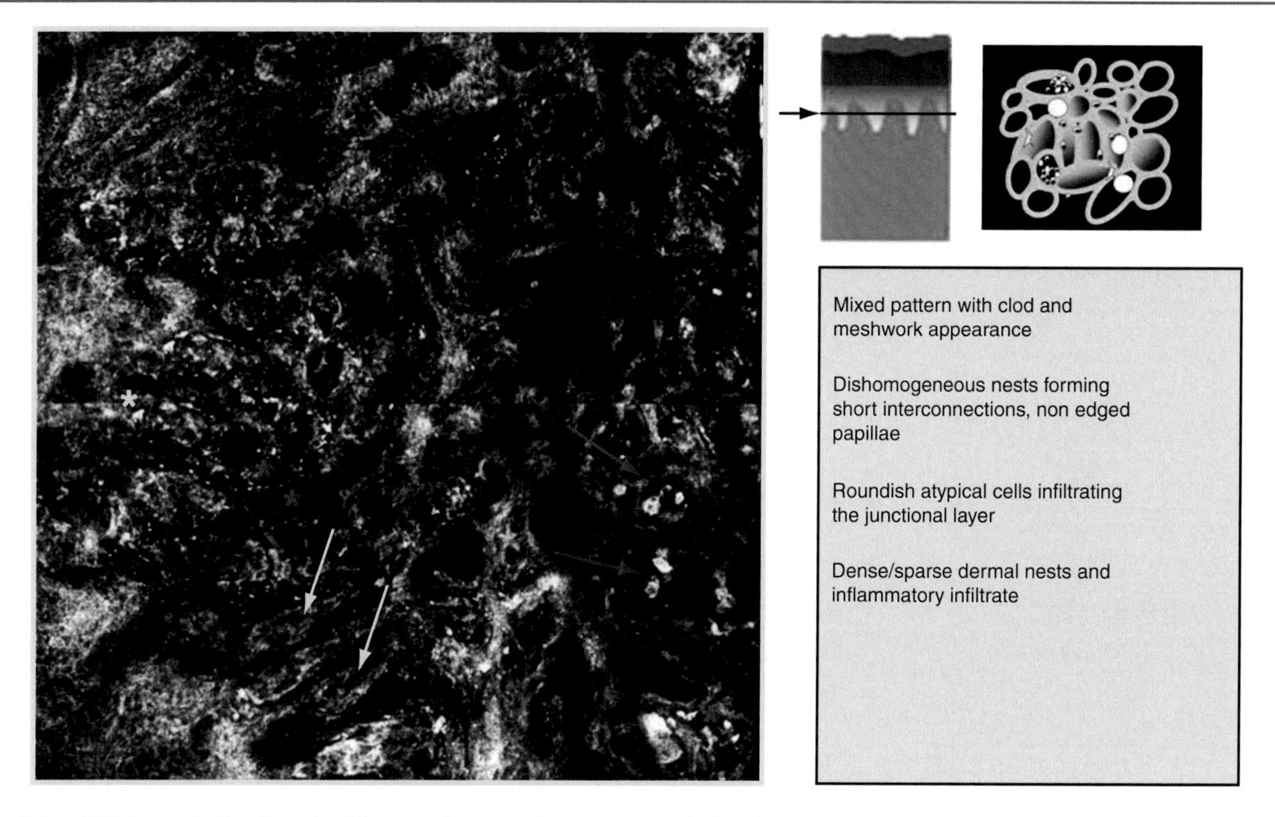

Fig. 9.3.1 RCM mosaic (1 × 1 mm) of the central area of the nevus shows nonedged papillae, irregular and dishomogeneous junctional nests, with short interconnections (*yellow* →), numerous roundish and bright atypical cells infiltrating the junctional layer (*yellow* *), in proximity of the nonspecific pattern area (*upper left corner*). In this section, the upper dermis is also visible, showing sparse nests and inflammatory cells (*red* →) including both melanophages and small bright spots (*red* *)

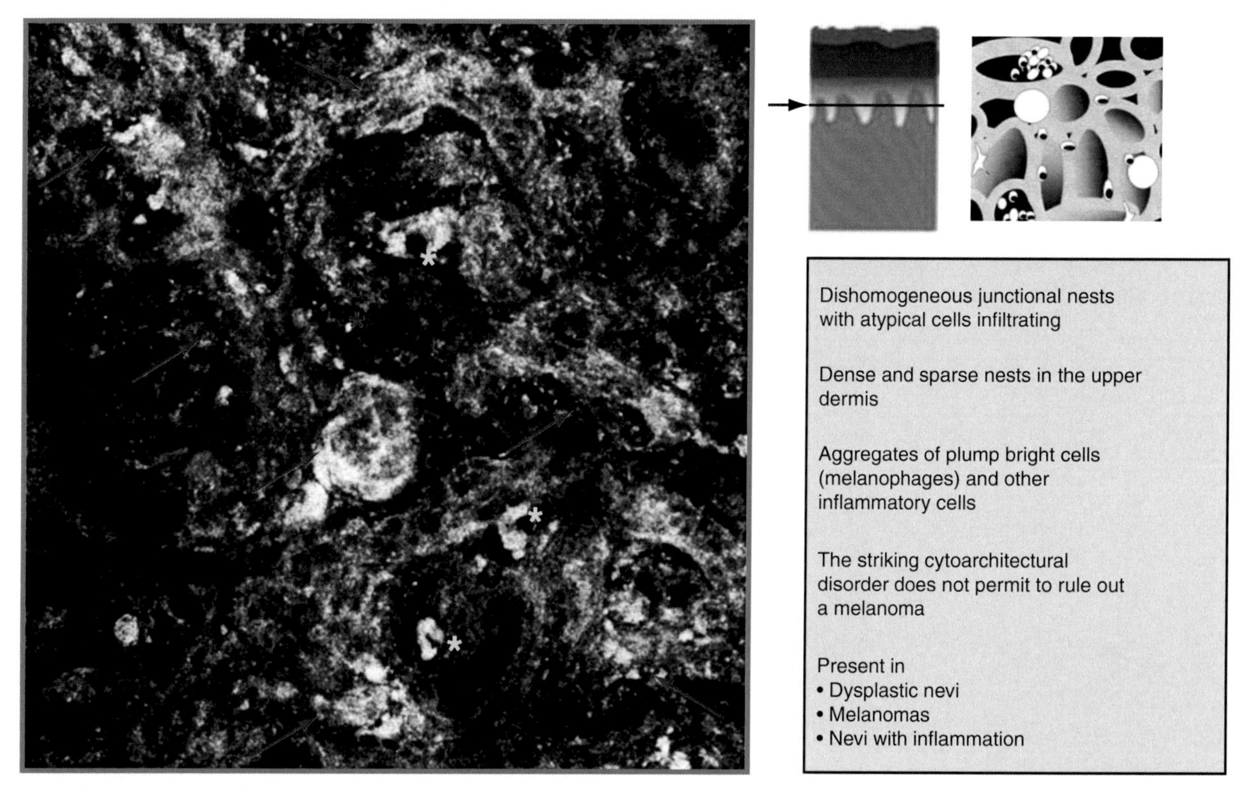

Fig. 9.3.2 Basic image (0.5 × 0.5 mm) of a central area of the nevus showing dishomogeneous and irregular junctional thickenings and nests surrounding nonedged papillae (*red* → and *). Within dermal papillae dense and dense & sparse nests are seen (*red* *), mixed with inflammatory infiltrate, including plump bright cells (*yellow* *) and small bright spots. Numerous atypical cells are detectable at the DEJ, in single cells or aggregated in nests

Core Messages

- Good correlation between confocal features and histologic criteria for dysplastic nevus characterization and grading is achieved.
- In RCM, dysplastic nevi are frequently characterized by a meshwork architecture, usually showing irregular, elongated and/or interconnected meshes, and by the presence of few atypical cells mostly located in the center of the lesion. Pagetoid spread is absent or very limited in its extent.
- Atypical/dysplastic nevi share some features with melanoma, making their differential diagnosis not easy. RCM enables to confidently detect the majority of mild to moderate dysplastic nevi, whereas in case of severe dysplasia a melanoma cannot be ruled out.

References

1. Clark WH Jr, Reimer RR, Greene M, Ainsworth AM, Mastrangelo MJ (1978) Origin of familial malignant melanomas from heritable melanocytic lesions. The B-K mole syndrome. Arch Dermatol 114:732–738
2. Ackerman AB (1988) What nevus is dysplastic, a syndrome and the commonest precursor of malignant melanoma? A riddle and an answer. Histopathology 13:241–256
3. Shea CR, Vollmer RT, Prieto VG (1999) Correlating architectural disorder and cytologic atypia in Clark (dysplastic) melanocytic nevi. Hum Pathol 30:500–505
4. Pellacani G, Farnetani F, Gonzalez S, Longo C, Cesinaro AM, Casari A, Beretti F, Seidenari S, Gill M (2011) In vivo confocal microscopy for detection and grading of dysplastic nevi: A pilot study. J Am Acad Dermatol Epub Jul 8 2011

Spitz Nevi

10

Sara Bassoli, Caterina Longo, and Giovanni Pellacani

The Spitz–Reed nevi family includes benign melanocytic tumors, generally acquired, characterized by a wide variety of clinical presentations, dermoscopic pattern and histopathologic features. The clinical differential diagnosis with melanoma is often considered due to its alarming clinical presentation. Spitz nevi are often described as pinkish-red papule suddenly arising in very young people, whereas Reed ones are commonly seen on the legs of adult patients. In both cases, patients often refer that the lesion suddenly appeared and is quickly growing. In this chapter, and often in the daily clinical experience, these two entities are joined in the same group, showing common histopathologic findings.

Histopathologically, Spitz nevi are defined by a set of characteristic features, although sometimes they cannot be differentiated from melanomas with certainty [1, 2]. Dermoscopy enabled the distinction of characteristic aspects of Spitz nevi, classified as a "starburst, globular and aspecific" subgroups [3, 4], nevertheless lacking of diagnostic clues for difficult lesions. In fact, one-third of pigmented Spitz nevi and all of nonpigmented Spitz nevi can be very challenging to diagnose as benign lesions, as well as there are some melanomas with a starburst or globular pattern that are dermoscopically indistinguishable from a Spitz nevus [3, 5, 6], and this led to a prophylactic surgical excision in most cases of lesions clinically and dermoscopically diagnosed as Spitz nevi.

S. Bassoli (✉) • G. Pellacani
Department of Dermatology and Venereology, University of Modena and Reggio Emilia, Modena, Italy
e-mail: sarabassoli79@gmail.com

C. Longo
Department of Dermatology, Arcispedale S Maria Nuova, Reggio Emilia, Reggio Emilia, Italy

The histopathologic diagnosis of Spitz nevus strongly relies on the assessment of the deeper parts of the lesion, including deep maturation and absence of mitotic figures [2].

Also considering the confocal features of Spitz nevi, though partially characteristic, they remain in most cases indistinguishable from melanoma [4, 7, 8]. A good correlation was found for some histopathologic aspects and RCM features, some of which considered characteristic of Spitz nevi, such as sharp lateral demarcation and presence of spindled cells, and other useful for diagnosis but not very specific, such as pagetoid infiltration, junctional and dermal nests, parakeratosis and trans-epidermal melanin elimination, and inflammatory infiltrate rich in melanophages. However, no correlates were found for other characteristic histologic aspects, such as Kamino's bodies, hyperkeratosis, acanthosis, mitoses and maturation with depth [8]. However, the frequent presence of features suggestive of malignancy in Spitz nevi, such as pagetoid and atypical cells, nonedged papillae and dishomogeneous nests, and the impossibility to explore the deeper parts of a given lesion, hamper a reliable diagnosis with confocal microscopy [7, 8].

10.1 RCM Features

Based on our experience the dermoscopic well-defined types of Spitz nevi correlate nicely with confocal microscopic counterparts (Table 10.1) [4, 7, 8]:

Group 1. Typical "Spitzoid" pattern, such as "starburst" or "globular".

Group 2. Peculiar "Spitzoid" aspects, such as "negative network" and "superficial black network".

Group 3. Simulators of atypical nevi or melanoma with "reticular", "homogeneous", "complex", or "multicomponent pattern".

Group 4. "Non specific" pattern.

R. Hofmann-Wellenhof et al. (eds.), *Reflectance Confocal Microscopy for Skin Diseases*,
DOI 10.1007/978-3-642-21997-9_10, © Springer-Verlag Berlin Heidelberg 2012

Table 10.1 Dermoscopic patterns of Spitz nevi and their respective confocal microscopic correlates

Dermoscopic pattern	RCM correlate	Differential diagnosis with melanoma
Starburst pattern	– Typical epidermis, sometimes a few pagetoid cells – Dense regular nests at dermal epidermal junction and within the papillary dermis – Sharp borders constituted by a peripheral rim of dense nests	Possible, based on specific confocal features
Globular pattern	– Nonedged papillae, atypical spindled or polygonal cells, and numerous melanophages in basal layer and dermis	
Inverse network pattern	– Thickened, frequently acanthotic epidermis, with a honeycombed or a cobblestone pattern	Possible when specific confocal features are visible
Superficial black network pattern	– Papillary contours often not clearly distinguishable	
Reticular/homogeneous/ multicomponent pattern	– Nonedged papillae and atypical cells at dermal–epidermal junction – Dishomogeneous nests with loss of cell cohesion in the dermis (sparse-cell nests)	Difficult for the presence of confocal features suggestive of malignancy
Nonspecific pattern	– Disarranged or broadened honeycombed epidermal pattern, few roundish pagetoid cells – Numerous large atypical cells, sometimes in sheet-like structures, at dermal–epidermal junction – Sparse cell and cerebriform clusters in the dermis	Impossible for lack of confocal features: always perform surgical excision

10.1.1 Group 1: Typical "Spitzoid" Lesions, such as "Starburst" or "Globular" Spitz Nevi

These are usually flat to palpable pigmented lesions, characterized by a rapid radial growth. The symmetry, frequently respected, is very suggestive of benignity. Upon confocal examination, in the superficial layer these lesions show a regular honeycombed or cobblestone pattern, although some dendritic and (most rarely) roundish pagetoid cells can be observed. At the dermal–epidermal junction, the general architecture is mainly showing a meshwork (for the "starburst" lesions) or clod pattern (for "globular" lesions). Both edged and nonedged papillae are visible, and it is possible to observe also spindled and polygonal cells, both at the junctional and upper dermal layer, although in a lower amount compared to melanomas; commonly, dense regular nests at the dermal–epidermal junction and within the papillary and sharp borders constituted predominantly by a peripheral rim of dense nests are seen (Fig. 10.1).

In this group of Spitz nevi the following features help in the distinction from melanoma: (a) the presence of none or rare pagetoid cells (either roundish and dendritic) mainly centrally located, (b) a prevalence of spindled atypical cells at the dermal–epidermal junction, and (c) numerous homogeneous dense nests in the DEJ and upper dermis. Sometimes, a high number of pagetoid cells or atypical cells at the junction are found widespread throughout the lesion. In these cases, the differentiation from melanoma is very challenging, or quite impossible.

10.1.2 Group 2: Lesions with Peculiar "Spitzoid" Aspects, such as "Negative Network" or "Superficial Black Network"

"Inverse" or "negative" network and superficial black network are dermoscopic features correlated to the diagnosis of Spitz nevus. These aspects characterize usually flat to palpable lesions that are either clinically and dermoscopically in differential diagnosis with melanoma. Despite different dermoscopic aspects, these lesions show similar features in confocal and in histopathology, such as thickened, frequently acanthotic epidermis. An atypical, sometimes broadened, honeycombed pattern is observed in lesions with inverse network, while a strongly bright cobblestone pattern is seen in the lesions with a superficial black network. Pagetoid cells are rarely observed. Exploration of the deeper layers is often difficult due to the increased epidermal thickness. In fact, in half of the cases, papillary contour is not clearly distinguishable and in most cases dermis is not visible. In these cases, the visualization of diagnostic features is impossible. When visible, DEJ usually shows an aspecific pattern with scattered and unevenly distributed papillae. Papillary contours are frequently not well defined (nonedged). Some large bright nucleated cells, spindled or polygonal in shape, can be detected, normally not showing a striking atypia (Fig. 10.2).

CASE 1 – Starburst pattern
Age: 28
Sex: M
Anatomical Site: Right thigh
History: New lesion rapidly growing
Histopathology: Reed nevus

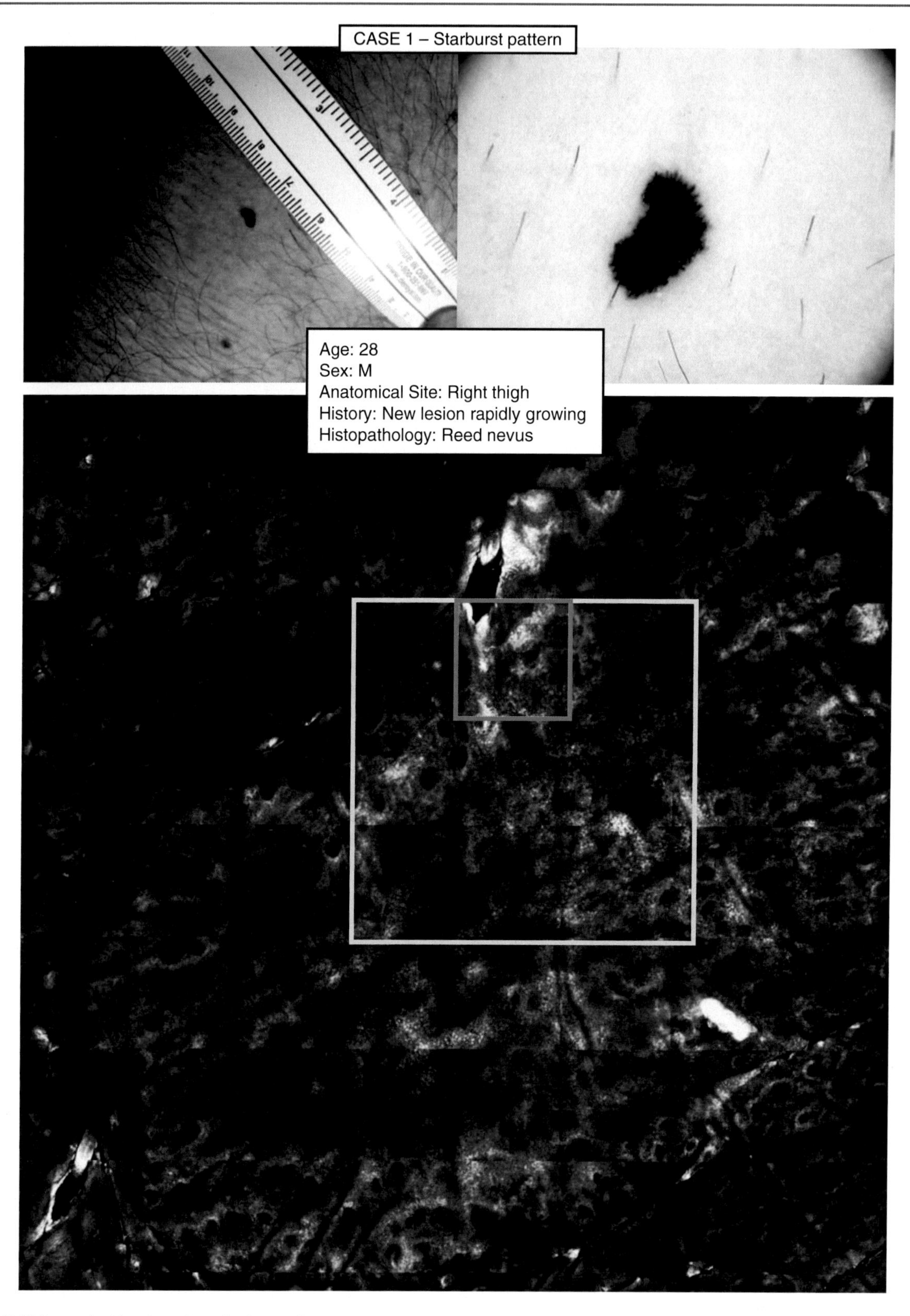

Fig. 10.1 RCM mosaic (4 × 4 mm) at the level of the DEJ reveals a variation of a meshwork pattern which is well defined and correlates with the dermoscopic shape of the lesion. Already at this magnification the texture of the lesion appears regular with evenly distributed papillae suggestive for a benign melanocytic lesion

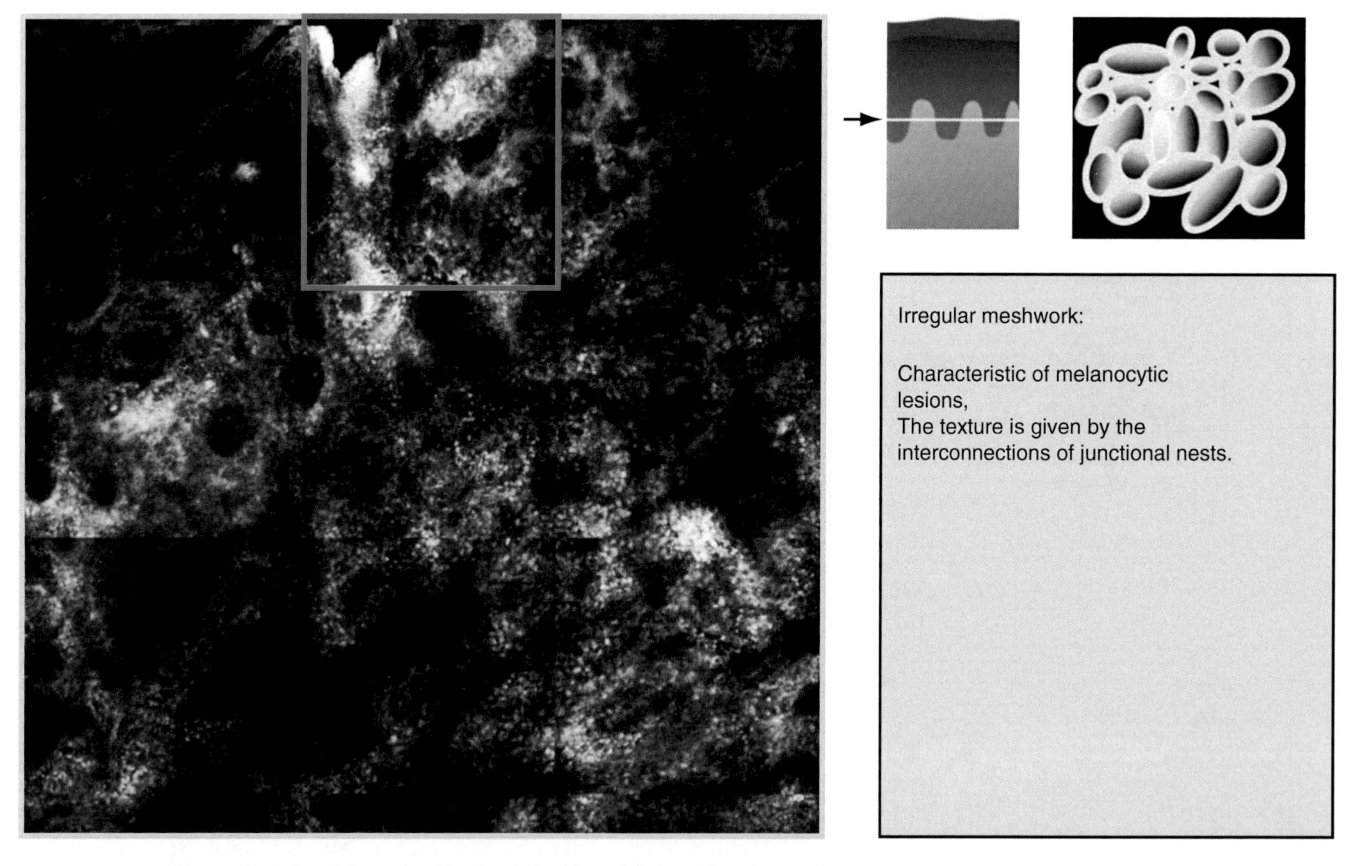

Fig. 10.1.1 RCM mosaic (1.5 × 1.5 mm) at the DEJ. At this resolution irregular meshwork pattern with both edged and nonedged papillae is clearly evident. Irregular meshwork is characterized by the interconnection of irregular and non homogeneous junctional nests

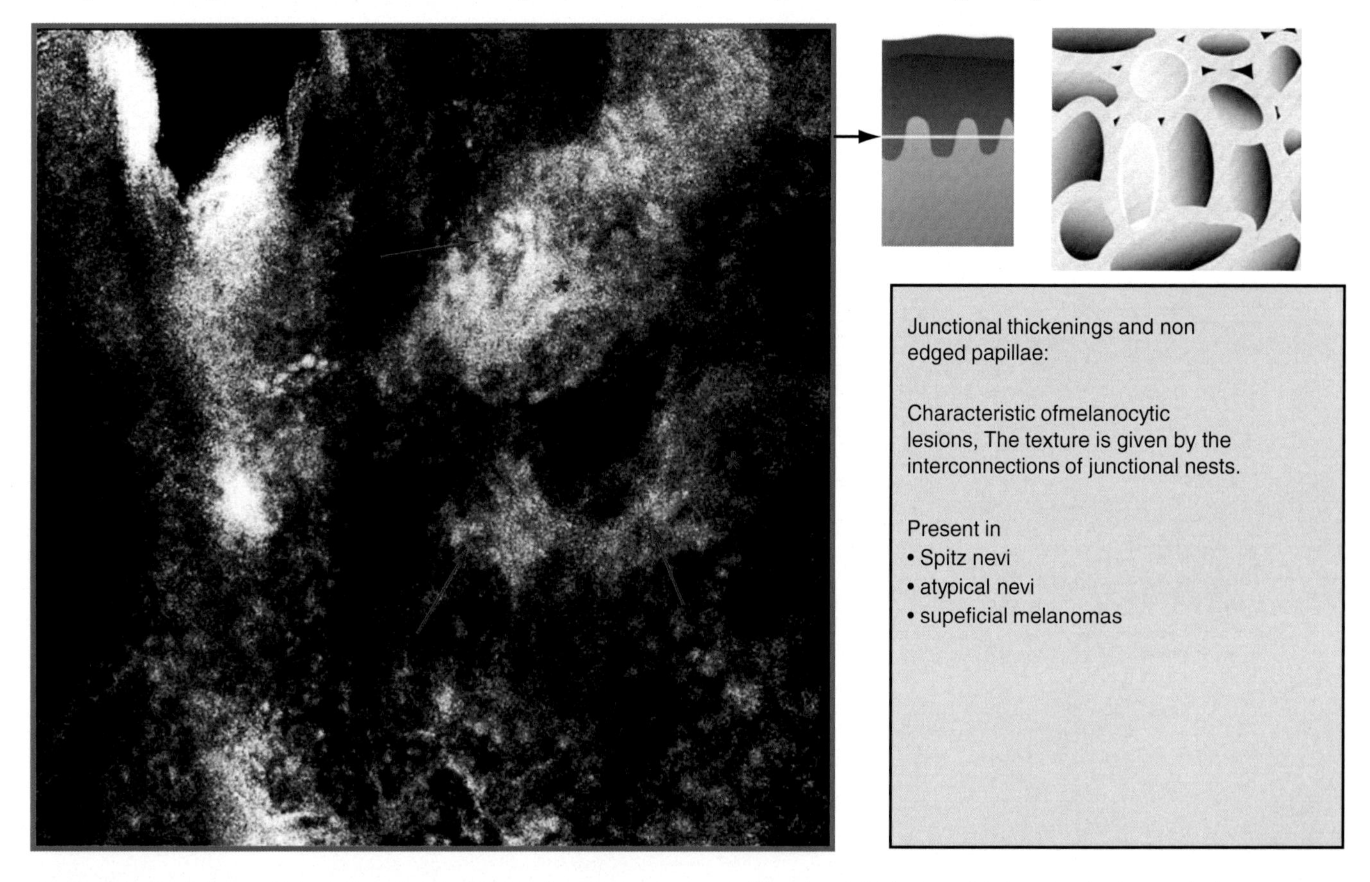

Fig. 10.1.2 Basic image (0.5 × 0.5 mm) at the DEJ depicts nicely two areas of junctional thickenings (*), irregular in shape, which present non-well-outlined borders, giving rise to non-edged-papillae. Few mildly atypical cells are visible within the nests (→)

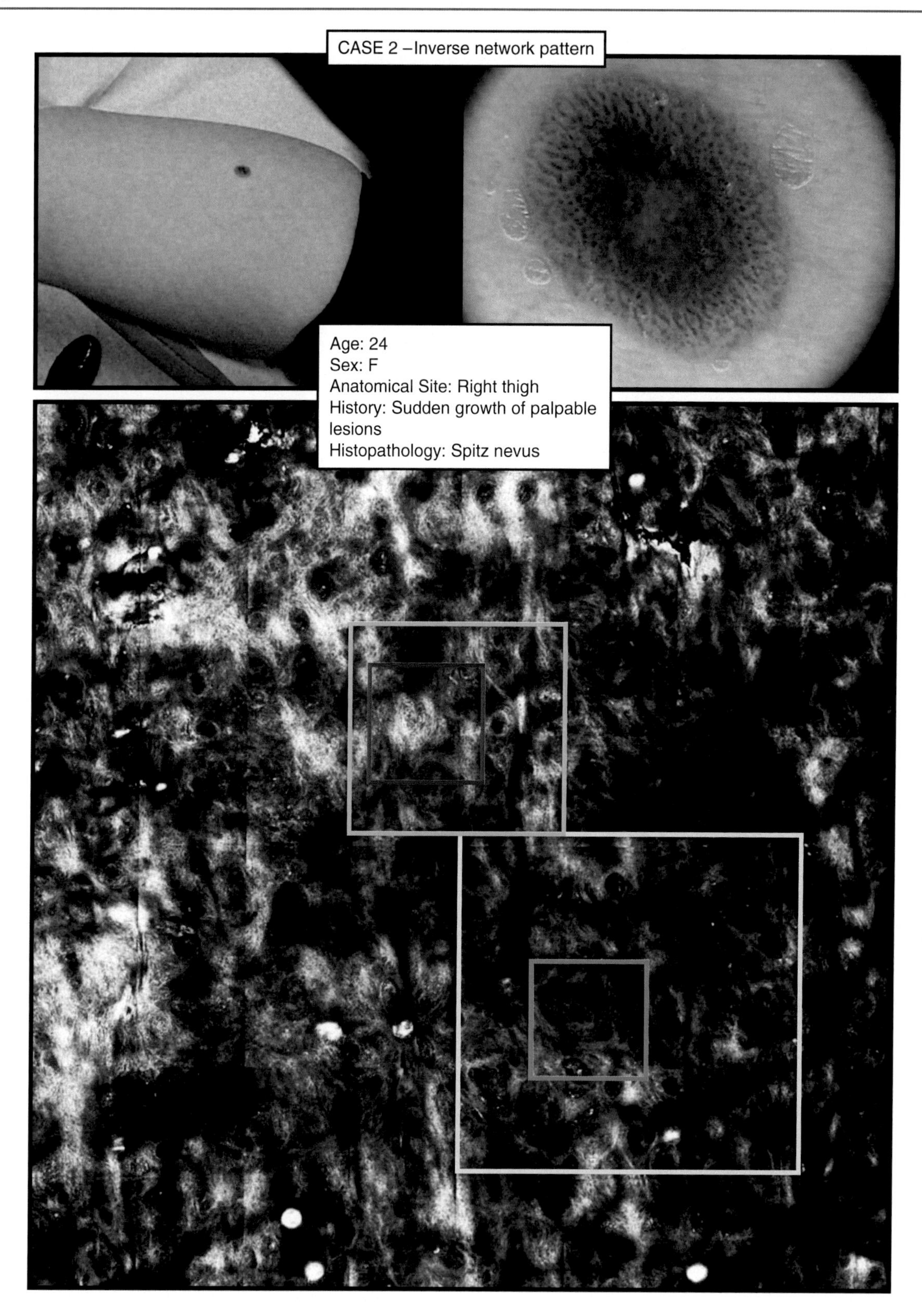

Fig. 10.2 RCM mosaic (4 × 4 mm) in the center of the lesion at the level of the DEJ reveals a nonspecific pattern mostly characterized by nonedged papillae unevenly distributed throughout the lesion, more evident in the right part of the image. In the left part of the lesion, a prominent bright epidermis intermingled with papillae is suggestive of acanthosis. The striking *white roundish* structures in the lower part of the image correspond to air bubbles

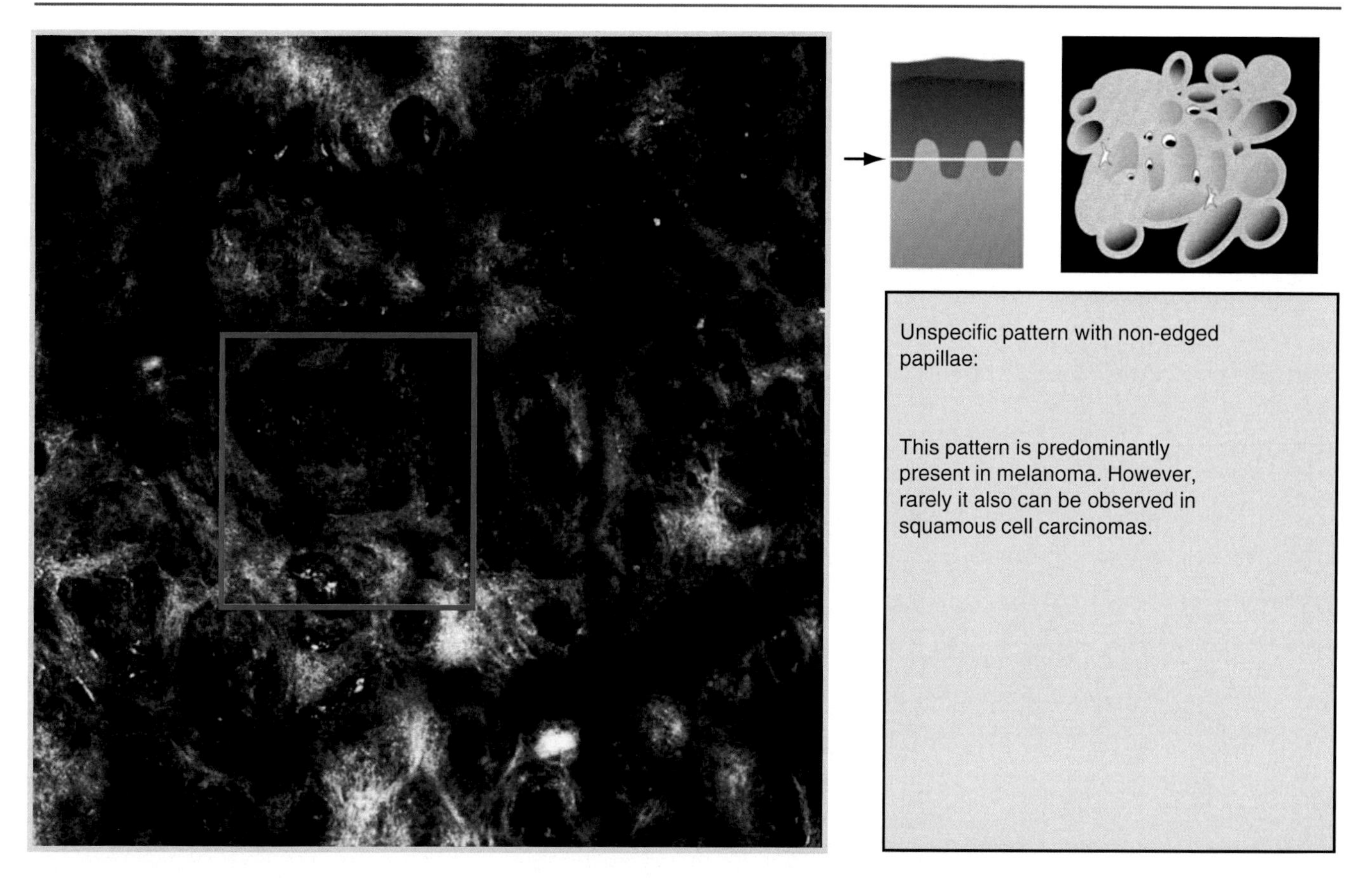

Fig. 10.2.1 RCM mosaic (1.5 × 1.5 mm) at the DEJ. Numerous nonedged papillae varying in size are forming a disorganized architecture. Already at this magnification, a cell cluster within a large nonedged papilla can be noted. Moreover, there are a few tiny bright particles within the papillae correlating to inflammatory cells

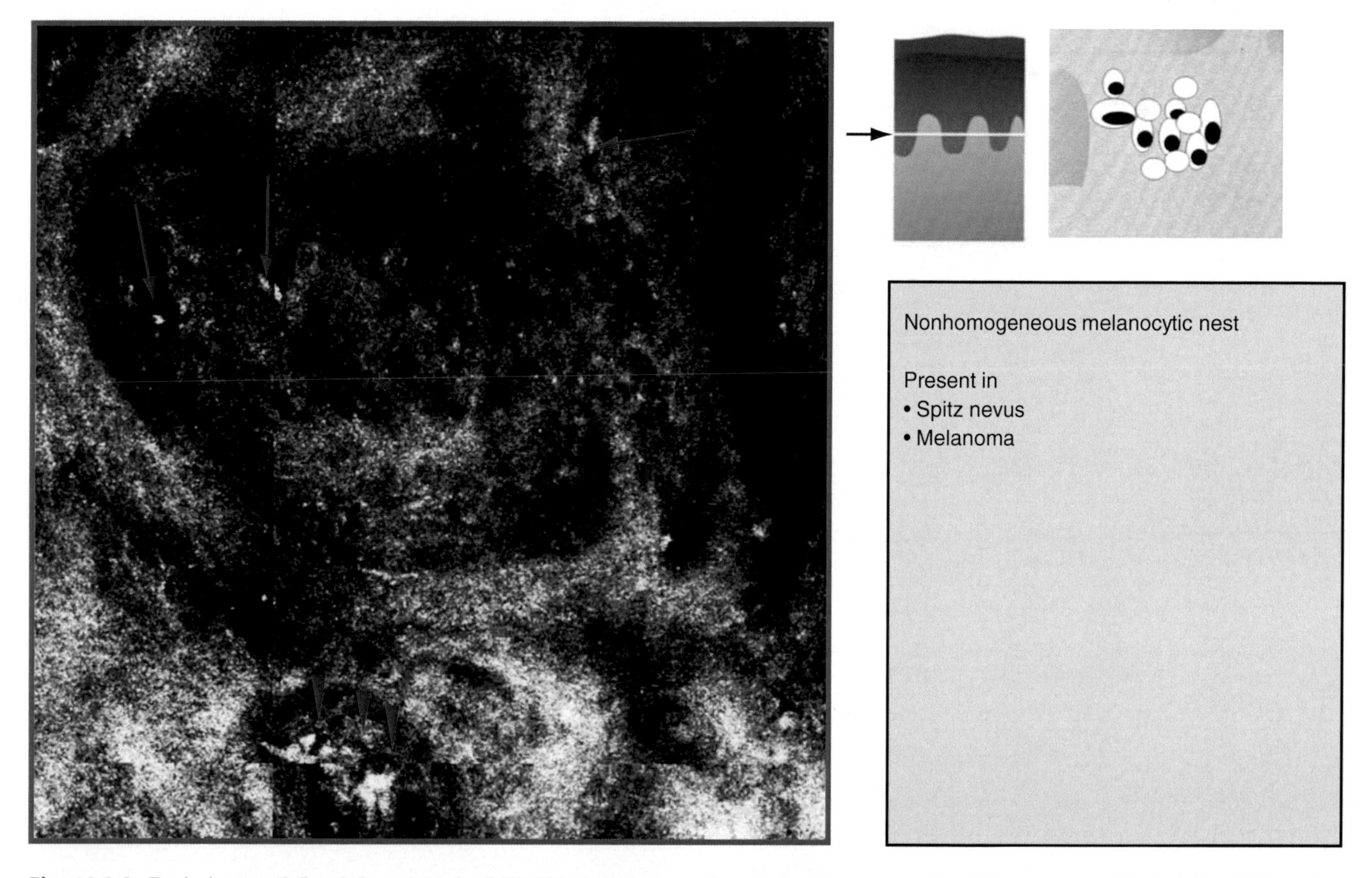

Fig. 10.2.2 Basic image (0.5 × 0.5 mm) at the DEJ. Within a large nonedged papilla there is an oval nonhomogeneously reflecting structure representing a melanocytic cell cluster with barely visible cell contours (*). Few *tiny white* particles are present within this nest and in the dermal papillae representing inflammatory cells (→). In addition, *tiny and larger white* particles can be noted within a papilla (▲) correlating to inflammatory cells and melanophages

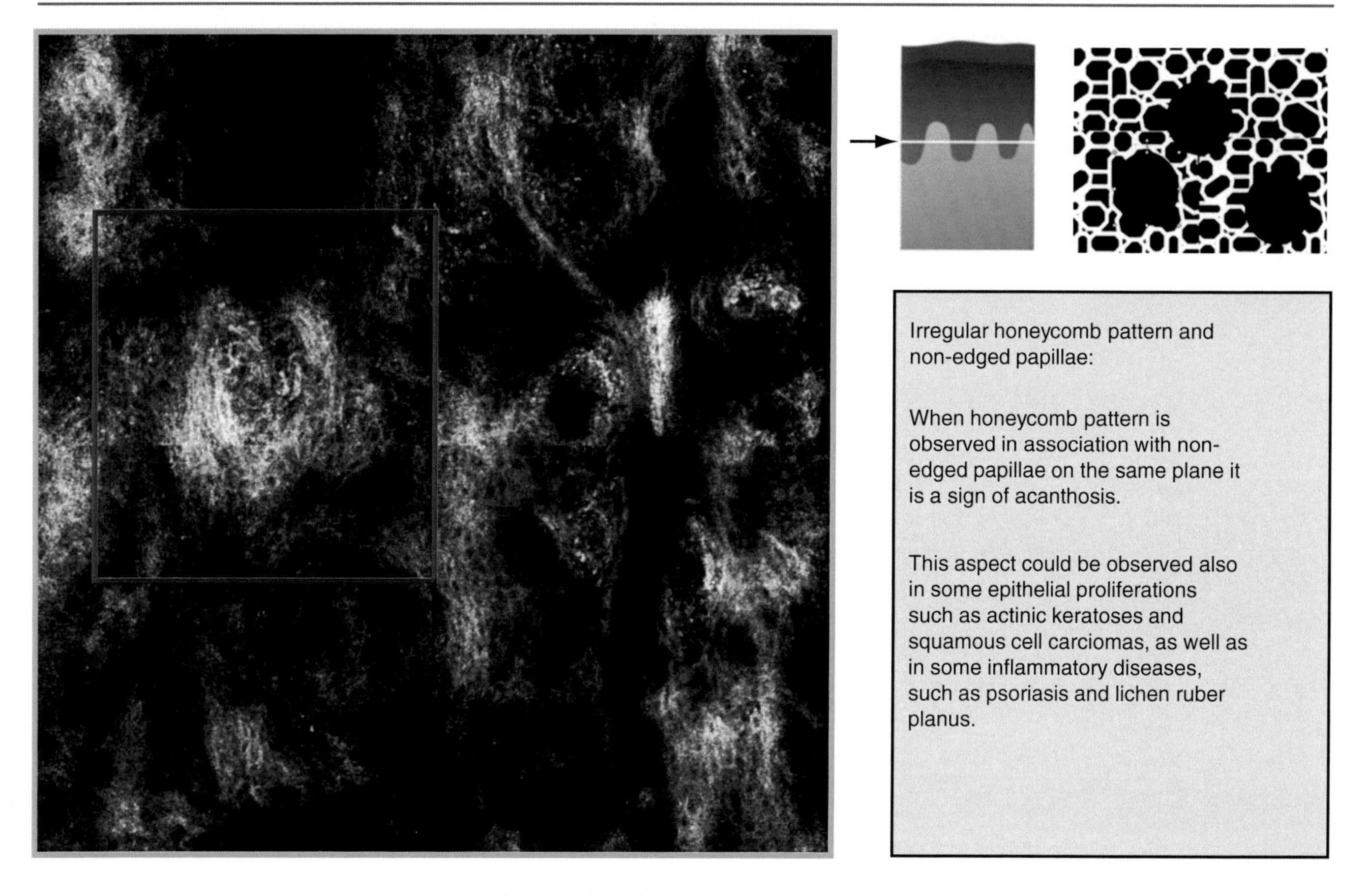

Fig. 10.2.3 RCM mosaic (1.5 × 1.5 mm) at the DEJ. This image shows patchy distribution of irregularly outlined honeycomb areas sometimes surrounding nonedged papillae corresponding to acanthosis

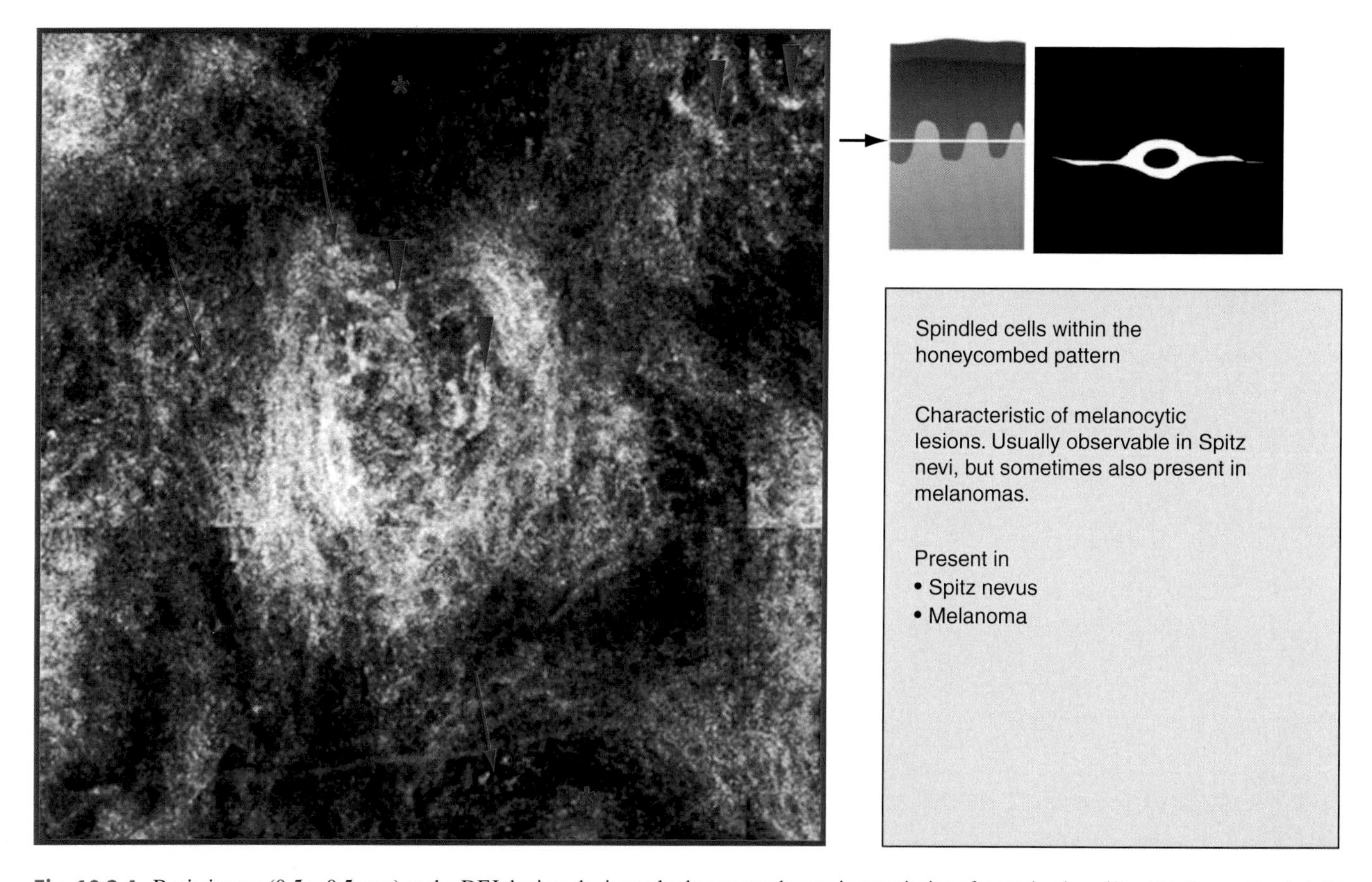

Fig. 10.2.4 Basic image (0.5 × 0.5 mm) at the DEJ depicts the irregular honeycomb area in proximity of nonedged papillae (*). Some *tiny bright* particles (→) and a few elongated (spindled) cells (▲), the latter consistent for a melanocytic lesion, are visible within the honeycomb pattern

10.1.3 Group 3: Simulators of Atypical Nevi or Melanoma with "Reticular", "Homogeneous", "Complex", or "Multicomponent Pattern"

This group represents a very heterogeneous population of Spitz nevi, frequently melanoma simulators in dermoscopy. Pagetoid scatter is frequently present. At the DEJ, irregular meshwork and/or aspecific pattern is usually present, as well as nonedged papillae and numerous atypical cells. Atypical cells at the DEJ and upper dermis tend to cluster into dishomogeneous (dense and sparse) nests. Sometimes, single nucleated cells are present in the papillary dermis. In sum,

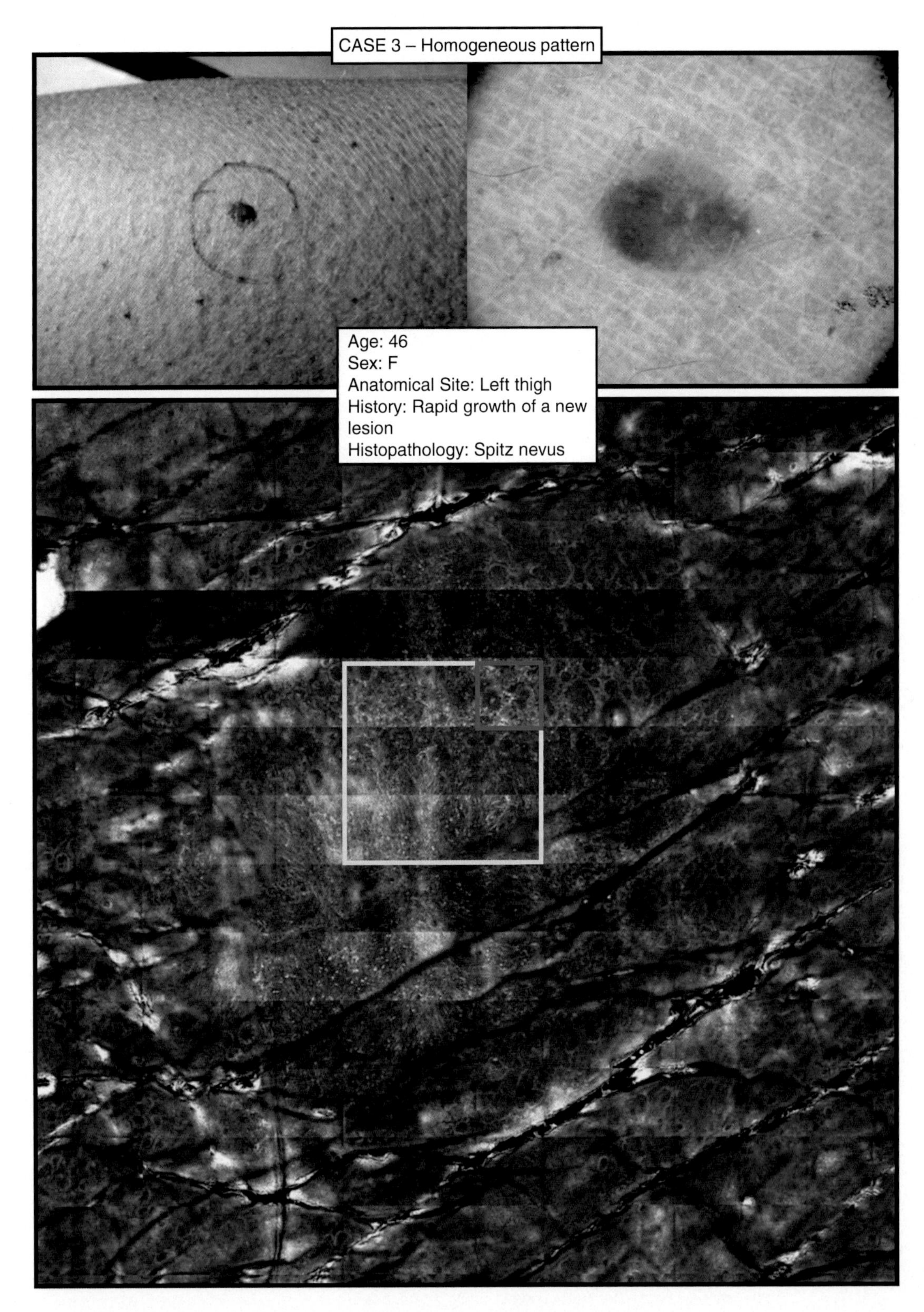

Fig. 10.3 RCM mosaic (6 × 6 mm) at the DEJ. The scanning RCM reveals a rather well-discriminated contour of a lesion with nonspecific pattern characterized by bright nonhomogeneous areas and scattered *bright dots* and *lines*

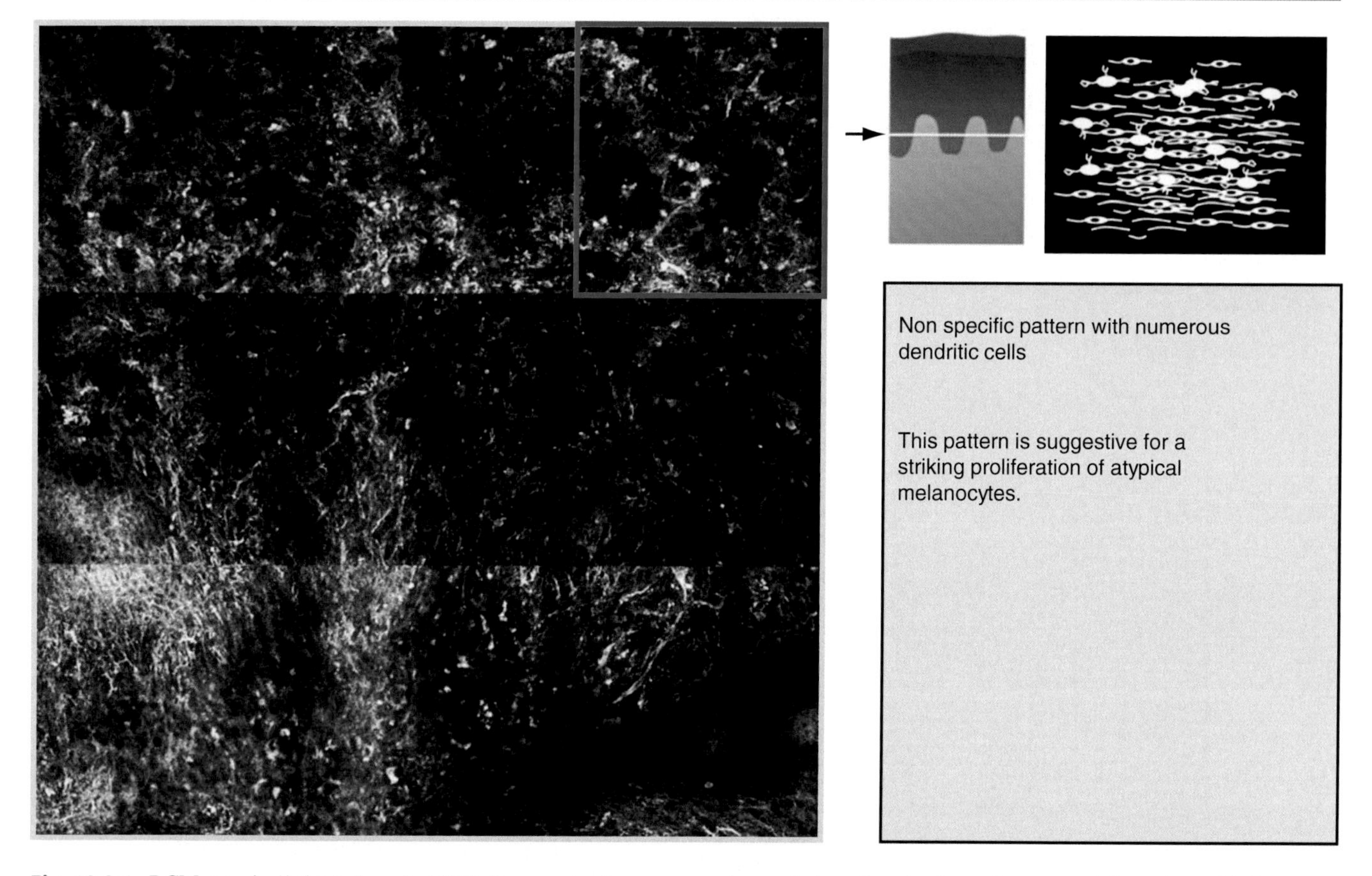

Fig. 10.3.1 RCM mosaic (1.5 × 1.5 mm) at DEJ. By zooming in numerous *dots* and *short lines* haphazardly arranged throughout this frame are strongly suggestive for an increased number of dendritic melanocytic cells at DEJ and in the suprabasal layer

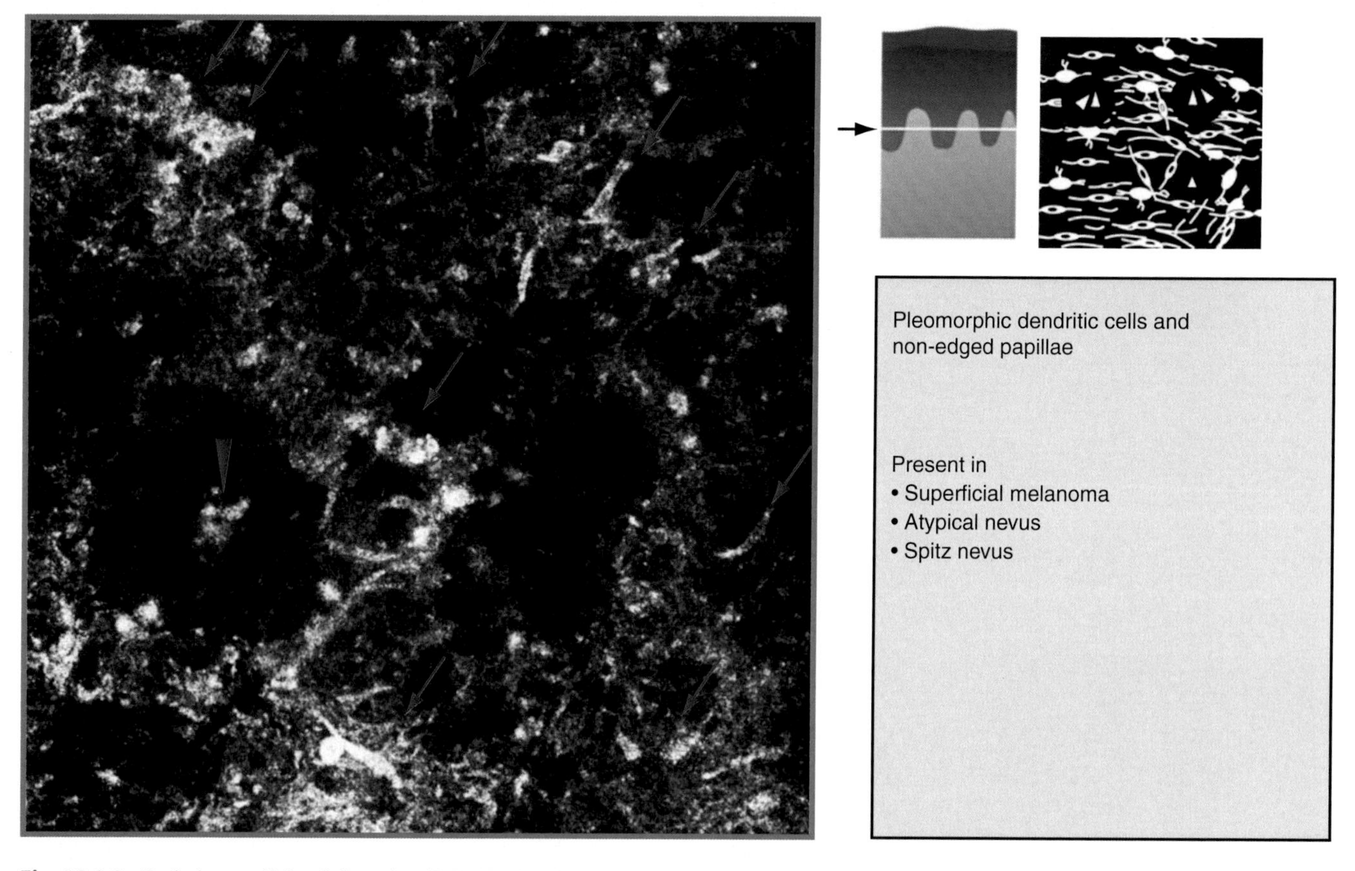

Fig. 10.3.2 Basic image (0.5 × 0.5 mm) at DEJ. Further zooming in exhibits pleomorphic dendritic cells mainly distributed in solitary units (→). Some nonedged papillae are visible. In the center of a nonedged papilla, a small cluster of plumb bright cells corresponding to melanophages can be clearly recognized (▲)

the confocal features observed in these lesions are strongly suggestive of malignancy, simulating melanoma (Figs. 10.3 and 10.4).

10.1.4 Group 4: "Nonspecific" Pattern

A minority of Spitz nevi are clinically nodular and nonspecific in dermoscopy, mimicking melanomas or other nonmelanocytic entities. In confocal, they may present in the epidermal layer a disarranged or a broadened honeycombed pattern, with a few roundish pagetoid cells. Frequently, DEJ is not visible due to the epidermal thickening. In these cases also a differentiation between melanocytic and nonmelanocytic lesion is not possible. When deeper layers are explorable, the architecture of papillae is disorganized. Numerous large atypical cells, roundish to polygonal in shape, are present at the DEJ and in the dermis. In addition, sheet-like structures or dishomogeneous (dense and sparse and/or cerebriform) nests can be observed in the superficial papillary dermis, simulating nodular melanomas (Fig. 10.5).

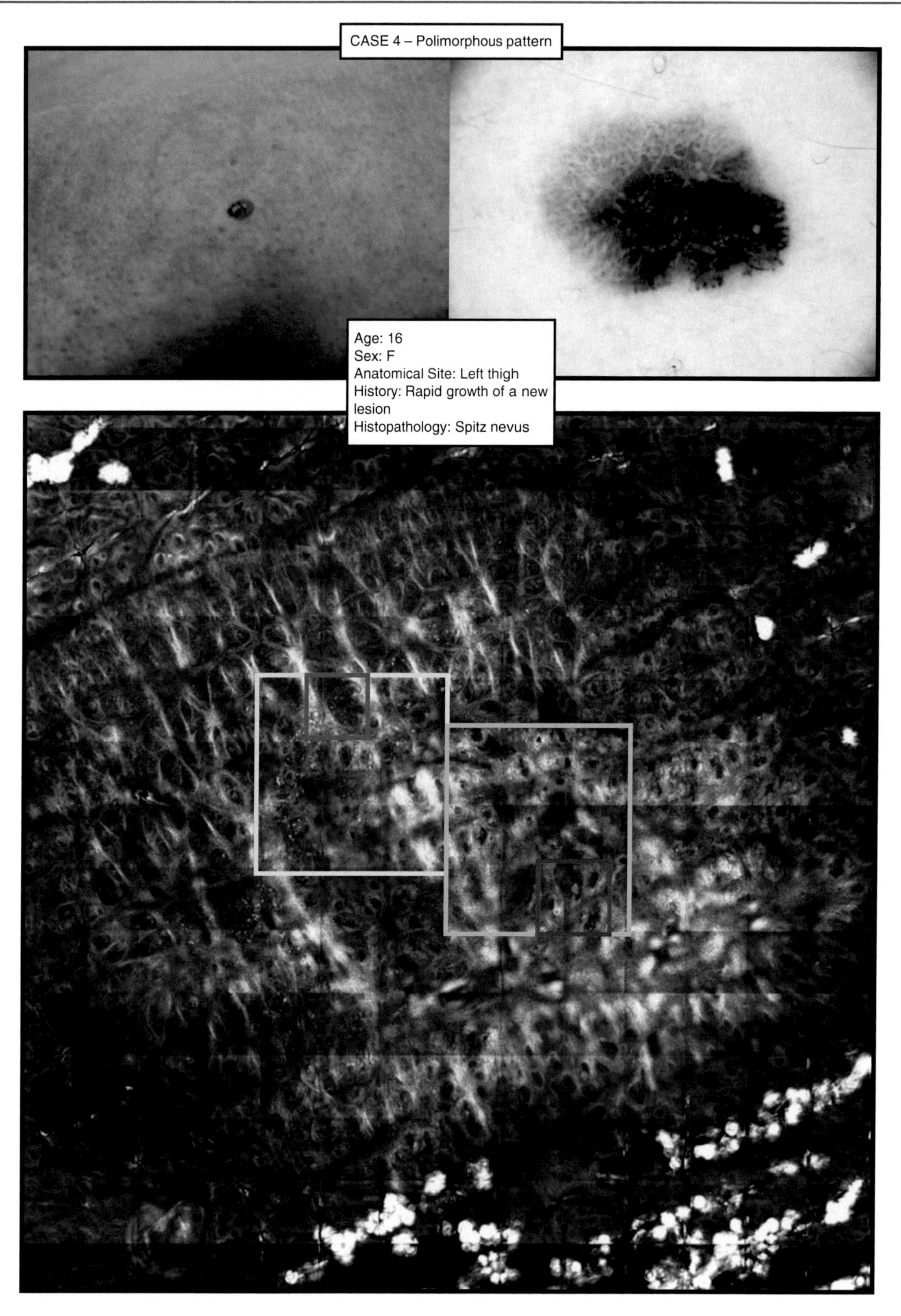

Fig. 10.4 RCM mosaic (7 × 7 mm) at DEJ. With scanning magnification two distinct parts can be differentiated. The central and lower right part of the lesion, corresponding to the pigmented one in dermoscopy, exhibits an irregular bright meshwork pattern, whereas the upper left portion is characterized by a nonspecific pattern with streaks and irregular papillae

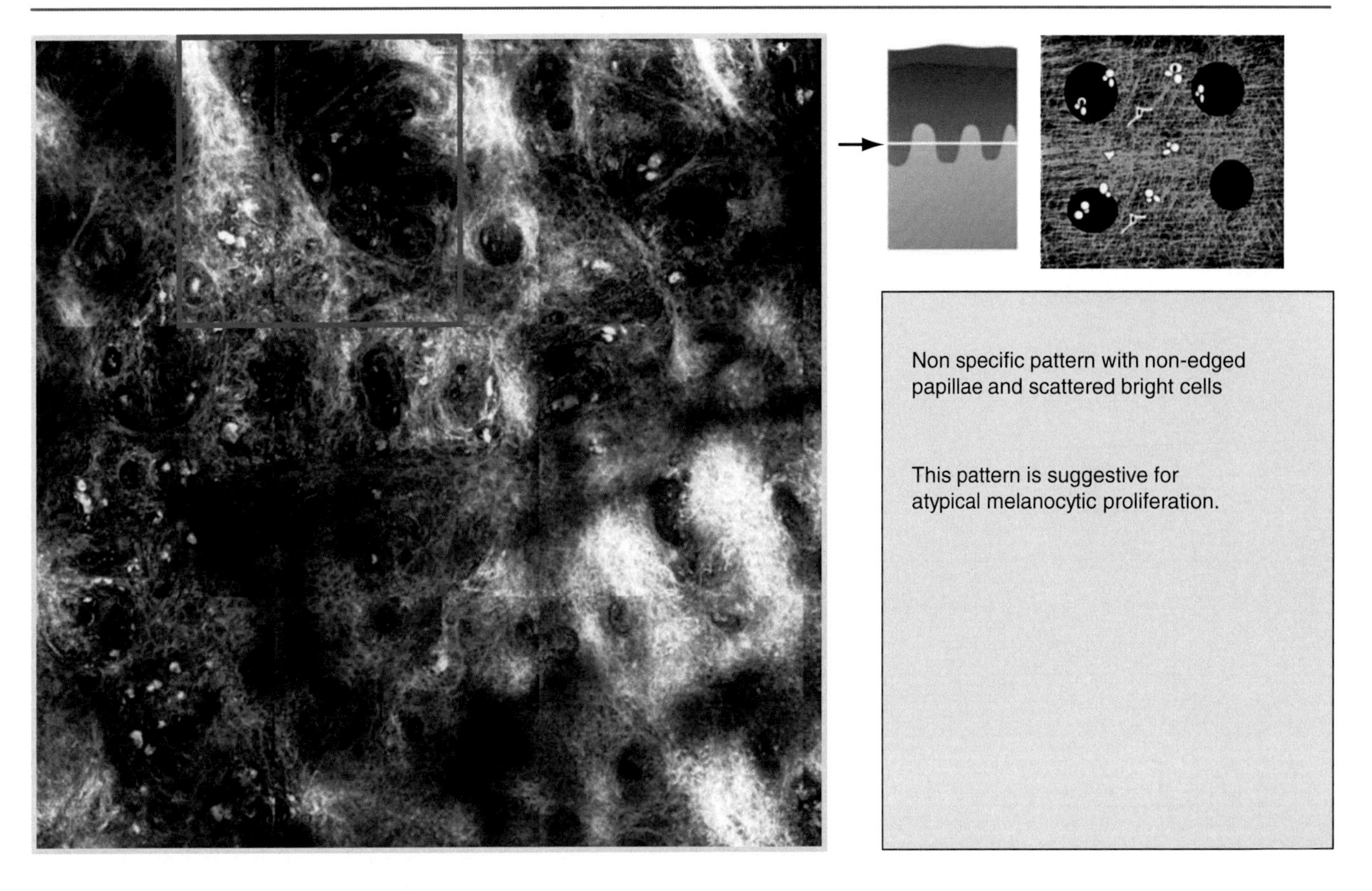

Fig. 10.4.1 RCM mosaic (1.5 × 1.5 mm) at DEJ. A nonspecific pattern with nonedged papillae and many bright cells unevenly distributed are detectable. Already at this resolution aggregates of faintly reflective cells are observed within the dermis (*blue inset*). In the lower right corner, patchy honeycombed areas surrounding some nonedged papillae, corresponding to acanthosis, are present

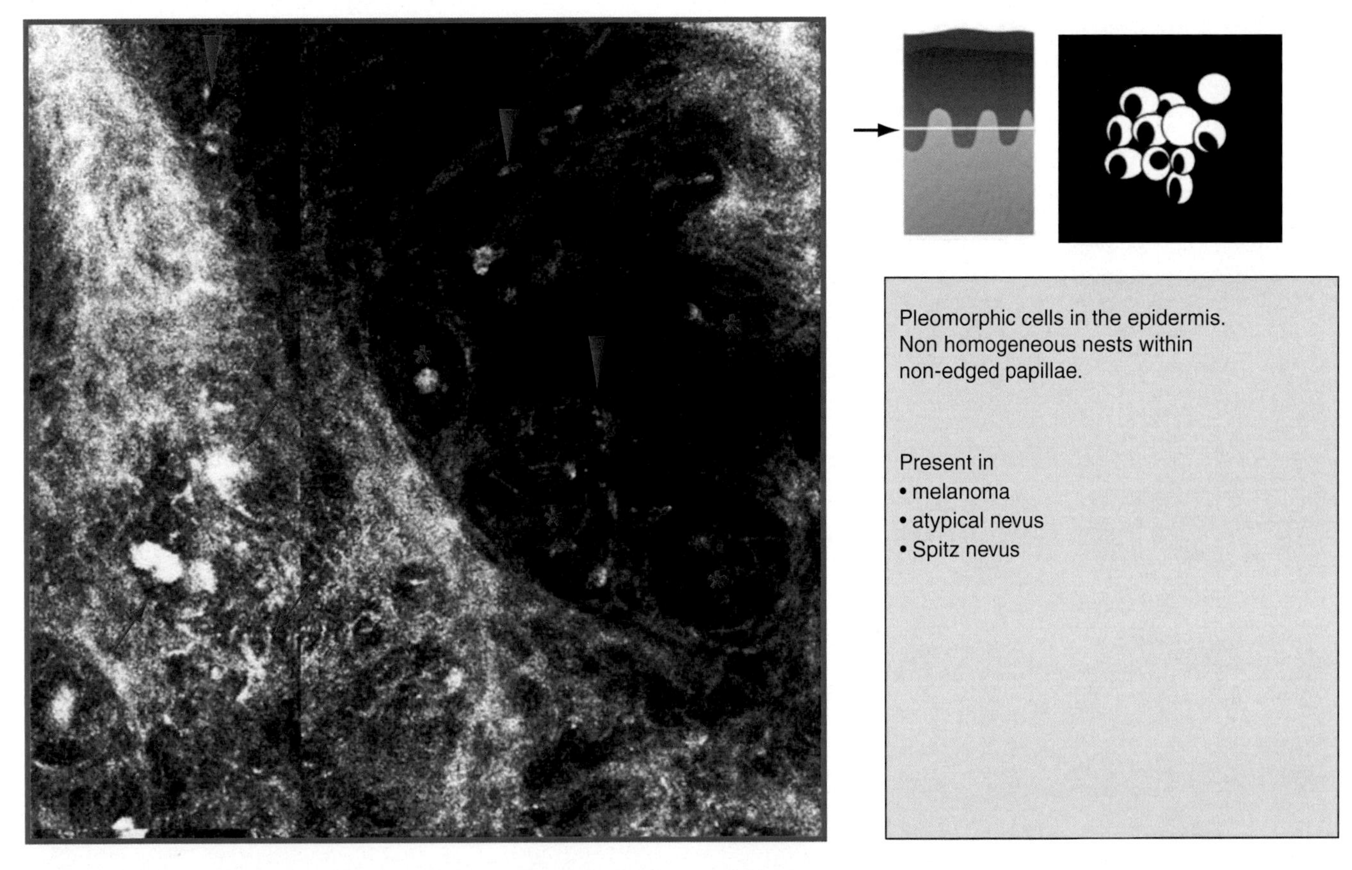

Fig. 10.4.2 Basic image (0.5 × 0.5 mm) at DEJ. This frame displays dendritic and polygonal bright cells within the epidermal layers (→) suggestive of atypical melanocytes. Within a non-well-defined nonedged papilla some oval nonhomogeneously reflecting structures probably corresponding to melanocytic cell clusters with barely visible cell contours (*) are observable. Few *small bright* particles corresponding to inflammatory cells are visible (▲)

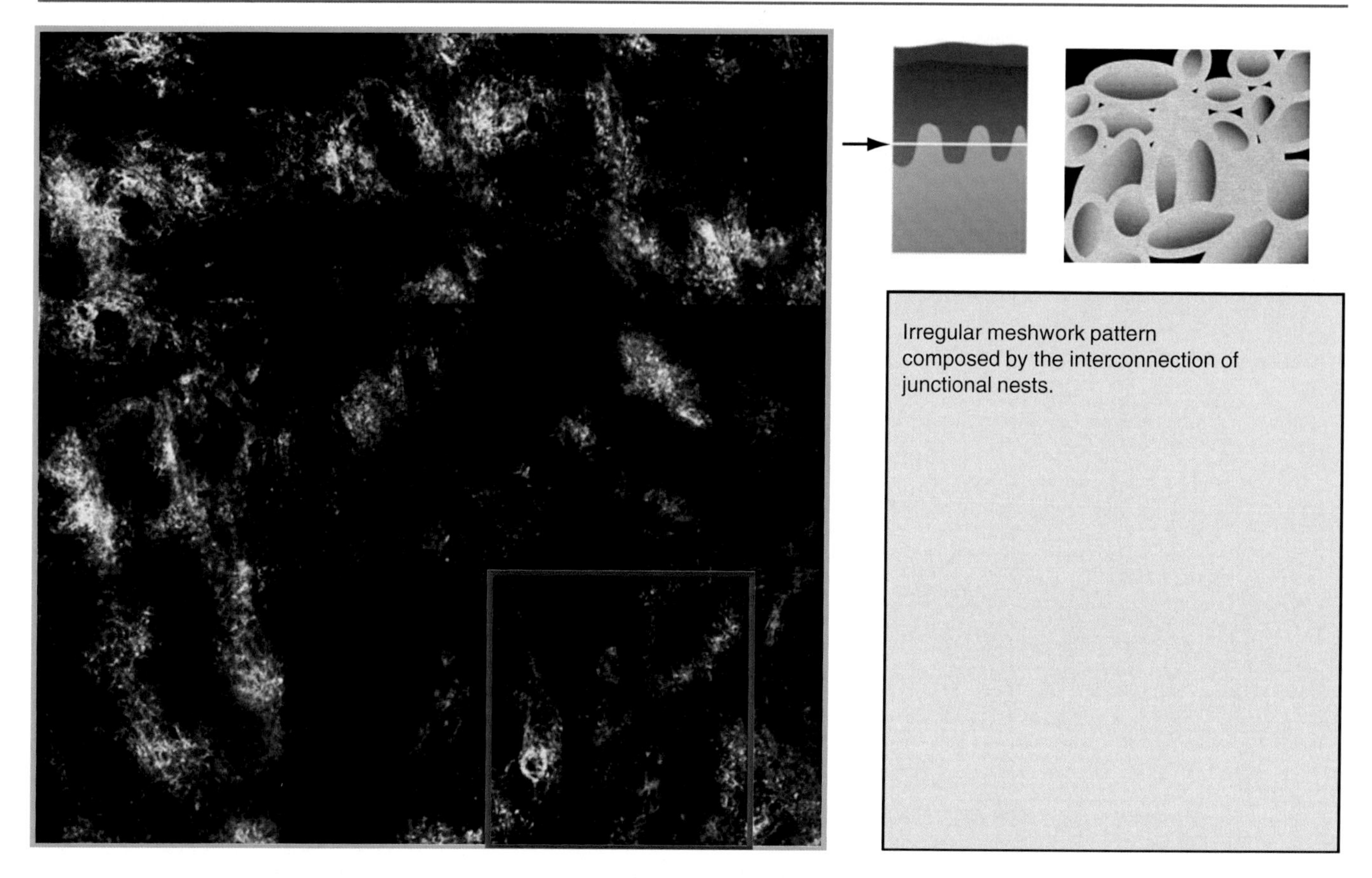

Fig. 10.4.3 RCM mosaic (1.5 × 1.5 mm) at DEJ. Irregular meshwork pattern with predominance of nonedged papillae is visible

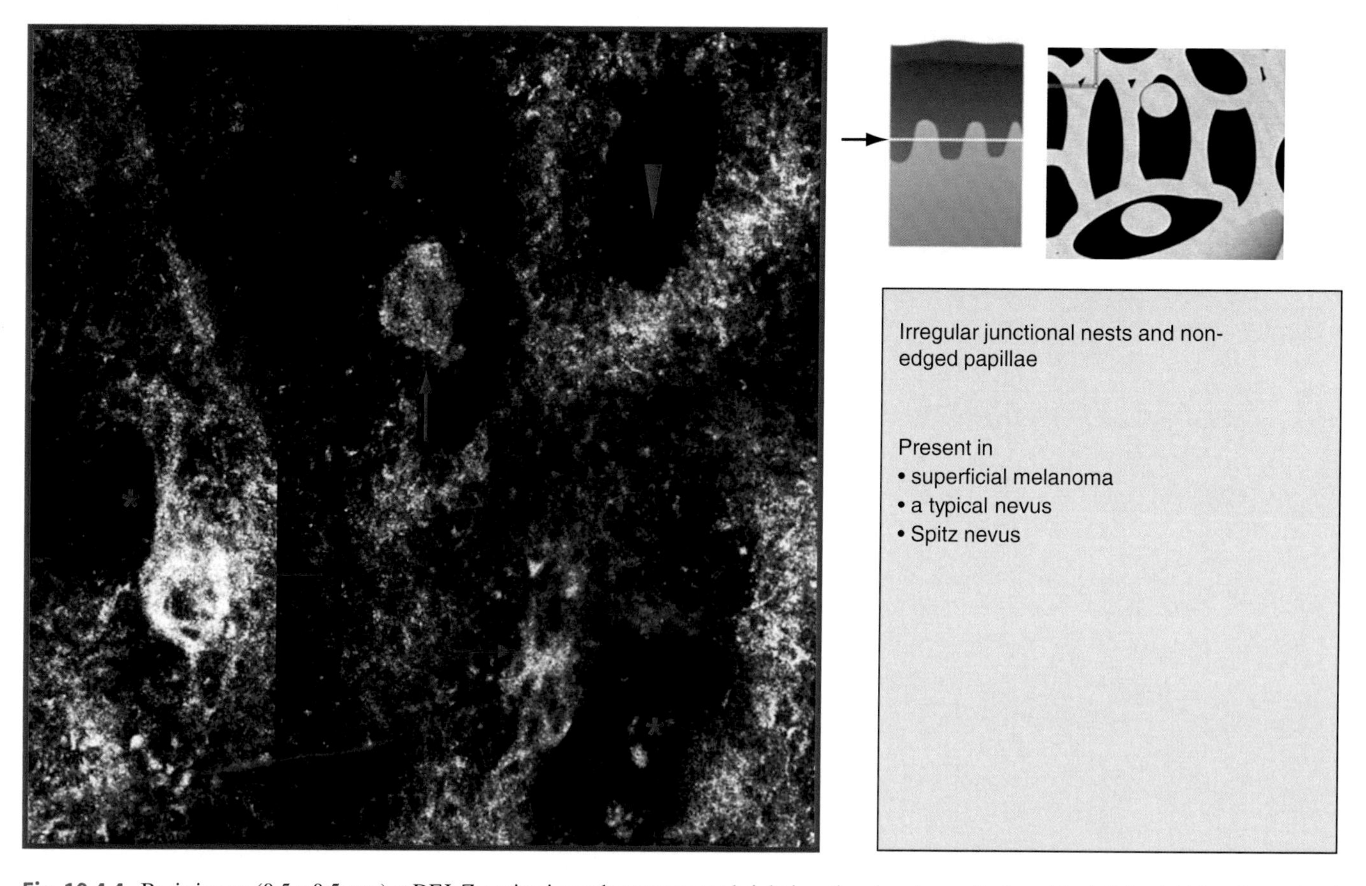

Fig. 10.4.4 Basic image (0.5 × 0.5 mm) at DEJ. Zooming in nonhomogeneous bright junctional nests are displayed (→). Edged (▲) and nonedged papillae (*) with few inflammatory cells are observable

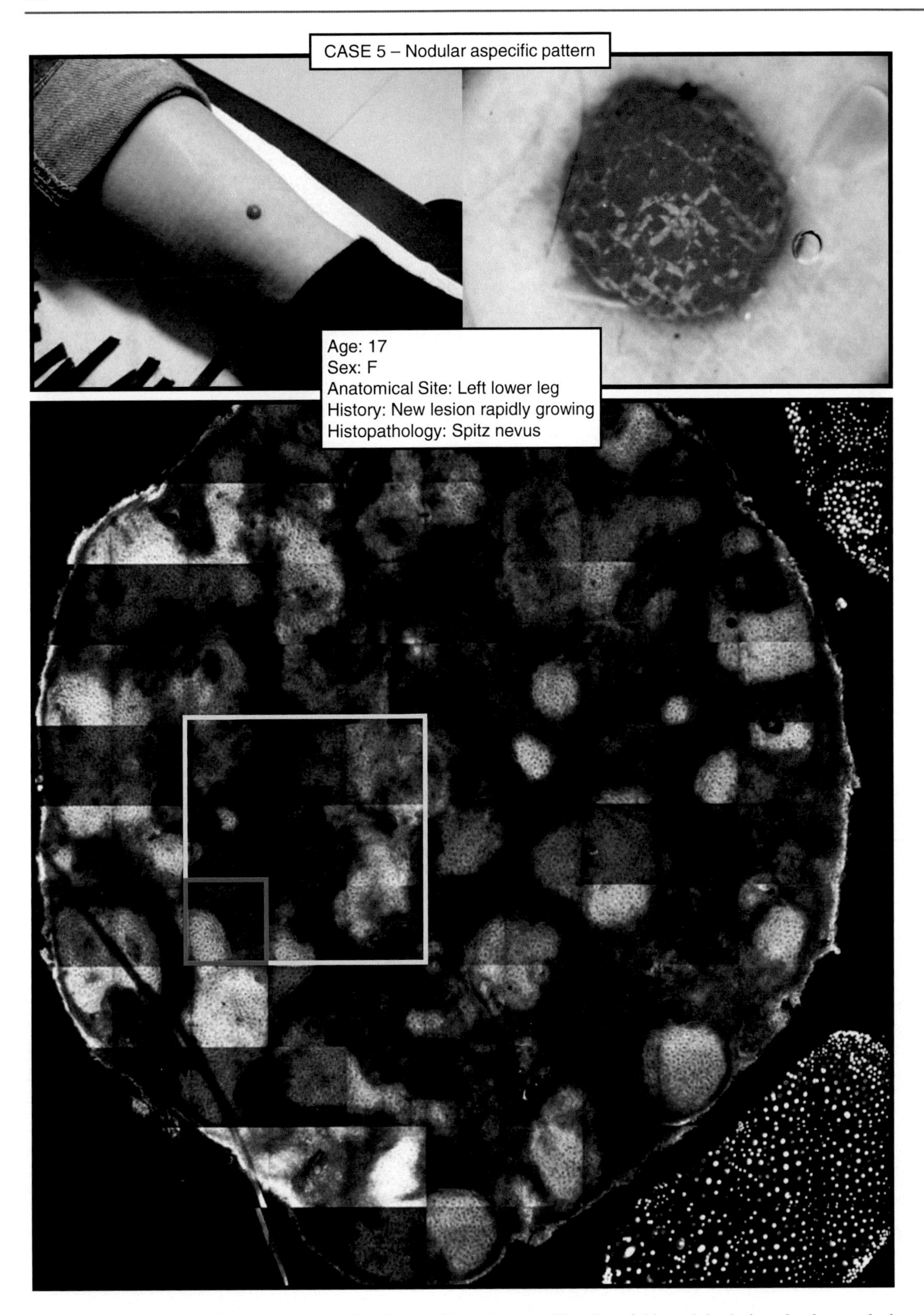

Fig. 10.5 RCM mosaic (6 × 6 mm) at suprabasal layer. Scanning magnification of this nodular lesion clearly reveals the contour. Patchy areas of honeycombed pattern are observable

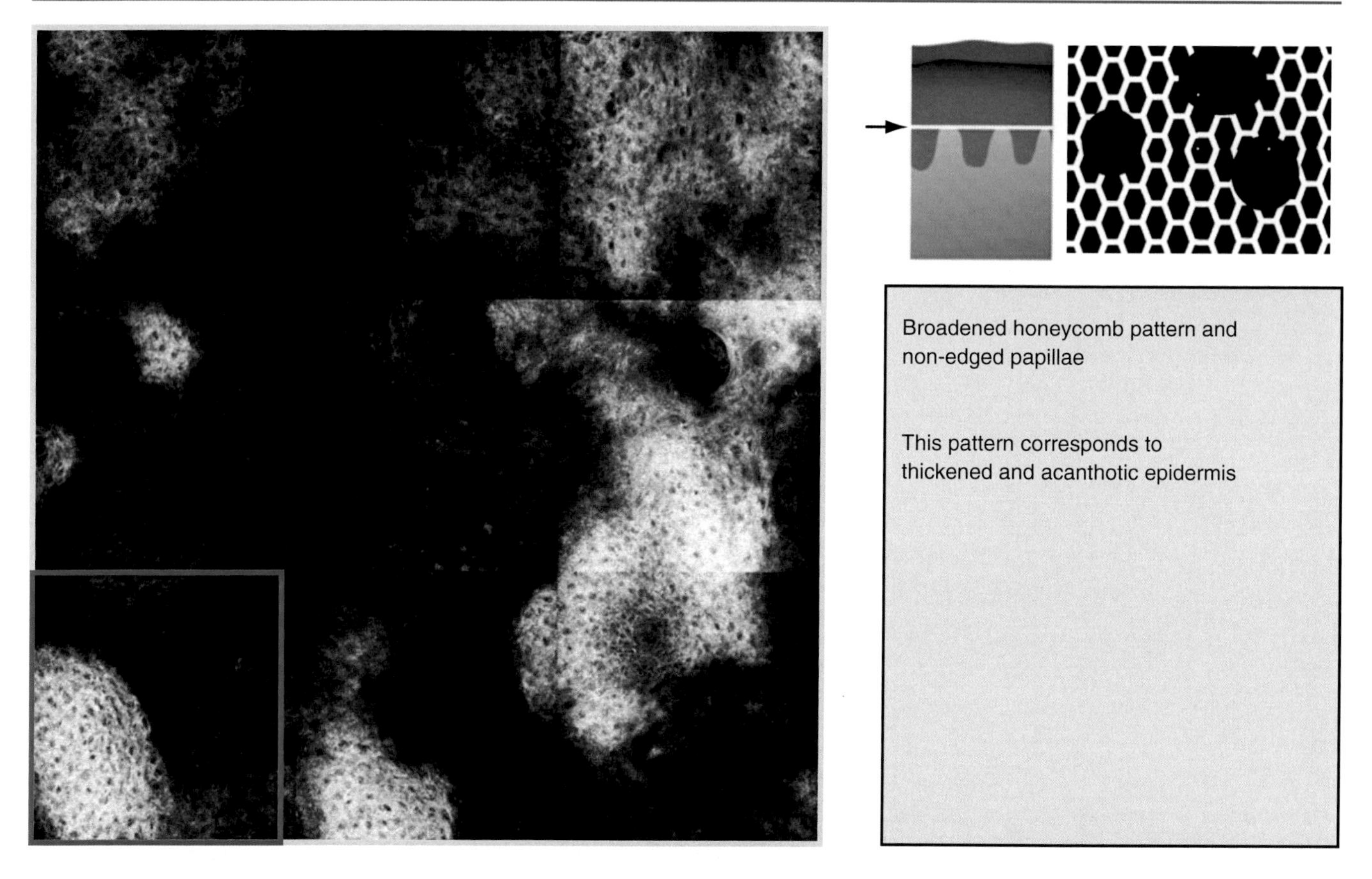

Fig. 10.5.1 RCM mosaic (1.5 × 1.5 mm) at suprabasal layer. Areas of broadened honeycomb pattern characterize the lesion. Because of the epidermal thickening, the DEJ cannot be clearly detected. Some nonedged papillae are barely visible in the darker areas

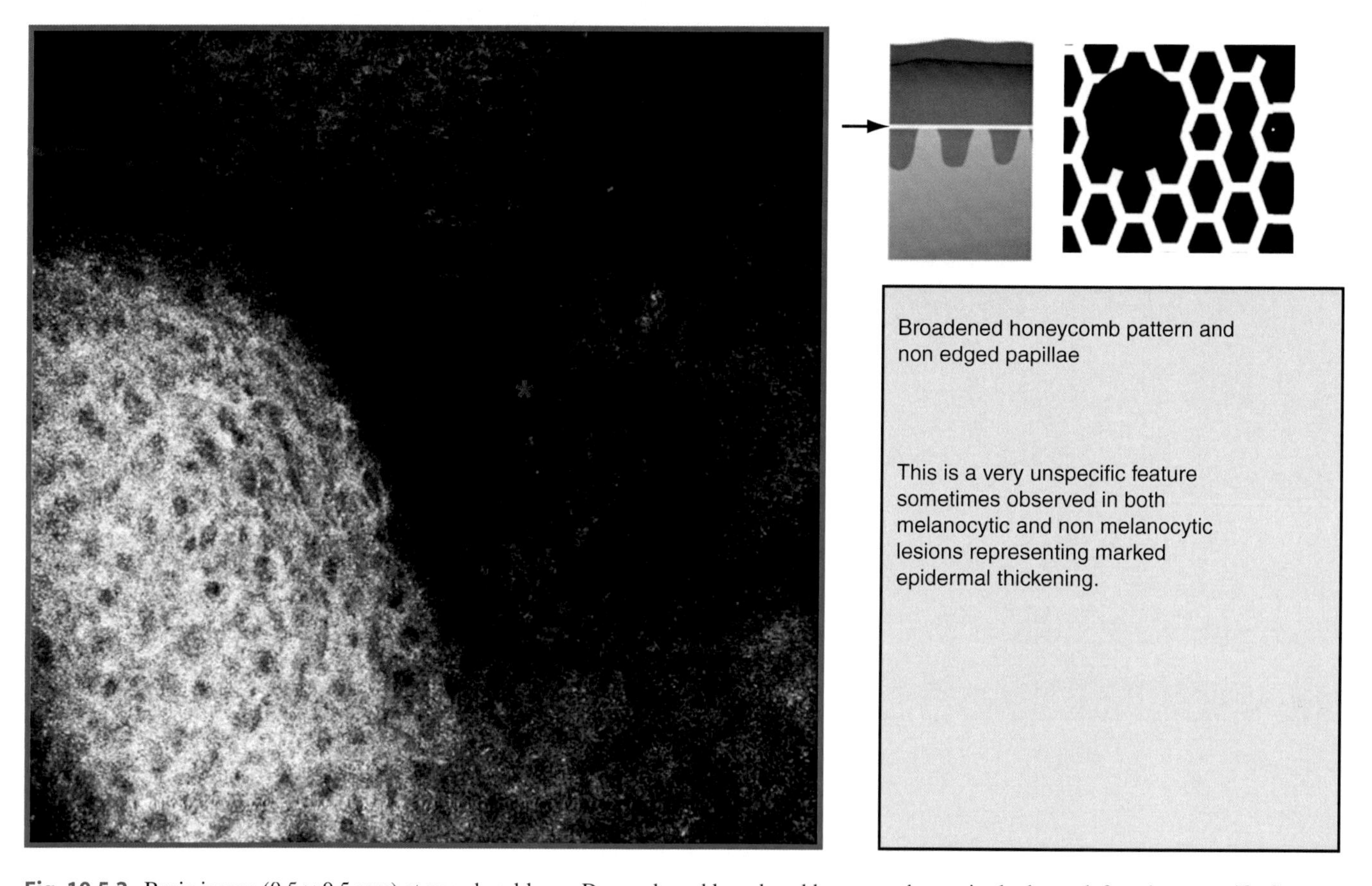

Fig. 10.5.2 Basic image (0.5 × 0.5 mm) at suprabasal layer. Dome-shaped broadened honeycomb area in the lower left and nonspecific features with a nonedge papilla are present (*). Single or nested melanocytes are nondetectable at this resolution

Core Messages

- A RCM diagnosis of Spitz nevus can only be rendered if the DEJ can be clearly visualized.
- In most cases, starburst and globular Spitz nevi have distinctive RCM correlates confirming the dermoscopic diagnosis.
- In atypical presentations, RCM does not add any significant input to the diagnosis.

References

1. Ackerman AB, Magana-Garcia M (1990) Naming acquired melanocytic nevi. Am J Dermatopathol 12:193–209
2. Barnhill RL (2006) The Spitzoid lesion: rethinking Spitz tumors, atypical variants, 'Spitzoid melanoma' and risk assessment. Mod Pathol 19:S21–S33
3. Ferrara G, Argenziano G, Soyer HP, Chimenti S, Di Blasi A, Pellacani G et al (2005) The spectrum of Spitz nevi: a clinicopathologic study of 83 cases. Arch Dermatol 141:1381–1387
4. Pellacani G, Cesinaro AM, Grana C, Seidenari S (2004) In vivo confocal scanning laser microscopy of pigmented Spitz nevi: comparison of in vivo confocal images with dermoscopy and routine histopathology. J Am Acad Dermatol 51:371–376
5. Pellacani G, Cesinaro AM, Seidenari S (2000) Morphological features of Spitz nevus as observed by digital videomicroscopy. Acta Derm Venereol 80:117–121
6. Argenziano G, Scalvenzi M, Staibano S, Brunetti B, Piccolo D, Delfino M et al (1999) Dermatoscopic pitfalls in differentiating pigmented Spitz naevi from cutaneous melanomas. Br J Dermatol 141:788–793
7. Pellacani G, Guitera P, Longo C, Avramidis M, Seidenari S, Menzies S (2007) The impact of in vivo reflectance confocal microscopy for the diagnostic accuracy of melanoma and equivocal melanocytic lesions. J Invest Dermatol 127:2759–2765
8. Pellacani G, Longo C, Ferrara G, Cesinaro AM, Bassoli S, Guitera P, Menzies SW, Seidenari S (2009) Spitz nevi: in vivo confocal microscopic features, dermoscopic aspects, histopathologic correlates and diagnostic significance. J Am Acad Dermatol 60(2):236–247

11 In Vivo Confocal Reflectance Microscopy of Congenital Melanocytic Nevi

Pantea Hashemi, Ashfaq A. Marghoob, Harold S. Rabinovitz, and Alon Scope

The presence of congenital melanocytic nevi (CMN) is determined in utero. CMN are neural crest-derived malformations, composed mainly of a benign proliferation of melanocytes. The most common method for the classification of CMN is based upon nevus size. Small CMN are defined as smaller than 1.5 cm in diameter, medium-sized CMN are 1.5–19.9 cm, large CMN are over 20 cm in diameter, and very large (i.e., giant CMN) are over 50 cm in diameter. Rational for the size-based classification is that there is an increased risk of developing melanoma, a larger cosmetic impact and a greater surgical complexity with increasing size of CMN. In addition, large and giant CMN are often intermixed with various other neural crest-derived elements such as neural tissue and may be associated with extra-cutaneous malformations such as neurocutaneous melanocytosis, dandy-walker malformation, and vascular anomalies [1]. While the risk of melanoma, as well as other rare tumors, is clinically correlated with the size of the CMN, size could simply be a surrogate for the biologic characteristics of the CMN which include the burden, degree of maturation, and depth of penetration of the melanocytes. Although most CMN are visible at birth, some may not become apparent until a variable period of time after birth; these nevi are considered tardive CMN [2].

Congenital nevi have been reported in 0.2–2.1% of newborn infants [3–5]. The vast majority are small and only one neonate per 20,000 has nevi larger than 20 cm in diameter [6]. Small CMN tend to be elevated lesions, with a mammillated surface, round to oval shape, sharply defined borders and hypertrichosis. Clinical distinction of small CMN from acquired nevi, whose presence is determined during postnatal life, often proves to be a futile exercise since the clinical, dermoscopic and histopathologic features of tardive CMN and acquired nevi overlap greatly. However, as a general rule, the larger the nevus and the earlier it becomes apparent on the skin, the greater the likelihood that it is a true CMN.

On dermoscopy, the five dominant dermoscopic patterns seen in CMN are reticular (patchy or diffuse), globular, reticular-globular (complex), diffuse homogenous brown pigmentation with or without sparsely distributed network or globules, and the multi-component pattern. Interestingly, dermoscopic patterns of CMN correlate with anatomic location. CMN on the extremities tend to be reticular in pattern, while those on the head, neck and trunk tend to be globular. Besides classic network and globules, other dermoscopic structures seen in CMN include hypertrichosis, milia-like cysts, perifollicular hypo- or hyper-pigmentation, cobblestone globules, target network, target globules, and blood vessels [7–9].

On histopathology, CMN fulfill general criteria for nevus including symmetric silhouette, sharp lateral circumscription, and "maturation" of nests and nuclei of melanocytes with progressive descent into the dermis. Histopathologic features that generally categorize a nevus as having congenital pattern include (1) melanocytes splaying between collagen bundles of the reticular dermis as single cells or as cords of cells; (2) extension of melanocytes around and within hair follicles, erector pili muscles, sebaceous glands, eccrine glands, blood vessels and nerves; (3) in large CMN, the presence

P. Hashemi (✉)
Dermatology Service, Memorial Sloan-Kettering Cancer Center, New York, NY, USA
e-mail: panteahashemi@gmail.com

A.A. Marghoob
Dermatology Service, Memorial Sloan-Kettering Cancer Center, Suffolk, Hauppauge, NY, USA
e-mail: marghooa@mskcc.org

H.S. Rabinovitz
Skin and Cancer Associates/ADM, Plantation, FL, USA
e-mail: harold@admcorp.com

A. Scope
Department of Dermatology, Sheba Medical Center, Ramat Gan, Israel
e-mail: scopea1@gmail.com

R. Hofmann-Wellenhof et al. (eds.), *Reflectance Confocal Microscopy for Skin Diseases*,
DOI 10.1007/978-3-642-21997-9_11, © Springer-Verlag Berlin Heidelberg 2012

Table 11.1 Key RCM features of CMN and their respective histologic and dermoscopic correlates

RCM features	Definition	Histologic correlate	Dermoscopic correlate
Dark holes or fissures	Roundish and linear structures, respectively, with lower refractivity than surrounding surface epidermis	Keratin-filled surface invagination	
Corneal cysts	Well-circumscribed large, round, highly refractive intra-epidermal structures	Horn pseudocysts	Milia-like cysts
Edged papillae	Dermal papillae demarcated by a rim of bright cells, giving the appearance of bright rings	Pigmented basal keratinocytes and melanocytes along the rete ridges	Pigment network
White papillae	Dermal papillae with a brighter content than in normal skin, however discrete nests and cells are not apparent. A "targetoid" appearance may be seen when dark areas are present at the center of the bright papilla	Brightness is thought to be due to the presence of melanocytes and/or melanophages within the papillary dermis	Fuzzy globules
Dense clusters expanding the dermal papillae	Compact aggregates of bright cells expanding and filling the dermal papillae	Dermal nests	Cobblestone globules

of melanocytes within the lower two-thirds of the dermis, and at times, the subcutaneous fat and deeper soft tissues [5, 10–12]. Other features may be the presence of terminal follicles and a papillated surface epidermis. The enumerated features can also be seen in nevi that appeared later in childhood, hence the term "nevus with congenital features" [13].

The risk of melanoma arising in association with CMN is well established but the exact rates vary based on nevus size, anatomic location and between publications. A recent review comparing the results of 14 studies with age-matched data from the Surveillance, Epidemiology and End Results database has estimated that patients with CMN carry approximately 465-fold increased relative risk of melanoma [14]. In large CMN, specifically, the absolute risk of melanoma has been estimated to be up to 10%. In general, small CMN are managed like any other type of small nevus, i.e. excision when suspicion arises based on clinical change or dermoscopic criteria for melanoma. When melanoma arises in association with small CMN, it usually arises at the DEJ where clinical detection via naked eye inspection and dermoscopic evaluation can be helpful in early diagnosis. In contrast, the utility of dermoscopy in evaluating large CMN is limited by the inability to visualize structures below the papillary dermis with dermoscopy; because melanoma in large CMN often arise within the dermis [15], early detection via dermoscopy is difficult. Focal changes in these lager nevi can be detected by patient (or parent) history, comparison to baseline clinical photography, palpation for new nodules and dermoscopy.

Reflectance confocal microscopy (RCM) can be used as an adjuvant in the bedside evaluation of CMN. Like dermoscopy, RCM imaging penetrates only as deep as the superficial dermis and thus RCM is likely to be useful in the evaluation of small CMN, or medium CMN that are flat. In larger CMN, particularly ones that are elevated/nodular, in which melanoma may arise in the dermis, RCM evaluation is less likely to be informative. In essence, the RCM evaluation of CMN is like that of any other nevus, the aim being to distinguish it from melanoma. In this chapter, we will focus on some of the RCM patterns that identify nevi as having congenital features on histopathology (Table 11.1).

At the level of the stratum corneum, a mosaic image may show dark holes and dark fissures, which are roundish and linear structures, respectively, with lower refractivity than surrounding surface epidermis (Fig. 11.1). These correlate with surface invaginations that are sometimes seen in CMN with mammillated surface. Starting from the suprabasal epidermis, CMN will often show "corneal cysts" seen as very bright round structures that maintain their reflectance with deeper imaging (acting like mirrors) (Fig. 11.2); these correlate with milia-like cysts seen on dermoscopy and with horn pseudocysts seen on histopathology. Like other nevus types, the suprabasal epidermis is expected to show a normal honeycomb pattern or normal cobblestone pattern. At the level of the DEJ, the dermal papilla (DP) may be seen on RCM as "edged papillae", with a ring of small bright basal cells around the darker DP (Fig. 11.3); edged papillae are seen on RCM particularly in CMN that show reticulation on dermoscopy. Edged papillae correlate on histopathology with pigmented basal keratinocytes and melanocytes along the rete ridges. Often, CMN show on RCM DP without a rim of bright cell around the DP; these cases will lack reticulation on dermoscopy and will show nonpigmented rete ridges on histopathology. The DP in CMN may appear wider than normal, being expanded by clusters (nests) of melanocytes (Fig. 11.4). These nests may appear as "dense" clusters – bright, compact aggregates of melanocytes. In CMN that show a cobblestone pattern on dermoscopy, the nests will be large on RCM and the DP greatly expanded [16–21] (Fig. 11.4). CMN may also present "white papillae" on RCM, meaning DP with content which is brighter than in normal skin (Fig. 11.5). "White papillae" are seen when dermal nests or aggregates of melanocytes are only mildly refractile [22]; these are seen in CMN that show a homogenous pattern or ill-descript (fuzzy) globules on dermoscopy.

The diameter, shape, and distribution of the dermal papillary rings or of the rete-ridge meshwork tend to appear uniform on RCM in nevi (Fig. 11.6). The presence of cell aggregates along adnexal or vascular structures on RCM can be occasionally seen [23].

Features on RCM that would be concerning for melanoma include the presence of bright nucleated or dendritic cells in pagetoid pattern, i.e. at the level of the suprabasal epidermis; pleomorphism of melanocytes (melanocytes with variable shapes, brightness and size) and the presence of atypical melanocytes in the basal layer. Atypical melanocytes on RCM are defined as nucleated or dendritic cells that are at least twice the size of basal keratinocytes, melanocytes having abnormal shape (like triangular or star shape) or melanocytes with large eccentric nucleus. The presence of large nucleated bright cells, polymorphic in size and shape, within the epidermis spreading upward in a pagetoid fashion appears to be a reliable RCM feature of melanoma [24]. However, the presence of melanocytes in a pagetoid pattern is not specific for melanoma, since melanocytes in a pagetoid pattern can be found in some CMN, spitz nevi, acral nevi, inflamed nevi or recurrent nevi [25–27]. Diagnosis of melanoma is favored when pagetoid spread is diffuse and involves the uppermost levels of the epidermis and lateral borders of the tumor. Nevi, on the other hand, show focal pagetoid spread of melanocytes (Fig. 11.1) and absence of cellular atypia [25–27]. In addition, Langerhans cells may appear as dendritic cells on RCM and may be difficult to distinguish from dendritic melanocytes [28]. Therefore, at present, RCM findings such as nucleated or dendritic cells in pagetoid pattern should be considered worrisome, particularly since histopathologic criteria such as maturation of melanocytes with descent into the dermis cannot be evaluated with RCM due to limitation in the imaging depth.

In summary, there are RCM features that suggest a congenital nevus pattern on histopathology. Given the depth limitation, RCM is useful as an adjuvant tool in the differentiation of small or flat CMN from melanoma within the context of the patient's history, lesion stability over time, palpation and dermoscopic features. Improvements in the penetration, resolution and possible combination with other imaging modalities may allow for better diagnostic accuracy in the near future [29].

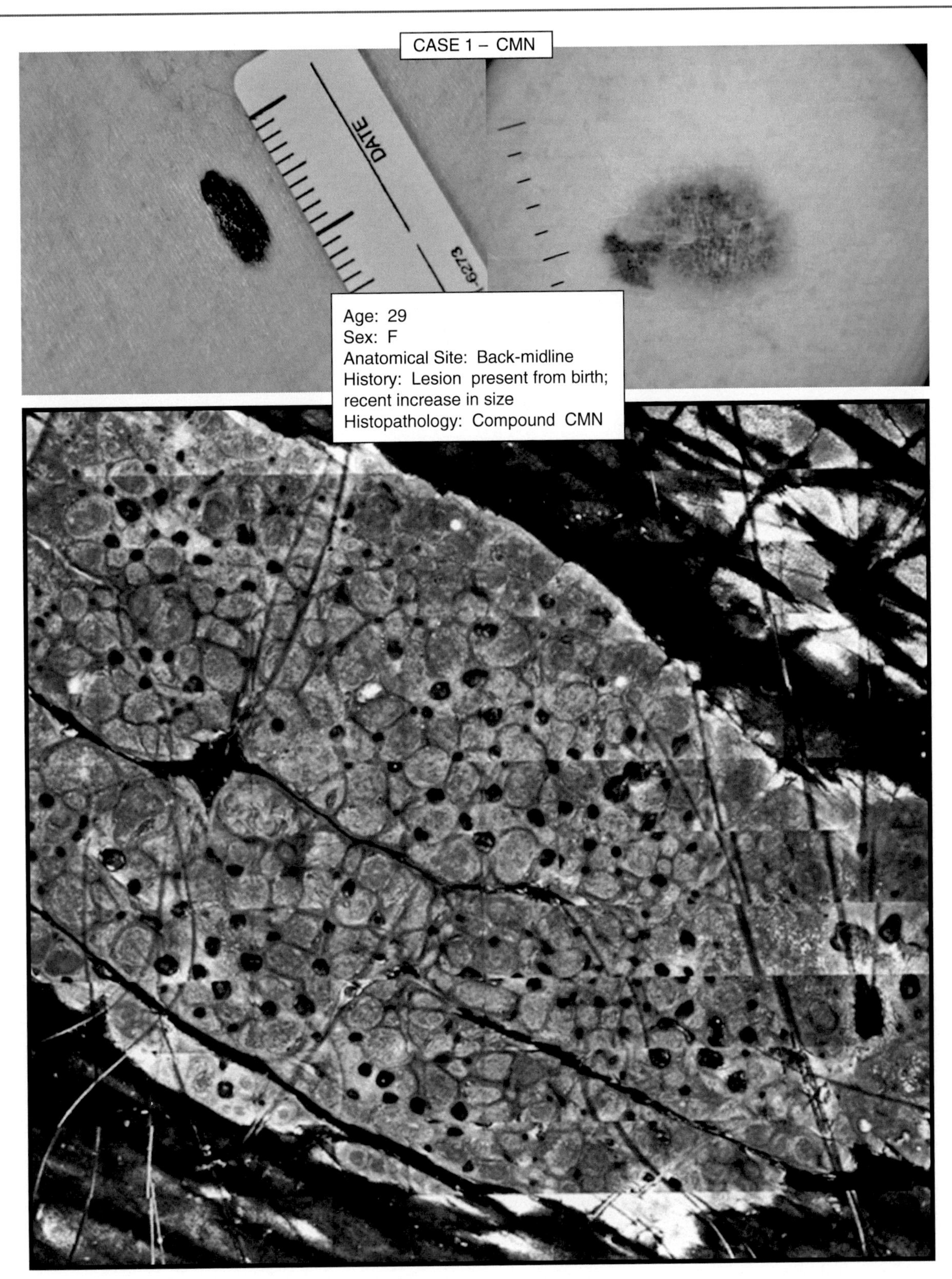

Fig. 11.1 RCM mosaic (6×6 mm) at suprabasal layer showing a clod pattern made of projections of large round and oval refractile structures (clods) separated by less refractile fissures and holes, seen as *dark linear and circular structures*, respectively. The clods correspond to exophytic projections of dermal nests of melanocytes in a papillated congenital nevus. The darker fissures and holes correspond to surface depressions in the epidermis. There are few bright corneal cysts in this mosaic, corresponding to horn pseudocysts

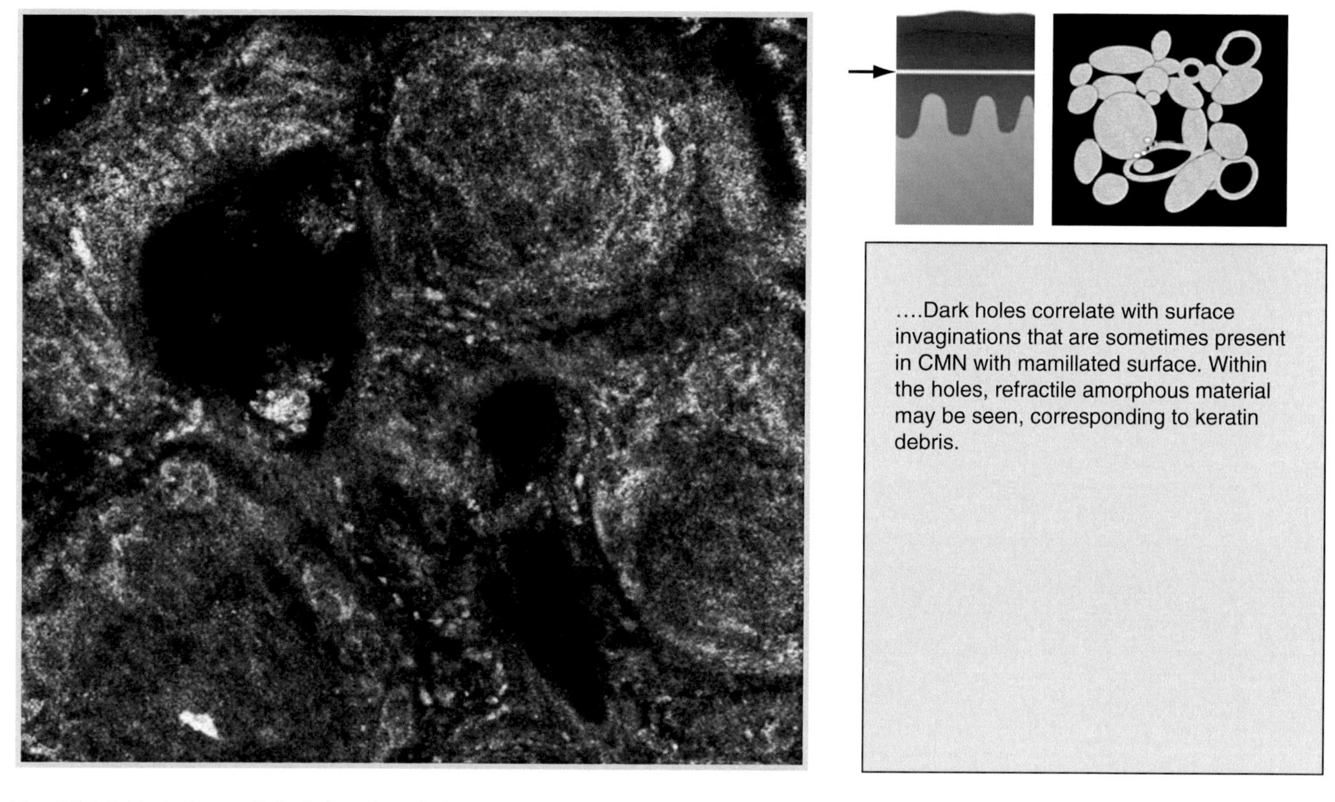

Fig. 11.1.1 Basic image (0.5×0.5 mm) at the level of the suprabasal epidermis depicts several dense clusters that project into the epidermis. The outline of individual cells within these dense clusters is inapparent. Dark holes between the clusters can be seen, corresponding to depressions in the surface epidermis

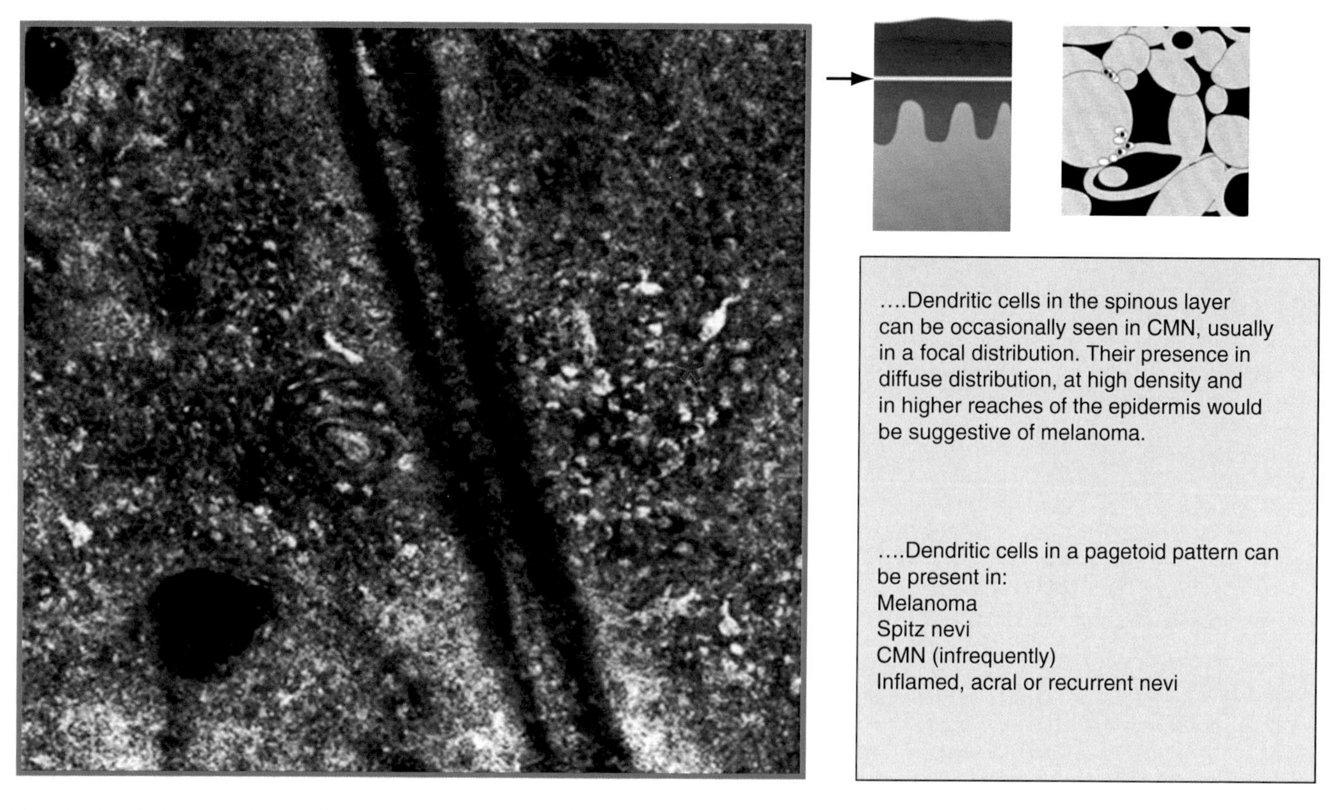

Fig. 11.1.2 Basic image (0.5×0.5 mm) at the spinous layer. Bright nucleated cells, some with dendritic processes can be seen

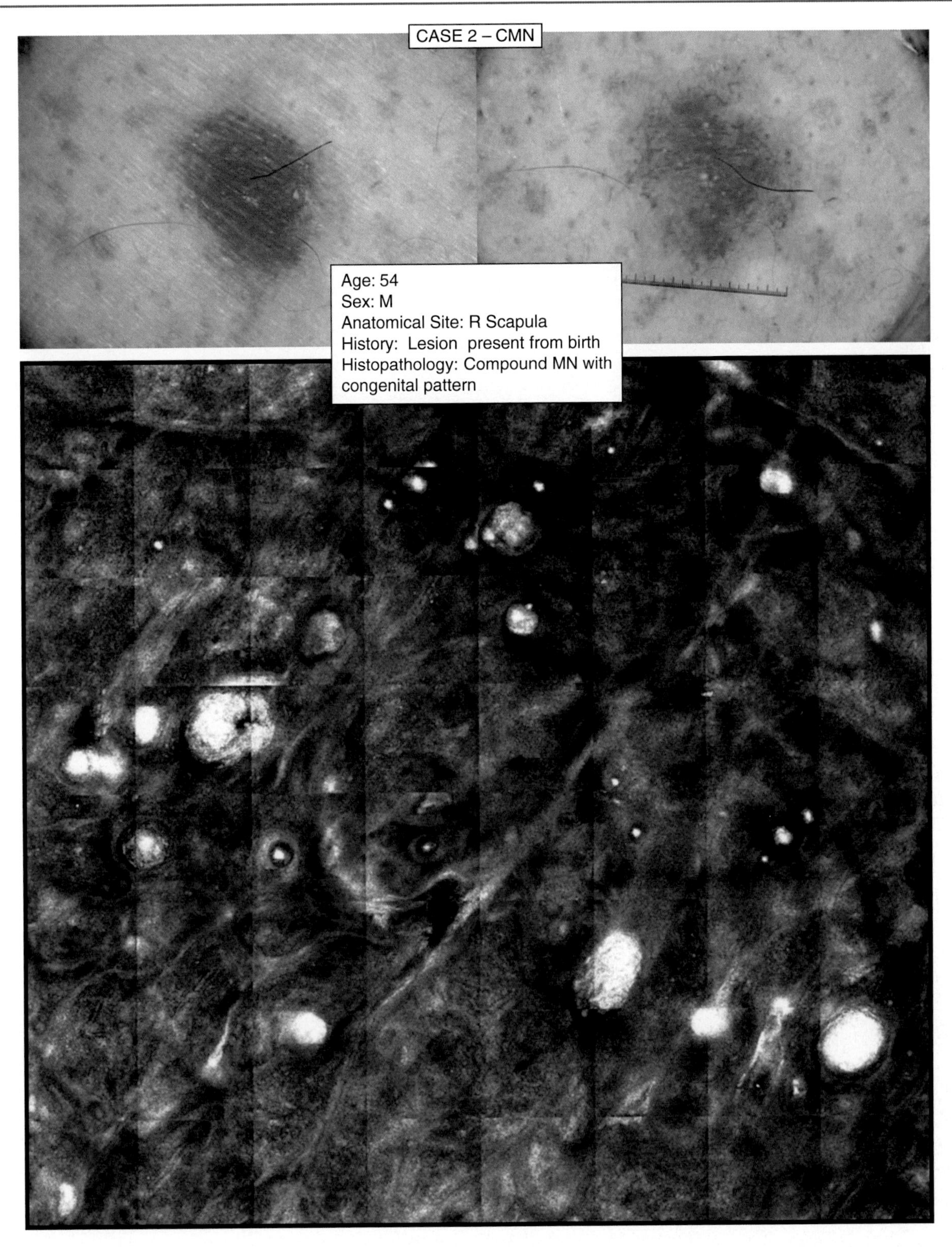

Fig. 11.2 RCM mosaic (4×4) at superficial dermis level reveals several corneal cysts, seen as well-circumscribed large, round to oval, highly refractive structures

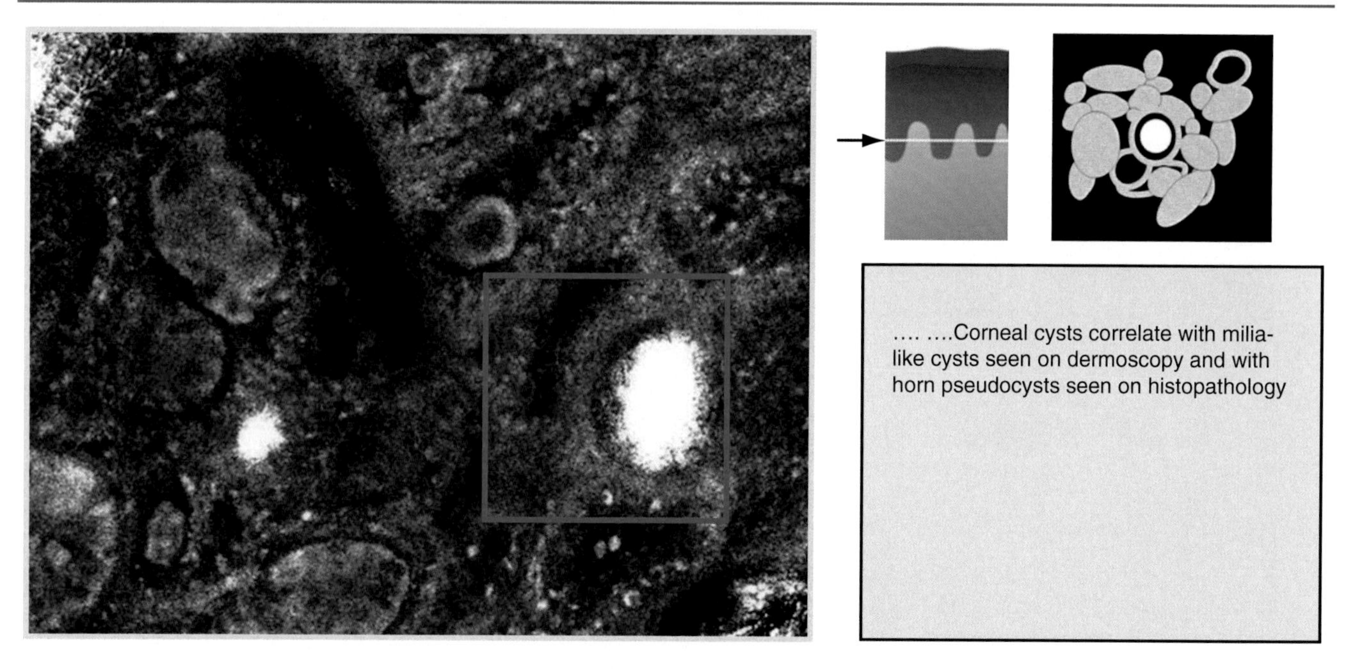

Fig. 11.2.1 Basic image (0.5 × 0.5 mm) at DEJ level showing two corneal cysts, seen as highly refractile structures. In addition, dense clusters (nests) are seen as less refractile polygonal to oval structures within the dermal papillae; these correlate with nests of melanocytes

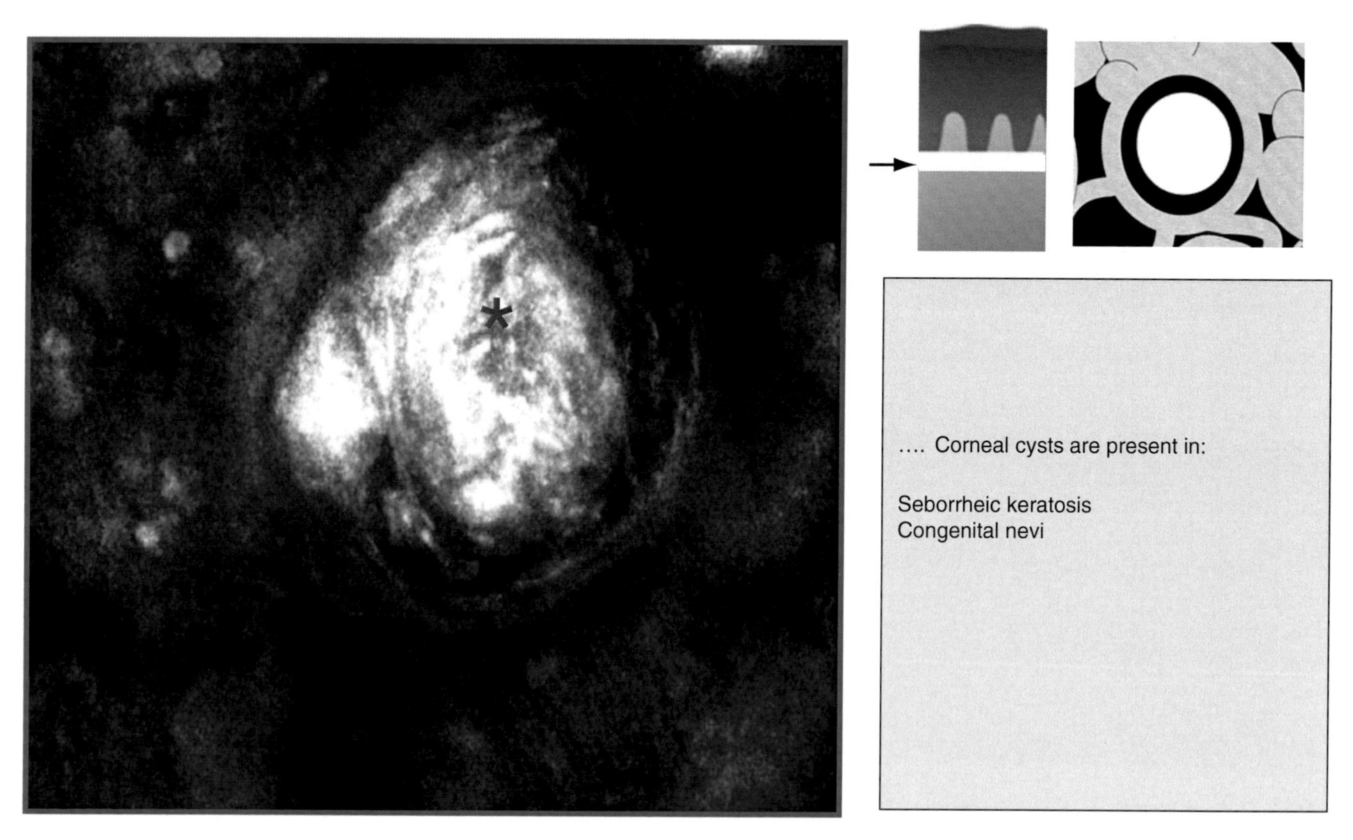

Fig. 11.2.2 Basic image (0.5 × 0.5 mm) at the level of the superficial dermis reveals a corneal cyst which consists of very bright, amorphous material; this correlates with a keratin-filled horn pseudocyst. Corneal cysts act like mirrors on RCM, maintaining high reflectivity even at deeper levels of imaging (*)

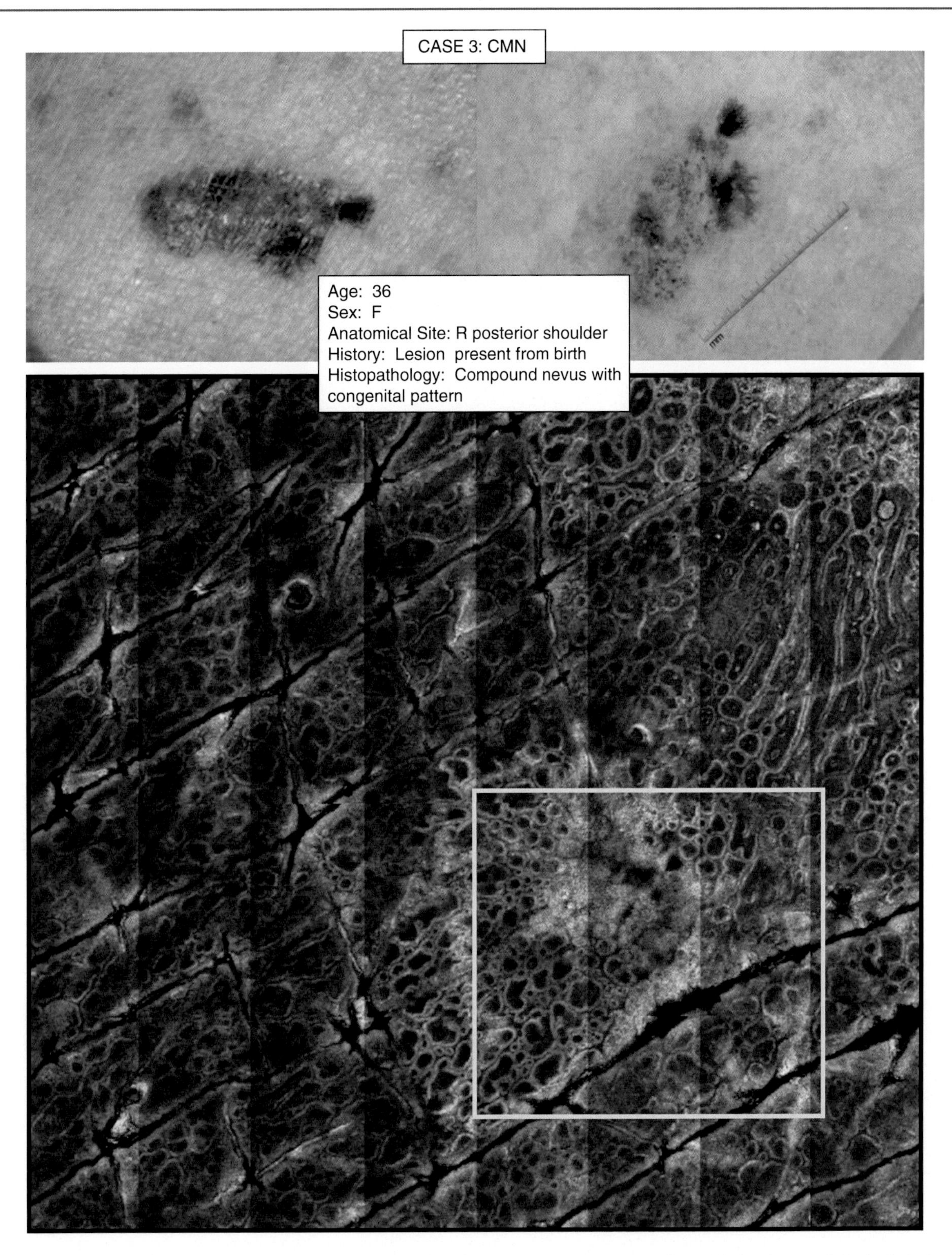

Fig. 11.3 RCM mosaic (4×4 mm) at DEJ level reveals a ringed pattern at the center corresponding with focal network (reticulation) seen on dermoscopy

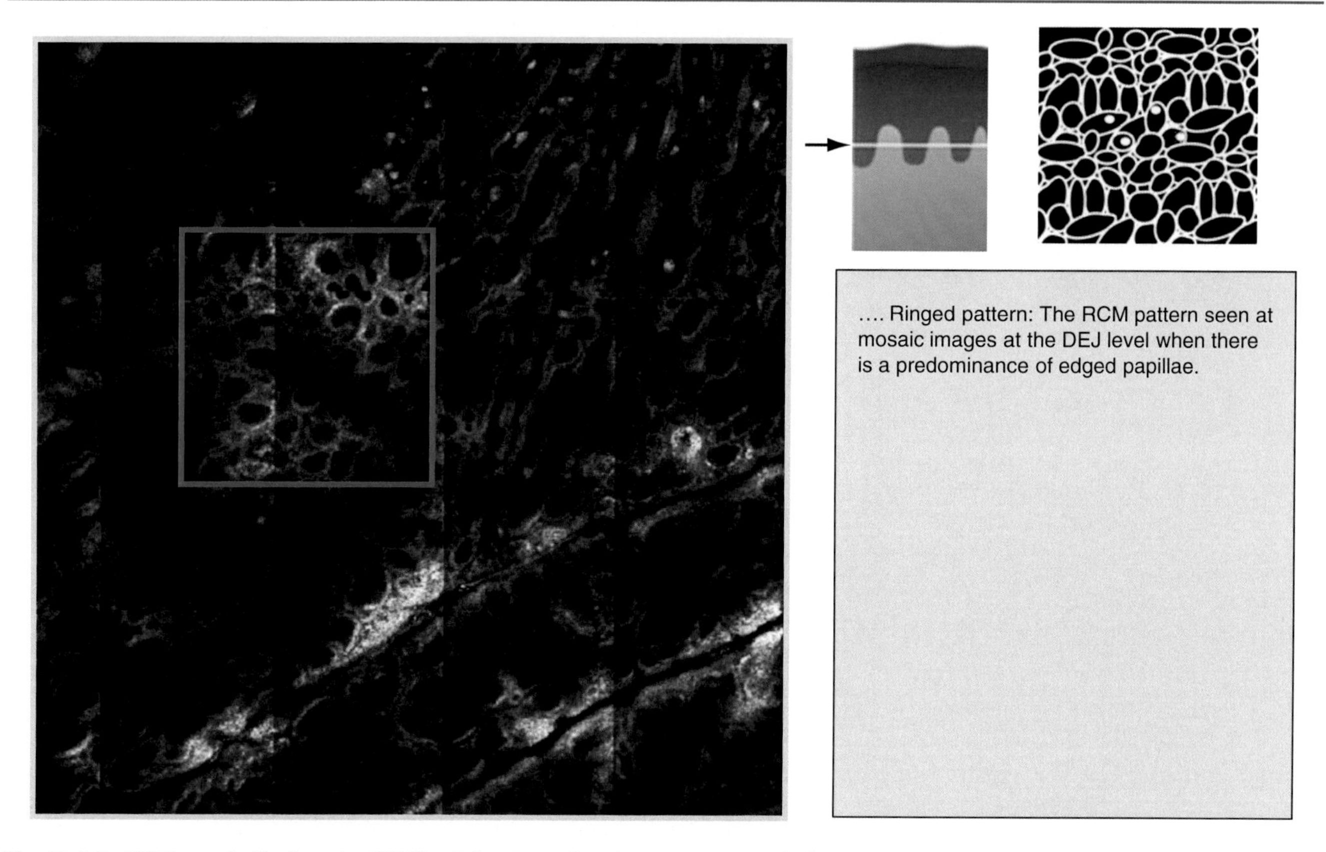

Fig. 11.3.1 RCM mosaic (2×2 mm) at DEJ level showing a ringed pattern composed of edged papillae in the center

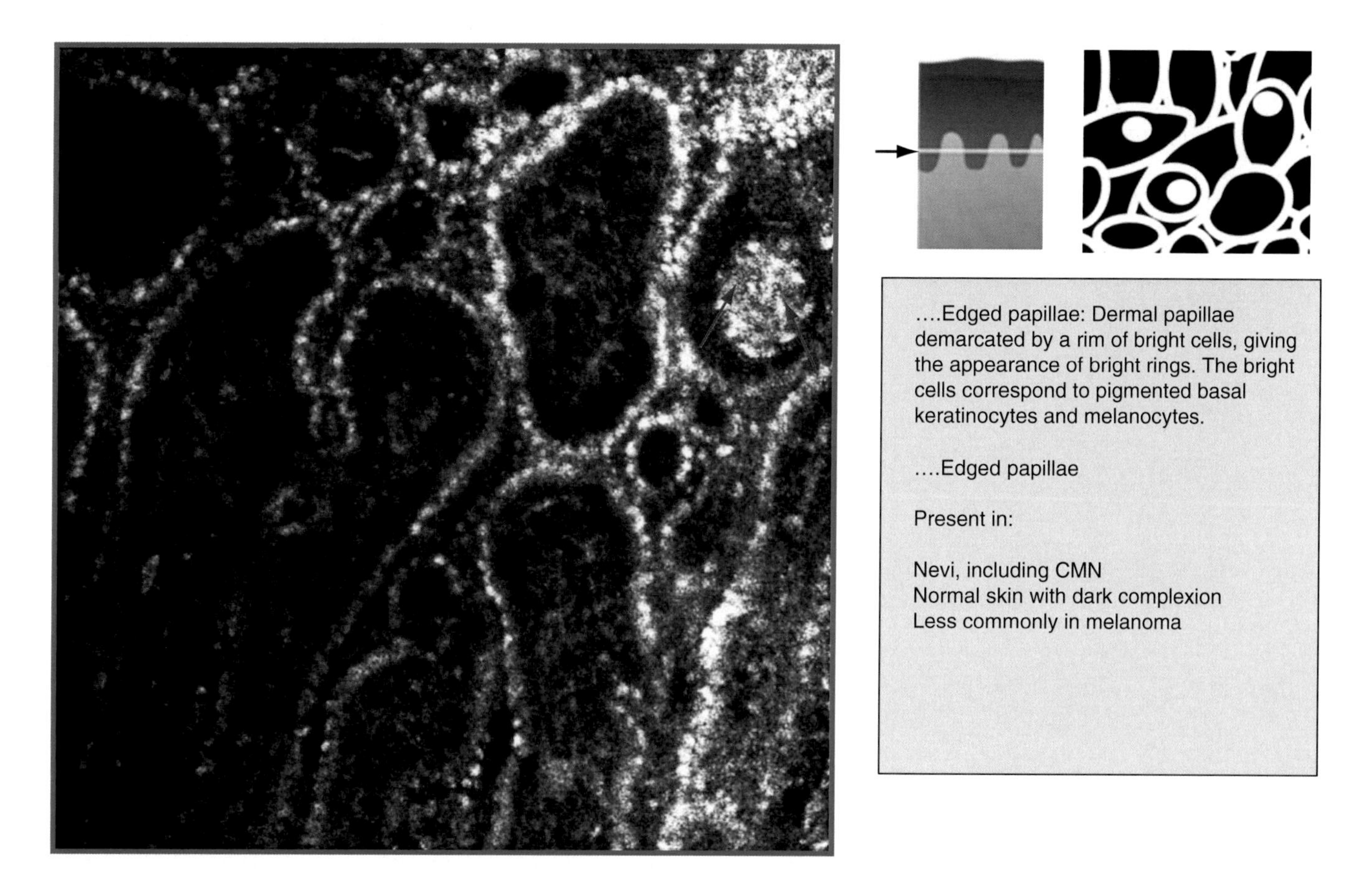

Fig. 11.3.2 Basic image (0.5 × 0.5 mm) disclosing edged papillae lined up by small, roundish, monomorphic cells without apparent nucleus; these correlate with pigmented keratinocytes and small melanocytes along the basal layer of the epidermis. Dense clusters can be seen within dermal papillae (→)

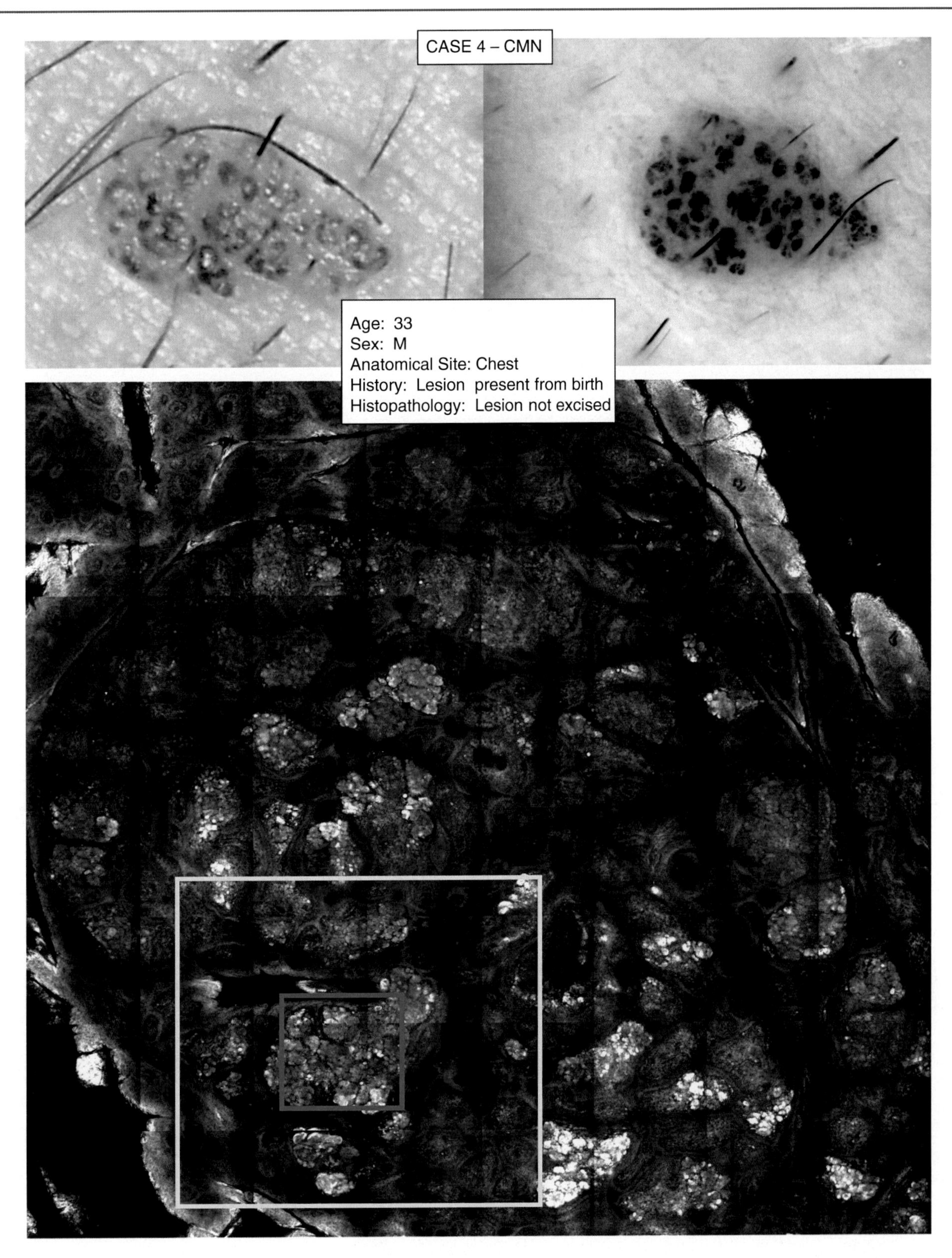

Fig. 11.4 RCM mosaic (4×4 mm) at the level of DEJ showing a clod pattern, composed of bright clusters expanding and filling the dermal papillae

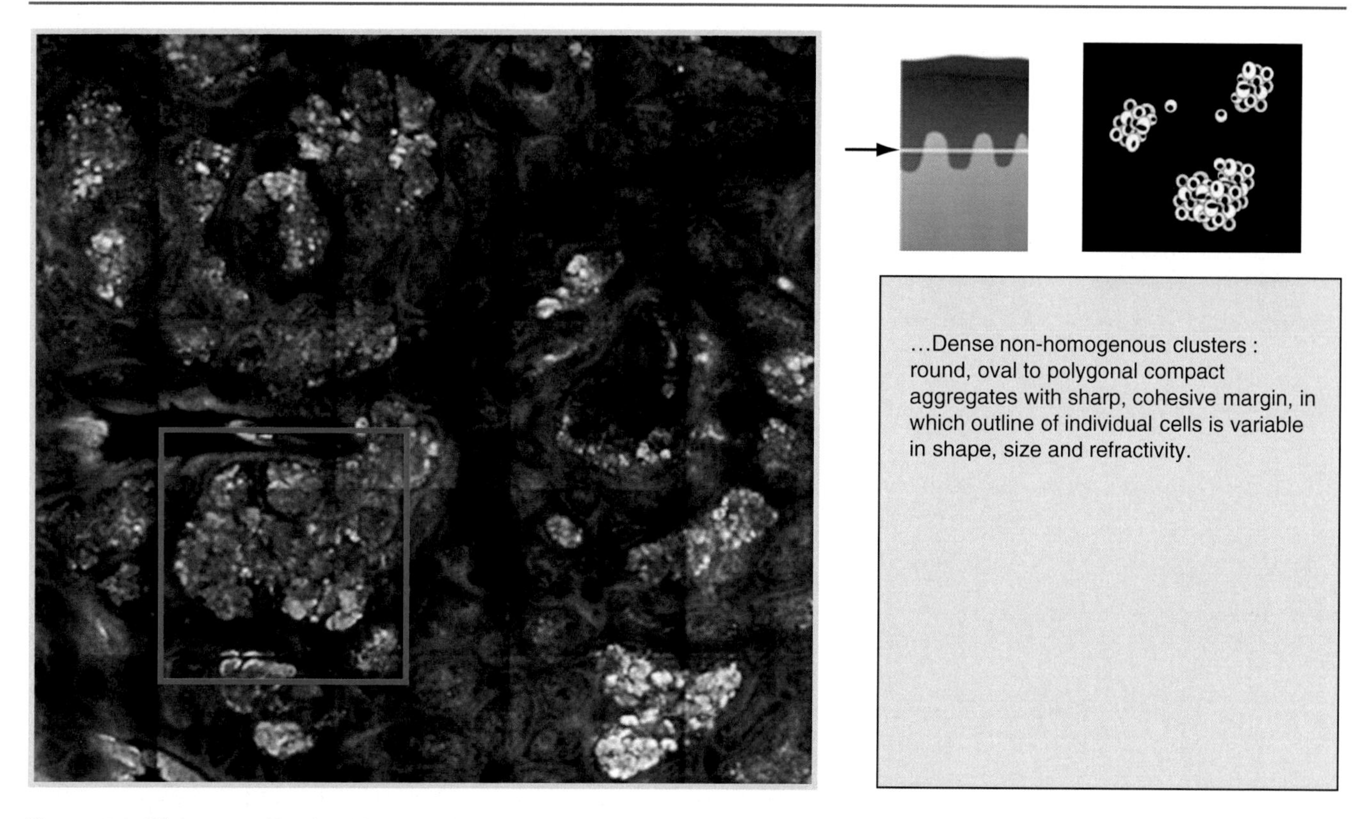

Fig. 11.4.1 Higher magnification RCM mosaic (2.5 × 2.5 mm) at the level of DEJ discloses bright dense clusters composed of cells with variable reflectivity (termed "dense nonhomogenous clusters")

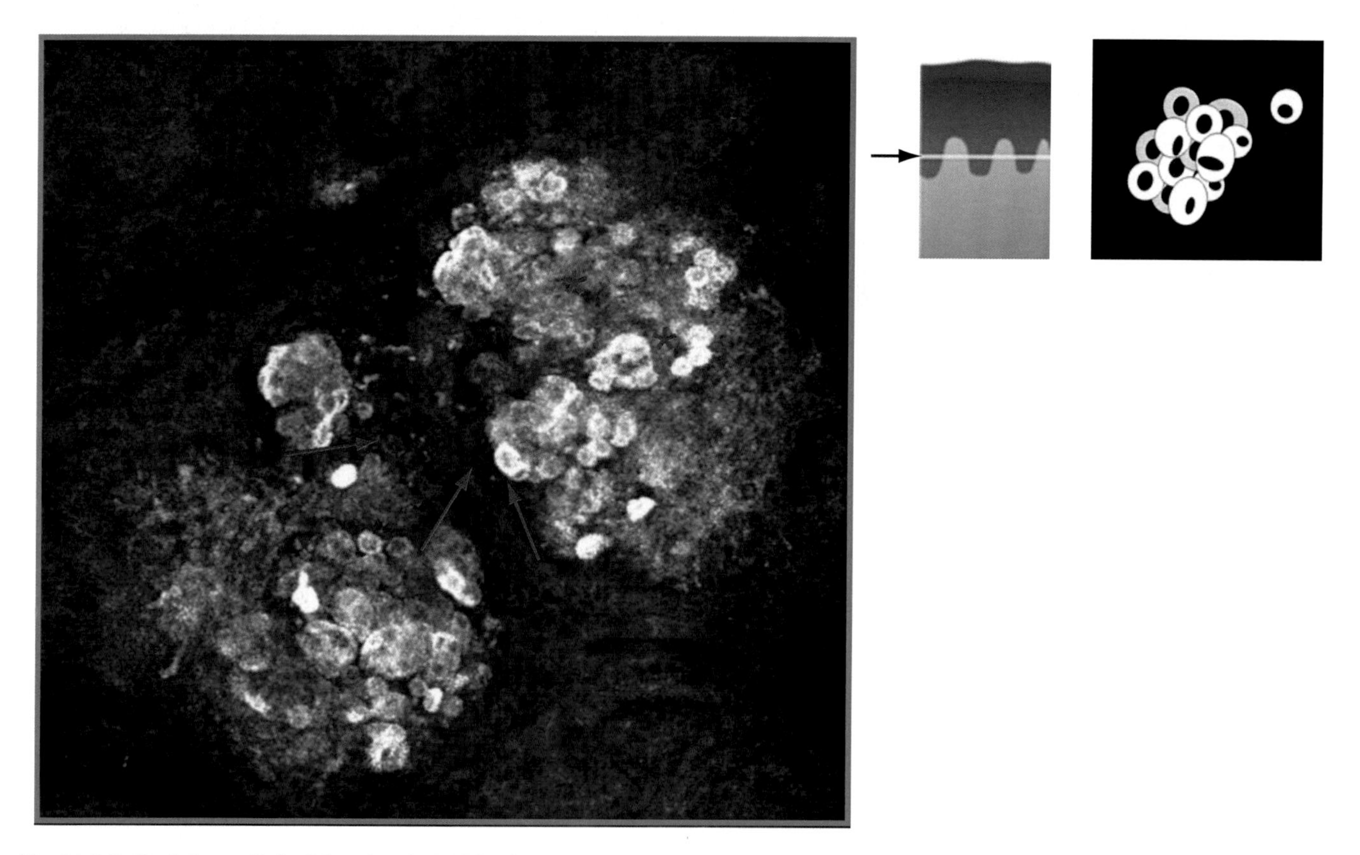

Fig. 11.4.2 Basic image (0.5 × 0.5 mm) at the DEJ level discloses bright round dense nonhomogenous clusters in which individual nucleated cells (melanocytes) of variable brightness can be appreciated. The clusters expand and fill the dermal papillae. They correspond to the globules seen on dermoscopy. The relatively darker spaces between the clusters (→) correspond to the rete ridges

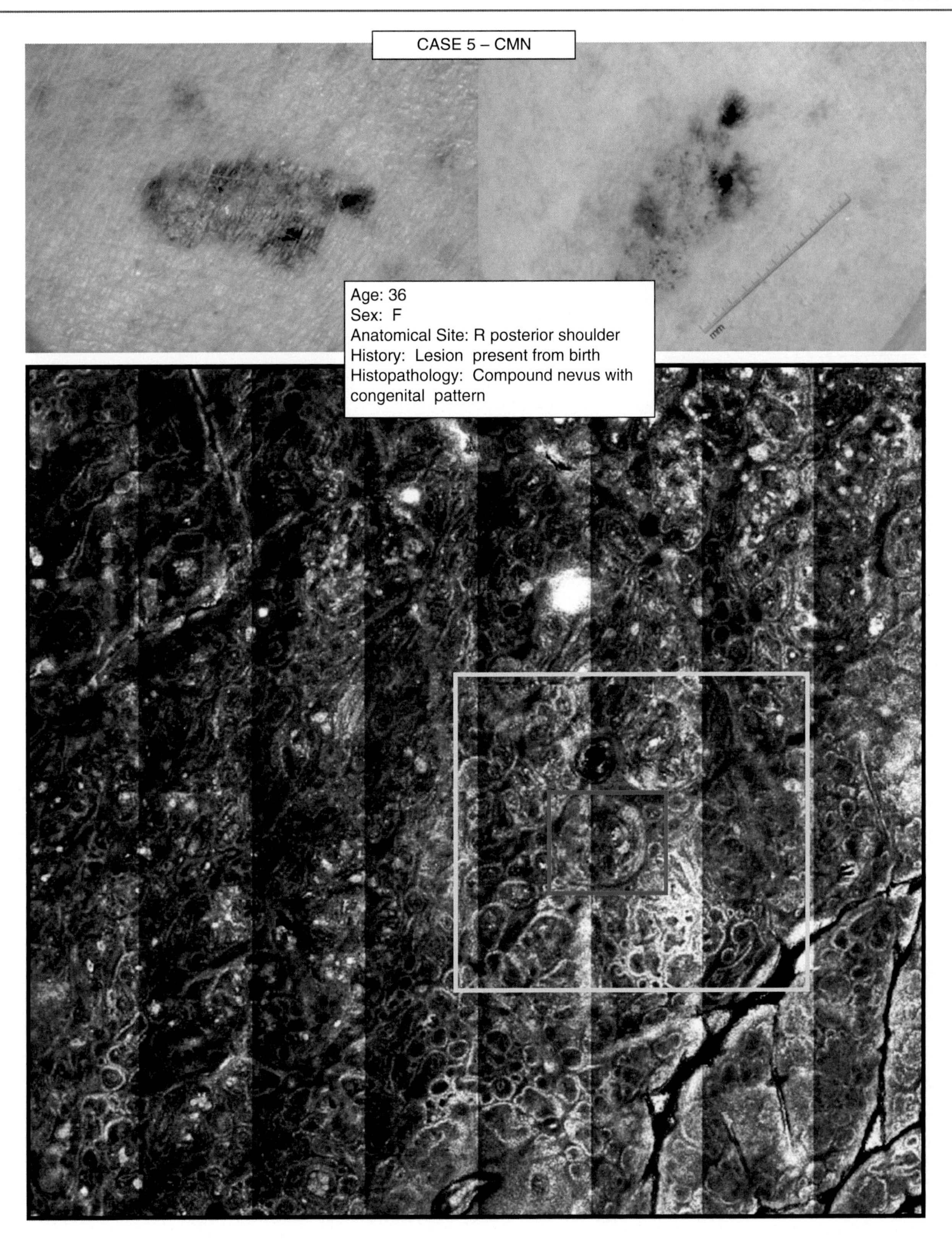

Fig. 11.5 RCM mosaic (4×4 mm) at the DEJ showing areas with clod pattern and other areas showing a ringed pattern. Few very bright corneal cysts can also be seen

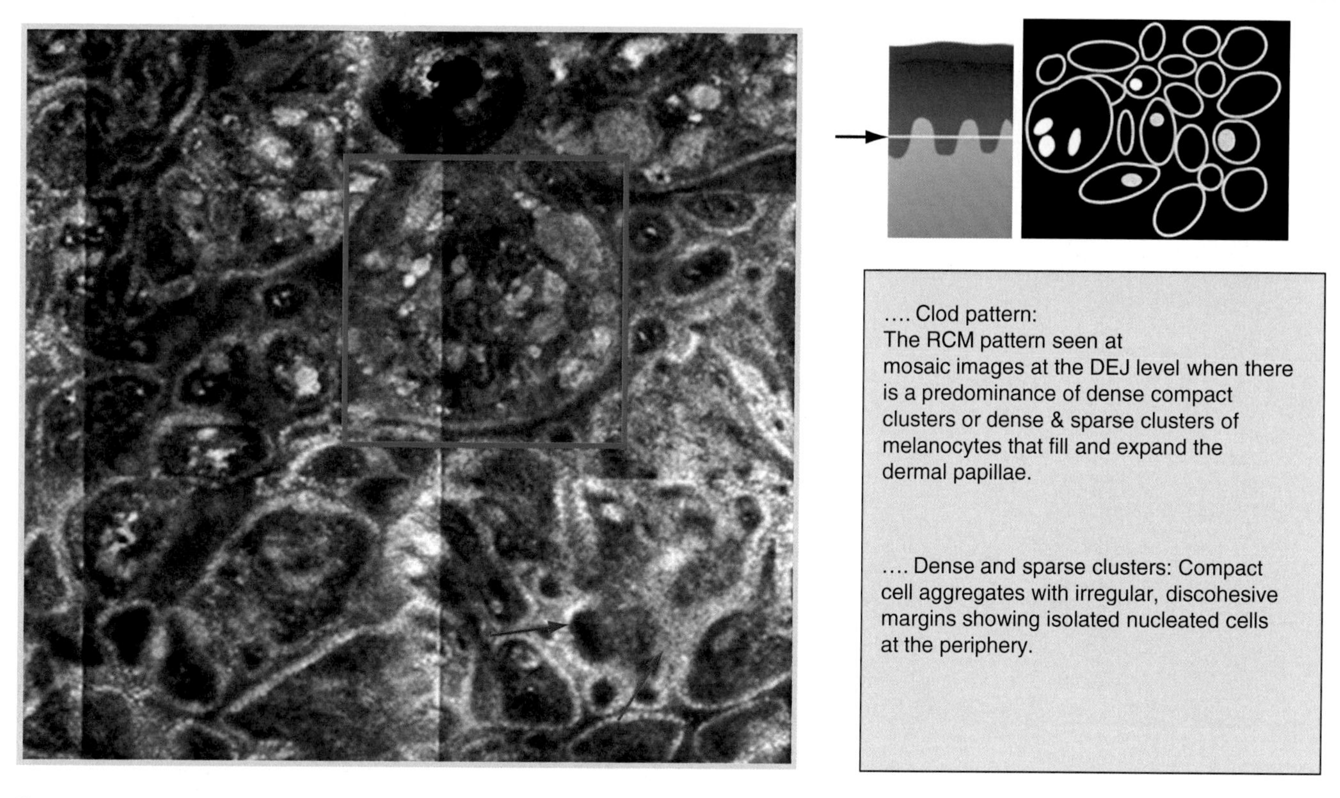

Fig. 11.5.1 RCM mosaic (1 × 1 mm) at DEJ showing that the clod pattern is made of dense and sparse clusters that fill and expand the dermal papillae. In addition, an area with ringed pattern displays edged papillae (*arrow*)

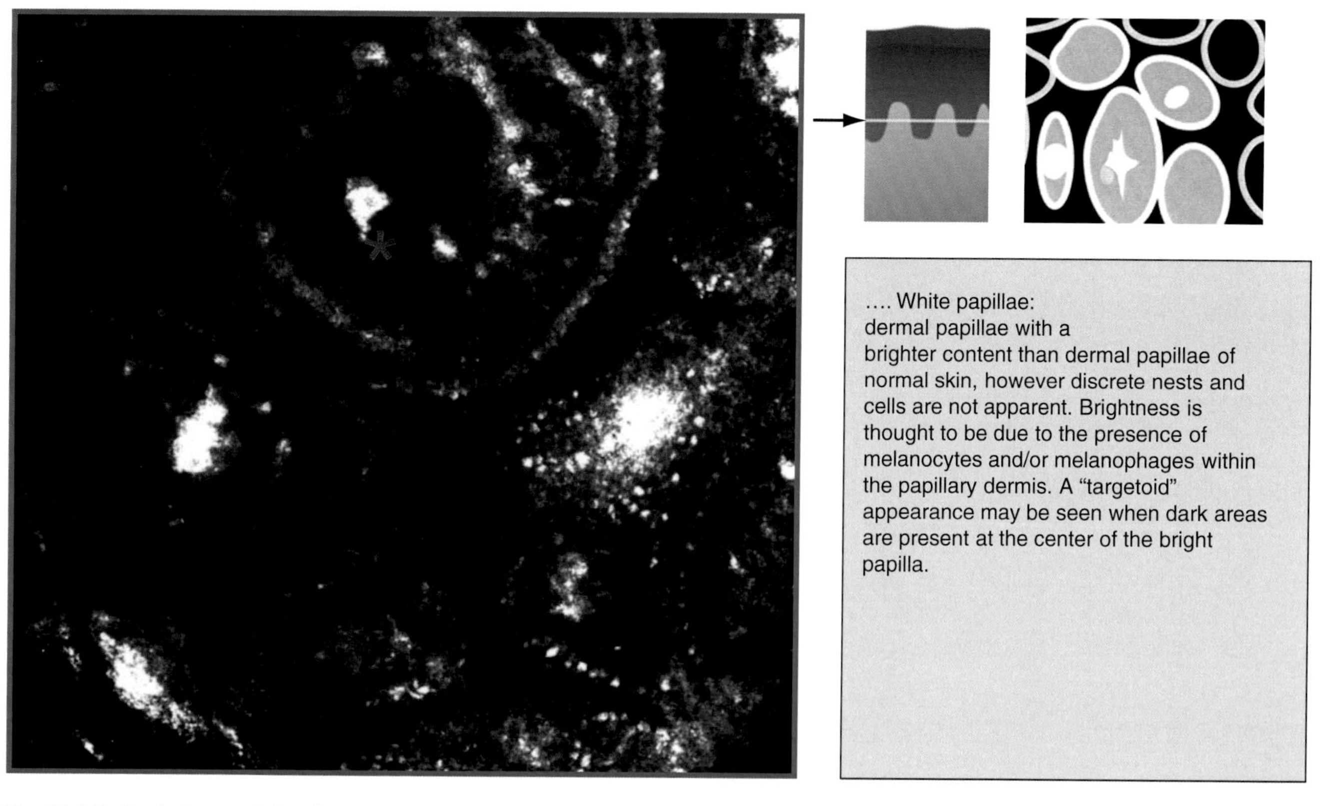

Fig. 11.5.2 Basic image (0.5 × 0.5 mm) at DEJ shows one of the "clods". In this case, the dermal papilla is expanded and appears more refractile than normal, but discrete nests and cells are less apparent. This pattern has been termed "white papillae". Dark round areas can be seen within the refractile papilla, and if central, may give the papilla a "targetoid" appearance (*)

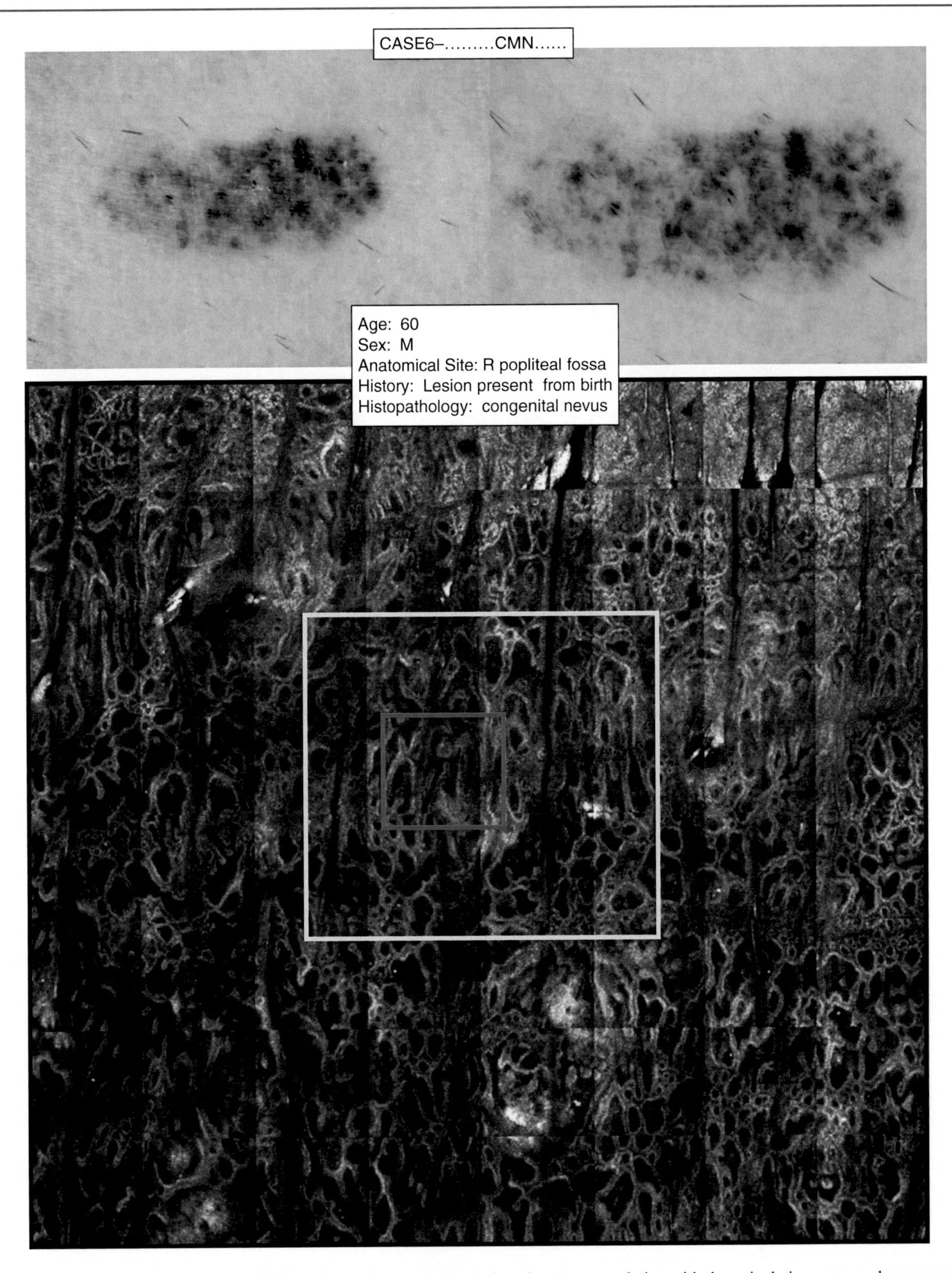

Fig. 11.6 RCM mosaic (4×4 mm) at DEJ level reveals a meshed and ringed pattern correlating with the reticulation seen on dermoscopy

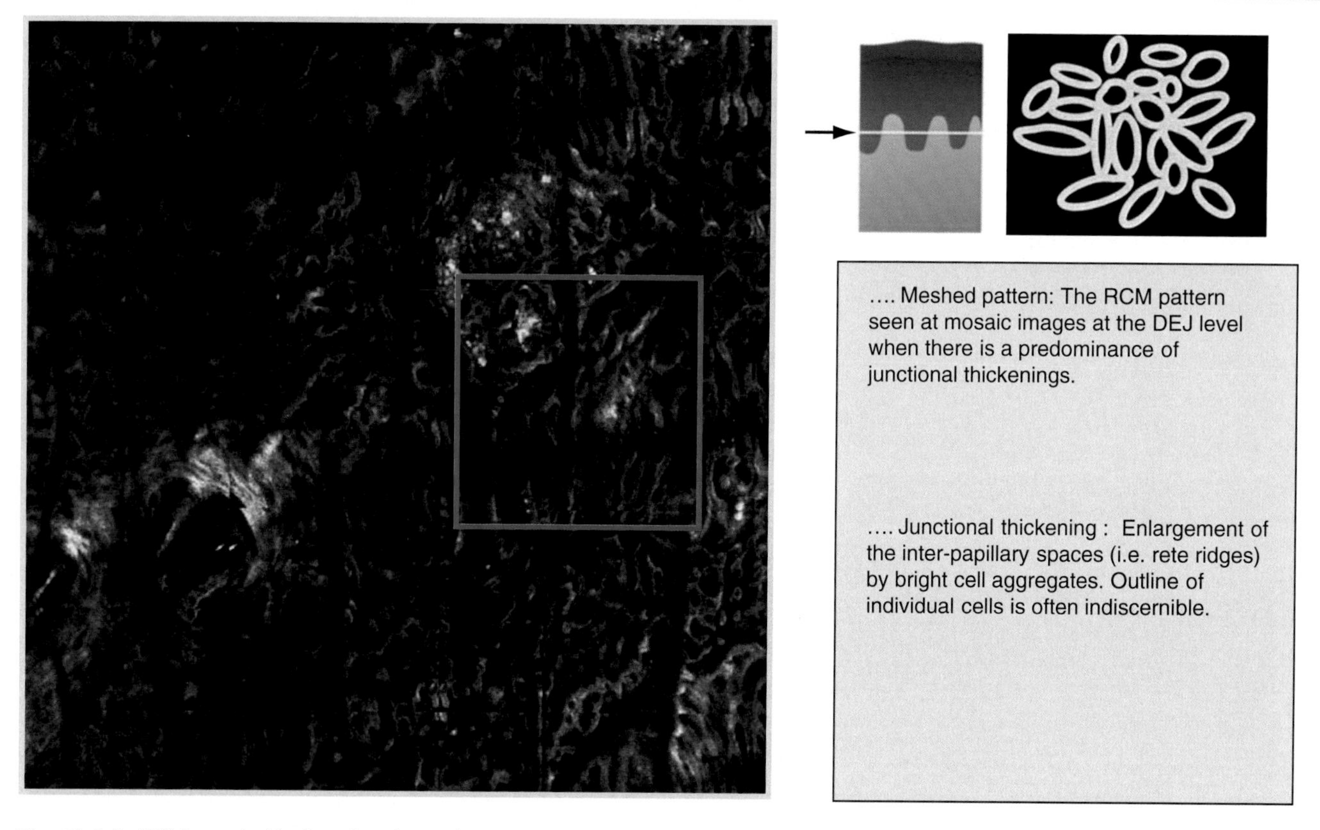

Fig. 11.6.1 RCM mosaic (4×4 mm) at deeper level of the DEJ showing a regular meshed pattern composed of bright interconnected rete ridges separated by darker, round to elongated dermal papillae

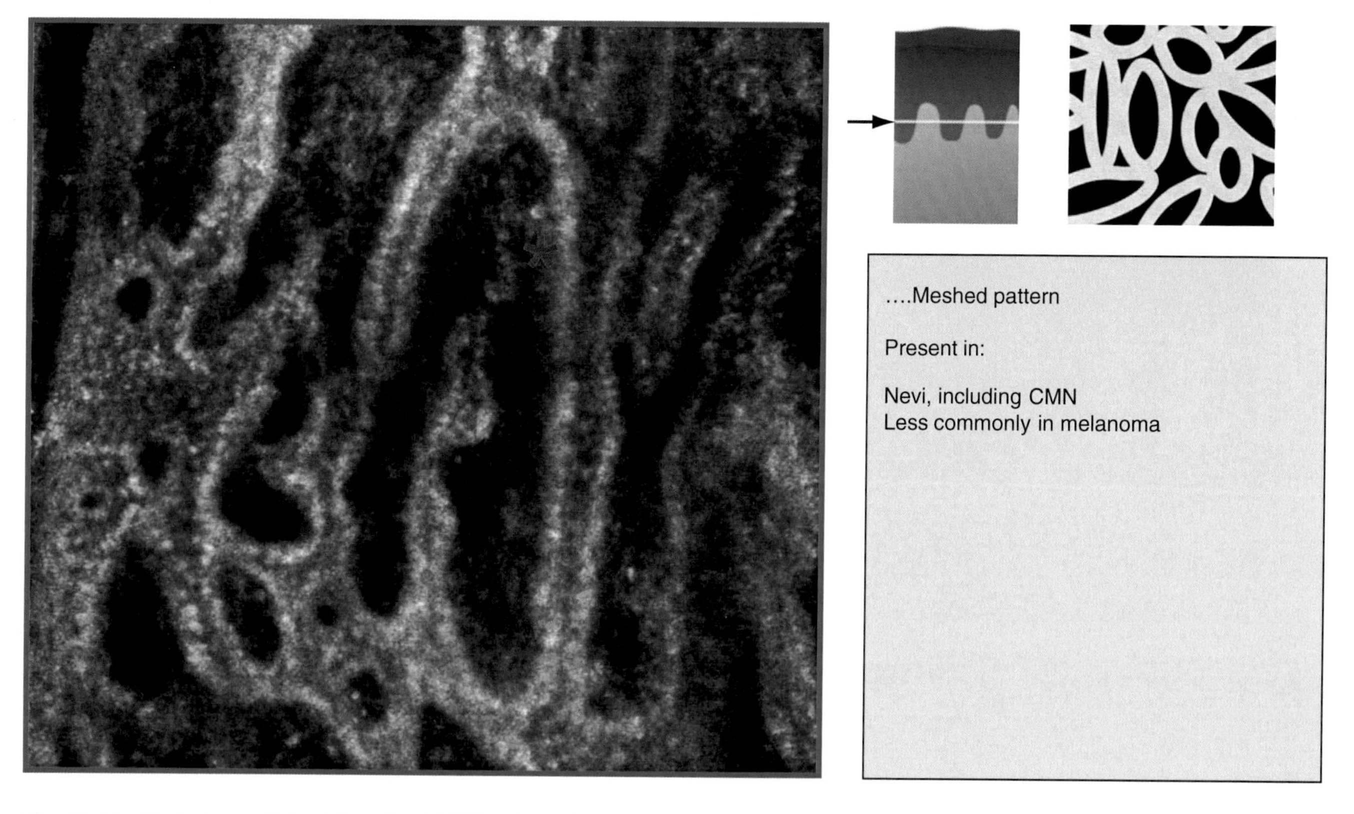

Fig. 11.6.2 Basic image (0.5×0.5 mm) at DEJ level showing edged papillae lined by small, roundish, monomorphic cells without apparent nucleus; these would correlate with pigmented keratinocytes and small melanocytes along the basal layer of the epidermis (*)

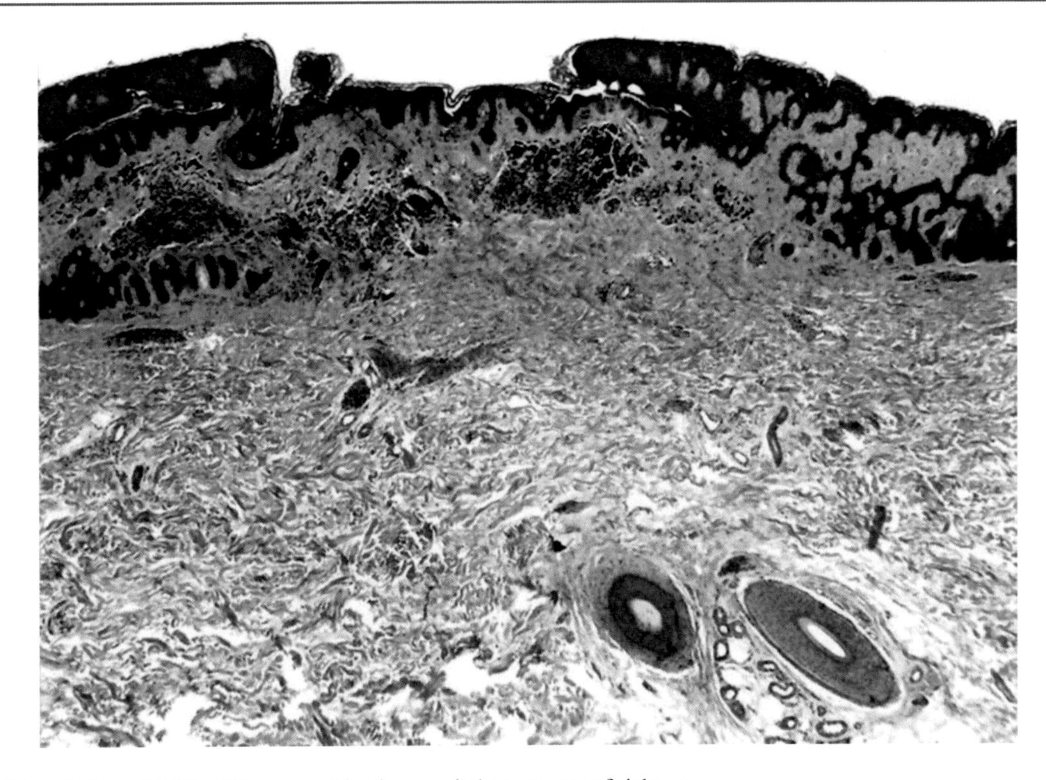

Fig. 11.6.3 Histopathology (H&E, ×50) of a combined congenital nevus, superficial type

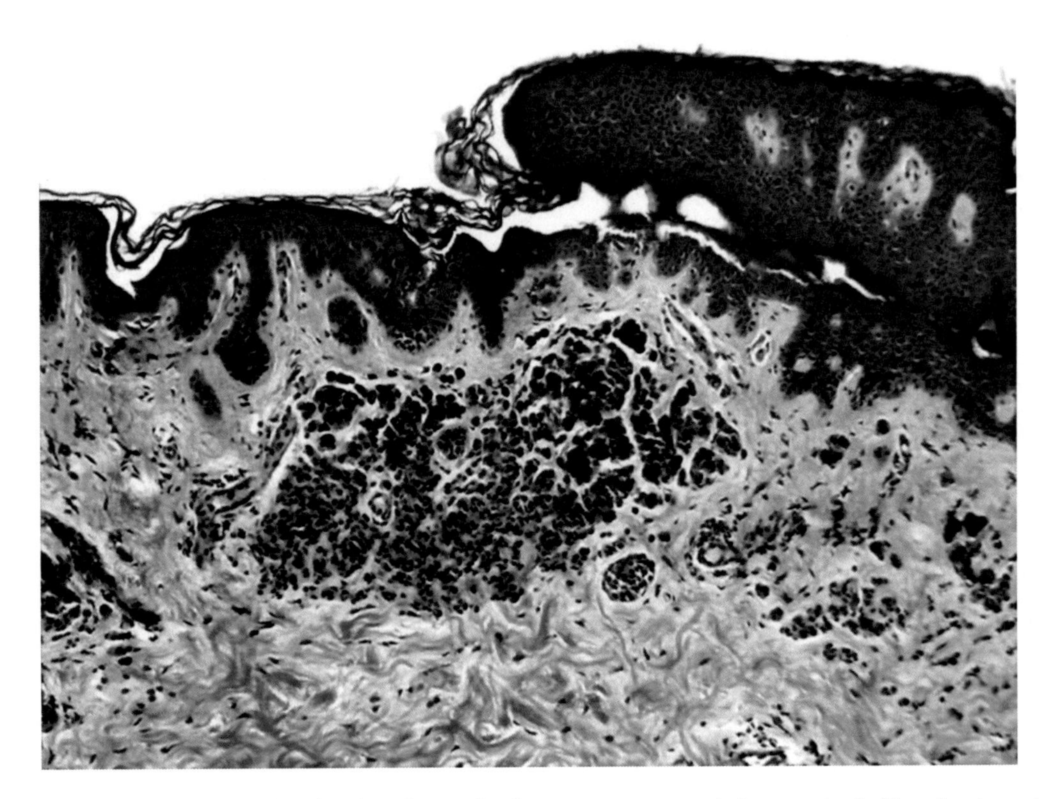

Fig. 11.6.4 Histopathology (H&E, ×100) showing dermal nest of melanocytes, some nests being composed of heavily pigmented melanocytes. Pigmentation of the basal keratinocytes and small melanocytes is apparent; this correlates with the edged-papillae pattern seen on RCM

Core Messages

- RCM imaging is useful in the evaluation of small and flat medium-sized CMN but has limited utility in the evaluation of large CMN.
- Dark holes or fissures, corneal cysts, edged papillae, white papillae, dense clusters of melanocytes filling and expanding the dermal papillae are RCM features suggestive of a congenital nevus.

Acknowledgment We would like to thank Itay Klaz, MD, for his assistance in the preparation of the figures.

References

1. Kopf AW, Bart RS, Hennessey P (1979) Congenital nevocytic nevi and malignant melanomas. J Am Acad Dermatol 1(2):123–130
2. Kinsler VA, Birley J, Atherton DJ (2009) Great Ormond Street Hospital for Children Registry for Congenital Melanocytic Naevi: prospective study 1988–2007. Part 2—Evaluation of treatments. Br J Dermatol 160(2):387–392
3. Berg P, Lindelof B (2002) Congenital nevocytic nevi: follow-up of a Swedish birth register sample regarding etiologic factors, discomfort, and removal rate. Pediatr Dermatol 19(4):293–297
4. Clemmensen OJ, Kroon S (1988) The histology of "congenital features" in early acquired melanocytic nevi. J Am Acad Dermatol 19(4):742–746
5. Walton RG, Jacobs AH, Cox AJ (1976) Pigmentedlesions in newborn infants. Br J Dermatol 95(4):389–396
6. Castilla EE, da Graca Dutra M, Orioli-Parreiras IM (1981) Epidemiology of congenital pigmented naevi: I. Incidence rates and relative frequencies. Br J Dermatol 104(3):307–315
7. Soyer HP et al (2001) Dermoscopy of pigmented skin lesions (Part II). Eur J Dermatol 11(5):483–498
8. Changchien L et al (2007) Age- and site-specific variation in the dermoscopic patterns of congenital melanocytic nevi: an aid to accurate classification and assessment of melanocytic nevi. Arch Dermatol 143(8):1007–1014
9. Marghoob AA, Fu JM, Sachs D (2005) Dermoscopic features of congenital melanocytic nevi. In: Marghoob AA, Braun RP, Kopf AW (eds) Atlas of dermoscopy. Taylor & Francis, Abingdon, pp 141–159
10. Tannous ZS et al (2005) Congenital melanocytic nevi: clinical and histopathologic features, risk of melanoma, and clinical management. J Am Acad Dermatol 52(2):197–203
11. Everett MA (1989) Histopathology of congenital pigmented nevi. Am J Dermatopathol 11(1):11–12
12. Clemmensen O, Ackerman AB (1984) All small congenital nevi need not be removed. Am J Dermatopathol 6(Suppl):189–194
13. Cribier BJ, Santinelli F, Grosshans E (1999) Lack of clinical-pathological correlation in the diagnosis of congenital naevi. Br J Dermatol 141(6):1004–1009
14. Krengel S, Hauschild A, Schafer T (2006) Melanoma risk in congenital melanocytic naevi: a systematic review. Br J Dermatol 155(1):1–8
15. Marghoob AA (2002) Congenital melanocytic nevi. Evaluation and management. Dermatol Clin 20(4):607–616, viii
16. Pellacani G et al (2007) The impact of in vivo reflectance confocal microscopy for the diagnostic accuracy of melanoma and equivocal melanocytic lesions. J Invest Dermatol 127(12):2759–2765
17. Langley RG et al (2001) Confocal scanning laser microscopy of benign and malignant melanocytic skin lesions in vivo. J Am Acad Dermatol 45(3):365–376
18. Gerger A et al (2005) Diagnostic applicability of in vivo confocal laser scanning microscopy in melanocytic skin tumors. J Invest Dermatol 124(3):493–498
19. Gerger A et al (2006) Sensitivity and specificity of confocal laser-scanning microscopy for in vivo diagnosis of malignant skin tumors. Cancer 107(1):193–200
20. Pellacani G, Cesinaro AM, Seidenari S (2005) Reflectance-mode confocal microscopy of pigmented skin lesions–improvement in melanoma diagnostic specificity. J Am Acad Dermatol 53(6): 979–985
21. Calzavara-Pinton P et al (2008) Reflectance confocal microscopy for in vivo skin imaging. Photochem Photobiol 84(6): 1421–1430
22. Ahlgrimm-Siess V et al (2008) In vivo confocal scanning laser microscopy of common naevi with globular, homogeneous and reticular pattern in dermoscopy. Br J Dermatol 158(5):1000–1007
23. Gill M, Lieb JA, Patel YG (2008) Congenital and common acquired melanocytic nevi. In: Gonzalez S, Gill M, Halpern AC (eds) Reflectance confocal microscopy of cutaneous tumors. Informa Healthcare, London, pp 86–98
24. Pellacani G, Cesinaro AM, Seidenari S (2005) Reflectance-mode confocal microscopy for the in vivo characterization of pagetoid melanocytosis in melanomas and nevi. J Invest Dermatol 125(3):532–537
25. Haupt HM, Stern JB (1995) Pagetoid melanocytosis. Histologic features in benign and malignant lesions. Am J Surg Pathol 19(7):792–797
26. Massi G (2007) Melanocytic nevi simulant of melanoma with medicolegal relevance. Virchows Arch 451(3):623–647
27. Stern JB, Haupt HM (1998) Pagetoid melanocytosis: tease or tocsin? Semin Diagn Pathol 15(3):225–229
28. Busam KJ, Marghoob AA, Halpern A (2005) Melanoma diagnosis by confocal microscopy: promise and pitfalls. J Invest Dermatol 125(3):vii
29. Li Y et al (2005) Dual mode reflectance and fluorescence confocal laser scanning microscopy for in vivo imaging melanoma progression in murine skin. J Invest Dermatol 125(4):798–804

The Many Faces of Nevi: Blue, "Black" and Recurrent Nevi

12

Verena Ahlgrimm-Siess, Edith Arzberger,
Rainer Hofmann-Wellenhof, and Alon Scope

The RCM criteria of most types of melanocytic nevi have been extensively described in the literature within the past years [1–4]. This chapter complements this body of knowledge by describing the RCM features of less frequent types of nevi, namely blue, "black" and recurrent nevi. Common to these nevus variants is that they are often the clinical outlier or "ugly duckling" among the patient's moles, and as such, these nevi tend to raise some clinical concern; moreover, their dermoscopic features are often equivocal. To this end, RCM can reveal additional architectural and cellular details about these nevi, and thus can serve as a helpful adjunct for diagnosis and management decision. In the following sections, we describe the RCM features of these nevi in the context of the current technical limitations of RCM, such as the restricted depth of penetration of light and the limited cellular details.

12.1 Common Blue Nevus

Many types of blue nevi have been described in the literature, including cellular, amelanotic and combined blue nevi to name just a few [5, 6] ; this variability probably reflects the fact that nevi described as "blue" on clinical grounds, actually represent different types of congenital nevi on histopathology. For simplicity, we describe herein only the RCM features of the so-called common blue nevus, defined below.

The common blue nevus usually appears as a solitary, blue-colored macule, papule or nodule on the head and neck or the dorsum of the hands and feet. On histopathology, there is a proliferation of markedly pigmented, bipolar dendritic melanocytes that are splayed as solitary units between thickened collagen bundles in the reticular dermis. In addition, scattered, pigment-laden melanophages are usually noted. While typically common blue nevi are long standing, patient history may be indecisive or even alluding to a recent change. In these cases, the clinical differential diagnosis may include a pigmented basal cell carcinoma, a nodular melanoma, a melanoma metastasis or melanoma arising within a preexisting blue nevus [7].

Dermoscopy is often helpful in the diagnosis of common blue nevus. The blue color noted clinically is also observed with dermoscopy; a steel-blue pigmentation lacking additional dermoscopic features is typically seen with nonpolarized dermoscopy. However, blue nevi may show at times color variegation on dermoscopy (e.g., blue-white, blue-brown or polychromatic structureless pigmentation), particularly when using polarized dermoscopy [8]. Such variegate blue nevi may be clinically and dermoscopically equivocal.

With confocal microscopy, common blue nevi characteristically show a typical honeycomb pattern of the epidermis and a preserved dermo-epidermal junction. Within the dermis, scattered bright dendritic cells corresponding to pigmented dendritic melanocytes can be observed. The demonstration of dermal melanocytes by RCM depends on their anatomic location. Only the most superficial portion of the reticular dermis is visualized by RCM at present. In addition, polygonal, plump-bright non-nucleated cells can be seen in the dermis, correlating to melanin-laden dermal melanophages; the dendritic melanocytes and the melanophages are often seen on RCM amidst thickened bright collagen bundles in the reticular dermis.

The main limitation of RCM in the assessment of common blue nevi is the restricted depth of penetration; the adequate evaluation of the entire depth of the lesion cannot be guaranteed. However, if RCM shows features that deviate from those described, the clinical diagnosis of blue nevus needs to be questioned. For example, the presence of

V. Ahlgrimm-Siess (✉) • E. Arzberger • R. Hofmann-Wellenhof
Department of Dermatology and Venerology,
Medical University of Graz, Graz, Austria
e-mail: v.ahlgrimm-siess@salk.at;
edith.arzberger@medunigraz.at; rainer.hofmann@medunigraz.at

A. Scope
Department of Dermatology, Sheba Medical Center,
Tel Hashomer, Israel
e-mail: scopea1@gmail.com

R. Hofmann-Wellenhof et al. (eds.), *Reflectance Confocal Microscopy for Skin Diseases*,
DOI 10.1007/978-3-642-21997-9_12, © Springer-Verlag Berlin Heidelberg 2012

melanocytes in pagetoid pattern within the epidermis, a disarranged DEJ and dermal cerebriform nests point to the diagnosis of melanoma[9, 10]. The detection of well-demarcated bright tumor islands at the DEJ/upper dermis, within thickened collagen with *en face* blood vessels, is diagnostic of pigmented basal cell carcinoma [11].

12.2 Black Nevus

The so-called black nevus is a recently described clinical entity [12]. On clinical examination, the black nevus presents as a dark brown to black macule or papule with an average diameter of 5 mm. This type of nevus is typically found in darker skin-typed patients (e.g., type IV skin) and is usually located on the trunk, predominantly on the back. With dermoscopy, black nevi usually display a central, sharply demarcated, dark-brown to black homogeneous area (black lamella) and a regular pigment network at the periphery; the partial removal of the black lamella with tape-stripping may enable the visualization of an underlying pigment network with dermoscopy. The dermoscopic finding of a black lamella correlates on histopathology with abundant melanin in a compact stratum corneum above a deeply pigmented junctional or compound nevus [13, 14].

Though benign, black nevi are often excised due to their worrisome clinical appearance; the black nevus is usually darker than the patient's other nevi and hence may be perceived clinically as an outlier, "ugly duckling" nevus [15]. Compounding the clinical concern are reports that the finding of black pigmentation in clinically atypical lesion may be a predictor of early melanoma [16]. Dermoscopy may alleviate the clinical concern with black nevi if there is a symmetric distribution of colors and structures; however, equivocal dermoscopic findings, such as an eccentric black lamella, irregular black dots (due to focally denser melanin deposits within the stratum corneum) or slight network irregularities, may lead to an unnecessary excision.

With RCM, black nevi usually show a thickened cornified layer with highly reflective, homogeneous areas of varying size and shape, correlating to pigmented scales. The underlying spinous-granular layers display a regular cobblestone pattern due to the high content of melanin granules within the keratinocytes. The DEJ typically shows a regular ringed pattern (i.e., edged-papillae) and small, predominantly junctional, nests.

Thus, RCM may point the clinician to the correct diagnosis in black nevi that are clinically and dermoscopically equivocal. Irregular black dots can be identified as bright melanin deposits within the cornified layer, and differentiated from nucleated or dendritic cells in pagetoid pattern that would be seen in melanoma. A regular epidermal and DEJ architecture can be visualized with RCM in black nevi despite the extent of epidermal pigmentation; this is similar to the reassuring effect of tape-stripping showing a regular underlying network with dermoscopy.

12.3 Recurrent Nevus

Recurrent nevi, following an incomplete removal of melanocytic nevi (e.g., by shave biopsy), may clinically and histopathologically simulate melanoma in situ [17, 18]. On clinical examination, irregularly pigmented, asymmetric macules with indistinct borders are characteristically seen in the surgical scar. Asymmetry of colors and structures, color variegation and concerning pigment structures, such as an irregular network, irregular dots or streaks, may be observed with dermoscopy [19]. On histopathology, recurrent nevus is characterized by the presence of irregularly distributed junctional nests and melanocytes disposed as solitary units, occasionally in pagetoid pattern, above the scar; peripheral and deep to the scar, remnants of the melanocytic nevus can often be seen. The presence of nevus nests beneath the scar, as well as review of the previous biopsy specimen, can assist the pathologist to arrive at the correct diagnosis of a recurrent nevus.

With RCM, a typical honeycomb or cobblestone pattern is usually observed at the spinous-granular layers of the epidermis; focal "streaming" of basal keratinocytes (i.e., distortion and elongation of keratinocytes along a longitudinal axis) may be present due to distortion caused by the underlying scar. Single bright, nucleated cells of varying sizes and shape may be seen at suprabasal epidermal layers, correlating to melanocytes in pagetoid pattern seen on histopathology. At the DEJ, a regular ringed pattern can be observed together with irregularly shaped dermal papillae, again due to distortion caused by the underlying scarring. The flattening of the DEJ over the scar may also result in a focal loss of the ringed pattern; the presence of irregularly distributed nests and single melanocytes of varying sizes and shape may also be seen. In the upper dermis, there is an increased density of bright and thickened collagen fibers, correlating to the fibrosis on histopathology.

RCM is particularly valuable for the differentiation of recurrent nevus from hyper-pigmentation which is occasionally seen within surgical scars. In cases of hyper-pigmentation, pigmented basal keratinocytes without nests or solitary melanocytes are characteristically observed. However, at present, in most cases of recurrent nevi, the differentiation from melanoma in situ with RCM is hindered by the limited penetration of light (inability to see the regular nests in the deeper dermis, underneath the scar) and the inability to visualize nuclear details. Thus, in cases showing melanocytic proliferation above the scar with RCM, the clinician will likely opt for an excision.

CASE 1 – Blue nevus

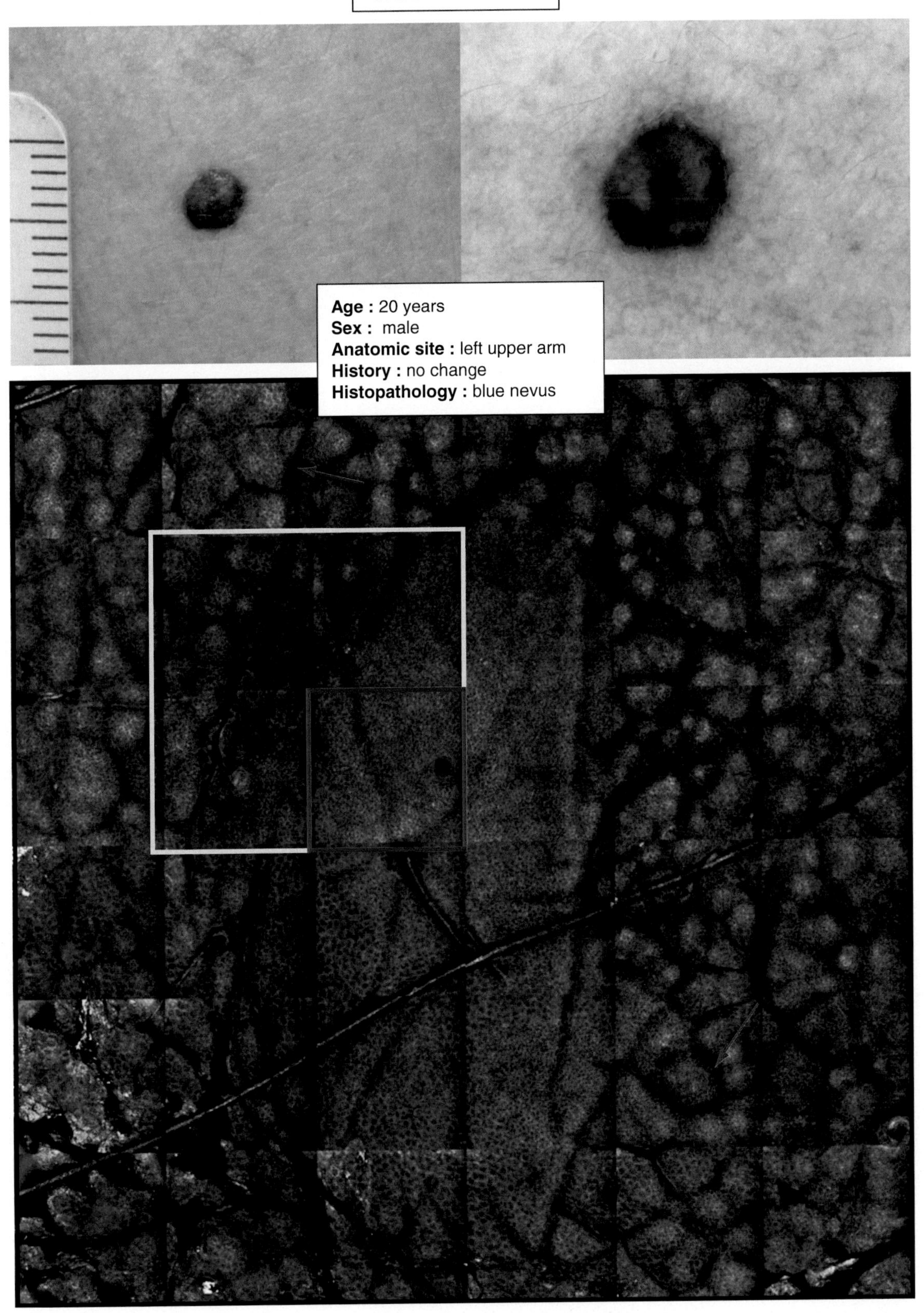

Fig. 12.1 RCM mosaic (3 × 3 mm) at the level of the spinous-granular layer displays a regular epidermal architecture with typical honeycomb pattern (*rectangles*). Epidermal bulbous projections (*arrows*) are observed at the lesion's periphery, correlating to the slightly papillomatous surface that is seen clinically

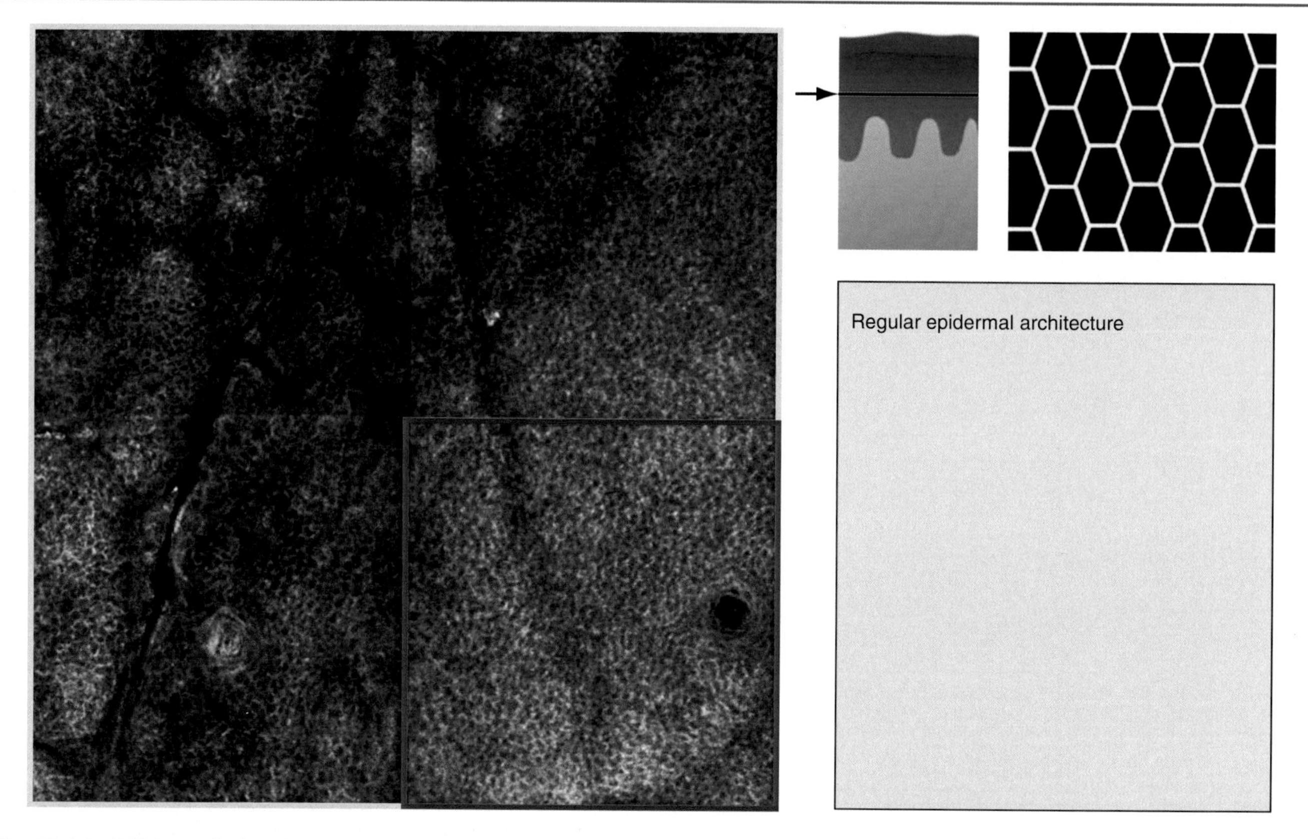

Fig. 12.1.1 RCM mosaic (1 × 1 mm) at the spinous-granular layer. A typical honeycomb pattern of the epidermis is seen

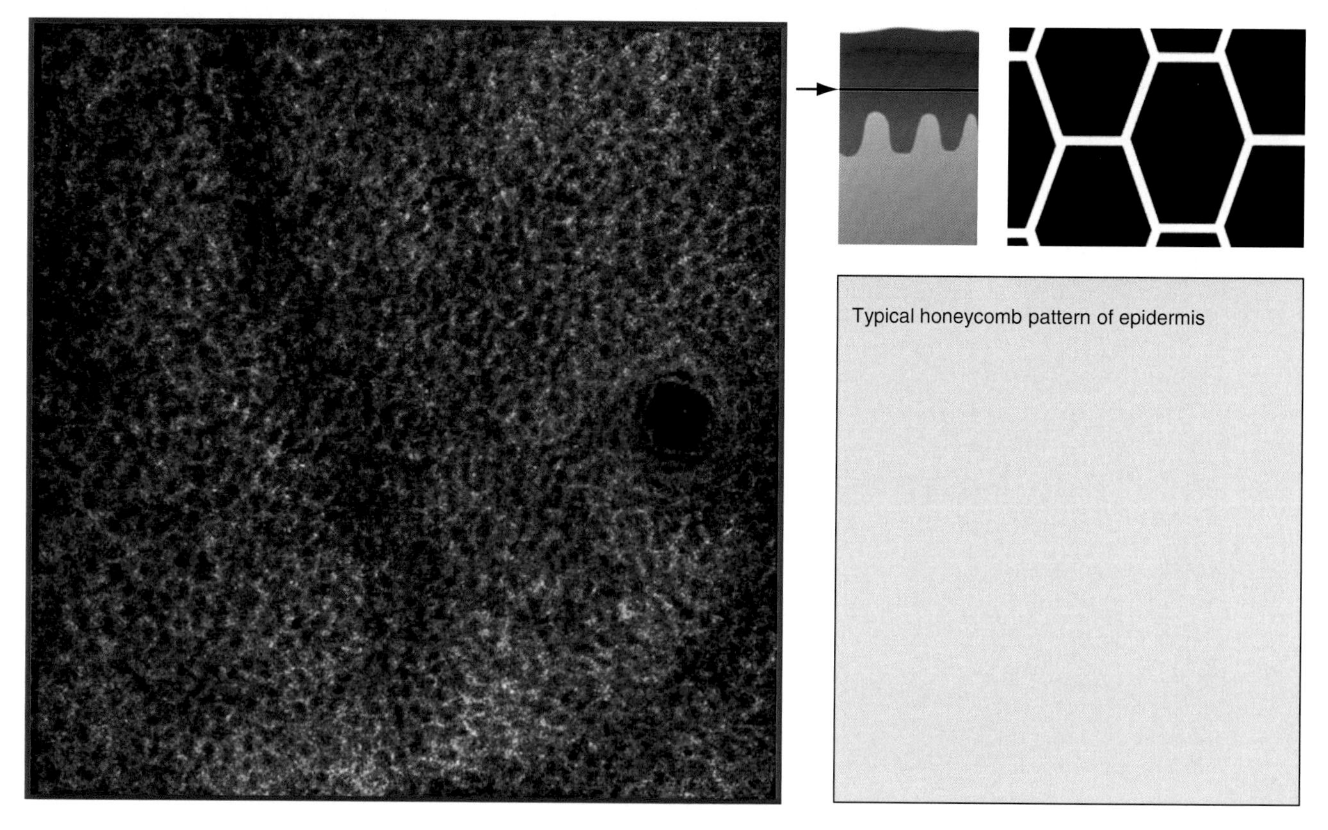

Fig. 12.1.2 Basic RCM image (0.5 × 0.5 mm) at the spinous-granular layer shows a typical honeycomb pattern of the epidermis; the dark nuclei are uniform in size, and the *bright lines* of the honeycomb are uniform in thickness, indicating that the keratinocytes are equal in size and spacing

CASE 1 – Blue nevus

Age: 20 years
Sex: male
Anatomic site: left upper arm
History: no change
Histopathology: blue nevus

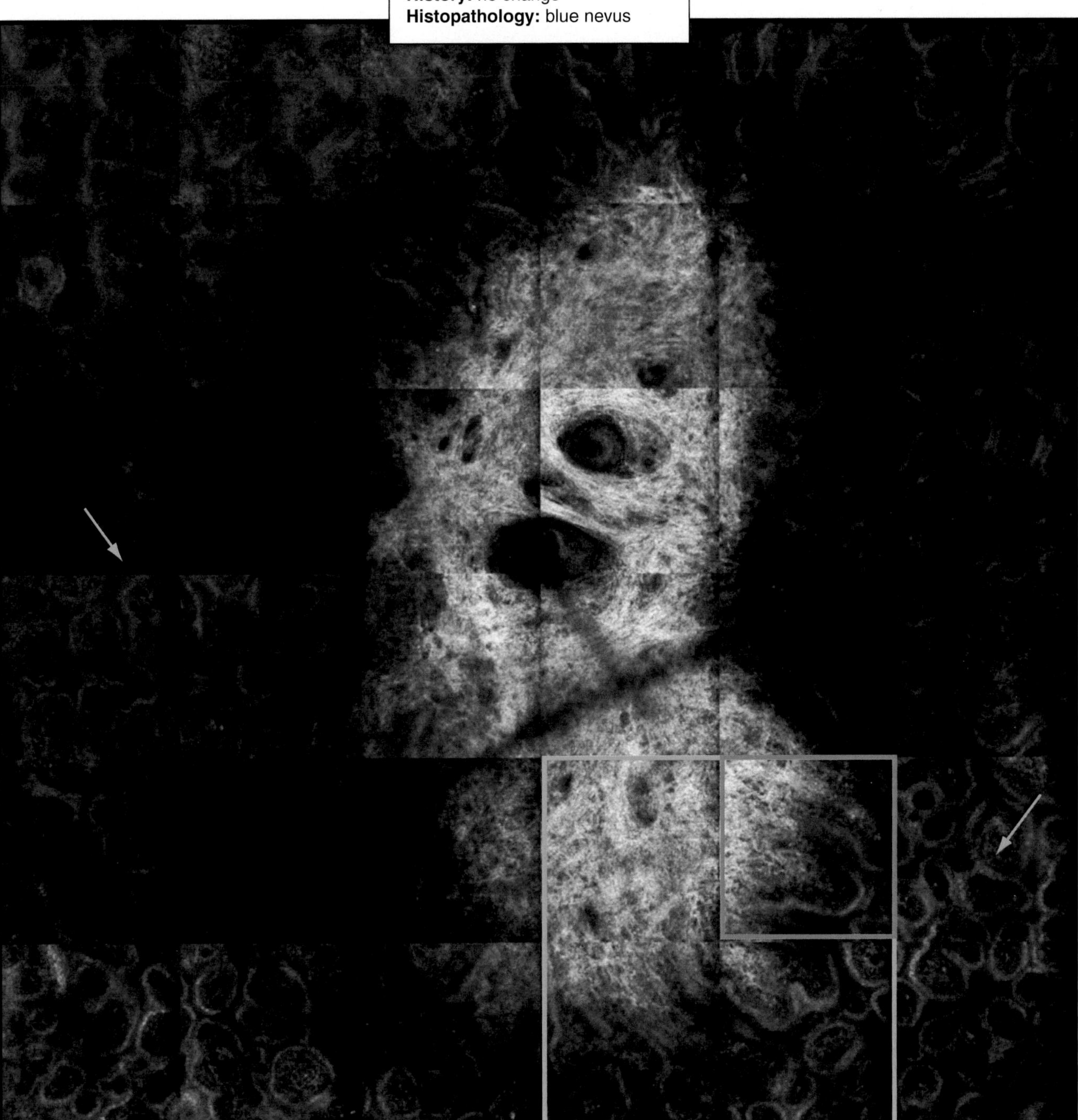

Fig. 12.2 RCM mosaic (3 × 3 mm) at the DEJ/upper dermis level. A bright area is seen at the lesion's center, correlating to fibrosis (*rectangles*). The lesion periphery displays a ringed pattern composed of back-to-back edged papillae (*arrows*)

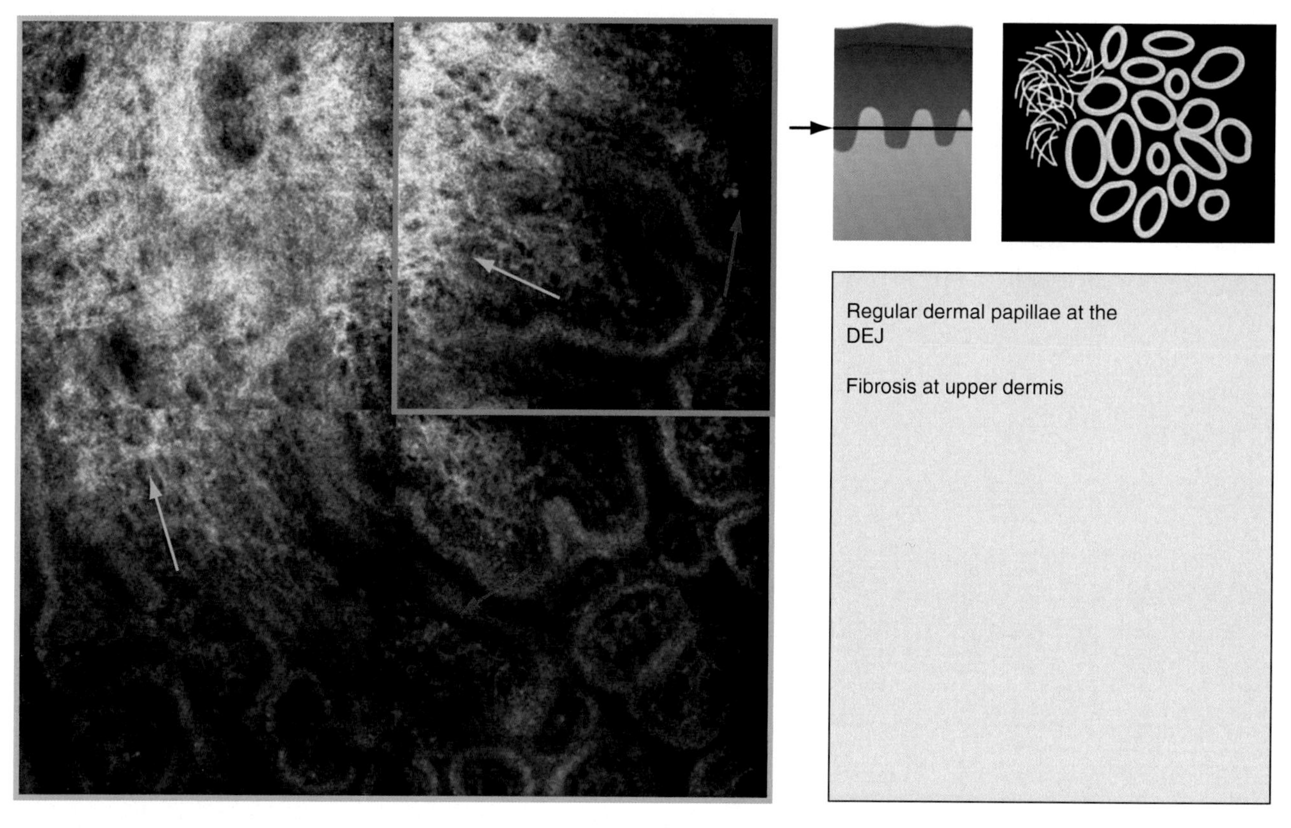

Fig. 12.2.1 RCM mosaic (1 × 1 mm) at the DEJ/upper dermis level displays focal increase of brightly reflecting reticulated fibers (*green arrows*) adjacent to densely packed edged papillae. Bright, round to triangular cells, singly or in aggregates, are observed within dermal papillae (*red arrows*), correlating to inflammatory cells including melanophages

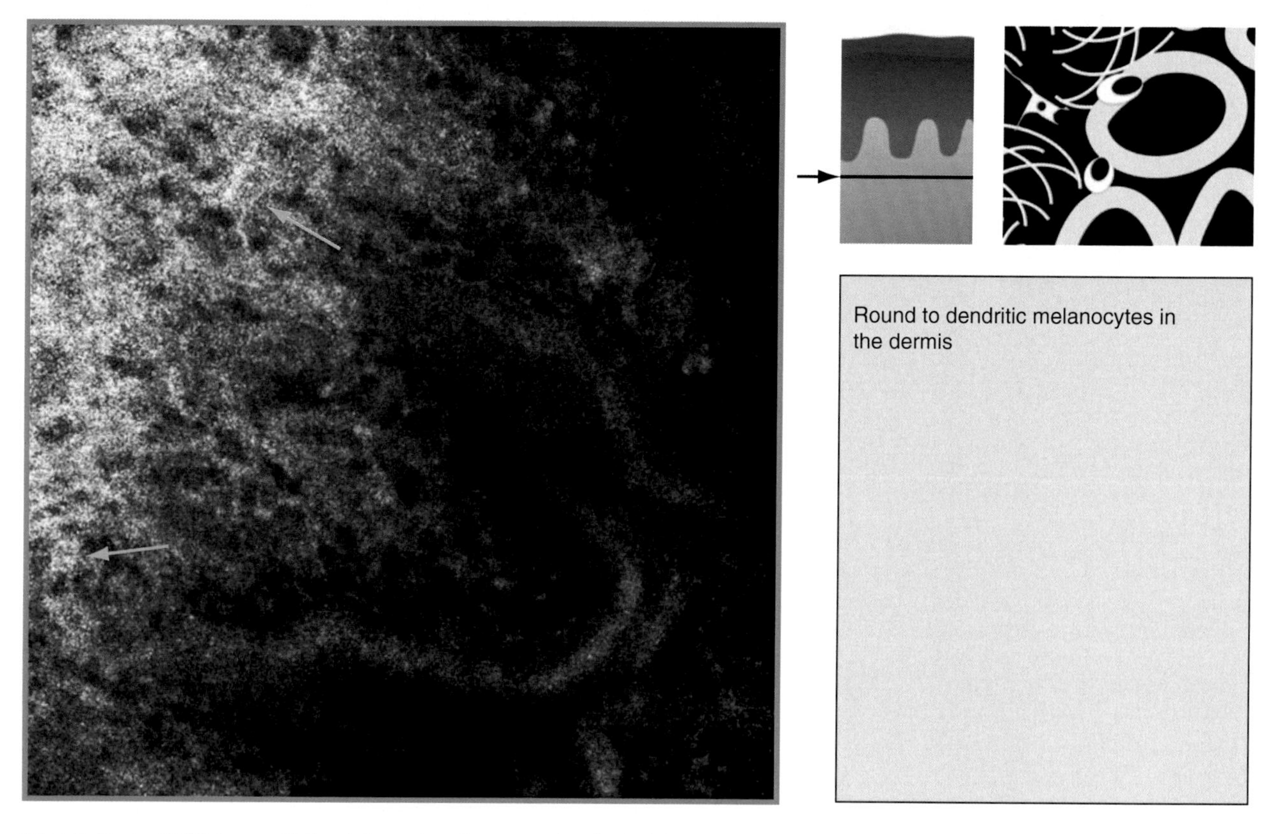

Fig. 12.2.2 Basic RCM image (0.5 × 0.5 mm) at the upper dermis. Bright round to dendritic nucleated cells (*green arrows*), correlating to melanocytes, are seen within the fibrotic dermis

CASE 2 – Black nevus

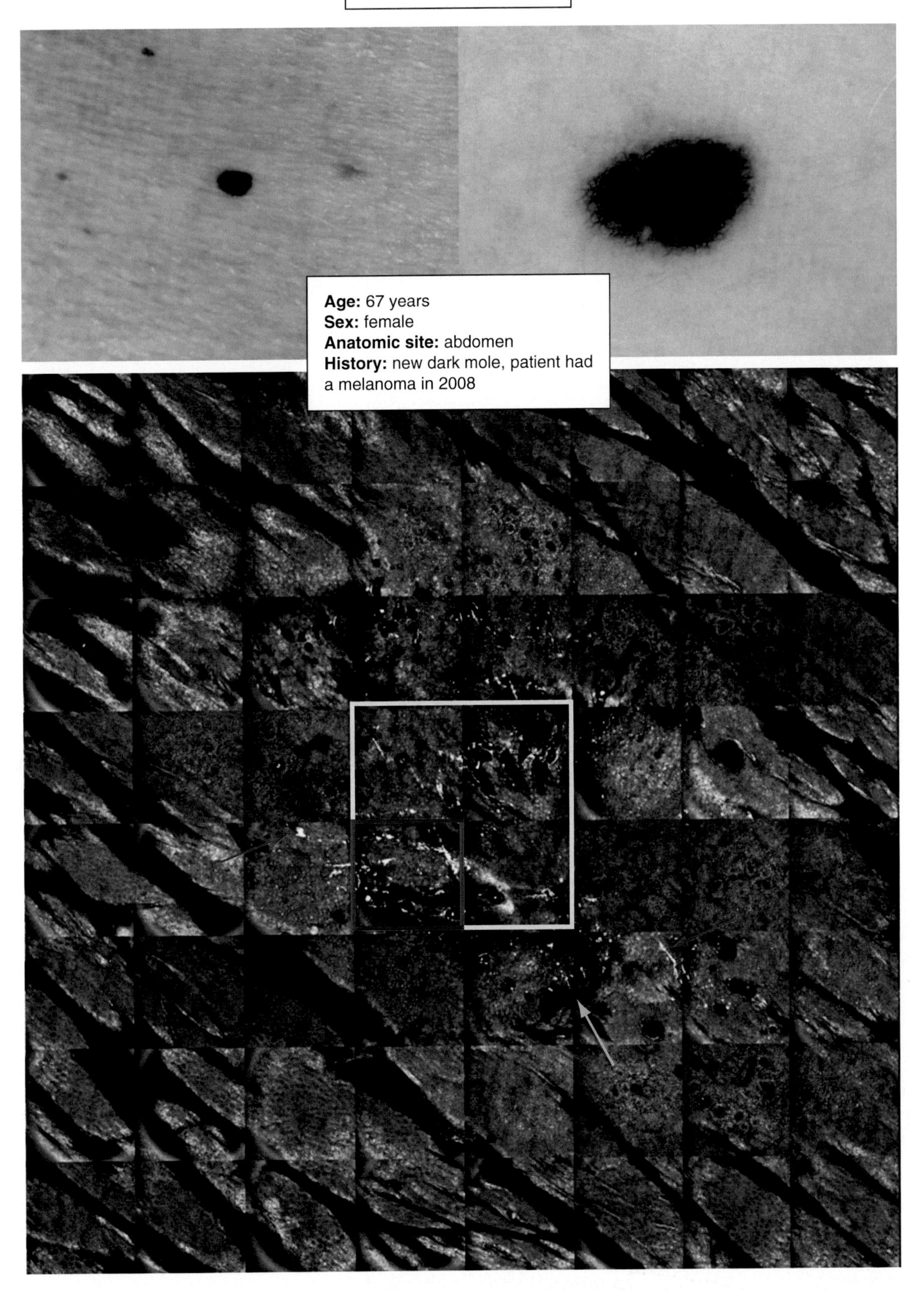

Fig. 12.3 RCM mosaic (3 × 3 mm) at the level of the epidermis shows an uneven skin surface with dark areas (*green arrow*) indicating foci of noncontact between the RCM lens and the skin surface. There are also round to polygonal areas of high reflectivity (*red arrows*) due to thickening of the stratum corneum with focal melanin deposition

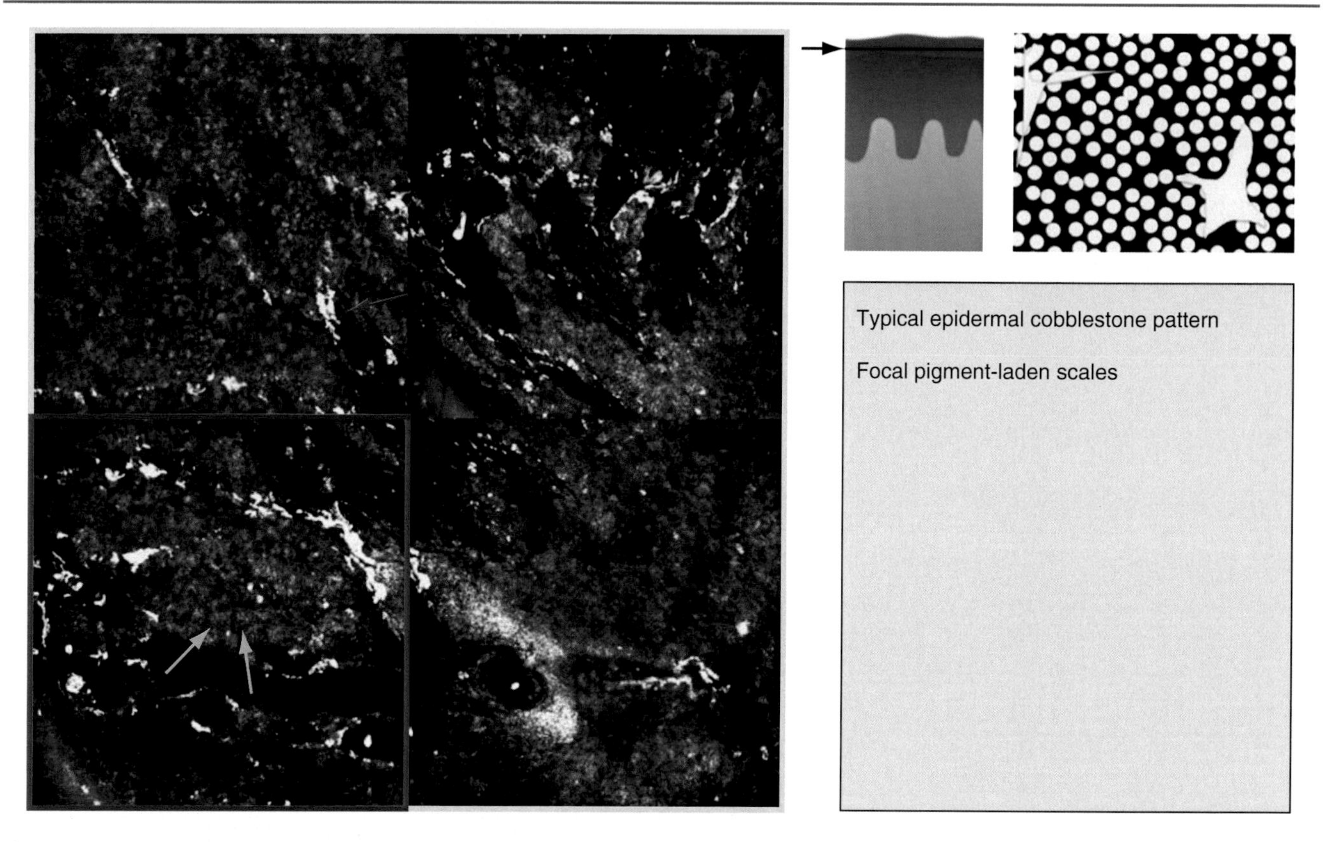

Fig. 12.3.1 RCM mosaic (1 × 1 mm) at the upper layers of the epidermis. A typical cobblestone pattern (*green arrows*) and homogeneously highly reflecting areas, correlating to pigment-laden scales are focally observed (*red arrow*)

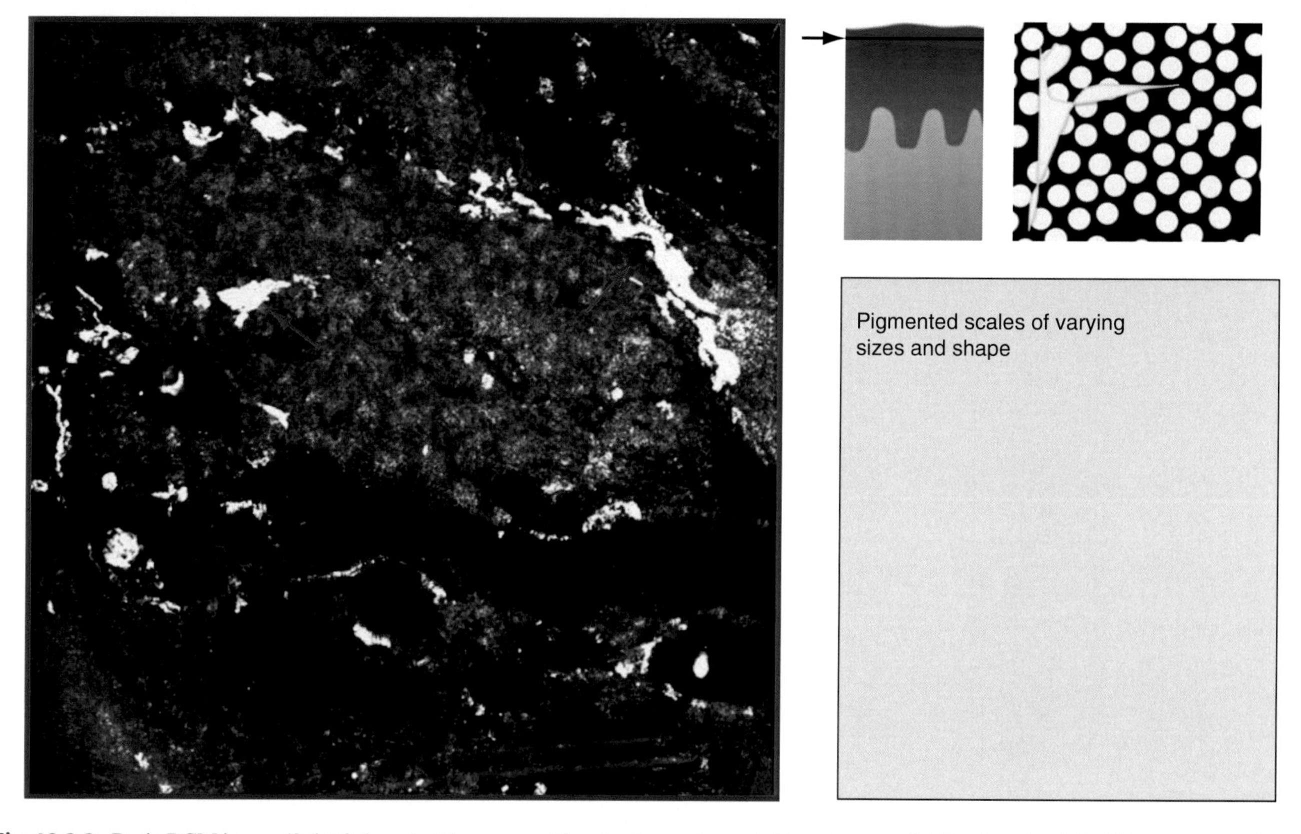

Fig. 12.3.2 Basic RCM image (0.5 × 0.5 mm) at the upper epidermis shows pigmented keratinocytes laid back-to-back (cobblestone pattern) and brightly reflecting scales of varying size and shape due to the high melanin content within keratinocytes

CASE 2 – Black nevus

Age: 67 years
Sex: female
Anatomic site: abdomen
History: new appearance of a dark mole, patient had a melanoma in 2008

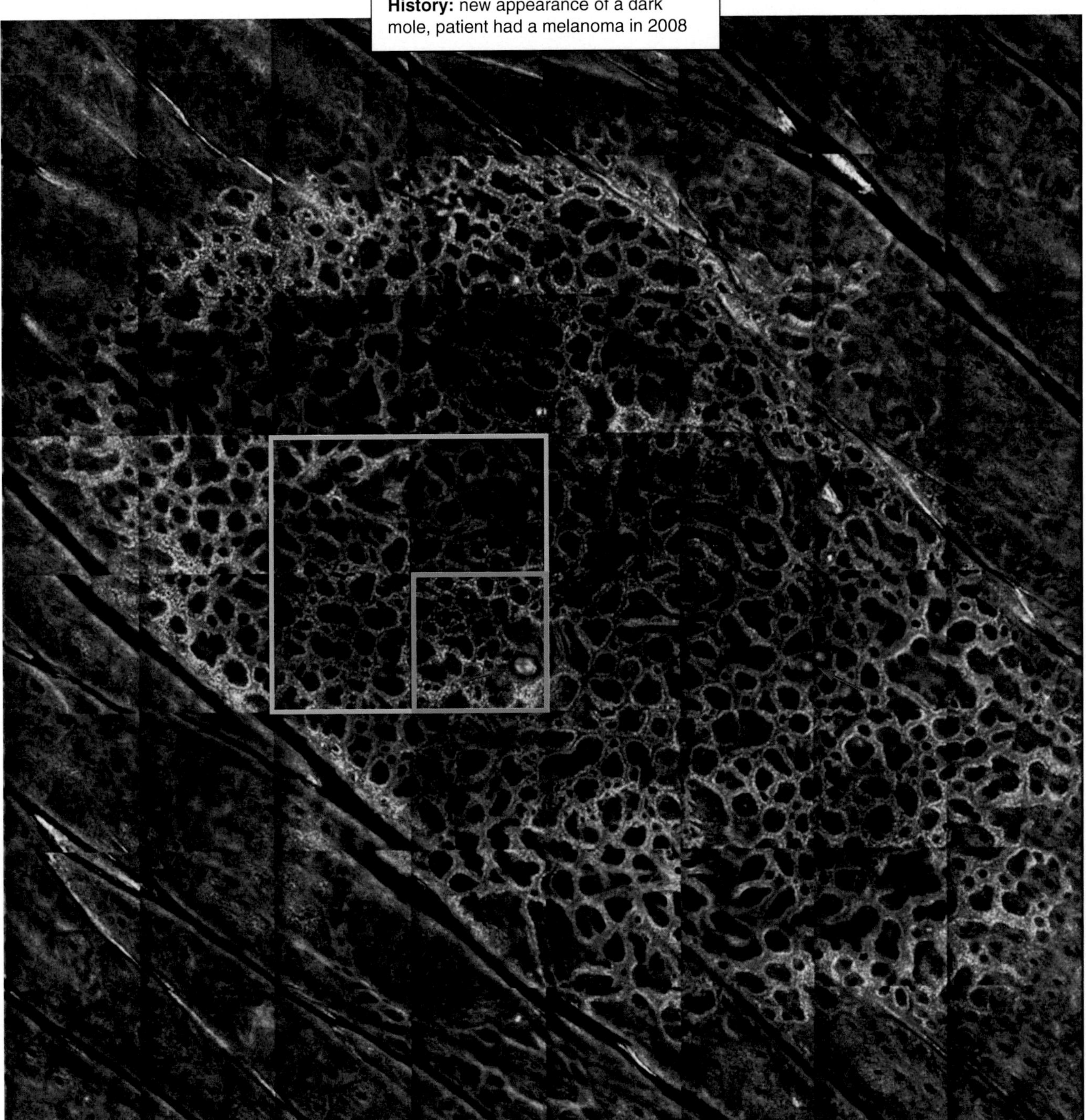

Fig. 12.4 RCM mosaic (4 × 4 mm) at the level of the DEJ. A regular DEJ architecture with densely packed, back-to-back edged papillae is observed (*rectangles*). Bright junctional and dermal round melanocytic nests (*arrows*) are focally noted

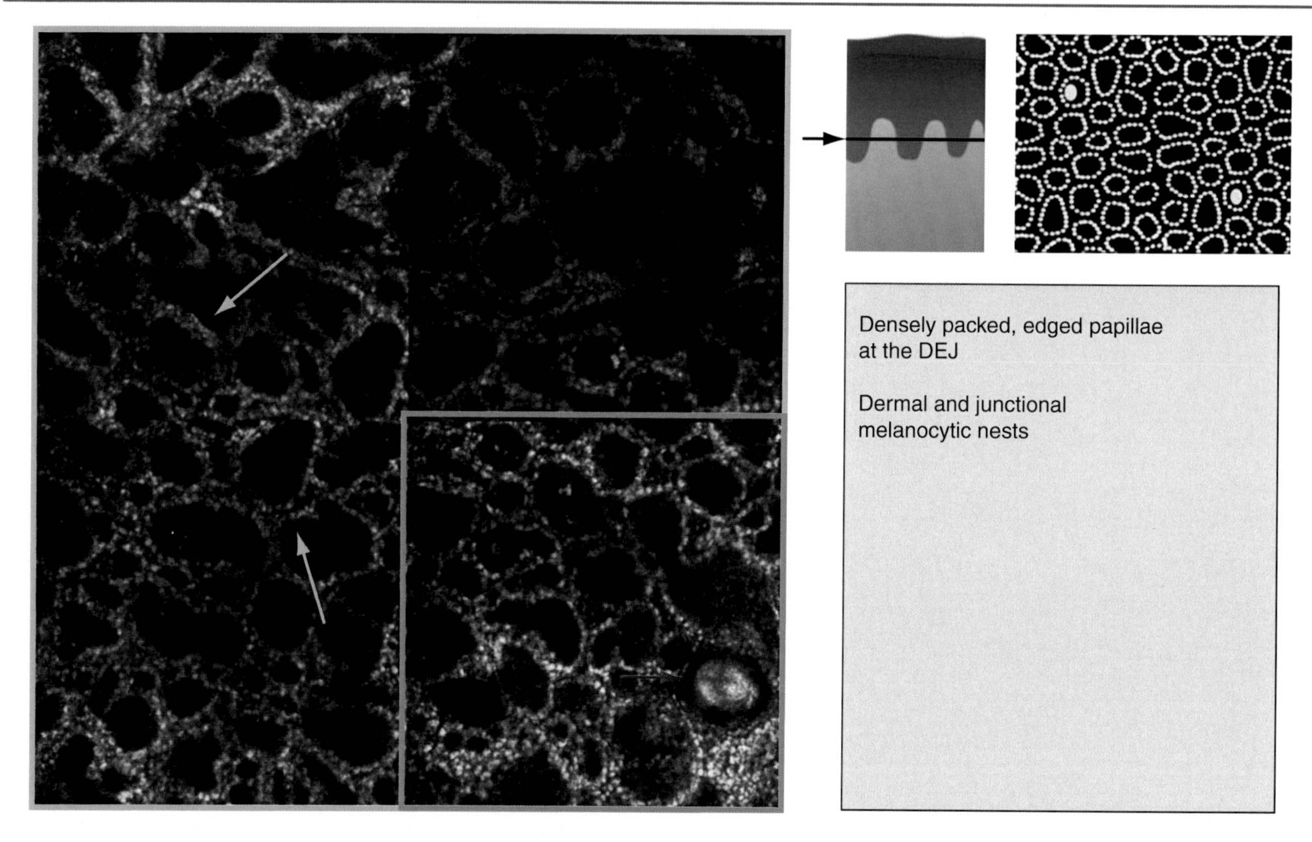

Fig. 12.4.1 RCM mosaic (1 × 1 mm) at the DEJ. A ringed pattern with edged papillae (*green arrows*) is observed throughout the image. A round, bright structure (*red arrow*), termed "dense nest", is seen within a dermal papilla; this structure correlates to a dermal melanocytic nest

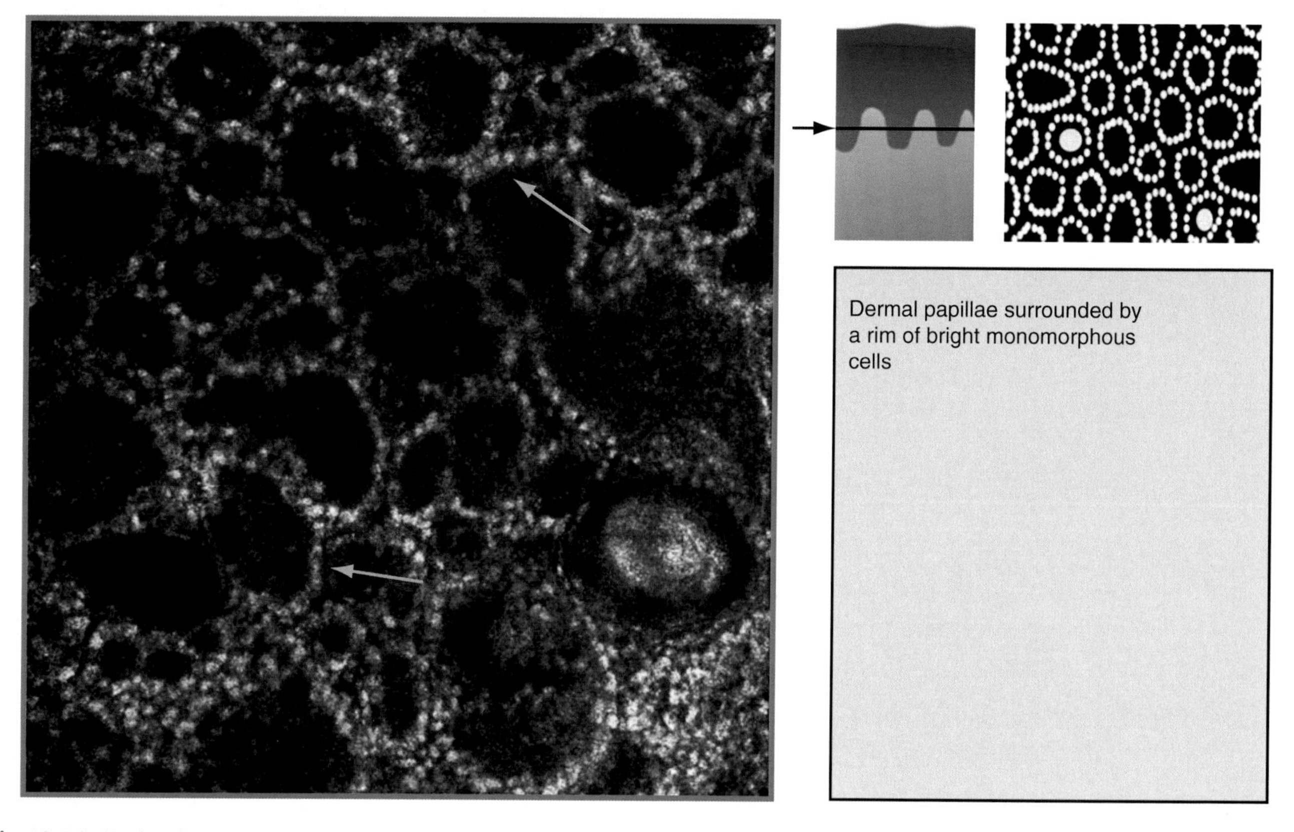

Fig. 12.4.2 Basic RCM image (0.5 × 0.5 mm) at the DEJ shows round to oval dermal papillae surrounded by a rim of monomorphous bright cells; these cells correlate to pigmented basal keratinocytes and melanocytes (*arrows*)

CASE 3 – Recurrent nevus

CM 1 2
Age: 34 years
Sex: female
Anatomic site: abdomen
History: recurrent pigmentation after shave biopsy of a mole
Histopathology: recurrent nevus

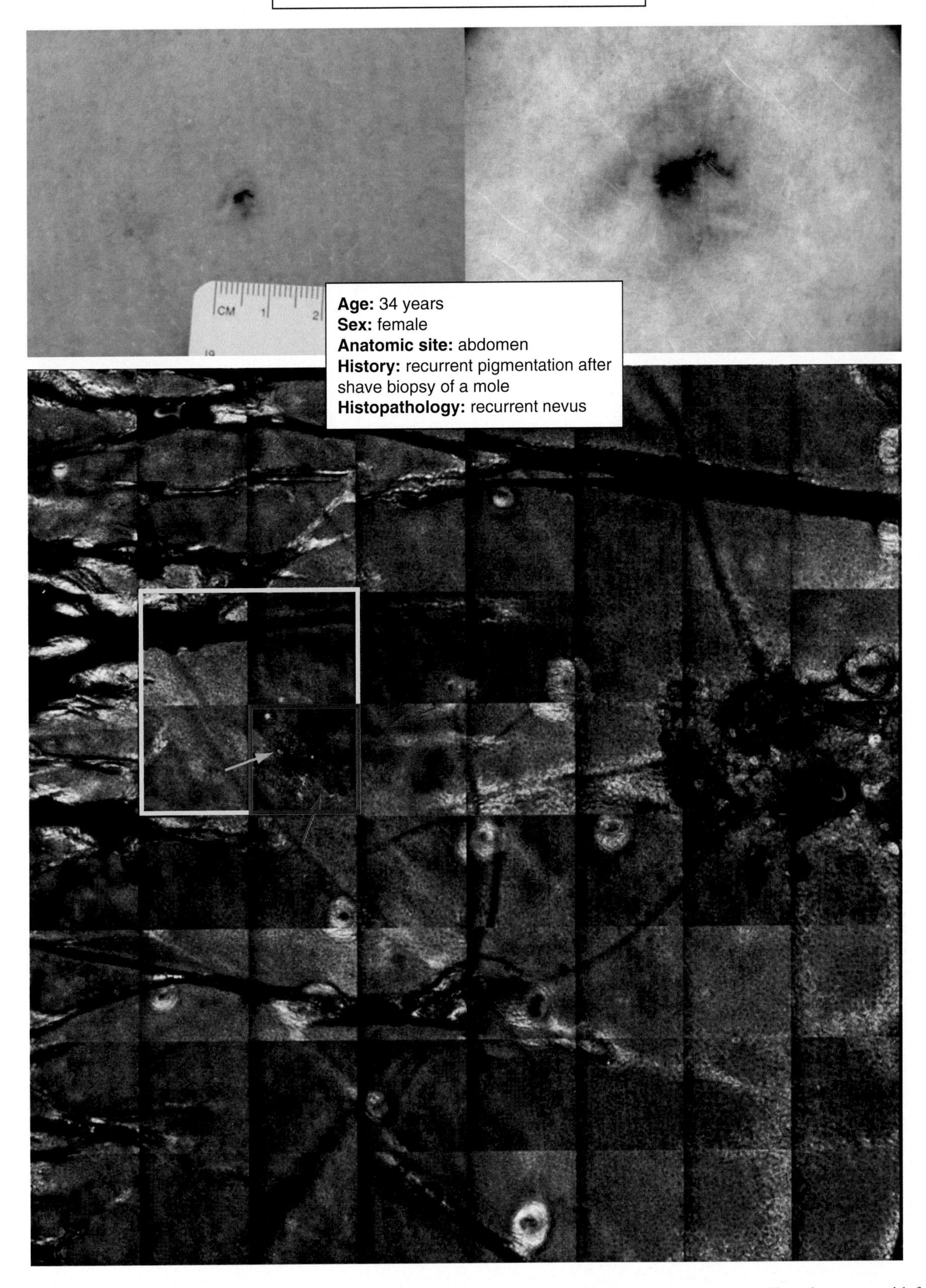

Fig. 12.5 RCM mosaic (4 × 4 mm) at the level of the upper epidermis showing mostly typical honeycomb pattern. There is an area with focal loss of the honeycomb pattern (*red arrows*), harboring single, bright cells (*green arrow*)

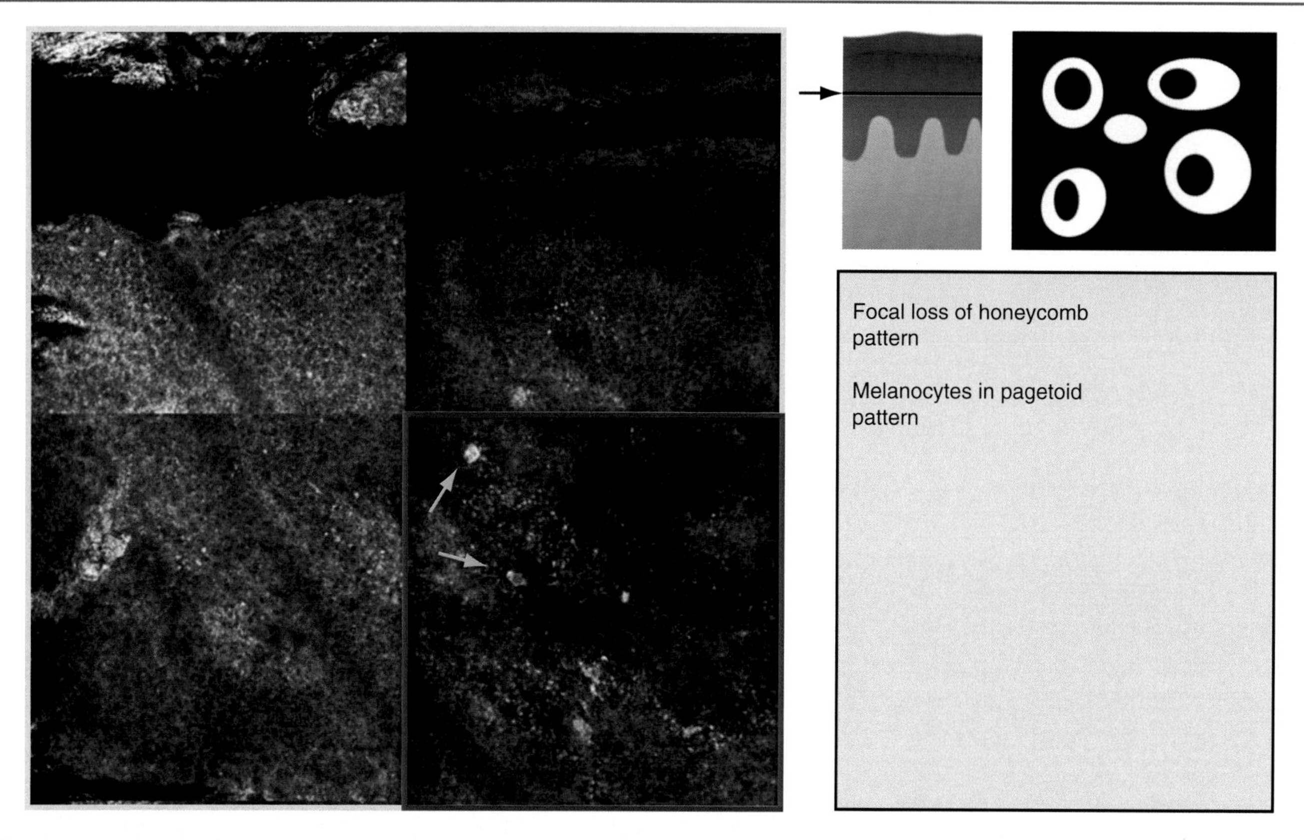

Fig. 12.5.1 RCM mosaic (1 × 1 mm) at the spinous-granular layers of the epidermis. Focal loss of the honeycomb pattern (*rectangle*) is observed with polymorphous, roundish and dendritic nucleated cells (*arrows*), correlating to melanocytes in pagetoid pattern

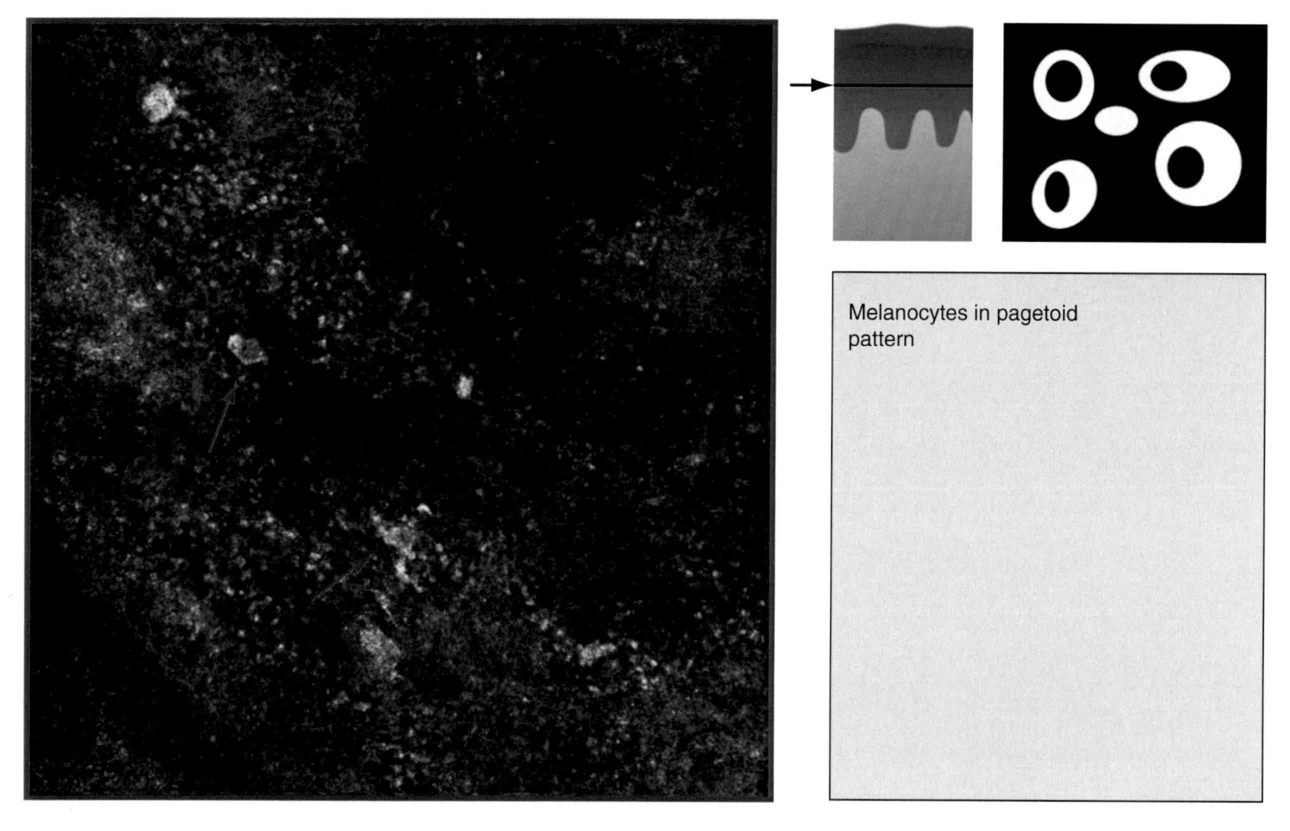

Fig. 12.5.2 Basic RCM image (0.5 × 0.5 mm) at the suprabasal epidermis displaying scattered, bright, nucleated cells of varying sizes, shape and reflectivity (*arrows*)

CASE 3 – Recurrent nevus

Age: 34 years
Sex: female
Anatomic site: abdomen
History: recurrent pigmentation after shave biopsy of a mole
Histopathology: recurrent nevus

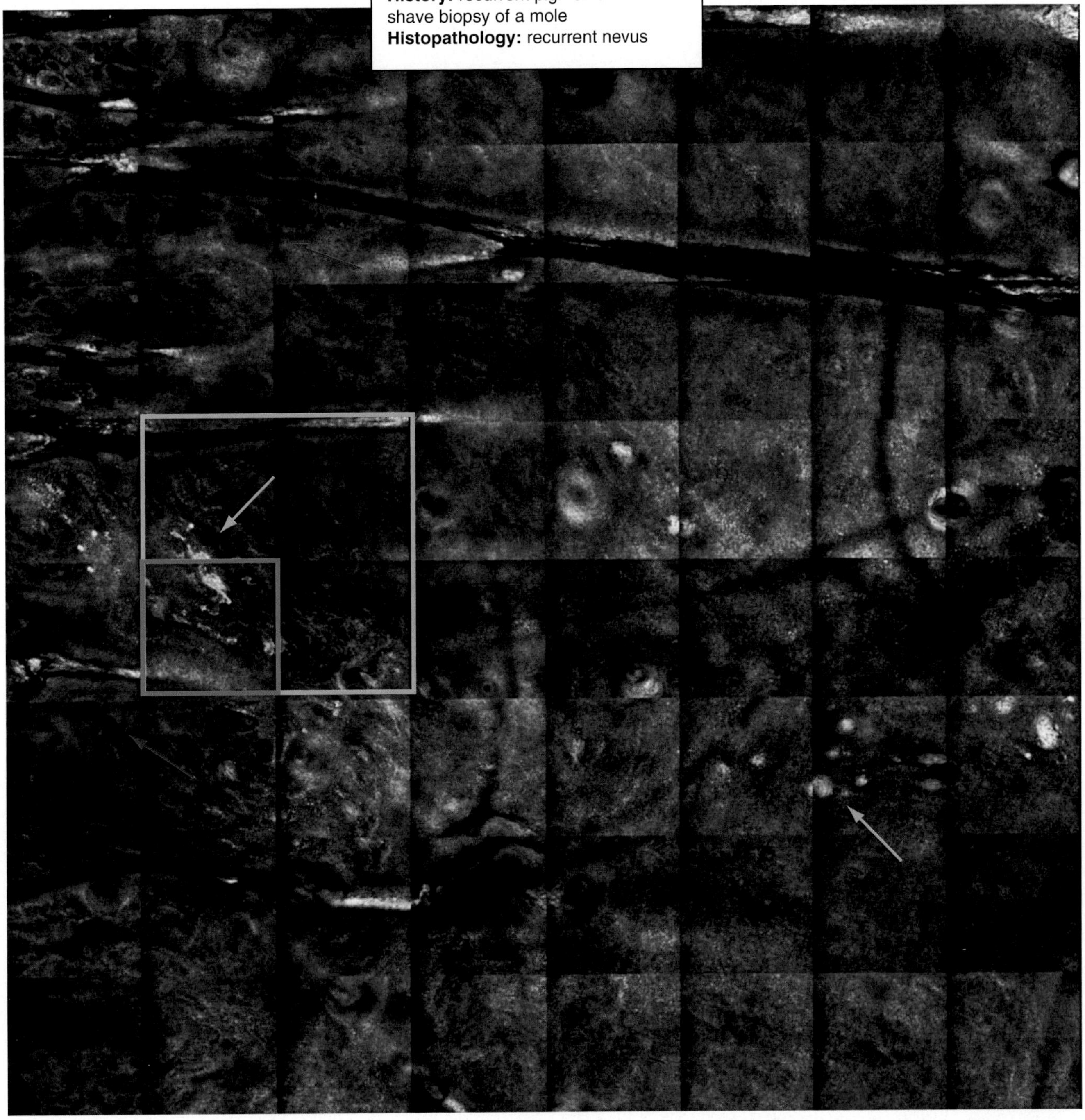

Fig. 12.6 RCM mosaic (4 × 4 mm) at the level of the DEJ. Flattening of the DEJ is evident by almost complete absence of dermal papillae, except for focally (*red arrows*); the flattening of the DEJ is probably due to scarring. Irregularly spaced and shaped bright structures are focally detected, correlating to junctional or dermal melanocytic nests (*green arrows*)

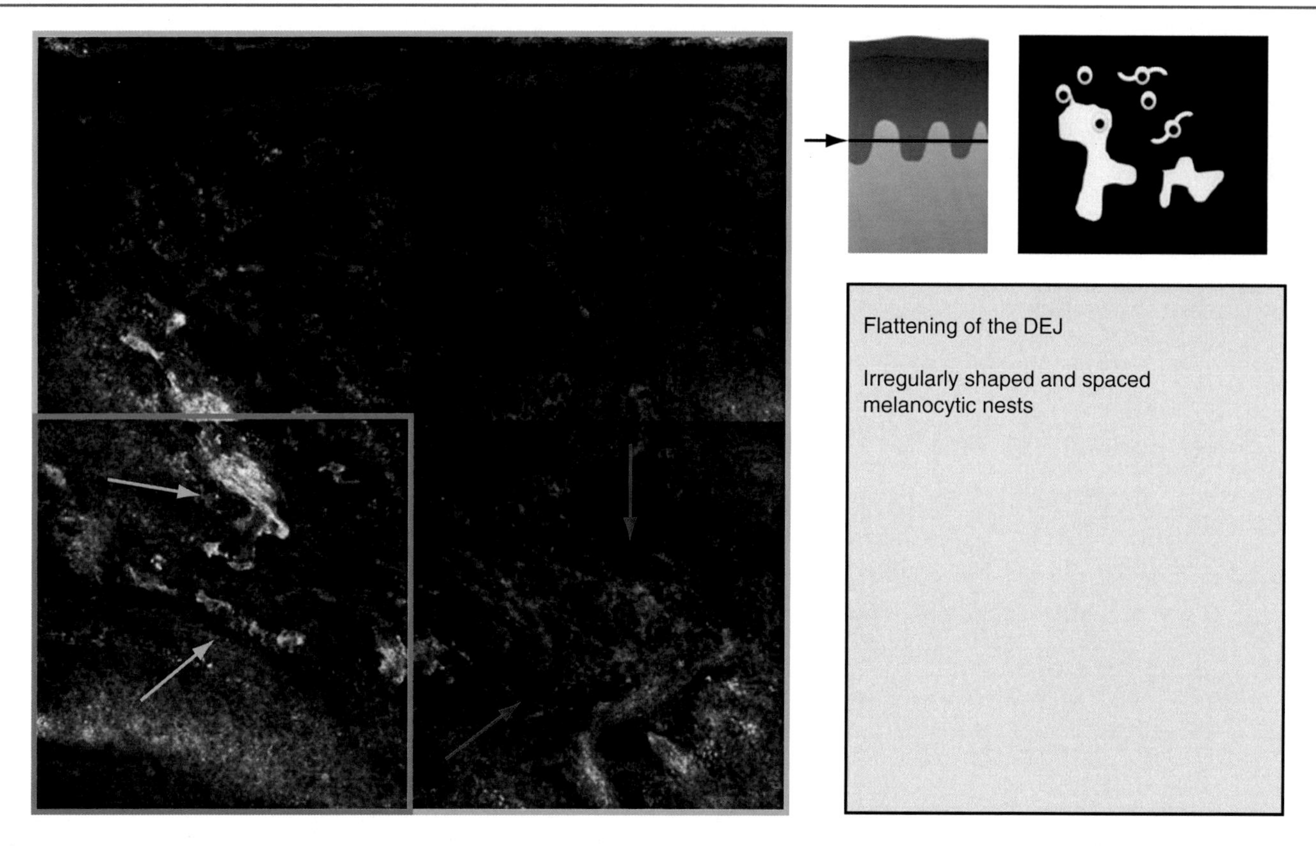

Fig. 12.6.1 RCM mosaic (1 × 1 mm) at the DEJ. A sharp demarcation between epidermis (honeycomb pattern) and dermis (collagen bundles, *red arrows*) is lacking due to flattening of the DEJ. Irregularly shaped bright melanocytic nests are focally seen (*green arrows*)

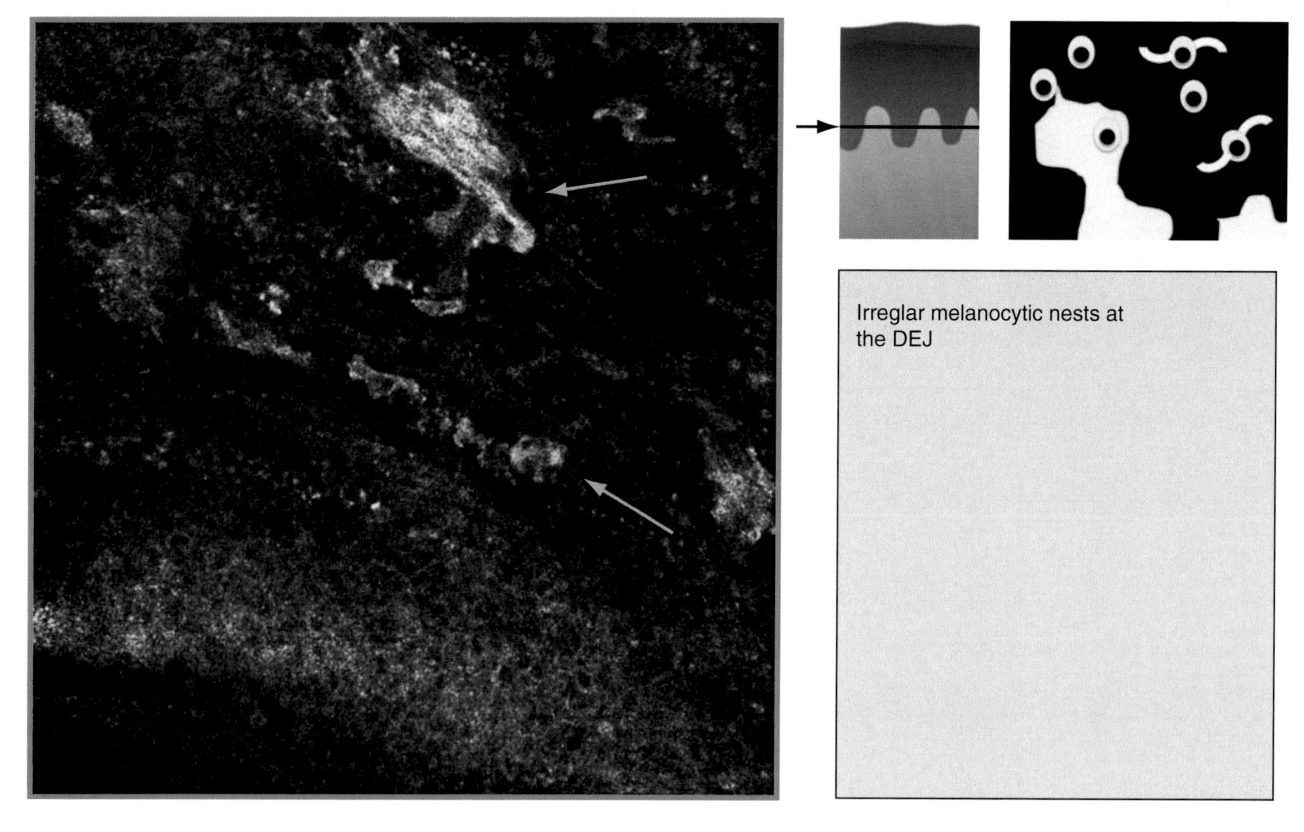

Fig. 12.6.2 Basic RCM image (0.5 × 0.5 mm) at the DEJ. Irregularly shaped melanocytic nests of various size, shape and reflectivity are noted (*green arrows*)

References

1. Ahlgrimm-Siess V, Massone C, Koller S, Fink-Puches R, Richtig E, Wolf I et al (2008) In vivo confocal scanning laser microscopy of common naevi with globular, homogeneous and reticular pattern in dermoscopy. Br J Dermatol 158(5):1000–1007
2. Scope A, Benvenuto-Andrade C, Agero AL, Malvehy J, Puig S, Rajadhyaksha M et al (2007) In vivo reflectance confocal microscopy imaging of melanocytic skin lesions: consensus terminology glossary and illustrative images. J Am Acad Dermatol 57(4):644–658
3. Pellacani G, Longo C, Malvehy J, Puig S, Carrera C, Segura S et al (2008) In vivo confocal microscopic and histopathologic correlations of dermoscopic features in 202 melanocytic lesions. Arch Dermatol 144(12):1597–1608
4. Pellacani G, Scope A, Ferrari B, Pupelli G, Bassoli S, Longo C et al (2009) New insights into nevogenesis: in vivo characterization and follow-up of melanocytic nevi by reflectance confocal microscopy. J Am Acad Dermatol 61(6):1001–1013
5. Ferrara G, Soyer HP, Malvehy J, Piccolo D, Puig S, Sopena J et al (2007) The many faces of blue nevus: a clinicopathologic study. J Cutan Pathol 34(7):543–551
6. Piccolo D, Altamura D, Lozzi GP, Peris K (2006) Blue-whitish veil-like structure as the primary dermoscopic feature of combined nevus. Dermatol Surg 32(9):1176–1178
7. Zalaudek I, Docimo G, Argenziano G (2009) Using dermoscopic criteria and patient-related factors for the management of pigmented melanocytic nevi. Arch Dermatol 145(7):816–826
8. Benvenuto-Andrade C, Dusza SW, Agero AL, Scope A, Rajadhyaksha M, Halpern AC, Marghoob AA (2007) Differences between polarized light dermoscopy and immersion contact dermoscopy for the evaluation of skin lesions. Arch Dermatol 143(3):329–338
9. Segura S, Pellacani G, Puig S, Longo C, Bassoli S, Guitera P et al (2008) In vivo microscopic features of nodular melanomas: dermoscopy, confocal microscopy, and histopathologic correlates. Arch Dermatol 144(10):1311–1320
10. Pellacani G, Bassoli S, Longo C, Cesinaro AM, Seidenari S (2007) Diving into the blue: in vivo microscopic characterization of the dermoscopic blue hue. J Am Acad Dermatol 57(1):96–104
11. Agero AL, Busam KJ, Benvenuto-Andrade C, Scope A, Gill M, Marghoob AA et al (2006) Reflectance confocal microscopy of pigmented basal cell carcinoma. J Am Acad Dermatol 54(4):638–643
12. Zalaudek I, Argenziano G, Mordente I, Moscarella E, Corona R, Sera F et al (2007) Nevus type in dermoscopy is related to skin type in white persons. Arch Dermatol 143(3):351–356
13. Cohen LM, Bennion SD, Johnson TW, Golitz LE (1997) Hypermelanotic nevus: clinical, histopathologic, and ultrastructural features in 316 cases. Am J Dermatopathol 19(1):23–30
14. Yadav S, Vossaert KA, Kopf AW, Silverman M, Grin-Jorgensen C (1993) Histopathologic correlates of structures seen on dermoscopy (epiluminescence microscopy). Am J Dermatopathol 15(4):297–305
15. Scope A, Dusza SW, Halpern AC, Rabinovitz H, Braun RP, Zalaudek I, Argenziano G, Marghoob AA (2008) The "ugly duckling" sign: agreement between observers. Arch Dermatol 144(1):58–64
16. Seidenari S, Pellacani G, Martella A (2005) Acquired melanocytic lesions and the decision to excise: role of color variegation and distribution as assessed by dermoscopy. Dermatol Surg 31(2):184–189
17. Sexton M, Sexton CW (1991) Recurrent pigmented melanocytic nevus. A benign lesion, not to be mistaken for malignant melanoma. Arch Pathol Lab Med 115(2):122–126
18. King R, Hayzen BA, Page RN, Googe PB, Zeagler D, Mihm MC Jr (2009) Recurrent nevus phenomenon: a clinicopathologic study of 357 cases and histologic comparison with melanoma with regression. Mod Pathol 22(5):611–617
19. Marghoob AA, Kopf AW (1997) Persistent nevus: an exception to the ABCD rule of dermoscopy. J Am Acad Dermatol 36(3 Pt 1):474–475

Part V

Melanocytic Lesions: Melanoma

Superficial Spreading Melanoma

13

Caterina Longo, Alice Casari, and Giovanni Pellacani

Superficial spreading melanoma (SSM) is the most common type of melanoma in Caucasian, accounting for about 70% of all diagnosed melanoma cases [1]. This type of melanoma can strike at any age and occurs slightly more often in females than males. SSM has two growth phases: the radial growth phase and the vertical ones [2]. The radial phase involves expansion of the lesion through the epidermis (upper skin layer). In the early radial phase, the lesion is thin, and it can remain in this phase for months or years. This is the less life threatening of the two phases because once the melanoma enters into the vertical growth stage, the prognosis worsens.

Clinically, it often appears as a dark, flat, or slightly raised mark on the skin with variegated colors. Its borders are irregular, with indentations or notches. Considering distinct microscopic hallmarks and epidemiologic data, two subtypes of SSM can be identified: pagetoid melanoma and solar melanoma.

13.1 Pagetoid Melanoma

Pagetoid melanoma usually occurs in adults with intermittent solar exposure history and numerous nevi (Figs. 13.1–13.4). Histopathologically, pagetoid melanoma is characterized by a prominent intraepidermal growth of large cells that often have abundant pale cytoplasm, with "dusty" (fine and evenly dispersed) melanin [3]. Pagetoid and buckshot scatter also describe this distribution of neoplastic cells and represent the hallmark of this melanoma type. A pre-existing naevus can be detected in some cases [4]. The most typical diagnostic alteration is an uneven epidermal contour in the area of the melanoma (or melanoma in situ) and elongated rete-ridges in an area in which a pre-existent naevus is present. If present, solar elastosis is very slight and no elastotic masses can be found.

Dermoscopically, pagetoid melanoma exhibits the classical global dermoscopic patterns such as reticular, globular, multicomponent and sometimes a nonspecific pattern [5, 6].

As a peculiar feature on RCM, pagetoid melanoma is predominantly constituted by melanocytes with roundish shape. Roundish-shaped melanocytes appear as large cells with abundant bright cytoplasm and sometimes showing a hyporeflective nucleus. They are scattered upwards in the epidermis (pagetoid melanocytosis) but they are also present at dermo-epidermal junction (DEJ) either as singe cells or in nests.

13.1.1 Superficial Layers (Epidermis)

The general pattern of superficial layer can be irregular honeycombed or cobblestone pattern in the majority of pagetoid melanomas. Usually, honeycombed patter is present in light pigmented cases whereas an atypical cobblestone pattern occurs when the pigmentation of the lesion is more pronounced. A disarray of the epidermis is present in some cases, usually in areas with abundant pagetoid spread. Pagetoid melanocytosis is present in almost all cases and it is represented by the presence of melanocytes with large diameter (>20 μm, twice than a neighboring keratinocyte) with an abundant refractive cytoplasm, and sometimes showing prominent hyporeflective nuclei [7]. The cell distribution

C. Longo (✉)
Department of Dermatology, Arcispedale S Maria Nuova, Reggio Emilia, Reggio Emilia, Italy
e-mail: longo.caterina@gmail.com

A. Casari • G. Pellacani
Department of Dermatology and Venereology, University of Modena and Reggio Emilia, Modena, Italy

R. Hofmann-Wellenhof et al. (eds.), *Reflectance Confocal Microscopy for Skin Diseases*,
DOI 10.1007/978-3-642-21997-9_13, © Springer-Verlag Berlin Heidelberg 2012

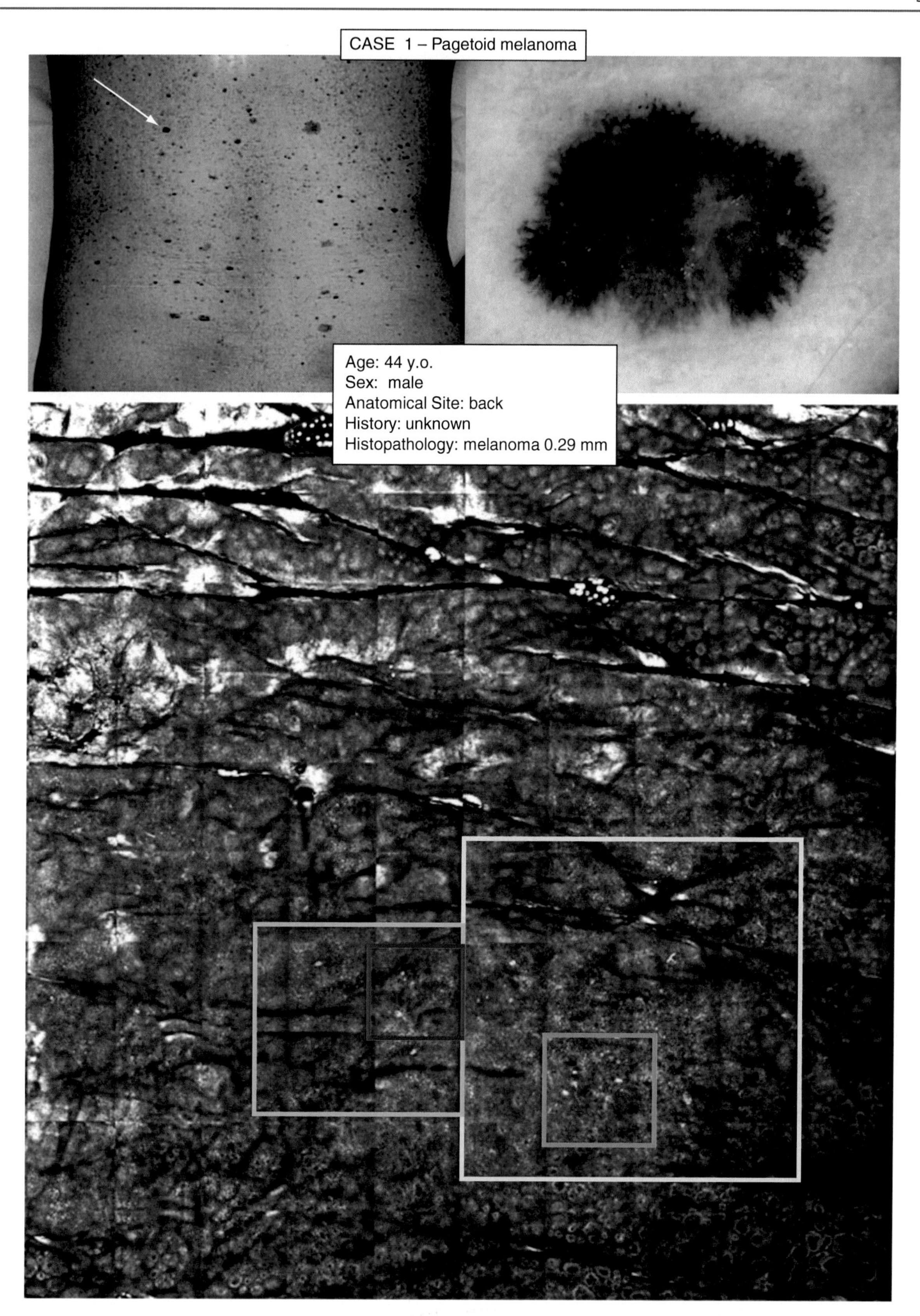

Fig. 13.1 RCM mosaic (5 × 5 mm) at stratum granulosum/spinosum highlighting bright cells in a context of a general cobblestone pattern. The lesion is slightly demarcated in respect to the surrounding skin

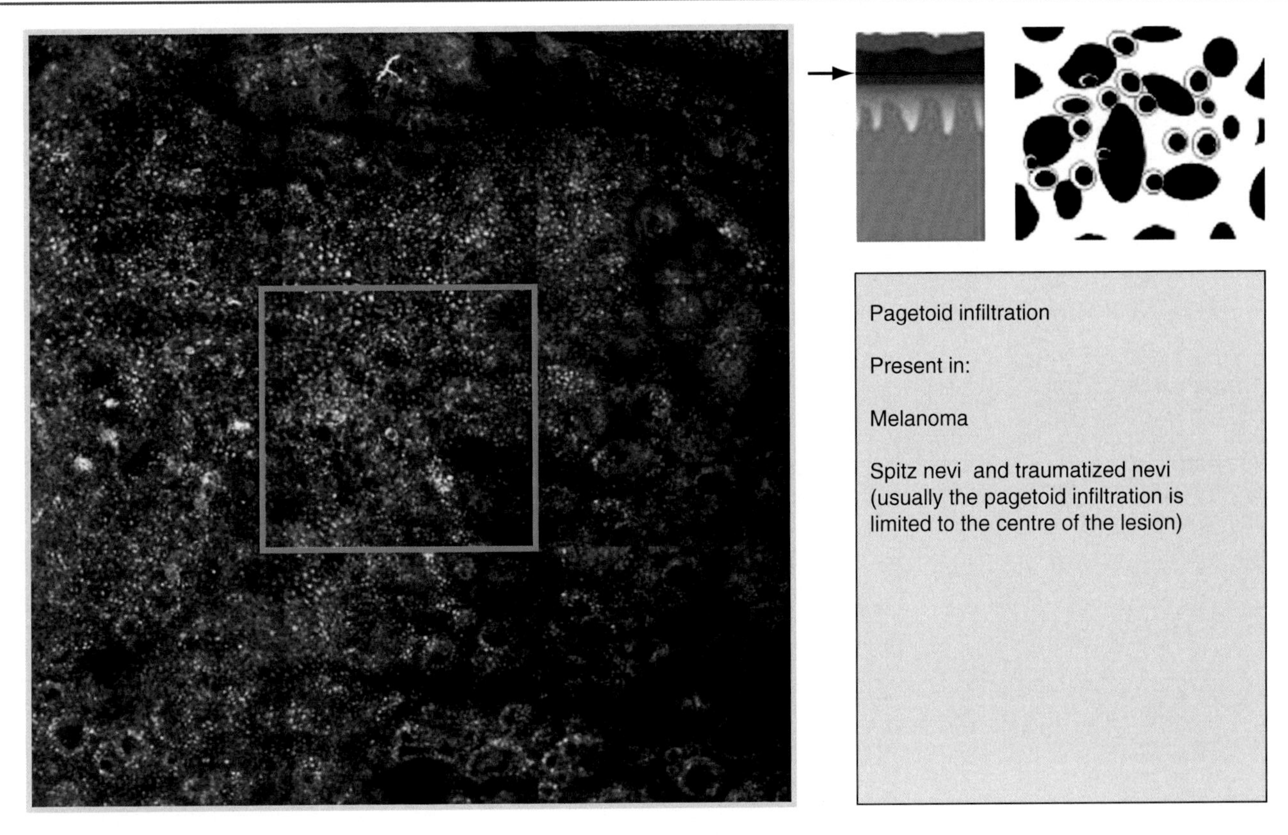

Fig. 13.1.1 RCM mosaic (1.5 × 1.5 mm) at stratum granulosum/spinosum showing the bright large elements corresponding to pagetoid infiltration located at the periphery of the lesion slightly demarcated in respect to the surrounding skin presenting edged papillae

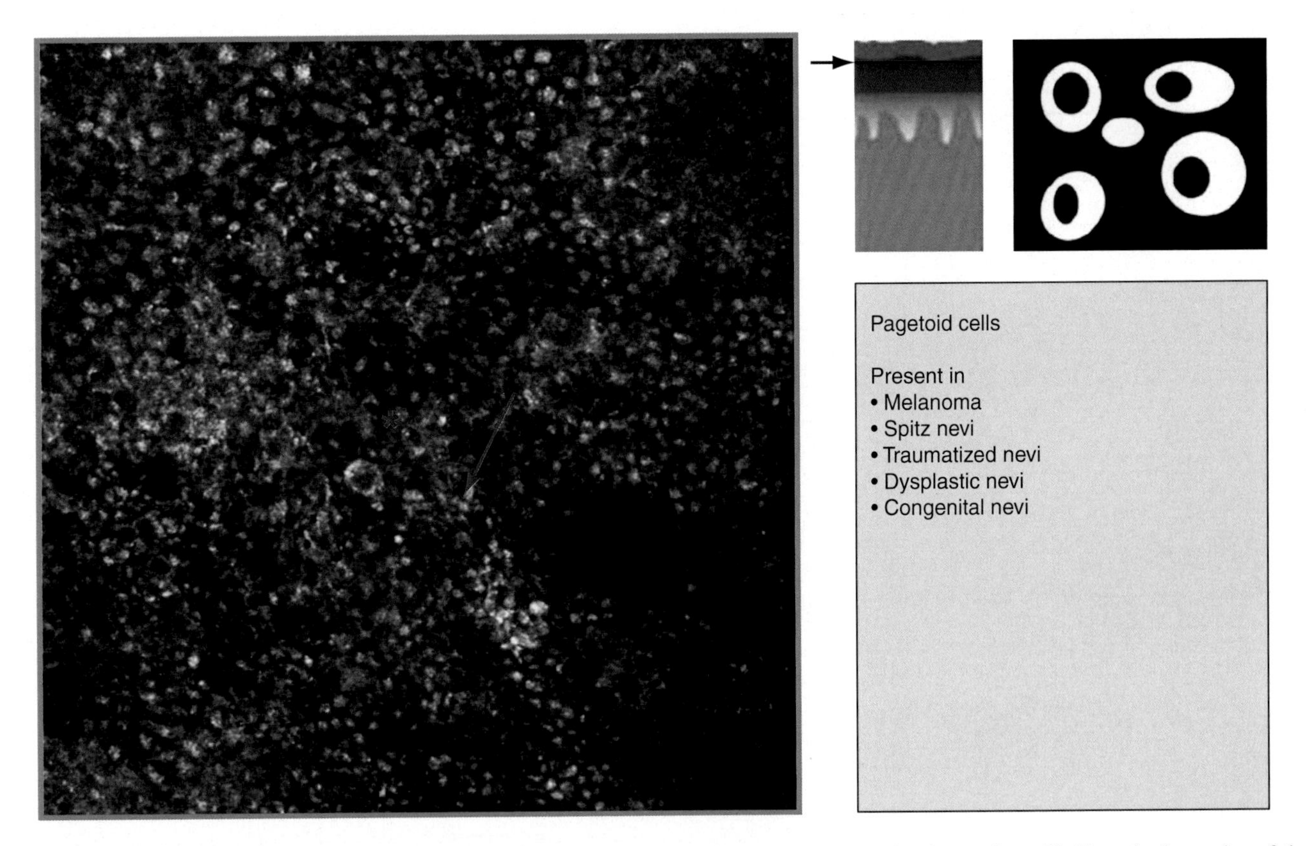

Fig. 13.1.2 Basic image (0.5 × 0.5 mm) large roundish cells with bright cytoplasm and hyporeflective nucleus (*). Note the large size of the pagetoid cells compared to the neighboring keratinocytes (*arrow*)

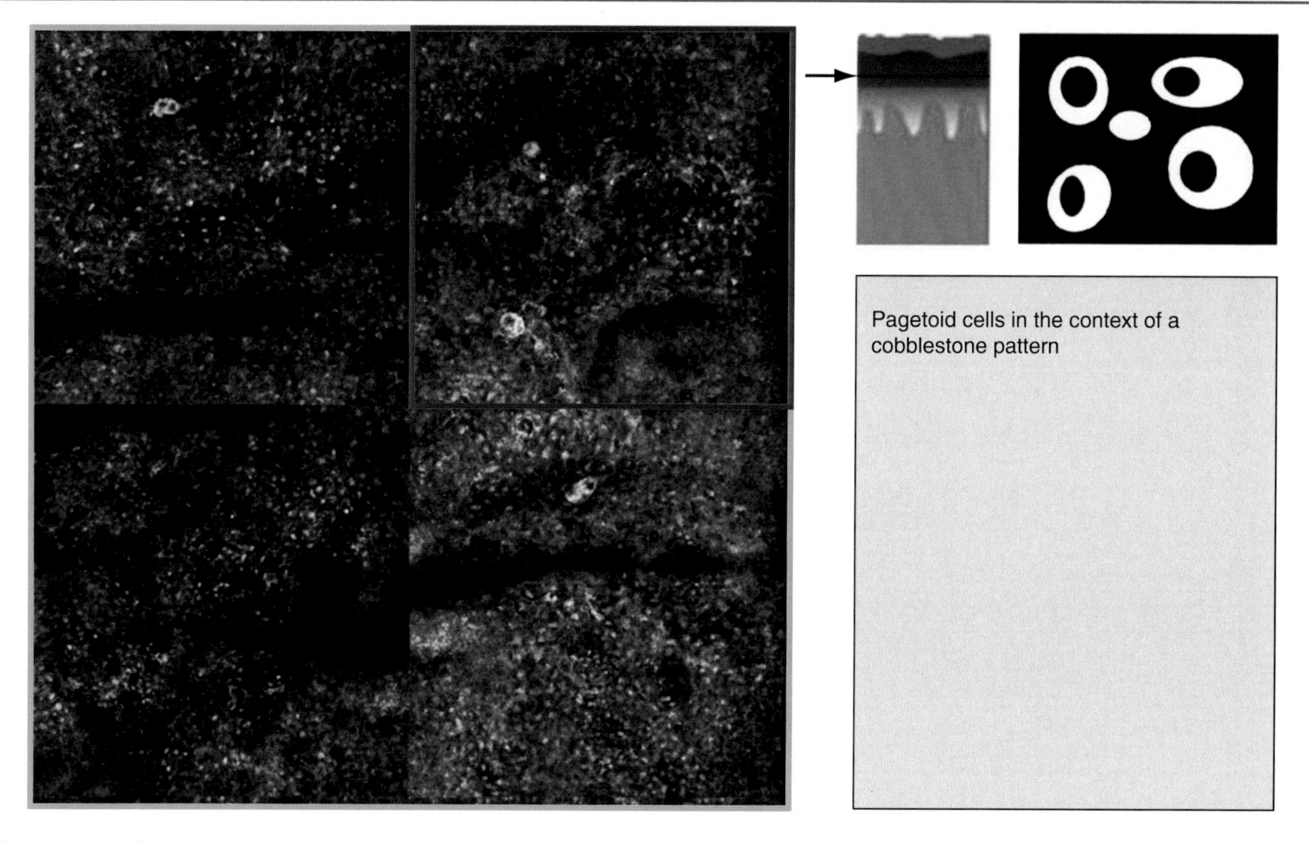

Fig. 13.1.3 RCM mosaic (1 × 1 mm) highlighting the roundish shape of these large pagetoid cells in the context of a cobblestone pattern

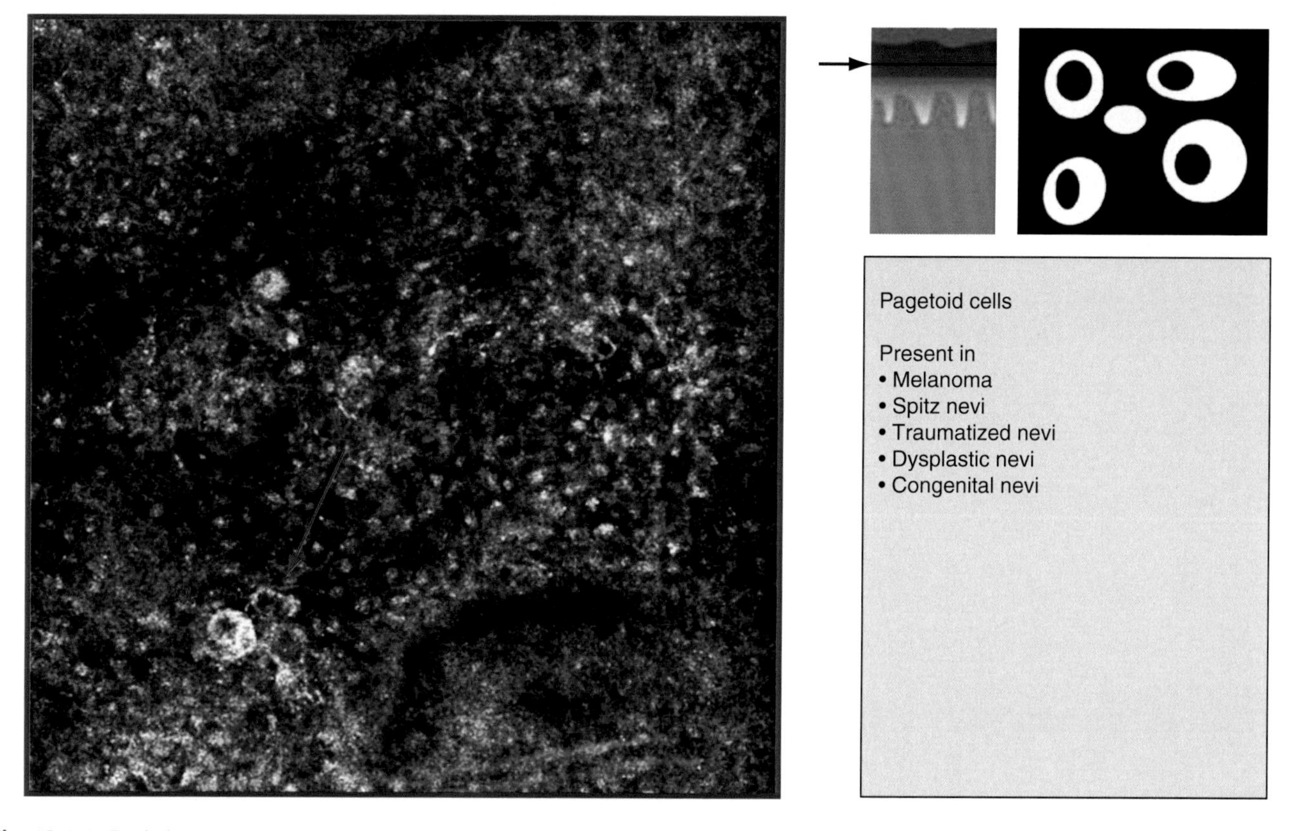

Fig. 13.1.4 Basic image (0.5 × 0.5 mm) showing the prominent hyporeflective nucleus of the pagetoid cells with large cell body (*) sometimes showing thick dendrites (→)

Fig. 13.1.5 RCM mosaic (5 × 5 mm) at DEJ level showing a meshwork pattern especially evident in the center of the lesion that turn into a more ringed pattern at the periphery

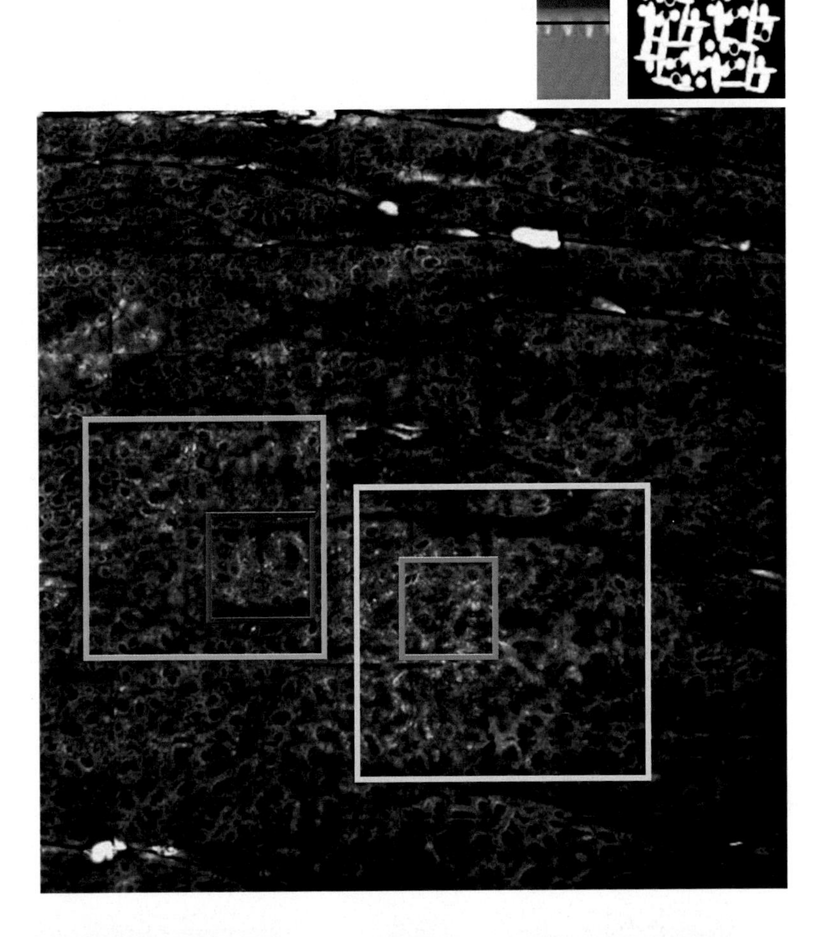

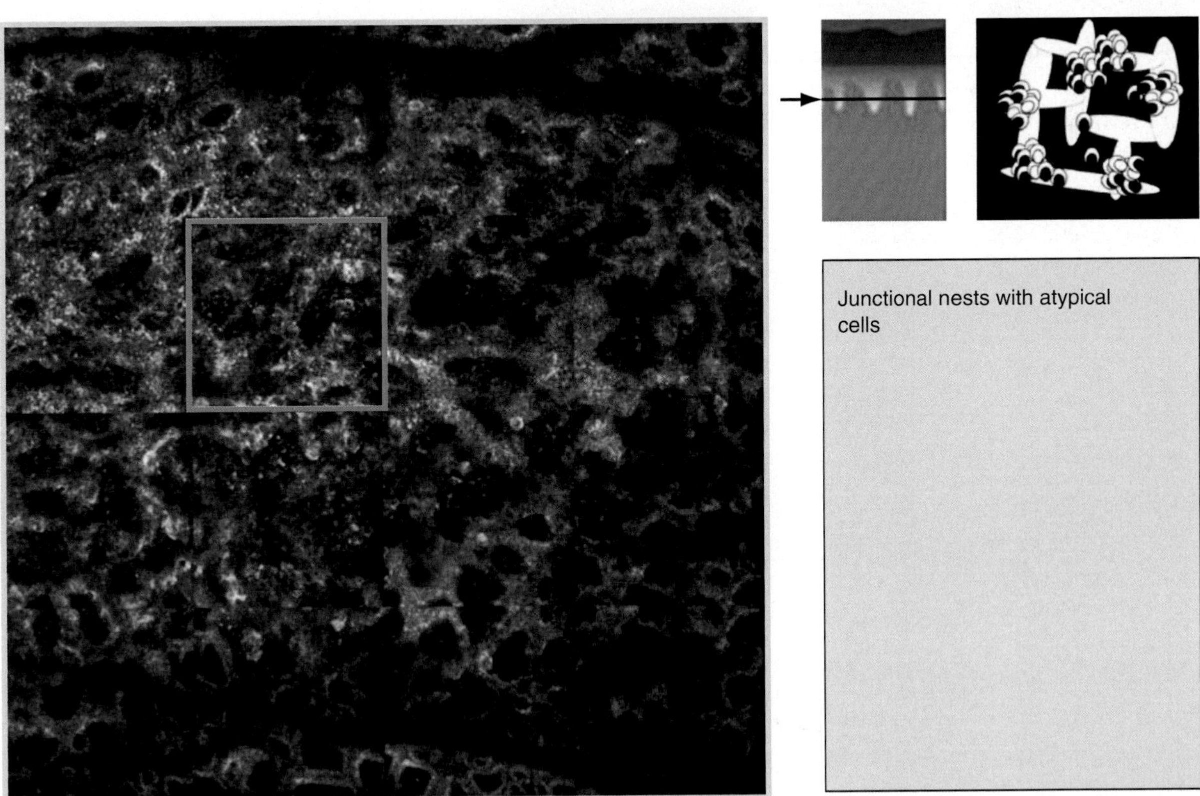

Fig. 13.1.6 RCM mosaic (2 × 2 mm) depicting an enlargement of the junctional space that appear populated by single bright cells

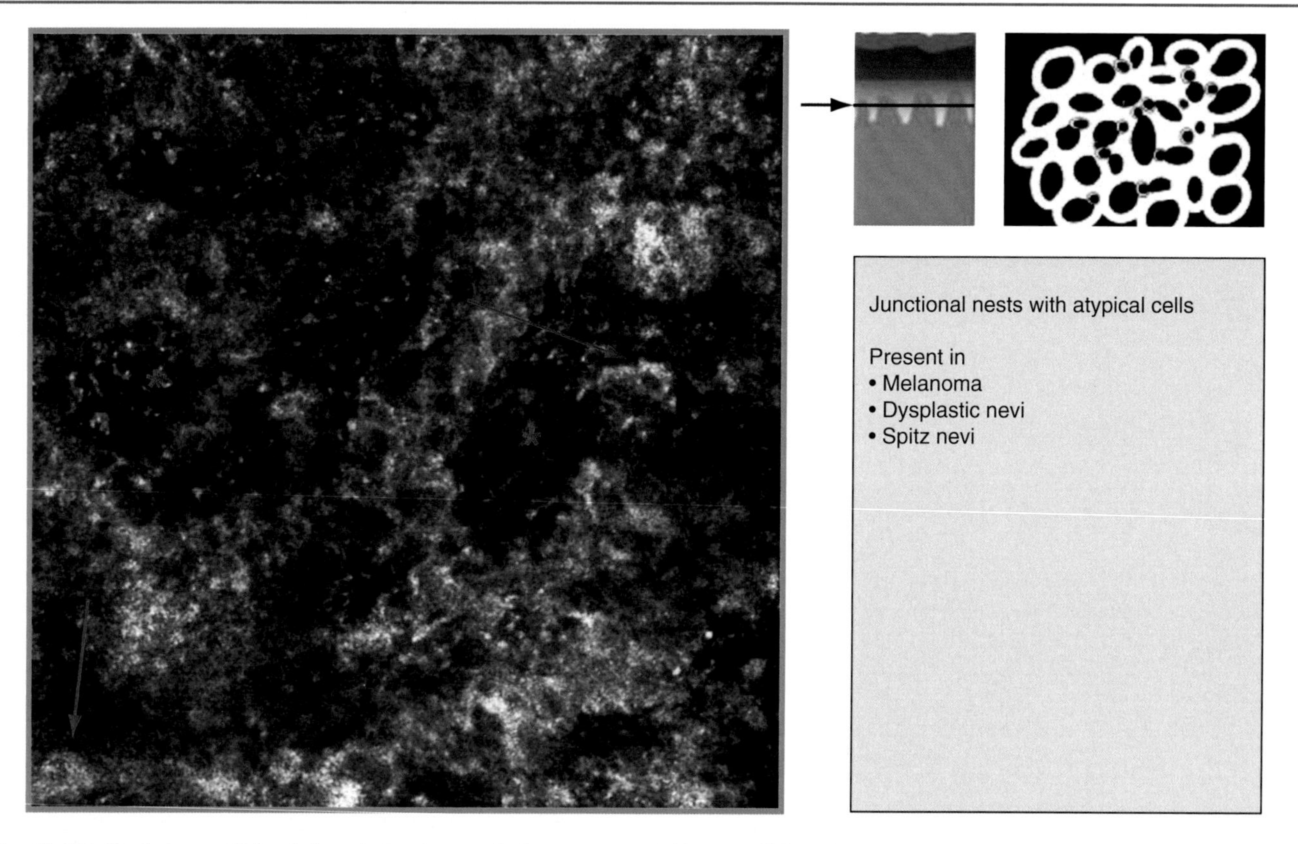

Fig. 13.1.7 Basic image (0.5 × 0.5 mm) showing atypical nests composed by roundish cells (→). The nests outline the hyporeflective dermal papillae (*). The dermo-epidermal junction contour results uneven and distorted for the presence of this junctional proliferation

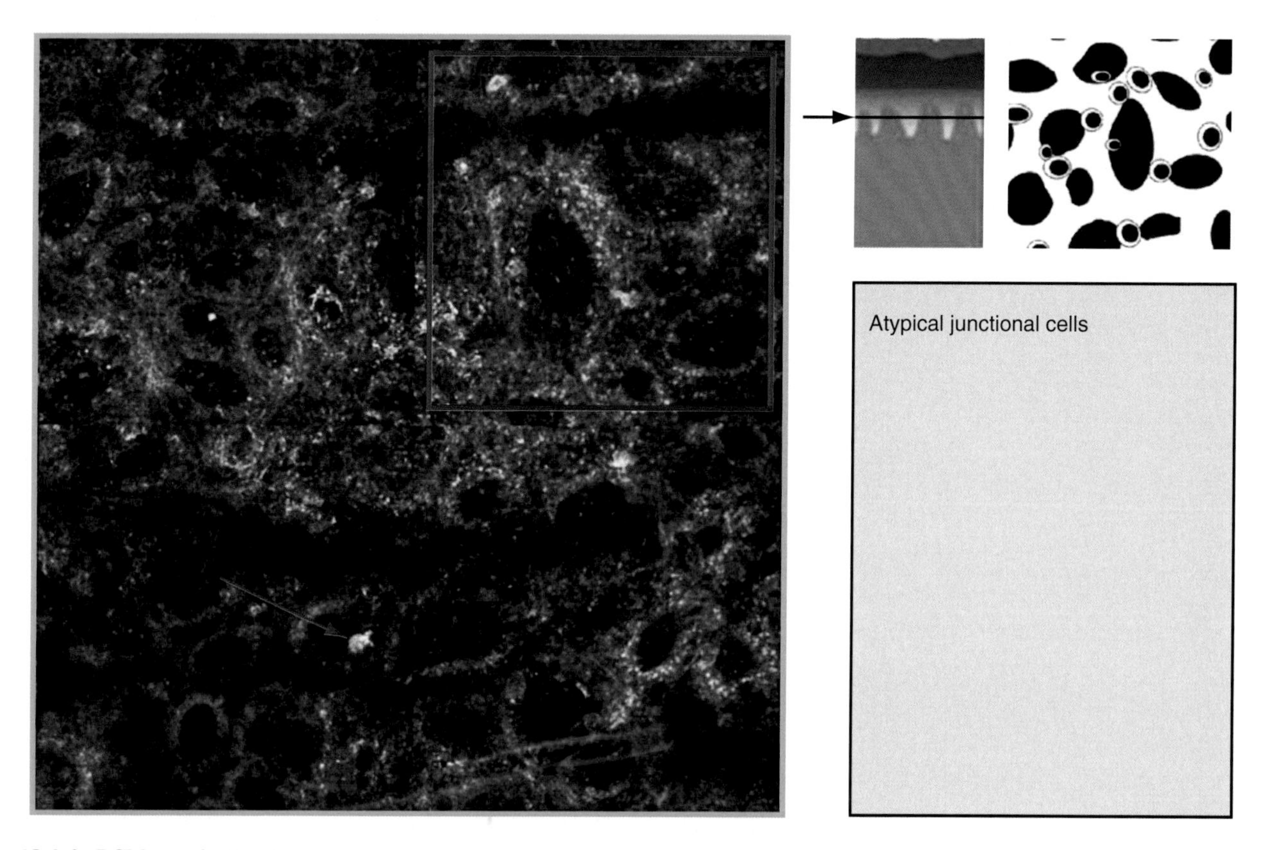

Fig. 13.1.8 RCM mosaic (1 × 1 mm) the atypical melanocytes with roundish cells show up as single/individual cells, not aggregated in nests, surrounding edged papillae. Sometimes it is possible to visualize short and thick dendrites

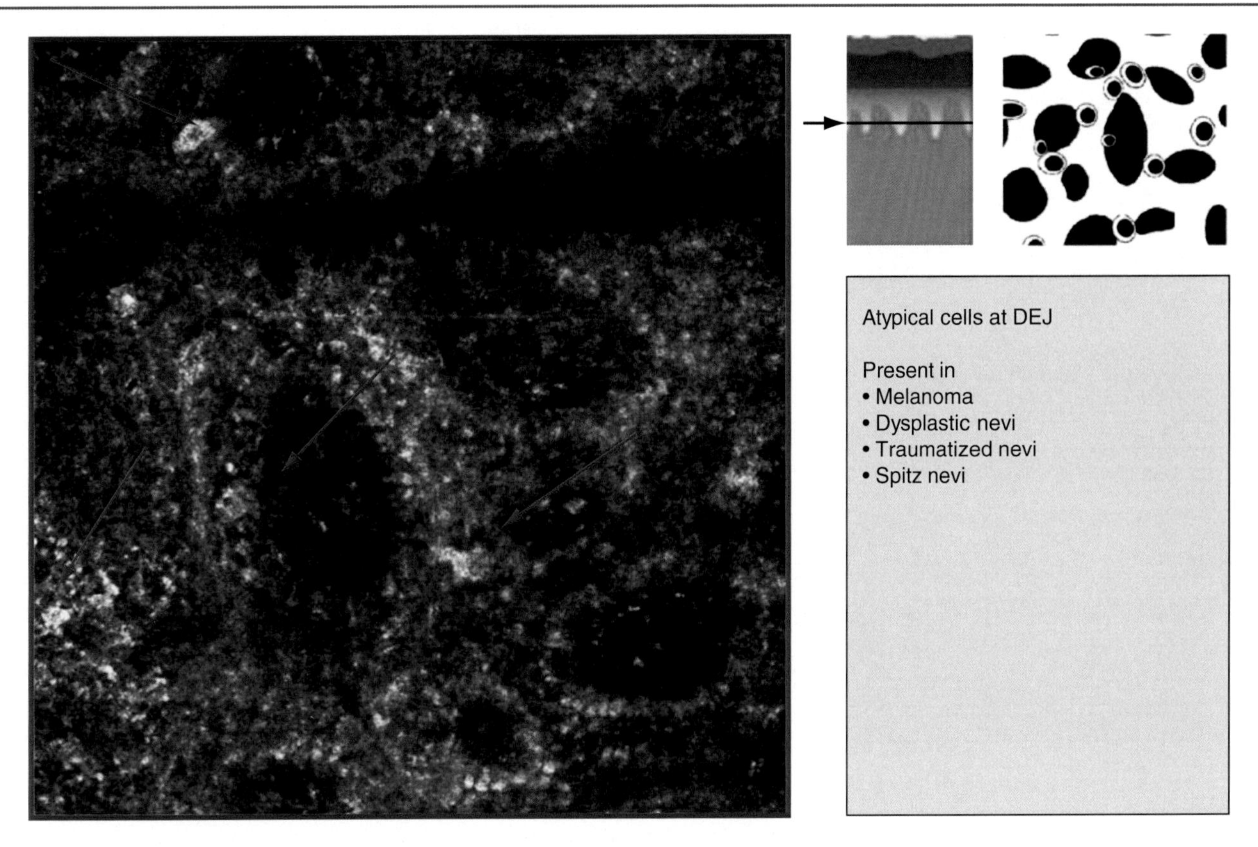

Fig. 13.1.9 Basic image (0.5 × 0.5 mm). Isolated atypical melanocytes with large refractive body sometimes with short and thick dendrites (→) surrounding edged dermal papillae

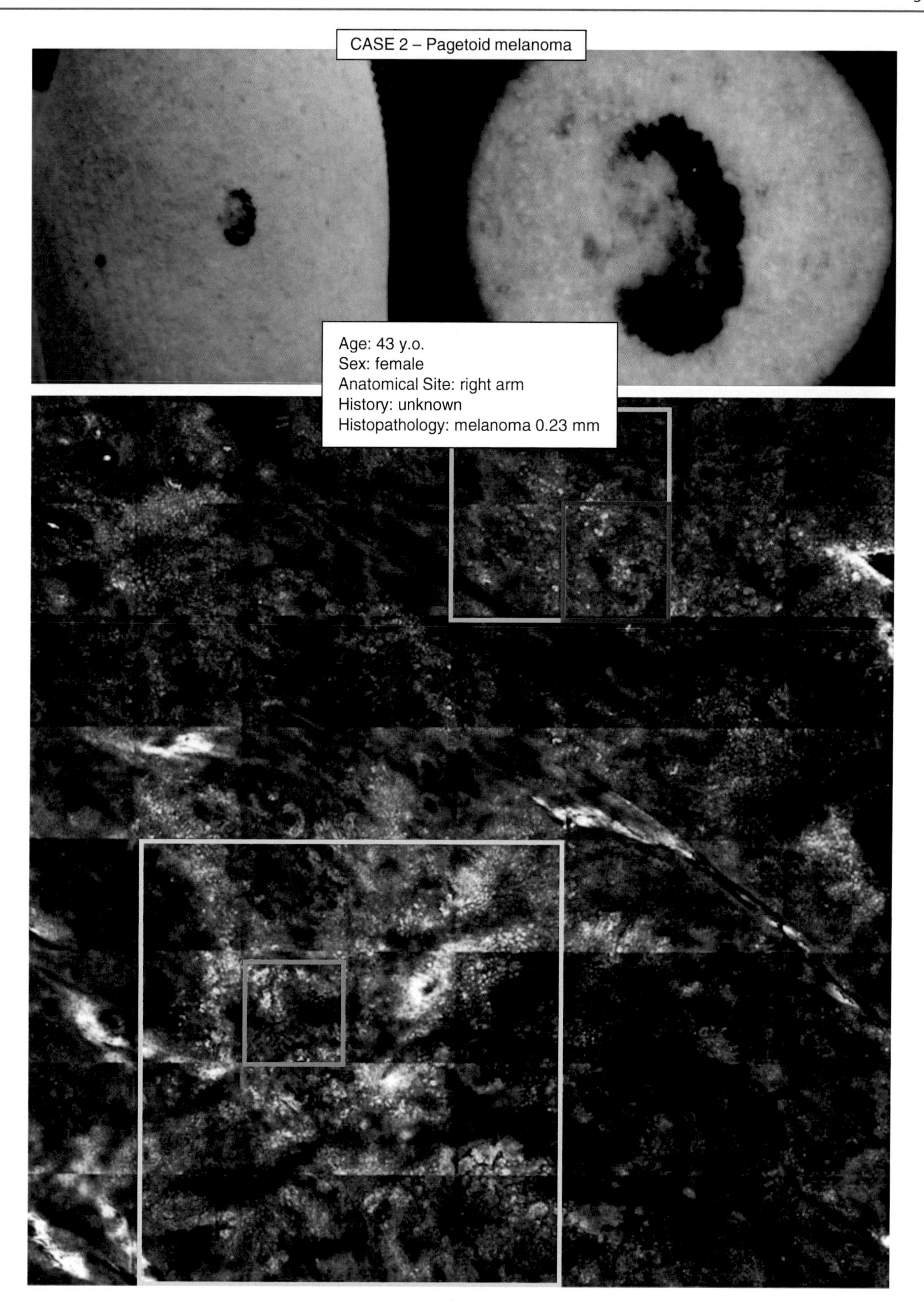

Fig. 13.2 RCM mosaic (4 × 4 mm) at stratum spinosum/granulosum show the disarrangement of the epidermal layer where numerous pagetoid cells are present throughout the entire lesion

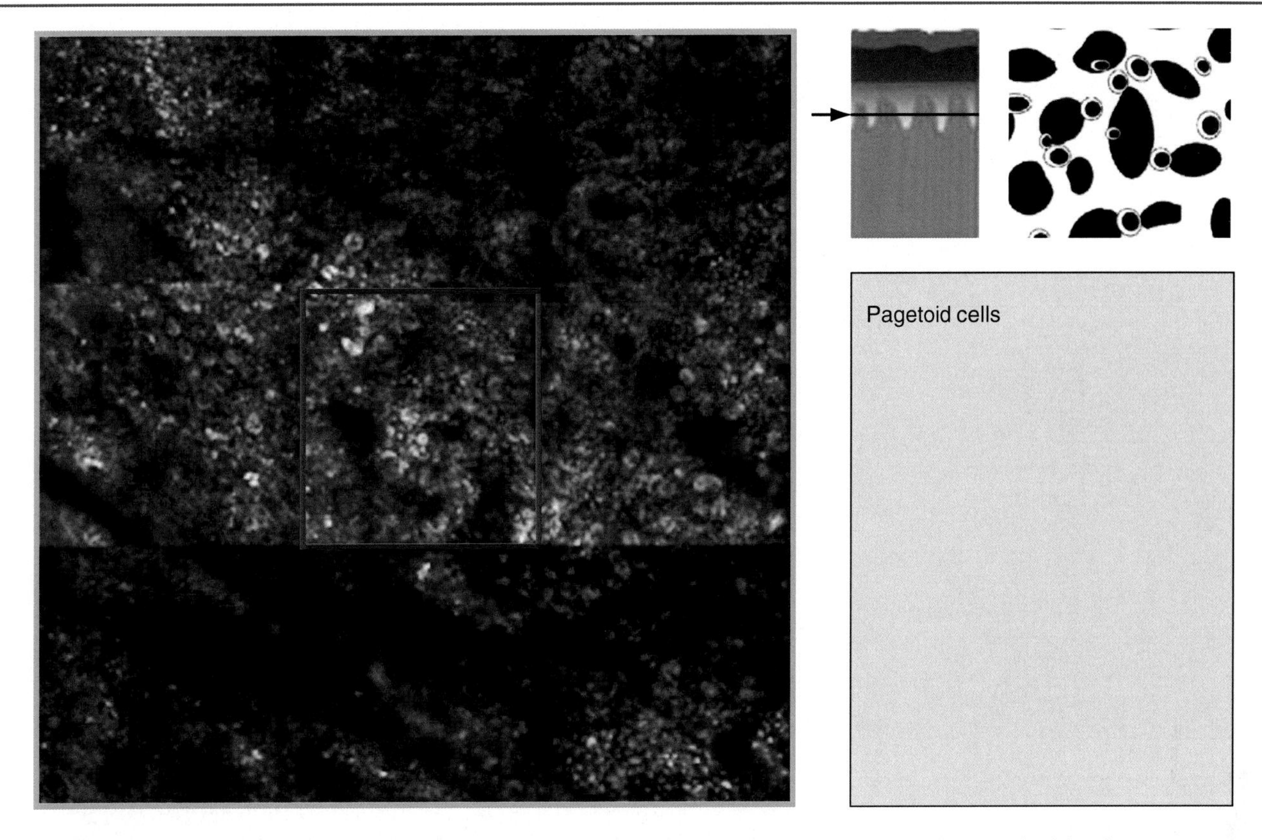

Fig. 13.2.1 RCM mosaic (1.5 × 1.5 mm) depicting a collection of bright pagetoid cells in a context of a disarrayed epidermis

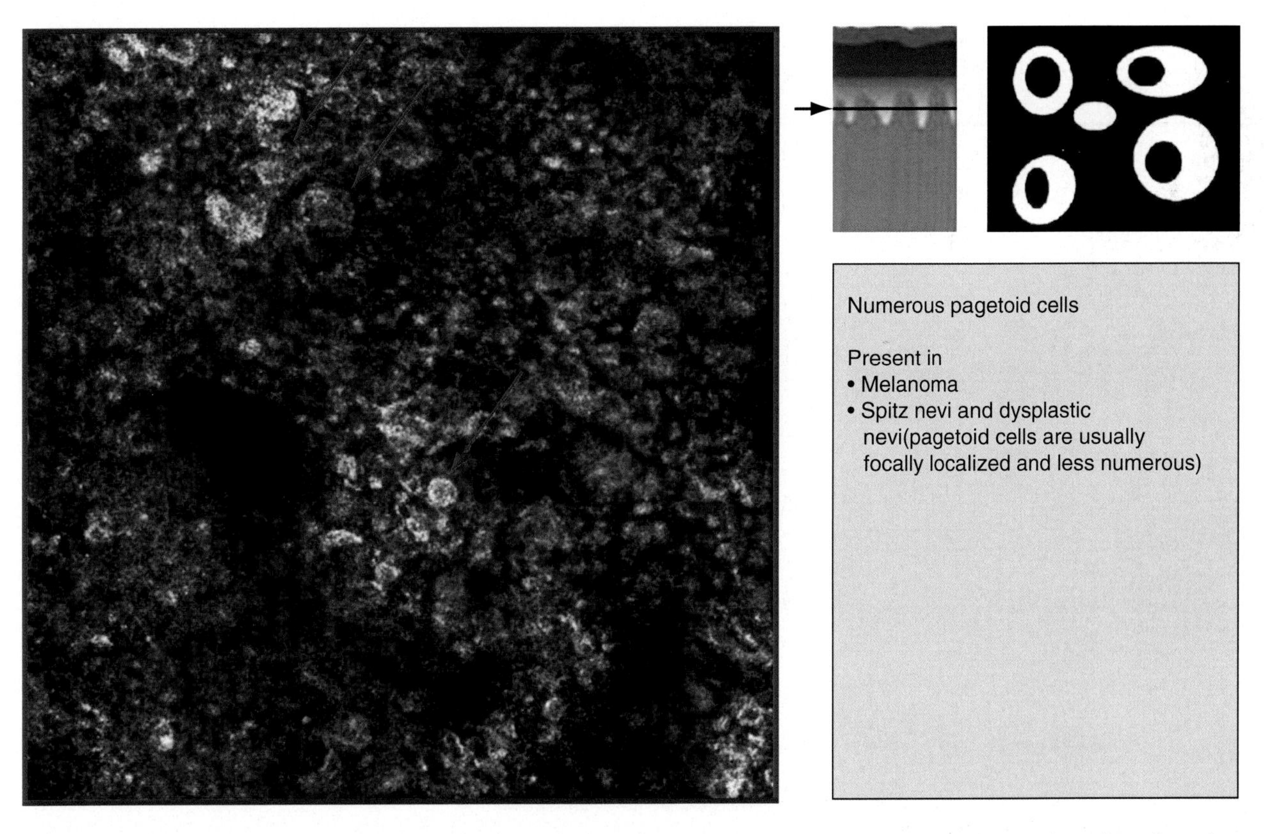

Fig. 13.2.2 Basic image (0.5 × 0.5 mm) showing the roundish shape of pagetoid cells (→) with an hyporeflective nucleus. Sometimes they tend to form clusters. The epidermis is completely disarrayed and populated by atypical melanocytes scattered throughout the entire compartment

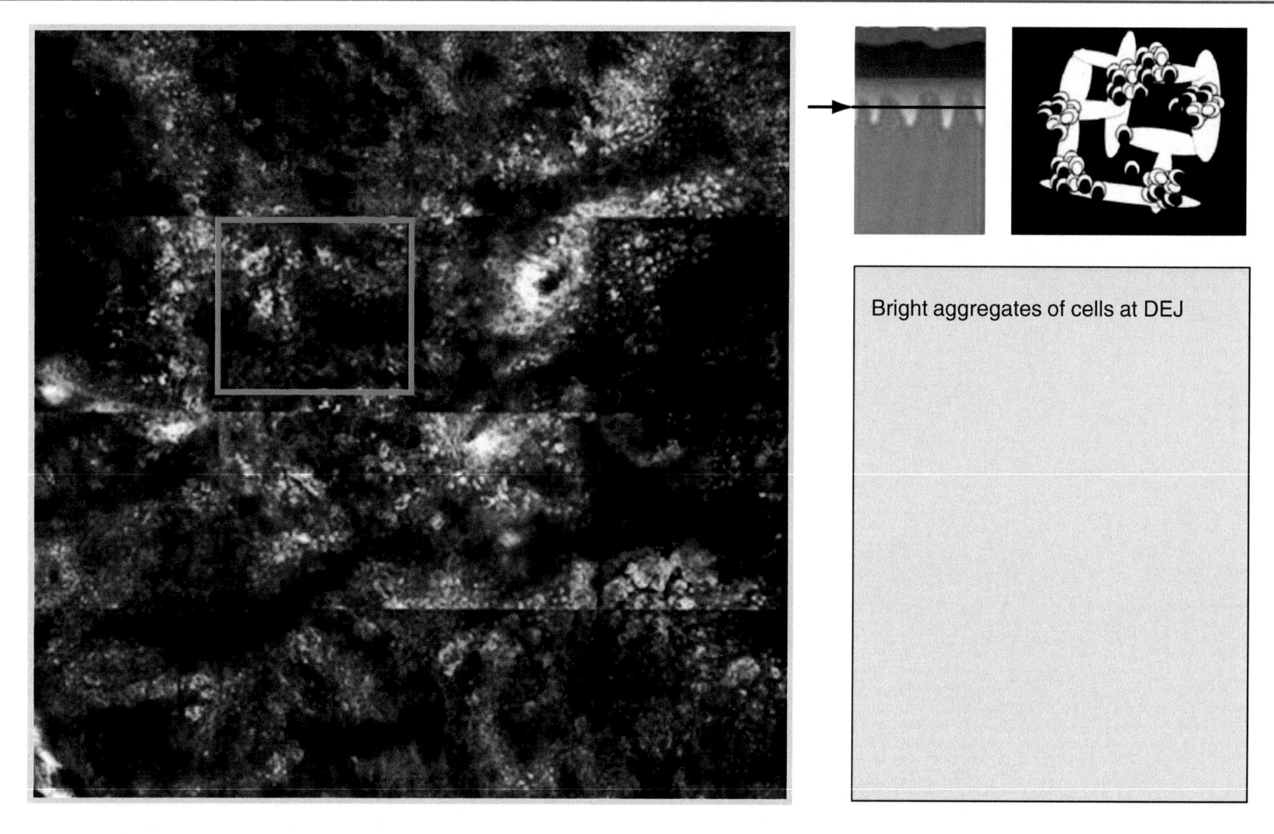

Fig. 13.2.3 RCM mosaic (2 × 2 mm) presenting a bright aggregate of cells at DEJ level where dermal papillae are no longer visible

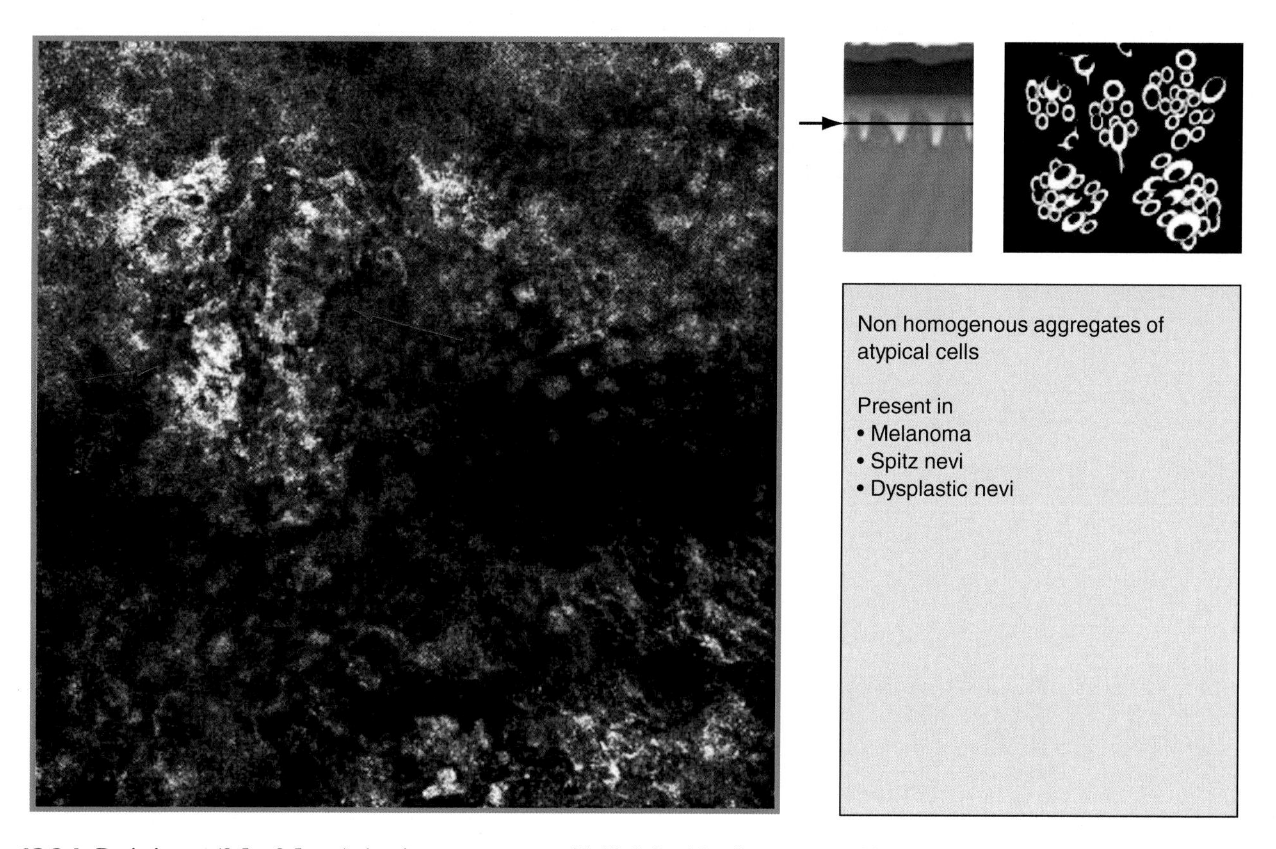

Fig. 13.2.4 Basic image (0.5 × 0.5 mm) showing an aggregate with ill-defined borders composed by atypical cells in the context of a disarrayed junctional profile (→)

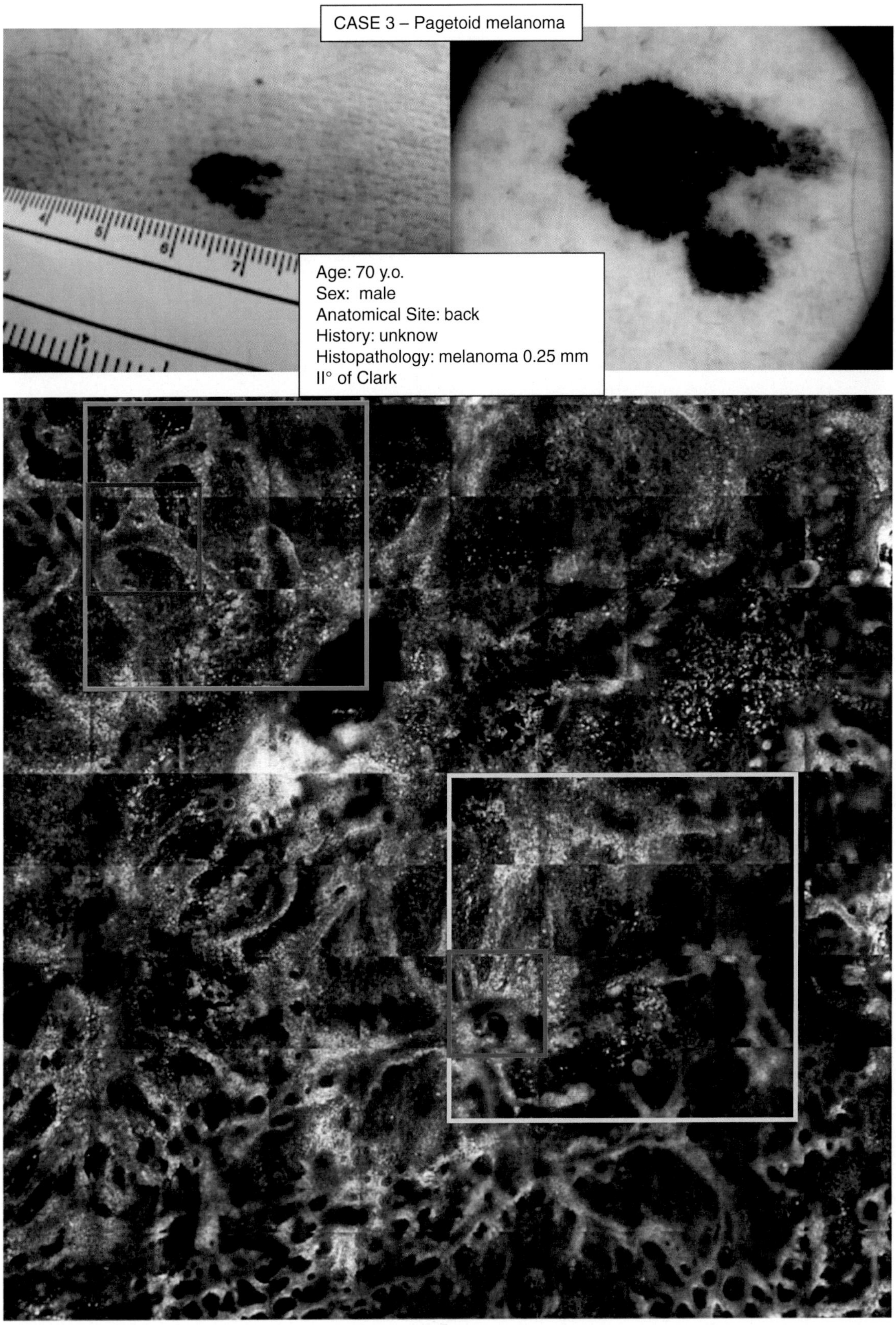

CASE 3 – Pagetoid melanoma

Age: 70 y.o.
Sex: male
Anatomical Site: back
History: unknow
Histopathology: melanoma 0.25 mm
II° of Clark

Fig. 13.3 RCM mosaic (5 × 5 mm) at DEJ level showing an atypical meshwork pattern constituted by irregularly spaced papillae and enlarged interpapillary spaces

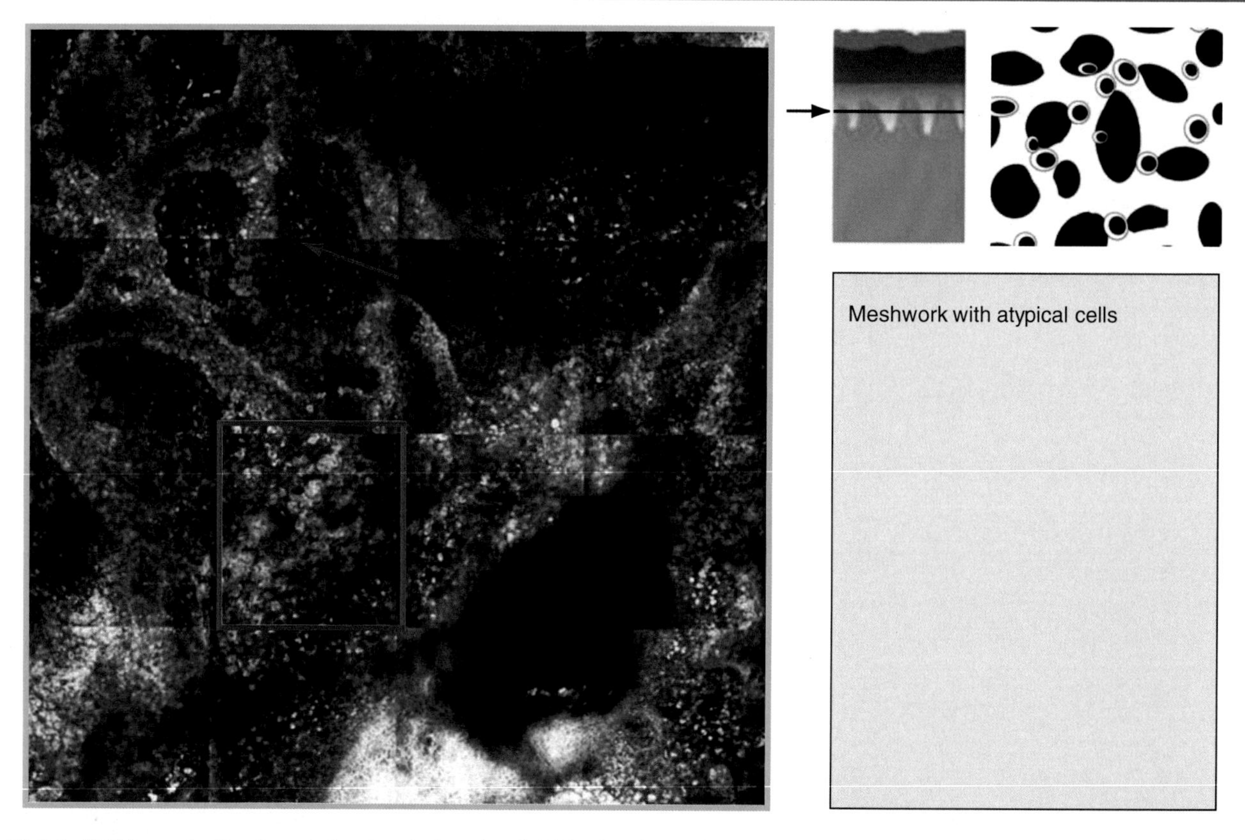

Fig. 13.3.1 RCM mosaic (2 × 2 mm) showing the junctional thickening due to the presence of crowded atypical melanocytes. At the periphery the meshwork pattern is more preserved (*arrow*) whereas it is replaced by the presence of sheet of cells (*red square*)

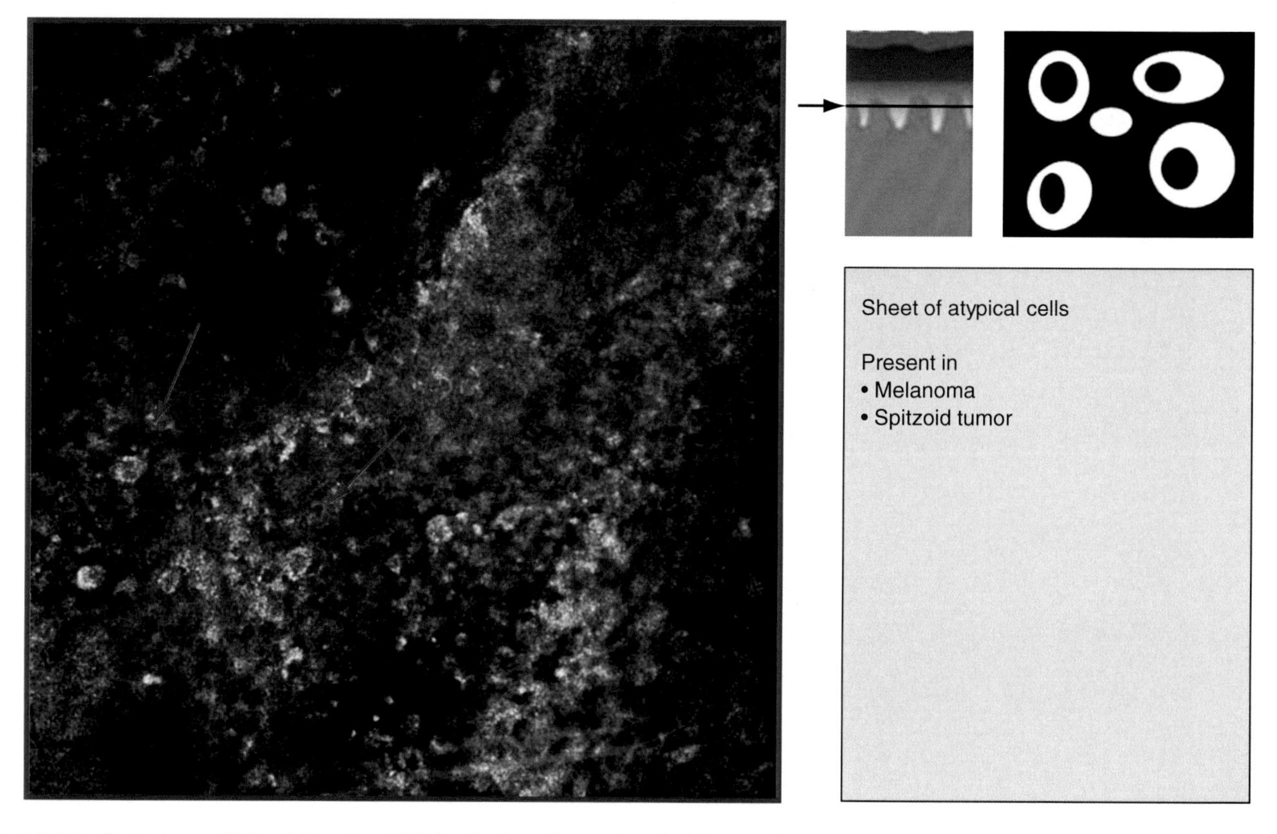

Fig. 13.3.2 Basic image (0.5 × 0.5 mm) at DEJ level where the meshwork silhouette is no longer present being replaced by sheet of roundish atypical melanocytes (→)

Meshwork with atypical cells

Fig. 13.3.3 RCM mosaic (2.5 × 2.5 mm) showing a meshwork pattern with a florid cellularity (*blue square*) and a more regularly spaced pattern in the remnant area

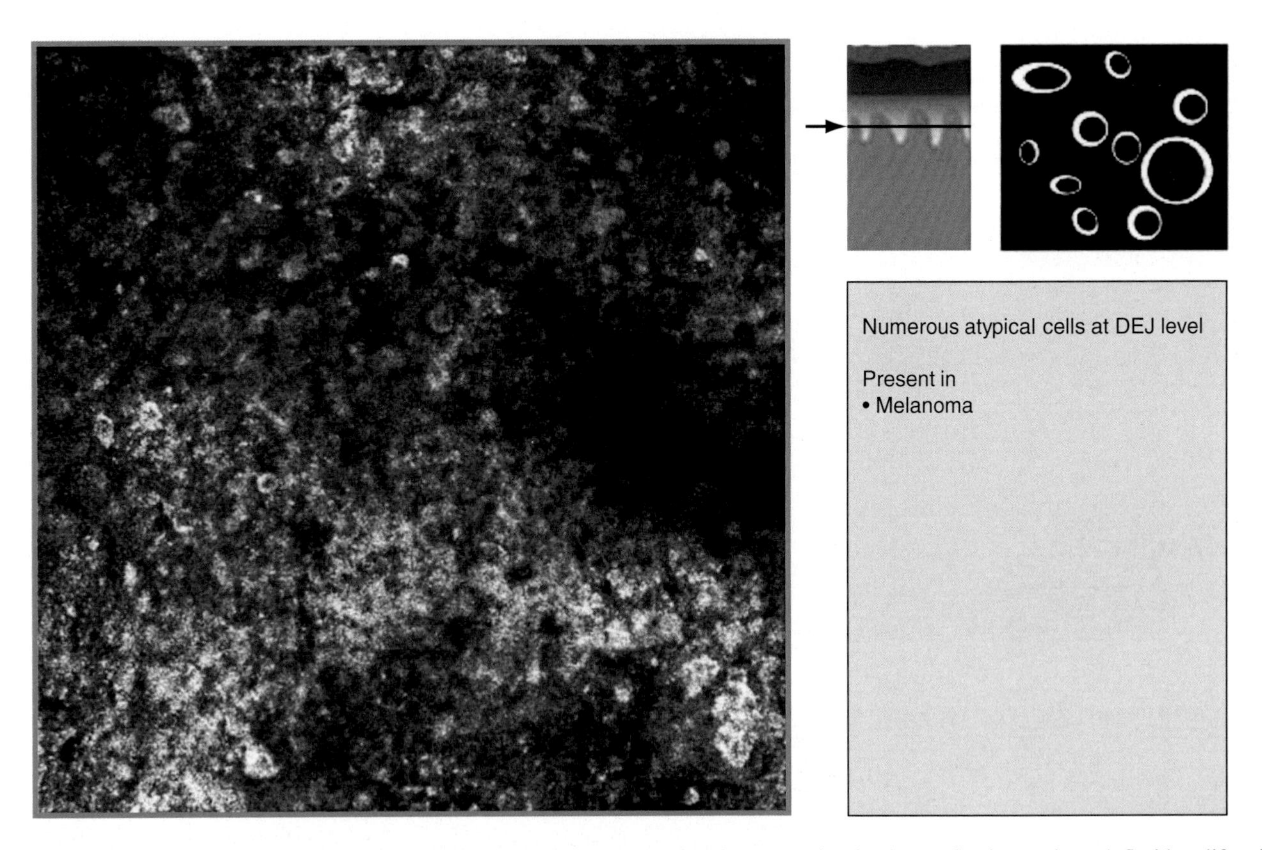

Fig. 13.3.4 Basic image (0.5 × 0.5 mm) showing numerous roundish atypical melanocytes showing hyporeflective nucleus. A florid proliferation of these cells is exclusively found in melanomas whereas in other instances they are less numerous

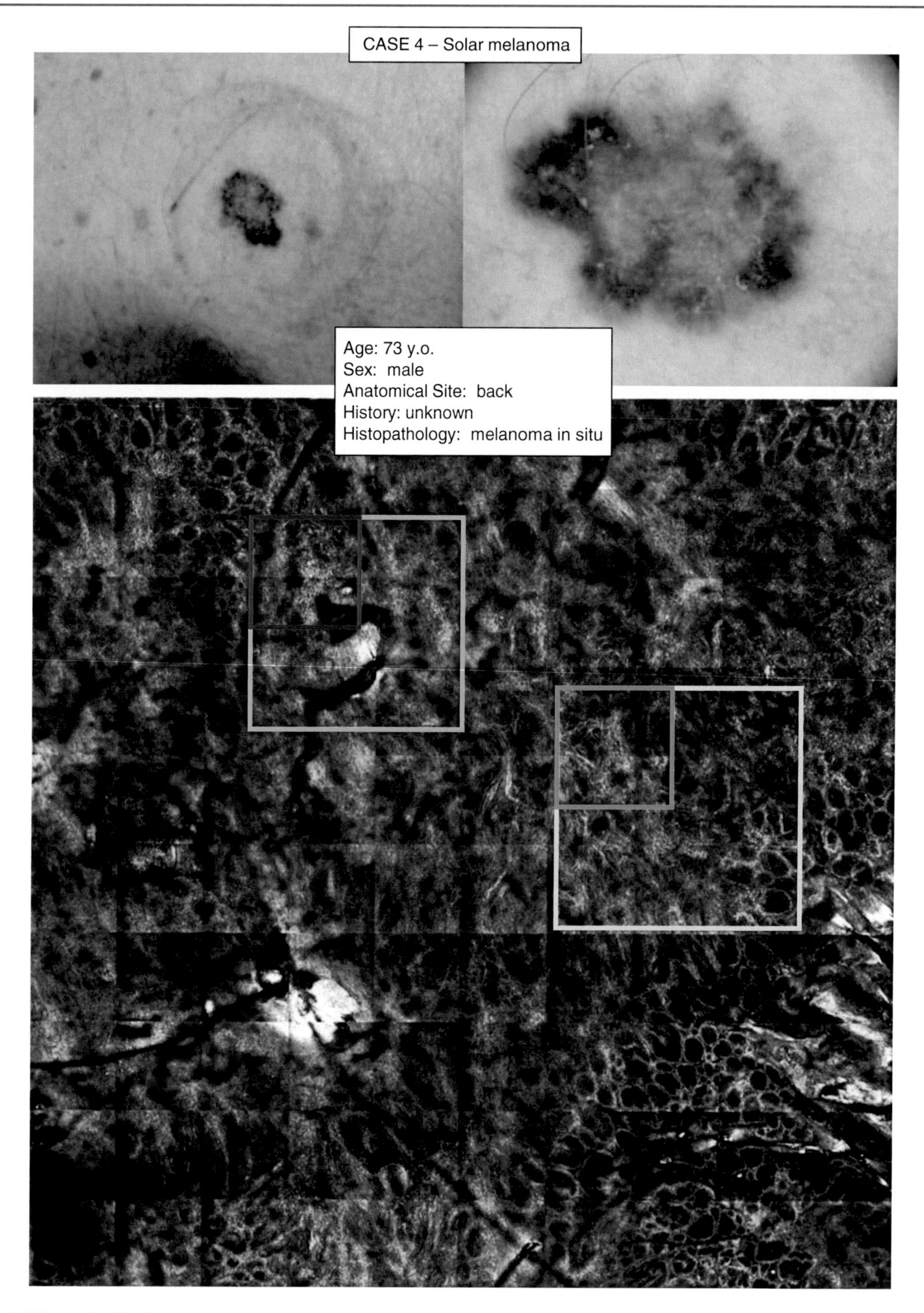

Fig. 13.4 RCM mosaic (5 × 5 mm) at stratum granulosum/spinosum showing a disarranged epidermal pattern. Numerous lines are visible in the *yellow* and *blue square*. The lesion is well demarcated in respect to the surrounding skin presenting an edged contour

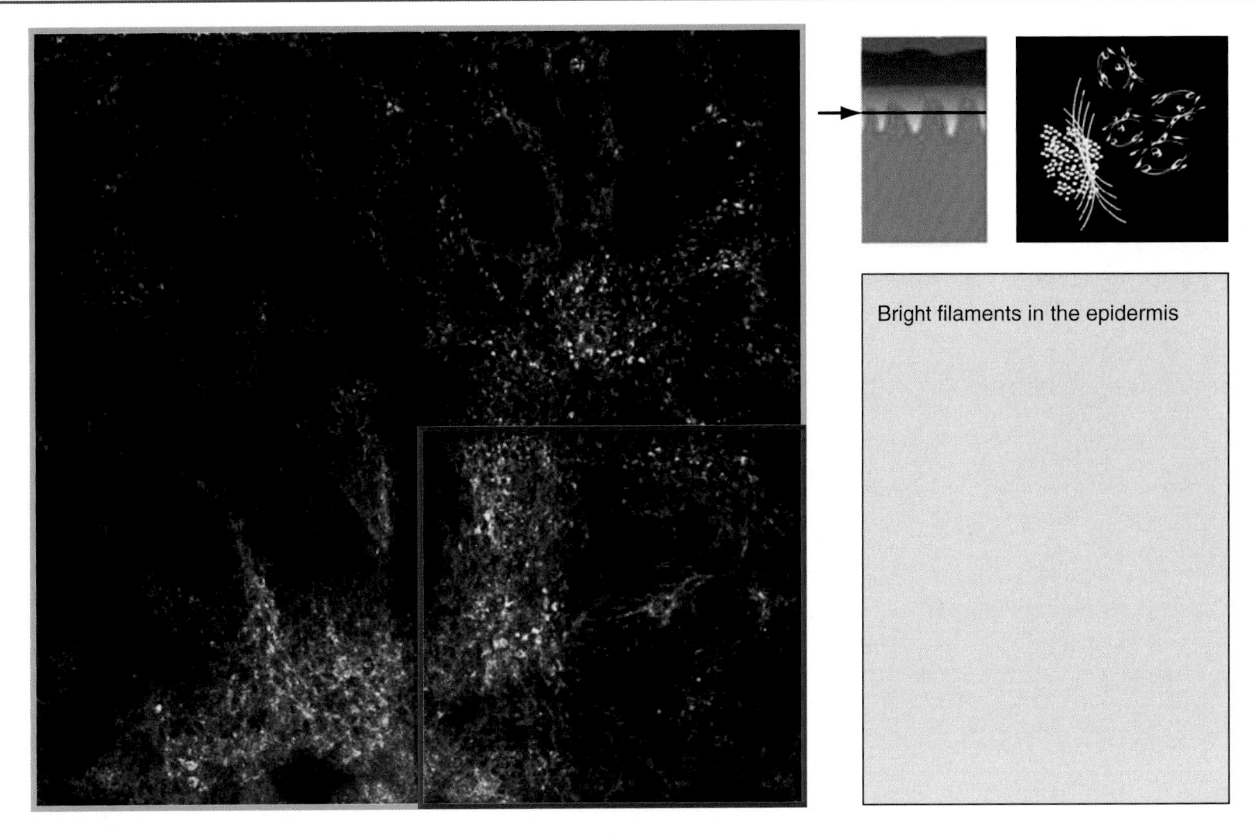

Fig. 13.4.1 RCM mosaic (1 × 1 mm). At first glance, the DEJ pattern is not showing marked disarray. However, in the epidermal component between the papillae is possible to observe bright filaments and dots irregularly distributed (*red square*) with nonedged papillae

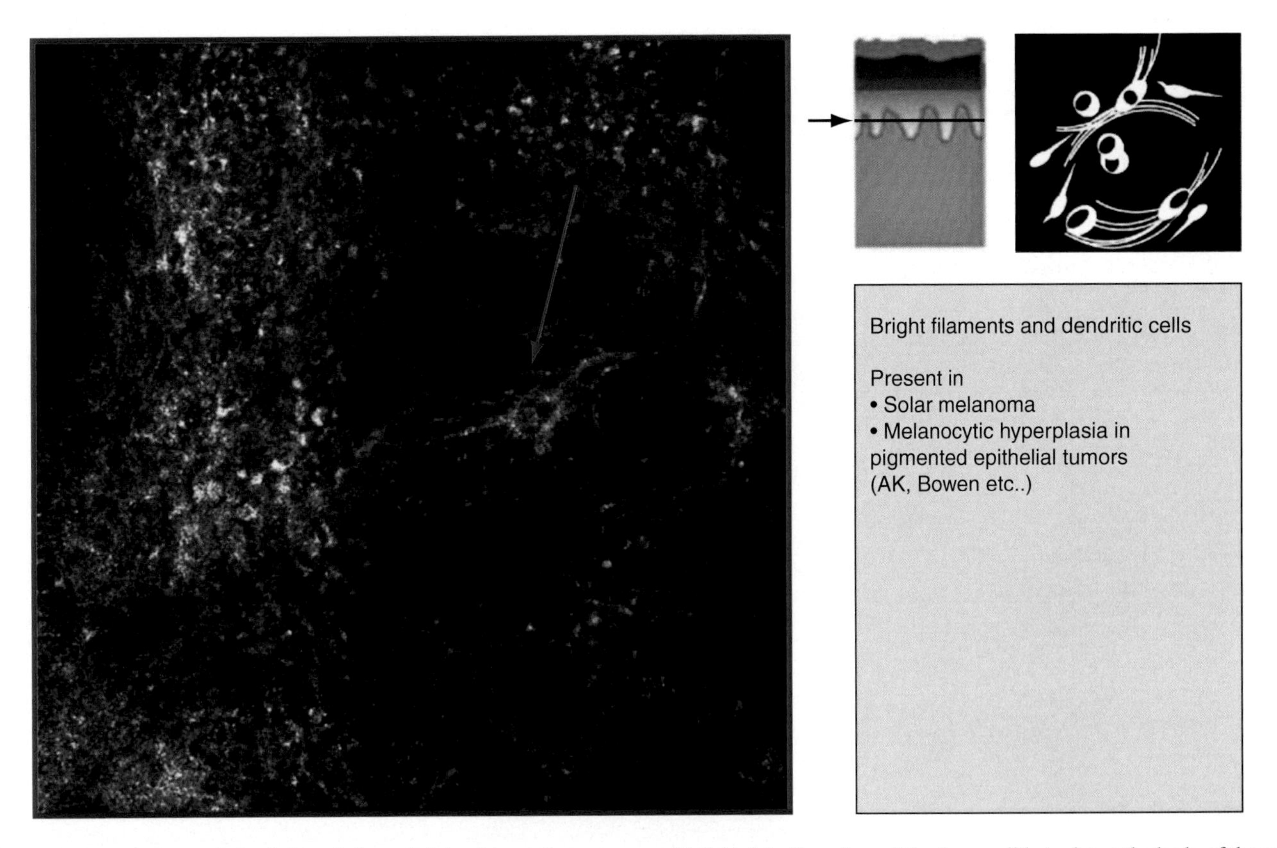

Fig. 13.4.2 Basic image (0.5 × 0.5 mm) shows bright elongated structures and bright dots. Sometimes it is also possible to detect the body of the cell corresponding to a dendritic melanocyte (→). Edged papillae could be defined as "nonedged" since it is not possible to readily outline the contour

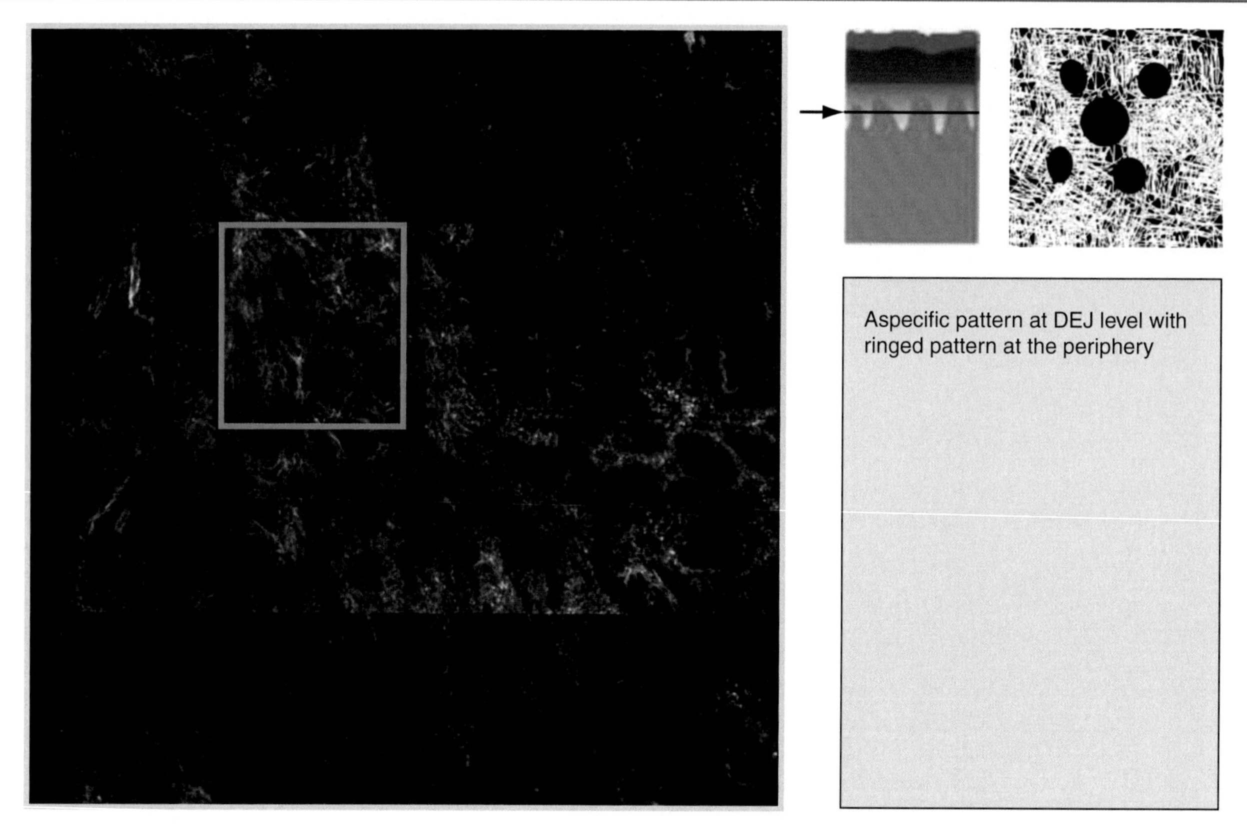

Fig. 13.4.3 RCM mosaic (2 × 2 mm) at DEJ level presenting numerous elongated structures in the context of an aspecific structure. At the periphery edged papillae, forming a ringed pattern, are still visible. This aspect corresponds to the flattening of the rete-ridge upon histopathology

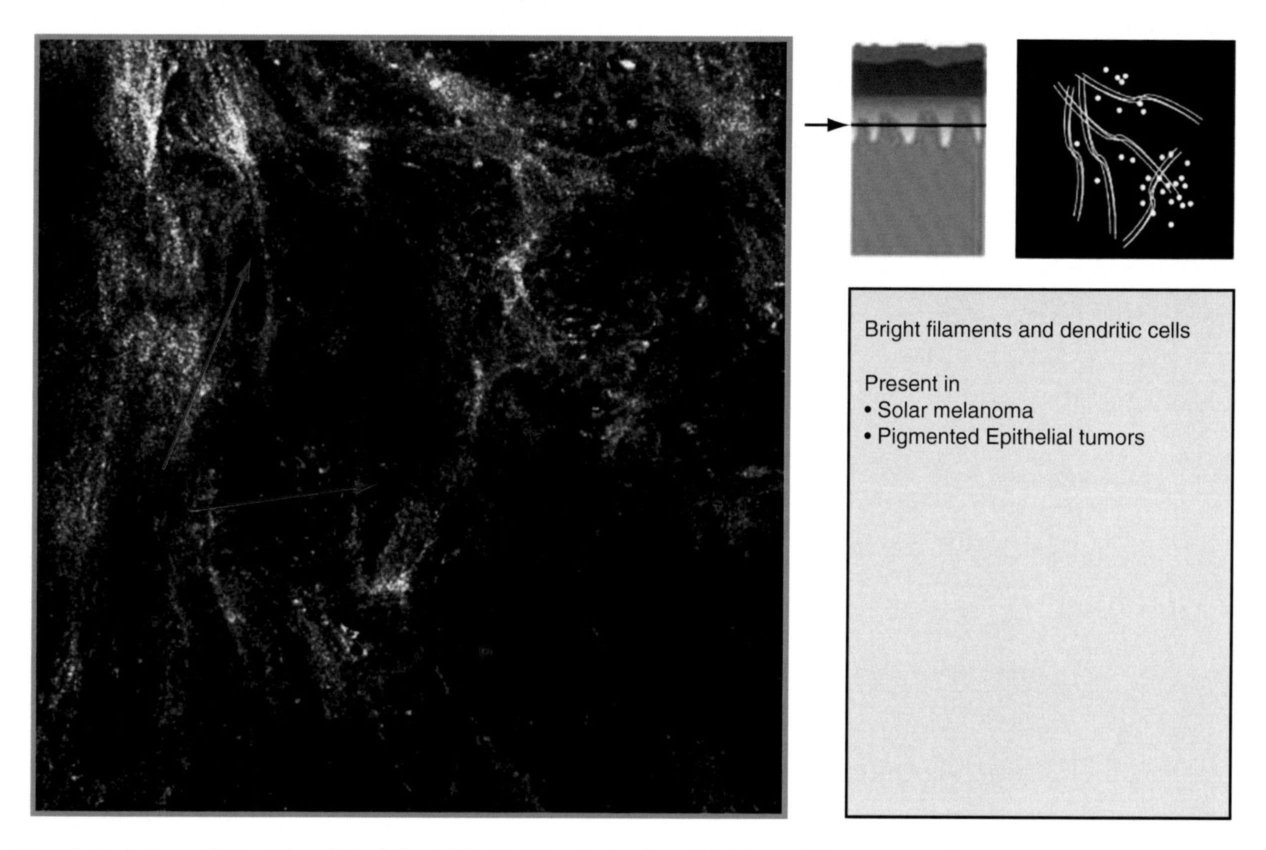

Fig. 13.4.4 Basic image (0.5 × 0.5 mm) depicting bright dendrites (→) and small bright particles corresponding to lymphocytes (*). In this image, the papillary contour is not readily detectable

throughout the lesion may vary from (i) localized, when the cells can be detected only in a small portion of the lesion, to (ii) a widespread distribution.

In the former (i), it can be sometimes difficult to discern the individual cells that can be very few and not so well-highlighted within the epidermal context. Notably, pagetoid cells mainly located in the center of the lesion can be occasionally found also in a variety of different entities such as Spitz nevi, congenital nevi, "traumatized" nevi and dysplastic nevi [8]. However, a careful exploration of the entire lesion is mandatory not to miss early melanomas that sometimes present as a unique sign of malignancy, the presence of few pagetoid cells peripherally located. When distributed onto the entire lesion, pagetoid cells are present either at the periphery and in the center of the melanoma and in this instance the diagnosis is easier than in cases with paucity of cells.

13.1.2 Dermo-Epidermal Junction

In two-third of the cases a meshwork pattern represents the predominant architecture at DEJ. RCM reveals confluent, junctional melanocytic aggregates that widen and distort the rete-ridges giving rise to junctional thickening and a meshwork pattern [9]. Evaluating the DEJ/basal layer, edged and nonedged papillae [10] can be recognized and atypical bright melanocytes are present as single cells or clustering into aggregates (junctional nests with atypical cells). In almost all cases, junctional nests appear as an enlarged interpapillary space where individual atypical roundish cells can be detected.

Pagetoid melanoma arising on a nevus is characterized by the presence of an abrupt transition between the two components, a localized distribution of junctional atypical cells and the presence of dense dermal nests that represent the most striking features [11].

13.1.3 Upper Dermis

When the melanoma is still in its inception, relatively uniform nests can be present immediately below the DEJ in the upper portion of the papillary dermis. In over the half of the cases, those nests are "dense and sparse nests" where individual pleomorphic roundish elements are loosely packed [12]. Inflammatory reaction is present as plump bright cells corresponding to melanophages and bright particles correlated with the presence of lymphocytes. Coarse collagen fibers can be occasionally found in few cases.

13.2 Solar Melanoma

The solar melanomas are first of all defined by their occurrence in the most sun-exposed areas in patients with low nevus count, and by the histologic presence of prominent solar elastosis (Figs. 13.5 and 13.6). No evidence of a pre-existing nevus is usually found. This melanoma type share many features and it is frequently undistinguishable from lentigo maligna that usually occurs on the face or heavily sun-exposed areas. Histologically, there is a linear proliferation of atypical melanocytes in the basal layer and a lymphocytic infiltrate is commonly present in the superficial portions of the dermis. In most cases, the adjacent skin exhibits marked solar degeneration with atrophy of the epidermis and moderate to marked elastosis of the dermis. Dermoscopically, solar melanoma often exhibit regression features such as white, scar-like depigmentation variably combined with blue-gray color and/or peppering (speckled blue-gray granules) [13, 14]. This melanoma type, when presenting blue-grayish coarse granules in a context of heavily sun-damage skin, can be in differential diagnosis with not melanocytic entities such as lichen-planus like keratosis.

13.2.1 Superficial Layers (Epidermis)

On confocal images, there is a striking basilar proliferation of atypical melanocytes with dendritic branches in both the epidermis and at dermo-epidermal junction level. The melanocytes may be so numerous forming an almost continuous melanocytic collection of atypical cells with numerous thin refractive branching structures. The superficial layers appear as atypical honeycombed or cobblestone pattern in two-third of cases and disarranged in approximately one-third. Pagetoid spread is constituted by pleomorphic cells with ovoidal or elongated body and variable morphology of the branches which can appear as thick and short dendrites or thin bright filamentous structures. When dendritic cells are few and not so pleomorphic, they can be morphologically undistinguishable from Langherans cells that may be present also in benign melanocytic and nonmelanocytic lesions. This striking dendritic cell proliferation is resembling the one present in lentigo maligna melanoma where in the latter they are preferentially located around hair follicles [15, 16].

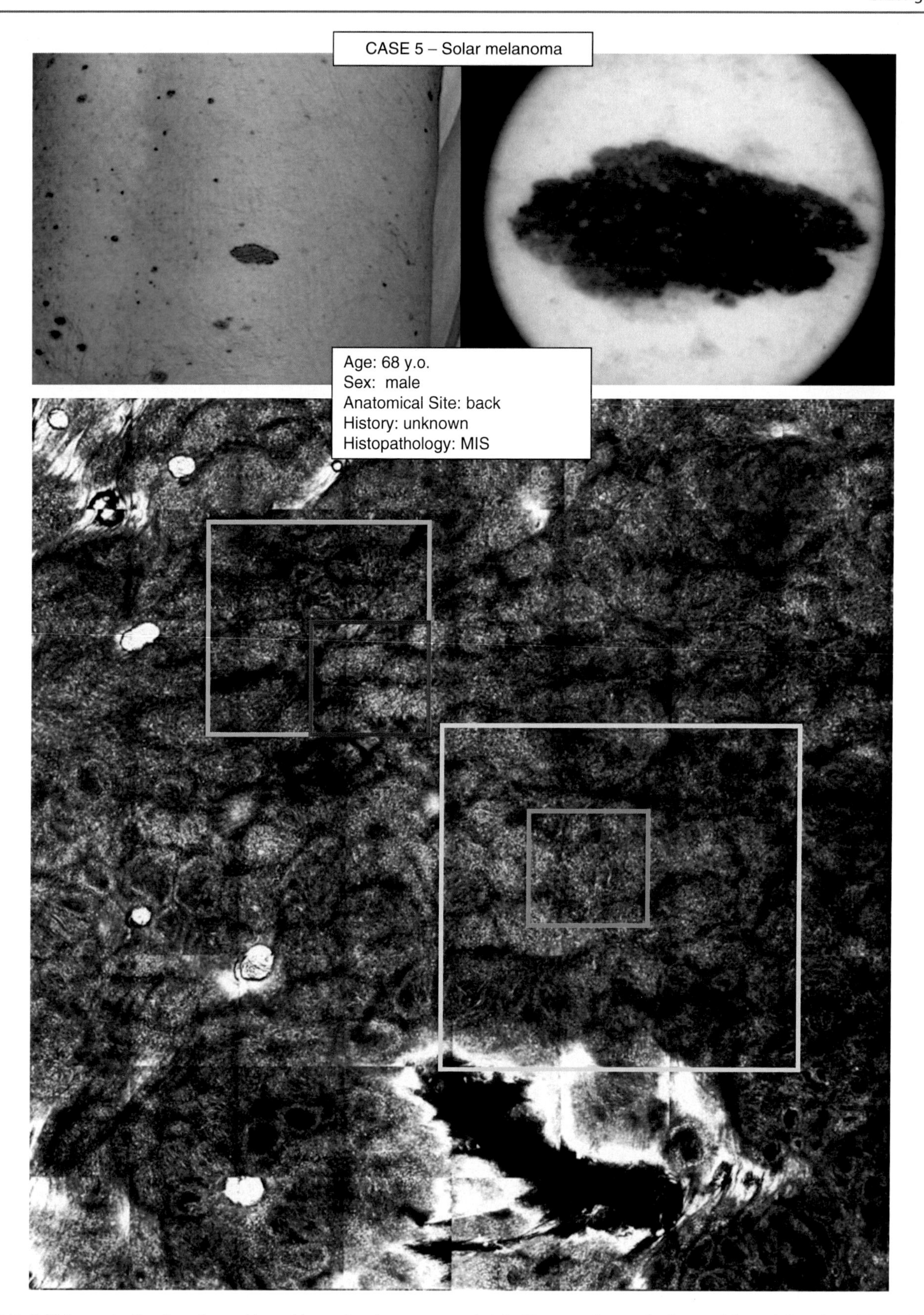

Fig. 13.5 RCM mosaic (5 × 5 mm) at epidermal layer showing numerous bright filaments that render impossible to define the epidermal pattern

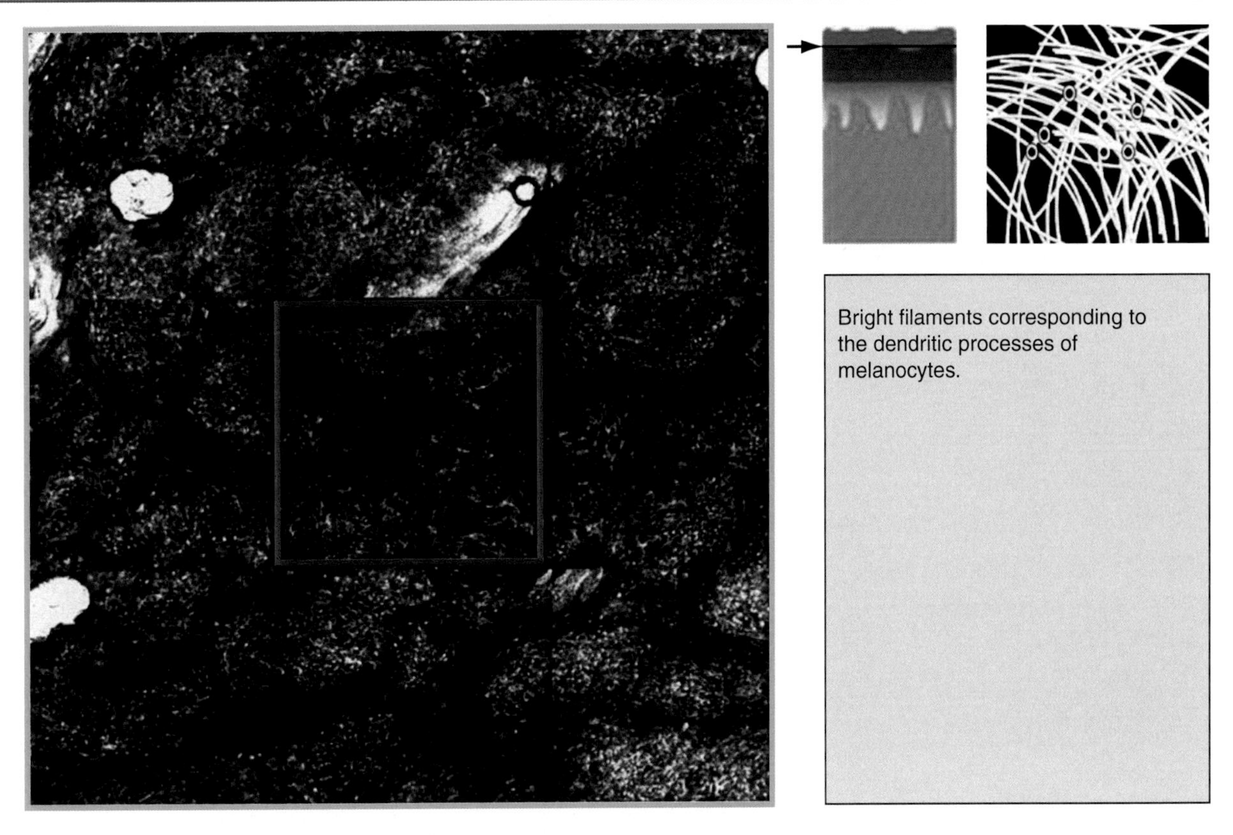

Fig. 13.5.1 RCM mosaic (1.5 × 1.5 mm) showing bright dendrites that obscure completely the keratinocytic population

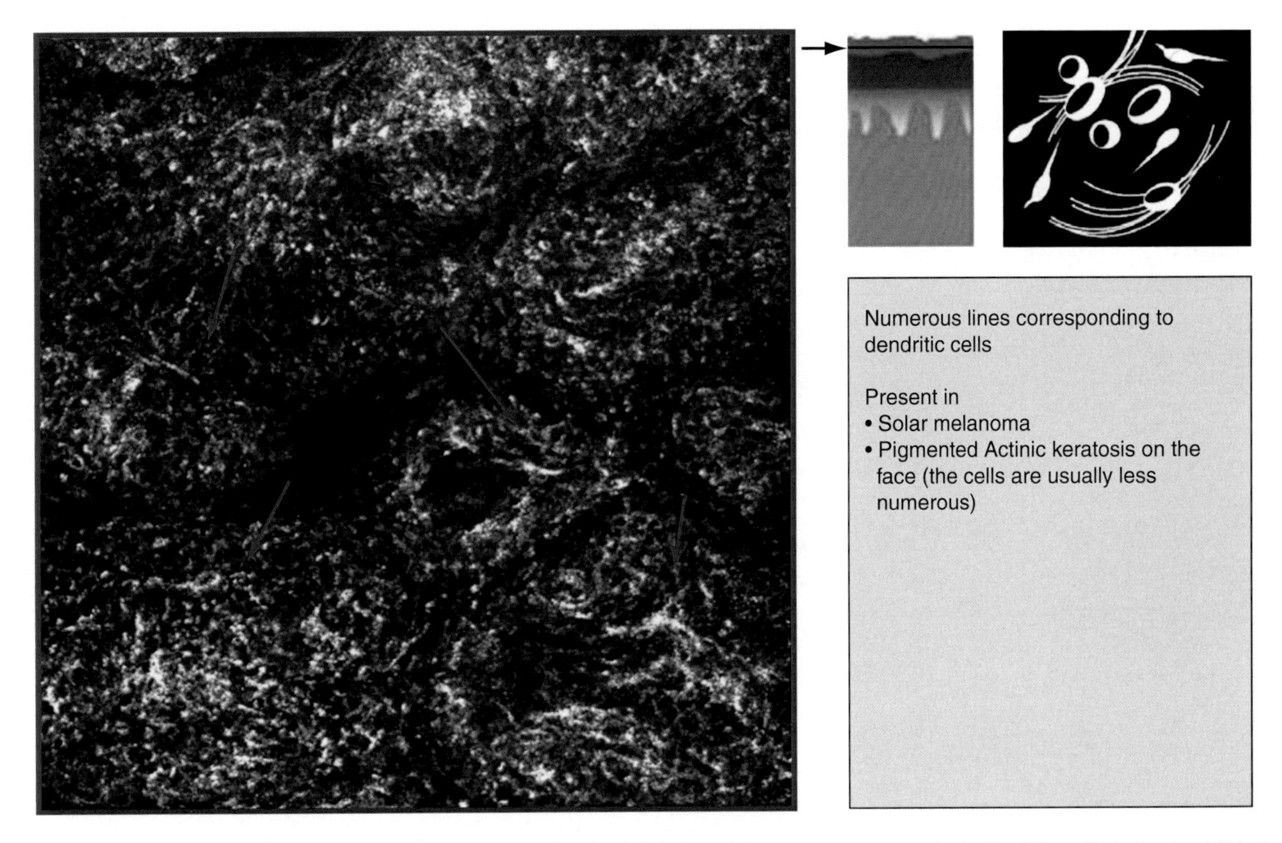

Fig. 13.5.2 Basic image (0.5 × 0.5 mm) showing dendritic cells with bright branching structures where the body of the cells is barely visible (→)

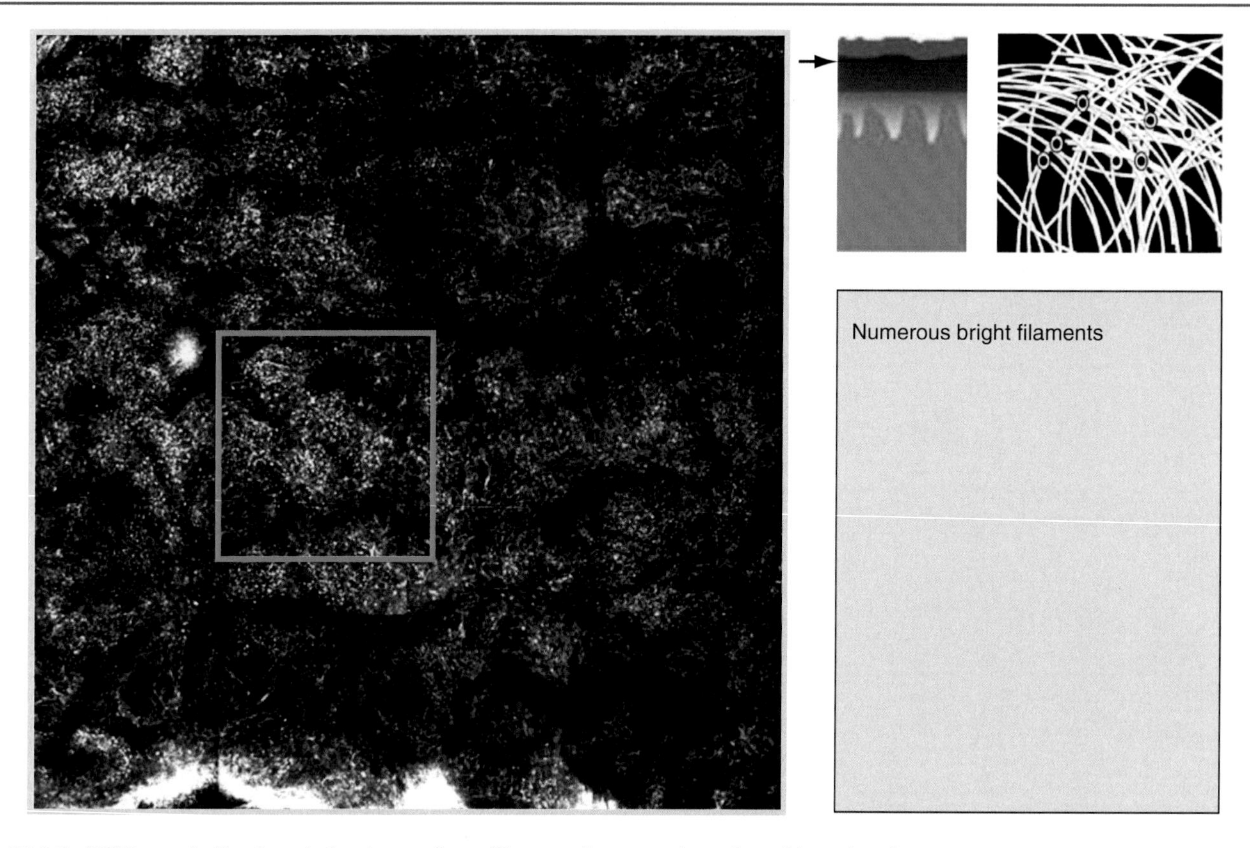

Fig. 13.5.3 RCM mosaic (2 × 2 mm) showing confluent filaments that cover the entire epidermal surface

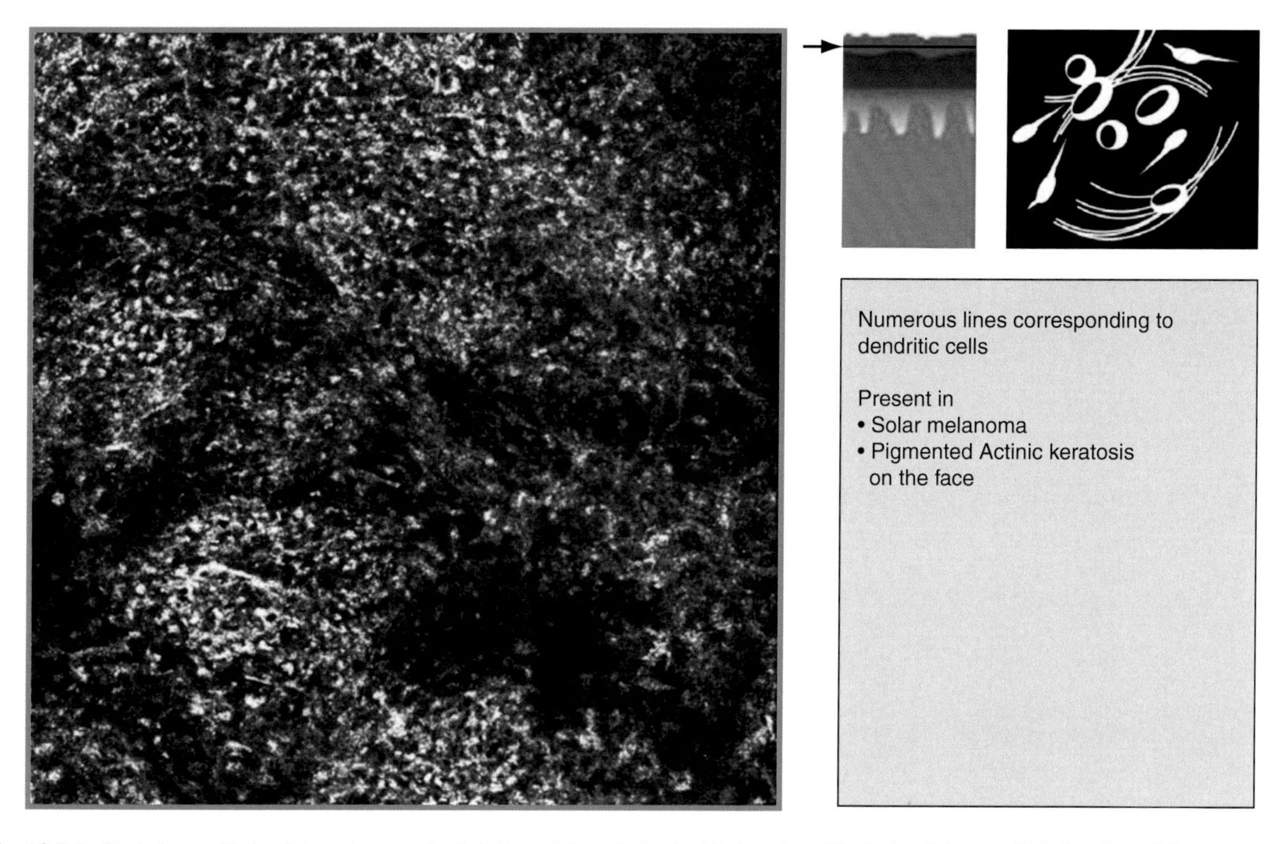

Fig. 13.5.4 Basic image (0.5 × 0.5 mm) presenting bright particles admixed with dendrites. The body of these cells is barely visible

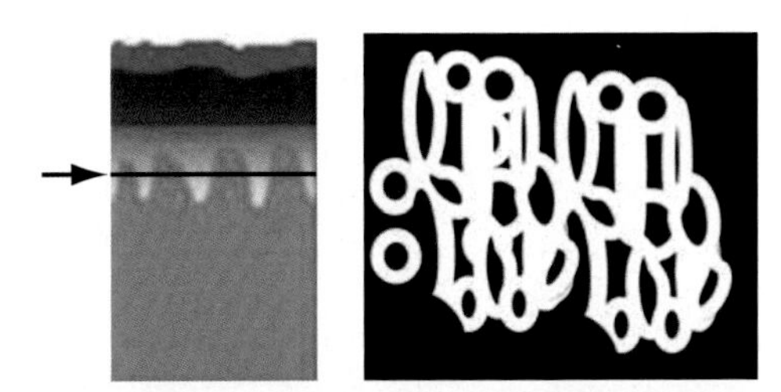

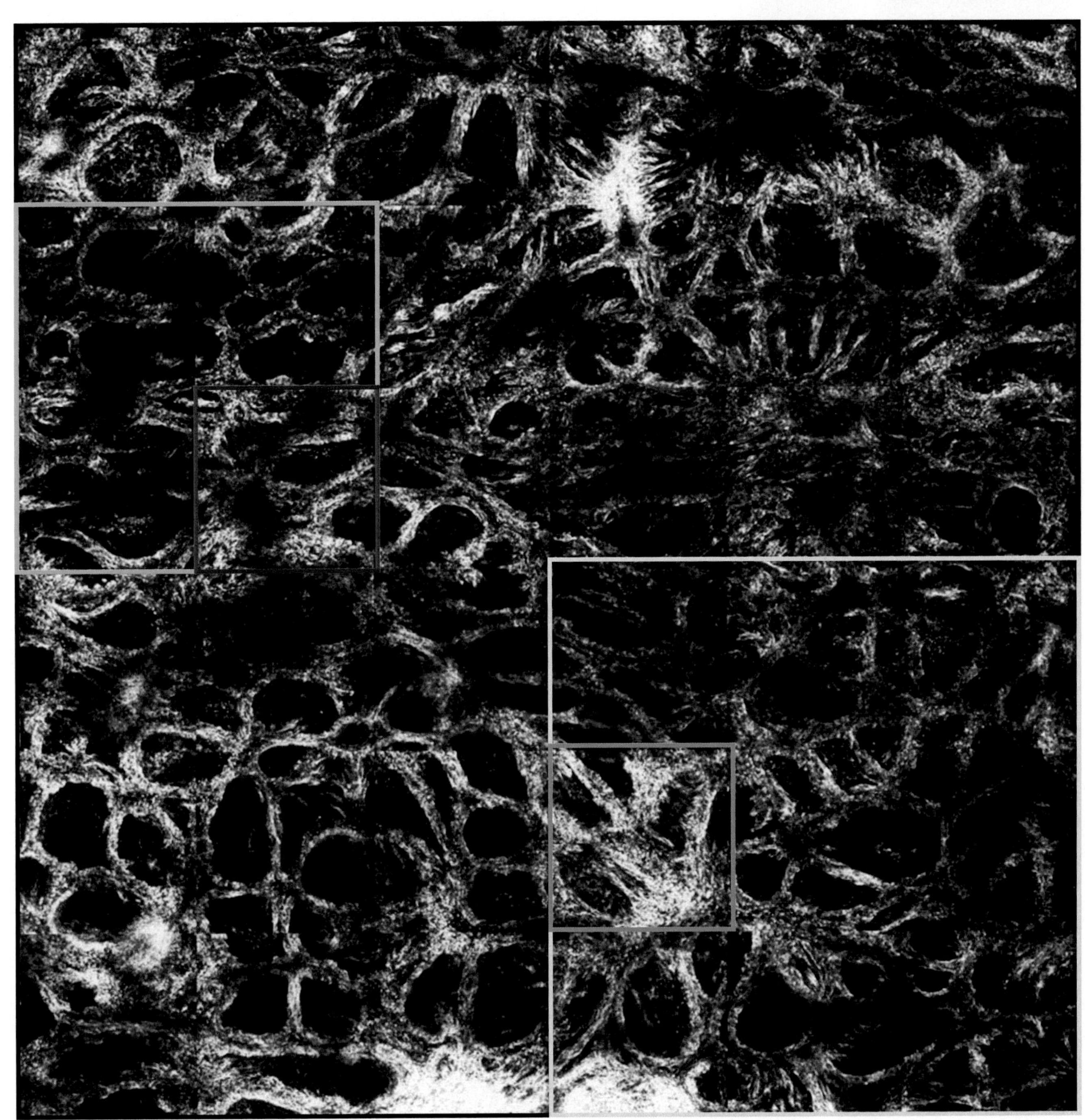

Fig. 13.5.5 RCM mosaic (3 × 3 mm) at DEJ level showing a meshwork pattern constituted by edged papillae. At a first glance, the pattern result orderly disposed throughout the entire area

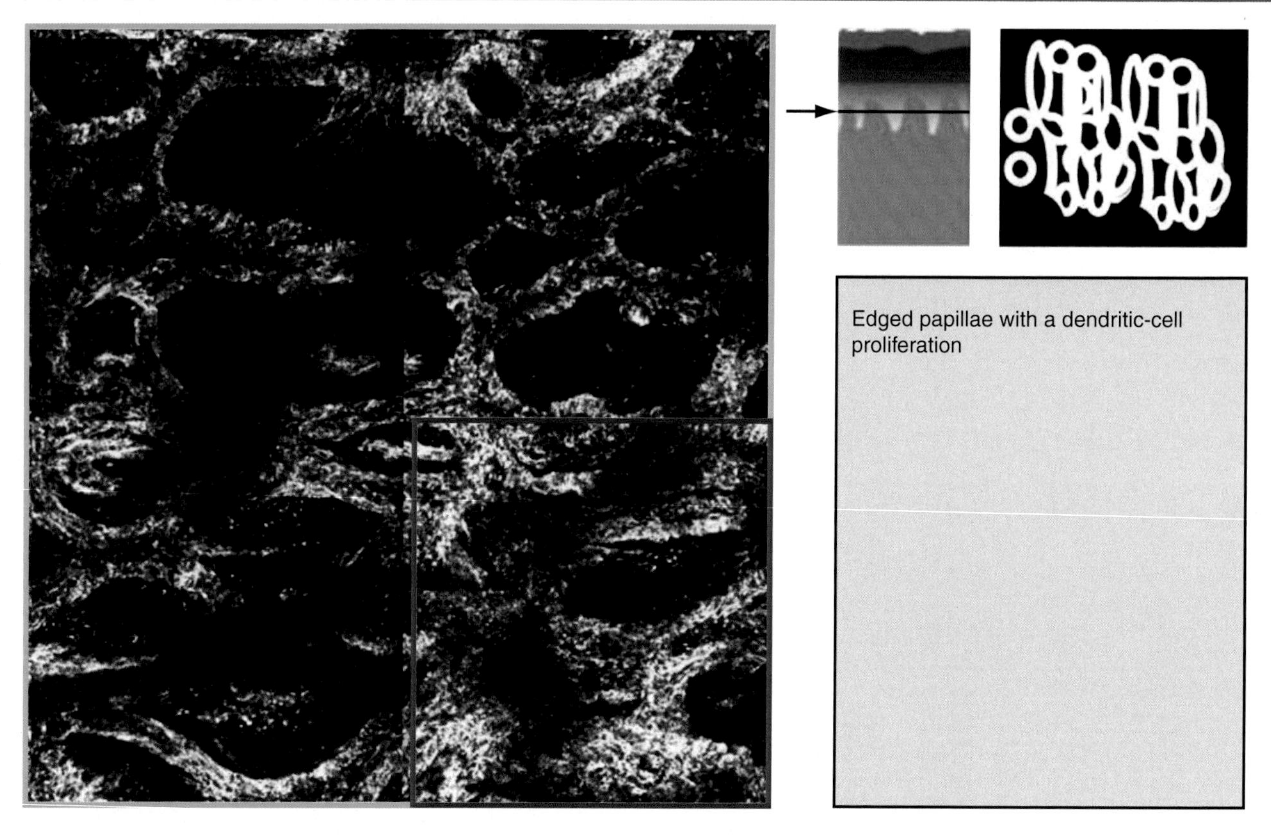

Fig. 13.5.6 RCM mosaic (1 × 1 mm) showing edged papillae. In the interpapillary space, numerous bright lines are seen. They correspond to dendritic melanocytes. Within the papillae, bright spots corresponding to inflammatory infiltrate are present

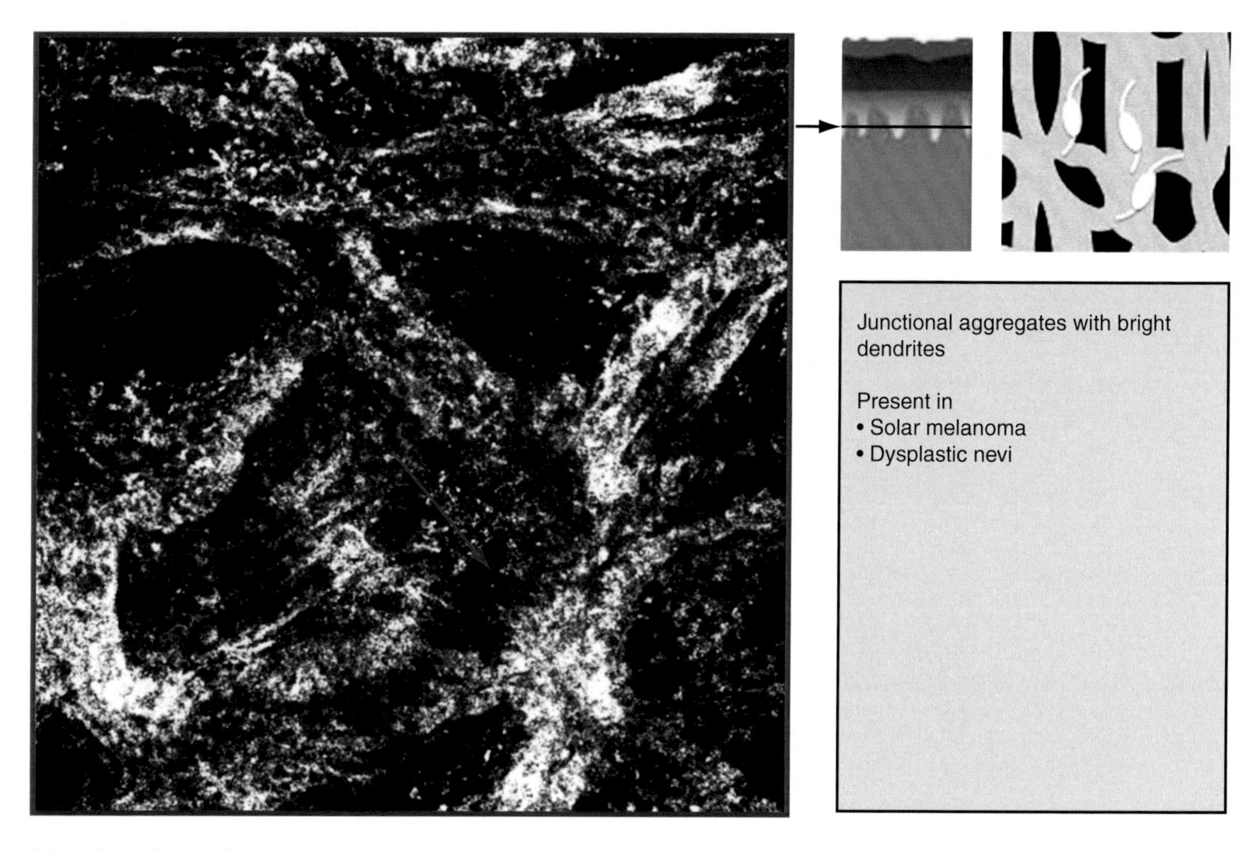

Fig. 13.5.7 Basic image (0.5 × 0.5 mm) showing dermal papillae surrounded by bright dendritic cells sometimes forming small junctional aggregates (*)

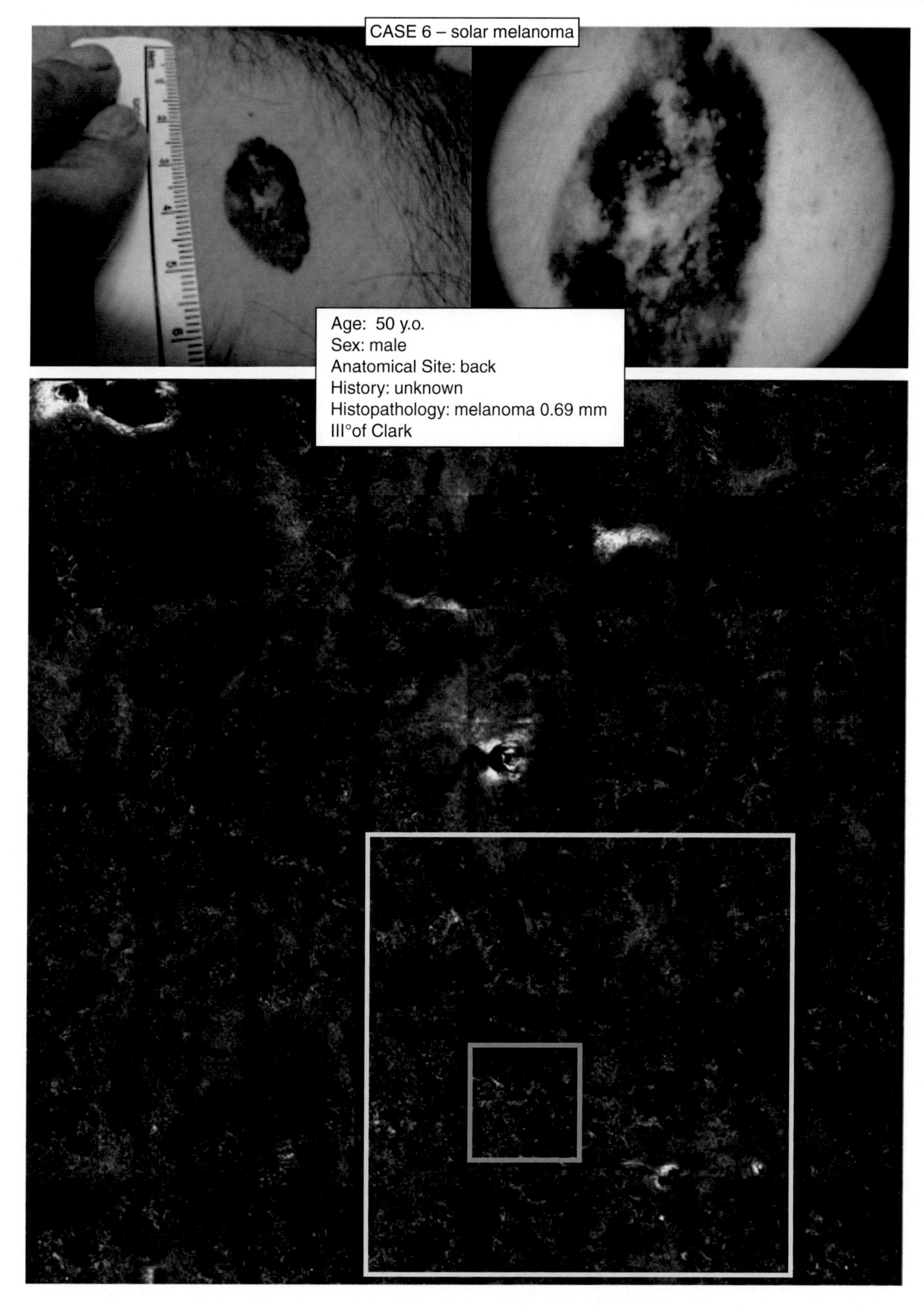

Fig. 13.6 RCM mosaic (4 × 4 mm). A disarrayed epidermis presenting bright aggregates covering the entire surface

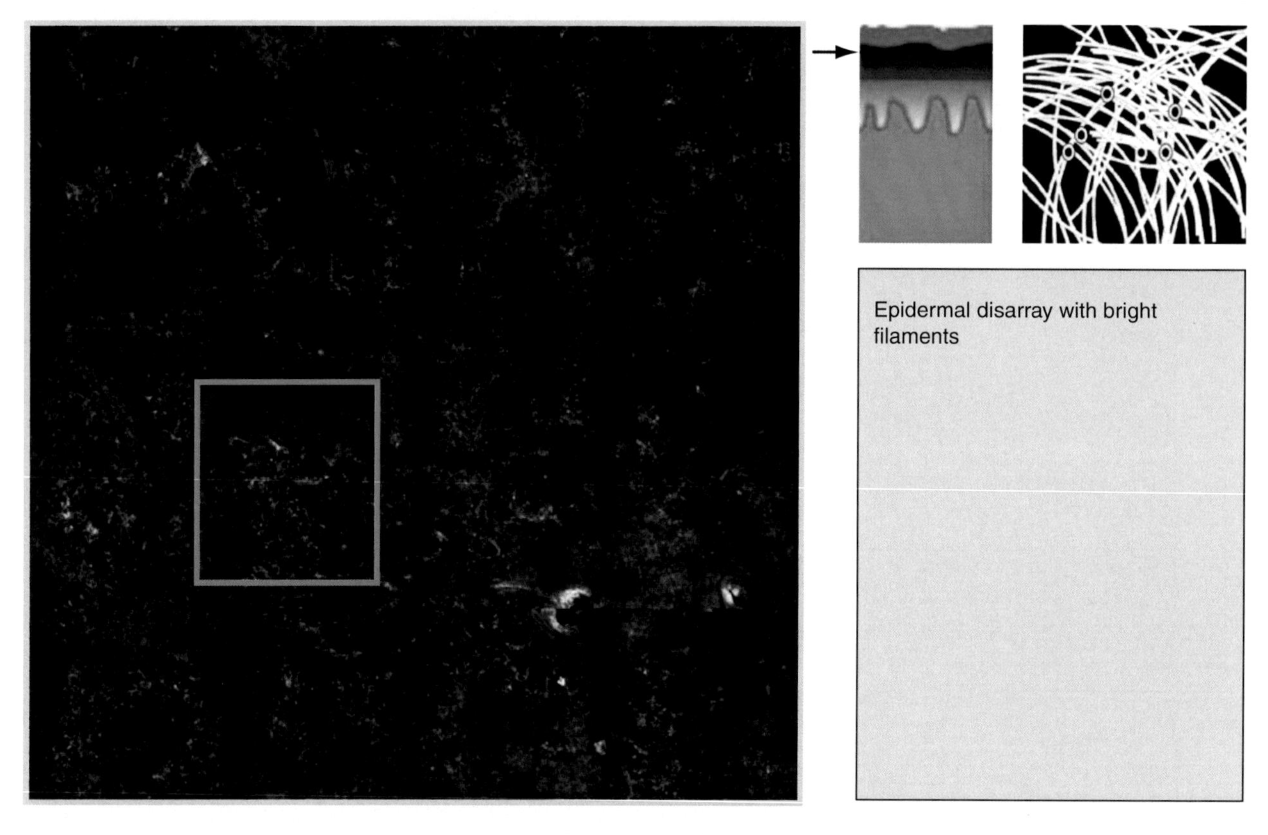

Fig. 13.6.1 RCM mosaic (2 × 2 mm) epidermal disarray where there are bright filaments with tendency to be aggregated

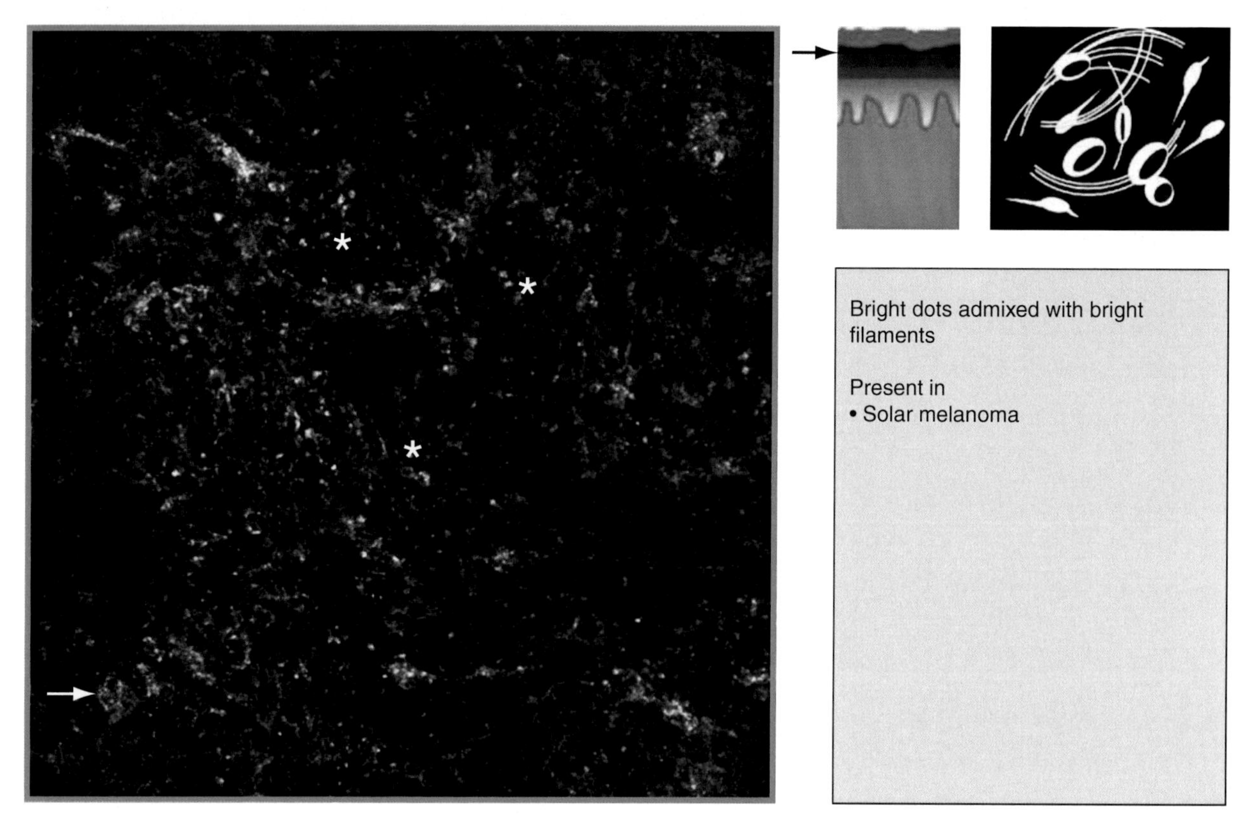

Fig. 13.6.2 Basic image (0.5 × 0.5 mm). Several bright dots (*) intermingled with bright filaments. Sometimes few roundish-shaped melanocytes can be found (→)

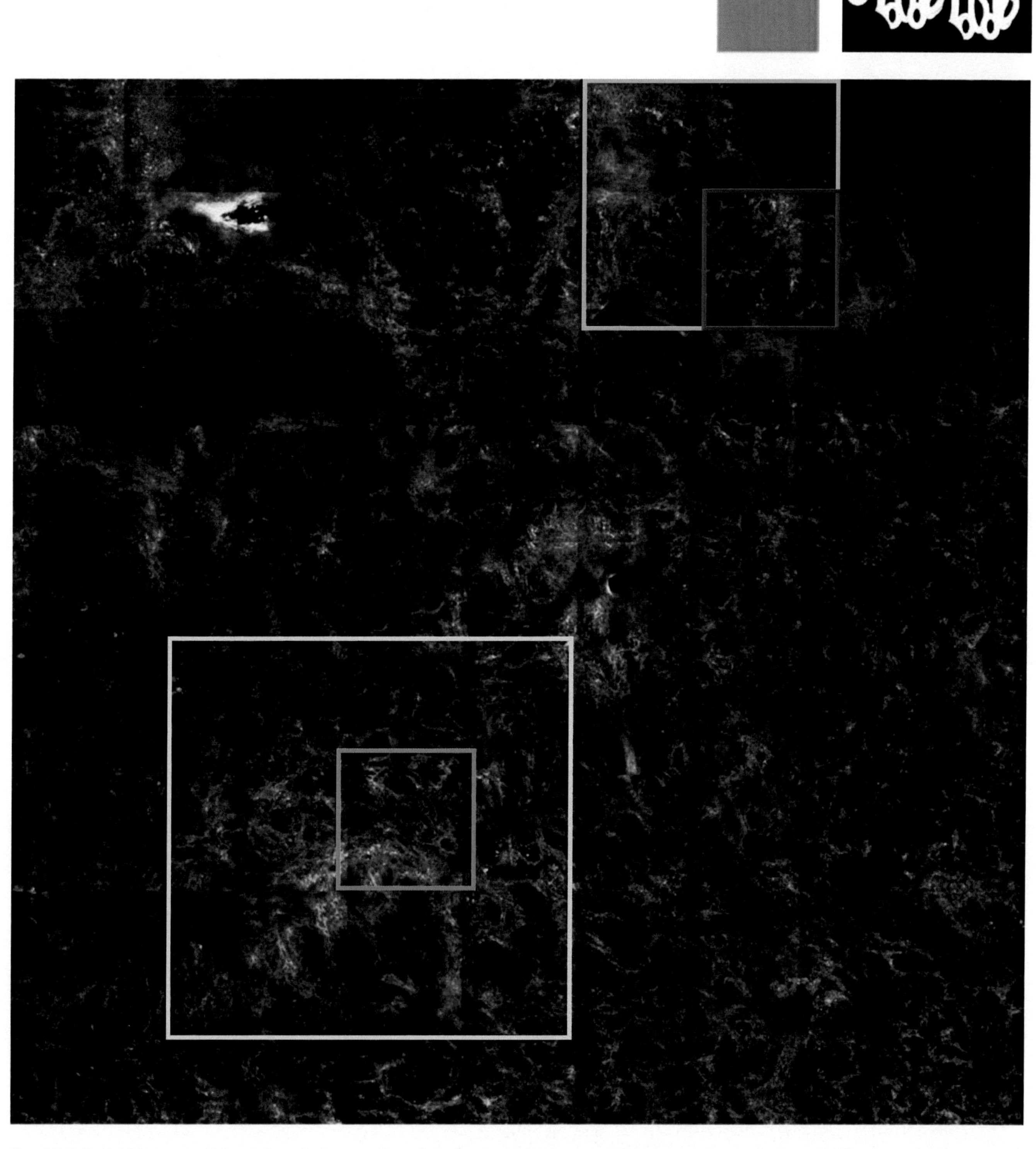

Fig. 13.6.3 RCM mosaic (4.5 × 4.5 mm). A general meshwork pattern (*blue square*) is present, along with an aspecific pattern (*yellow square*) occupying a limited portion of the lesion

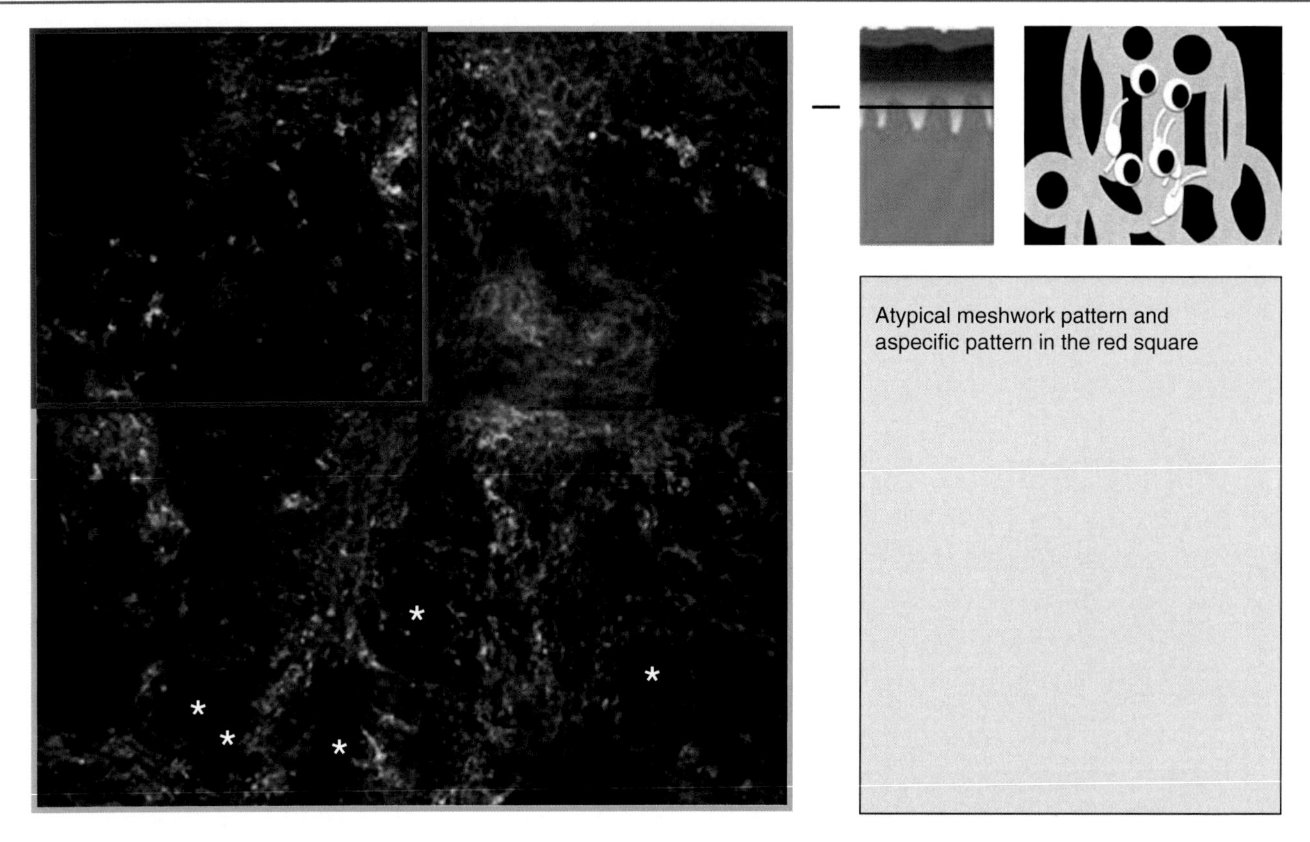

Fig. 13.6.4 RCM mosaic (1 × 1 mm). Isolated cells (*red square*) sometimes forming aggregates where the body of the cells are not visible. The dermal papillae are barely visible (*) and numerous bright filaments enlarge the interpapillary space to give rise to a meshwork pattern

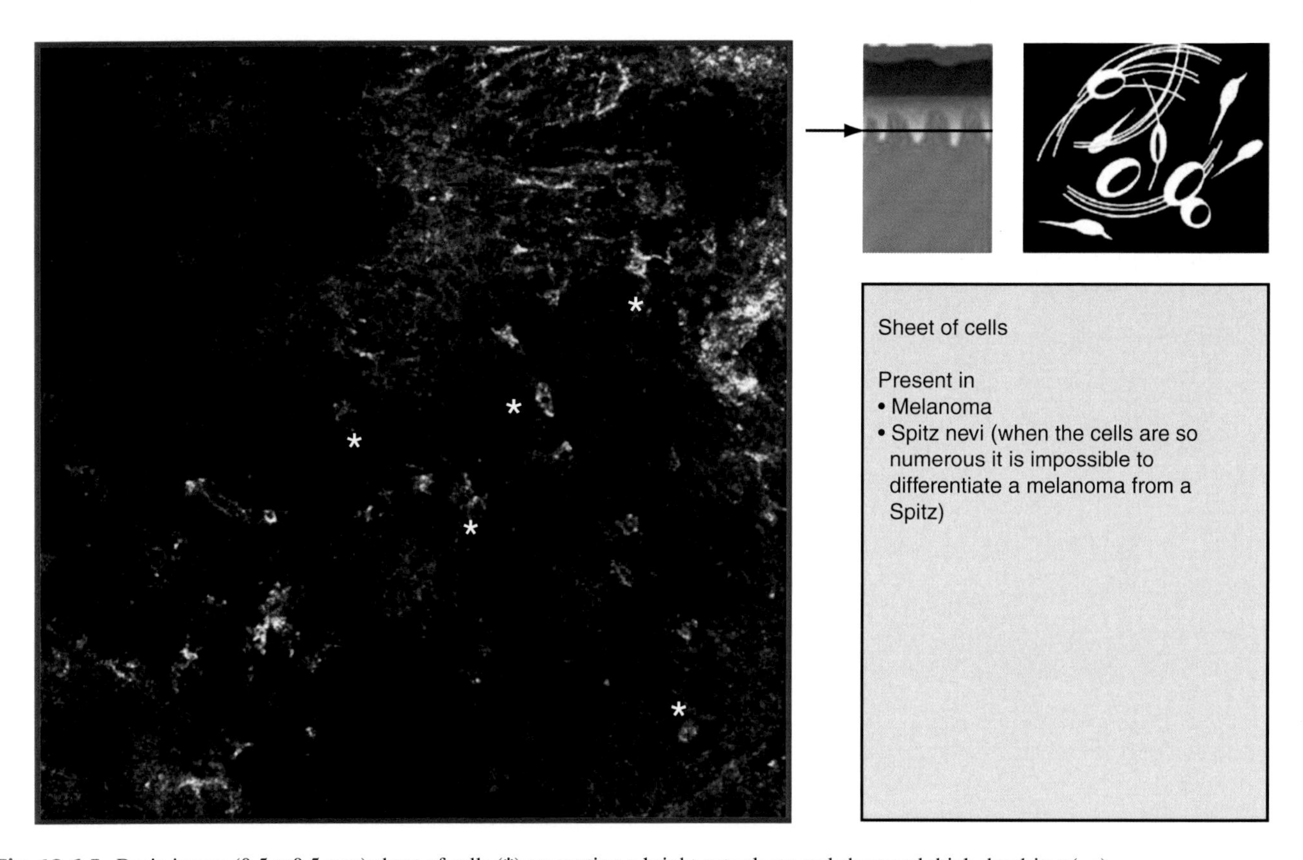

Fig. 13.6.5 Basic image (0.5 × 0.5 mm) sheet of cells (*) presenting a bright cytoplasm and short and thick dendrites (→)

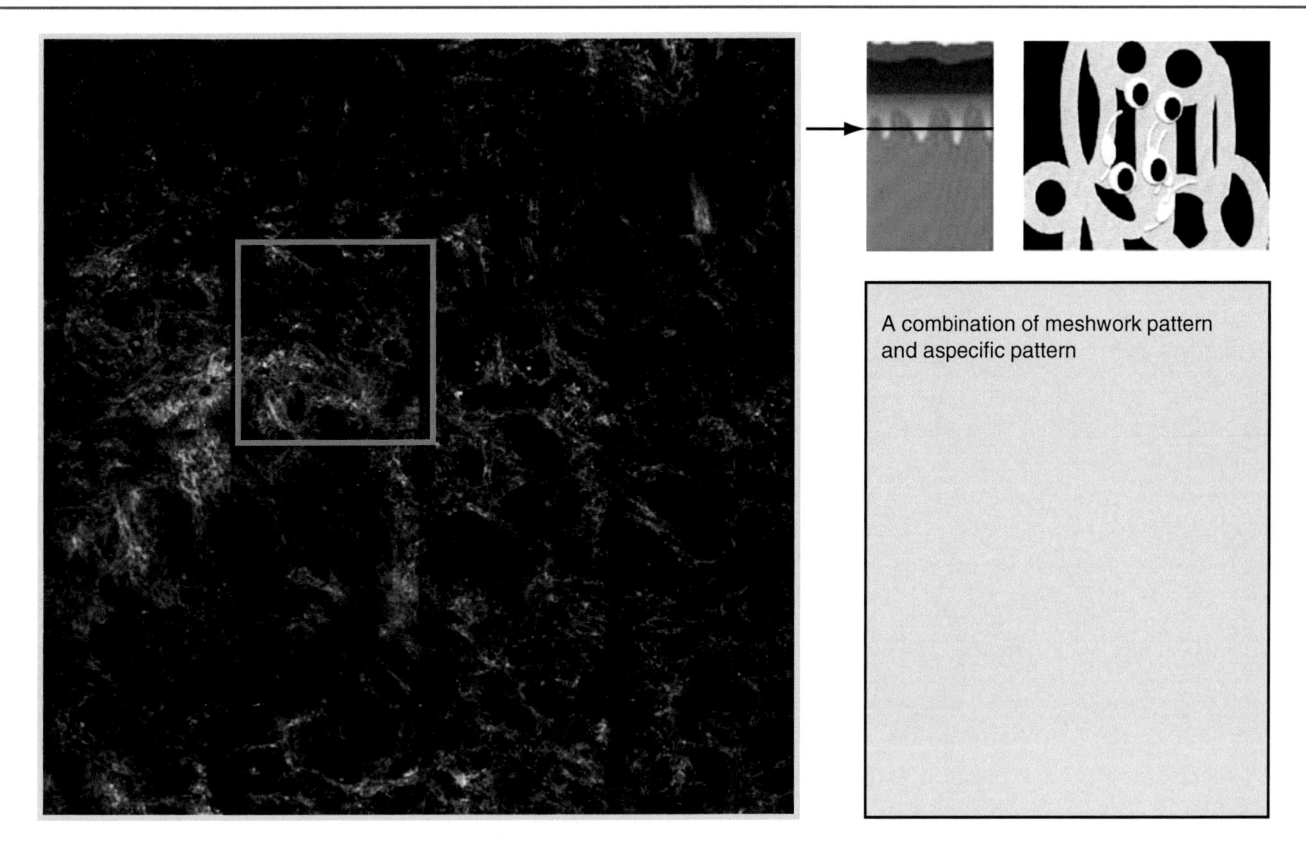

Fig. 13.6.6 RCM mosaic (2 × 2 mm). A general meshwork pattern with areas where the pattern is no longer visible (*blue square*)

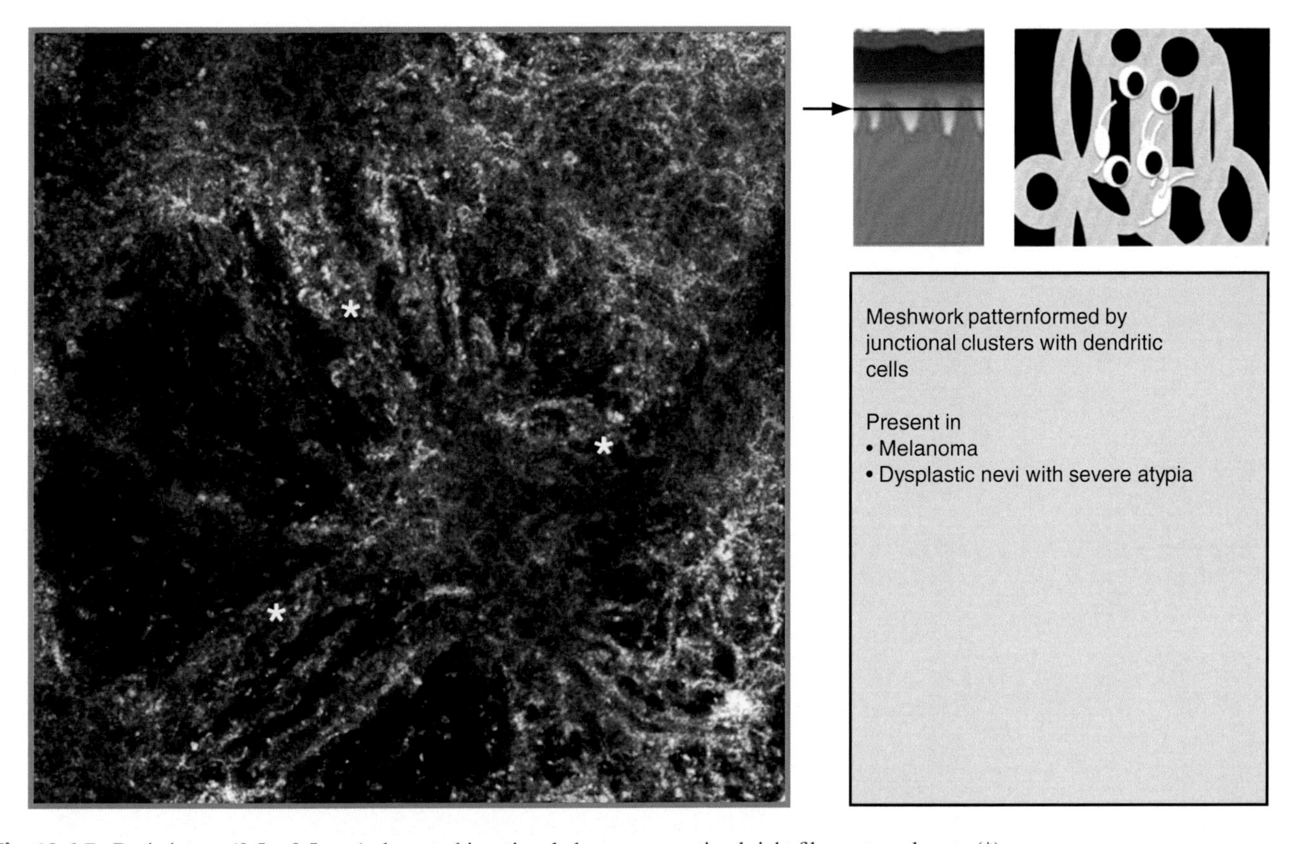

Fig. 13.6.7 Basic image (0.5 × 0.5 mm) elongated junctional clusters presenting bright filaments and spots (*)

13.2.2 Dermo-Epidermal Junction

A ringed or meshwork pattern is observable with atypical cells mainly seen as individual elements. The effacement of the dermo-epidermal contour and the thinning of the epidermis give rise to the progressive disappearing of the ringed pattern in favor of an aspecific/undefined architecture where the dermal papillae cannot be appreciated. In this melanoma type, at DEJ level, the cells are usually seen as individual elements, and when in aggregates, they tend to form junctional clusters or sort of sheets of cells where the body of the cells is not clearly observable and dendrites appear tightly close each other.

13.2.3 Upper Dermis

In the upper dermis, a marked solar elastosis corresponding to coarse and huddle collagen is present [17]. Highly refractive curled fibers corresponding to fragmented elastic fibers are seen in the presence of severe solar elastosis. Admixed with the bright collagen fibers, there are inflammatory cells as plump bright cells and bright stellate spots. It is not infrequent to find some areas presenting polycyclic papillary contours and bulbous projections that may lead to a misdiagnosis when the lesion is not analyzed *in toto* especially if it is large in diameter. The presence of those structures is related to the actinic damage in which this melanoma arise that also render difficult to outline the borders on the tumors from the surrounding skin.

References

1. Jemal A, Siegel R, Ward E et al (2008) Cancer statistics, 2008. CA Cancer J Clin 58:71–96
2. Clark WH Jr, Elder DE, Van Horn M (1986) The biologic forms of malignant melanoma. Hum Pathol 17:443–450
3. Barnhill RL, Mihm MC Jr (1993) The histopathology of cutaneous malignant melanoma. Semin Diagn Pathol 10:47–75
4. Crucioli V, Stilwell J (1982) The histogenesis of malignant melanoma in relation to pre-existing pigmented lesions. J Cutan Pathol 9:396–404
5. Argenziano G, Soyer HP, Chimenti S et al (2003) Dermoscopy of pigmented skin lesions: results of a consensus meeting via the Internet. J Am Acad Dermatol 48:679–693
6. Soyer HP, Kenet RO, Wolf IH, Kenet BJ, Cerroni L (2000) Clinicopathological correlation of pigmented skin lesions using dermoscopy. Eur J Dermatol 10:22–28
7. Pellacani G, Cesinaro AM, Seidenari S (2005) Reflectance-mode confocal microscopy for the in vivo characterization of pagetoid melanocytosis in melanomas and nevi. J Invest Dermatol 125:532–537
8. Pellacani G, Longo C, Ferrara G et al (2009) Spitz nevi: in vivo confocal microscopic features, dermatoscopic aspects, histopathologic correlates, and diagnostic significance. J Am Acad Dermatol 60:236–247
9. Pellacani G, Scope A, Ferrari B et al (2009) New insights into nevogenesis: in vivo characterization and follow-up of melanocytic nevi by reflectance confocal microscopy. J Am Acad Dermatol 61:1001–1013
10. Pellacani G, Cesinaro AM, Longo C, Grana C, Seidenari S (2005) Microscopic in vivo description of cellular architecture of dermoscopic pigment network in nevi and melanomas. Arch Dermatol 141:147–154
11. Longo C, Rito C, Beretti F, Cesinaro AM, Piñeiro-Maceira J, Seidenari S, Pellacani G. De novo melanoma and melanoma arising from pre-existing nevus: *In vivo* morphologic differences as evaluated by confocal microscopy. J Am Acad Dermatol. 2011 Sep;65(3): 604–14
12. Pellacani G, Cesinaro AM, Seidenari S (2005) *In vivo* assessment of melanocytic nests in nevi and melanomas by reflectance confocal microscopy. Mod Pathol 18:469–474
13. Zalaudek I, Argenziano G, Ferrara G et al (2004) Clinically equivocal melanocytic skin lesions with features of regression: a dermoscopic-pathological study. Br J Dermatol 150:64–71
14. Seidenari S, Ferrari C, Borsari S, et al (2010) Reticular grey-blue areas of regression as a dermoscopic marker of melanoma in situ. Br J Dermatol. doi:10.1111/j.1365-2133.2010.09821.x
15. Ahlgrimm-Siess V, Massone C, Scope A et al (2009) Reflectance confocal microscopy of facial lentigo maligna and lentigo maligna melanoma: a preliminary study. Br J Dermatol 161:1307–1316
16. Guitera P, Pellacani G, Crotty KA et al (2010) The impact of in vivo reflectance confocal microscopy on the diagnostic accuracy of lentigo maligna and equivocal pigmented and nonpigmented macules of the face. J Invest Dermatol 130:2080–2091
17. Longo C, Casari A, Beretti F, Cesinaro AM, Pellacani G. Skin aging: *in vivo* microscopic assessment of epidermal and dermal changes by means of confocal microscopy. J Am Acad Dermatol 2011 In Press

Melanoma Progression

14

Caterina Longo, Alice Casari, Giuseppe Argenziano,
Iris Zalaudek, and Giovanni Pellacani

Melanoma arises by a process of stepwise progression in which the transition from melanocytes to metastatic melanoma involves several histologic intermediates. According to the "three-step tumor progression model", these intermediates include radial growth phase melanoma (RGP), microinvasive radial growth phase and vertical growth phase melanoma (VGP) [1, 2].

Histologically, cells of the RGP are present within the epidermis and capable of local superficial microinvasion but not metastasis, whereas VGP cells grow in expansile groups within the dermal layer of the skin and are metastasis competent.

In this chapter, we provide a schematic representation of the salient melanoma features along the progression pattern of growth as they appear under confocal microscopy examination.

Despite the two main melanoma types, pagetoid and solar melanomas, differ in their early phase, when they become microinvasive and invasive, no striking differences can be found.

C. Longo (✉) • G. Argenziano
Department of Dermatology, Arcispedale S Maria Nuova,
Reggio Emilia, Modena, Italy
e-mail: longo.caterina@gmail.com

A. Casari • G. Pellacani
Department of Dermatology and Venereology,
University of Modena and Reggio Emilia, Modena, Italy

I. Zalaudek
Department of Dermatology,
Medical University of Graz, Graz, Austria

The cell population become quite pleomorphic in size and shape being constituted by both roundish and variably dendritic cells. There is a lack of predominance of one cell type in respect of the other as seen in early growth phase of melanoma distinct types.

14.1 Microinvasive Phase of Growth

Clinically, the tumor is raised and palpable. Histopathologically, atypical melanocytes invade the dermis from the basal layer where they are usually located. Melanomas showed an irregularly thickened epidermis with distortion of the rete-ridge pattern.

Upon RCM examination, the epidermis show pagetoid infiltration that is quite consistent in number of cells (Fig. 14.1). The overall epidermal pattern can be either honeycombed, cobblestone or disarrayed. Atypical melanocytes are packed along DEJ and superficial dermis to form irregular dense and sparse nests (Fig. 14.1). A nested proliferation of atypical melanocytes is predominant over individual elements. Confluent nests are present going deeper into dermis and melanocytes tend to form sheet-like structures. The presence of this massive cell proliferation produces a "nonspecific" pattern, which correspond on H&E sections to a prominent nested proliferation in the upper dermis and a disarray of the rete-ridge (Fig. 14.2). Atypical nucleated cells tend to infiltrate the dermal papillae. Regression is present in almost 50% of melanoma with microinvasion and it can show up as a grossly arranged coarse collagen fibers intermingled with inflammatory infiltrate, variably composed by plump bright cells and bright spots.

R. Hofmann-Wellenhof et al. (eds.), *Reflectance Confocal Microscopy for Skin Diseases*,
DOI 10.1007/978-3-642-21997-9_14, © Springer-Verlag Berlin Heidelberg 2012

CASE 1 – Microinvasive phase of growth
Age: 51 y.o.
Sex: female
Anatomical Site: left shoulder
History: unknown
Histopathology: melanoma of 0.69 mm III° of Clark

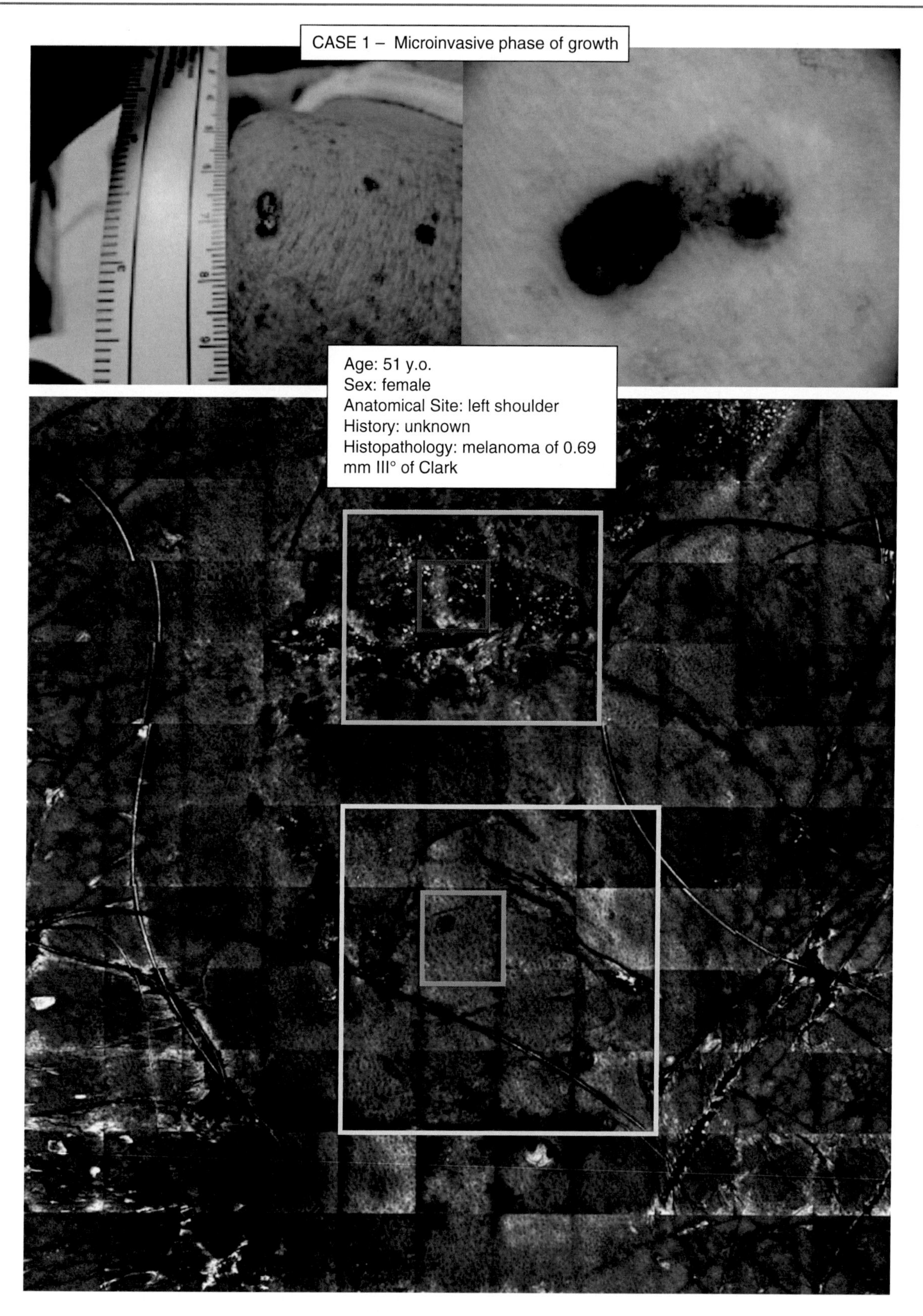

Fig. 14.1 RCM mosaic (6.5 × 6.5 mm) at granulosum spinosum layer. The upper part (*green and red insets*) is located at the border between the flat area and the nodule and is showing at this magnification marked disarrangement with numerous irregularly distributed bright spots. The lower part of the image (*yellow-blue insets*) corresponds to the nodular portion of the lesion showing a blue veil at dermoscopy, not displaying significant alteration at RCM

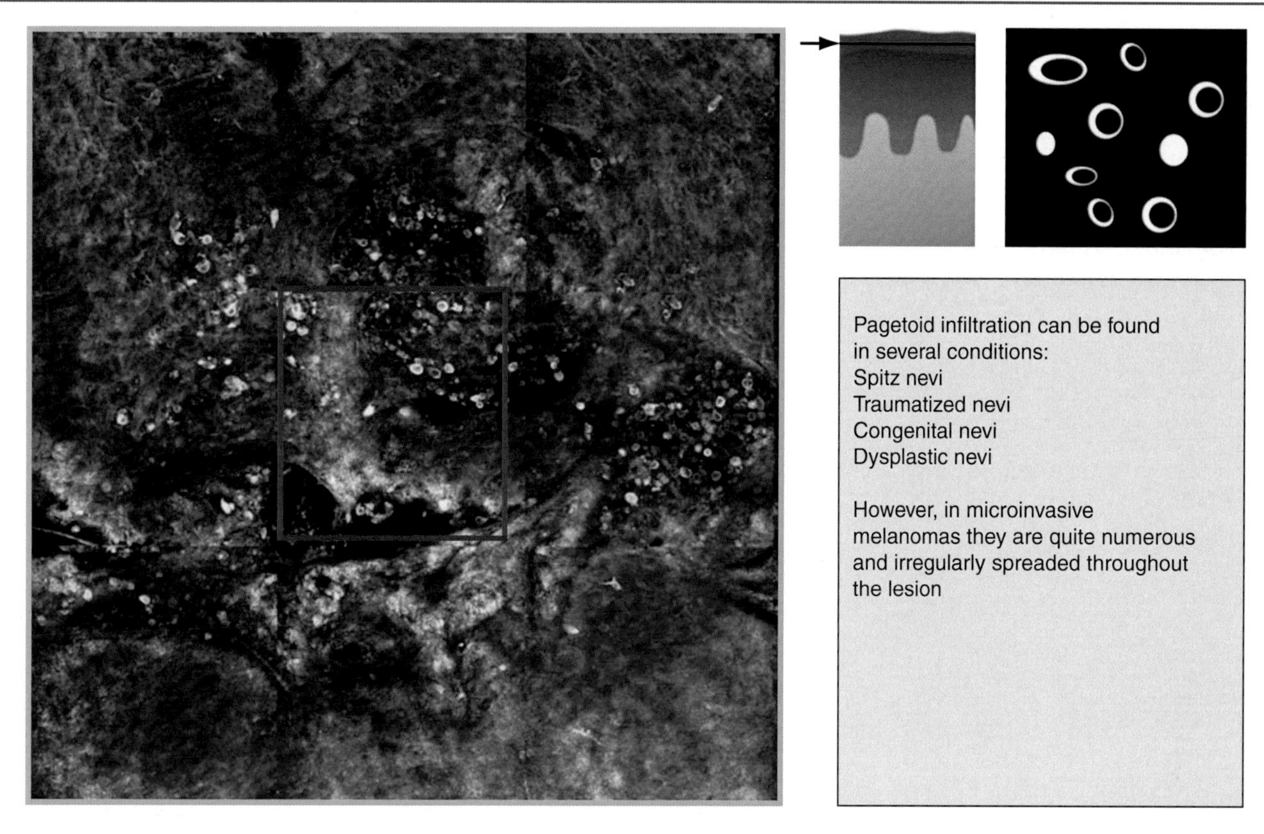

Fig. 14.1.1 RCM mosaic (1.5 × 1.5 mm) at granulosum spinosum layer is exhibiting numerous bright cells in a context of disarranged epidermal pattern

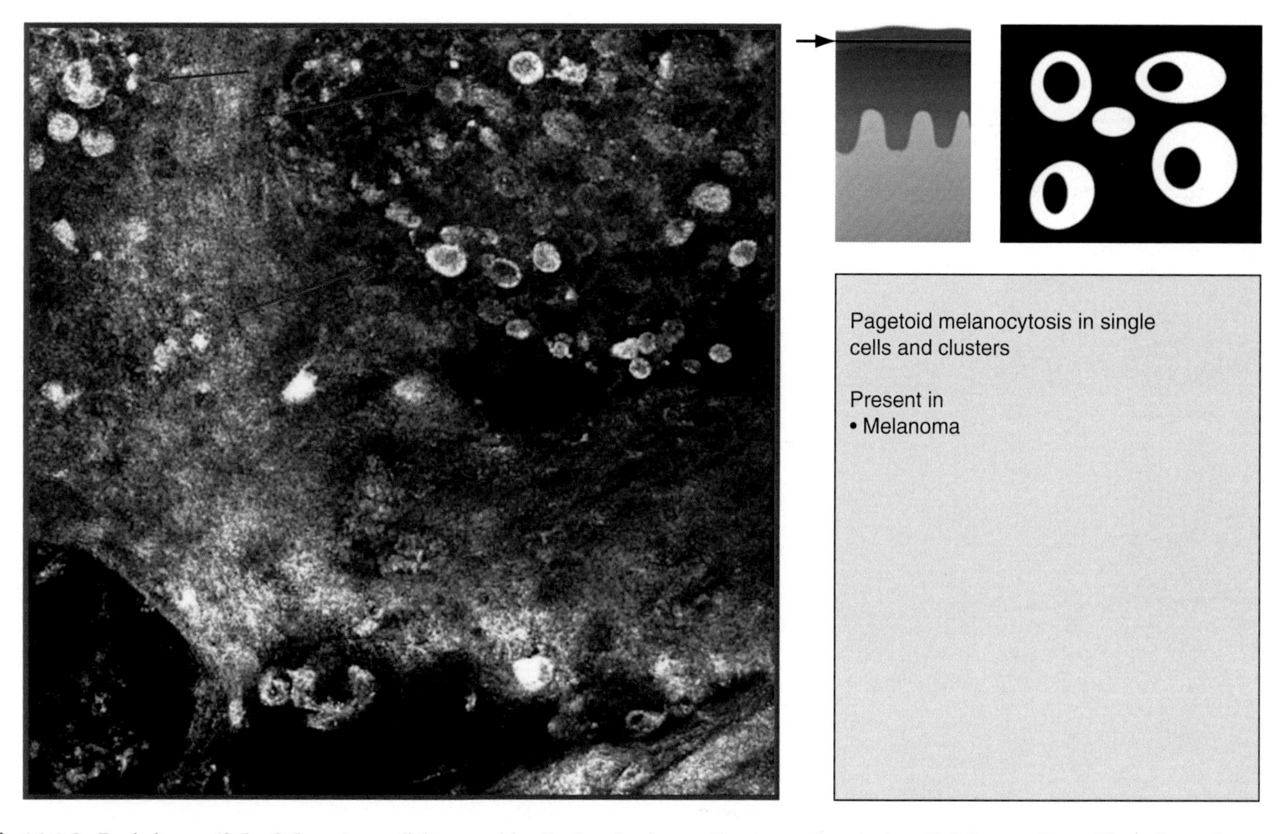

Fig 14.1.2 Basic image (0.5 × 0.5 mm) roundish pagetoid cells showing hyporeflective nucleus (→) and bright cytoplasm. The cells are large and pleomorphic and are also visible as large aggregates pushing and thinning the epidermis

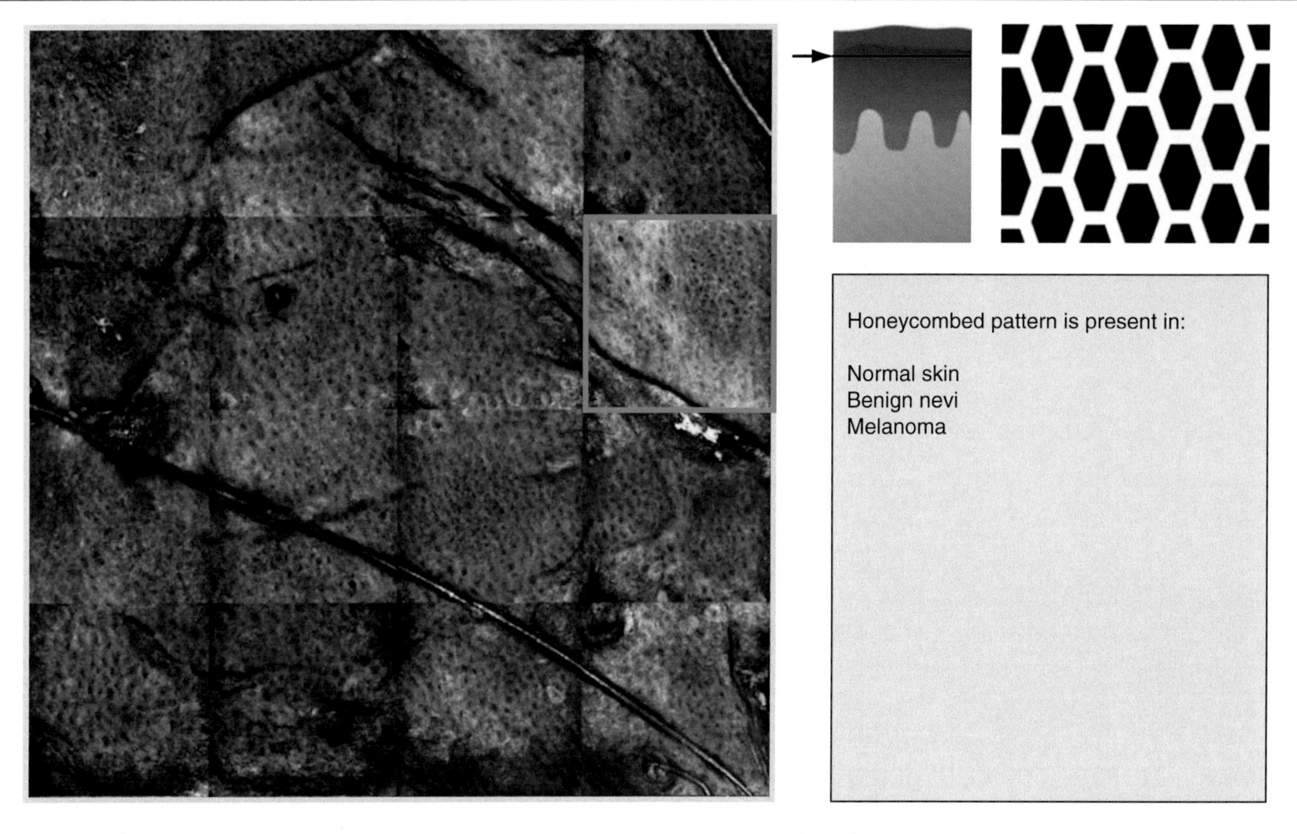

Fig. 14.1.3 RCM mosaic (2 × 2 mm) at granulosum/spinosum layer on the nodular portion of the tumor shows a honeycombed pattern. In this area no striking alteration nor atypical pagetoid cells are visible

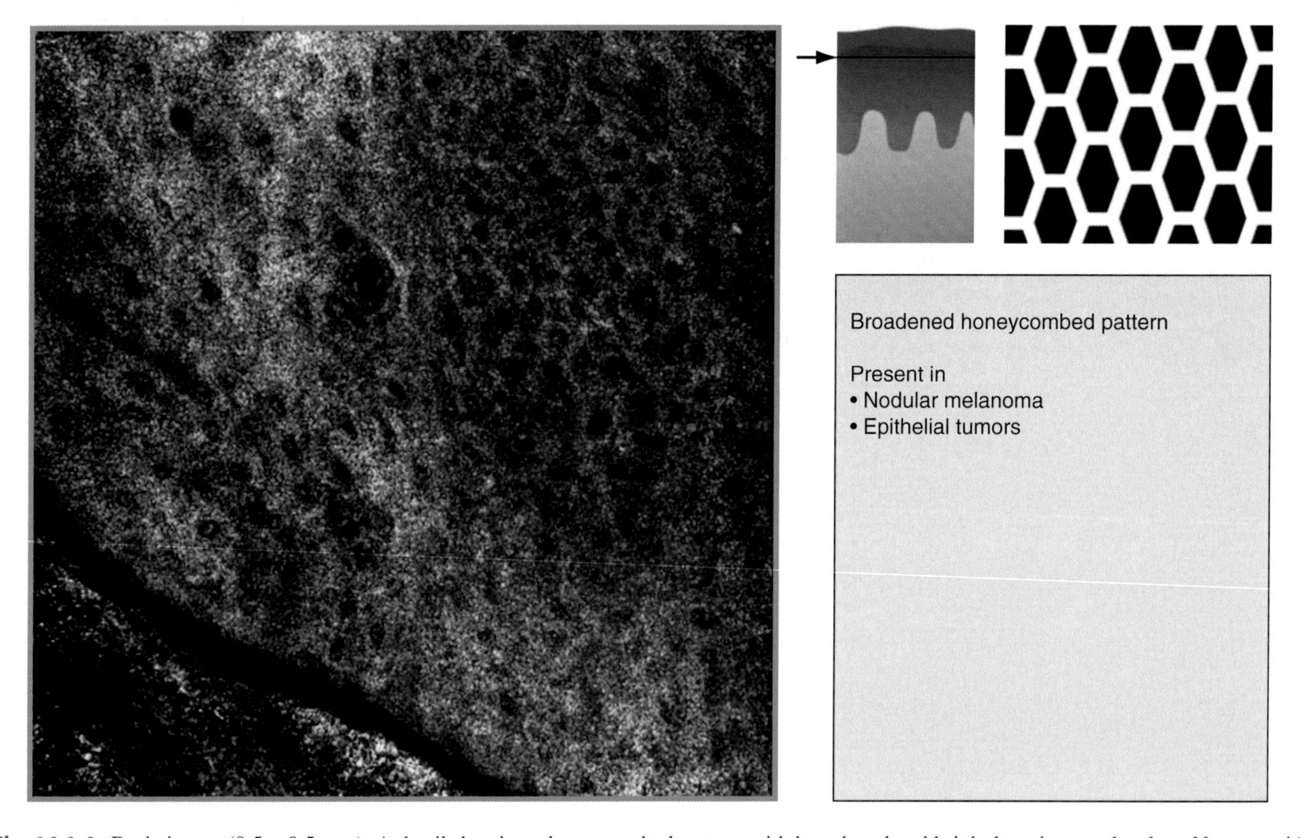

Fig. 14.1.4 Basic image (0.5 × 0.5 mm). A detail showing a honeycombed pattern with broadened and bright keratinocyte borders. No pagetoid cells are visible

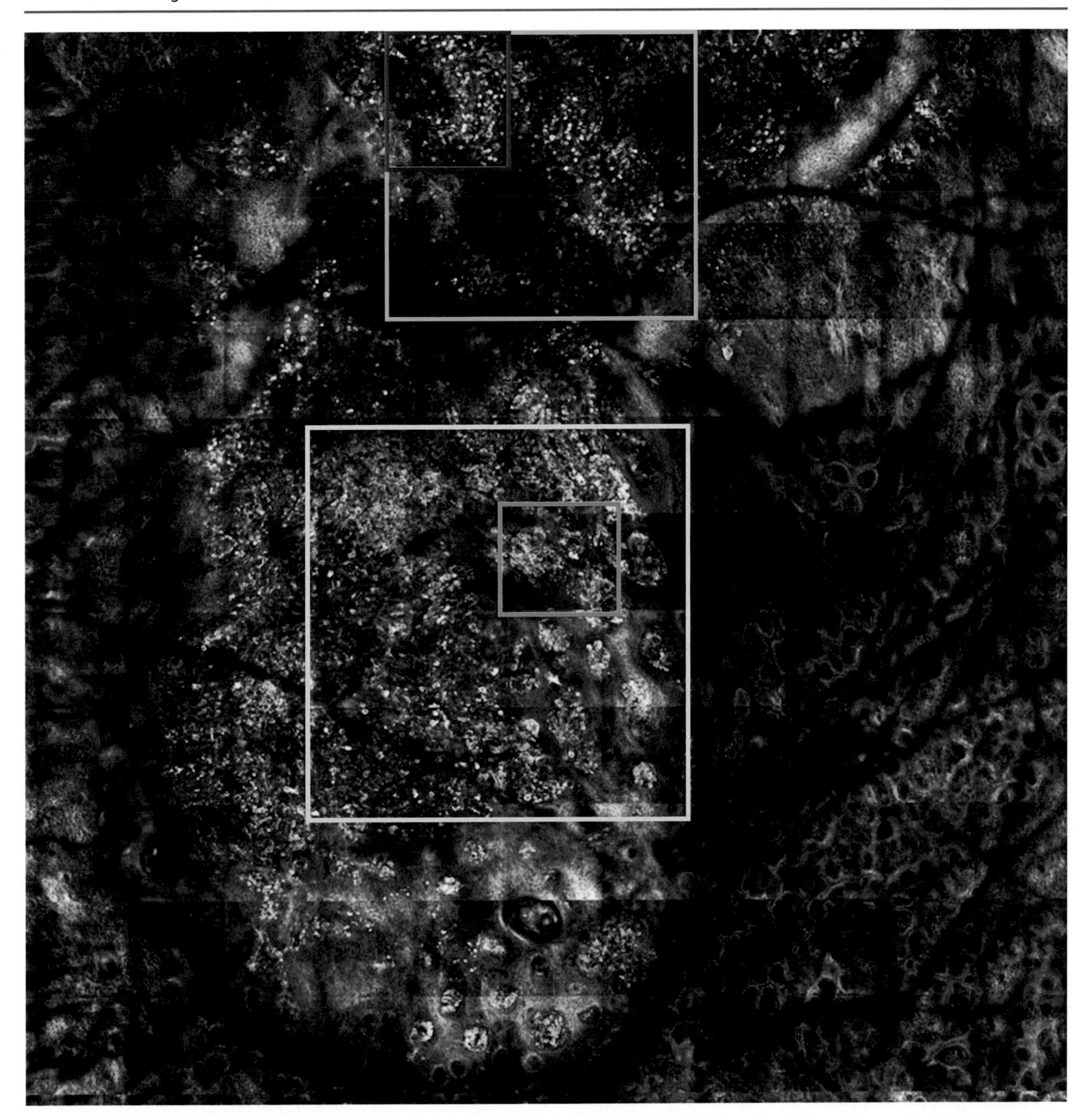

Fig. 14.1.5 RCM mosaic (6.5 × 6.5 mm) at DEJ level showing a non-specific pattern due to the prominent cell proliferation. The diffuse brightness which outline the lesion is constituted by bright structures. Some roundish areas, corresponding to papillae, are still detectable at the borders of the lesion, though infiltrated by bright structures. Whereas in the center of the lesion a more compact proliferation is obscuring the dermal papillae

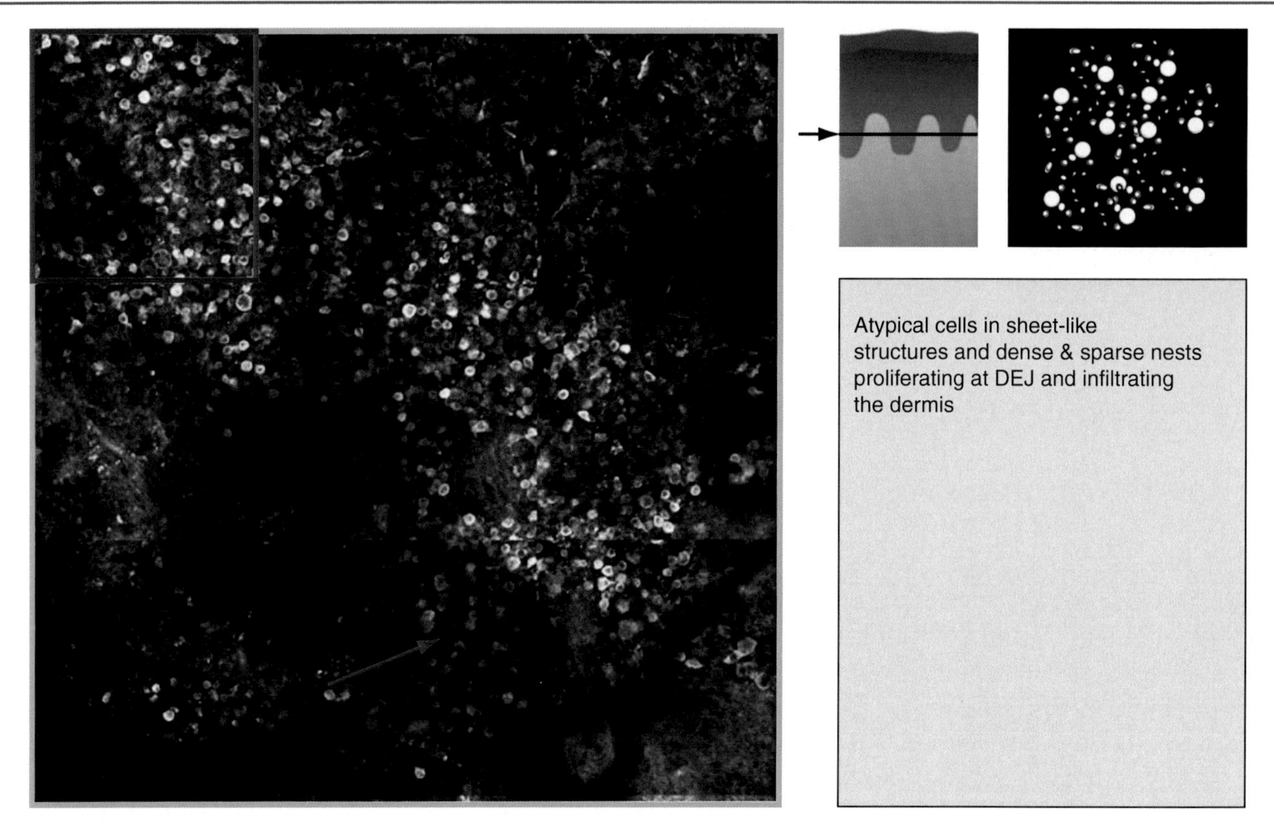

Fig. 14.1.6 RCM mosaic (1.5 × 1.5 mm) with confluent atypical melanocytes at the DEJ, where the papillary contour is no longer visible. Numerous cells extend at the DEJ in loosely aggregates also infiltrating the dermis (→)

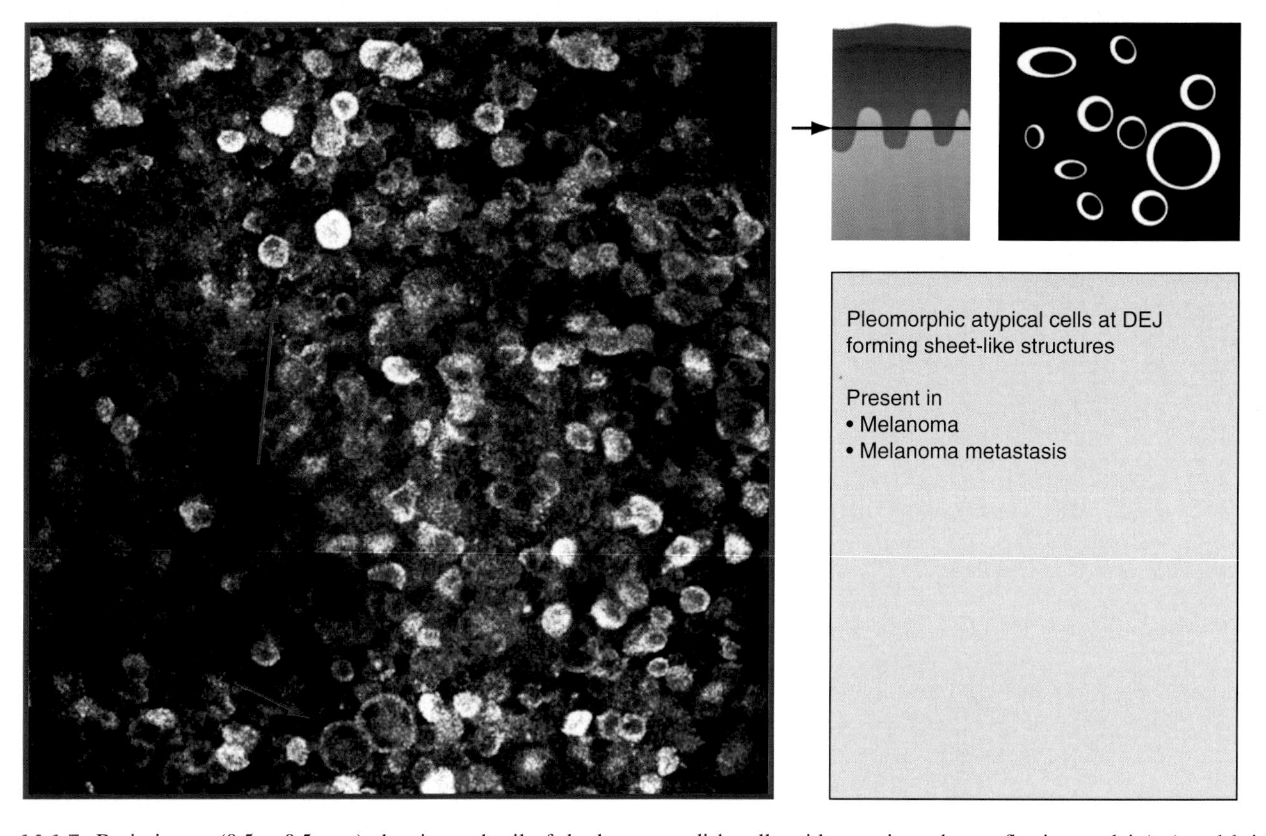

Fig. 14.1.7 Basic image (0.5 × 0.5 mm) showing a detail of the large roundish cells with prominent hyporeflective nuclei (→) and bright cytoplasm, forming sheet-like structures

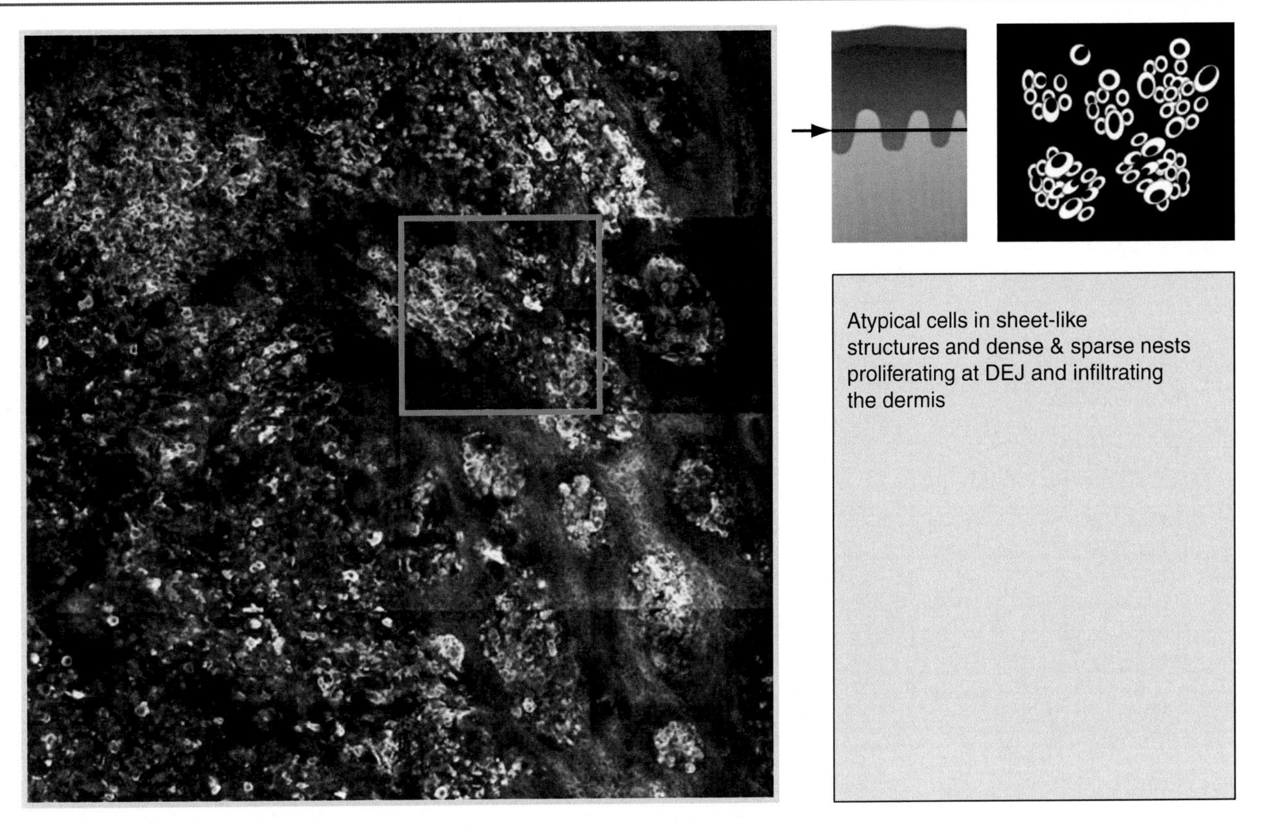

Fig. 14.1.8 RCM mosaic (2 × 2 mm) at the DEJ in correspondence of the nodular portion of the lesion displays pleomorphic cells with tendency to form sheet-like structures or dense and sparse nests

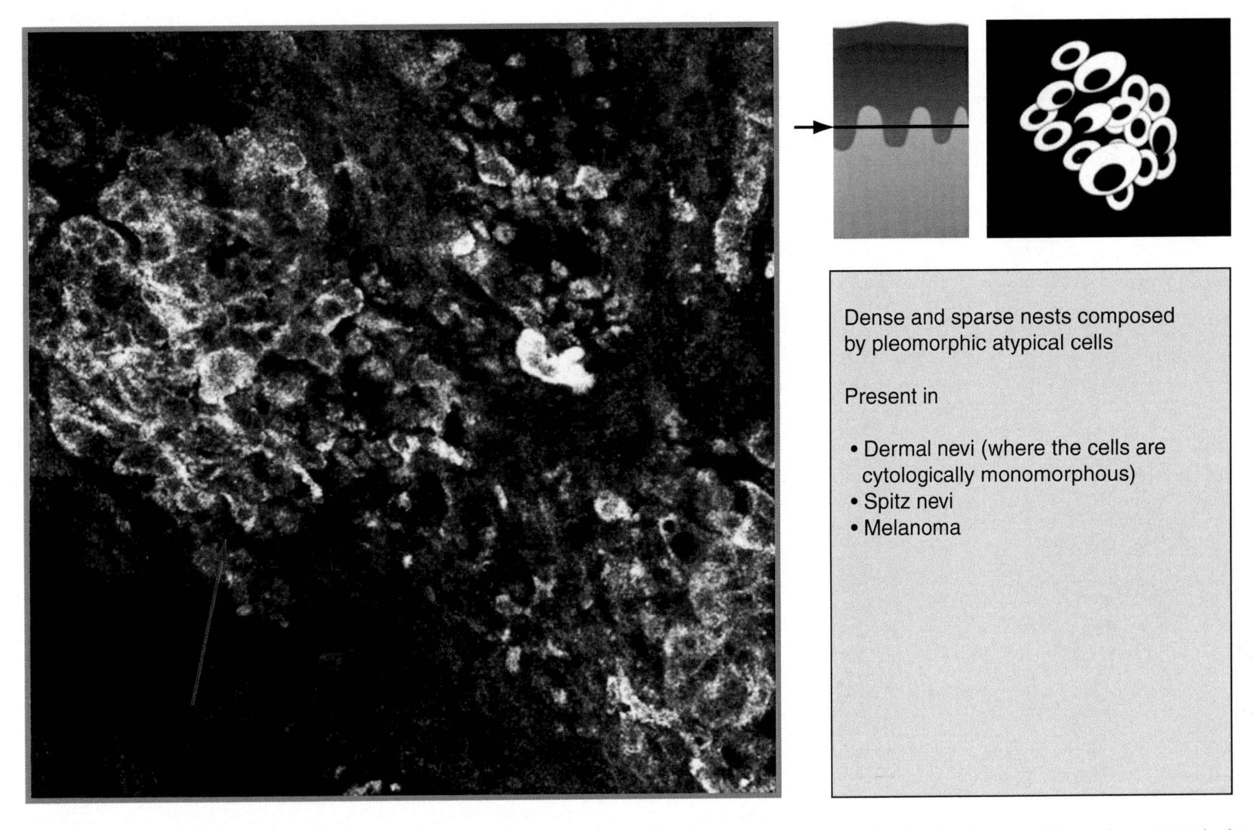

Fig. 14.1.9 Basic image (0.5 × 0.5 mm) showing a detail of a dense and sparse nest composed by large pleomorphic melanocytes (→) with prominent hyporefrective nucleus. The DEJ disruption does not permit to detect the border between the epidermis and the dermis

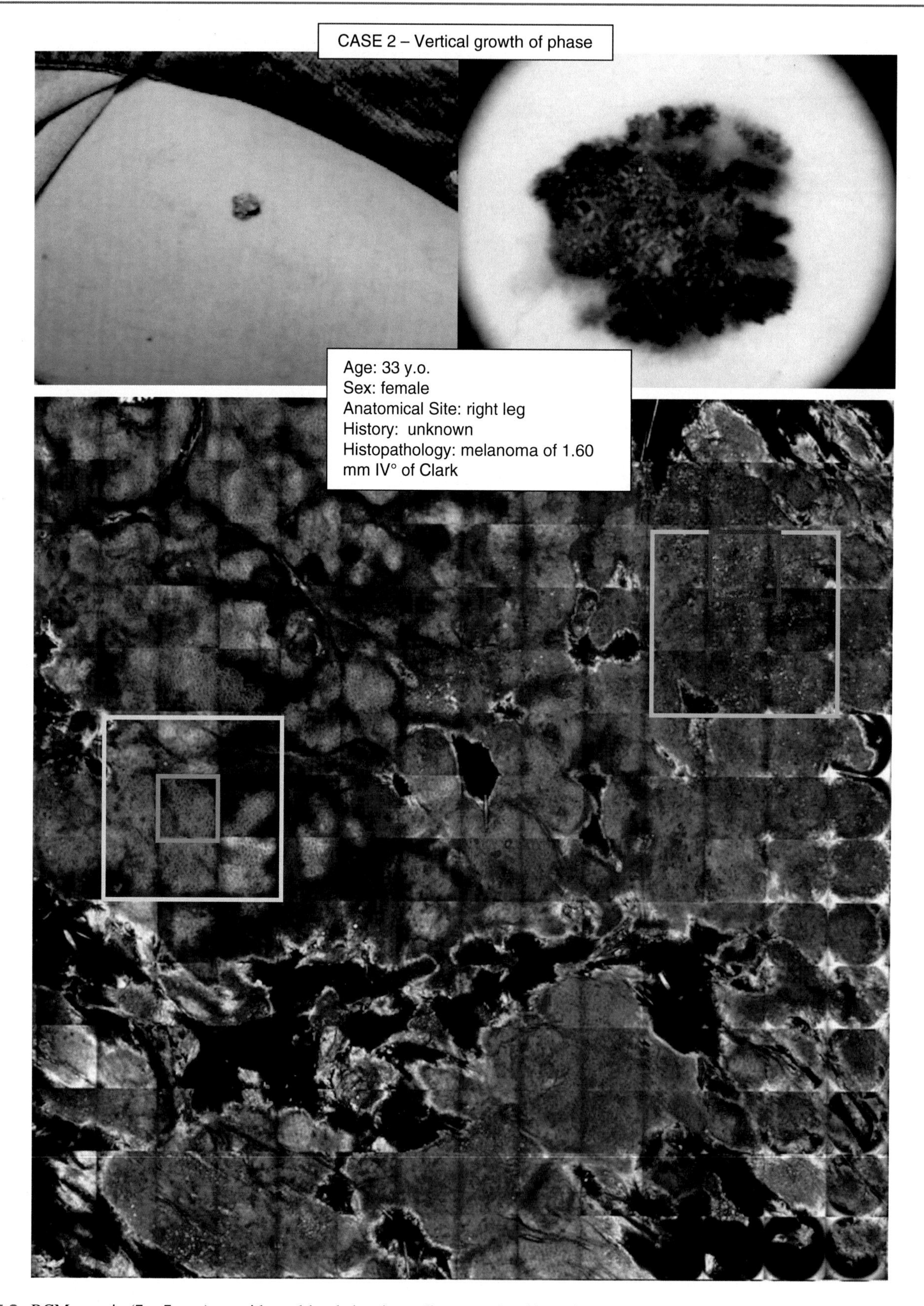

Fig. 14.2 RCM mosaic (7 × 7 mm) at epidermal level showing a disarranged epidermal pattern with disruption of the stratum corneum. In the *green* and *red square* bright spots are visible whereas in the *yellow* and *blue square* no bright spots are detectable

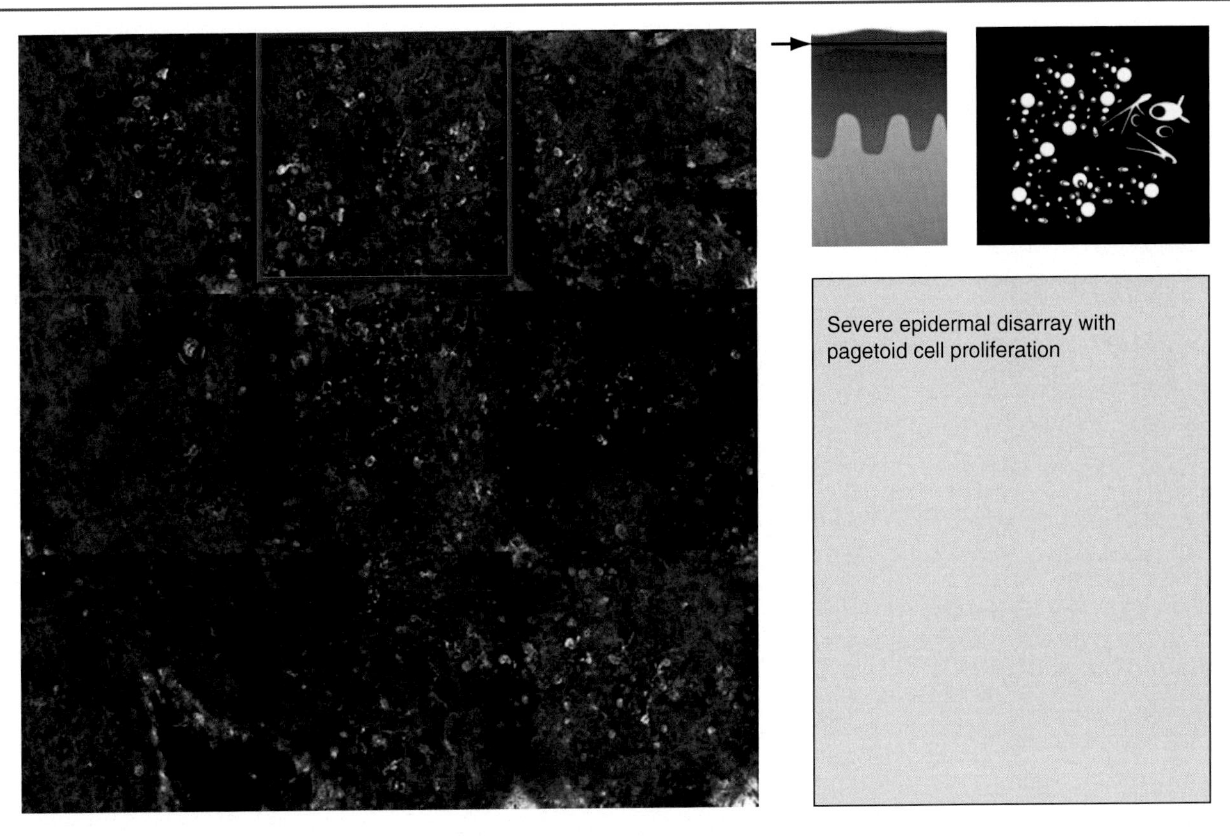

Fig. 14.2.1 RCM mosaic (1.5 × 1.5 mm) disarranged pattern with pagetoid spread constituted by variably bright cells

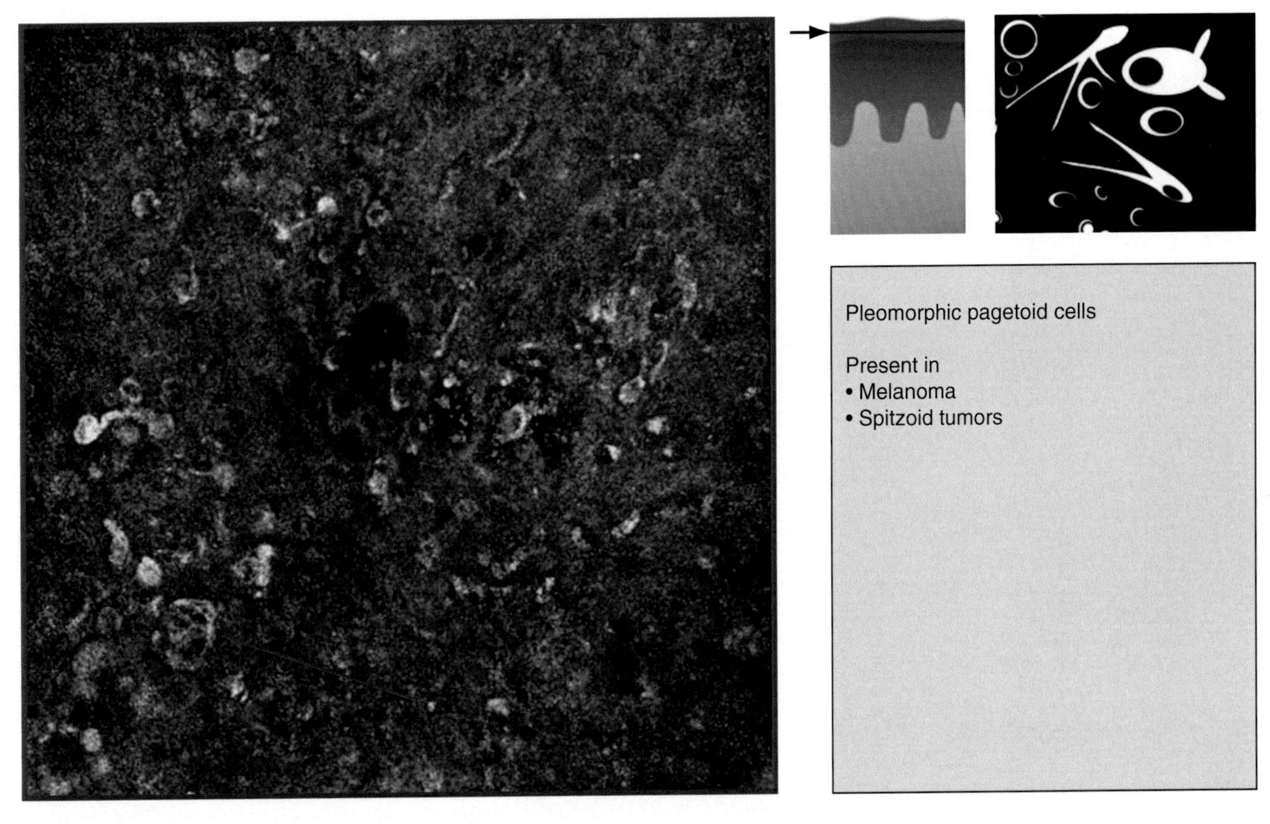

Fig. 14.2.2 Basic image (0.5 × 0.5 mm) pagetoid cells with dendritic shape (*) admixed with roundish large pagetoid cells with prominent and multiple nucleoli (→)

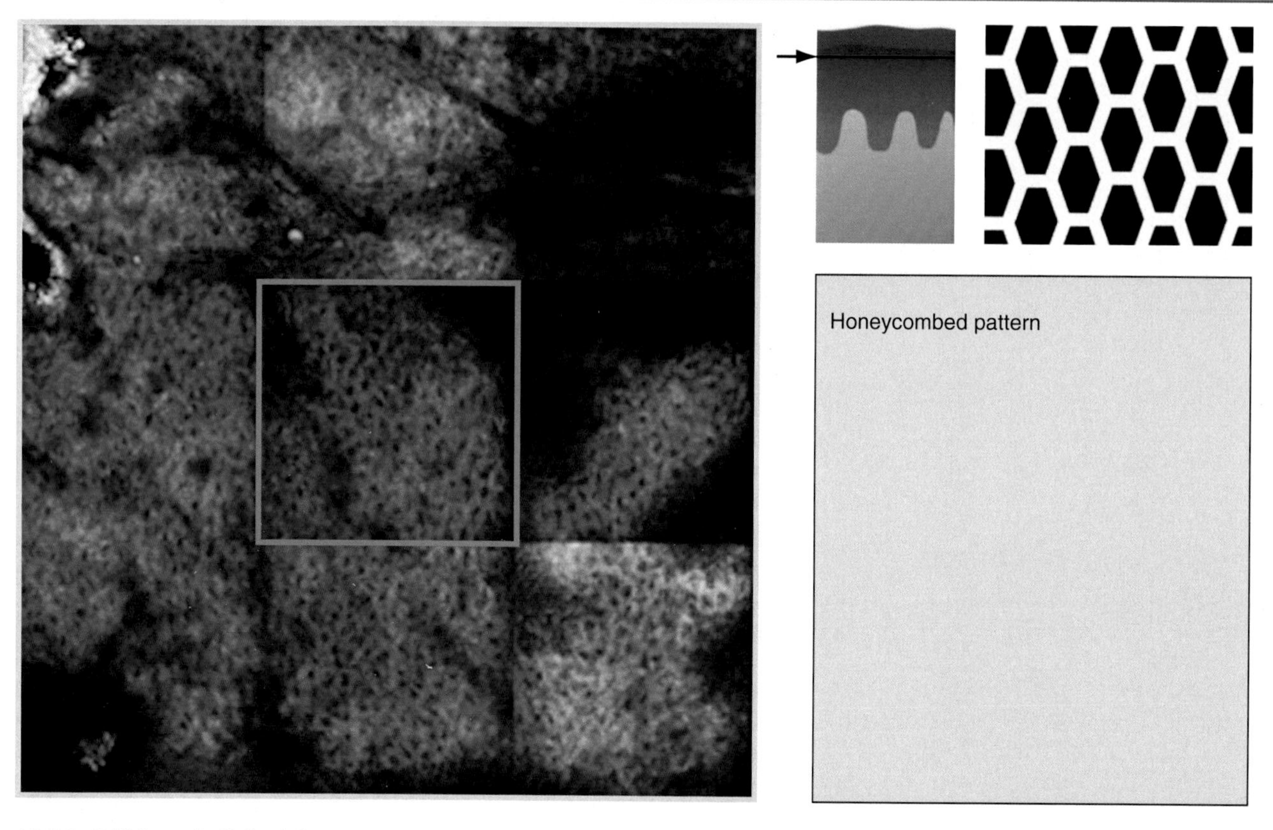

Fig. 14.2.3 RCM mosaic (1.5 × 1.5 mm) at epidermal level showing a portion of honeycombed pattern and absence of cellularity, corresponding to the whitish area of the veil seen under dermoscopy

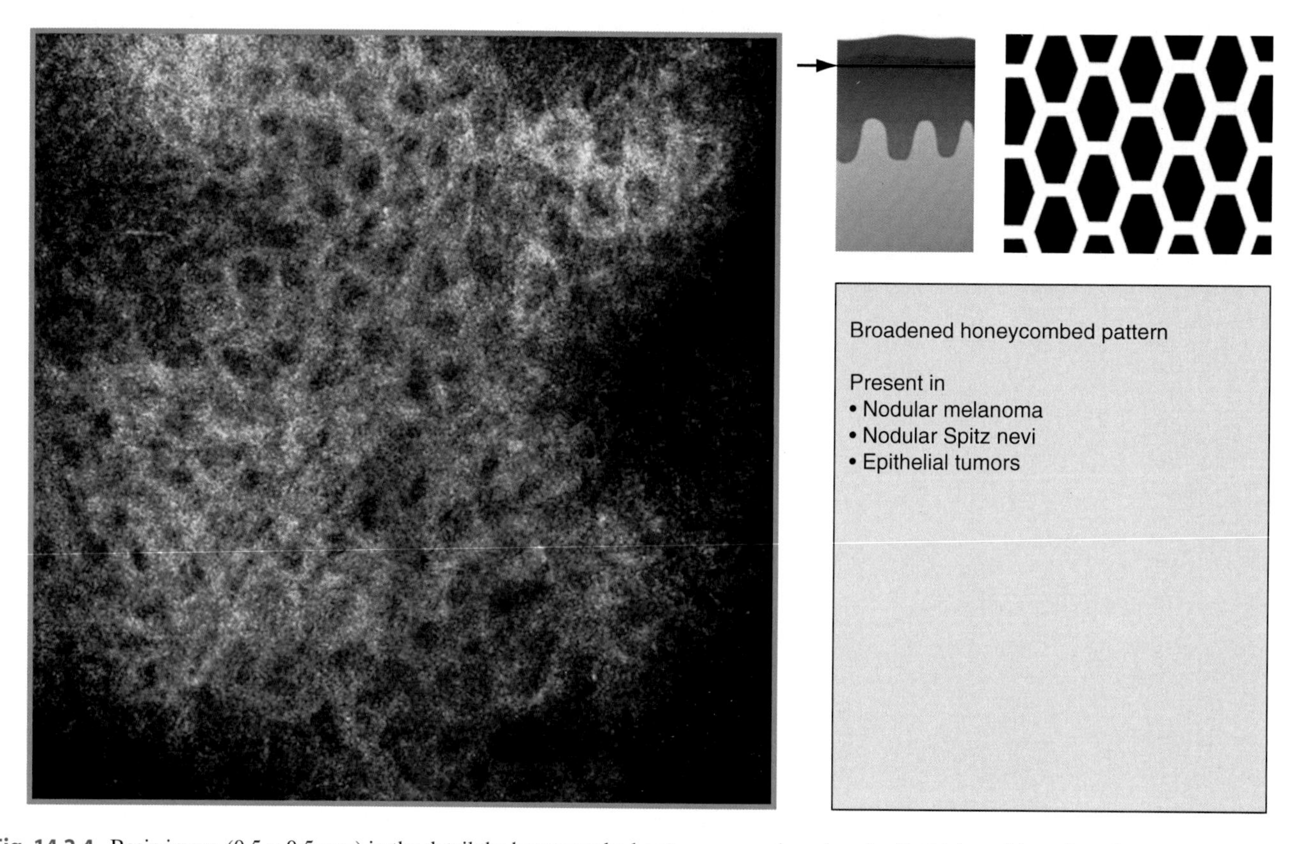

Fig. 14.2.4 Basic image (0.5 × 0.5 mm) in the detail the honeycombed pattern appear broadened with thickened inter-keratinocyte space

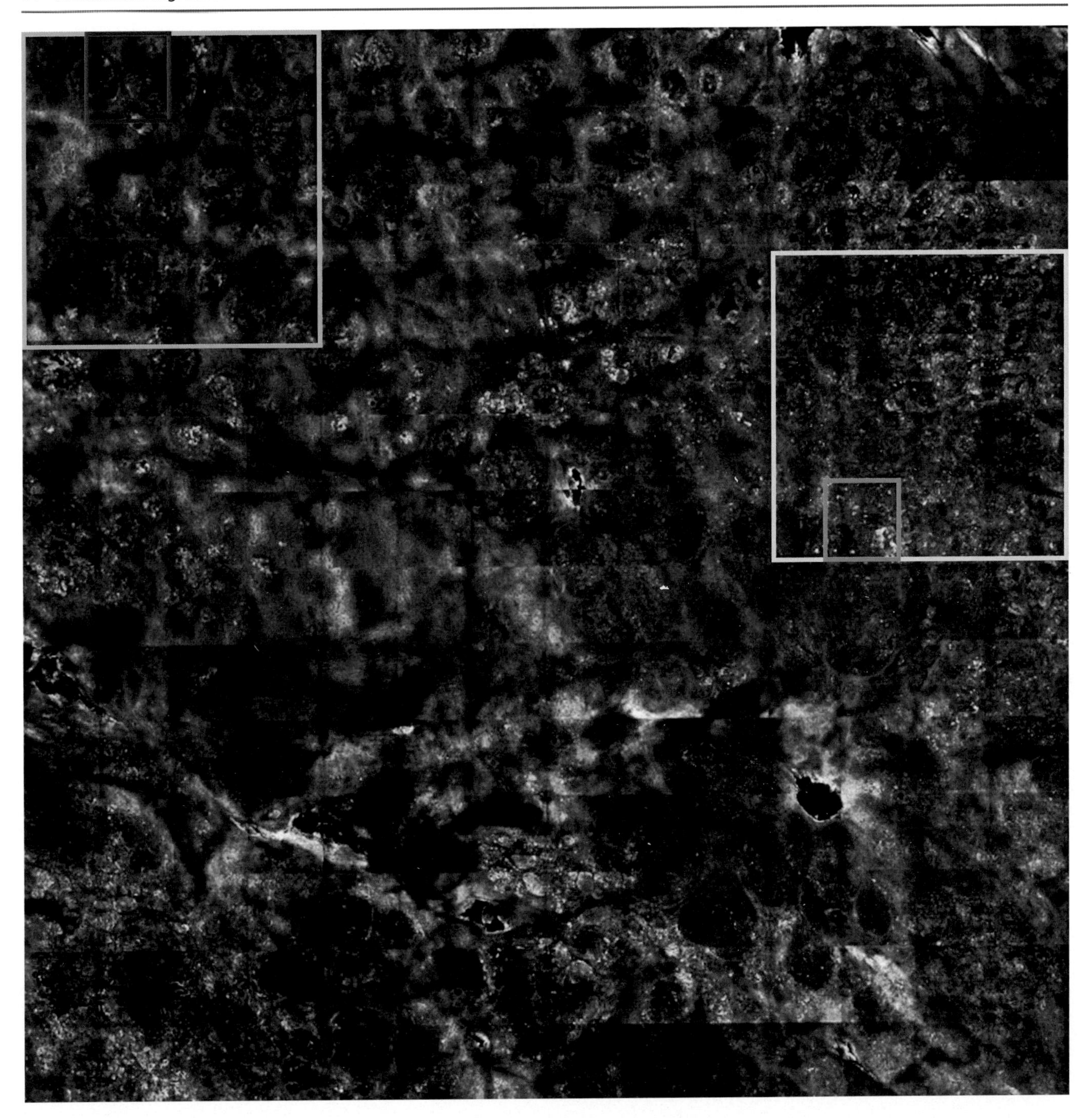

Fig. 14.2.5 RCM mosaic (7 × 7 mm) at DEJ level. The overall architecture is an aspecific pattern because the dermal papillae or a meshwork pattern is not detectable. Numerous bright aggregates occupy large areas of the lesion (*yellow and green square*)

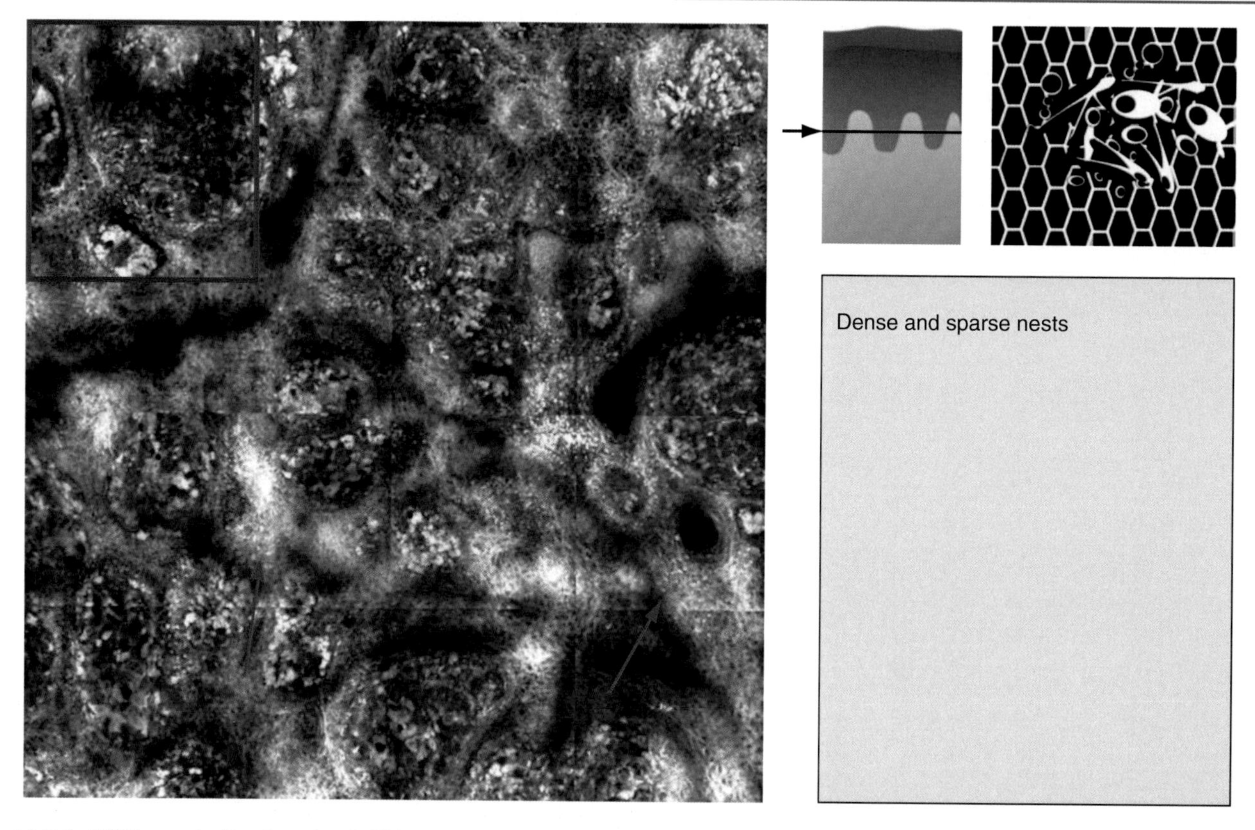

Fig. 14.2.6 RCM mosaic (2 × 2 mm) at DEJ level. Nests of cells are visible within honeycomb pattern (→). This is due to the thinning of the epidermis and the massive presence of a nested proliferation pushing from the dermal compartment

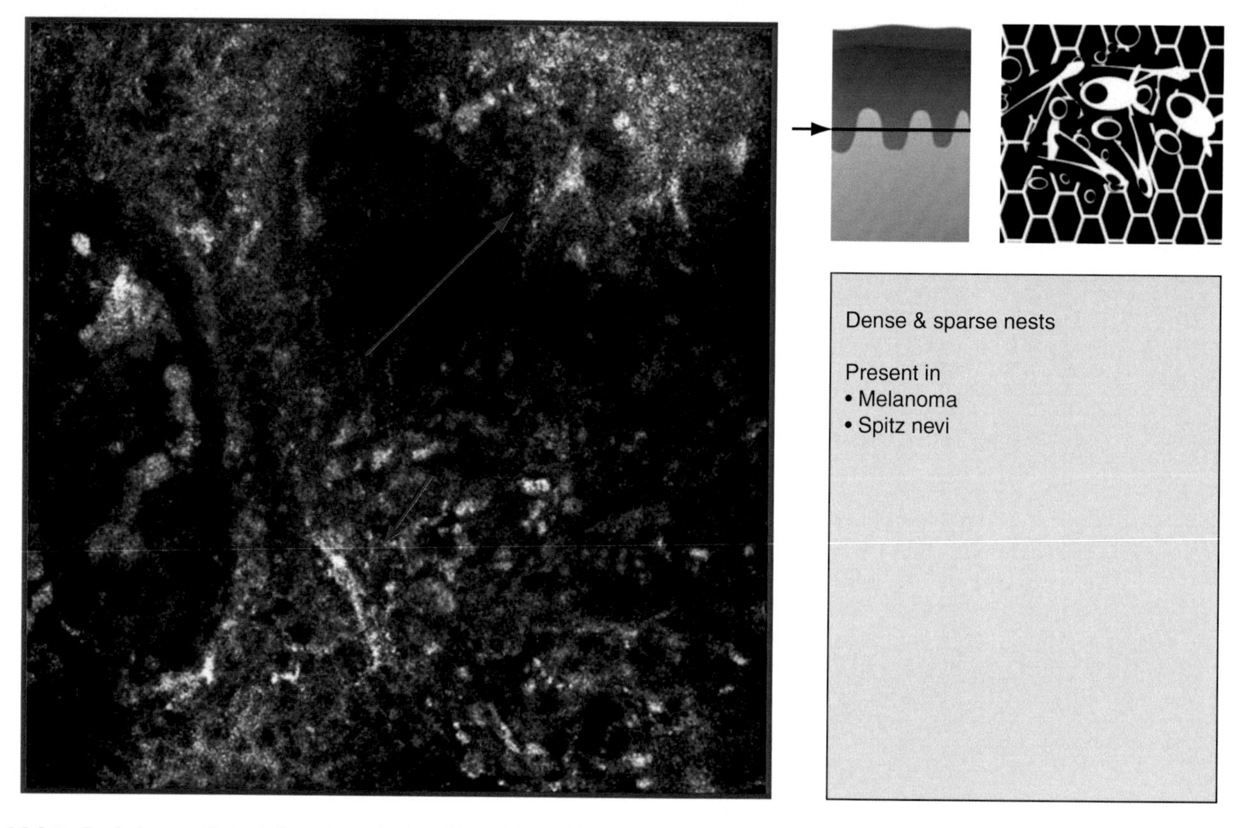

Fig. 14.2.7 Basic image (0.5 × 0.5 mm) dendritic cells with branching structures and the tendency to form aggregates (→)

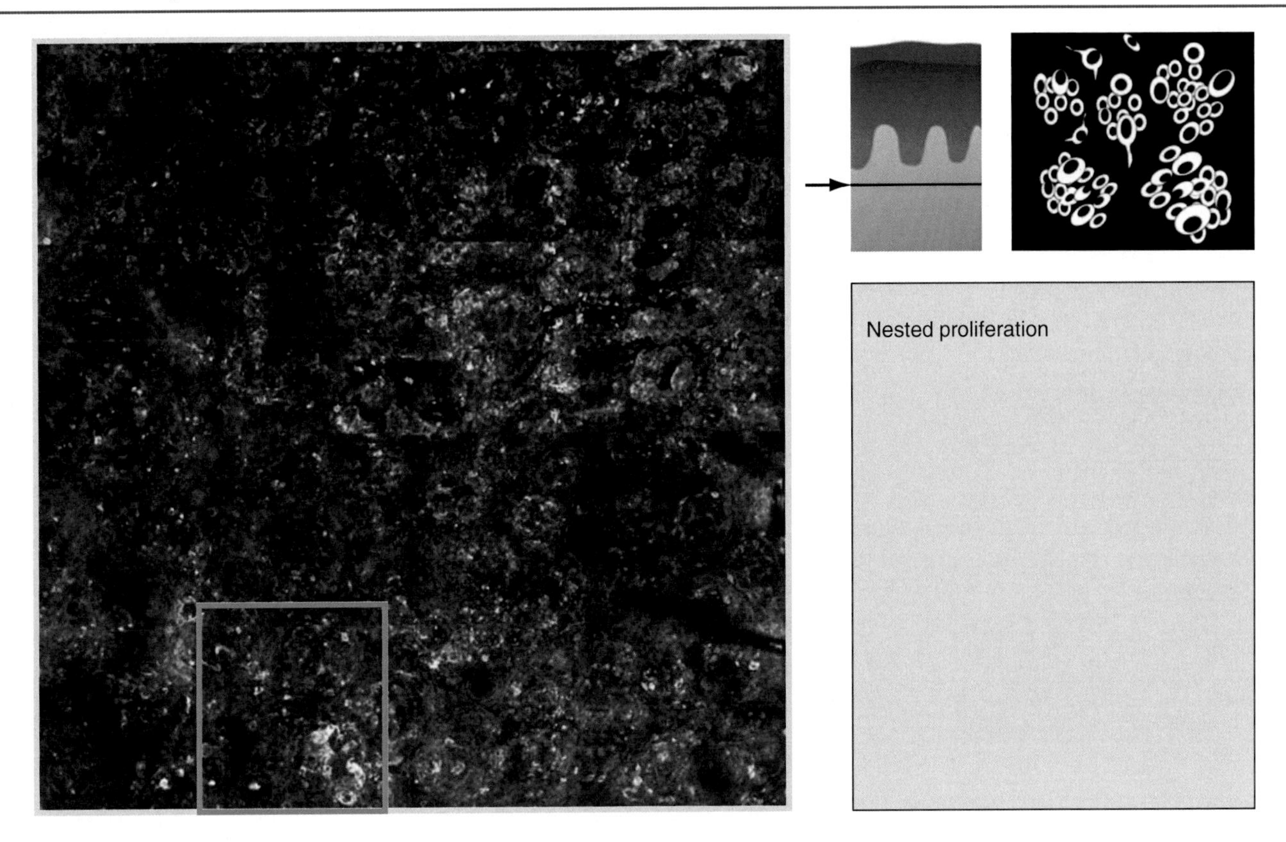

Fig. 14.2.8 RCM mosaic (2 × 2 mm) at papillary dermis. Nested cell proliferation occupying the entire dermal compartment

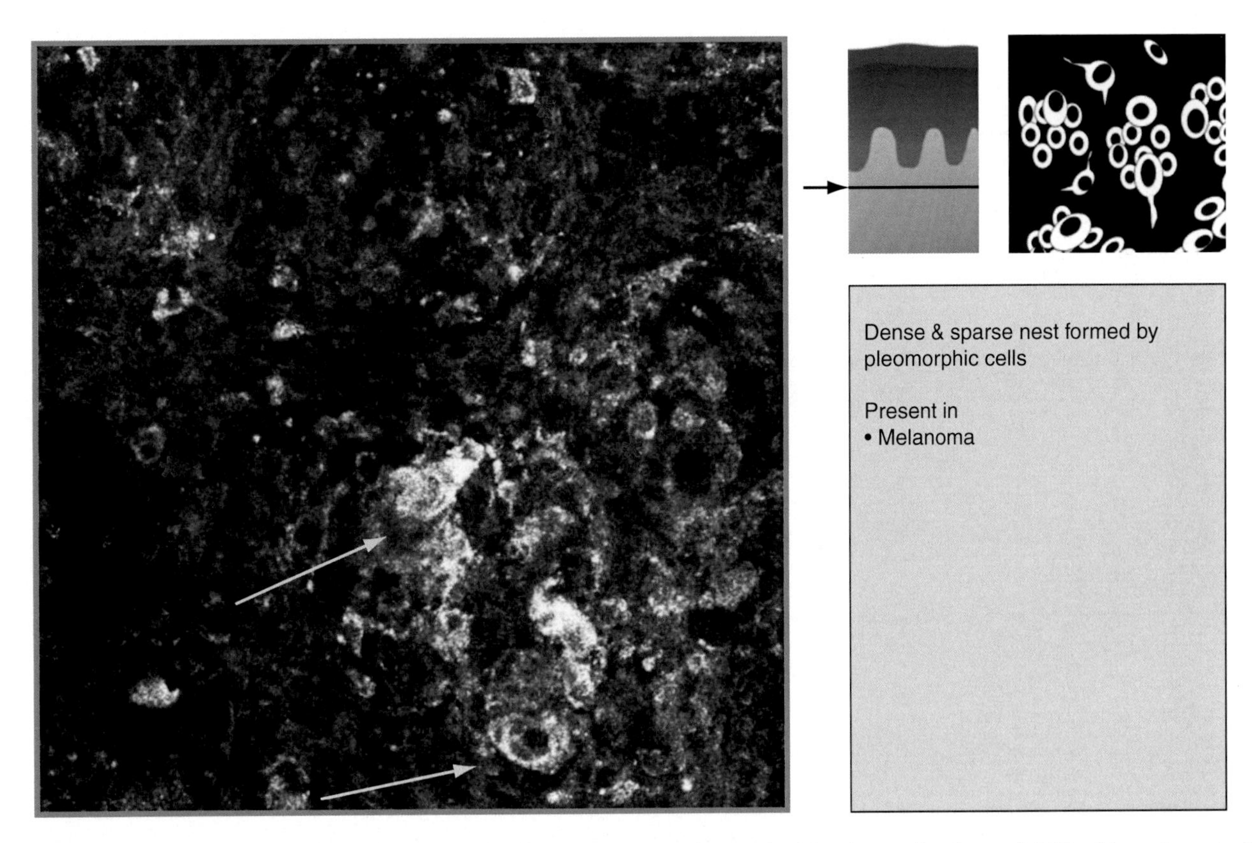

Fig. 14.2.9 Basic image (0.5 × 0.5 mm) pleomorphic cells with large cytoplasm and evident hyporefrective nuclei (*) with tendency to form aggregates (→)

14.2 Vertical Growth Phase

Clinically, a palpable or nodular portion is visible in the context of a flat lesion or remnants of it. The vertical growth, matter of this chapter, concerns the invasion occurring in a context of radial growth phase. This is a different situation in respect of "pure" nodular lesion, not presenting a radial growth from the beginning but representing a distinct melanoma subgroup [3, 4], which will be discussed later in this book.

Histologically, the epidermis over the nodular portion of the tumor is usually thin and effaced and, not rarely, ulcerated. The dermal component is typified by a cohesive nodule or smaller nests of malignant melanocytes that have a pushing or expansile pattern of growth.

On RCM images, epidermal layers are characterized by honeycombed or, sometimes, broadened honeycombed pattern. Pagetoid cells, either roundish or dendritic in shape, can be detectable (Fig. 14.3). Conversely, in "pure" nodular melanomas the pagetoid infiltration is usually not present or limited to few cells focally distributed.

As a peculiar finding, cells arranged in sheet-like structures or forming sparse nests are visualized as soon as there is the transition from epidermal to dermal compartment. In fact, at this stage of growth, the epidermis is very thin and the DEJ is completely destroyed by melanocytic atypical proliferation. At the periphery of the lesion it is still possible to observe dermal papillae, usually nonedged and surrounded by atypical junctional proliferation corresponding to the RGP whereas in the nodular portion. However, a complete papillary contour is not visible due to the epidermal effacement and prominent cell proliferation. Rarely, cerebriform nests showing up as hyporefrective aggregates of small cells outlined by bright collagen septae can be visualized at the deepest dermal level. The presence of cerebriform nest is highly specific of malignancy and suggestive of deep dermal invasion. Overall, the dermal component of nodules arising on a SSM is undistinguishable from the ones observable in pure nodular melanomas.

A prominent vascularization with convolute and tortuous vessels is a frequent finding at this stage of invasion. The vessels can be found in proximity of tumoral proliferation or even admixed to malignant cell growth. The vessels usually show a large calibres and fast blood flow easily observable during live imaging. Ulceration represents a common findings and it appear as dark areas, usually with sharp borders and irregular contours, filled with amorphous material and/or clotted bright small particles. The nodular portion of SSM and pure nodular melanomas share morphologic findings with dermal metastasis, especially when they are epidermotropic.

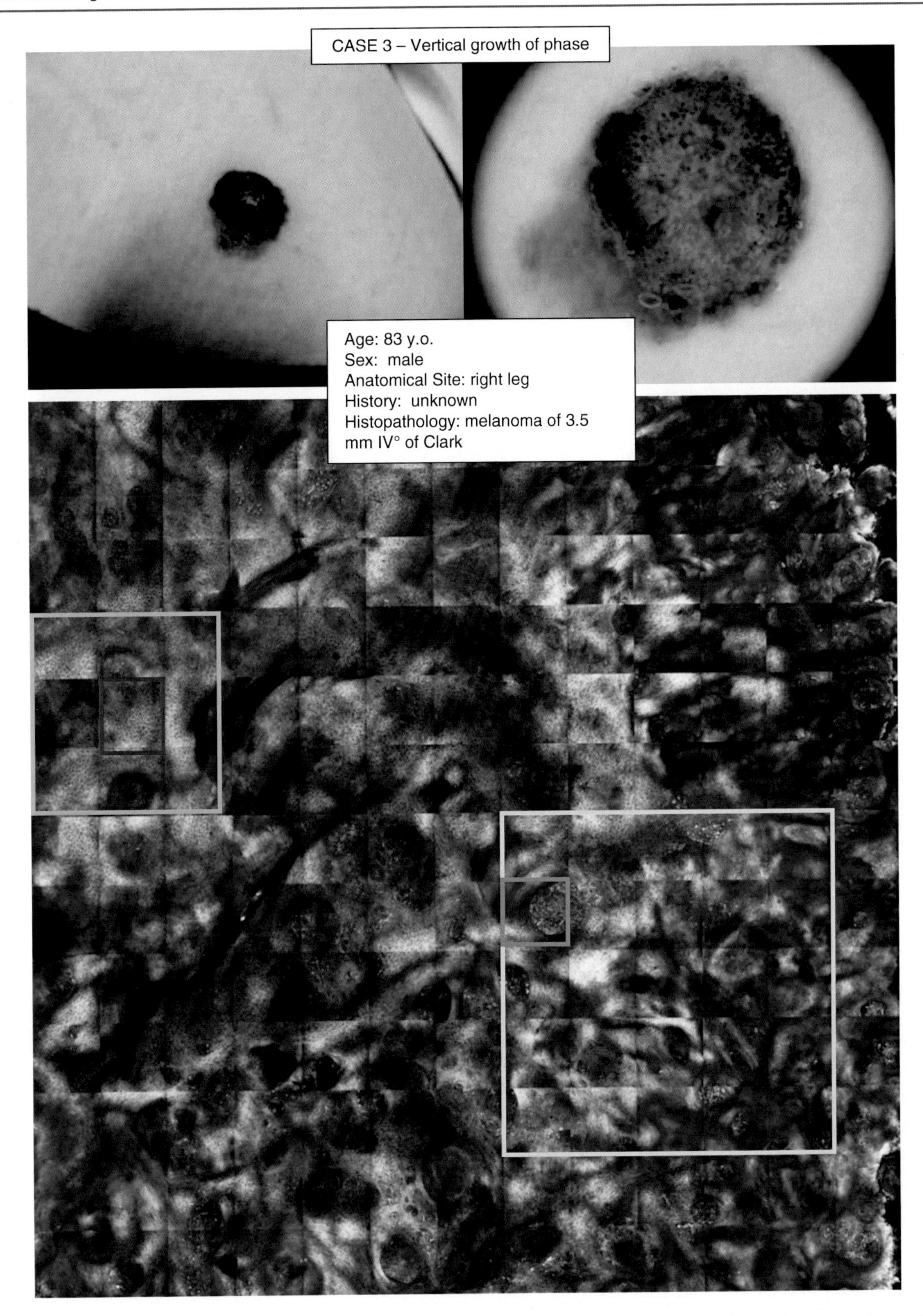

Fig. 14.3 RCM mosaic (7.5 × 7.5 mm) at epidermal level. Broadened honeycombed pattern (*green and red square*) corresponding to the most acanthotic area of the nodule without cell proliferation. Bright aggregates (*yellow square*) in the context of the honeycombed pattern

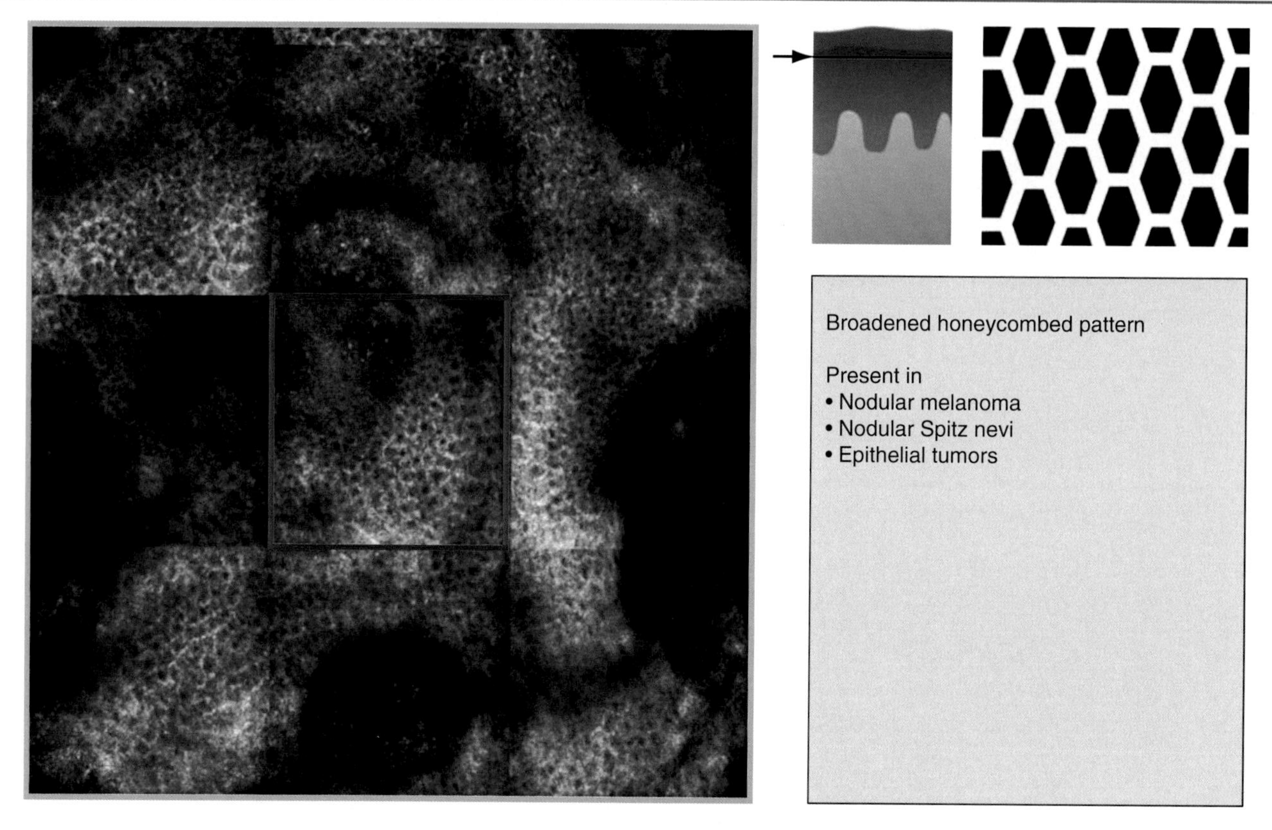

Fig. 14.3.1 RCM mosaic (1.5 × 1.5 mm) broadened honeycombed pattern not presenting pagetoid cells

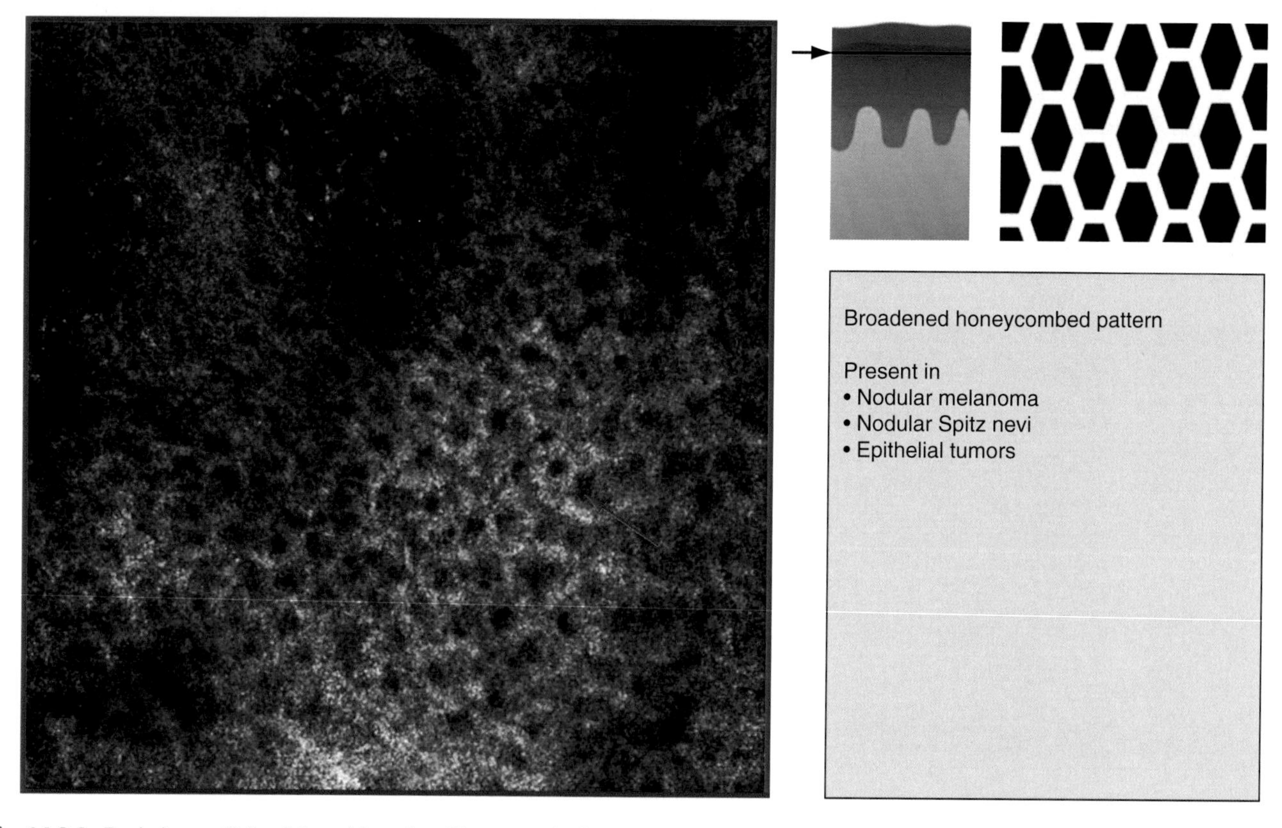

Fig. 14.3.2 Basic image (0.5 × 0.5 mm) broadened honeycombed pattern with bright enlarged keratinocyte borders (→)

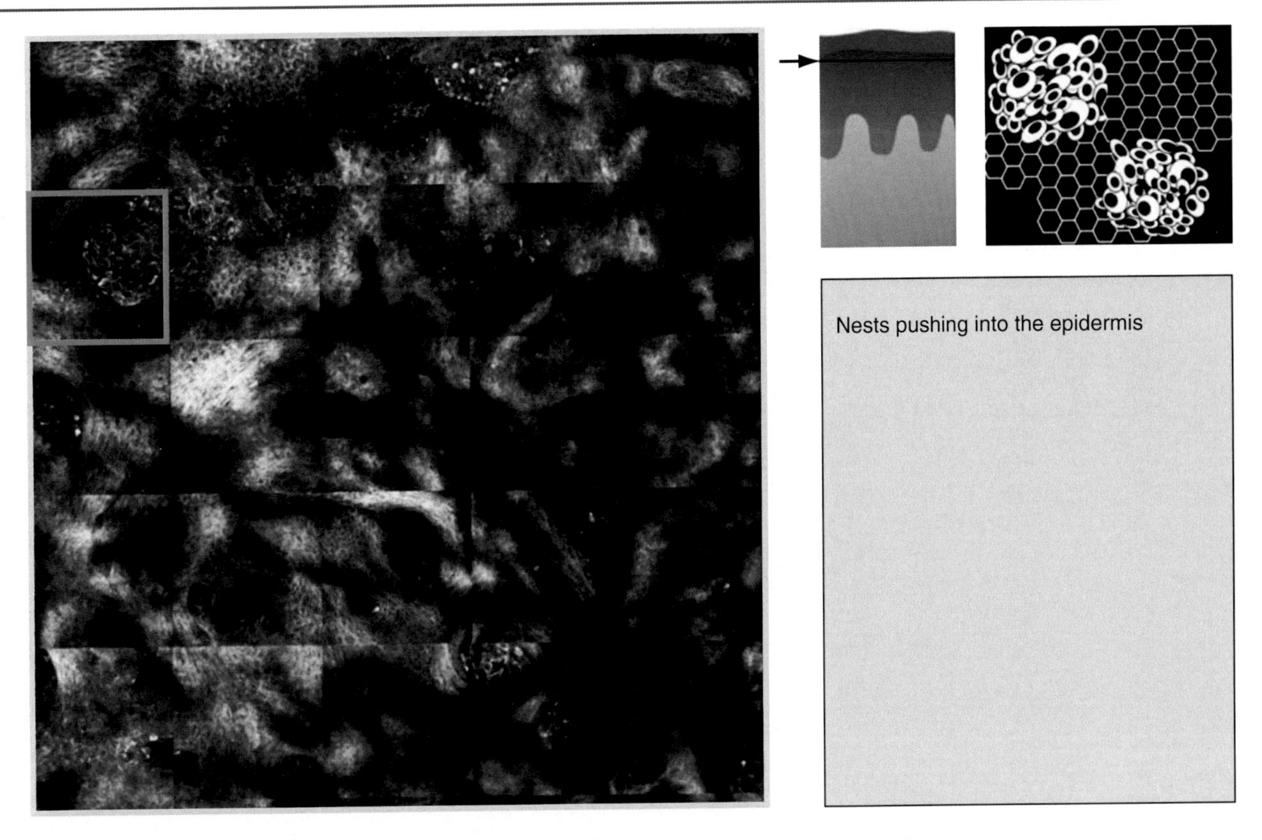

Fig. 14.3.3 RCM mosaic (2.5 × 2.5 mm) showing a bright roundish aggregate

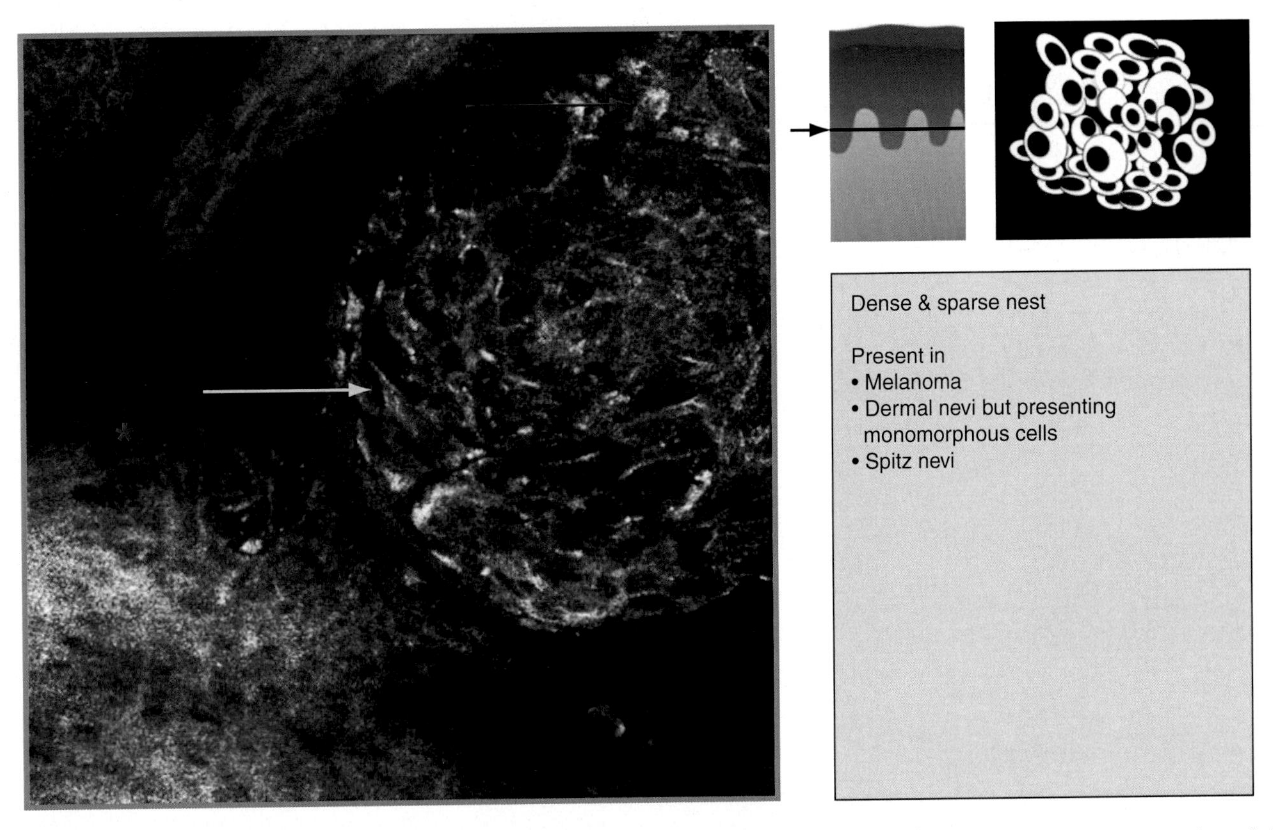

Fig. 14.3.4 Basic image (0.5 × 0.5 mm). Dense and sparse nests formed by either dendritic (*white arrow*) and roundish cells (*red arrow*) in a honeycombed epidermal pattern (*). The presence of these nests in the epidermis is indicative of a thinning and consumption of the epidermis as showed upon histopathology

Core Messages

- Pagetoid and solar melanomas show similar confocal features in their microinvasive and vertical growth phase.
- Microinvasive phase is characterized by pagetoid infiltration, usually composed by numerous cells with a widespread distribution. The rete-ridge profile is not visible and an aspecific architecture characterize all lesions. Cells tend to be aggregated in sheet like structures or dense and sparse nests.
- Nodular component on SSM present distinctive features in respect of pure nodular melanoma. More specifically, pagetoid spread is remarkably present in the vertical growth of phase of SSM compared to pure nodular melanomas. The dermal component is similar in both tumors. Sheet-like structures and cerebriform nests can be found at the deepest dermal layer along with prominent vascularization.

References

1. Clark WH Jr, From L, Bernardino EA, Mihm MC (1969) The histogenesis and biologic behavior of primary human malignant melanomas of the skin. Cancer Res 29:705–727
2. Guerry Dt, Synnestvedt M, Elder DE, Schultz D (1993) Lessons from tumor progression: The invasive radial growth phase of melanoma is common, incapable of metastasis, and indolent. J Invest Dermatol 100:342S–345S
3. Segura S, Pellacani G, Puig S, Longo C, Bassoli S, Guitera P, Palou J, Menzies S, Seidenari S, Malvehy J (2008) In vivo microscopic features of nodular melanomas: dermoscopy, confocal microscopy, and histopathologic correlates. Arch Dermatol 144:1311–1320
4. Clark WH Jr, Elder DE, Van Horn M (1986) The biologic forms of malignant melanoma. Hum Pathol 17:443–450

Nodular Melanoma

15

Joseph Malvehy, Susana Puig, Cristina Carrera, and Sonia Segura

Nodular melanoma is the second most common type of melanoma responsible for about 9–15% of invasive melanomas and up to 50% of melanomas thicker than 2 mm. It is most commonly seen in elderly men but can occur at any age and in both sexes [1]. Nodular melanoma arises in normal skin or in a precursor lesion but without the presence of a radial growth phase. Thus, nodular melanoma, even in its early stages, has the potential to metastasis. The classification of melanoma by subtype is based on anatomic, epidemiological and pattern of progression features. However, recent research has shown that there may also be molecular and genetic differences between melanoma subtypes. These differences may explain the difference in the natural evolution of melanoma subtypes [2–5]. Diagnosis of nodular melanoma may be challenging and misdiagnosis at the first time of consultation is not infrequent [6]. In nodular melanoma, classical clinical criteria of the ABCDE rule for diagnosis of melanoma, with the exception of change, fail in initial stages because these tumors are often small, round shaped, symmetric and with regular borders. The color is often quite homogeneous compared with superficial malignant melanoma and may be pink or reddish rather than black, bluish or brown [7, 8]. A significant percentage of nodular melanoma are hypocromic or amelanotic [9]. The clinical findings of nodular melanoma are similar to the aspect of nodular part in other variants including superficial malignant melanoma.

Confocal-histopathological correlation is good, enabling the in vivo visualization of some characteristic histologic features in the epidermis and superficial dermis, whereas aspects deeper than 300 μm are not valuable due to limited resolution of microscopes [10].

Within epidermis, nodular melanoma lack characteristic melanoma features, such as epidermal disarrangement and pagetoid melanocytosis, usually showing a honeycombed pattern or a peculiar broadened pattern, consisting of polygonal cells with black nuclei and bright thick cytoplasm that probably correspond to the presence of a compact eosinophilic corneal layer over a thin epidermis [11] (Figs. 15.1.1, 15.2, 15.4, 15.5). Differently superficial malignant melanomas usually exhibit, despite their different evolution stage, mostly disarranged pattern and the presence of moderate to intense pagetoid cells by RCM (Fig. 15.3).

At dermoepidermal junction, the nodular component in both nodular melanomas and nodules of superficial malignant melanomas exhibit similar features: lack of typical papillary architecture, corresponding to the epidermal flattening and presence of pleomorphic cells with bright cytoplasm and dark nucleus in basal layer, sometimes distributed in sheet-like structures, and in papillary dermis, isolated or aggregated in dishomogeneous clusters (Figs. 15.1–15.4).

Deep, amorphous, hyporefractive nests, called cerebriform nests, are more characteristic of nodular melanomas, correlating with deep tumoral infiltration (Fig. 15.2.2). In superficial malignant melanomas with blue coloration, the rete-ridge are markedly disarranged, but grossly preserved, resulting in the frequent observation of nonedged papillae of irregular size and shape in combination with a marked cytological atypia (Fig. 1.3). Nucleated cells corresponding to malignant melanocyte infiltration are also observable in blue superficial malignant melanomas, usually in combination with dishomogeneous aggregates of atypical cells (Figs. 15.3.2 and 15.5.4).

As a new RCM feature almost exclusively seen in pure nodular melanoma, in upper dermis some bright fibrillar structures (called collagen bundles) bunched in large bundles and delimitating aggregates of atypical cells are seen

J. Malvehy (✉) • S. Puig • C. Carrera
Department of Dermatology, Melanoma Unit, Hospital Clinic of Barcelona, Barcelona, Spain
e-mail: jmalvehy@clinic.ub.es

S. Segura
Department of Dermatology, Hospital del Mar, Barcelona, Spain

R. Hofmann-Wellenhof et al. (eds.), *Reflectance Confocal Microscopy for Skin Diseases*,
DOI 10.1007/978-3-642-21997-9_15, © Springer-Verlag Berlin Heidelberg 2012

(Fig. 15.4.2). Its histopathologic correlation is probably corresponding to compacted collagen surrounding tumoral mass. Plump cells are also present in most of the lesions and correlate with dermal macrophages, usually in association to a moderate degree of inflammation. Moreover, nodular melanoma and nodular areas of superficial malignant melanoma exhibit enlarged and tortuous vessels in most of the cases being less frequent in blue superficial malignant melanoma, indicating the presence of prominent neovascularization in thicker tumors (Figs. 15.1.2 and 15.2.1).

Interestingly, nodular melanoma and nodular superficial malignant melanoma show similar confocal and histopathologic features in the dermal component, characterized by prominent cellularity and moderate inflammatory infiltrate with the absence of regression, probably for the similarity of the biological aggressive behavior in the presence of a weak immunological response (Fig. 15.1.4).

15.1 Conclusions

1. Nodular melanoma by means of RCM exhibits differential features respect nodular areas of superficial malignant melanoma.
2. Nodular melanoma exhibits a honeycombed pattern at epidermal layers with no significant pagetoid cells in most of the cases, differing from superficial malignant melanoma.
3. At the dermo-epidermal junction, rarely dermal papilla are seen in both nodular melanoma and nodular areas from superficial malignant melanoma.
4. Nonagregated diffuse atypical cells, variable number of dense dishomogeneous cell clusters, atypical nucleated cells and plump cells are noted in the upper dermis.
5. In nodular melanoma, characteristic cerebriform clusters are often seen.

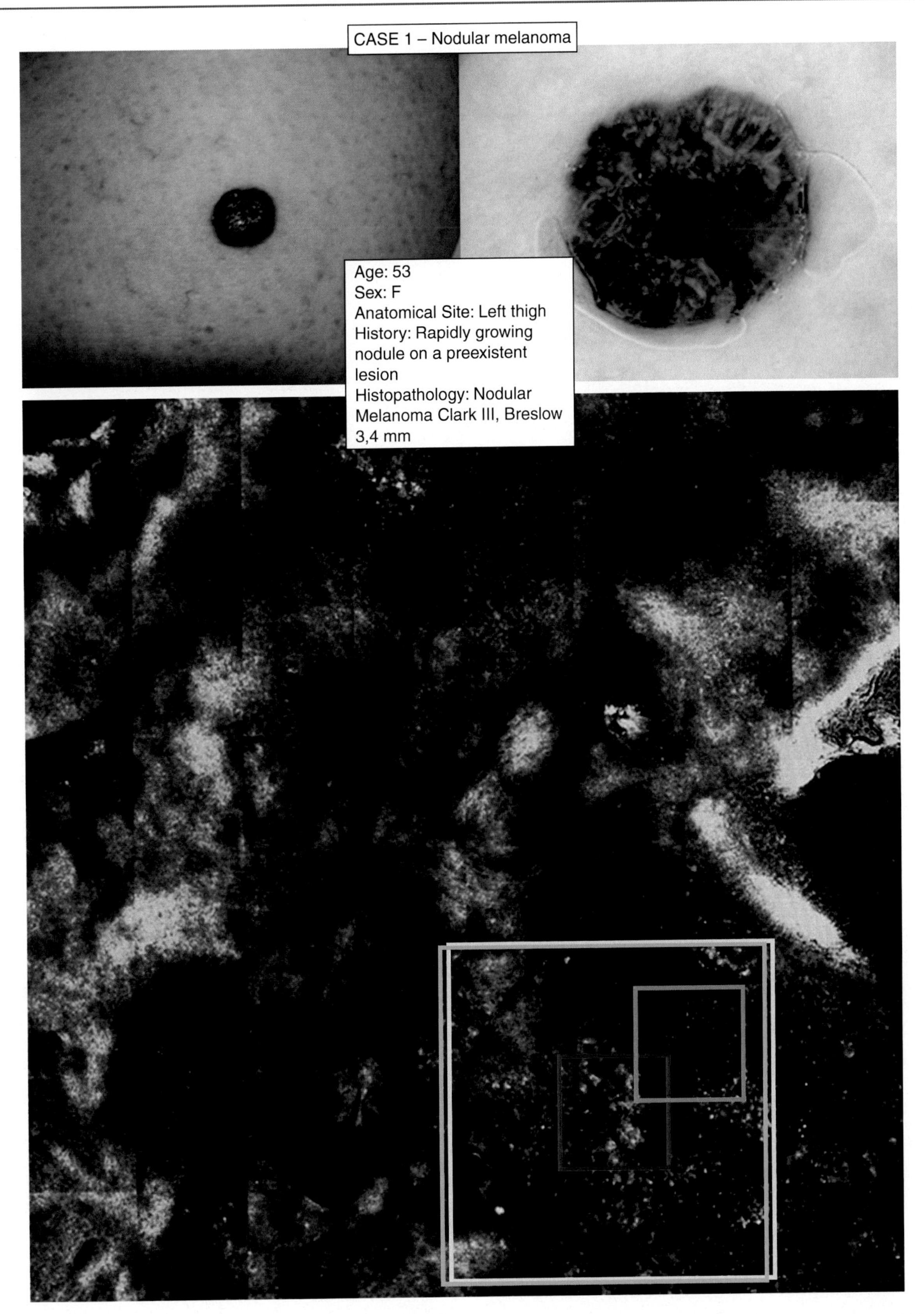

Fig. 15.1 RCM mosaic (4 × 4 mm). Nodular lesion with irregular surface in which different skin layers are represented. We can observe some areas showing a honeycombed pattern corresponding to epidermis. The darker areas of the mosaic represent DEJ and upper dermis and exhibit bright irregular cells distributed in a sheet-like manner and in some areas aggregated forming irregular nests

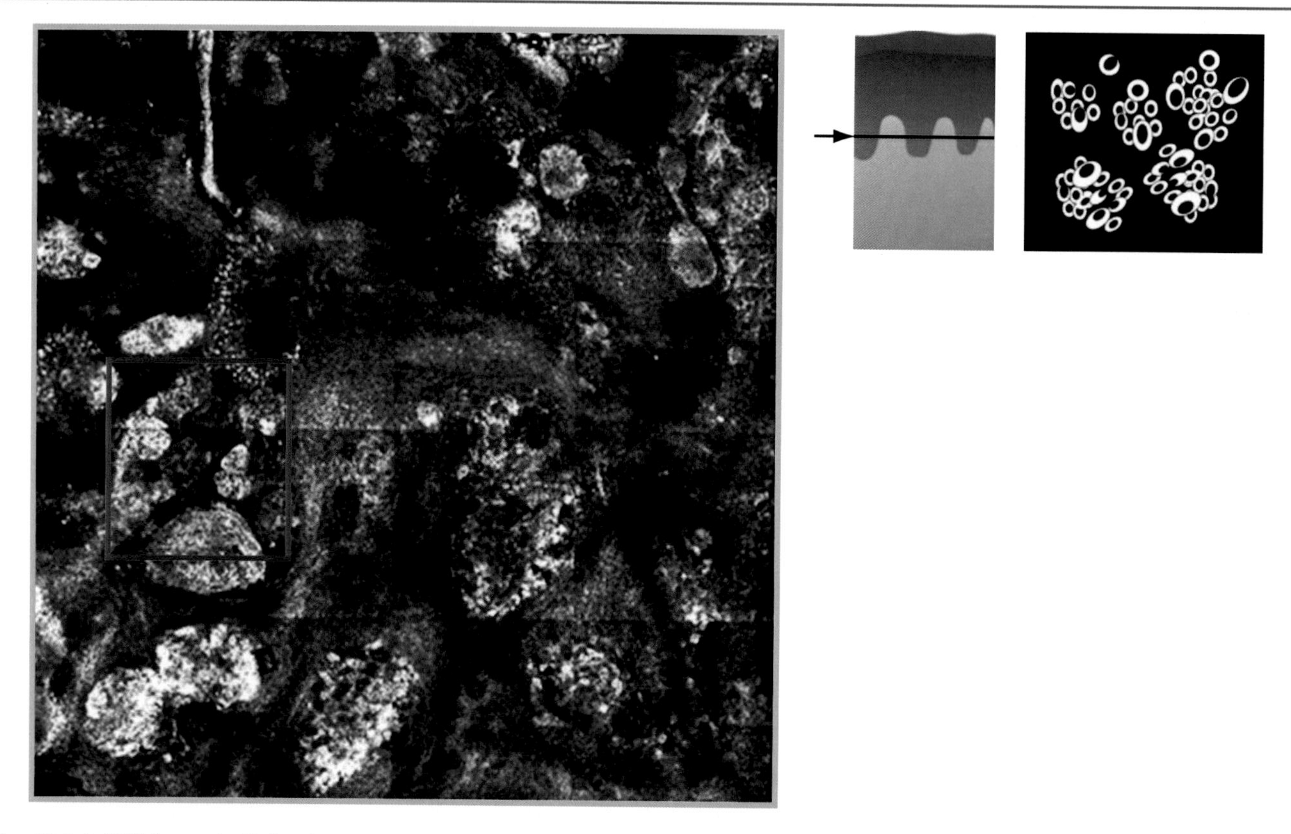

Fig. 15.1.1 RCM mosaic (1.5 × 1.5 mm) at DEJ. Proliferation of sheet-like cells, aggregates of cells forming nonhomogeneous nests and increased vascular structures

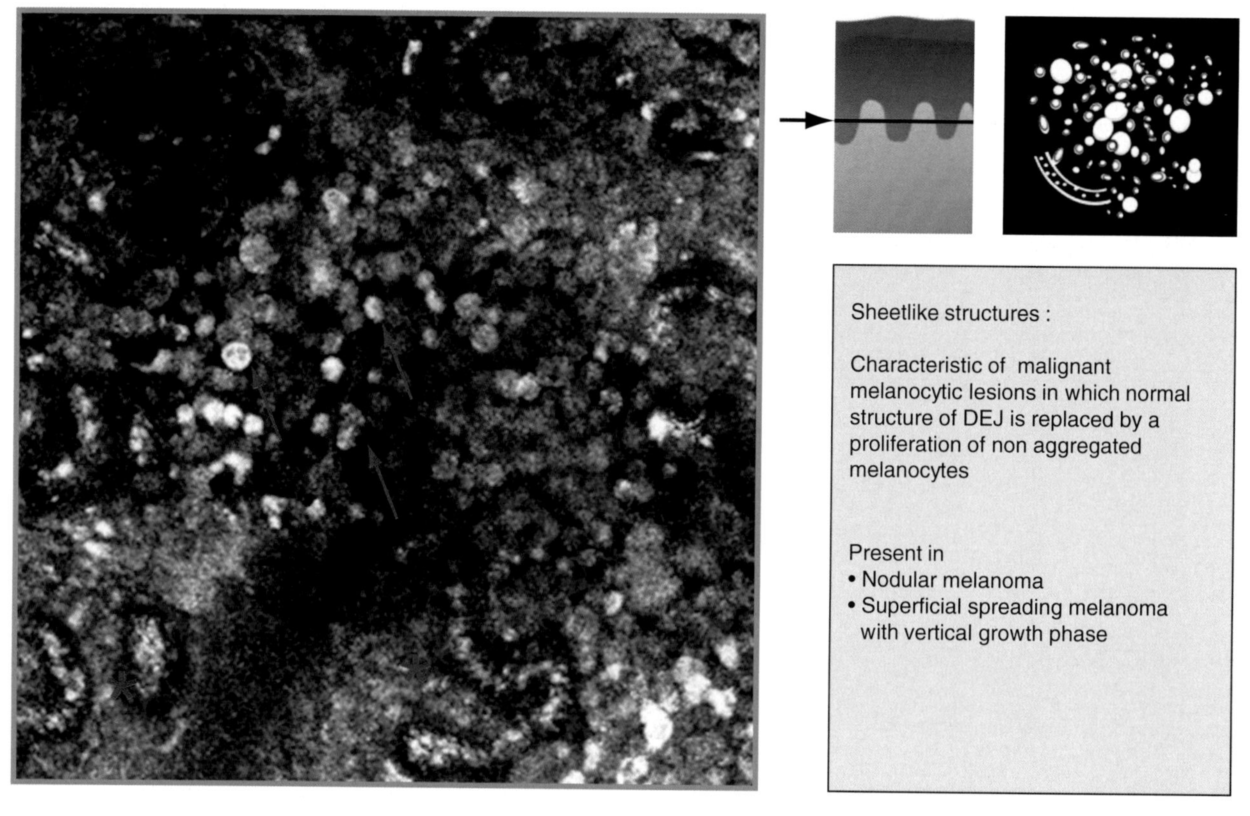

Fig. 15.1.2 Basic image (0.5 × 0.5 mm) at the DEJ. Proliferation of nonaggregated nucleated atypical cells distributed in a sheet-like manner (→) associated to enlarged tortuous vessels (*)

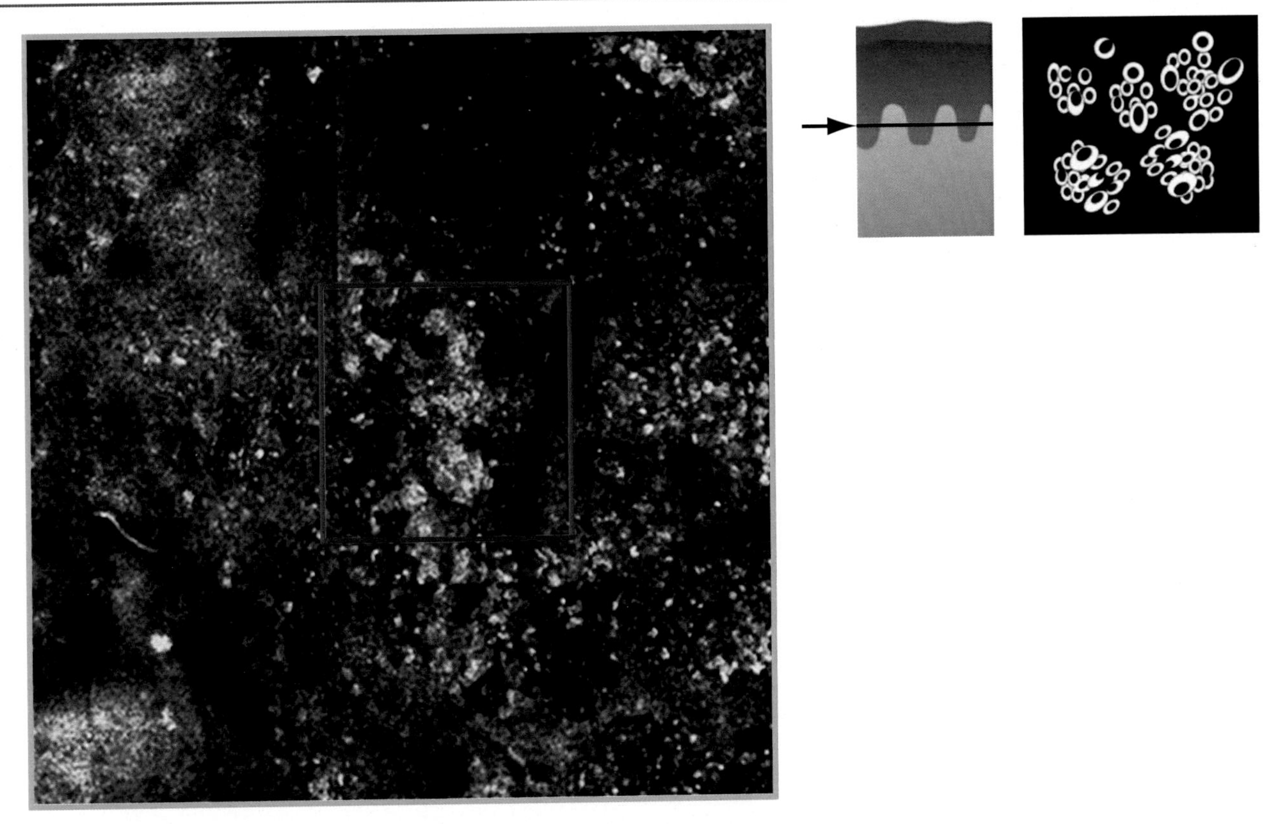

Fig. 15.1.3 RCM mosaic (1.5 × 1.5 mm) at DEJ. Proliferation of sheet-like cells, aggregates of cells forming nonhomogeneous nests and increased vascular structures

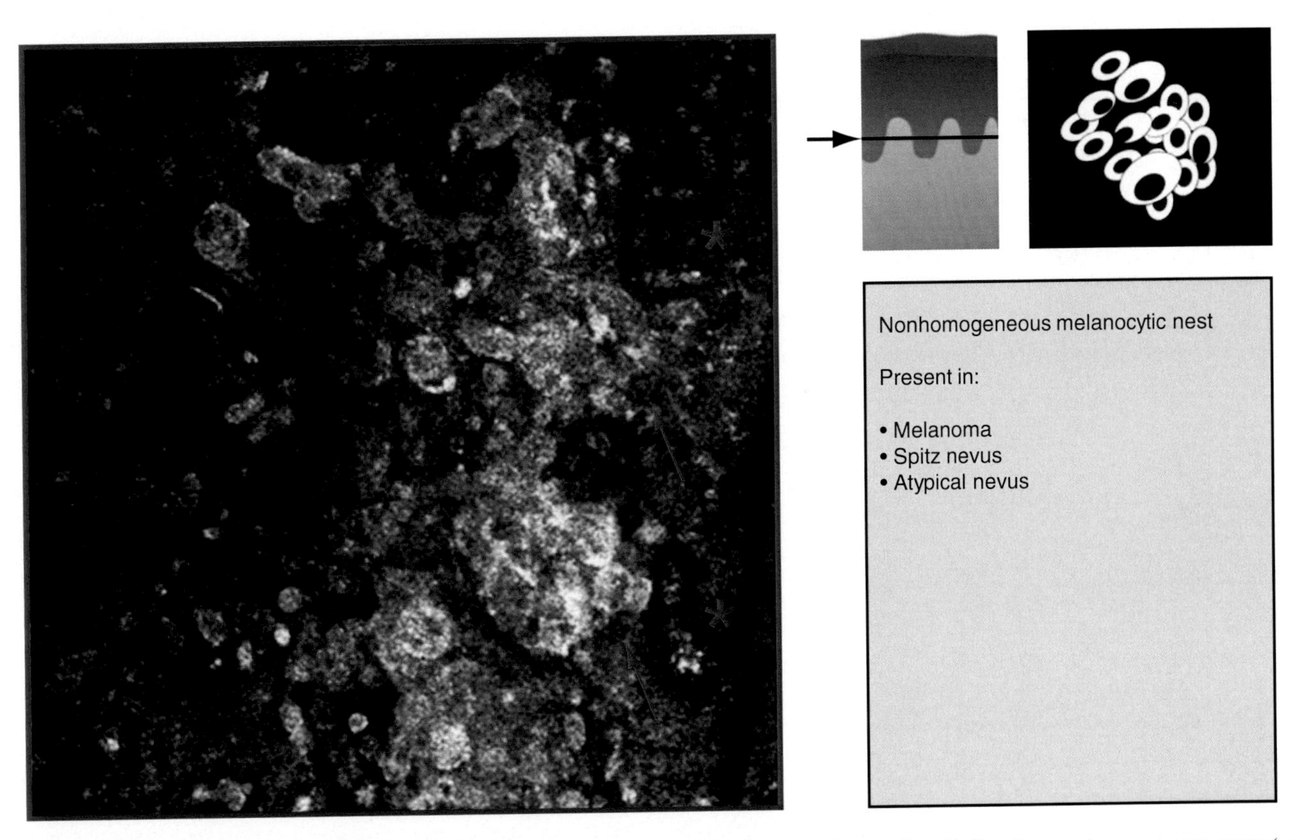

Fig. 15.1.4 Basic image (0.5 × 0.5 mm) at DEJ-upper dermis. Aggregates of atypical melanocytic cells forming nonhomogeneous nests (→) associated to tortuous vessels (*)

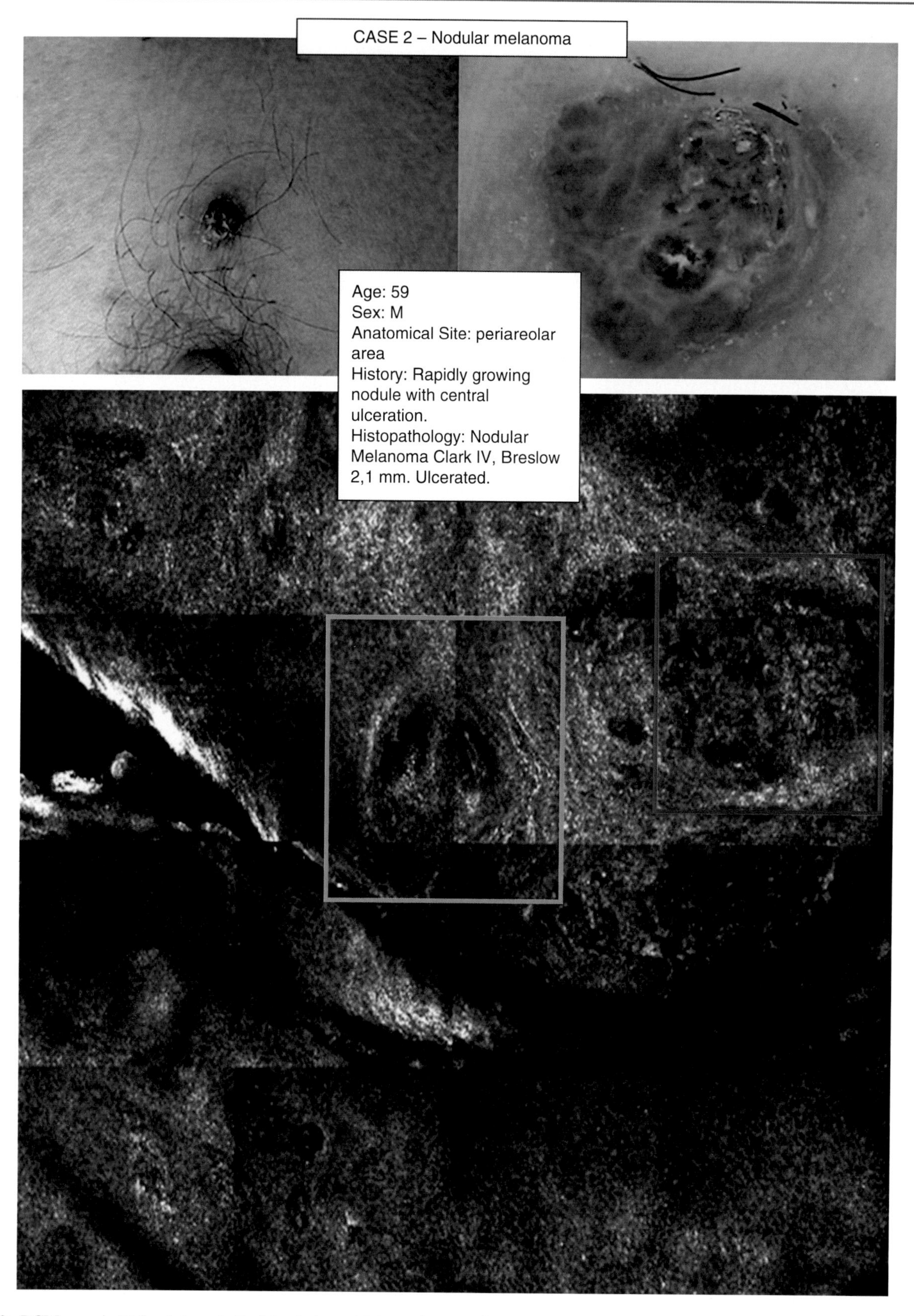

Fig. 15.2 RCM mosaic (1.9 × 1.4 mm). Nodular lesion with irregular surface in which different skin layers are represented. Patchy atypical honeycombed pattern associated to focal dermal cellular aggregates and prominent vessels. This latter feature correlates with the clinical vascular appearance and the dermoscopic findings with multiple colors (*brown, red, blue*), large globules with atypical vessels

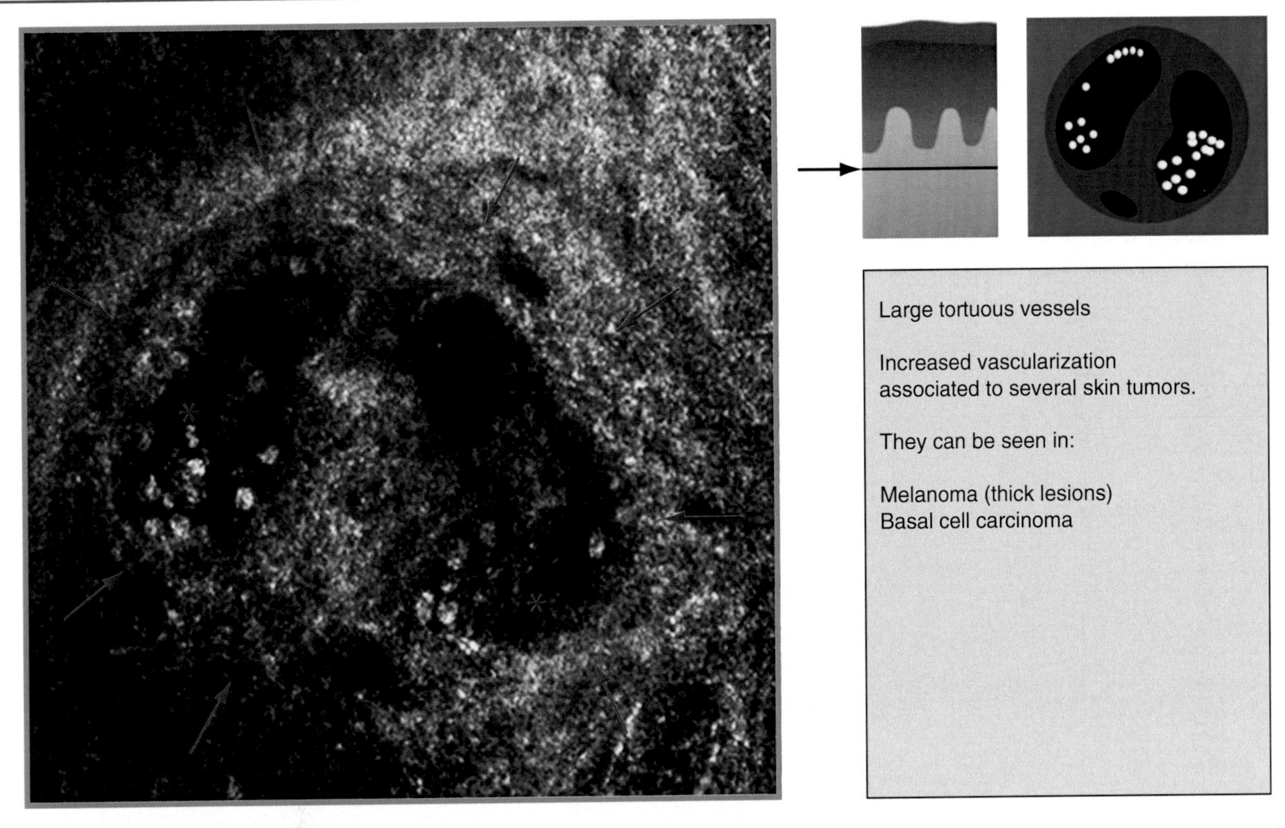

Fig. 15.2.1 Basic image (0.350 × 0.350 mm) at upper dermis. Horizontal section of a large tortuous vessels with a thick wall (→) showing circulating blood cells inside (*)

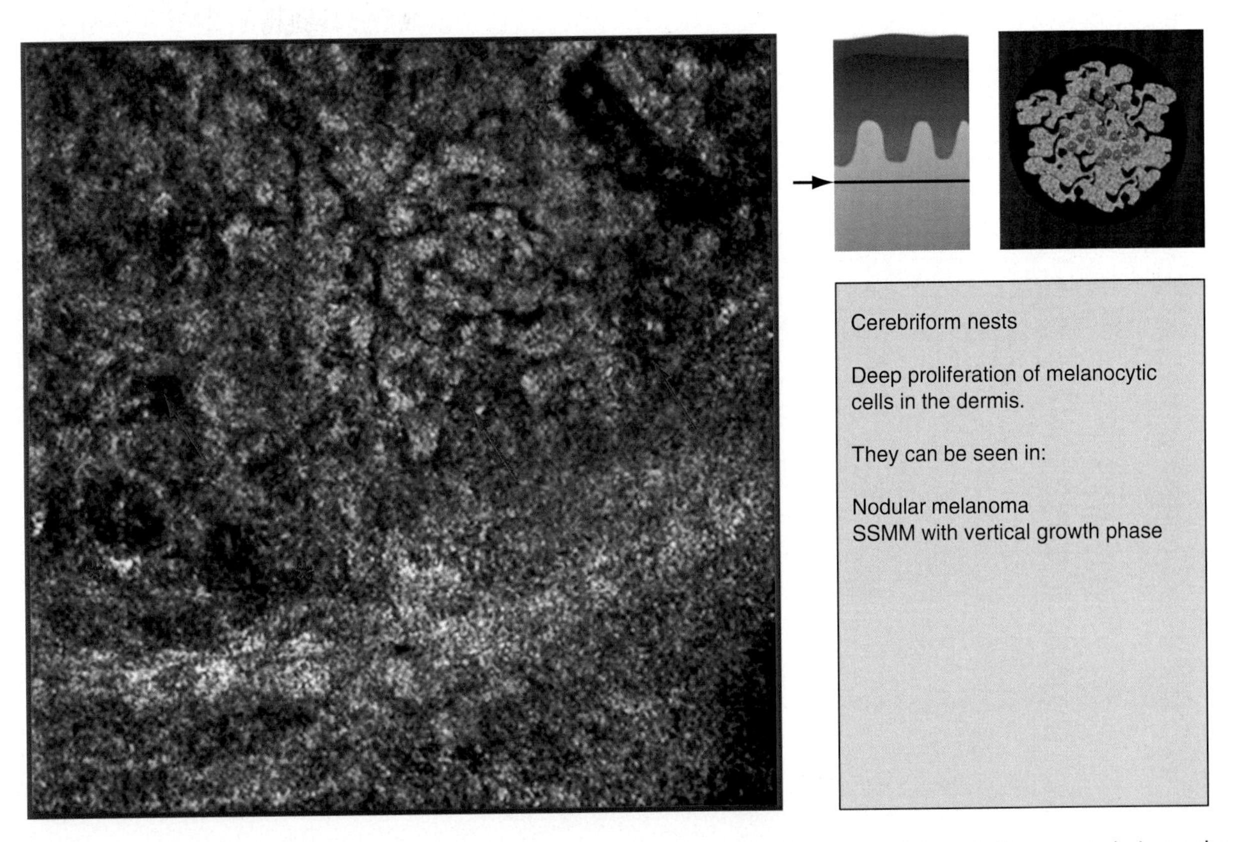

Fig. 15.2.2 Basic image (0.350 × 0.350 mm) at upper dermis. Amorphous, hyporeflective nests, called cerebriform nests, (→) associated to enlarged dermal vessels (*)

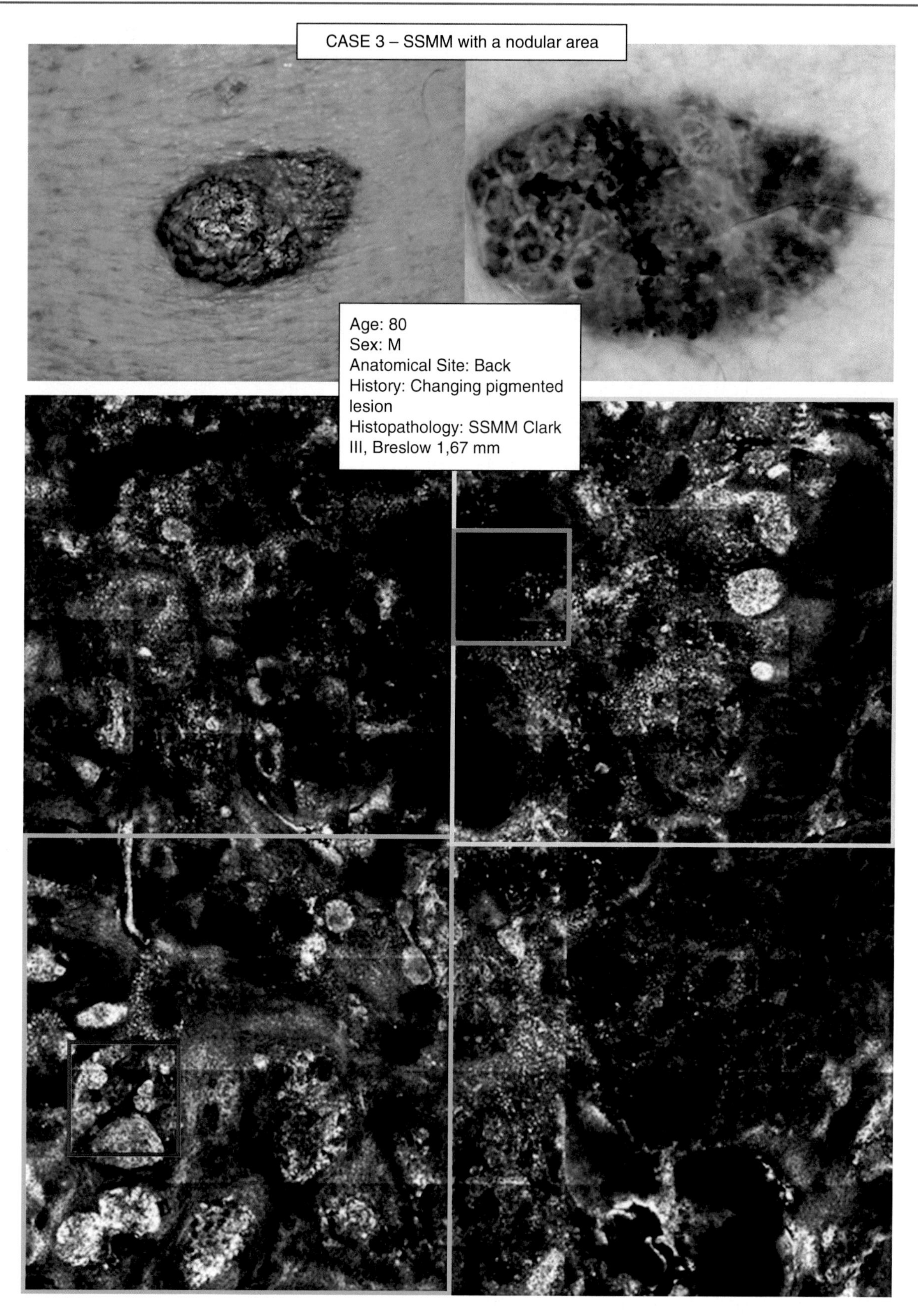

Fig. 15.3 RCM mosaic (4 × 4 mm) at DEJ. Scan image of the more pigmented and nodular part of the lesion where we can observe cellular aggregates irregular in size and distribution associated to areas exhibiting nonaggregated cells forming sheet-like structures. On the right lower corner we can see an irregular meshwork corresponding to the flat part of the lesion

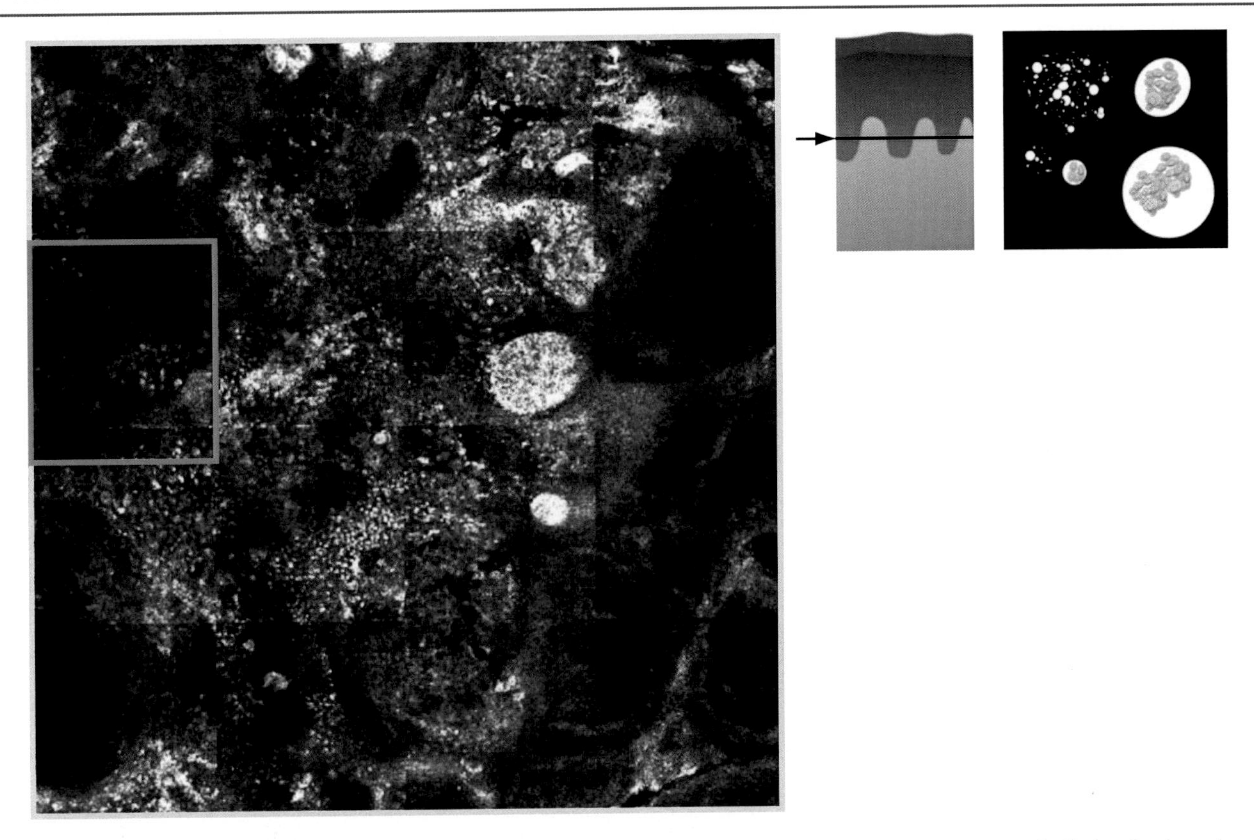

Fig. 15.3.1 RCM mosaic (1 × 1 mm) at DEJ showing a diffuse proliferation of polymorphous cells and focal aggregates of cells forming irregular nests in size and reflectivity

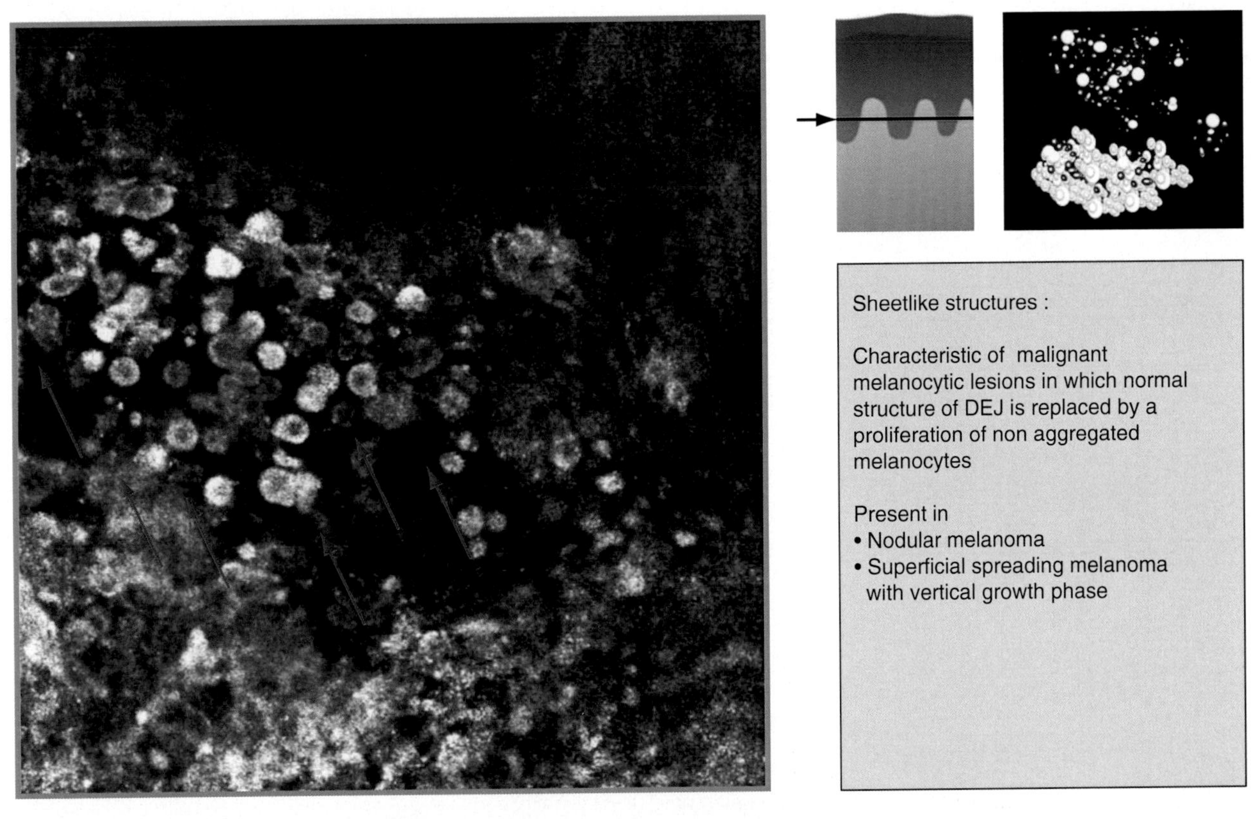

Fig. 15.3.2 Basic image (0.5 × 0.5 mm) at the DEJ. Proliferation of nonaggregated nucleated atypical cells distributed in a sheet-like manner (→)

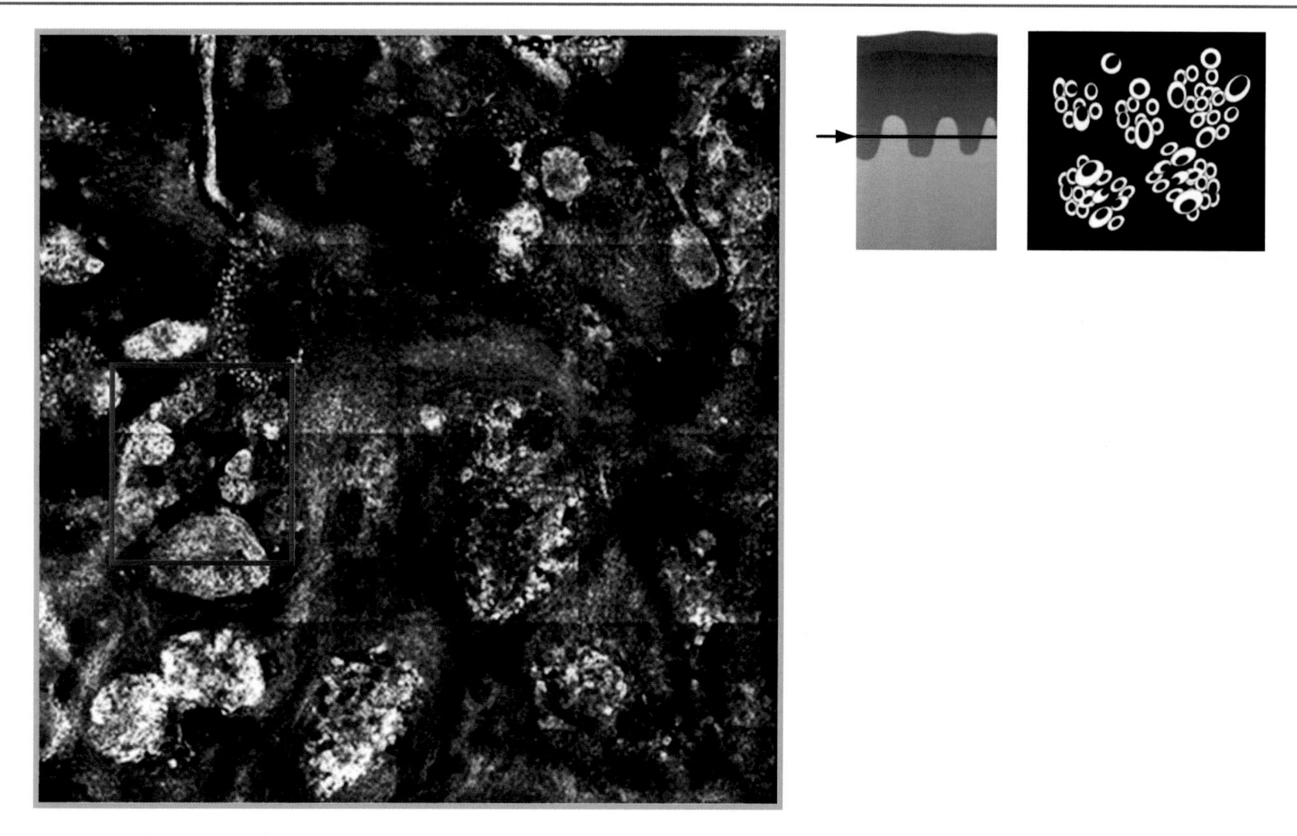

Fig. 15.3.3 RCM mosaic (1 × 1 mm) at DEJ. Aggregates of cells forming nonhomogeneous nests with focal areas of nonaggregated cells

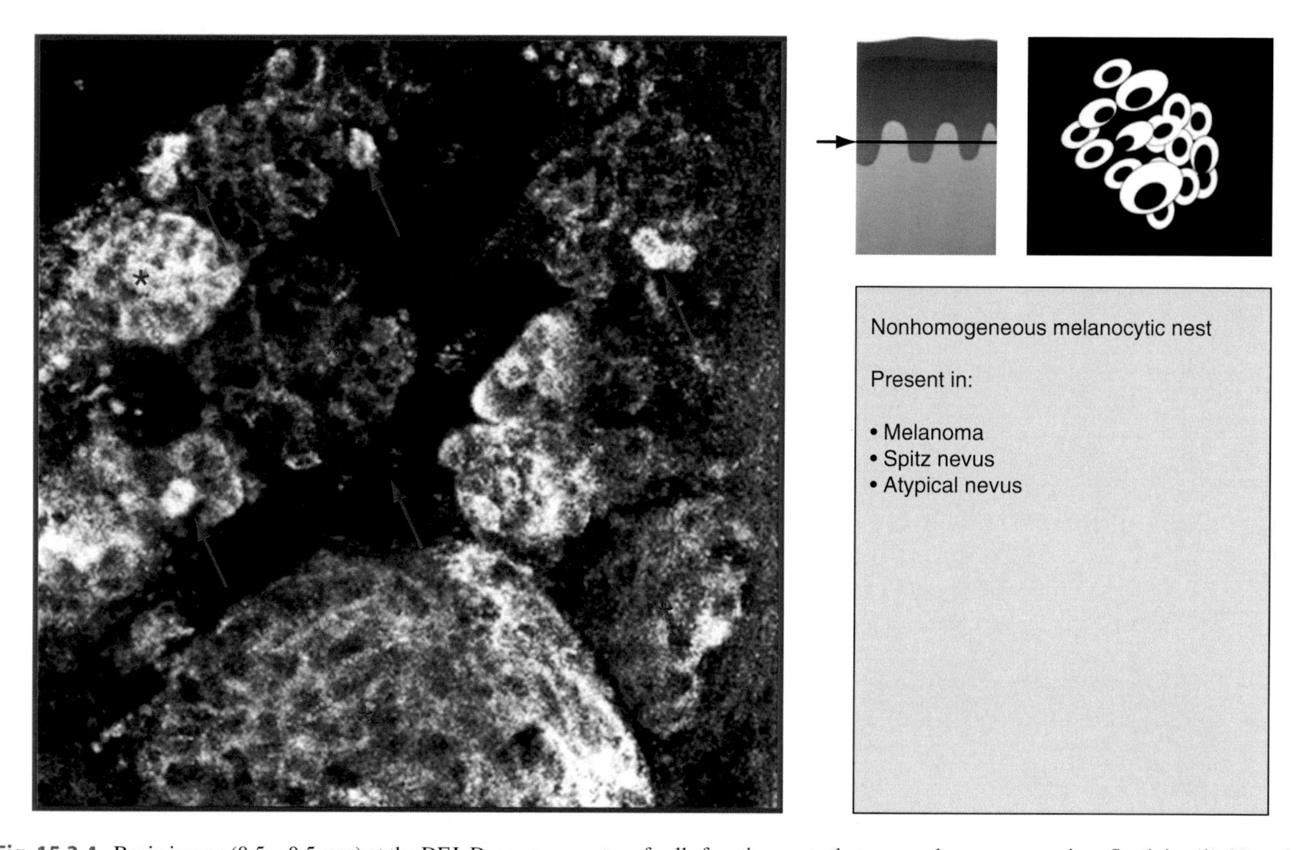

Fig. 15.3.4 Basic image (0.5 × 0.5 mm) at the DEJ. Dense aggregates of cells forming nests that are nonhomogeneous in reflectivity (*). Note the presence large atypical cells (→)

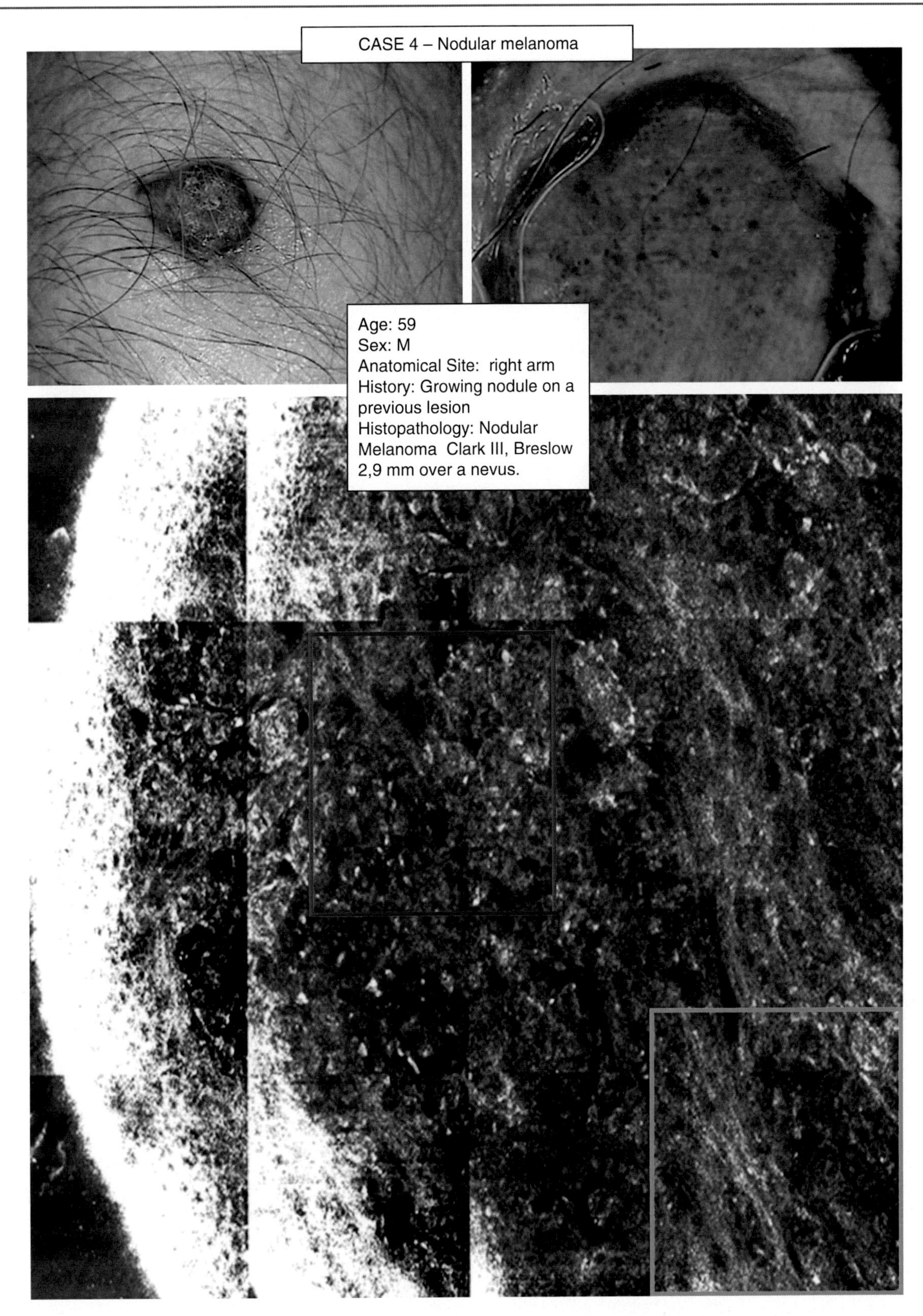

Fig. 15.4 RCM mosaic (1.9 × 1.4 mm). Nodular lesion in which different skin layers are represented. Honeycombed pattern at the periphery of the image corresponding to epidermal layers. In the center we can observe amorphous hypo-reflective cellular aggregates associated to focal dense nests and fibrous collagen tracts. Note the presence of isolated bright cells throughout the lesion

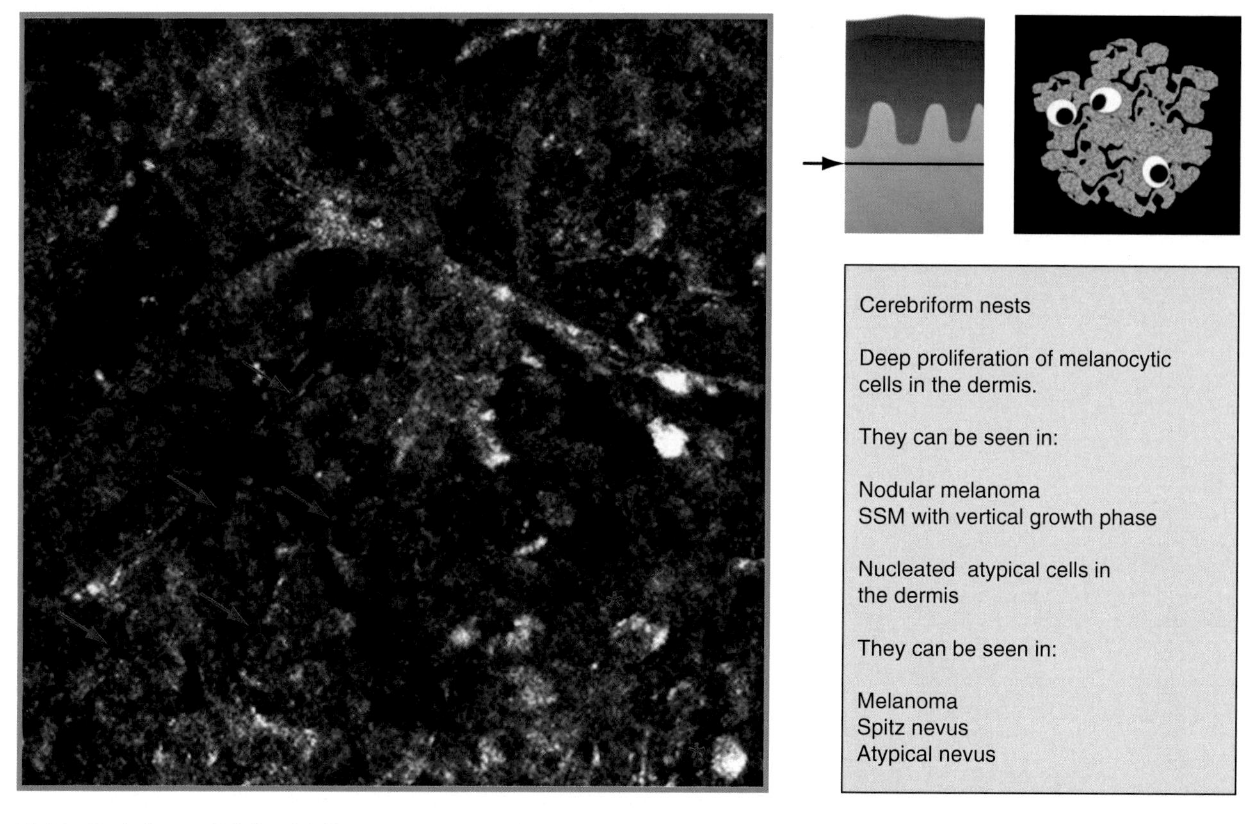

Fig. 15.4.1 Basic image (0.350 × 0.350 mm) at upper dermis. Amorphous, hypo-reflective nests (→) associated to nucleated atypical cells (*)

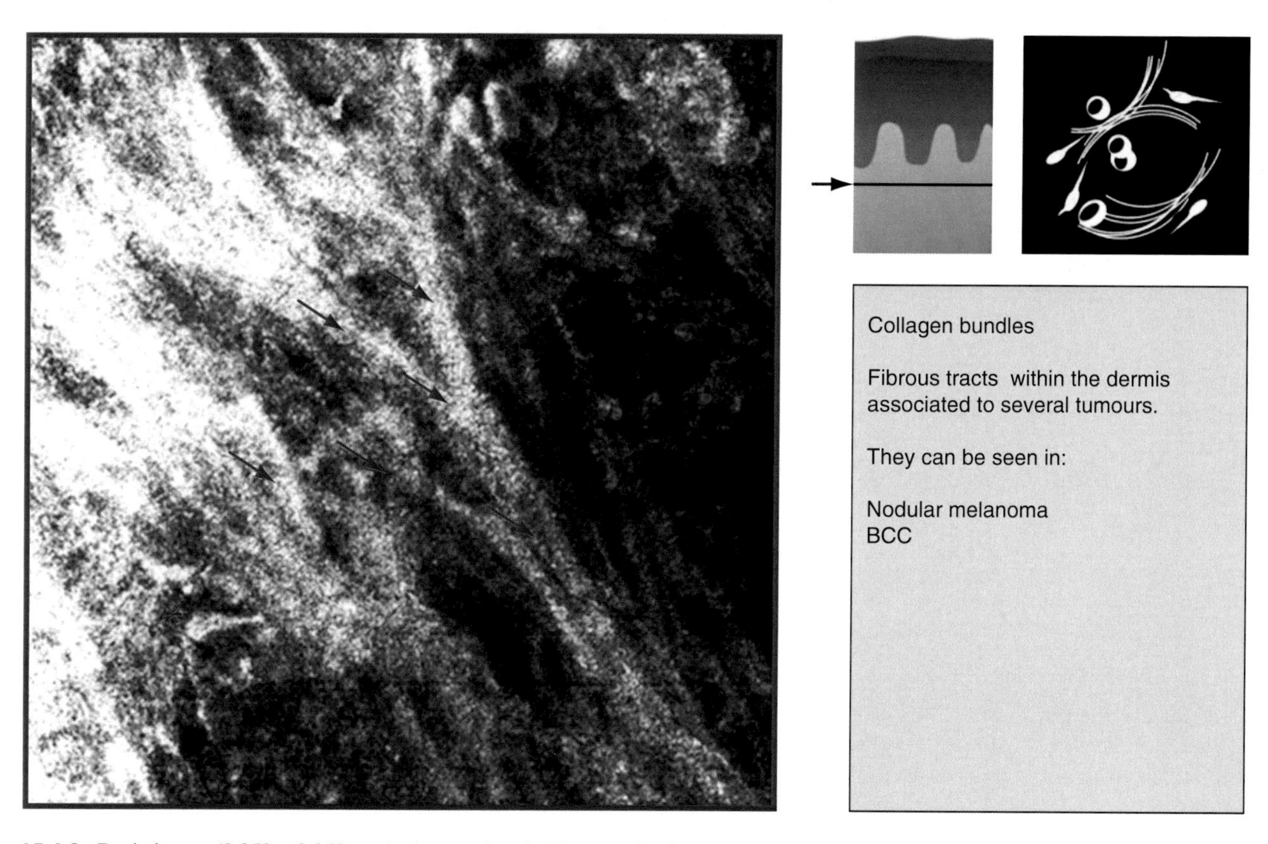

Fig. 15.4.2 Basic image (0.350 × 0.350 mm) at upper dermis. Hyper-reflective tracts within the dermis (→) associated to some spindle cells (*)

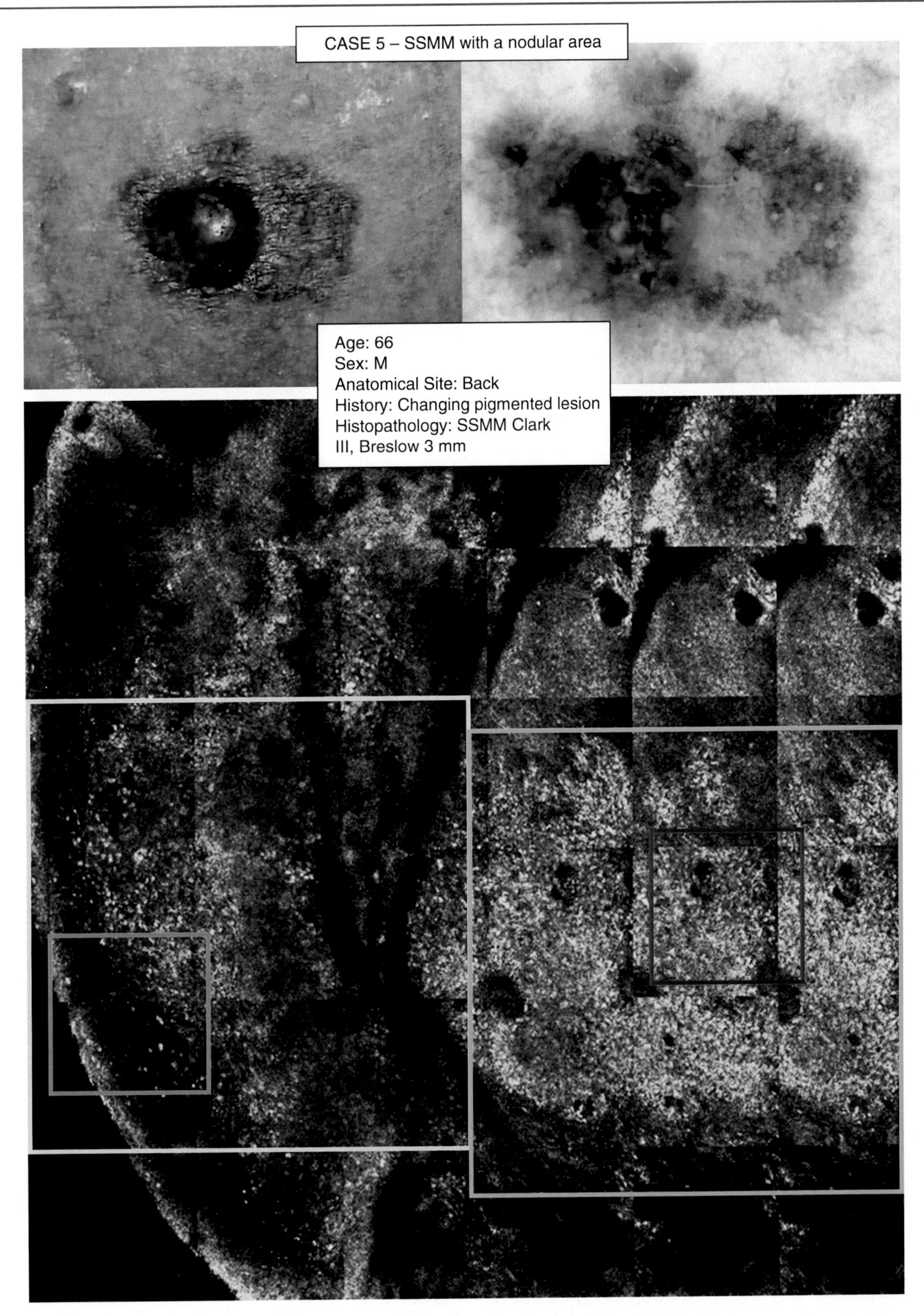

Fig. 15.5 RCM mosaic (3 × 3 mm). Scan image of the more pigmented and nodular part of the lesion. On the left central part we have a representation of suprabasal layers where we can observe a disarranged pattern with intraepidermal round cells. The right central part of the mosaic corresponds to DEJ where we observe nonaggregated cells forming sheet-like structures

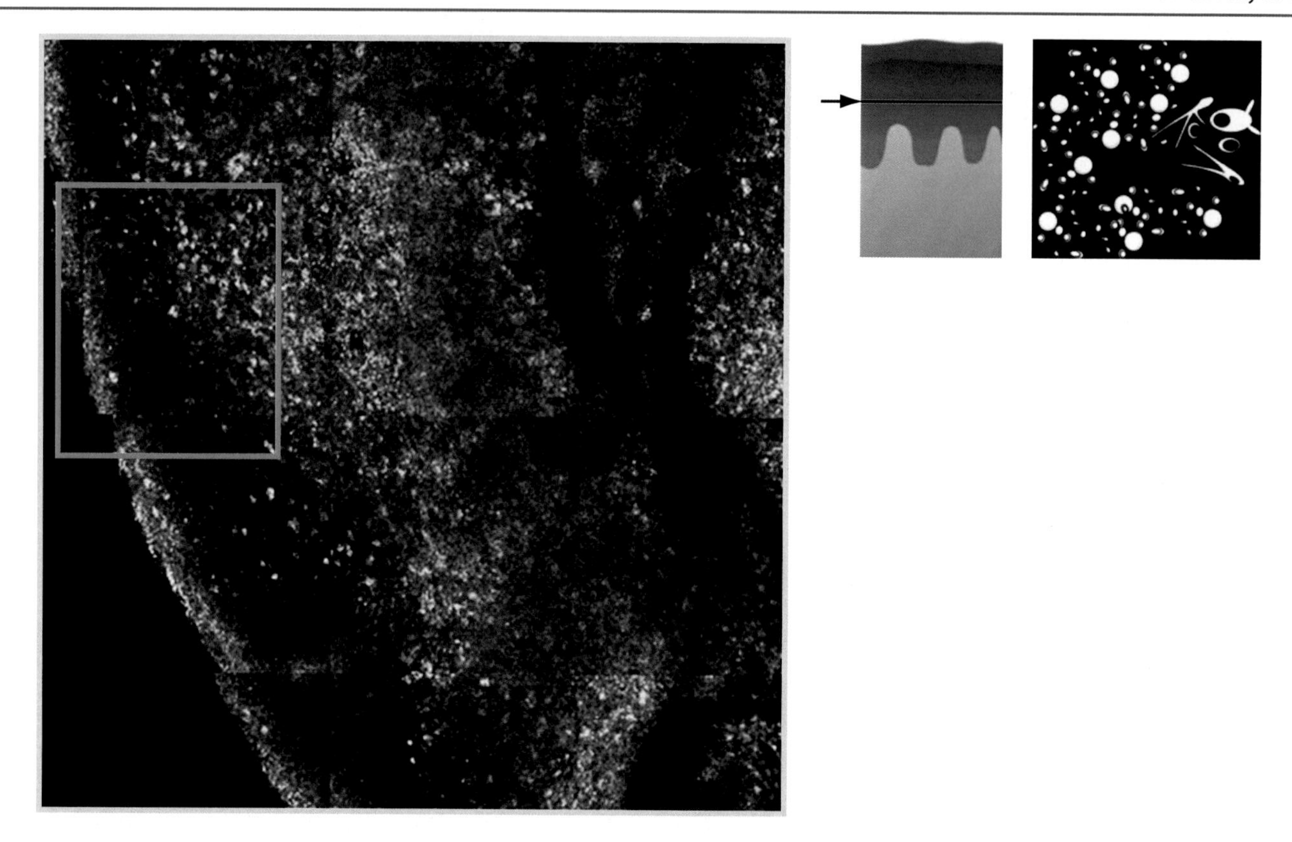

Fig. 15.5.1 RCM mosaic (1.5 × 1.5 mm) at spinous layer. Absence of honeycombed pattern at suprabasal layers, exhibiting disarrangement and presence of pagetoid spreading

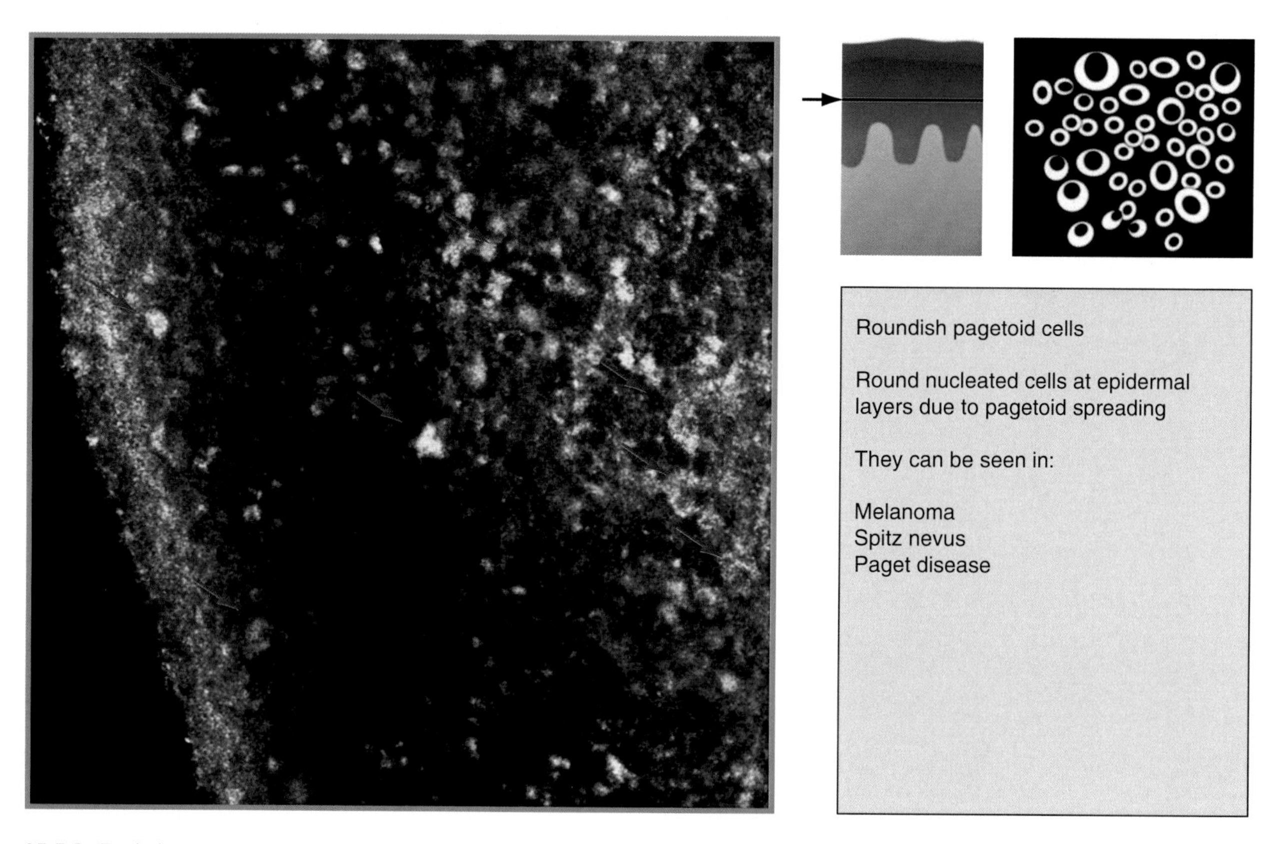

Fig. 15.5.2 Basic image (0.5 × 0.5 mm) at spinous layer. Disarranged epidermal pattern with roundish pagetoid cells (→)

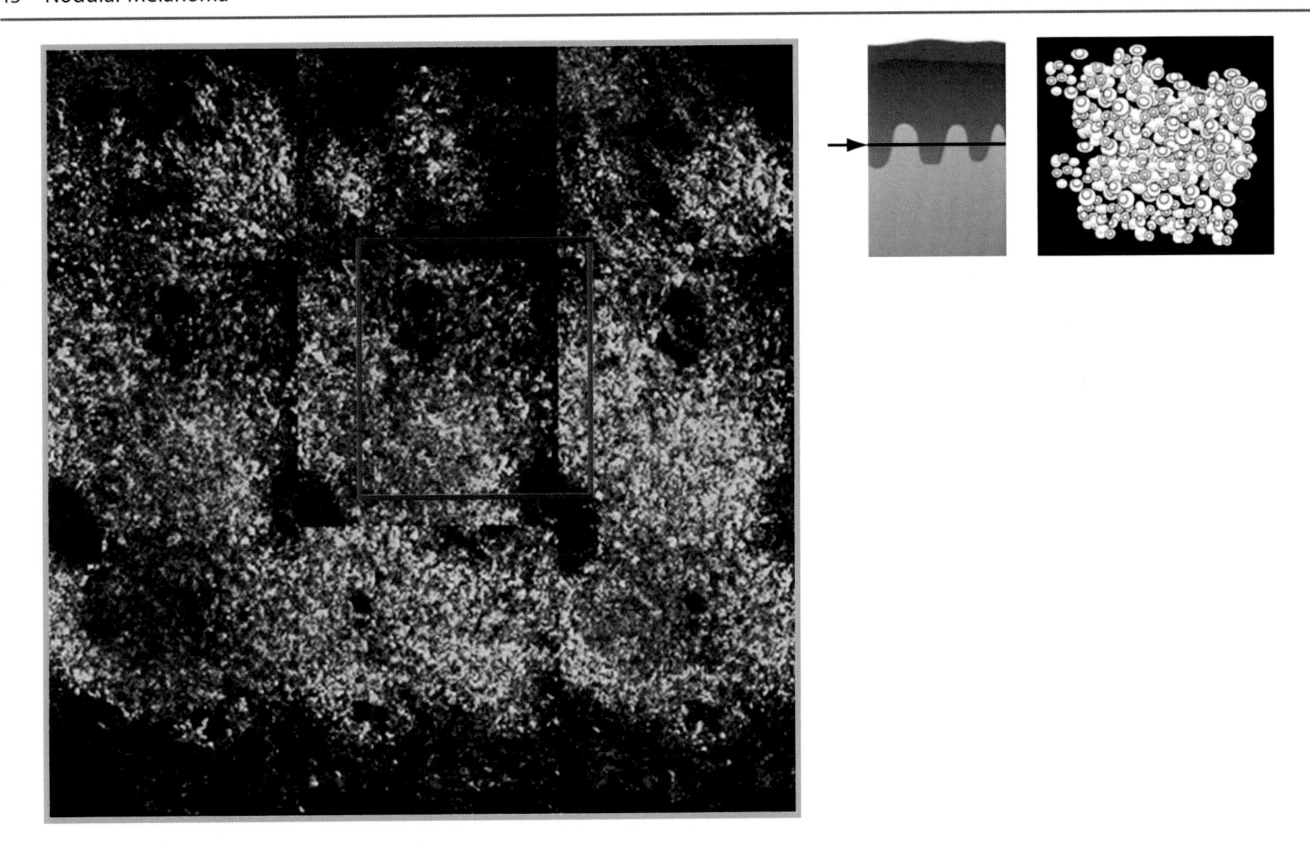

Fig. 15.5.3 RCM mosaic (1.5 × 1.5 mm) at DEJ showing a diffuse proliferation of nonaggregated reflective cells distributed in a sheet-like manner

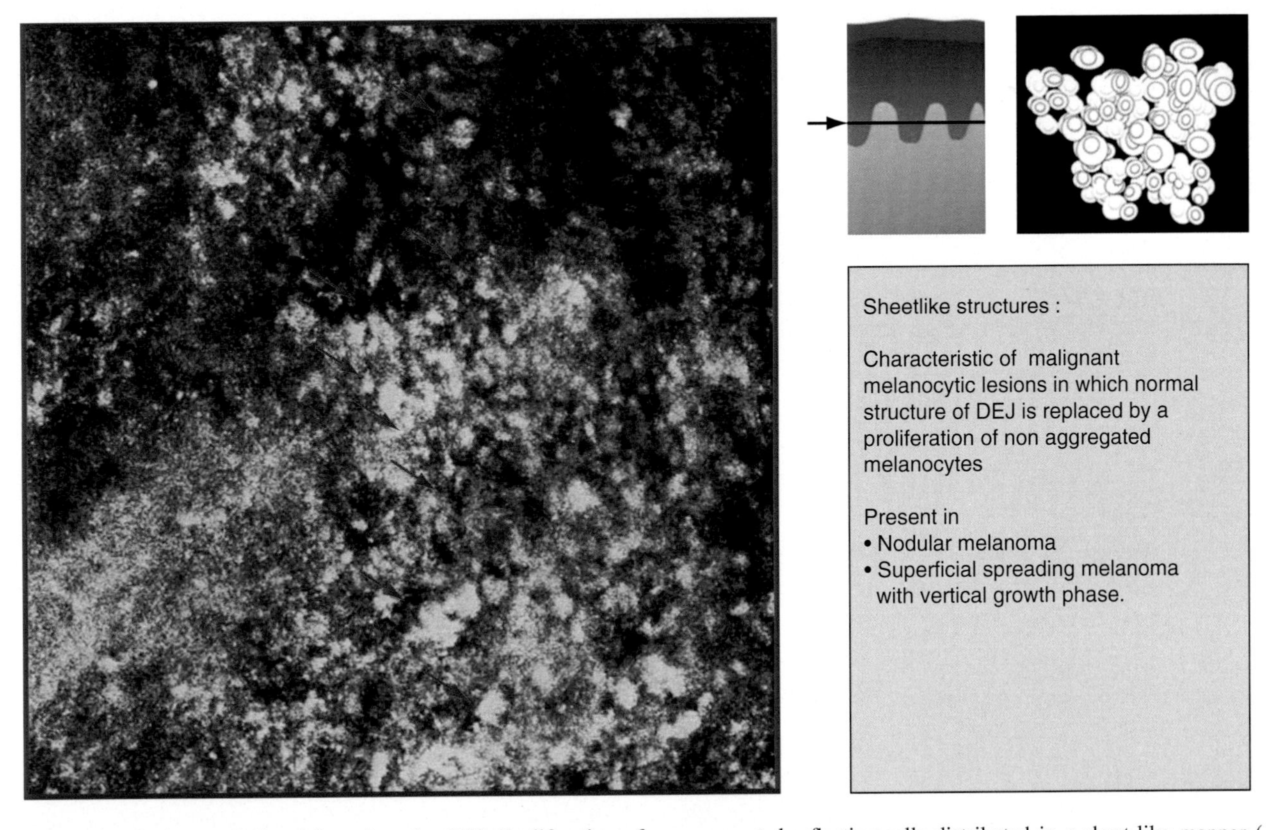

Fig. 15.5.4 Basic image (0.5 × 0.5 mm) at the DEJ. Proliferation of nonaggregated reflective cells distributed in a sheet-like manner (→) corresponding to malignant melanocytes and probably macrophages

References

1. Chang AE, Karnell LH, Menck HR (1998) The National Cancer Data Base report on cutaneous and noncutaneous melanoma: a summary of 84,836 cases from the past decade. The American College of Surgeons Commission on Cancer and the American Cancer Society. Cancer 83:1664–1678
2. Demierre MF, Chung C, Miller DR, Geller AC (2005) Early detection of thick melanomas in the United States: beware of the nodular subtype. Arch Dermatol 141:745–750
3. Clark WH Jr, From L, Bernardino EA, Mihm MC (1969) The histogenesis and biologic behaviour of primary human malignant melanomas of the skin. Cancer Res 29:705–727
4. Poetsch M, Dittberner T, Woenckhaus C (2003) Can different genetic changes characterize histogenetic subtypes and biologic behaviour in sporadic malignant melanoma of the skin? Cell Mol Life Sci 60:1923–1932
5. Curtin JA, Fridlyand J, Kageshita T et al (2005) Distinct sets of genetic alterations in melanoma. N Engl J Med 353:2135–2147
6. Richard MA, Grob JJ, Avril MF et al (2000) Delays in diagnosis and melanoma prognosis, II: the role of doctors. Int J Cancer 89:280–285
7. Brochez L, Verhaeghe E, Bleyen L, Naeyaert JM (2001) Diagnostic ability of general practitioners and dermatologists in discriminating pigmented skin lesions. J Am Acad Dermatol 44:979–986
8. Chamberlain AJ, Fritschi L, Kelly JW (2003) Nodular melanoma: patients' perceptions of presenting features and implications for earlier detection. J Am Acad Dermatol 48:694–701
9. Pizzichetta MA, Talamini R, Stanganelli I et al (2004) Amelanotic/hypomelanotic melanoma: clinical and dermoscopic features. Br J Dermatol 150:1117–1124
10. Rajadhyasksha M, González S, Zavislan JM, Anderson RR, Webb RH (1999) In vivo confocal scanning laser microscopy of human skin II: advances in instrumentation and comparison with histology. J Invest Dermatol 113:293–303
11. Segura S, Pellacani G, Puig S, Longo C, Bassoli S, Guitera P, Palou J, Menzies S, Seidenari S, Malvehy J (2008) In vivo microscopic features of nodular melanomas: dermoscopy, confocal microscopy, and histopathologic correlates. Arch Dermatol 144(10):1311–1320

Lentigo Maligna

16

Pascale Guitera

16.1 Introduction

Lentigo maligna (LM) is a frequent diagnostic challenge for clinicians because it occurs on exposed sun-damaged skin (often the face) of elderly people with diverse pigmentation types [1]. It is also a challenge for pathologists, as there is often great heterogeneity in the histopathologic features of LM in different parts of the lesion [2] and, in the early stages, it may be difficult to differentiate LM from melanocytic hyperplasia in sun-damaged skin [3–5]. LM also represents a therapeutic challenge because of its usual large size and face location. The recurrences are estimated to be between 8 and 31% after conventional surgery [6–8]. It can spread far beyond the visible margins [8]. In vivo reflectance confocal microscopy (RCM) provides a horizontal view (8 × 8 mm), so it is possible to assess more of the lesion using this technique compared with pathologic assessment of vertically orientated small biopsy specimens (even with step sectioning).

16.2 RCM Features

Preliminary reports showed that RCM can be used to differentiate LM from other pigmentations of the face [9–11] and can assist in defining peripheral margins of LM [12], even amelanotic tumors [13].

Recently, RCM features that can distinguish LM from benign macules (BM) of the face, such as solar lentigo, ephelis, actinic keratosis and flat seborrhoeic keratosis, have been determined and different algorithms have been tested for diagnosing LM on a large series of 110 LM and 247 BM of the face [14].

Epidermal features

- Epidermal disarray (Figs. 16.1.2, 16.2.2, 16.3.2, 16.4.2) was frequently observed in LM (56%), although it was also present in 18% of BM of the face. On the contrary, a regular honeycombed pattern was strongly correlated to BM (92%). Of note, a broadened honeycomb was more frequently observed in BM of the face (16%) – and in particular actinic keratoses and seborrheic keratoses.
- Pagetoid infiltration (Figs. 16.1.2, 16.2.2, 16.3.2, 16.4.2) was reported in 75% of LM and 28% of BM of the face. This high level of pagetoid cells seen in BM maybe explained by melanocytic hyperplasia and/or hyperpigmented keratinocytes, interpreted under confocal microscopy as small pagetoid cells. Therefore, to be "significant", pagetoid cells have to be:
  - round (dendritic ones are often seen in actinic keratosis and inflammatory lesions),
  - large (>20 μm), and
  - numerous.

At the dermo-epidermal junction level

- Nonedged papillae (dermal papillae without a demarcated rim of bright cells, but separated by a series of large reflecting cells) were observed in 68% of LM and in 17% of BM of the face.
  Of note, although highly significant, nonedged papillae are difficult to assess [15], particularly on the face where "non visible" papillae are a common and pathologically well-known feature. To clarify:
  - when the papillae are "non visible" (Figs. 16.1, 16.3, 16.4), the confocal field of view contains – without transition – epidermal feature (like honeycomb) and dermal feature (collagen bundles).
  - when the papillae are "edged" (Fig. 16.3.1), there can be with a ring of pigmented cells (phototype skin >2) or a distinct hole (phototype I and II), but the edge itself is well demarcated.
  - when the papillae are "non-edged" (Figs. 16.1.4 and 16.2.1), they are distorted by atypical reflective cells.

P. Guitera
Melanoma Institute Australia, North Sydney, Australia

Discipline of Dermatology, Sydney University
Syndey Melanoma Diagnostic Centre,
RPA, Sydney, Australia
e-mail: pascale.guitera@melanoma.org.au

R. Hofmann-Wellenhof et al. (eds.), *Reflectance Confocal Microscopy for Skin Diseases*,
DOI 10.1007/978-3-642-21997-9_16, © Springer-Verlag Berlin Heidelberg 2012

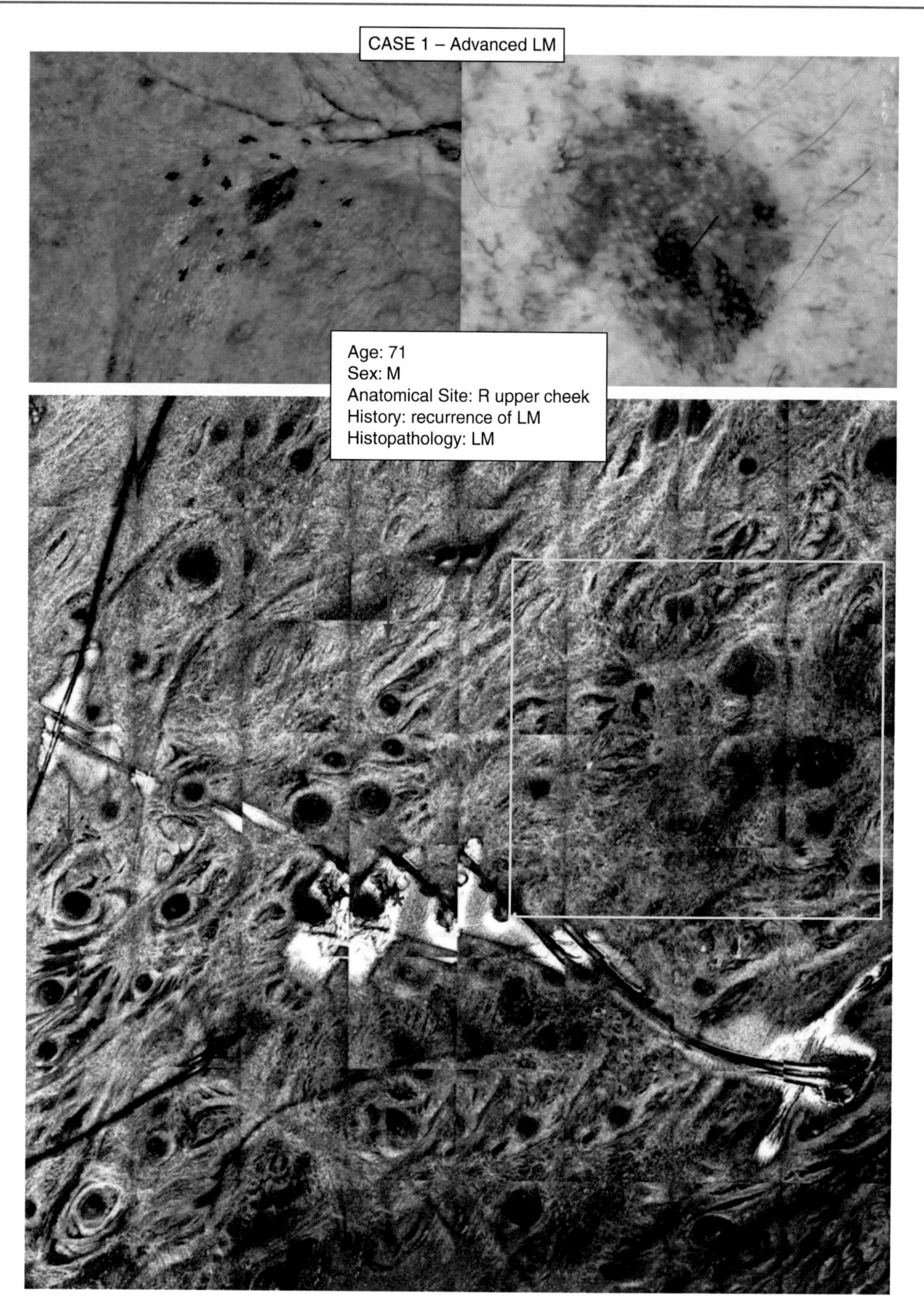

Fig. 16.1 RCM mosaic (4 × 4 mm) at the level of the DEJ reveals a variation of a meshwork pattern due to colonization of atypical cells around the hair and glandular openings with some junctional thickening (→). It corresponds to rhomboidal structures described in dermoscopy. The area marked by a star (*) is an artifact (air bubble)

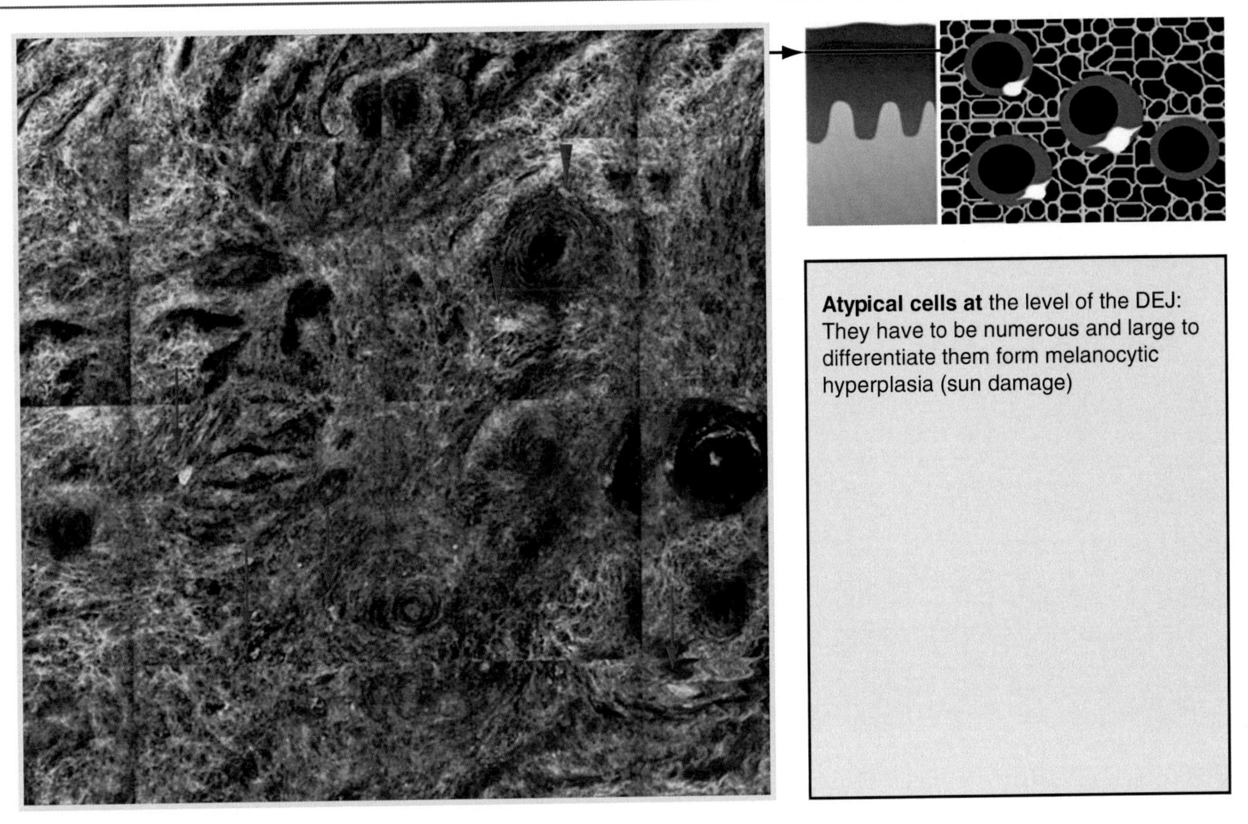

Fig. 16.1.1 RCM mosaic (1.5 × 1.5 mm) at the level of the DEJ reveals multiple atypical large cells (→), some of them are around the follicular opening (▲)

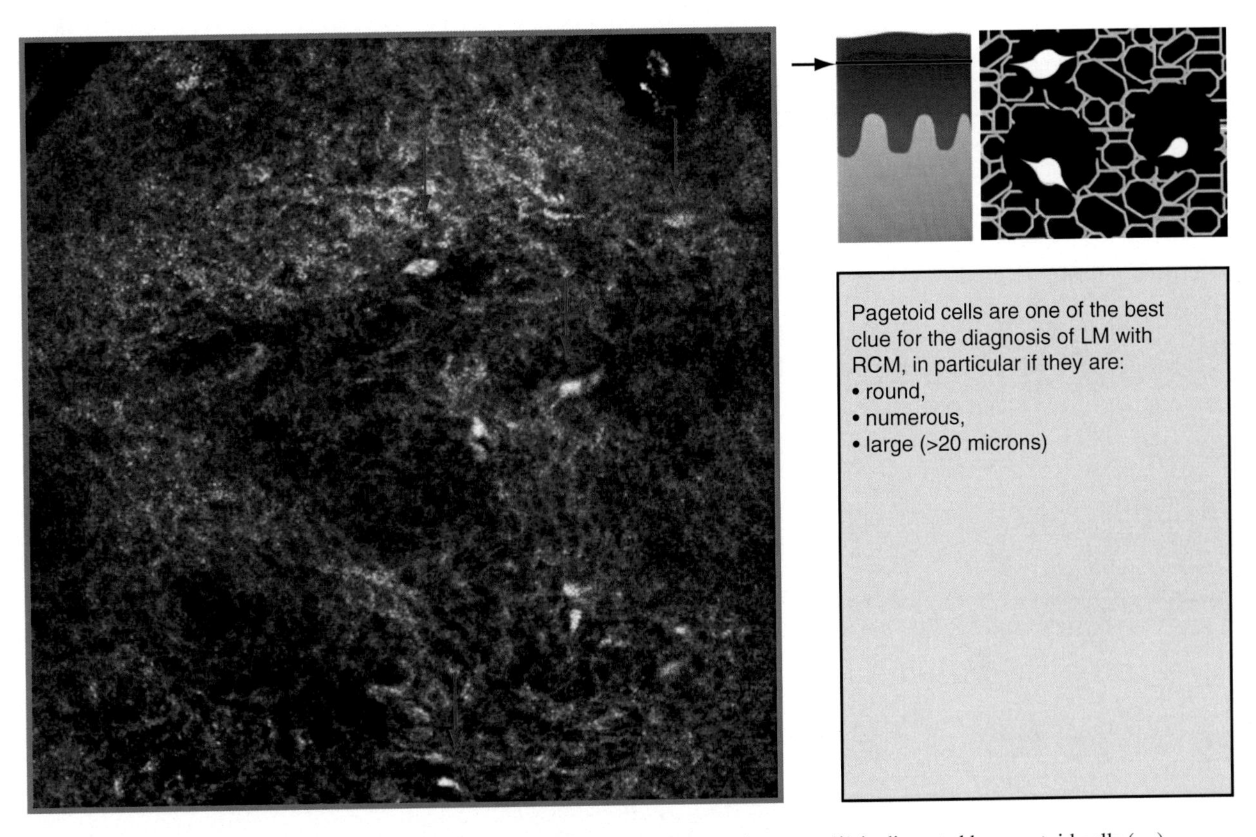

Fig. 16.1.2 Basic image (0.5 × 0.5 mm) at the epidermis level where the honeycomb pattern (*) is disrupted by pagetoid cells (→)

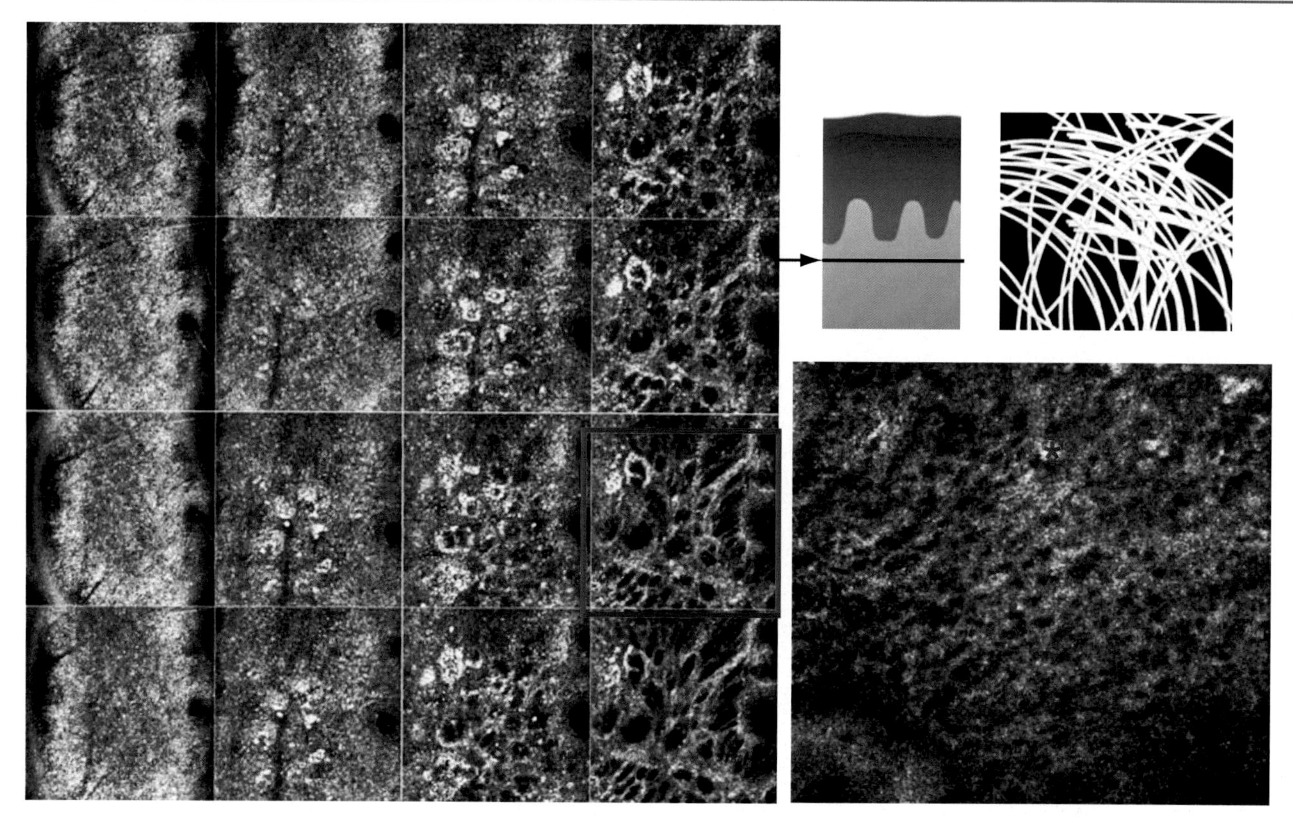

Fig. 16.1.3 RCM stack from the stratum corneum to the upper dermis. The epidermis layer is thin (45 μm) due to the face location and solar damaged. In the dermis, coarse refractive structures corresponding solar elastosis are seen (*)

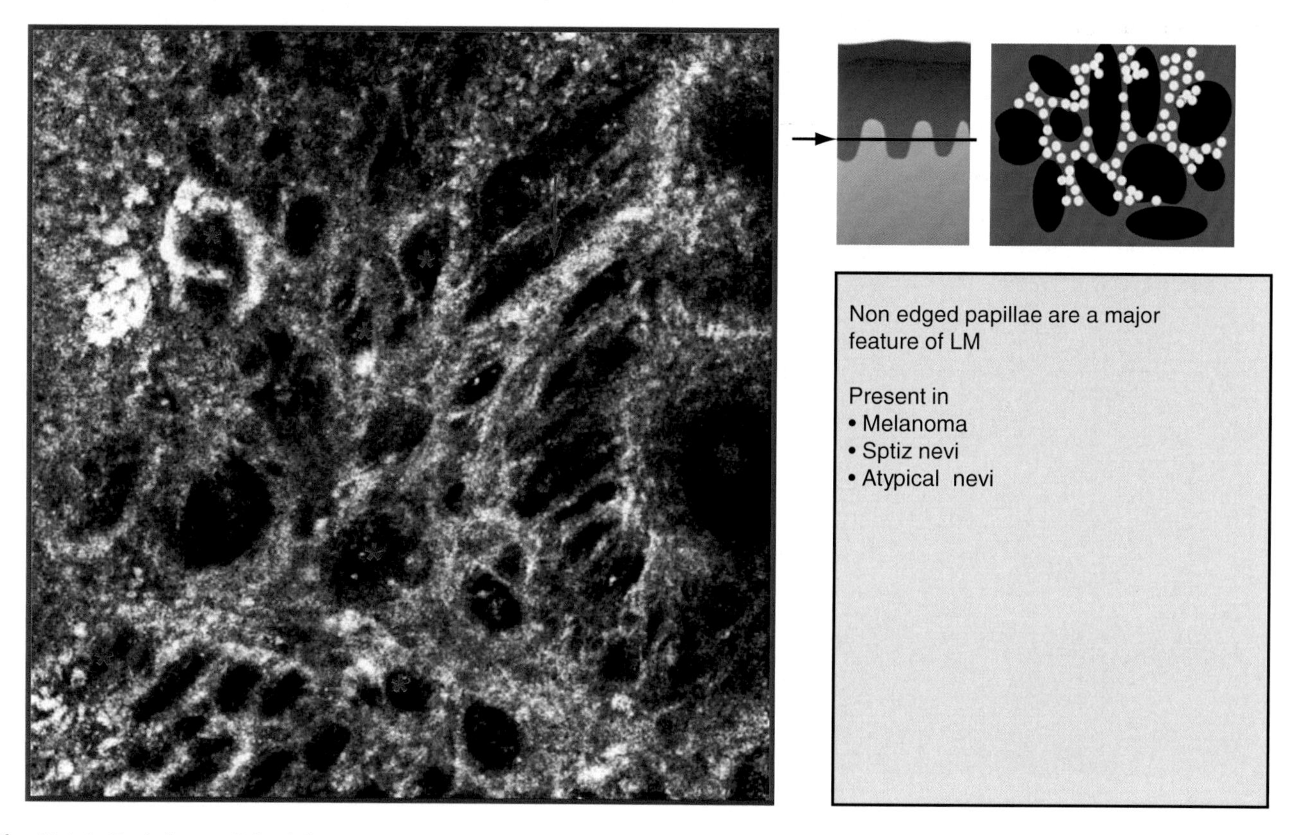

Fig. 16.1.4 Basic image (0.5 × 0.5 mm) shows nonedged papillae (*) distorted by atypical reflective cells. Junctional thickenings (→) are typical of more advanced LM with rhomboidal structures

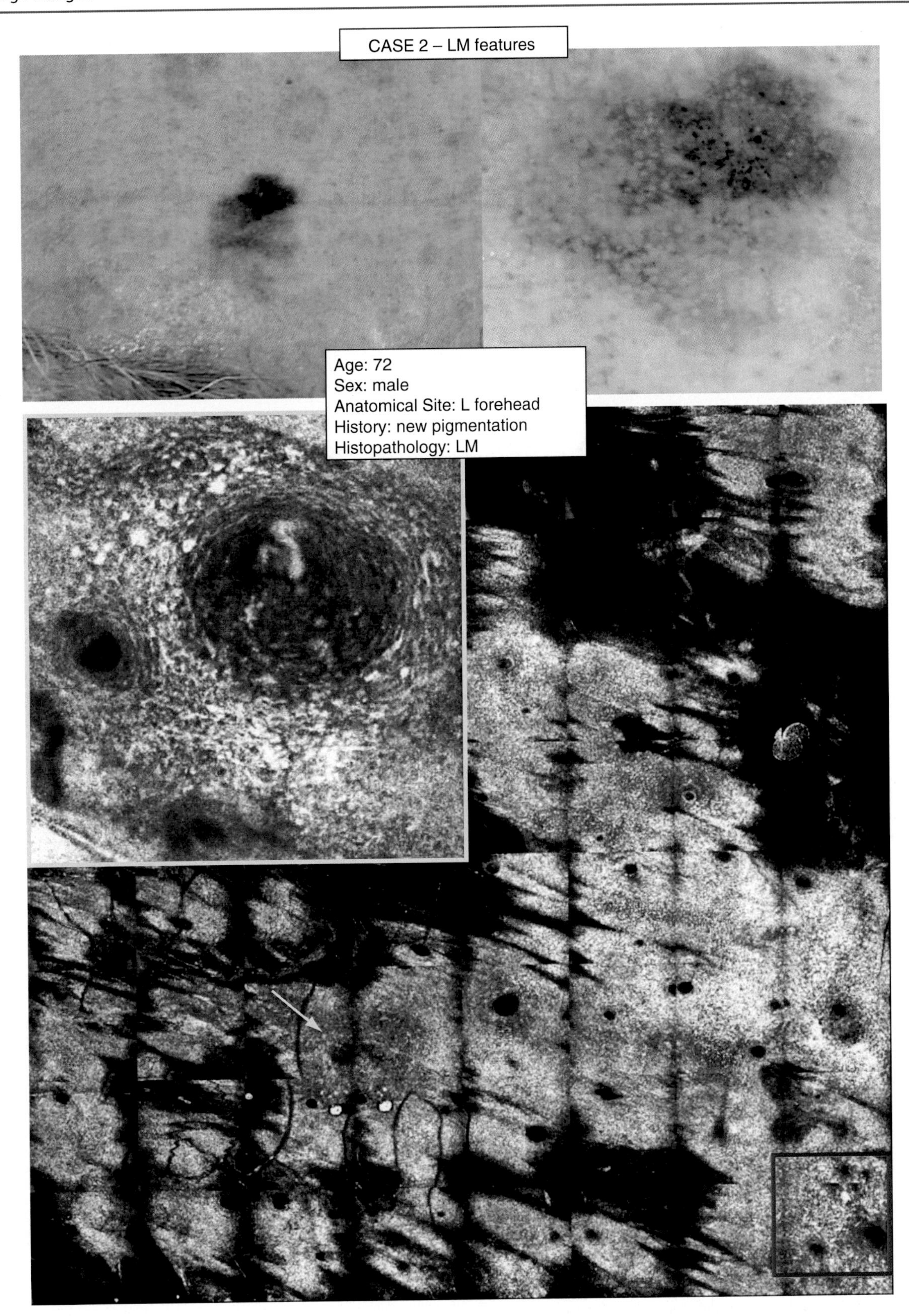

Fig. 16.2 RCM mosaic (4 × 4 mm) at the level of the DEJ showing less advanced features with involvement of atypical cells in the follicular opening (typically seen as asymmetric follicular opening in dermoscopy) – see *yellow square* with a basic image (0.5 × 0.5 mm)

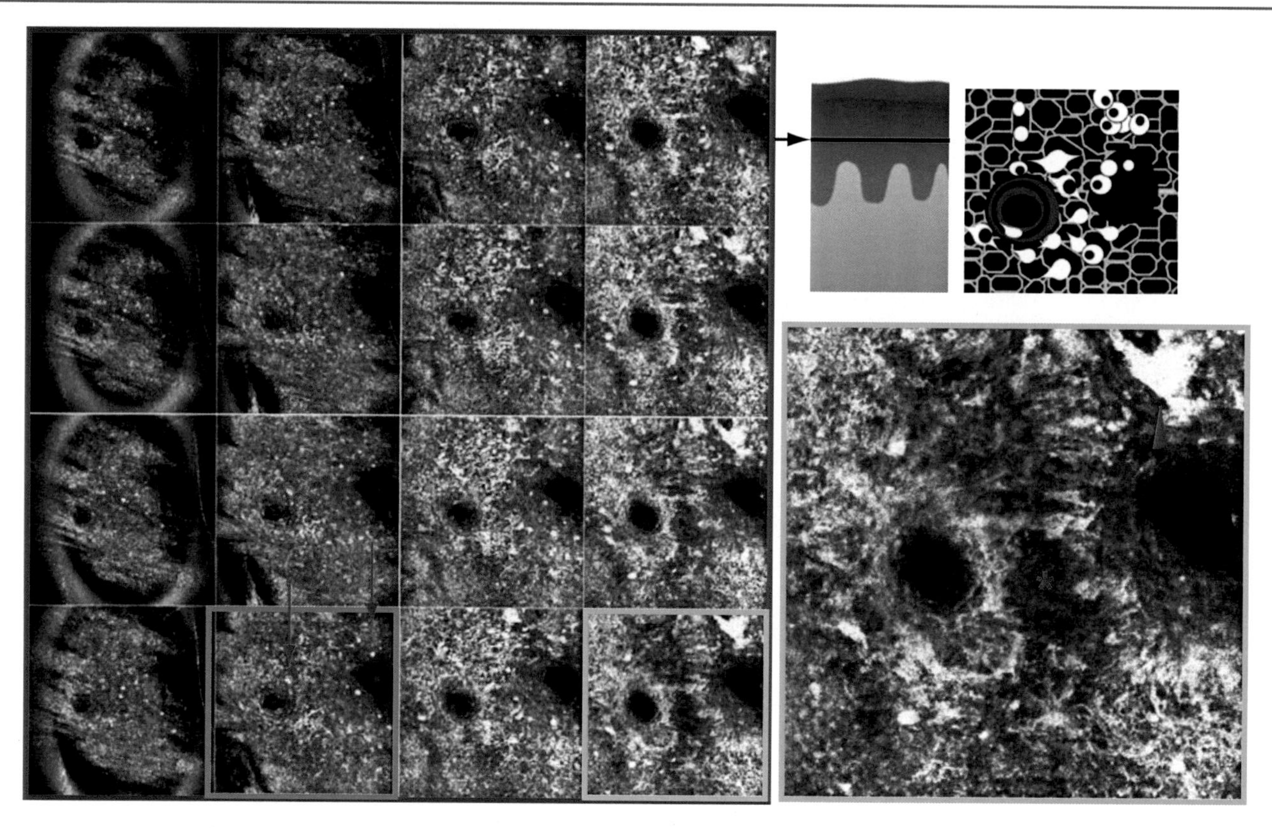

Fig. 16.2.1 RCM stack from the stratum corneum to DEJ layer showing pagetoid cells (→) in the epidermis layer (*blue square*) and then atypical cells even in small nests (▲) and nonedge papillae (*) at the junction (*green square*)

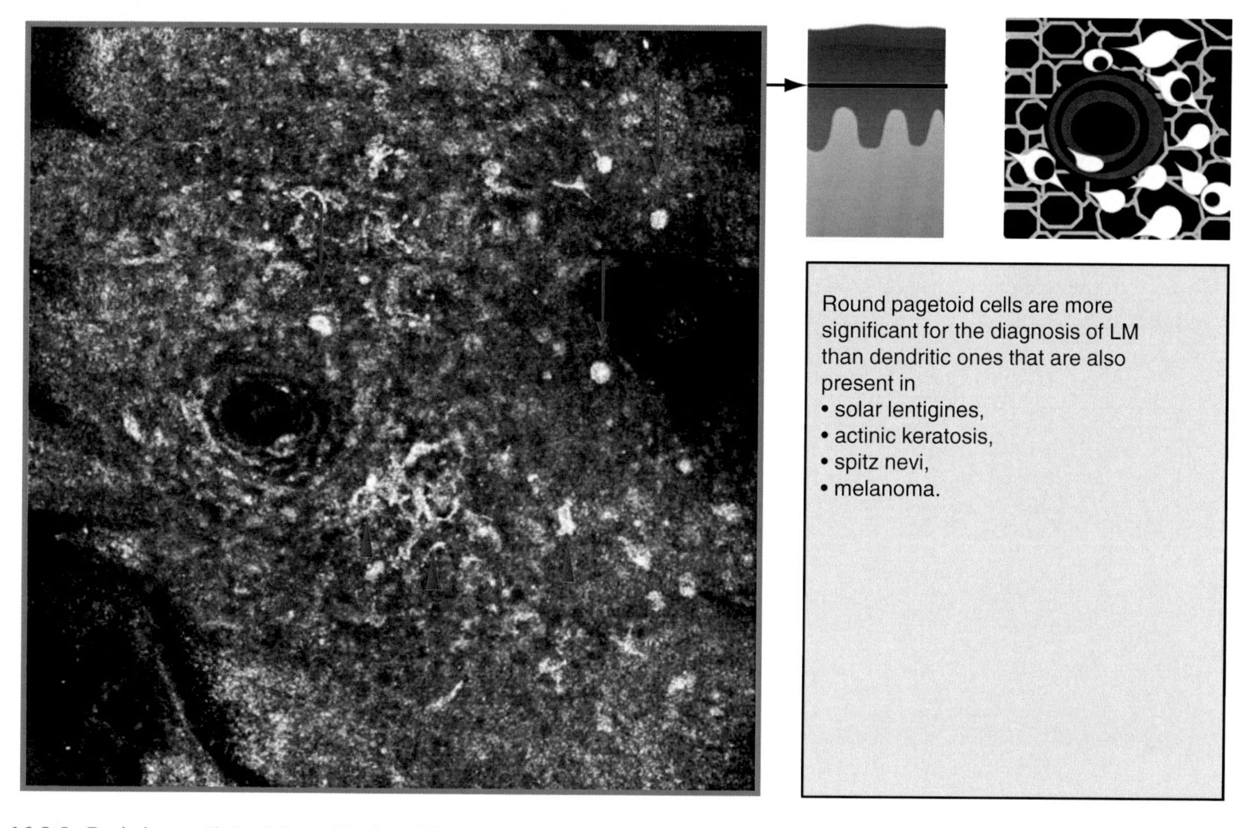

Fig. 16.2.2 Basic image (0.5 × 0.5 mm) in the epidermis with round (→) and dendritic pagetoid cells (▲) disrupting the normal epidermis

CASE 3 – Target biopsy
Age: 31
Sex: m
Anatomical Site: L cheek
History: solar lentigine (biopsied)
changing under monitoring
2nd Histopathology: LM

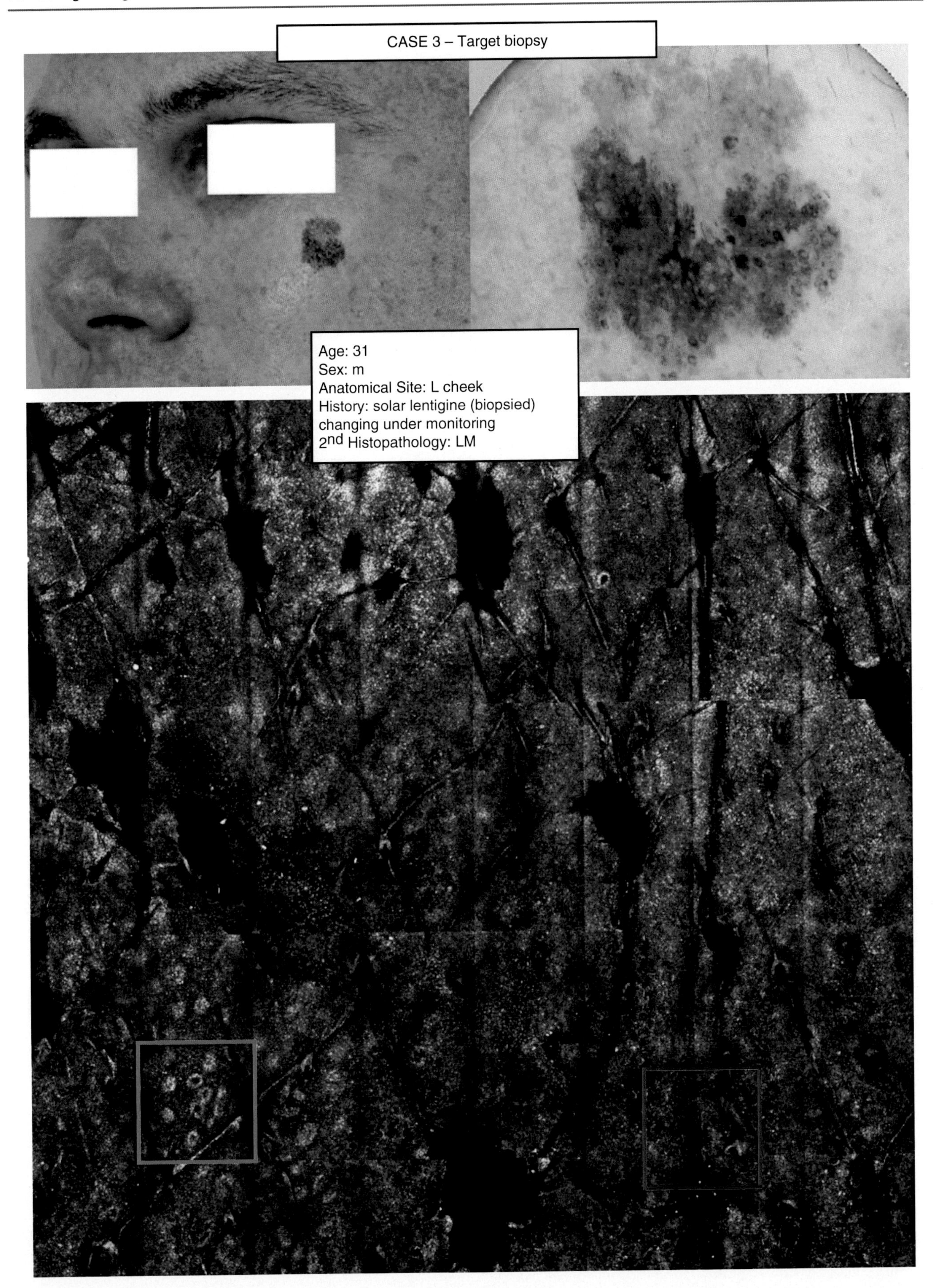

Fig. 16.3 RCM mosaic (4 × 4 mm) at the level of the DEJ showing two types of features – see *blue and red squares*

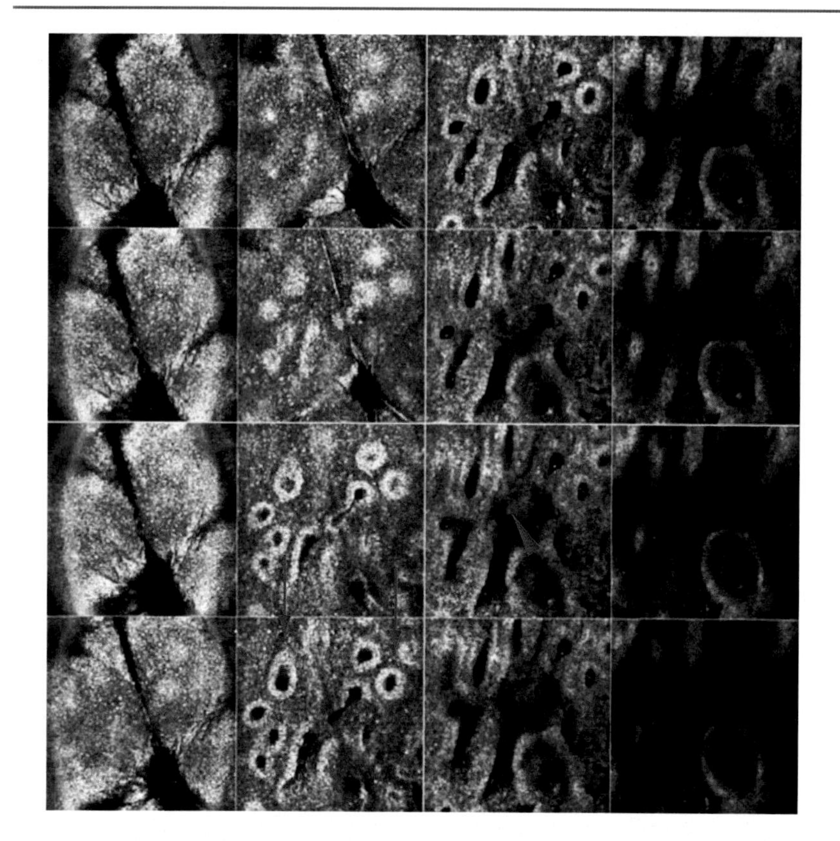

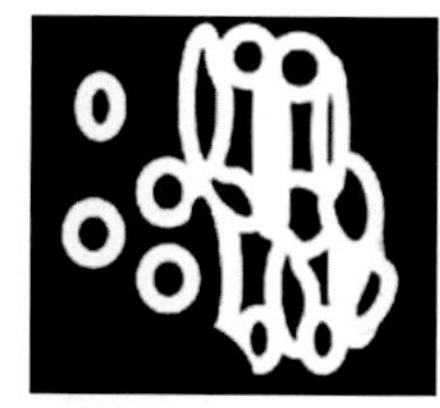

Benign pigmented macules of the face are typicaly with

- a regular honey comb or broadened honeycomb pattern in the epidermis
- monomorpheous, small, round cells at the junction following regular papillae
- No pigmented cells are seen in the dermis.

Fig. 16.3.1 RCM stack from the stratum corneum to the upper dermis layer showing lentiginous pigmented cells and edged papillae (→) at the junction. This feature is often found in solar lentigines and flat seborhereic keratosis (▲)

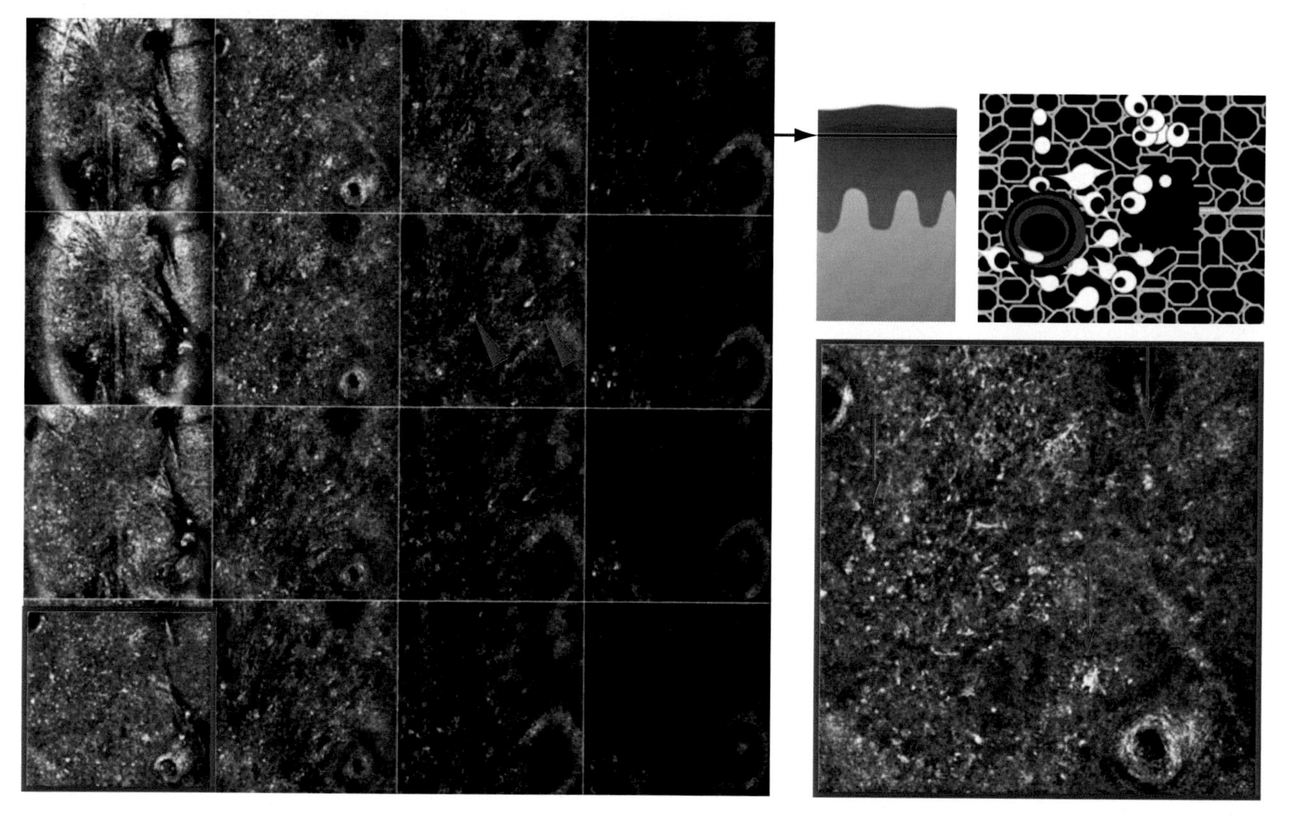

Fig. 16.3.2 RCM stack from the stratum corneum to the upper dermis layer showing pagetoid cells (→) and epidermal disarray at the epidermal layer (see basic image (0.5 × 0.5 mm) in the *red square*)) and atypical cells at the junction (▲). When targeted on this area the diagnosis was changed to LM

CASE 4 – Define the area to treat
Age: 51
Sex: male
Anatomical Site: L cheek
History: new pigmentation
Histopathology: LM

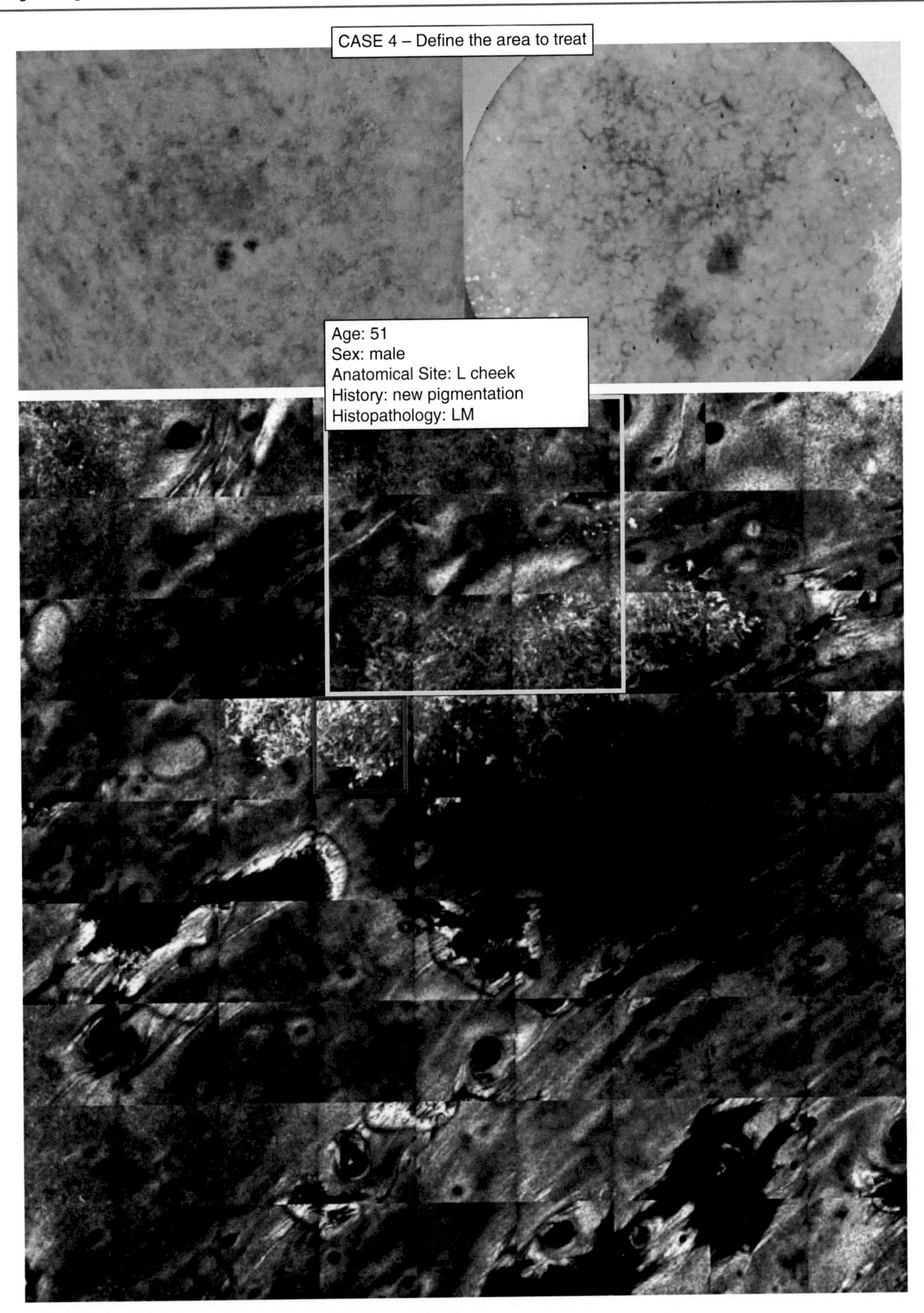

Fig. 16.4 RCM mosaic (4 × 4 mm) at the level of the DEJ showing some atypical reflective cells. Note the absence of visible papillae that is a frequent feature of face lesions

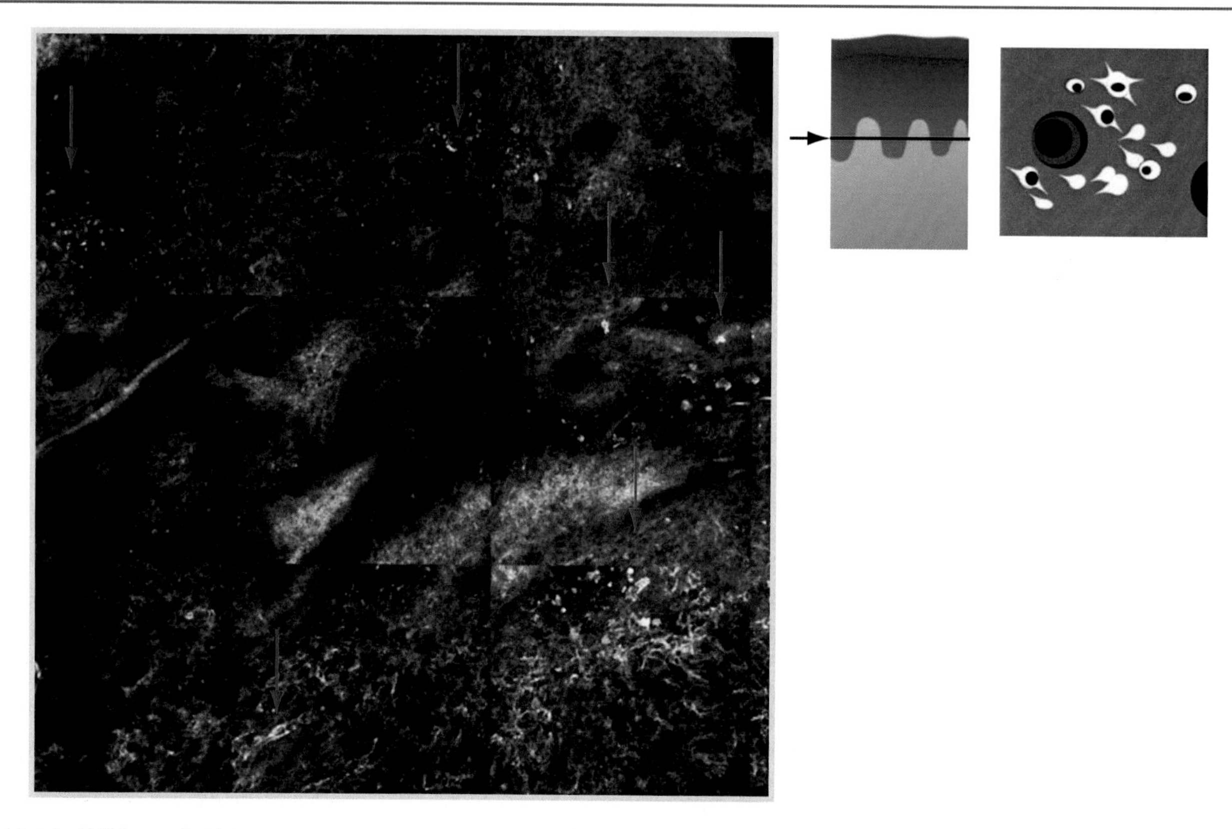

Fig. 16.4.1 RCM mosaic (1.4 × 1.4 mm) at the level of the DEJ with multiple atypical reflective cells

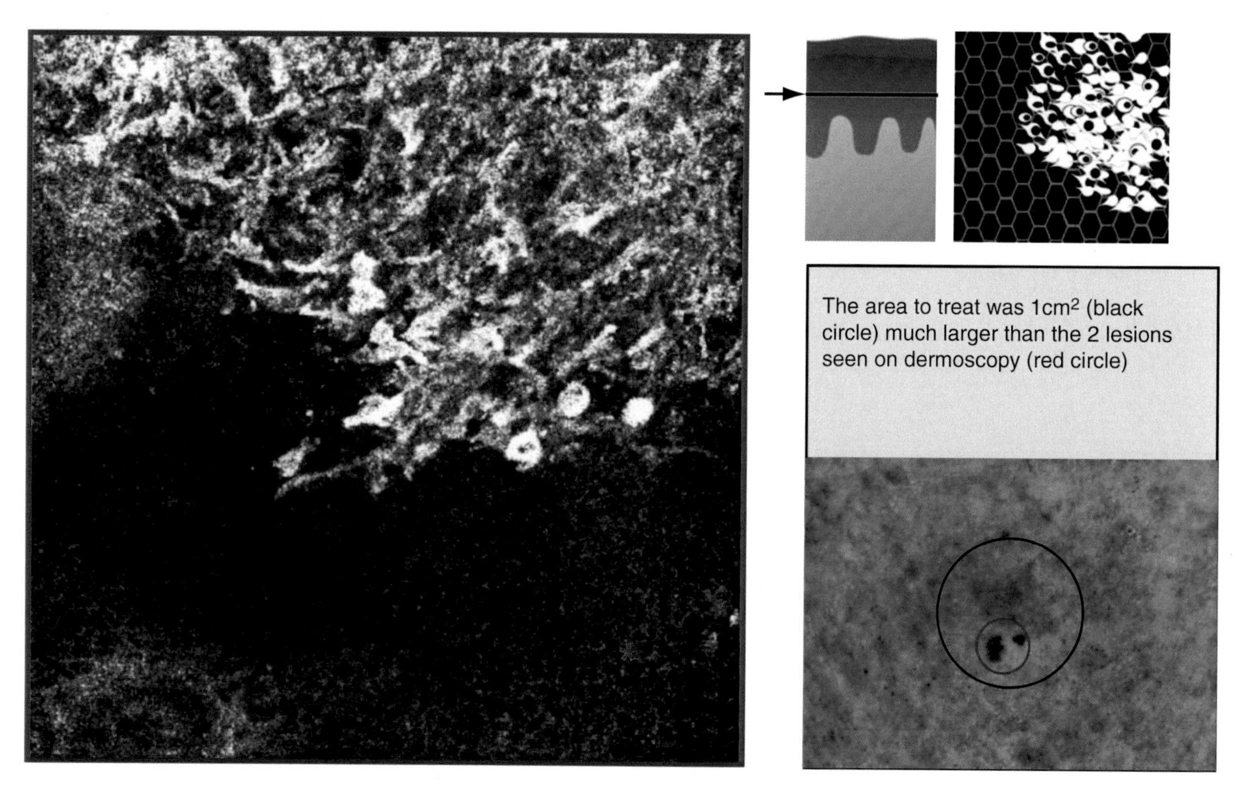

Fig. 16.4.2 Basic image (0.5 × 0.5 mm) of pagetoid cells disrupting the normal epidermis (*)

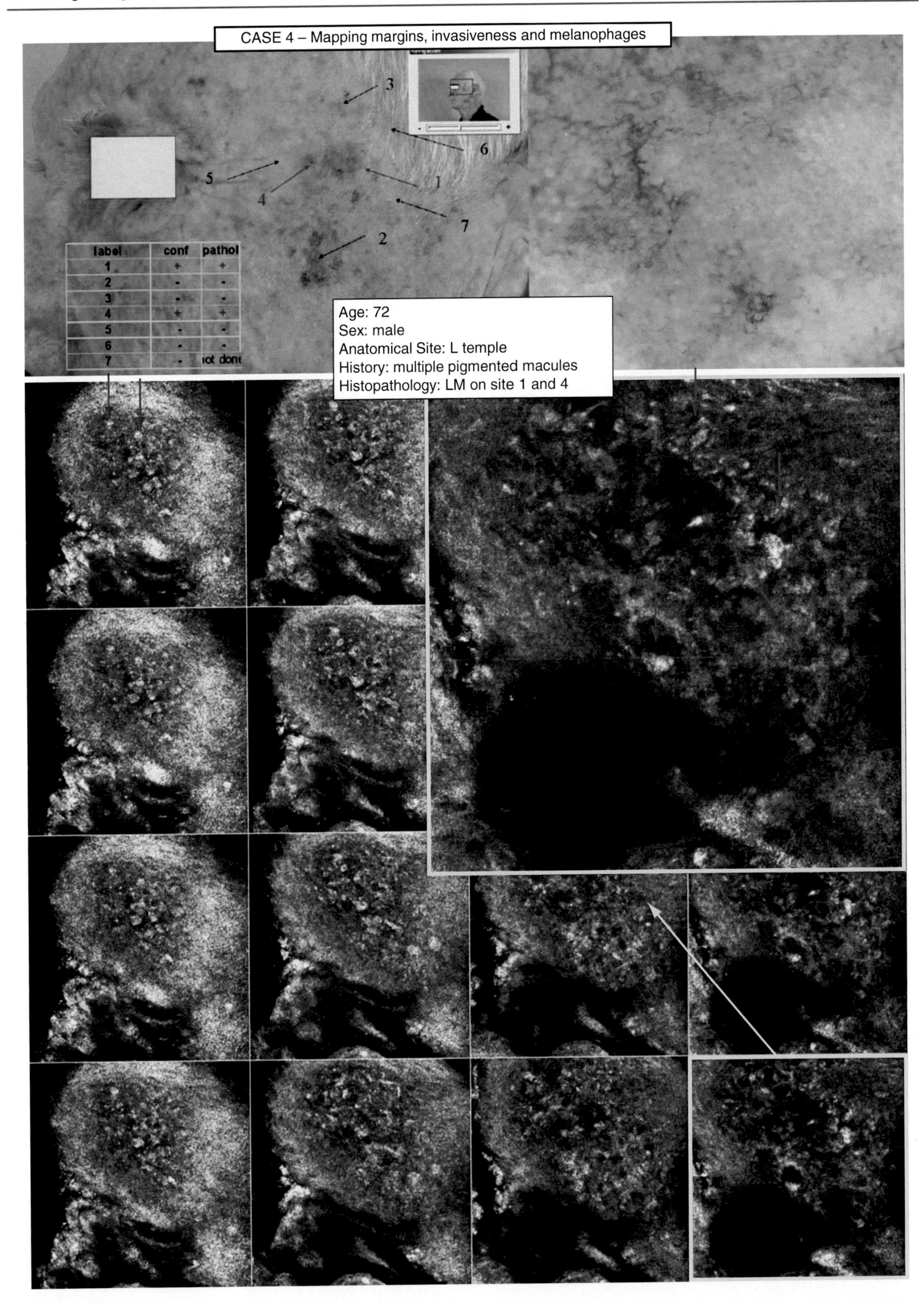

Fig. 16.5 RCM stack RCM stack from the stratum corneum to the upper dermis layer showing atypical cells (→) throughout the lesions. *Yellow square* at the DEJ

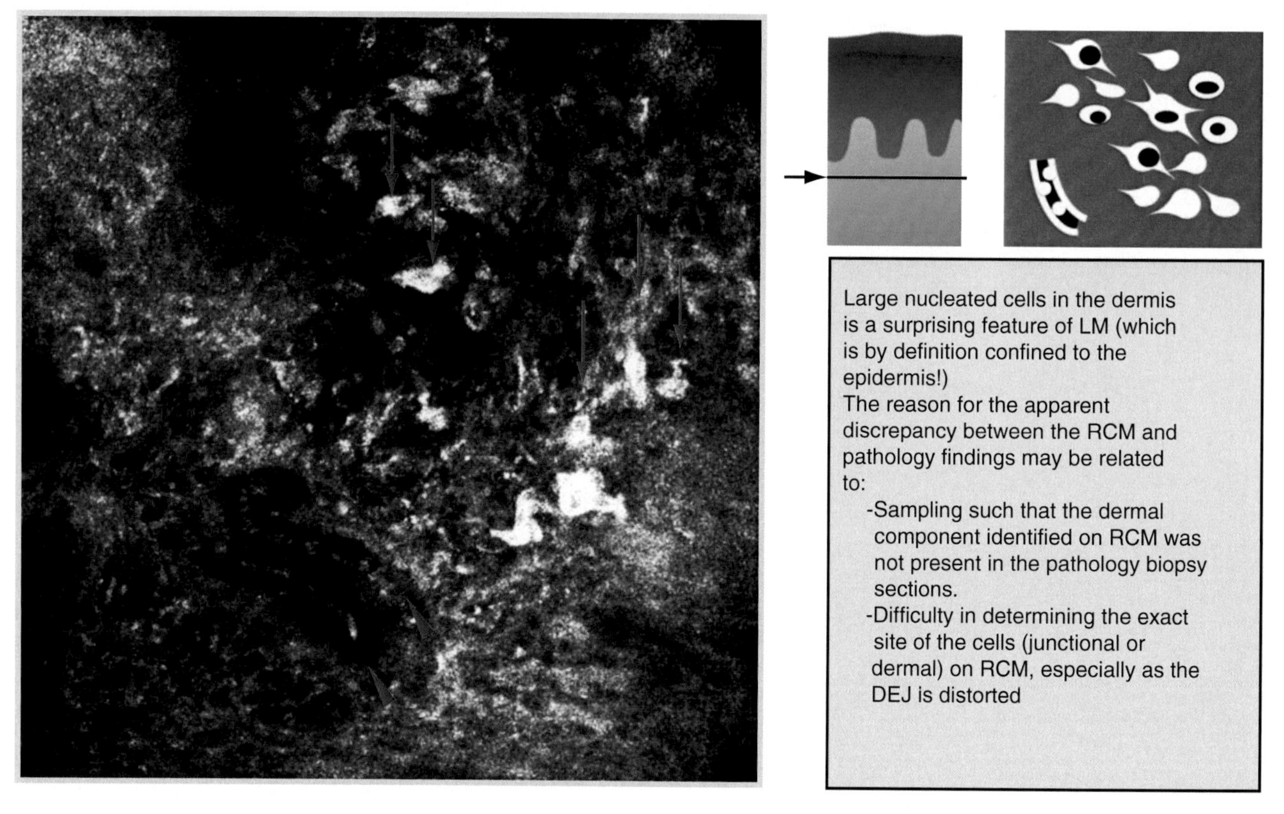

Fig. 16.5.1 Basic image (0.5 × 0.5 mm) in the upper dermis with nucleated atypical cells (→). Note the vessels indicating the dermis layer and (▲) and we can wonder if this LM was in fact micro invasive (?)

Thus, the interpretation difficulties arise when the field of view is not actually horizontal and the "ring" of cells appear incomplete or when "non-edged" and "edged" are present in a different area (Fig. 16.3). Numerous follicular and glandular openings can also be confusing with papillae. It is important to investigate the lesion in all *x*, *y* and *z* planes until the diagnosis can be made confidently.

- Atypical cells at the junction (defined as reflective cells with size of more than twice the keratinocytes around and/or with irregular shapes) are one of the common features of LM (Figs. 16.1.1, 16.1.4, 16.2.1, 16.4.1, 16.5). They have to be numerous to be significant. In advanced LM, they can be organized in small nests (Fig. 16.2.1) and even create some junctional thickening or cord-like rete ridges (Figs. 16.1, 16.1.1, 16.3) corresponding to rhomboidal features under dermoscopy.
- Follicular localization of atypical cells in the epidermis and/or at the JED level was seen in 59% of LM. It is a well-known criterion in dermoscopy and the macro image can help target this area of interest (Fig. 16.2).

Dermal features

- Fifteen percent of the LM showed large nucleated cells within the dermal papillae (Fig. 16.5.1) compared with 2% of BM of the face. While the presence of nucleated cells in the dermis is a minor criterion in the previous melanocytic RCM score determined on melanocytic lesions excluding LM [15], it is surprising that this feature is important in the diagnosis of LM which is, by definition, confined to the epidermis! The reason for the apparent discrepancy between the RCM and pathology findings may be related to:
  - sampling, such that the dermal component identified on RCM was not present in the pathology biopsy sections.
  - difficulty in determining the exact site of the cells (junctional or dermal) on RCM is another possible explanation, especially as the dermo-epidermal junction is partially distorted in many cases of LM.

  Of note, RCM could be particularly interesting to target small biopsy in the area where cells "seem to be" in the dermis in order to demonstrate the invasiveness of the tumor, but there is still insufficient evidence to support this notion.
- Plump bright cells, particularly sparse within the papillary dermis, described as melanophages, were strongly associated with the LM (grey dots, corresponding to melanophages are also a useful dermoscopy feature for the diagnosis of LM). Distinguishing nuclei in cells or nest of cells in the dermis where the features are blurred due to attenuation of the reflective signal is sometimes very challenging. Nevertheless, it has recently be demonstrated

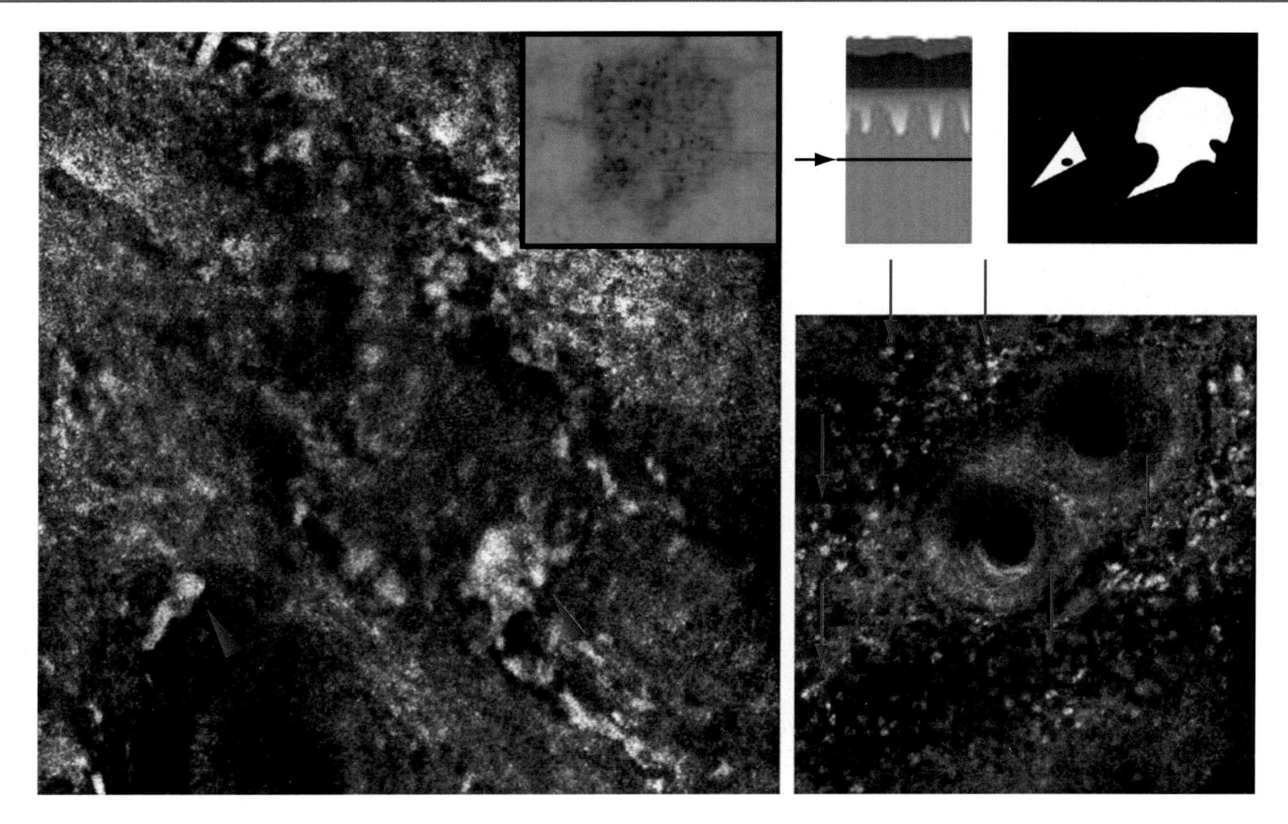

Fig. 16.6 Basic images (0.5 × 0.5 mm) of a lichen planus like keratosis (see dermoscopy in the *black square* with typical *grey dots*). Melanophages (→) are typically more ill-defined, smaller, with less visible nuclei and aggregated in more ill-defined nests (▲) but they can be difficult to distinguish from dermal melanocytes seen in the figure above

[16] that melanophages tend to be significantly smaller than melanocytes (mean cell diameter 13.6 μm: SD 1.6 versus 18.2 μm; SD 2.9 for melanocytes; $p= 0.006$) and visible nuclei (intracellular low reflectance round-oval structures) were identified in only 15% of cells (versus 57% in dermal melanocytes; $p< 0.001$) (Fig. 16.6). When they could be identified, the nuclei were smaller in melanophages (mean diameter 3.2 μm, SD 1.2 versus 6.4 μm; SD 0.7; $p< 0.001$). Melanophages were also significantly more ill-defined (76% of cells versus 18% for melanocytes; $p< 0.001$), less round (23% versus 69%; $p< 0.001$) and less dendritic (1% versus 12%; $p< 0.001$). They were also aggregated into some ill-defined edge nest (Fig. 16.6) in contrast to the dense or sparse or cerebriform nests described with melanocytes [17].

LM score: An algorithm was developed (LM score) to distinguish LM from BM [14],

- two major features
  - nonedged papillae (+2)
  - pagetoid cells round + >20 μm (+2)
- four minor ones
  - 3 positive

    >3 atypical cells at the junction in five fields (0.5 mm 2) (+1)

    follicular localization of pagetoid cells and/or atypical junctional cells (+1)

    nucleated cells within the papilla (+1)
  - 1 negative

    broadened honeycomb pattern (−1)

Sensitivity and specificity

- A LM score of ≥2 resulted in a sensitivity of 85% and specificity of 76% for the diagnosis of LM (OR for LM 18.6; 95% CI: 9.3–37.1). In an independent test set of 29 LM and 44 BM, the OR for LM was 60.7 (95% CI: 11.9–309) (93% sensitivity, 82% specificity).
- The LM score showed a similar sensitivity for six invasive LM melanomas (median Breslow thickness 0.34 mm). In contrast, it showed a poor sensitivity on LM that were classified as uncertain or "early" LM by pathology (22%). It has to be emphasized that LM is often a subtle diagnosis on RCM, as with pathology slides, and clinicians have to deal with an imperfect gold standard.
- Differential diagnosis: Solar lentigines present typically with an increase in the density of dermal papillae surrounded by a bright monomorphic layer of cells, forming regular geometric shapes (Fig. 16.3.1). They are quite easy to diagnose and have been described in Ref. [10].

Flat seborrheic keratosis can have the same confocal aspect. Of note, with a specificity of the LM score around 64%, keratoses were less easy to differentiate from LM than other BMs of the face, perhaps due to the distortion of pigmented keratinocytes that had a similar reflectance signal under RCM to atypical (small) melanocytes. Clinical and dermoscopy features should help and be taken into account as they can rule out the diagnosis. In the author's opinion, punch biopsy and digital monitoring remain the best alternative tools in doubtful cases.

Margin and recurrence determination

- RCM could be particularly useful not only to provide a LM diagnosis but also to assess margins:
  Clinically, LM is often amelanotic peripherally and can spread far beyond the visible margins [8]. Delineating the extent of disease is a major challenge to avoid recurrence. Surgical treatment is the preferred option when possible but margins of 5 mm are inadequate in 30–80% of LM [18]. Mohs surgery or staged excision has been proposed as techniques to more precisely delineate the margins of LM, but both are expensive and the procedures require a high degree of expertise.
- Moreover, surgery may be contraindicated due to the extent of disease, comorbidities or patient preference for a more conservative approach. Radiotherapy, cryosurgery and other medical treatments (imiquimod) have also been proposed to treat larger field, hoping to decrease recurrence rates while having less cosmetic issues. Nevertheless, clinical follow up is unreliable: pigmentation after inflammation due to treatment, and in particular pigment incontinence, is a well-known pitfall of clinical detection of false-positive recurrence [19]. On the other hand, amelanotic recurrences have also been well documented [20]. Thus, RCM could provide the best approach for mapping the area to be treated and for detecting recurrences.
  On a large series of 110 LM and 247 BM of the face [14], the LM score performed as well on peripheral LM margins (n= 20) as on biopsies from the lesions themselves (n= 61), even though the peripheral sites were often completely amelanotic (9 out of 20). Targeting punch biopsies to the middle of the confocal field seemed to afford better histological-confocal correlation in LM, which often contain irregular margins of scattered cells. Of note in this study, the LM algorithm was equally effective in the diagnosis of amelanotic lesions compared to pigmented lesions. The reader should refer to Chap.17 for a more detailed account on amelanotic melanoma.

Core Messages

1. The main LM features are:
   - nonedged papillae (dermal papillae separated by a series of large reflecting cells);
   - round and large (>20 µm) pagetoid cells.

   Minor features are numerous atypical cells at the dermoepidermal junction; follicular localization of atypical cells; nucleated cells within the dermal papillae, and no broadened honeycomb pattern.
2. RCM is useful for:
   - diagnosis of difficult cases: amelanotic, recurrences, large or cosmetically challenging…
   - Search of margins;
   - Follow up of treatment (radiotherapy, imiquimod, short surgical margins…).

   The down sides:
   - time consuming, in particular when mapping large area;
   - pathology challenges = confocal challenges.

References

1. Ackerman AB, Briggs PL, Bravo F (1993) Differential diagnosis in dermopathology III. Lea & Febiger, Philadelphia, pp 166–169
2. Dalton SR, Gardner TL, Libow LF, Elston DM (2005) Contiguous lesions in lentigo maligna. J Am Acad Dermatol 52:859–862
3. Klauder JV, Beerman H (2005) Melanotic freckle (Hutchinson), mélanose circonscrite précancéreuse (Dubreuilh). AMA Arch Derm 71:2–10
4. Weyers W, Bonczkowitz M, Weyers I, Bittinger A, Schill WB (1996) Melanoma in situ versus melanocytic hyperplasia in sun-damaged skin. Assessment of the significance of histopathologic criteria for differential diagnosis. Am J Dermatopathol 18: 560–566
5. Cohen LM (1996) The starburst giant cell is useful for distinguishing lentigo maligna from photodamaged skin. J Am Acad Dermatol 35:962–968
6. Agarwal-Antal N, Bowen GM, Gerwels JW (2002) Histologic evaluation of lentigo maligna with permanent sections: implications regarding current guidelines. J Am Acad Dermatol 47:743–748
7. Osborne JE, Hutchinson PE (2002) A follow-up study to investigate the efficacy of initial treatment of lentigo maligna with surgical excision. Br J Plast Surg 55:611–615
8. McKenna JK, Florell SR, Goldman GD, Bowen GM (2006) Lentigo maligna/lentigo maligna melanoma: current state of diagnosis and treatment. Dermatol Surg 32:493–504
9. Tannous ZS, Mihm MC, Flotte TJ, Gonzalez S (2002) In vivo examination of lentigo maligna and malignant melanoma in situ, lentigo maligna type by near-infrared reflectance confocal microscopy: comparison of in vivo confocal images with histologic sections. J Am Acad Dermatol 46:260–263

10. Langley RG, Burton E, Walsh N, Propperova I, Murray SJ (2006) In vivo confocal scanning laser microscopy of benign lentigines: comparison to conventional histology and in vivo characteristics of lentigo maligna. J Am Acad Dermatol 55:88–97
11. Chen CS, Elias M, Busam K, Rajadhyaksha M, Marghoob AA (2005) Multimodal in vivo optical imaging, including confocal microscopy, facilitates presurgical margin mapping for clinically complex lentigo maligna melanoma. Br J Dermatol 153: 1031–1036
12. Curiel-Lewandrowski C, Williams CM, Swindells KJ, Tahan SR, Astner S, Frankenthaler RA et al (2004) Use of in vivo confocal microscopy in malignant melanoma: an aid in diagnosis and assessment of surgical and nonsurgical therapeutic approaches. Arch Dermatol 140:1127–1132
13. Ahlgrimm-Siess V, Massone C, Scope A, Fink-Puches R, Richtig E, Wolf IH, Koller S, Gerger A, Smolle J, Hofmann-Wellenhof R (2009) Reflectance confocal microscopy of facial lentigo maligna and lentigo maligna melanoma: a preliminary study. Br J Dermatol 161:1307–1316
14. Guitera P, Pellacani G, Crotty KA, Scolyer RA, Li LX, Bassoli S, Vinceti M, Rabinovitz H, Longo C, Menzies SW (2010) The impact of in vivo reflectance confocal microscopy on the diagnostic accuracy of lentigo maligna and equivocal pigmented and nonpigmented macules of the face. J Invest Dermatol 130:2080–2091
15. Pellacani G, Vinceti M, Bassoli S, Braun R, Gonzalez S, Guitera P, Longo C, Marghoob AA, Menzies SW, Puig S, Scope A, Seidenari S, Malvehy J (2009) Reflectance confocal microscopy and features of melanocytic lesions: an internet-based study of the reproducibility of terminology. Arch Dermatol 145(10):1137–1143
16. Guitera P, Li LX, Scolyer RA, Menzies SW (2010) Morphologic features of melanophages under in vivo reflectance confocal microscopy. Arch Dermatol 146(5):492–498
17. Pellacani G, Cesinaro AM, Seidenari S (2005) In vivo confocal reflectance microscopy for the characterization of melanocytic nests and correlation with dermoscopy and histology. Br J Dermatol 152(2):384–386
18. Hazan C, Dusza SW, Delgado R, Busam KJ, Halpern AC, Nehal KS (2008) Staged excision for lentigo maligna and lentigo maligna melanoma: a retrospective analysis of 117 cases. J Am Acad Dermatol 58(1):142–148
19. Cotter MA, McKenna JK, Bowen GM (2008) Treatment of lentigo maligna with imiquimod before staged excision. Dermatol Surg 34(2):147–151
20. Fisher GH, Lang PG (2003) Treatment of melanoma in situ on sun-damaged skin with topical 5% imiquimod cream complicated by the development of invasive disease. Arch Dermatol 139(7): 945–947

17 Amelanotic Melanoma

Pascale Guitera

17.1 Introduction

Diagnosis of a melanocytic lesion that is clinically barely visible or nonpigmented is particularly difficult. A list of simulators of amelanotic melanoma [1] has been published. It is also a rare condition, with an estimated occurrence between 2 and 8% of the melanomas [2]. These issues lead to a delay in the diagnosis and a subsequently worse prognosis.

Because evidence of melanin is usually found in amelanotic melanoma pathologically, the difficulty in diagnosing these lesions lies with the clinician and not the pathologist. A new dermoscopic method has recently been described, which achieved a sensitivity of 70% and specificity of 56% (96% sensitivity, 37% specificity alternate model) in a large set (n = 105) of hypo/amelanotic melanomas [3]. Thus, dermoscopy performs quite poorly on these types of lesions whereas RCM is more effective for diagnosing hypo/amelanotic melanocytic lesions.

17.2 RCM Features

The specificity for melanoma diagnosis of the RCM score was significantly superior for amelanotic and light-colored melanocytic lesions compared with partially and completely pigmented ones. It achieves a sensitivity of 85% and specificity of 84% [4]. Langley et al. also reported a series of lesions where two of four melanomas misclassified by dermoscopy and correctly identified by RCM were hypo/amelanotic lesions [5].

This may be explained by the fact that melanin appears very bright under RCM, even if it is present in very small quantities [6]. Immunohistochemical and ultrastructural studies show that amelanotic melanoma cells contain melanosomes and rare melanin granules even if they are not visible clinically [7, 8]. When the lesion is heavily pigmented, the background of keratinocytes is bright and atypical cells may be more difficult to identify.

A case report of amelanotic LM diagnosed with RCM has been described [9]. The LM score is a method to differentiate LM from benign macules of the face described recently in a large study [10]. Of note, the specificity of the LM score was higher when the benign macules were amelanotic (90%, n = 67), or lightly pigmented (87%, n = 53) compared with partially or darkly pigmented cases (59%, n = 83) ($p < 0.001$). The sensitivity of the method varied, with 93% for amelanotic LM (n = 14), 78% for the light-colored lesions (n = 9) (Fig. 17.1) and 84% for the partially or darkly pigmented lesions (n = 49) (Fig. 17.2).

Vessels' shape is a major dermoscopy feature for the diagnosis of amelanotic lesions. Vessels' presence is not included in the RCM score proposed by Pellacani et al. as the best method to differentiate melanoma (excluding LM) from nevi [4]. They are likewise not included in the LM score [10]. Nevertheless, they are often described in melanoma, particularly in deep ones (Fig. 17.1.2) [11].

P. Guitera
Melanoma Institute Australia,
North Sydney, Australia

Discipline of Dermatology, Sydney University Sydney Melanoma Diagnostic Centre, RPA, Sydney, Australia
e-mail: pascale.guitera@melanoma.org.au

R. Hofmann-Wellenhof et al. (eds.), *Reflectance Confocal Microscopy for Skin Diseases*,
DOI 10.1007/978-3-642-21997-9_17, © Springer-Verlag Berlin Heidelberg 2012

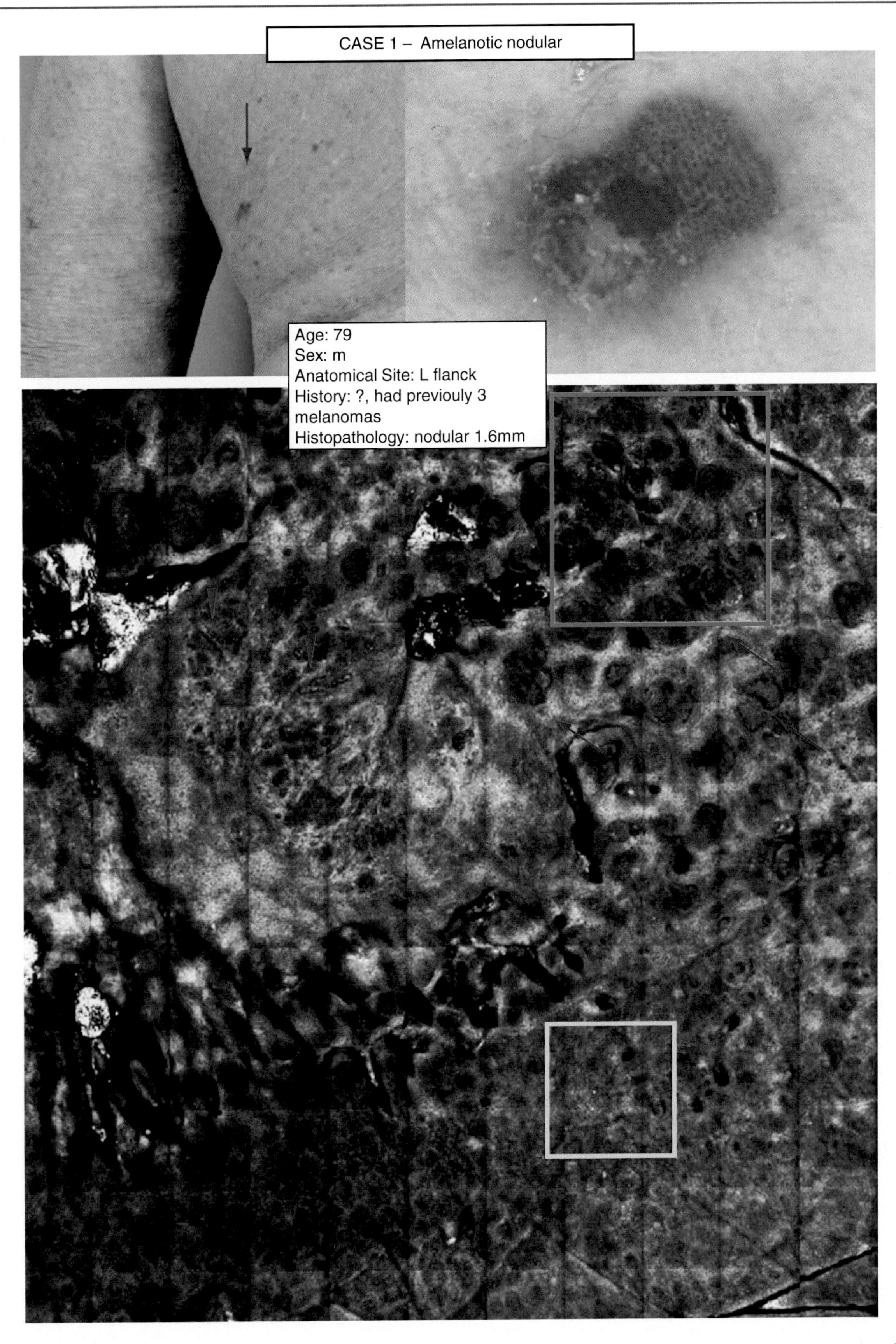

Fig. 17.1 RCM mosaic (5.5 × 5.5 mm) at the epidermal layer (*lower part*) and junctional layer (*upper part*) with large nests (→) and multiple large vessels (▲)

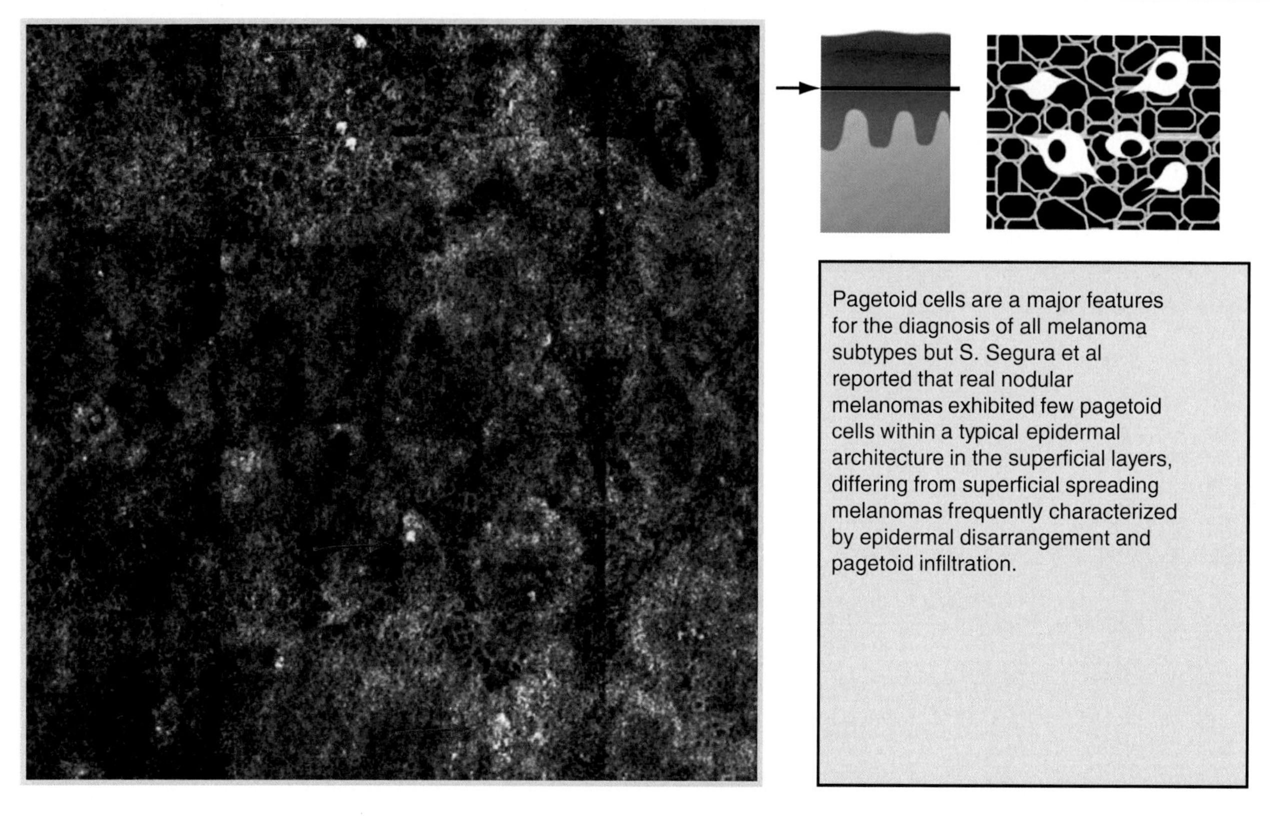

Fig. 17.1.1 RCM mosaic (1 × 1 mm) at the epidermis level: round and large bright pagetoid cells are visible (→), the background of karatinocytes is dark because nonpigmented

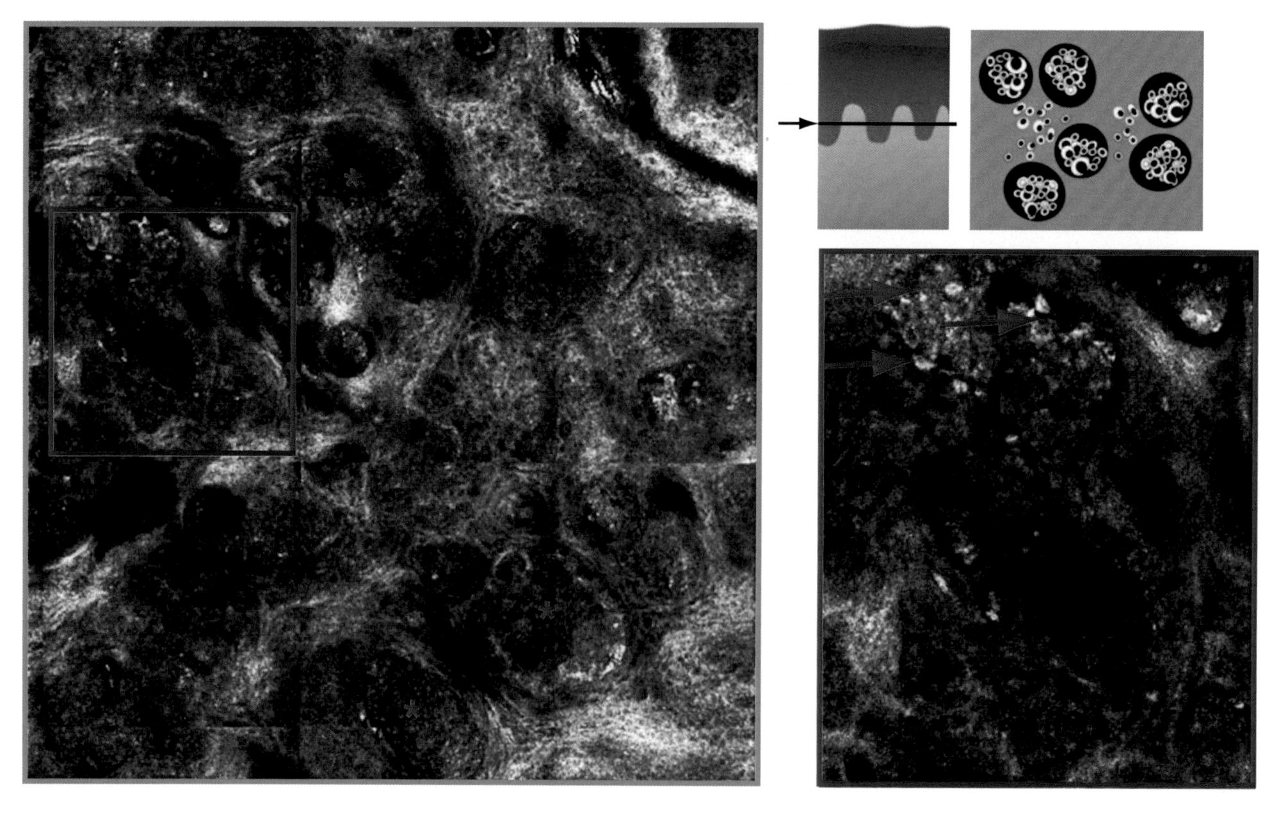

Fig. 17.1.2 RCM mosaic (1 × 1 mm) in the *blue square* showing lare nests (*) containing atypical bright cells (→) better seen in the *red square*. Basic image (0.5 × 0.5 mm)

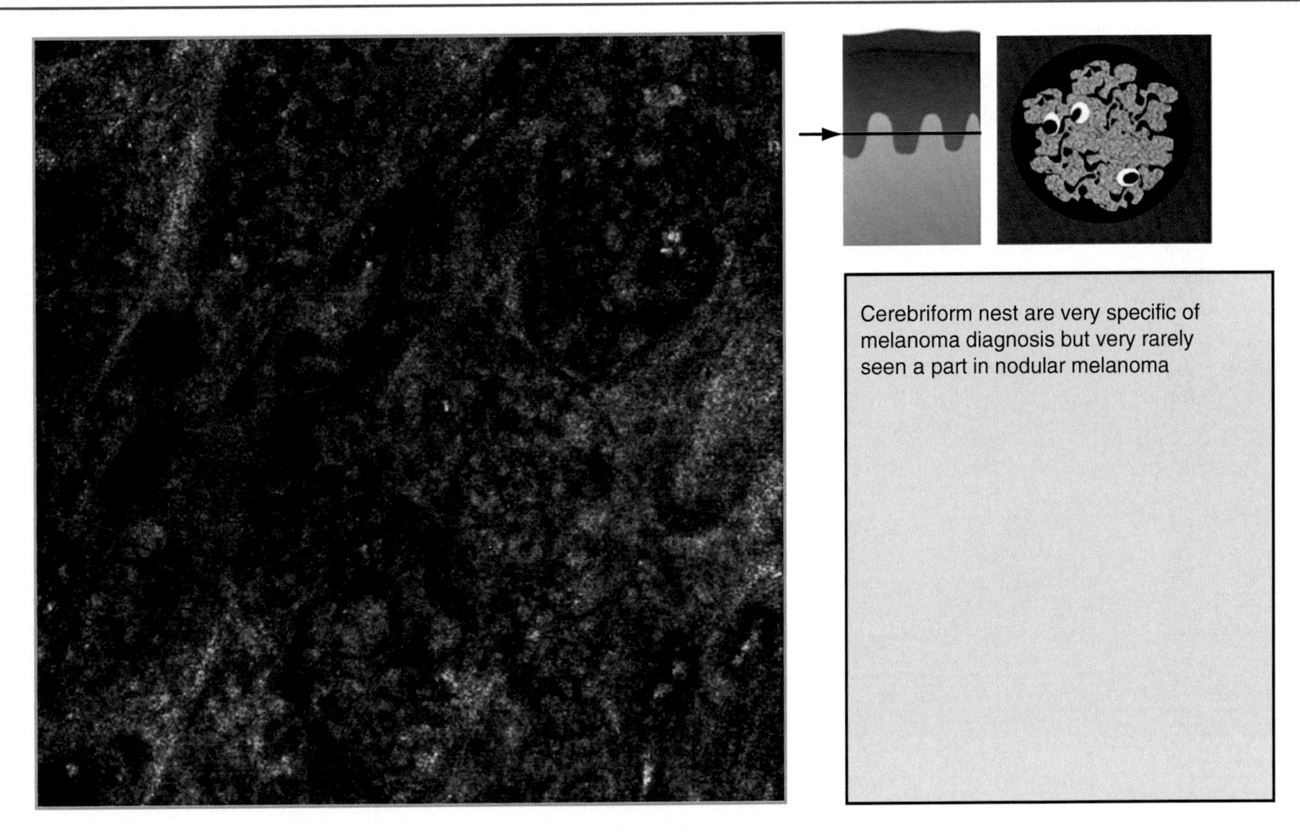

Fig. 17.1.3 Multiple cerebriform nests were seen in this nodular melanoma

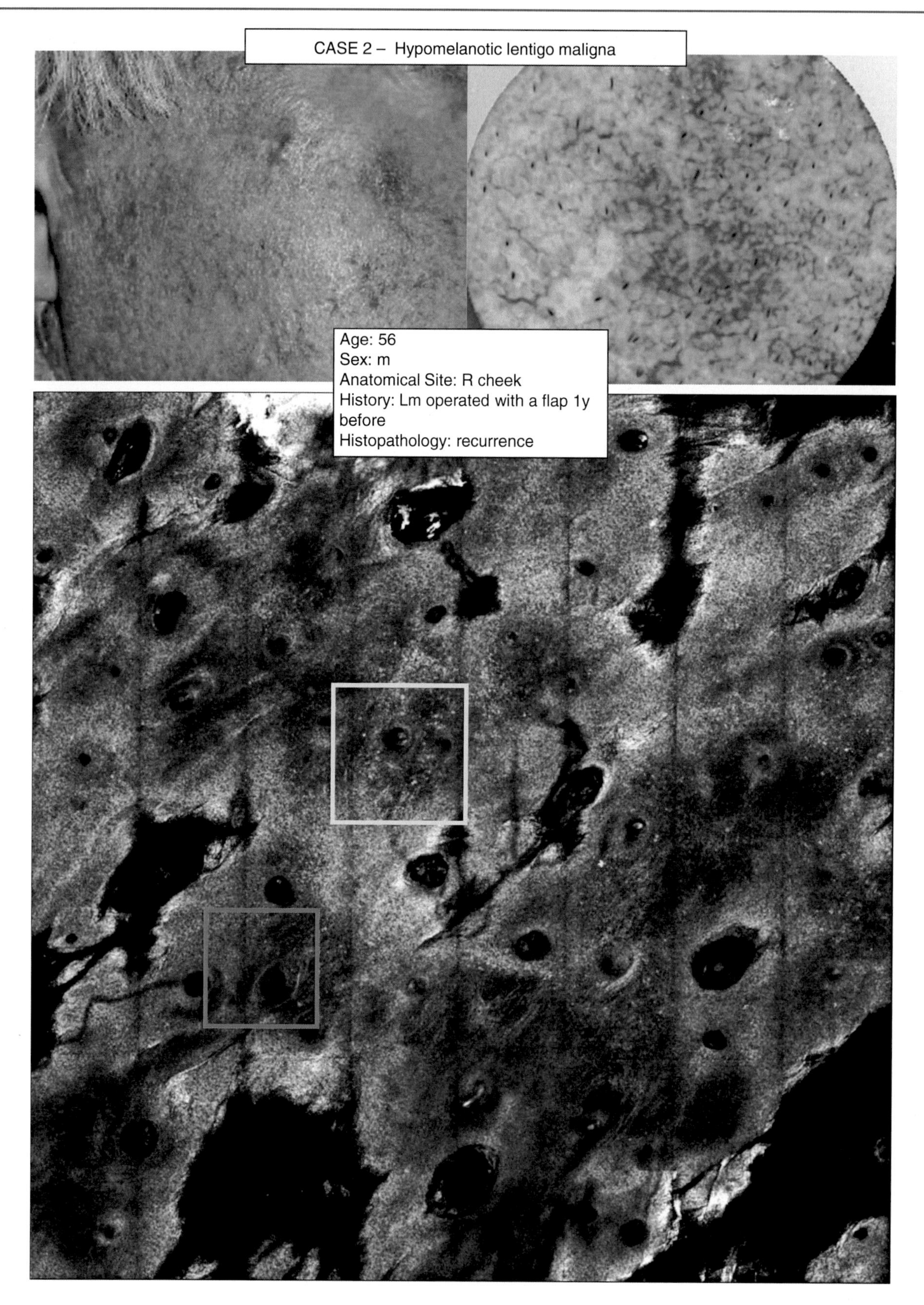

Fig. 17.2 RCM mosaic (4 × 4 mm) at the level of the DEJ reveals numerous follicular opening but no visible papillae

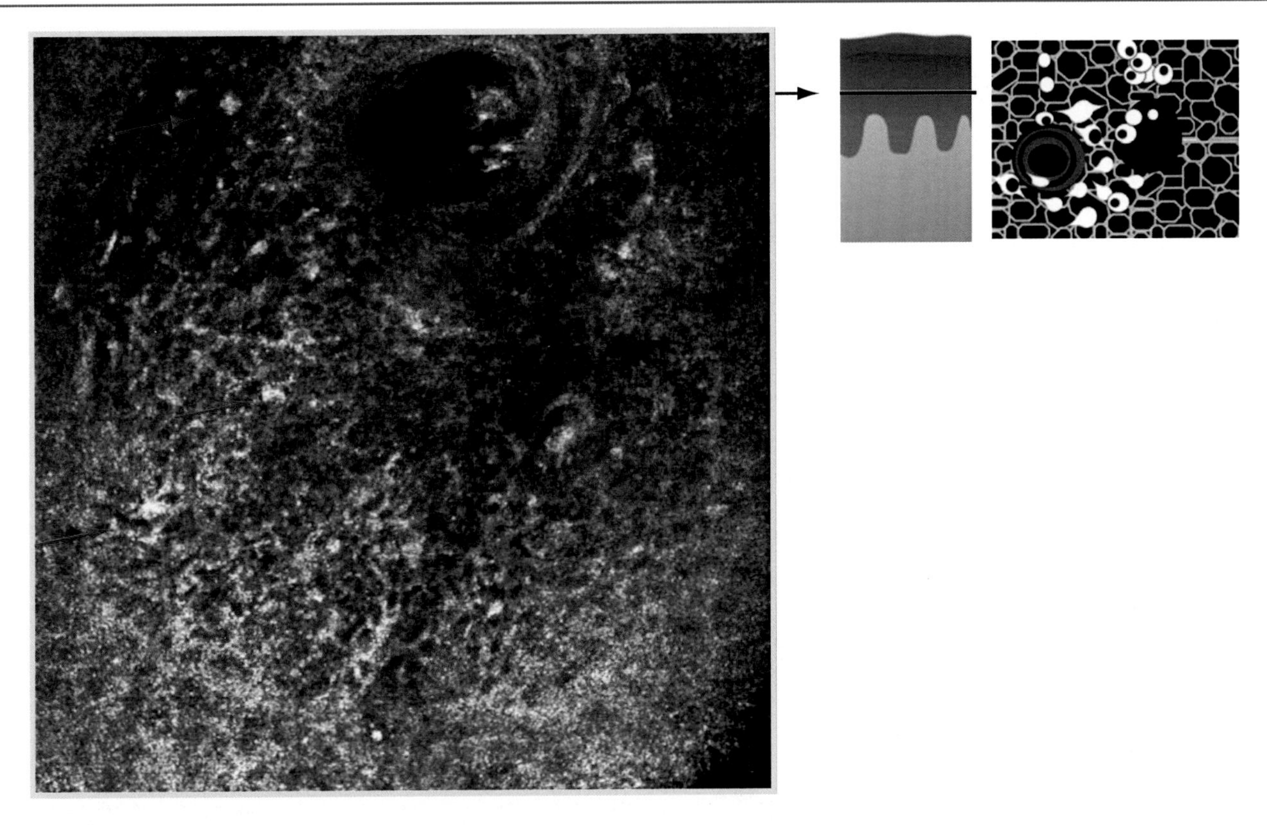

Fig. 17.2.1 Basic image (0.5 × 0.5 mm) with epidermal disarray and large round bright pagetoid cells (→)

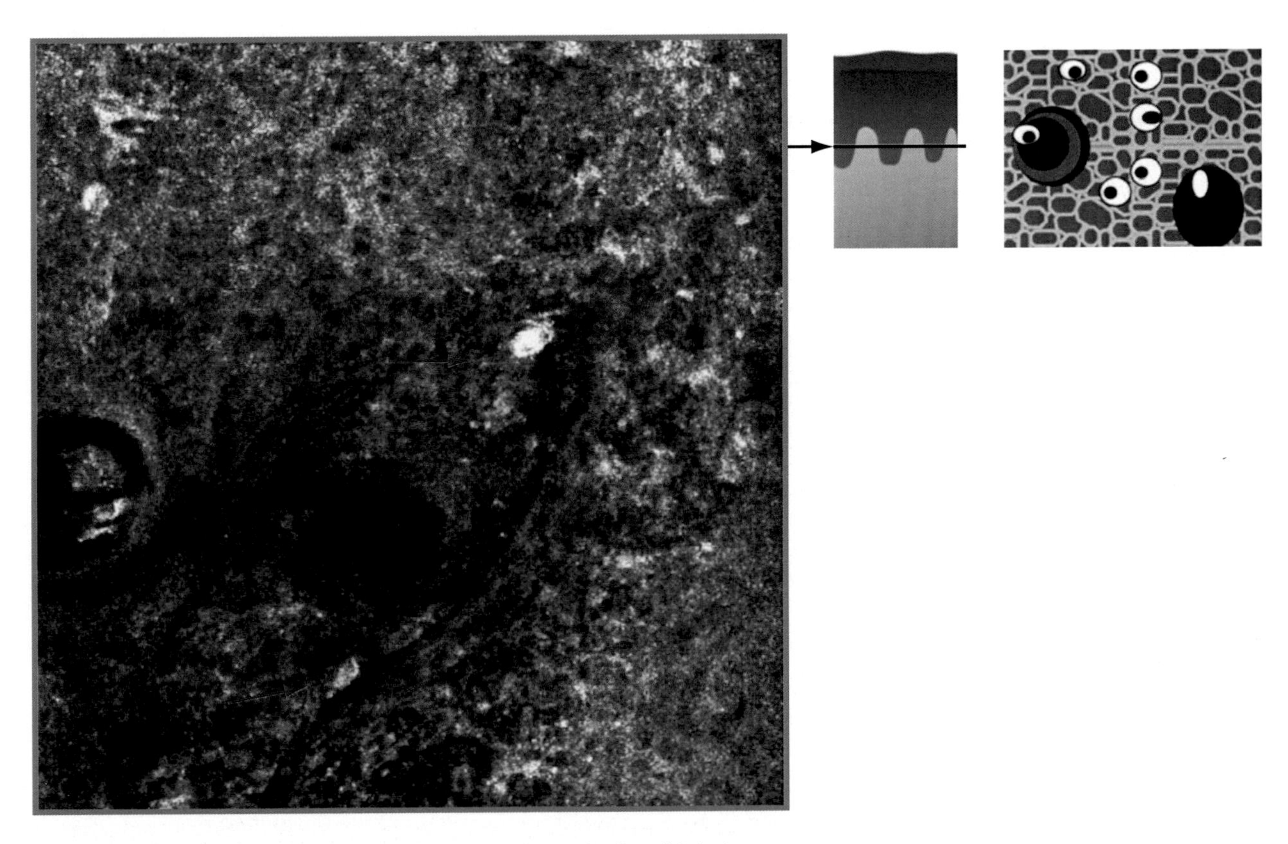

Fig. 17.2.2 Basic image (0.5 × 0.5 mm) with atypical cells (marked atypia) (→)

Core Messages

- Amelanotic melanomas present the same features than pigmented ones and are even often easier to diagnose. It is a major indication to perform RCM.

References

1. Koch SE, Lange JR (2000) Amelanotic melanoma: the great masquerader. J Am Acad Dermatol 42(5 Pt 1):731–734
2. Ariel M (1981) Amelanotic malignant melanoma. In: Ariel M (ed) Malignant melanoma. Appleton Century-Crofts, New York, pp 259–263
3. Menzies SW, Kreusch J, Byth K, Pizzichetta MA, Marghoob A, Braun R, Malvehy J, Puig S, Argenziano G, Zalaudek I, Rabinovitz HS, Oliviero M, Cabo H, Ahlgrimm-Siess V, Avramidis M, Guitera P, Soyer HP, Ghigliotti G, Tanaka M, Perusquia AM, Pagnanelli G, Bono R, Thomas L, Pellacani G, Langford D, Piccolo D, Terstappen K, Stanganelli I, Llambrich A, Johr R (2008) Dermoscopic evaluation of amelanotic and hypomelanotic melanoma. Arch Dermatol 144(9): 1120–1127
4. Guitera P, Pellacani G, Longo C, Seidenari S, Avramidis M, Menzies SW (2009) In vivo reflectance confocal microscopy enhances secondary evaluation of melanocytic lesions. J Invest Dermatol 129(1): 131–138
5. Langley RG, Walsh N, Sutherland AE, Propperova I, Delaney L, Morris SF et al (2007) The diagnostic accuracy of in vivo confocal scanning laser microscopy compared to dermoscopy of benign and malignant melanocytic lesions: a prospective study. Dermatology 215:365–372
6. Rajadhyaksha M, Grossman M, Esterowitz D, Webb RH, Anderson RR (1995) In vivo confocal scanning laser microscopy of human skin: melanin provides strong contrast. J Invest Dermatol 104: 946–952
7. Gibson LE, Goellner JR (1988) Amelanotic melanoma: cases studied by Fontana stain, S-100 immunostain, and ultrastructural examination. Mayo Clin Proc 63(8):777–782
8. Erlandson RA (1987) Ultrastructural diagnosis of amelanotic malignant melanoma: aberrant melanosomes, myelin figures or lysosomes? Ultrastruct Pathol 11(2–3):191–208
9. Curiel-Lewandrowski C, Williams CM, Swindells KJ, Tahan SR, Astner S, Frankenthaler RA et al (2004) Use of in vivo confocal microscopy in malignant melanoma: an aid in diagnosis and assessment of surgical and nonsurgical therapeutic approaches. Arch Dermatol 140:1127–1132
10. Guitera P, Pellacani G, Crotty KA, Scolyer RA, Li LX, Bassoli S, Vinceti M, Rabinovitz H, Longo C, Menzies SW (2010) The impact of in vivo reflectance confocal microscopy on the diagnostic accuracy of lentigo maligna and equivocal pigmented and nonpigmented macules of the face. J Invest Dermatol [Epub ahead of print]
11. Segura S, Pellacani G, Puig S, Longo C, Bassoli S, Guitera P, Palou J, Menzies S, Seidenari S, Malvehy J (2008) In vivo microscopic features of nodular melanomas: dermoscopy, confocal microscopy, and histopathologic correlates. Arch Dermatol 144(10):1311–1320

Part VI

Nonmelanocytic Skin Lesions

Semiology and Pattern Analysis in Nonmelanocytic Lesions

18

Josep Malvehy, Myrna Hanke-Martinez, Joanne Costa, Gabriel Salerni, Cristina Carrera, and Susana Puig

Confocal microscopy has been used in the study of nonmelanocytic tumors since the beginning of the technology [1]. Numerous publications have provided criteria and descriptors for different neoplasms such as basal cell carcinoma, keratinizing tumors, angioma and dermatofibroma among others. The limits of resolution and depth of the microscope make impossible the observation of the tumor component in the reticular dermis and hypodermis and therefore RCM is not useful for the study of the deep component of thick lesions of the skin. Likewise RCM cannot provide reliable information in deep recurrences or surgical margins in the case of carcinoma prior to surgery [2]. Moreover, RCM can be very sensible and specific in the detection of the superficial part of the tumor that is sufficient for a correct diagnosis in many cutaneous neoplasms. In the case of basal cell carcinoma (BCC) and squamous cell carcinoma (SCC), different application of RCM in the ex vivo modality with the use of specific staining products for RCM such as acridine has been reported. Ex vivo RCM has been postulated to be useful in MOHS surgery in theses tumors [3].

RCM has been proved to be a valuable tool for the noninvasive monitoring of response to treatments in BCC, SCC or actinic keratosis with imiquimoid, photodynamic therapy or cryotherapy [4]. This has been found of special interest in patients with multiple sporadic tumors or in genodermatosis like Gorlin-Goltz syndrome or xeroderma pigmentosum [5].

A two-step algorithm for the evaluation of skin tumors with RCM has been reported [6]. In the first step, differentiation between melanocytic and nonmelanocytic tumors is achieved based on the absence or presence in RCM of melanocytic criteria: cobblestone pattern, pagetoid cells, dermal nests and dermal papilla (widespread) (Fig. 18.1.1).

J. Malvehy (✉) • M. Hanke-Martinez • J. Costa • G. Salerni
C. Carrera • S. Puig
Department of Dermatology, Melanoma Unit,
Hospital Clinic of Barcelona, Barcelona, Spain
e-mail: jmalvehy@clinic.ub.es

In this chapter, a glossary of the main findings observed in some of the most frequent nonmelanocytic neoplasms will be presented. In the following chapters, a detailed description of basal cell carcinoma, actinic keratosis, squamous cell carcinoma, lymphoma and a final potpourri of tumors will be found but the list of findings in different skin tumors certainly will be increased in the future.

18.1 Basal Cell Carcinoma

Reflectance confocal microscopy is a very useful tool for the noninvasive evaluation of pigmented and nonpigmented varieties of BCC. The clinical detection of early BCC is often a clinical challenge when these lesions are seen on the face and the differential diagnosis includes benign and malignant tumors that can be distinguished with a correct biopsy. RCM in our experience provides very useful information and in many situations a clear confirmation of a BCC can be obtained in a few minutes. In the case of BCC with clinical indication for treatment with imiquimoid or other noninvasive options, the confocal microscopy has additional value with the identification of the tumor prior to the treatment and monitoring of response and detection of subclinical recurrences [7].

In the case of pigmented BCC, the presence of dendritic cells corresponding to melanocytes in the tumor islands is also a major finding [8].

Criteria for the recognition of [9] BCC in RCM include the presence of the following criteria:

1. *Tumor islands:* Round to oval, cord-like or lobulated structures at the level of DEJ or superficial dermis that can be either darker than the surrounding epidermis or dermis ("dark silhouettes") or bright well-demarcated structures.
2. *Polarization of nuclei (streaming):* cells within the tumor islands, or overlying basal or spinous keratinocytes, display nuclei that are elongated and distorted into alignment along the same axis.

R. Hofmann-Wellenhof et al. (eds.), *Reflectance Confocal Microscopy for Skin Diseases*,
DOI 10.1007/978-3-642-21997-9_18, © Springer-Verlag Berlin Heidelberg 2012

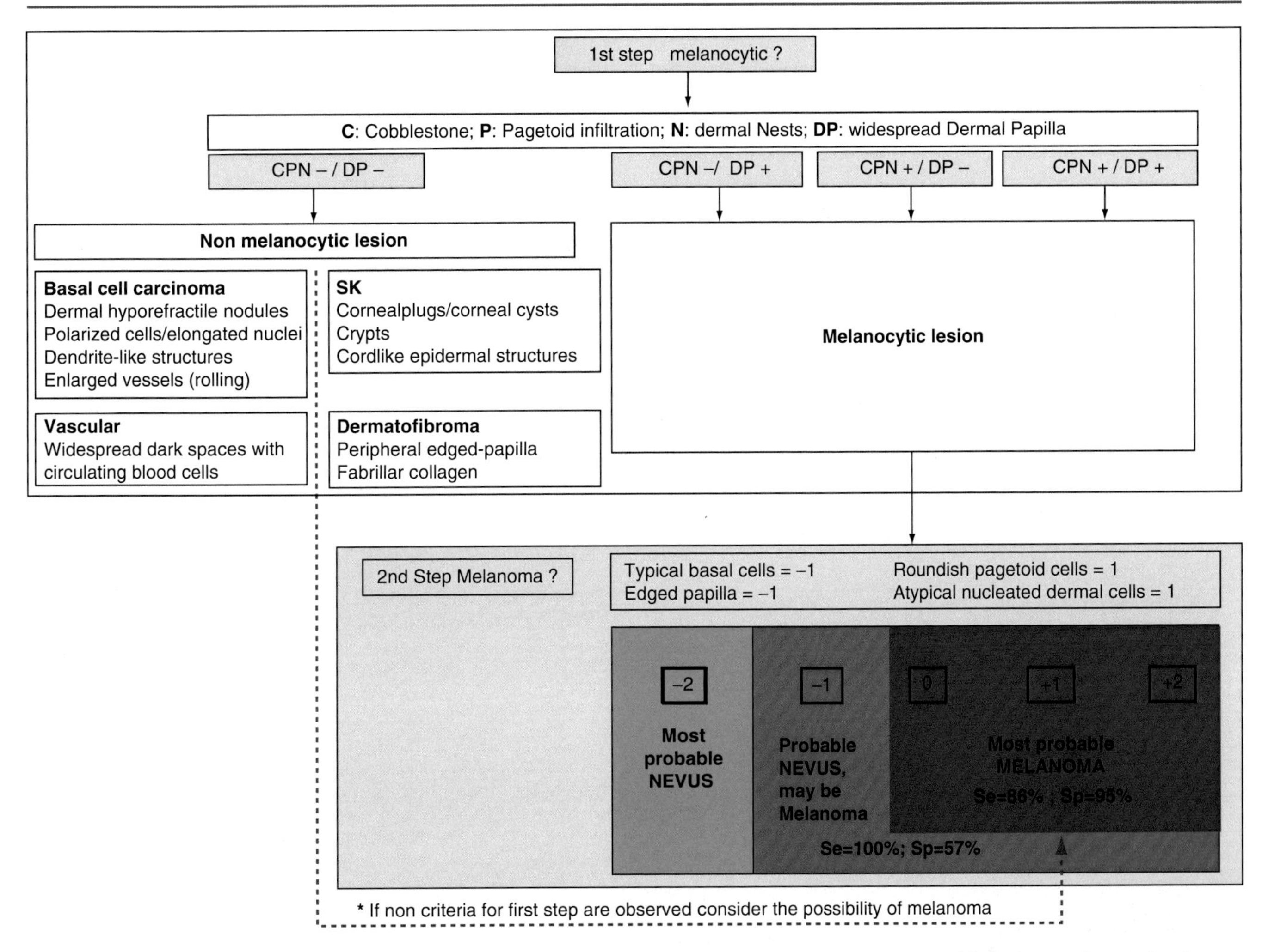

Fig. 18.1.1 Algorithm for confocal diagnosis of skin tumors. In first step, decision is made if lesion is melanocytic or not according to presence or absence of DP and CPN criteria. Lesions that are nonmelanocytic must fulfill known confocal features for basal cell carcinoma, seborrheic keratosis, angioma, or dermatofibroma. If absent, they must be considered melanocytic and might represent melanoma (*). In second step, melanocytic lesions are assessed for presence of protective features (score –1) and/or risk features (score + 1) for melanoma diagnosis. Final score gives probability of melanoma depending on established threshold. *CPN* presence of cobblestone pattern, pagetoid cells, or dermal nests; *DP* widespread dermal papilla; *Se* sensitivity; *Sp* specificity

3. *Dark cleft (clefting):* dark slit-like space observed between tumor island and surrounding dermis.
4. *Canalicular blood vessels:* thickened, elongated or tortuous dark structures, oriented parallel to the skin surface, containing moving small, round bright structures (white blood cells).

Figures 18.1.2–18.1.5 illustrate the main findings in BCC. In Chap. 19 confocal findings of BCC are covered in detail.

18.2 Actinic Keratosis and Squamous Cell Carcinoma

Actinic keratoses (AK) are the most frequent malignant cutaneous tumors and have been considered cutaneous squamous carcinoma in situ. In patients with skin sun damage, AK are very frequent and large areas of the skin exhibit an "actinic field of cancerization" with keratinocytic dysplasia at some degree. RCM makes visible many of the characteristic architectural and cellular alterations of AK with a good correlation with histopathology [10]. Again RCM allows the objective evaluation of AK previously to treatment of AK with imiquimoid, cryotherapy, photodynamic therapy, diclofenac or with other options and it makes evidenced when the resolution of the epithelial dysplasia is obtained.

RCM findings in AK and SCC are [11]:

1. *Parakeratosis*: individual highly-refractile round cells in the stratum corneum.
2. *Scale (hyperkeratosis):* increase of thickness of stratum corneum seen as refractile amorphous material.
3. *Irregular (atypical) honeycomb pattern:* abnormal pattern of the spinous-granular layers formed by bright cellular outlines which vary in size and shapes and in the thickness and brightness of the lines.

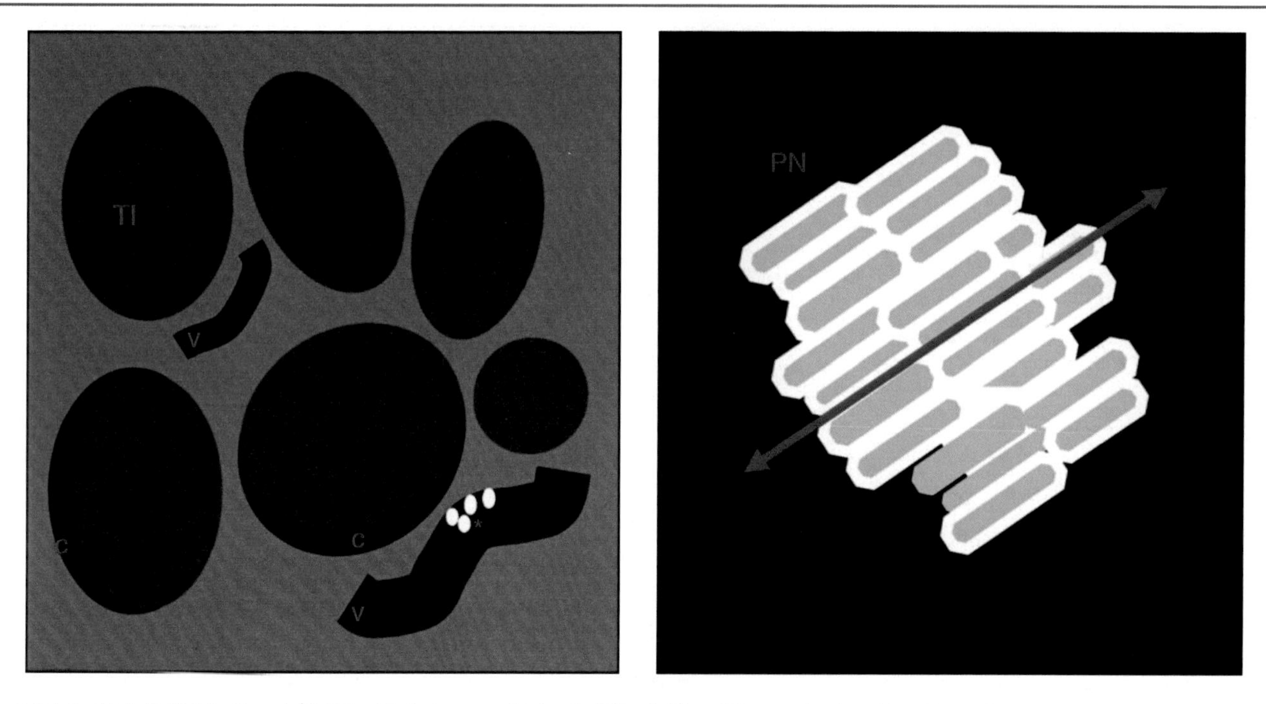

Fig. 18.1.2 Main RCM findings in BCC with dark tumoral islands (TI), clefting (C); vessels (*) with rolling of leukocytes (*); Polarization of nuclei (streaming) (PN)

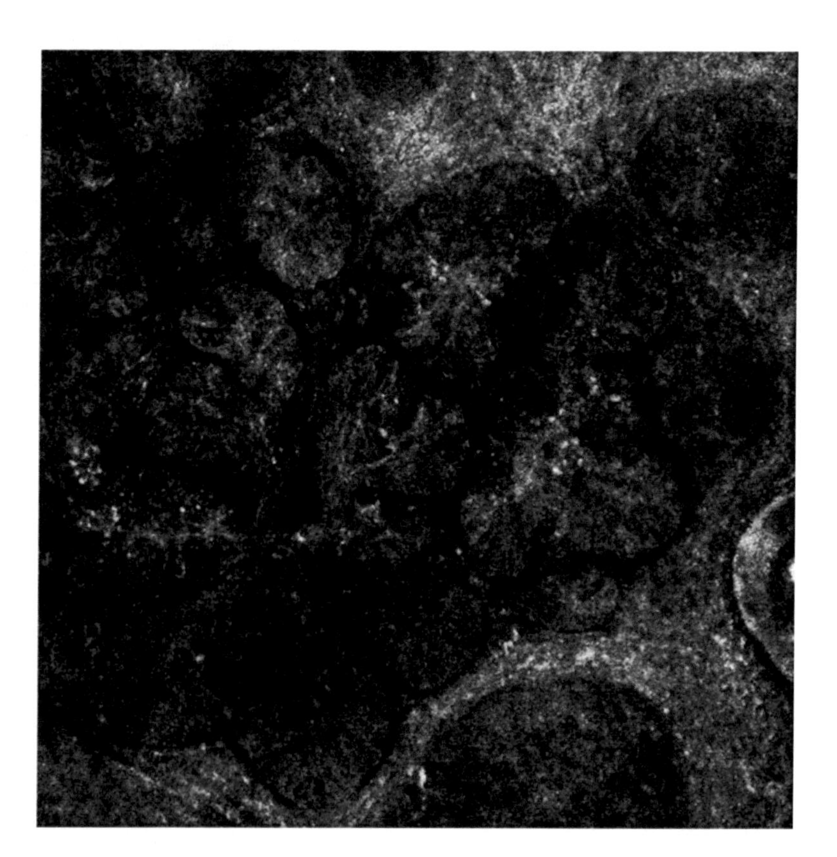

Fig. 18.1.3 Tumoral islands and dark clefting in a basal cell carcinoma

Fig. 18.1.4 Polarization of nuclei in a BCC

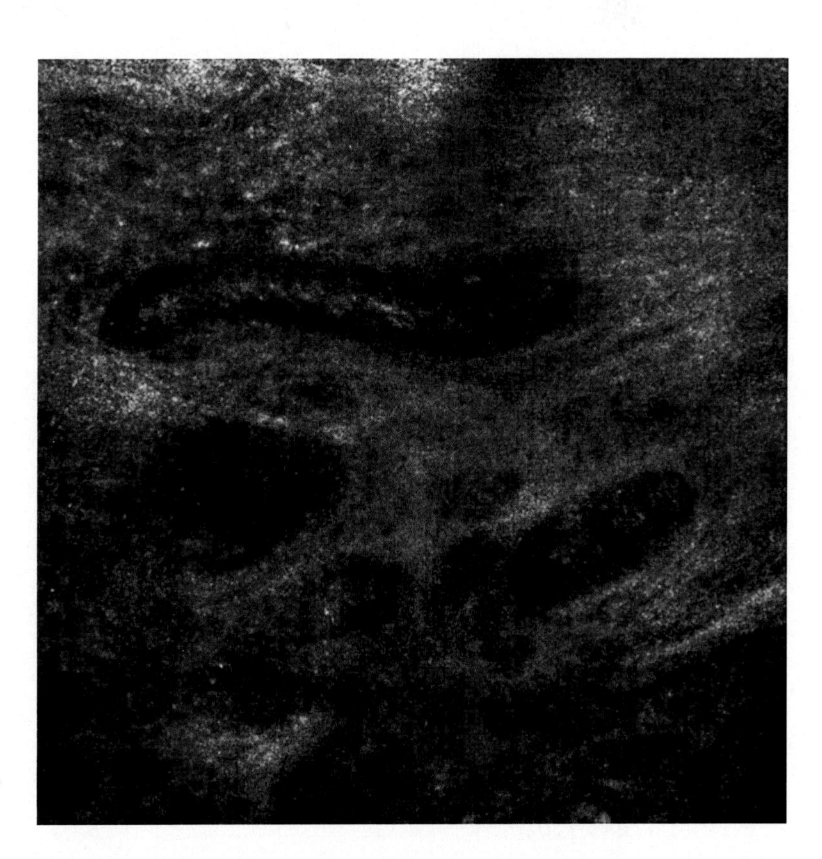

Fig. 18.1.5 Large vessels with blood cells and rolling of leukocytes

4. *Round blood vessels:* dilated blood vessels within the dermal papillae that run perpendicular to the horizontal RCM plane of imaging.

An increasing frequency of abnormal RCM features can be observed across the spectrum of keratinocytic neoplasias and therefore SCC exhibits more severe alterations than AK in epithelial architecture and cell morphology. The presence of an atypical honeycomb or a disarranged pattern of the spinous-granular layer, round nucleated cells at the spinous-granular layer, and round blood vessels traversing through the dermal papilla are the key RCM features of SCC. These vessels that correspond to the "glomerular vessels" under dermoscopy are seen in SCC by RCM even when they are not visible with other imaging technology. In general, AK alterations tend to be focally distributed and round vessels are less frequent. Anyhow clear differentiation by RCM between AK and in situ SCC or between in situ and invasive SCC has not been established.

Figures 18.1.6–18.1.9 illustrate the main findings in AK and SCC. In Chaps. 20 and 21 RCM findings in AK and SCC will be presented in more detail.

18.3 Seborrheic Keratosis

In the case of seborrheic keratosis (SK), a wide spectrum of clinical presentations and dermoscopic findings can be seen in lesions according to tumor type, skin type and anatomical locations. Findings of RCM of seborrheic keratosis are: [12, 13]

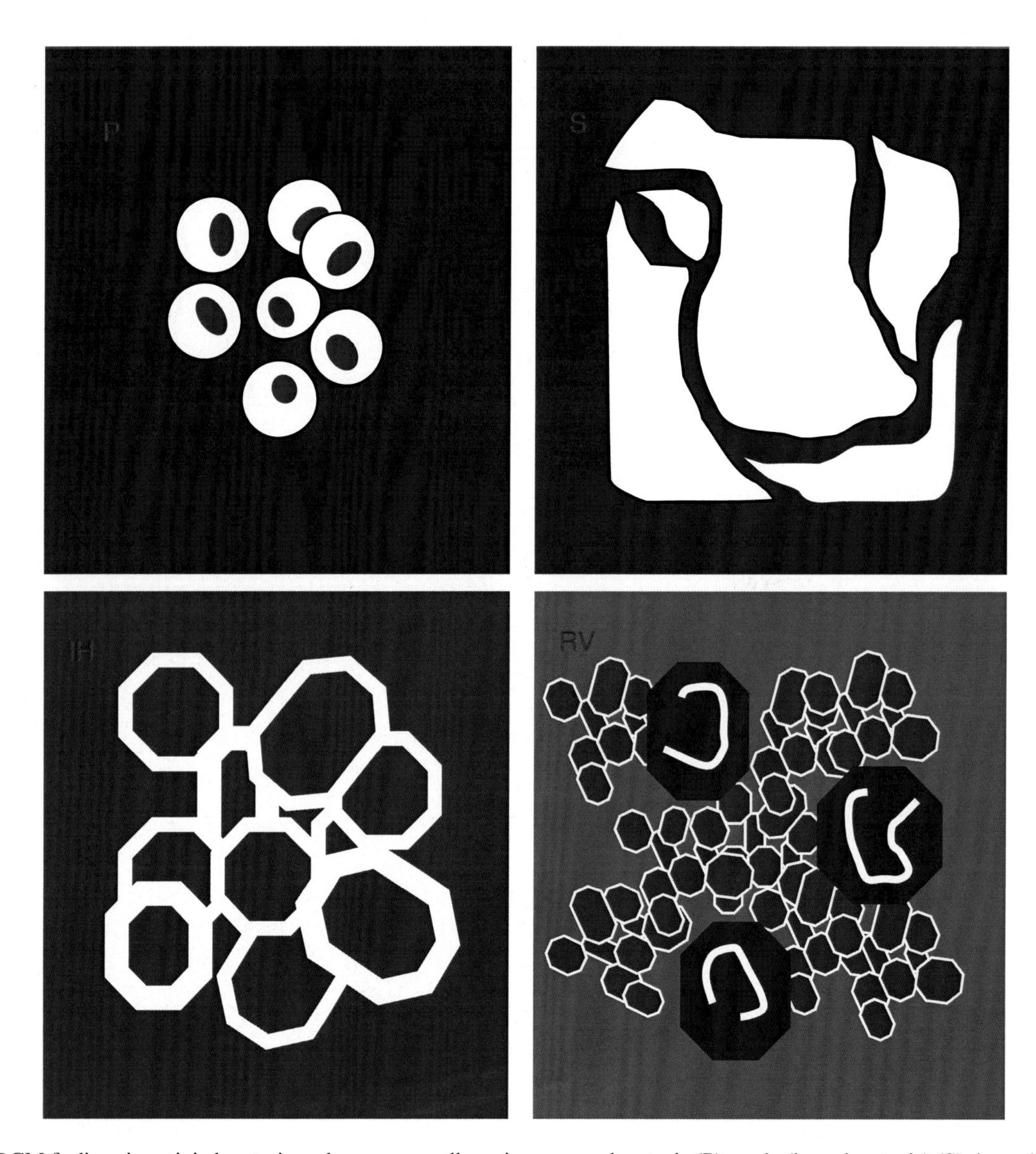

Fig. 18.1.6 RCM findings in actinic keratosis and squamous cell carcinoma: parakeratosis (P); scale (hyperkeratosis) (S); irregular (atypical) honeycomb pattern (IH); round blood vessels (RV)

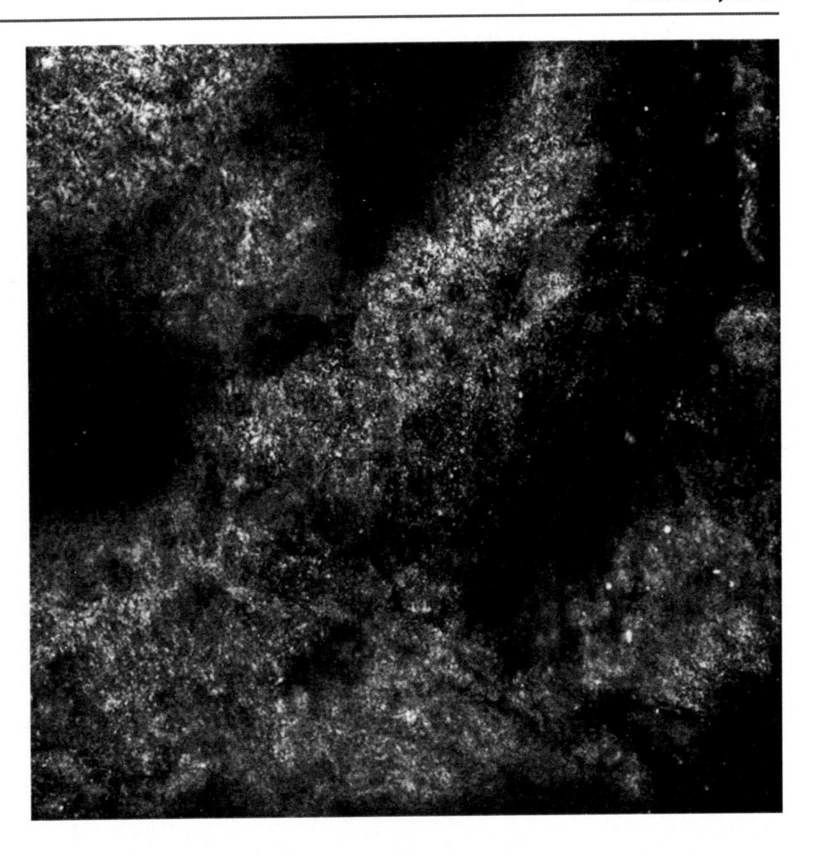

Fig. 18.1.7 Parakeratosis in an actinic keratosis

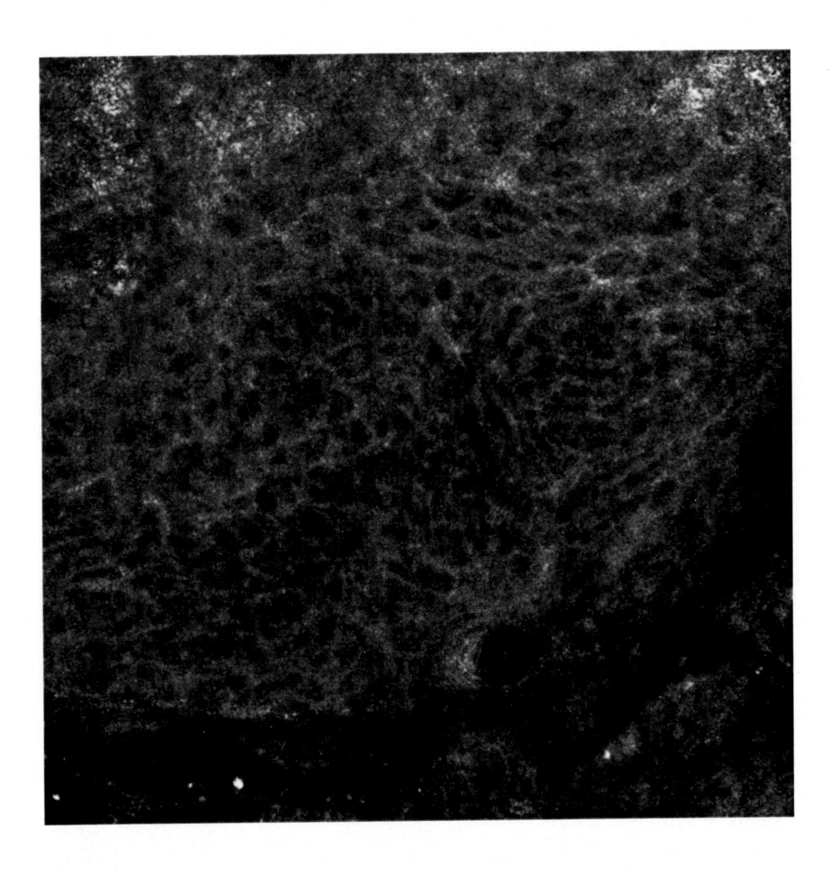

Fig. 18.1.8 Irregular honeycomb in an actinic keratosis

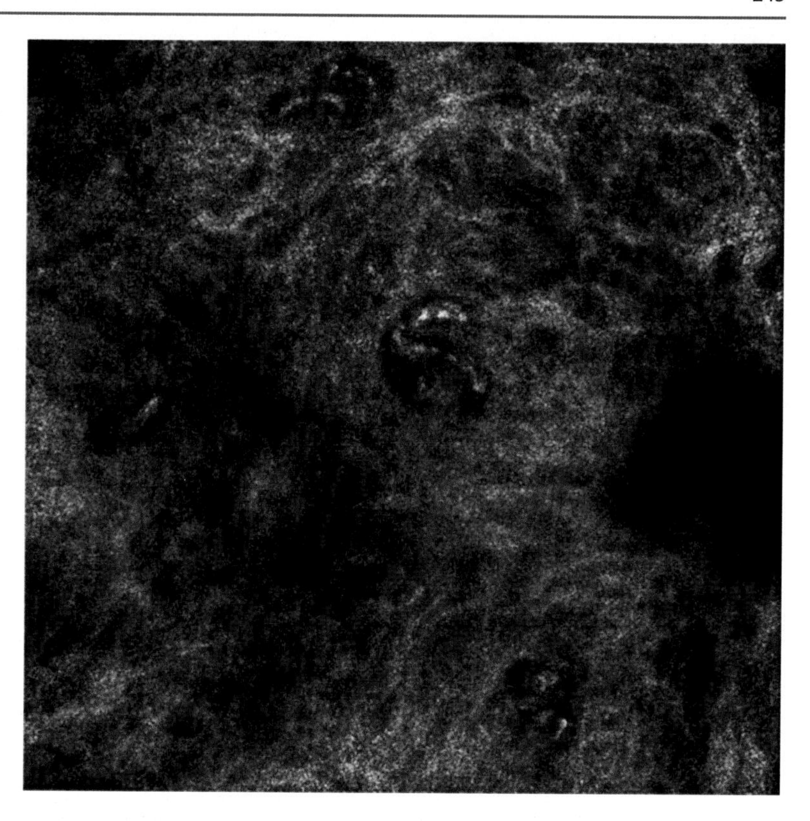

Fig. 18.1.9 Round blood vessels in a squamous cell carcinoma

1. *Corneal plugs:* bright laminar onion-like structures on epidermal surface.
2. *Corneal cysts:* well-circumscribed large, round, highly refractive intra-epidermal structures.
3. *Surface holes and fissures (crypts):* round to linear structures, darker than the surrounding epidermal surface.
4. *Elongated cords:* thickened interwoven or parallel bright tubular structures at the DEJ, containing aggregated bright, monomorphic cells with ill-defined borders.
5. *Bulbous projections:* round to oval structures contiguous with or adjacent to the elongated cords.

In reticulated SK, elongated cords are the predominant findings whereas in thicker SK fissures and crypts, acanthosis and changes related to keratinization such as follicular plugs or keratin cysts are the predominant findings. When SK are strongly pigmented, numerous dendritic cells corresponding to melanocytes and plumb cells corresponding to macrophages are seen in the epidermal and in the dermis, respectively. In some SK vessels with a hairpin shape most of them of fine diameter can be distinguished. This finding is also frequently found in inflamed SK.

In seborrheic keratosis exhibiting "fat fingers" under dermoscopy, RCM shows in the mosaics the digitate linear and curvilinear structures that directly correlate with the gyri [14]. Furthermore, when imaging deeper, the roundish dermal papillae projecting can be appreciated upward into the "fat fingers."

Figures 18.1.10–18.1.13 illustrate the main findings in SK. In Chap. 24 confocal microscopy of seborrheic keratosis and other nonmelanocytic tumors is presented.

18.4 Solar Lentigo

Unique RCM characteristics of lentigines have been described, facilitating rapid in vivo discrimination from malignant melanoma.

The most striking finding in solar lentigo by RCM is observed at the dermoepidermal junction with increase in the density of dermal papillae surrounded by a bright monomorphic layer of cells [15, 17]. Distinct patterns can be distinguished, as these papillae assume irregular geometric shapes with a rim of bright, highly refractile, monomorphic, and cytologically benign-appearing cells. These findings are absent in lentigo maligna melanoma. Lentigines exhibit an absence of atypical melanocytes, whereas the melanomas show atypical, bright, polymorphous cells present in a pagetoid pattern with coarse, branching dendrites or pleomorphic nucleated round cells observed throughout the epidermis.

Figures 18.1.14 and18.1.15 illustrate the main findings in solar lentigo.

18.5 Dermatofibroma

Dermatofibromas (DF) are very frequent benign cutaneous tumors with numerous clinical and pathological faces. By dermoscopy different patterns have been described in DF [18]. The stereotypical form of DF with central white patch and delicate reticulation at the periphery has a perfect

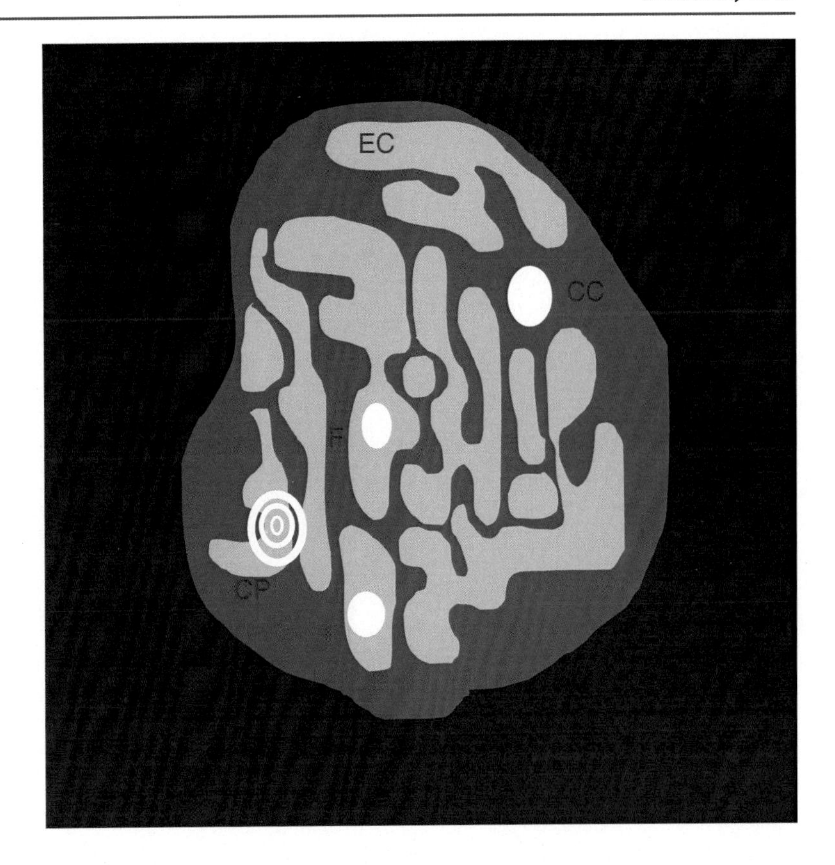

Fig. 18.1.10 RCM findings in seborrheic keratosis: corneal plugs; corneal cysts (CC); surface holes and fissures (crypts) (F); elongated cords and bulbous projections (EC)

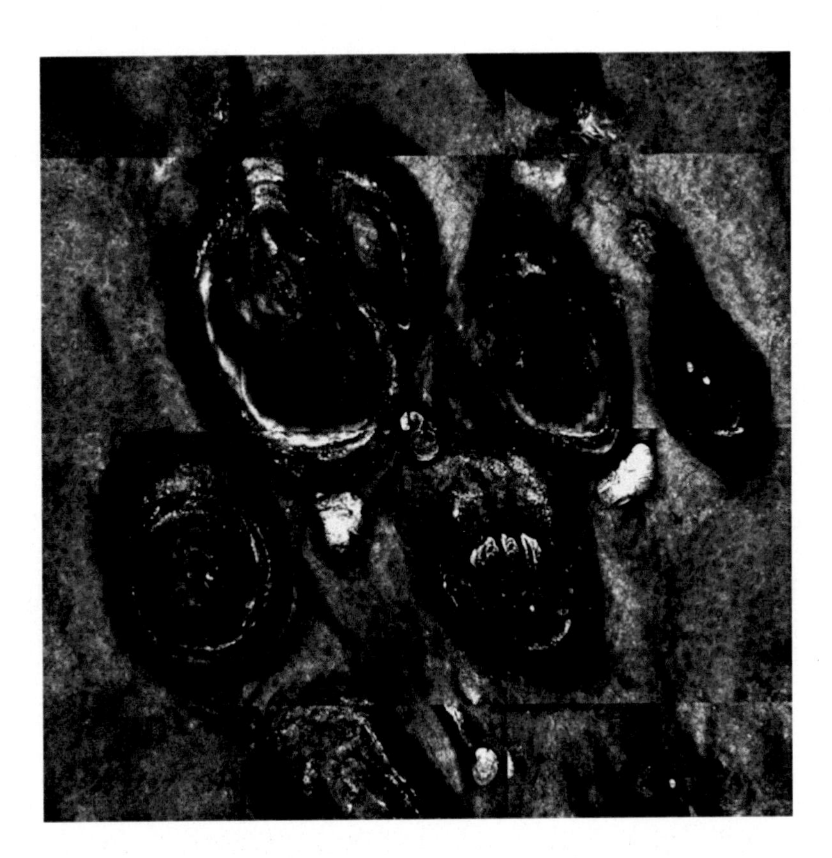

Fig. 18.1.11 Corneal plugs and cysts in a seborrheic keratosis

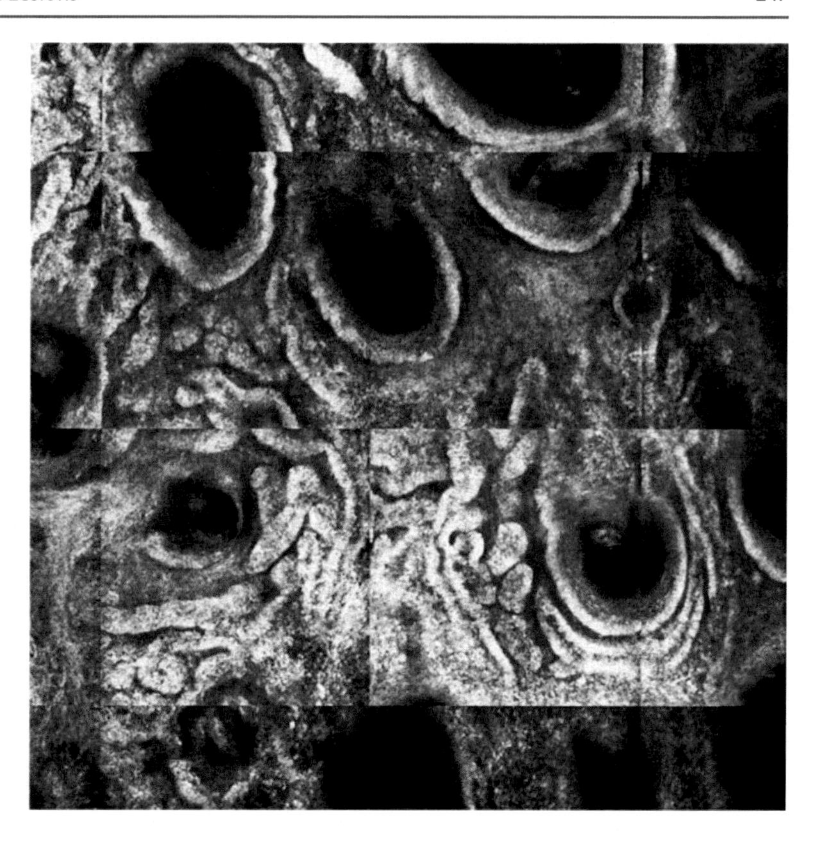

Fig. 18.1.12 Typical pattern of elongated cords and bulbous projections in a seborrheic keratosis

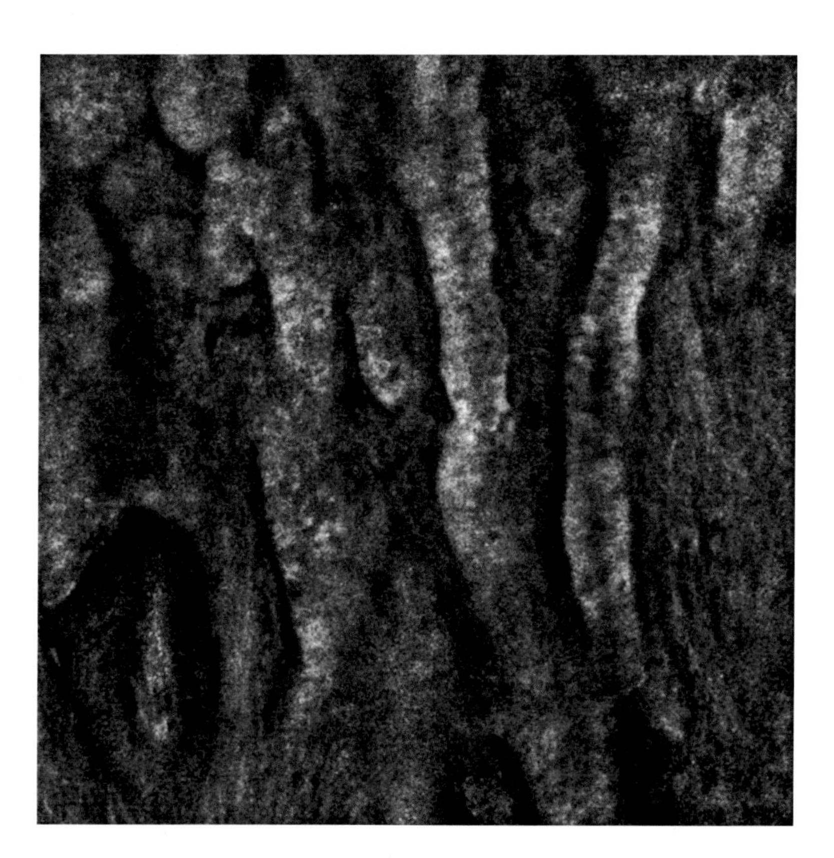

Fig. 18.1.13 Detail of elongated cords in a reticulated seborrheic keratosis of the face

Fig. 18.1.14 RCM findings in solar lentigo with increase in the density of dermal papillae surrounded by a bright monomorphic layer of cells

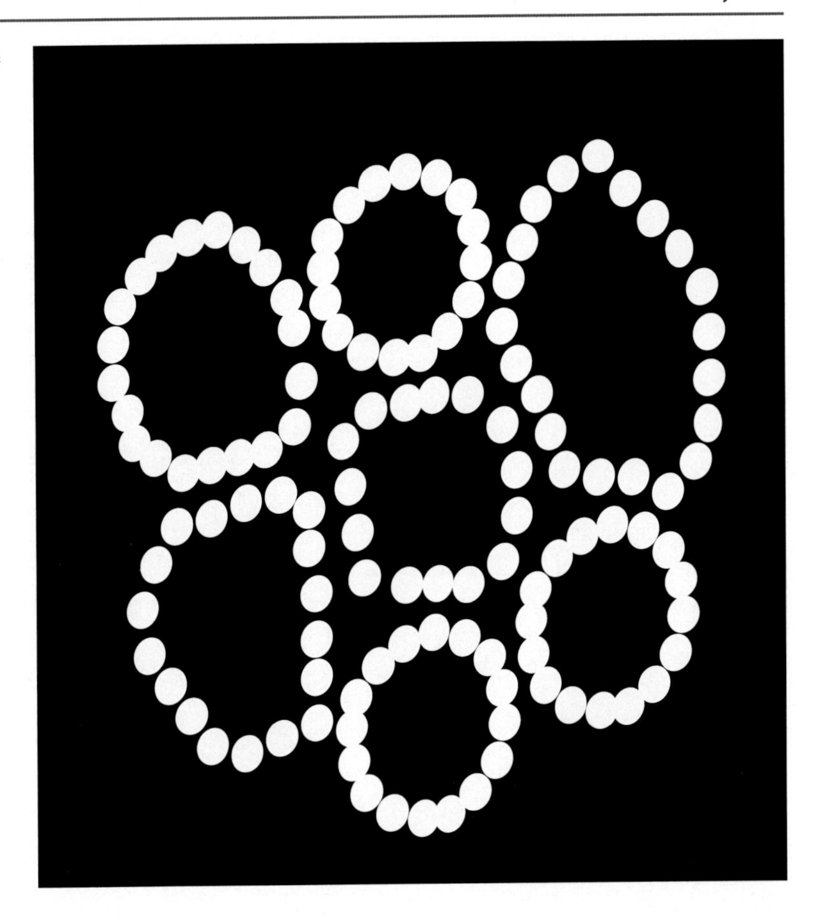

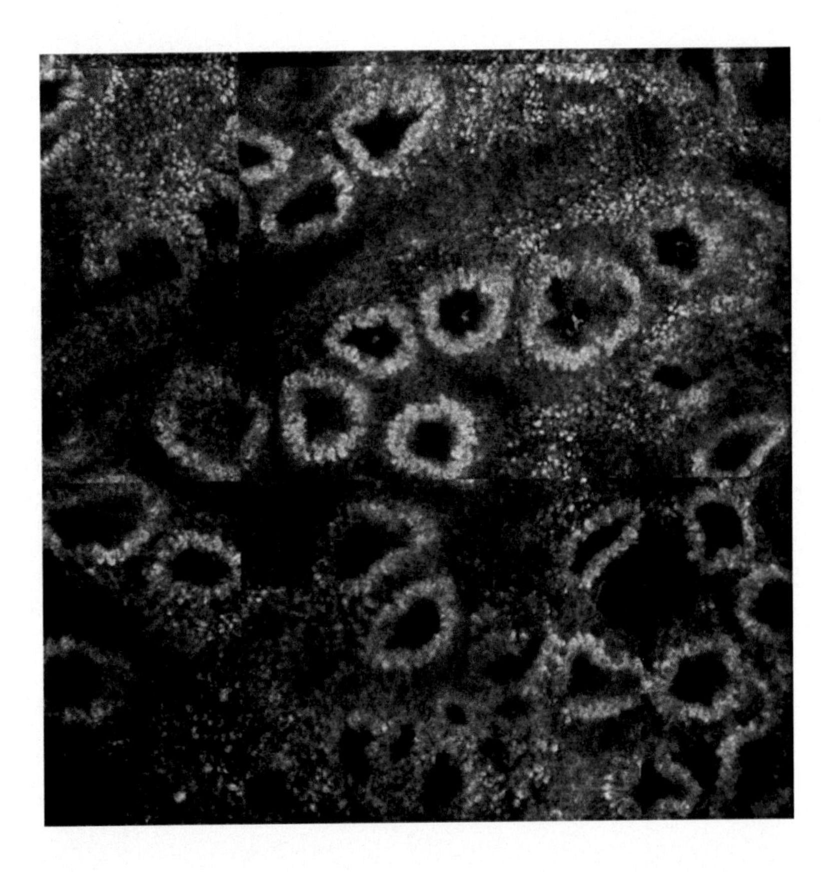

Fig. 18.1.15 Typical pattern of a solar lentigo

correlation under RCM with mosaics. When DF are pigmented dermoscopy usually show a typical delicate reticulation with typical globule-like structures [19]. These structures correspond on RCM to*wide bright rings* composed of pigmented basal keratinocytes around dermal papillae without melanocytic proliferation.*Collagen bundles* with thin spaces separate the bright rings. The epidermis in DF exhibits a typical honeycomb pattern and in some DF acanthosis can be observed. A high-magnification RCM optical section (0.5 × 0.5 mm) at the dermal-epidermal junction level focusing on globule-like structures shows wider rings composed of monomorphic bright, round cells (arrows), around a darker dermal papilla. At the center of the lesion, even if pigment is not seen by dermoscopy, there are similar bright rings, albeit wider and more spaced apart. Notably, the rings at the center of the lesion are separated by bright thick fibrillar structures, compatible with dermal collagen that is present in the fibrotic area of DF seen as a white patch by dermoscopy. In many DF vessels usually of fine calibre are also frequently seen by dermoscopy and RCM.

Major findings of DF by RCM are the following:

1. Increased density of bright papillary rings.
2. Bright thick fibrillar structures in the center.

Figure 18.1.16 illustrates the main findings in DF.

18.6 Sebaceous Hyperplasia

Sebaceous hyperplasia (SH) is a frequent benign tumor that can mimic BCC by clinical examination. Under dermoscopy SH exhibit crown vessels and yellow globules corresponding to the gland with lipid contend. Like dermoscopy confocal scanning laser microscopy may help to discriminate between BCC and SH [20, 21]. In SH, imaging reveals an enlarged sebaceous lobule consisting of cuboidal cells with bright speckled cytoplasm and centrally located nuclei and a dilated central follicular infundibulum. Bands of collagen that separate the lobules can be seen if they are superficial but in some SH only the duct can be clearly distinguished when the gland is too deep for RCM resolution. Vessels are distinguished in SH embracing the sebaceous lobules at the periphery.

Figure 18.1.17 illustrates the main findings in SH.

18.7 Angioma and Angiokeratoma

In cherry angioma the predominant findings of RCM are vascular spaces in the superficial dermis seen as wide dark spaces with thin septa displaying moving small, round bright and brisk structures (blood cells) [22].

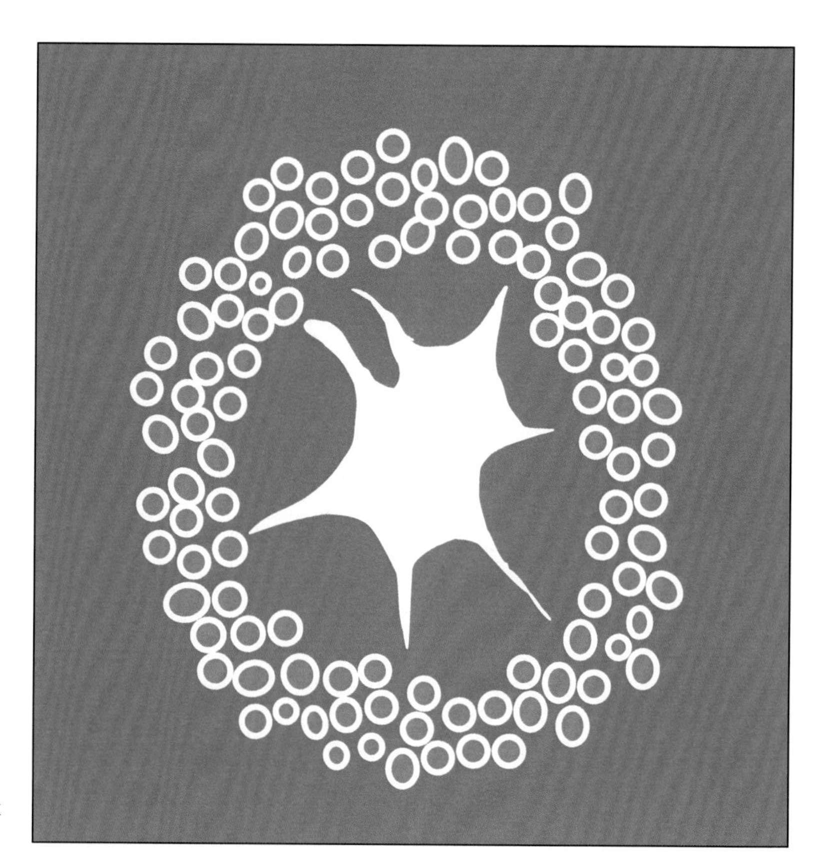

Fig. 18.1.16 Major findings in dermatofibroma are increased density of bright papillary rings and bright thick fibrillar structures in the center

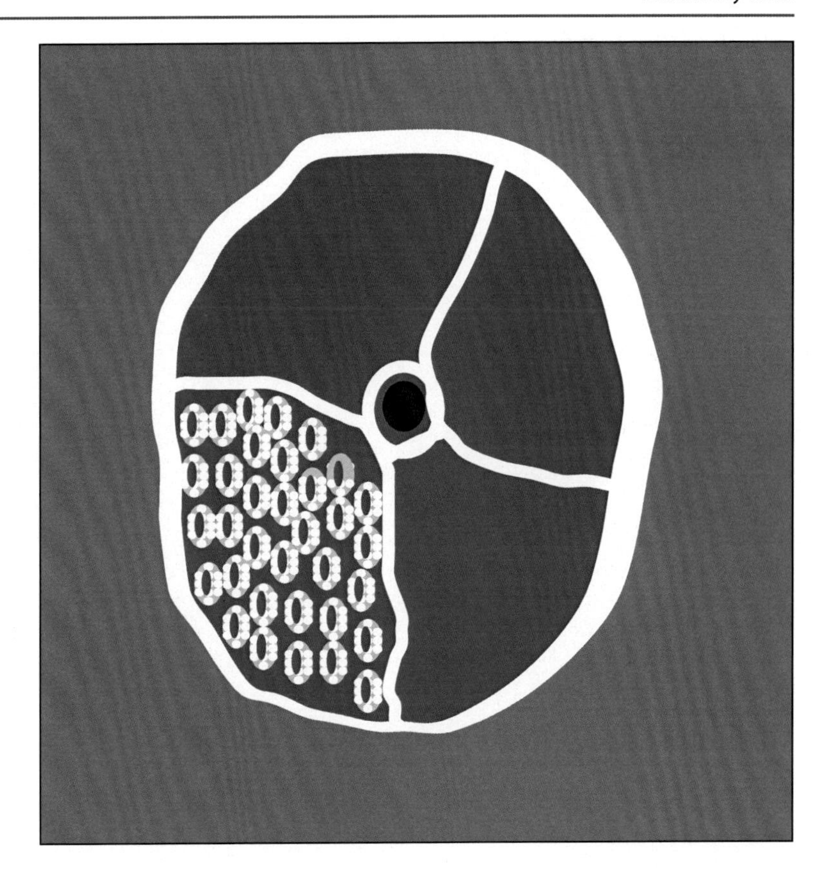

Fig. 18.1.17 Main findings in sebaceous hyperplasia: enlarged sebaceous lobules consisting of cuboidal cells with bright speckled cytoplasm and centrally located nuclei and a dilated central follicular infundibulum

In the case of angiokeratoma, the tumor exhibits thrombosed vascular spaces and findings of keratoma. By RCM in addition to the findings seen in cherry angioma a thickened stratum corneum and epidermis are found. The existence of thrombosis in the vascular spaces is seen as blood cells packing the vascular lumina.

Figures 18.1.18 and18.1.19 illustrate the main findings in vascular lesions.

18.8 Other Nonmelanocytic Tumors

RCM has been used to study different nonmelanocytic tumors such as clear-cell acanthoma, trichoepithelioma, adult xanthogranuloma or cutaneous Paget disease.

In *trichoepithelioma tumor* islands shown to be connected with follicular structures, [23] dark spaces with refractile material in the center and brightly refractile parallel bundles wrapping the tumor islands, corresponding to the collagen bundles surrounding the tumor.

In *adult xanthogranuloma*, the stereotypical Touton cells are seen as large highly refractive atypical cells, some of them exhibiting pleomorphic nuclei, present in the upper dermis [24]. A dense amorphous stromal component with some poorly refractive cells exhibiting mild demarcation is also present.

Pigmented cutaneous Paget disease has been described with clinical, dermoscopical, confocal and histopathological study [25-27]. In this case, clinical and dermoscopic findings were consistent with melanoma. Confocal microscopic features, such as large reflecting cells with dark nuclei spreading upward in pagetoid fashion, were also suggestive of melanoma.

In *clear-cell acanthoma* RCM is able to identify most of the established diagnostic histological features for this tumor: well-circumscribed lesions, often edged by a hyperkeratotic collarette with parakeratosis; inflammatory cells in the spinous layer; large keratinocytes; acanthosis with papillomatosis; epidermal disarray; and dilated capillaries forming glomeruloid shapes in the upper dermis. In conclusion, RCM appears to be a useful tool for in vivo diagnosis of clear cell acanthoma and may help avoid unnecessary biopsies [28].

In Chap. 25, a poutpourri of skin tumors with images can be found. In future the number of criteria in RCM for other skin neoplasms will grow and new studies with larger number of cases will make more accurate those criteria already described.

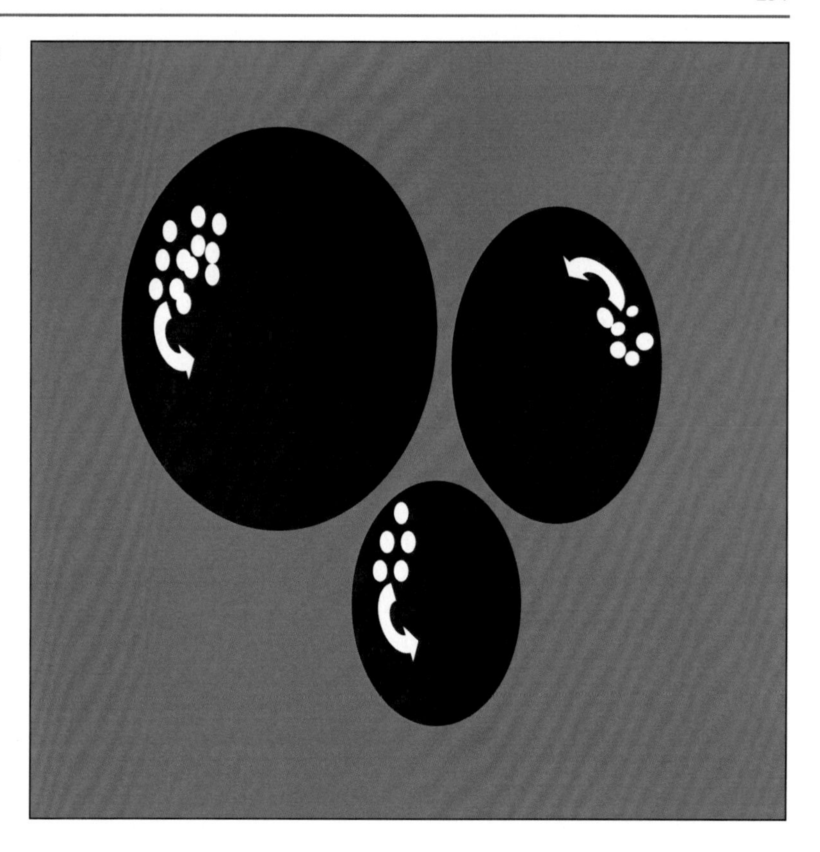

Fig. 18.1.18 Main findings in vascular lesions with wide dark spaces with thin septa displaying moving small, round bright and brisk structures (blood cells)

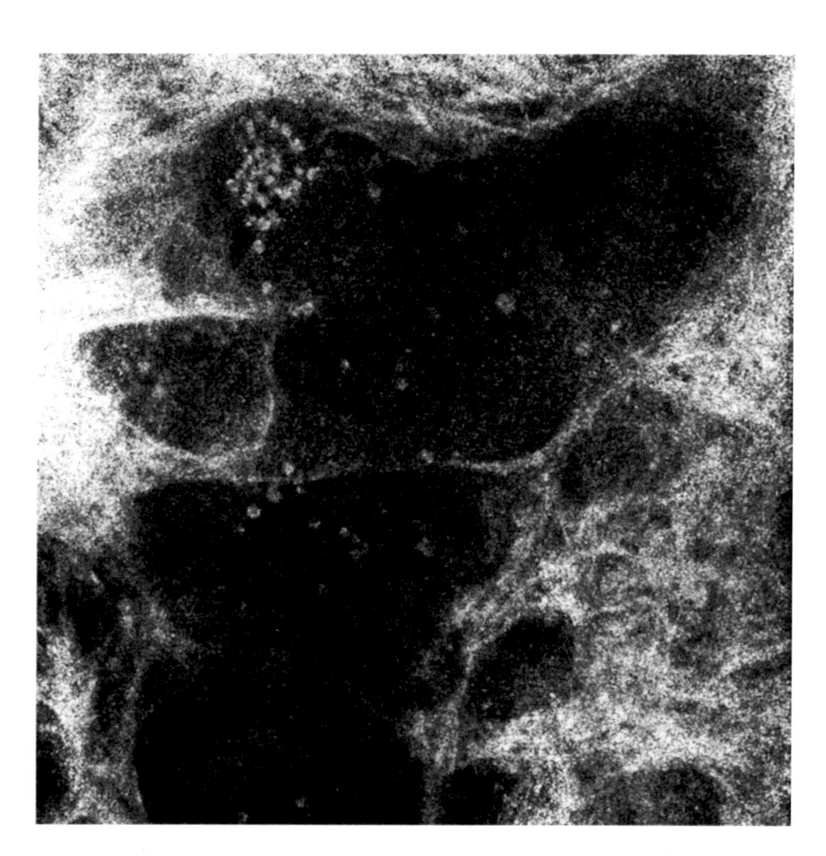

Fig. 18.1.19 Confocal microscopy of an angioma. Wide dark spaces with thin septa. In real-time imaging moving small, round bright and brisk structures (blood cells) are seen

References

1. González S, Tannous Z.Real-time, in vivo confocal reflectance microscopy of basal cell carcinoma.J Am Acad Dermatol. 2002 Dec;47(6):869-74.
2. Tannous Z, Torres A, González S.In vivo real-time confocal reflectance microscopy: a noninvasive guide for Mohs micrographic surgery facilitated by aluminum chloride, an excellent contrast enhancer. Dermatol Surg. 2003 Aug;29(8):839-46.
3. Karen JK, Gareau DS, Dusza SW, Tudisco M, Rajadhyaksha M, Nehal KS. Detection of basal cell carcinomas in Mohs excisions with fluorescence confocal mosaicing microscopy.Br J Dermatol. 2009 Jun;160(6):1242-50.
4. Ahlgrimm-Siess V, Horn M, Koller S, Ludwig R, Gerger A, Hofmann-Wellenhof R. Monitoring efficacy of cryotherapy for superficial basal cell carcinomas with in vivo reflectance confocal microscopy: a preliminary study. J Dermatol Sci. 2009;53(1):60-4.
5. Segura S, Puig S, Carrera C, Lecha M, Borges V, Malvehy J.Non-invasive management of non-melanoma skin cancer in patients with cancer predisposition genodermatosis: a role for confocal microscopy and photodynamic therapy.J Eur Acad Dermatol Venereol. 2011;25(7):819-27.
6. Segura S, Puig S, Carrera C, Palou J, Malvehy J.Development of a two-step method for the diagnosis of melanoma by reflectance confocal microscopy.J Am Acad Dermatol. 2009;61(2):216-29.
7. Astner S, Dietterle S, Otberg N, Röwert-Huber HJ, Stockfleth E, Lademann J. Clinical applicability of in vivo fluorescence confocal microscopy for noninvasive diagnosis and therapeutic monitoring of nonmelanoma skin cancer. J Biomed Opt. 2008;13(1):014003.
8. Segura S, Puig S, Carrera C, Palou J, Malvehy J.Dendritic cells in pigmented basal cell carcinoma: a relevant finding by reflectance-mode confocal microscopy.Arch Dermatol. 2007;143(7):883-6.
9. Nori S, Rius-Díaz F, Cuevas J, Goldgeier M, Jaen P, Torres A, González S.Sensitivity and specificity of reflectance-mode confocal microscopy for in vivo diagnosis of basal cell carcinoma: a multicenter study. J Am Acad Dermatol. 2004;51(6):923-30.
10. Ulrich M, Maltusch A, Rius-Diaz F, Röwert-Huber J, González S, Sterry W, Stockfleth E, Astner S.Clinical applicability of in vivo reflectance confocal microscopy for the diagnosis of actinic keratoses.Dermatol Surg. 2008;34(5):610-9.
11. Rishpon A, Kim N, Scope A, Porges L, Oliviero MC, Braun RP, Marghoob AA, Fox CA, Rabinovitz HS. Reflectance confocal microscopy criteria for squamous cell carcinomas and actinic keratoses. Arch Dermatol. 2009;145(7):766-72.
12. Braga JC, Scope A, Klaz I, Mecca P, González S, Rabinovitz H, Marghoob AA. The significance of reflectance confocal microscopy in the assessment of solitary pink skin lesions. J Am Acad Dermatol. 2009;61(2):230-41.
13. Ahlgrimm-Siess V, Cao T, Oliviero M, Hofmann-Wellenhof R, Rabinovitz HS, Scope A.The vasculature of nonmelanocytic skin tumors in reflectance confocal microscopy, II: Vascular features of seborrheic keratosis. Arch Dermatol. 2010;146(6):694-5.
14. "Fat fingers:" a clue in the dermoscopic diagnosis of seborrheic keratoses. Kopf AW, Rabinovitz H, Marghoob A, Braun RP, Wang S, Oliviero M, Polsky D.J Am Acad Dermatol. 2006;55(6):1089-91.
15. Richtig E, Hofmann-Wellenhof R, Kopera D, El-Shabrawi-Caelen L, Ahlgrimm-Siess V. In vivo analysis of solar lentigines by reflectance confocal microscopy before and after Q-switched ruby laser treatment. Acta Derm Venereol. 2011 ;91(2):164-8.
16. In vivo microscopic approaches for facial melanocytic lesions after quality-switched ruby laser therapy: time-sequential imaging of melanin and melanocytes of solar lentigo in Asian skin.Yamashita T, Negishi K, Hariya T, Yanai M, Iikura T, Wakamatsu S. Dermatol Surg. 2010;36(7):1138-47.
17. Langley RG, Burton E, Walsh N, Propperova I, Murray SJ. In vivo confocal scanning laser microscopy of benign lentigines: comparison to conventional histology and in vivo characteristics of lentigo maligna. J Am Acad Dermatol. 2006;55(1):88-97.
18. Zaballos P, Puig S, Llambrich A, Malvehy J. Dermoscopy of dermatofibromas: a prospective morphological study of 412 cases. Arch Dermatol. 2008 Jan;144(1):75-83.
19. Scope A, Ardigo M, Marghoob AACorrelation of dermoscopic globule-like structures of dermatofibroma using reflectance confocal microscopy.. Dermatology. 2008;216(1):81-2.
20. Propperova I, Langley RG. Reflectance-mode confocal microscopy for the diagnosis of sebaceous hyperplasia in vivo. Arch Dermatol. 2007 Jan;143(1):134.
21. Aghassi D, González E, Anderson RR, Rajadhyaksha M, González S. Elucidating the pulsed-dye laser treatment of sebaceous hyperplasia in vivo with real-time confocal scanning laser microscopy. J Am Acad Dermatol. 2000 Jul;43(1 Pt 1):49-53.
22. Astner S, González S, Cuevas J, Röwert-Huber J, Sterry W, Stockfleth E, Ulrich M.Preliminary evaluation of benign vascular lesions using in vivo reflectance confocal microscopy. Dermatol Surg. 2010 ;36(7):1099-110.
23. Ardigo M, Zieff J, Scope A, Gill M, Spencer P, Deng L, Marghoob AA. Dermoscopic and reflectance confocal microscope findings of trichoepithelioma. Dermatology. 2007;215(4):354-8.
24. Lovato L, Salerni G, Puig S, Carrera C, Palou J, Malvehy J.Adult xanthogranuloma mimicking basal cell carcinoma: dermoscopy, reflectance confocal microscopy and pathological correlation. Dermatology. 2010;220(1):66-70.
25. Longo C, Fantini F, Cesinaro AM, Bassoli S, Seidenari S, Pellacani G. Pigmented mammary Paget disease: dermoscopic, in vivo reflectance-mode confocal microscopic, and immunohistochemical study of a case. Arch Dermatol. 2007;143(6):752-4.
26. Pan ZY, Liang J, Zhang QA, Lin JR, Zheng ZZ. In vivo reflectance confocal microscopy of extramammary Paget disease: Diagnostic evaluation and surgical management. J Am Acad Dermatol. 2011 May 25.
27. Richtig E, Ahlgrimm-Siess V, Arzberger E, Hofmann-Wellenhof Noninvasive differentiation between mamillary eczema and Paget disease by in vivo reflectance confocal microscopy on the basis of two case reports. R. Br J Dermatol. 2011;165(2):440-1.
28. Ardigo M, Buffon RB, Scope A, Cota C, Buccini P, Berardesca E, Pellacani G, Marghoob AA, Gill M. Comparing in vivo reflectance confocal microscopy, dermoscopy, and histology of clear-cell acanthoma. Dermatol Surg. 2009.

Dermoscopic and Histopathologic Correlations

19

Harold S. Rabinovitz, Margaret Oliviero, Joseph Malvehy, and Susana Puig

RCM is the perfect tool to establish optimal correlation between dermoscopic features and histopathology as it offers the ability to view skin structures as well as cell and microscopic components [1–3]. RCM findings to be understood and properly applied need to be correlated with histopathology. In this chapter, some of the most important RCM structures in nonmelanocytic neoplasms are briefly discussed with their dermoscopic and/or histologic correlates.

19.1 Basal Cell Carcinoma [2–6] (Fig. 19.1)

19.1.1 Superficial Horizontal Branched Vessels [2, 7]

Prominent vasculature that is enlarged, horizontal, branched, with a slow flow and sometimes white blood cells are seen hugging the lumen wall (traffic rolling phenomena).

- Dermoscopic correlation: Arborizing vessels thick and thin (serpentine branched) and in-focus branched vessels
- Histopathological correlation: Vessels in cross section are located between epidermis and dermal tumor nodules

19.1.2 Tumor Nodules/Islands

Dermal reflective tumor islands surrounded by a dark space (see clefting) and that may be delineated at the periphery by cells elongated and streaming (polarization of the nuclei—see palisade).

- Dermoscopy correlation: Ovoid nests and blue globules.
- Histopathological correlation: Tumor islands, basaloid islands with melanin.

Tumor islands may be hypo-reflective in nonpigmented BCC and then are identified by the presence of collagen bundles around them.

- Dermoscopy correlation: Nonpigmented pink areas.
- Histopathological correlation: Nests of basaloid cells without pigment

19.1.3 Dendritic Cells [6]

Sometimes, dendritic-shape structures can be identified within the tumor nodules, particularly noted at the periphery.

- Histopathological correlation: Benign melanocytes that are in association with the tumor island.

Dendritic-shape structures can be also identified in the overlying epidermis in some BCCs.

- Histopathological correlation: Langerhans cells.

19.1.4 Bright Plump Cells and Bright Dots

These structures are also located between tumor nodules.

- Dermoscopy correlation: Gray dots.
- Histopathology correlation: Melanophages and free melanin.

19.1.5 Nuclei Palisade [3]

Presence of elongated monomorphic basaloid nuclei, also described as polarization of these nuclei along the same axis of orientation.

- Histopathology correlation: Polarization of basal cells.

H.S. Rabinovitz (✉) • M. Oliviero
Skin and Cancer Associates/ADM, Plantation, FL, USA
e-mail: harold@admcorp.com

J. Malvehy • S. Puig
Department of Dermatology, Melanoma Unit,
Hospital Clinic of Barcelona, Barcelona, Spain
e-mail: jmalvehy@clinic.ub.es; susipuig@gmail.com

R. Hofmann-Wellenhof et al. (eds.), *Reflectance Confocal Microscopy for Skin Diseases*,
DOI 10.1007/978-3-642-21997-9_19, © Springer-Verlag Berlin Heidelberg 2012

19.1.6 Clefting [4]

Tumor islands are tightly packed in the papillary dermis. They may be oval, polycyclic or appear as elongated cordlike structures surrounded by a cleft-like space.
- Histopathology correlation: Peritumoral cleft-like spaces are also seen in BCC on histopathology and correspond to the peritumoral mucin deposition.

19.2 Actinic Keratosis, Squamous Cell Carcinoma and Bowen Disease [2, 8] (Fig. 19.2)

19.2.1 Nucleated Corneocytes

RCM nucleated corneocytes may be seen as the presence of black nuclei shadows in the stratum corneum.
- Dermoscopy: Scale is better visualized with noncontact polarized light.
- Histopathology correlation: parakeratosis.

19.2.2 Broadened and Atypical Honeycomb

In keratinocytic neoplasms, the honeycomb is atypical, broadened and with individual cells that vary in size and shape. In some areas the honeycomb features are not visualized and the pattern is disarranged.
- Histopathology correlation: Atypical keratinocytes in the epidermis.

19.2.3 Round Blood Vessels Traversing Through the Dermal Papilla

In SCCs the epidermal proliferation tend to diminish the diameter of the dermal papilla where small vessels (dotted vessels in dermoscopy) may be seen. In larger papillae, vessels may be coiled (glomerular vessels).
- Dermoscopy: Clusters of glomerular vessels (coiled vessels) or vessels seen as red dots.
- Histopathology correlation: Acanthosis with vessels visible in the center of dermal papillae.

19.3 Seborrheic Keratosis [2, 9]

19.3.1 Corneal Plugs and Corneal Cysts

Corneal plugs are bright laminar onion-like structures on the epidermal surface and corneal cysts are bright round homogeneous intraepidermal structures.
- Dermoscopy: Comedo-like openings and milia cysts.
- Histopathology correlation: corneal plugs are keratin-filled invaginations of the epidermis and corneal cysts are keratin-filled structures inside the epidermis without connection to the exterior.

19.3.2 Crypts

Crypts are deep hyporeflective folds on the epidermal surface.
- Dermoscopy: Fissures.
- Histopathology correlation: Invaginations of the seborrheic keratosis surface.

19.3.3 Cordlike Structures

They are monomorphic bright epidermal cords characterized by monomorphous cells at the dermoepidermal junction
- Dermoscopy: Fingerprint-like structures.
- Histopathology correlation: Elongation of the rete ridges is characteristic of solar lentigines and early seborrheic keratoses.

19.4 Angiomas [2]

19.4.1 Vascular Spaces

Large dark spaces with blood cells inside and slow flow.
- Dermoscopy: Red lagoons (lacunae).
- Histopathology correlation: Dermal vascular proliferation with vascular spaces.

19.5 Dermatofibromas [2]

19.5.1 Broadened Bright Dermal Fibers

- Dermoscopy: Central White patch.
- Histopathology correlation: Thickening of the dermal collagen.

19.6 Paget Disease

19.6.1 Bright Roundish Pagetoid Cells

- Histopathology correlation: Neoplastic cells showing glandular differentiation.

19.7 Ocronosis [10]

19.7.1 Banana Bodies

With RCM multiple banana-shaped nonrefractile structures are seen in dermis.

- Dermoscopy: Irregular brown-gray globular, annular and arciform structures.
- Histopathology correlation: focal deposition of ochronotic pigment (yellow to brown material) in the papillary and middle dermis.

19.8 Xanthogranuloma [11]

19.8.1 Multinucleated Giant Cells

- Histopathology correlation: Touton cells.

19.8.2 Large Highly Refractive Atypical Cells

Large cells some of them exhibiting pleomorphic nuclei.

- Histopathology correlation: Cells with foamy xanthomatous cytoplasm

	RCM	Dermoscopy	Histopathology
BCC	– Superficial horizontal branched vessels	– Arborizing vessels	– Vessels between epidermis and dermal tumor nodules
	– Reflective tumor islands surrounded by a dark space	– Maple leaf like structures and blue ovoid nests	– Basaloid tumor islands with melanin
	– Hypo-reflective tumor islands surrounded by collagen bundles	– Nonpigmented pink areas	– Nests of basaloid cells without pigment
	– Dendritic-shape structures within the tumor nodules	–	– Benign melanocytes
	– Dendritic cells in the overlying epidermis	–	– Langerhans cells
	– Bright plump cells and bright dots	– Gray dots	– Melanophages and free melanin
	– Nuclei palisade	–	– Polarization of basal cells
	– Clefting	–	– Peritumoral cleft-like spaces corresponding to the peritumoral mucin deposition
AK, SCC and Bowen disease	– Nucleated corneocytes	– Scale	– Parakeratosis
	– Broadened and atypical honeycomb	–	– Atypical keratinocytes in the epidermis
	– Round blood vessels traversing through the dermal papilla	– Dotted and glomerular vessels	– Acanthosis with vessels visible in the center of dermal papillae
SK	– Corneal plugs and corneal cysts	– Comedo-like openings and millia like cysts	
	– Crypts	– Fissures	– Invaginations
	– Cordlike structures	– Fingerprint-like structures	– Elongation of the rete ridges
Angioma	– Vascular spaces with slow flow	– Red lagoons	– Dermal vascular proliferation with vascular spaces
Dermatofibroma	– Broadened bright dermal fibers	– Central white patch	– Thickening of the dermal collagen
Paget diseases	– Bright roundish pagetoid cells	–	– Neoplastic cells showing glandular differentiation
Ocronosis	– Banana bodies	– Irregular brown-gray globular, annular and arciform structures	– Banana bodies. Focal deposition of ochronotic pigment (yellow to brown material) in the papillary and middle dermis
Xanthogranuloma	– Multinucleated giant cells		– Touton cells
	– Large highly refractive atypical cells		– Cells with foamy xanthomatous cytoplasm

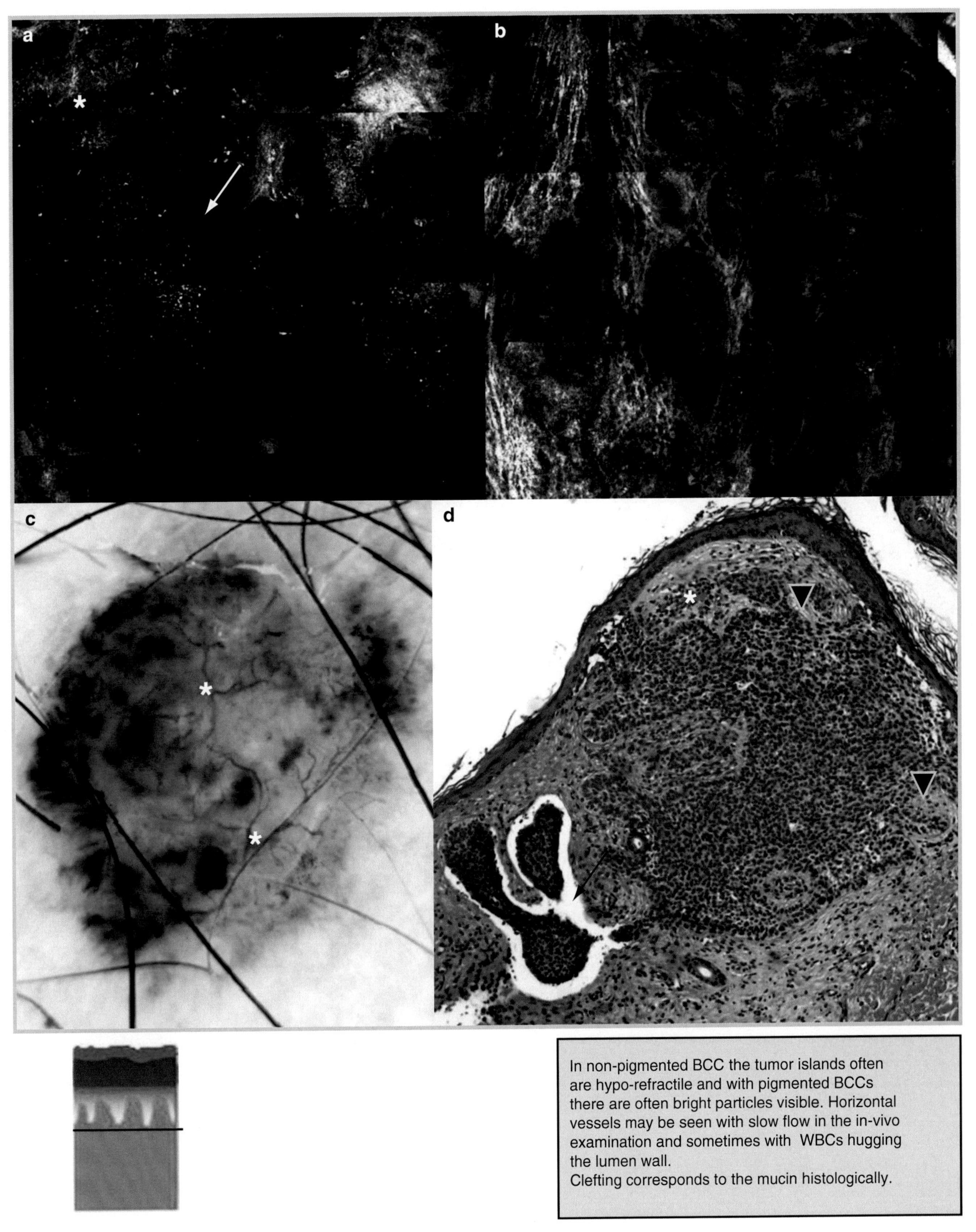

Fig. 19.1 Correlation of BCC RCM criteria with dermoscopy and histopathology. (**a**) Mosaic at reticular dermis (1.5 × 1.5 mm) with superficial horizontal vessels (*), tumor island with bright particles, palisading of the nuclei at the periphery and clefting (*arrow*). (**b**) Mosaic at dermis of other less pigmented area (1.5 × 1.5 mm) showing tumor island surrounded by collagen boundaries. (**c**) Dermoscopy of a BCC showing arborizing vessels (*), brown-gray globules and maple leaf like areas at the periphery. (**d**) Corresponding histopathology- with tumor nodules in dermis, with clefting (*arrow*), and mucin (*arrow head*) surrounding them. Superficial vessels (*)

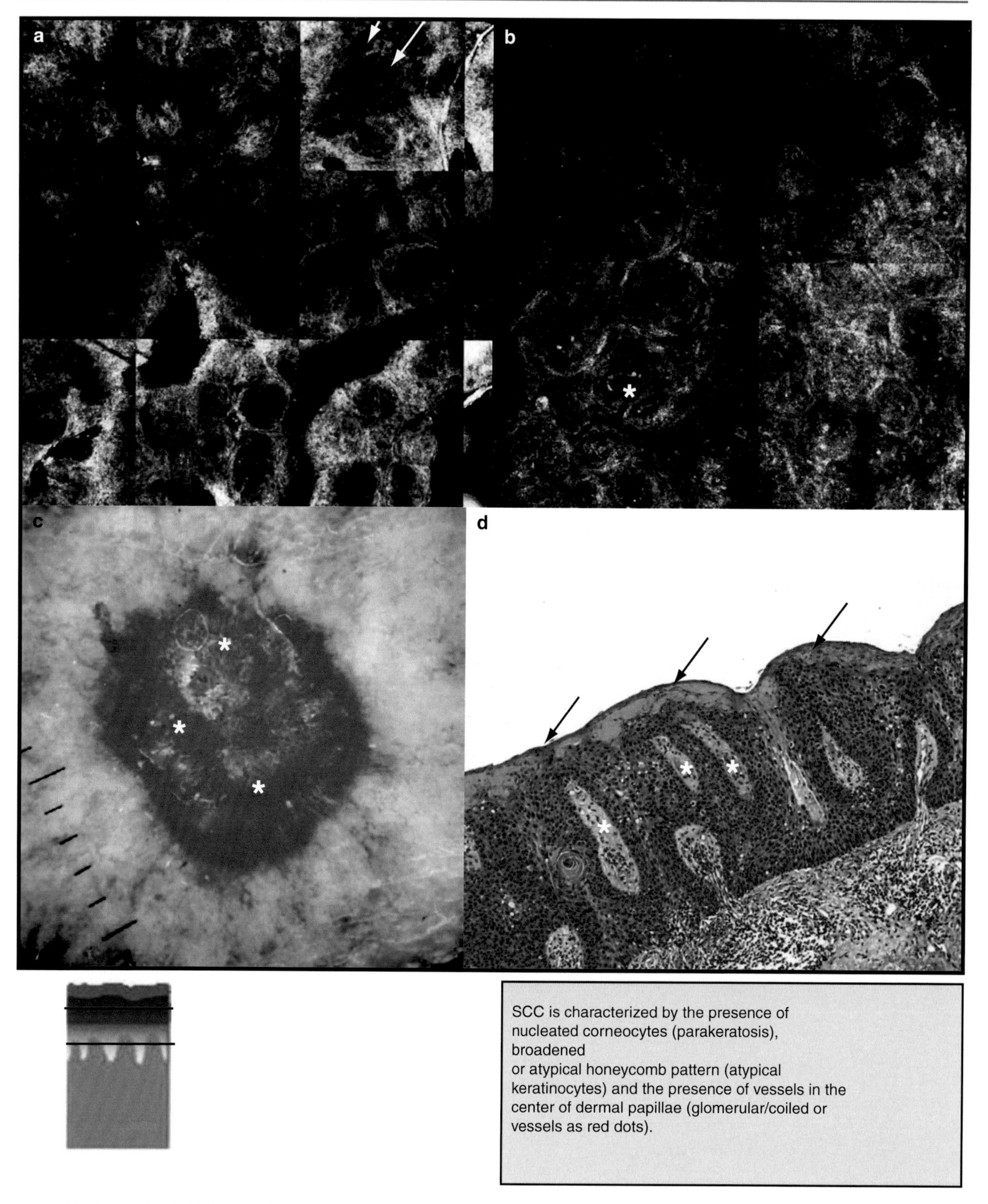

Fig. 19.2 Correlation of SCC RCM criteria with dermoscopy and histopathology. (**a**) Mosaic at upper epidermis (1.5 × 1.5 mm) with nucleated corneocytes seen as black nuclei shadows, atypical honeycomb, broadened and with individual cells that varies in size and orientation (*arrow*). (**b**) Mosaic at dermoepidermal junction (1 × 1 mm) showing vessels (*) in the center of the papillae surrounded by atypical keratinocytes. (**c**) Dermoscopy of a SCC showing glomerular vessels (*) and scales. (**d**) Corresponding histopathology with parakeratosis (*arrow*) atypical keratinocytes (*arrow head*) and vessels (*) in the center of the dermal papillae

References

1. Rajadhyasksha M, González S, Zavislan JM, Anderson RR, Webb RH (1999) In vivo confocal scanning laser microscopy of human skin II: advances in instrumentation and comparison with histology. J Invest Dermatol 113:293–303
2. Segura S, Puig S, Carrera C, Palou J, Malvehy J (2009) Development of a two-step method for the diagnosis of melanoma by reflectance confocal microscopy. J Am Acad Dermatol 61(2):216–229
3. González S, Tannus Z (2002) Real-time in vivo confocal reflectance microscopy of basal cell carcinoma. J Am Acad Dermatol 47: 869–874
4. Ulrich M, Roewert-Huber J, González S, Rius-Diaz F, Stockfleth E, Kanitakis J (2011) Peritumoral clefting in basal cell carcinoma: correlation of in vivo reflectance confocal microscopy and routine histology. J Cutan Pathol 38(2):190–195
5. Segura S, Puig S, Carrera C, Palou J, Malvehy J (2007) Dendritic cells in pigmented basal cell carcinoma: a relevant finding by reflectance-mode confocal microscopy. Arch Dermatol 143(7):883–886
6. Salerni G, Lovatto L, Carrera C, Palou J, Alos L, Puig-Butille JA, Badenas C, Malvehy J, Puig S (2011) Correlation among dermoscopy, confocal reflectance microscopy, and histologic features of melanoma and basal cell carcinoma collision tumor. Dermatol Surg 37(2):275–279
7. Ahlgrimm-Siess V, Cao T, Oliviero M, Hofmann-Wellenhof R, Rabinovitz HS, Scope A (2010) The vasculature of nonmelanocytic skin tumors in reflectance confocal microscopy: vascular features of basal cell carcinoma. Arch Dermatol 146(3):353–354
8. Ulrich M, Maltusch A, Rius-Diaz F, Röwert-Huber J, González S, Sterry W, Stockfleth E, Astner S (2008) Clinical applicability of in vivo reflectance confocal microscopy for the diagnosis of actinic keratoses. Dermatol Surg 34(5):610–619, Epub 2008 Feb 8
9. Ahlgrimm-Siess V, Cao T, Oliviero M, Hofmann-Wellenhof R, Rabinovitz HS, Scope A (2010) The vasculature of nonmelanocytic skin tumors in reflectance confocal microscopy, II: vascular features of seborrheic keratosis. Arch Dermatol 146(6):694–695
10. Gil I, Segura S, Martínez-Escala E, Lloreta J, Puig S, Vélez M, Pujol RM, Herrero-González JE (2010) Dermoscopic and reflectance confocal microscopic features of exogenous ochronosis. Arch Dermatol 146(9):1021–1025
11. Lovato L, Salerni G, Puig S, Carrera C, Palou J, Malvehy J (2010) Adult xanthogranuloma mimicking basal cell carcinoma: dermoscopy, reflectance confocal microscopy and pathological correlation. Dermatology 220(1):66–70

Solar Lentigo, Seborrheic Keratosis and Lichen Planus-Like Keratosis

20

Verena Ahlgrimm-Siess, Richard G.B. Langley, and Rainer Hofmann-Wellenhof

20.1 Introduction

Solar lentigo, seborrheic keratosis and lichen planus-like keratosis represent a spectrum of benign skin neoplasms with common clinical, dermoscopic and histopathologic findings [1]. Despite their variable clinical and dermoscopic appearances, the diagnosis can often be done on clinical grounds alone. The differentiation from malignant skin neoplasms, however, can be difficult in irritated, regressive or highly pigmented lesions. RCM may enable a non-invasive diagnosis in clinically and dermoscopically equivocal cases by visualizing key RCM features, which usually correlate well with histopathologic findings [2].

20.2 Solar Lentigo

Solar lentigines (SL) appear clinically as tan to dark brown macules of varying sizes and shape. Dermoscopy typically shows sharply demarcated lesion borders ("moth-eaten borders"), a regular pigment network, fingerprinting or a so-called pseudo-network in facial lesions. On the background of chronically sun-damaged skin, the clinical differentiation from lentigo maligna or pigmented actinic keratosis may be difficult; the presence of gray-blue areas in irritated SL and the lack of regular network structures in facial SL may hinder a correct diagnosis with dermoscopy.

V. Ahlgrimm-Siess (✉) • R. Hofmann-Wellenhof
Division of Dermatology and Venerology,
Medical University of Graz, Graz, Austria
e-mail: v.ahlgrimm-siess@salk.at; rainer.hofmann@medunigraz.at

R.G.B. Langley
Division of Dermatology, QE2 Health Science Center,
Dalhousie University, Halifax, Canada
e-mail: rgblangl@dal.ca

Confocal microscopy shows distinct findings in SL; a regular honeycomb pattern is usually visualized at epidermal layers and densely packed, round to polymorphous dermal papillae as well as branching tubular structures with bulbous projections (cord-like rete ridges) are observed at the DEJ [3]. The cord-like rete ridges correlate well with the elongated rete ridges seen in histopathology. Edged dermal papillae and highly reflective cord-like rete ridges may be visualized as network structures and fingerprinting with dermoscopy.

20.3 Seborrheic Keratosis

On clinical examination, seborrheic keratoses (SK) usually present as sharply demarcated plaques, papules or nodules; a peripheral macular portion may be observed in SK arising from a solar lentigo. Most SK are clinically tan to dark brown or flesh colored, whereas irritated or regressive SK often display a focal or universal pink or gray-blue hue. With dermoscopy, sharply demarcated borders, a gyrated surface, network-like structures, milia-like cysts and comedo-like openings are characteristically observed [4]. Irritated or regressive SK may show dermoscopic features suggestive of malignancy, such as gray-blue or milky-red areas and irregular vessels. Heavily pigmented seborrheic keratoses may even lack distinct dermoscopic criteria.

With confocal microscopy, a regular epidermal architecture is characteristically observed. Most SK display a typical honeycomb pattern that may be focally broadened in evolving or irritated SK. Heavily pigmented SK may show a typical cobblestone pattern due to the high content of melanin within basal and suprabasal keratinocytes. At the DEJ, densely packed round to polymorphous papillae are typically observed; cord-like rete ridges are seen in approximately one third of SK. Additional RCM criteria observed in SK correlate well with dermoscopic findings; epidermal projections

R. Hofmann-Wellenhof et al. (eds.), *Reflectance Confocal Microscopy for Skin Diseases*,
DOI 10.1007/978-3-642-21997-9_20,

and keratin-filled invaginations of the lesion surface, sharply demarcated horn cysts at epidermal layers and dilated blood vessels as well as melanophages within the upper dermis correlate with the gyri and sulci, comedo-like openings, milia-like cysts, looped/dotted vessels and gray-blue areas observed in dermoscopy. Most of these features are detected with higher sensitivity with RCM [2, 5].

20.4 Lichen Planus-Like Keratosis

Lichen planus-like keratosis (LPLK) is supposed to be either a SL or a SK undergoing regression; clinical, dermoscopic and histopathologic findings suggestive of SK or SL are therefore observed along with characteristic findings of LPLK. Clinically, LPLK appear as solitary macules or flat plaques with subtle scaling of the lesion surface. The lesion coloration may vary from pink-violaceous to blue-gray or black [6]. With dermoscopy, a localized or diffuse granular pattern with coarse, gray-blue granules is typically observed; dermoscopic structures of SL or SK may be additionally detected [7]. The differentiation of LPLK from melanoma, Bowen's disease or superficial basal cell carcinoma may be challenging clinically and with dermoscopy.

With confocal microscopy, a regular epidermal architecture as well as densely packed round to polymorphous papillae and/or cord-like rete ridges at the DEJ are seen. The upper dermis typically displays an inflammatory infiltrate composed of scattered bright spots, correlating to lymphocytes, and single or aggregated bright, triangular, non-nucleated cells, correlating to melanophages. The inflammatory infiltrate seen with RCM correlates well with the band-like lymphocytic infiltrate and melanophages in histopathology. Aggregates of melanophages are visualized as gray-blue granules with dermoscopy. Additional RCM features suggestive of SK, such as bright horn cysts, epidermal projections and keratin-filled invaginations of the lesion surface may be focally detected with RCM.

20.5 Conclusion

The detection of key RCM features of SL, SK and LPLK in the absence of confocal criteria suggestive of malignancy (e.g. pagetoid nucleated cells, disarrangement of the DEJ, cerebriform/basaloid dermal nests) may enable a non-invasive differentiation of clinically and dermoscopically equivocal cases from melanoma, squamous cell carcinoma or basal cell carcinoma.

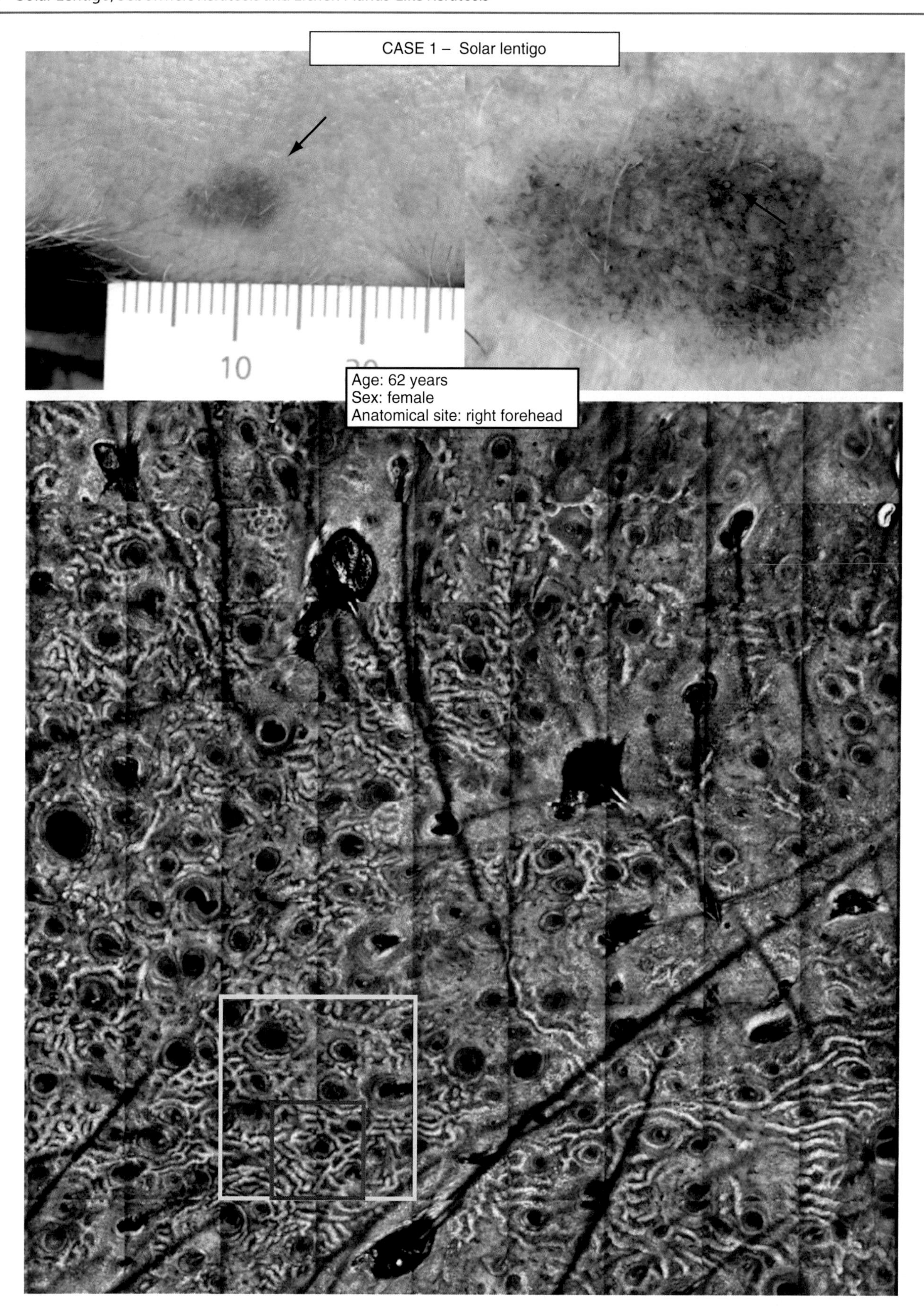

Fig. 20.1 RCM mosaic (4.5 × 4.5 mm) at the DEJ. Bright, branching tubular structures with bulbous projections are observed at the DEJ

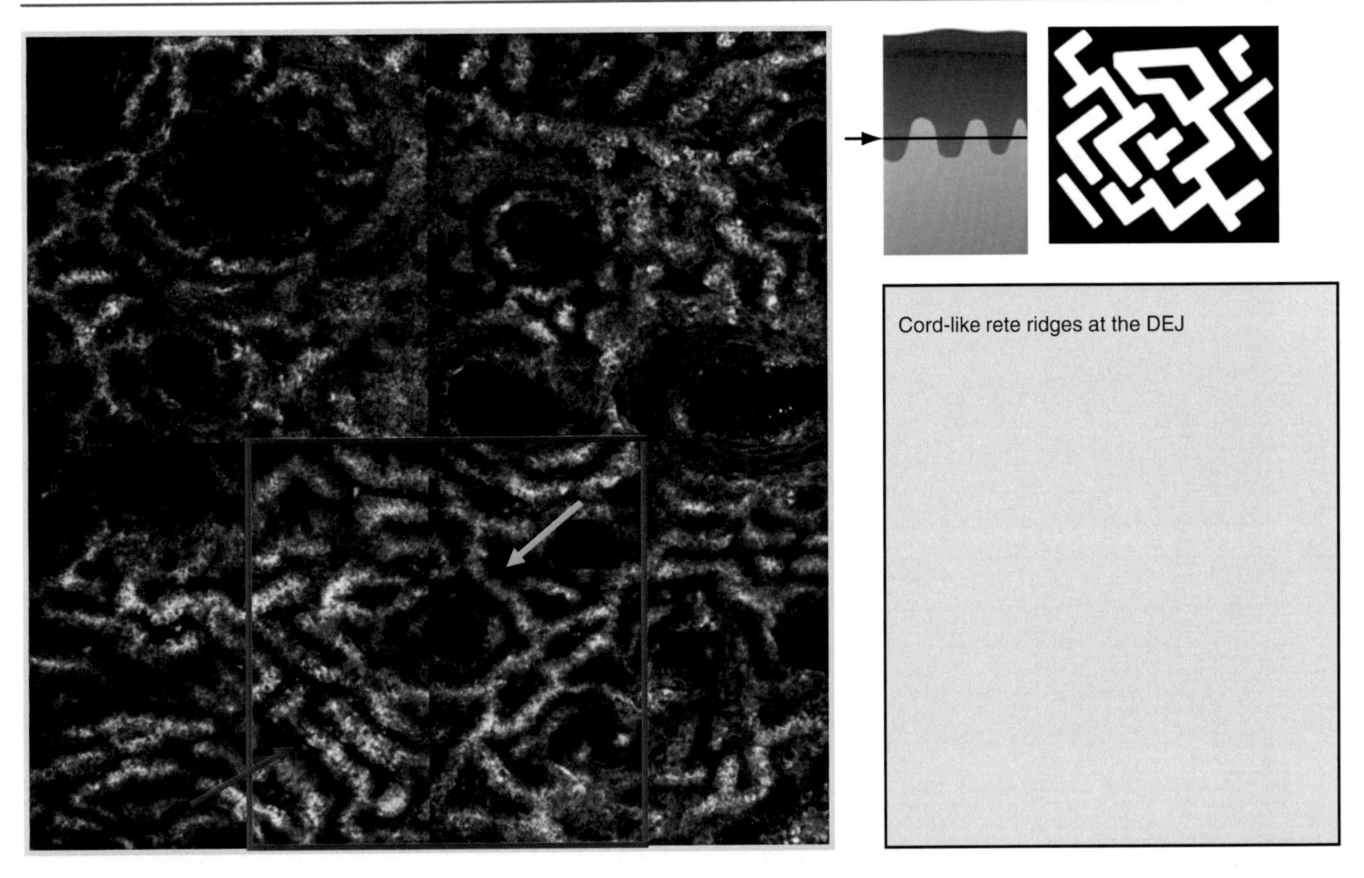

Fig. 20.1.1 RCM mosaic (1 × 1 mm) at the DEJ shows densely packed, bright cord-like rete ridges (*red arrow*), which may be visualised as fingerprinting with dermoscopy. Cord-like rete ridges surrounding adnexal openings are additionally seen (*green arrow*)

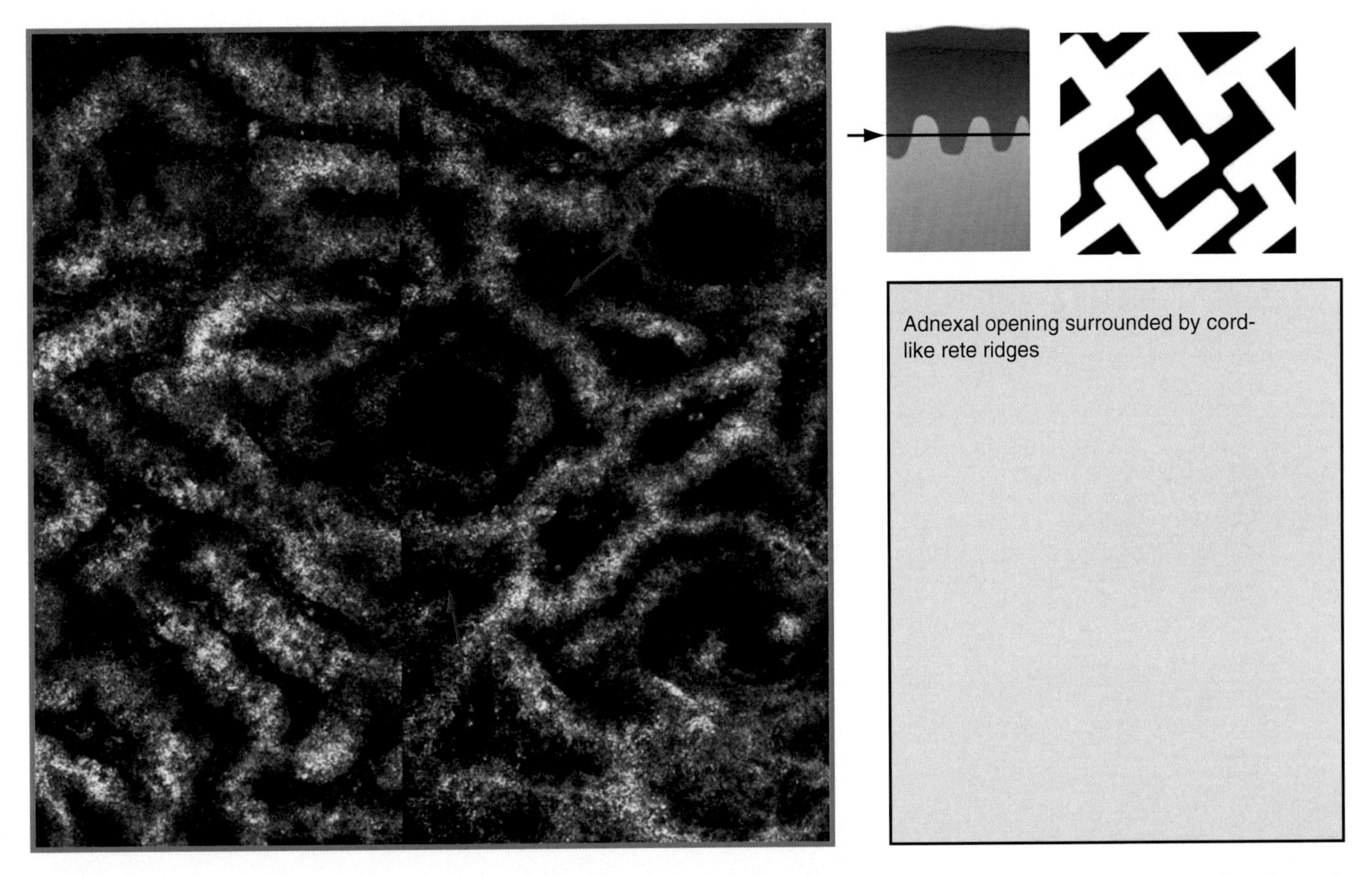

Fig. 20.1.2 Detail RCM image (0.5 × 0.5 mm) at the DEJ. An adnexal opening surrounded by cord-like rete ridges (*red arrows*) is observed, correlating to the pigmented follicular openings visualized with dermoscopy

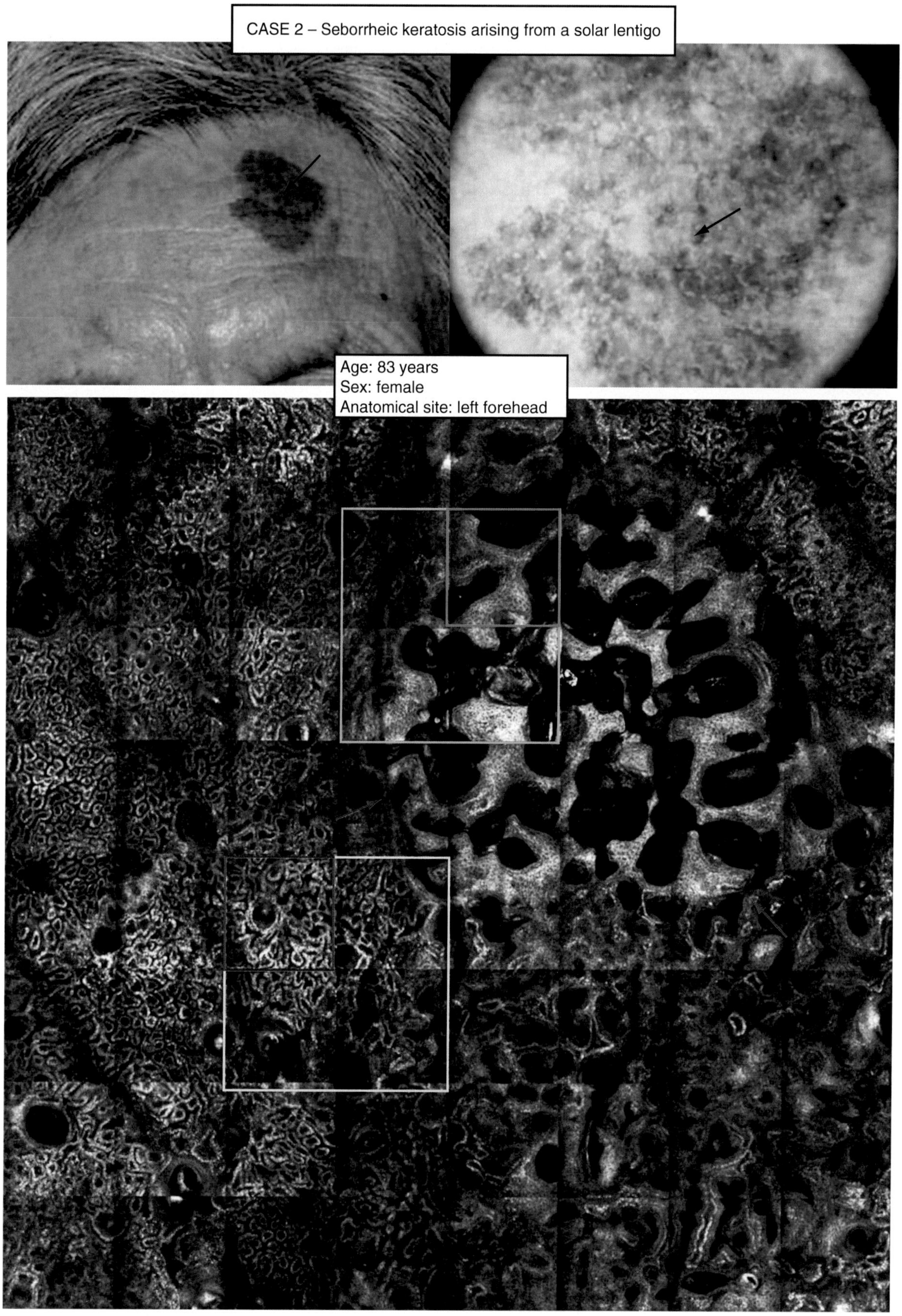

CASE 2 – Seborrheic keratosis arising from a solar lentigo

Age: 83 years
Sex: female
Anatomical site: left forehead

Fig. 20.2 RCM mosaic (4 × 4 mm) at the DEJ shows bright, cord-like rete ridges and edged dermal papillae (*yellow and red rectangles*). In the upper-right corner, an area displaying epidermal bulbous projections and keratin-filled invaginations (*arrows, green and blue rectangles*) is observed

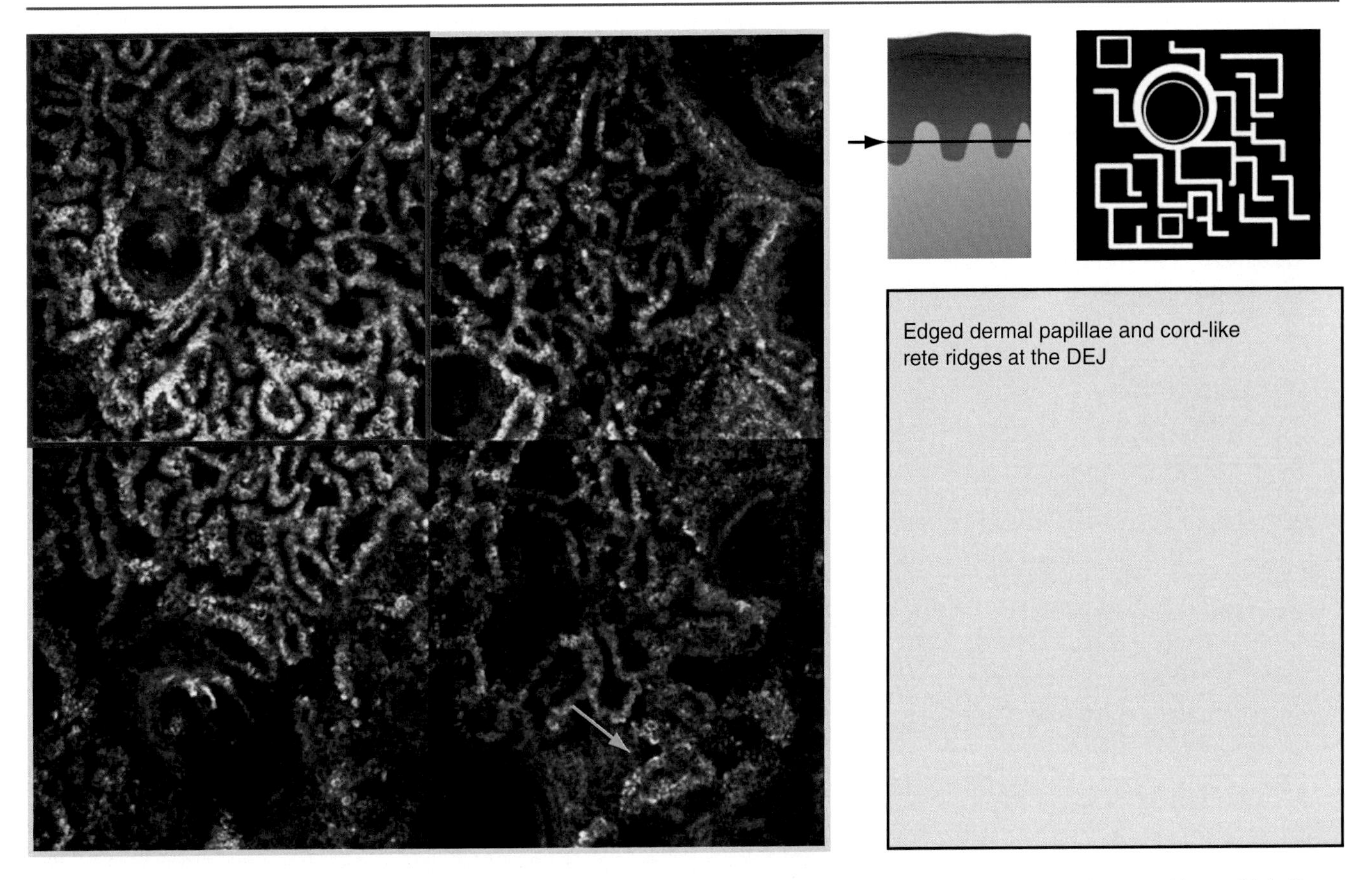

Fig. 20.2.1.1 RCM mosaic (1 × 1 mm) at the DEJ. Polymorphous, edged dermal papillae (*green arrow*) and cord-like rete ridges with bulbous projections (*red arrow*) are observed

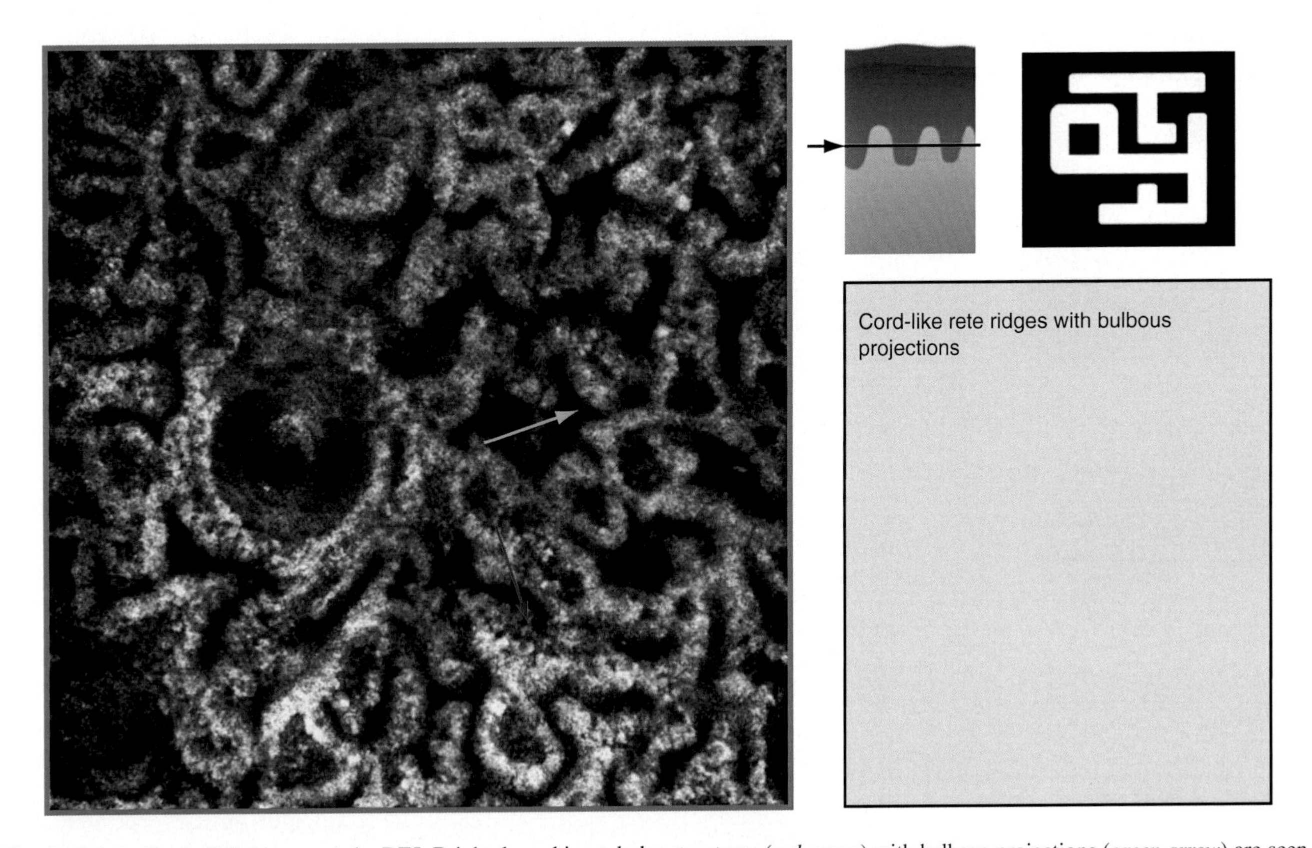

Fig. 20.2.1.2 Single RCM image at the DEJ. Bright, branching tubular structures (*red arrow*) with bulbous projections (*green arrow*) are seen, correlating to elongated rete ridges in histology

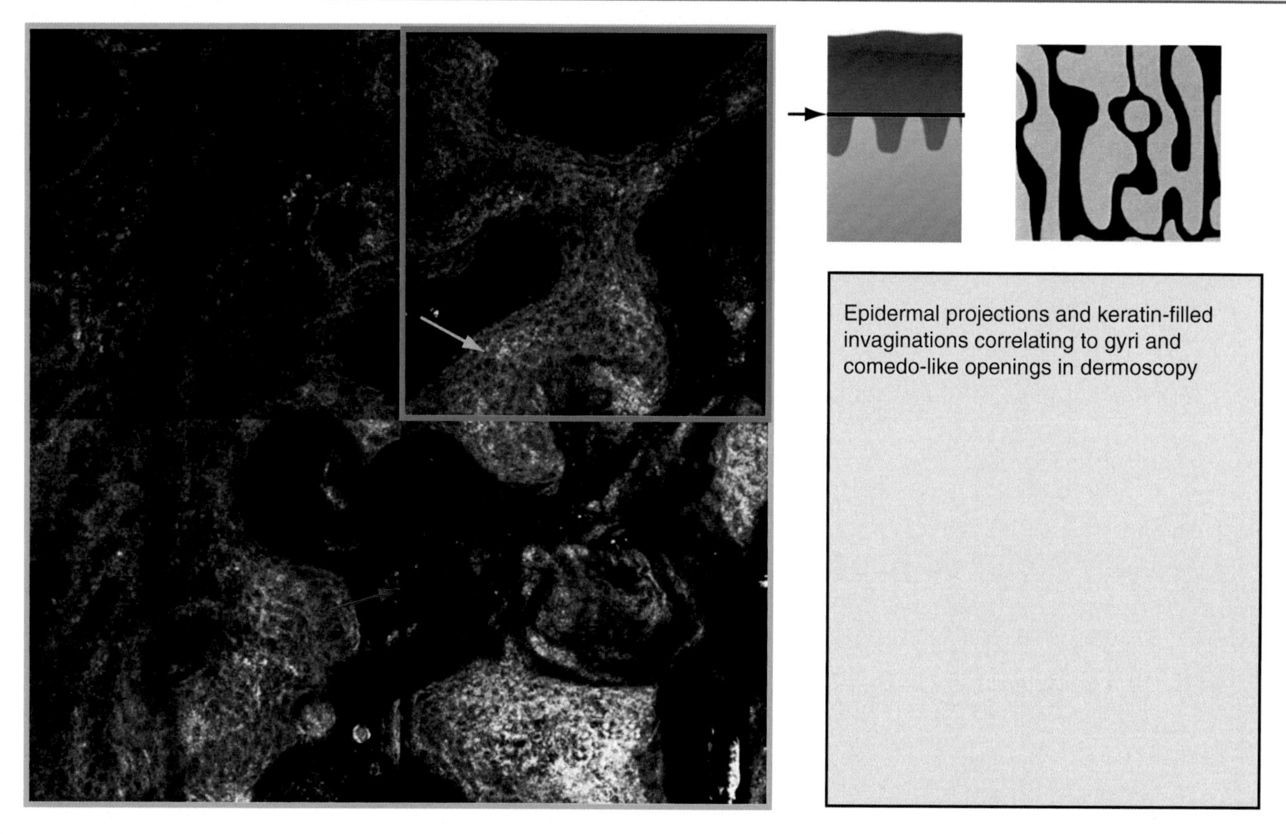

Fig. 20.2.2.1 RCM mosaic (1 × 1 mm) at the DEJ. Epidermal projections with a typical honeycomb pattern (*green arrow*) and keratin-filled invaginations (*red arrow*) suggestive of a seborrheic keratosis are seen

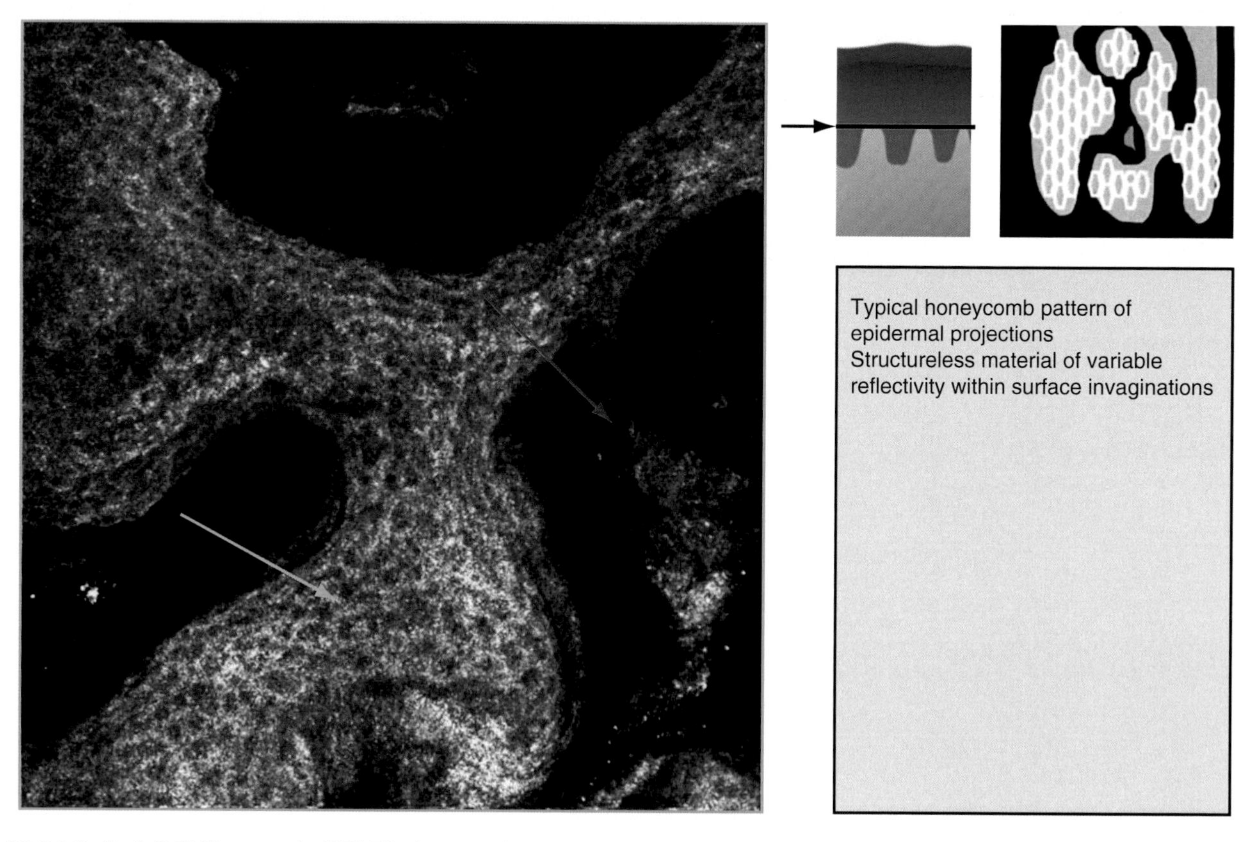

Fig. 20.2.2.2 Basic RCM image at the DEJ. The honeycomb pattern of epidermal projections shows regular size of nuclei and thickness of intercellular connections (*green arrow*). Structureless material of variable reflectivity is observed within the round and elongated invaginations of the lesion surface (*red arrow*)

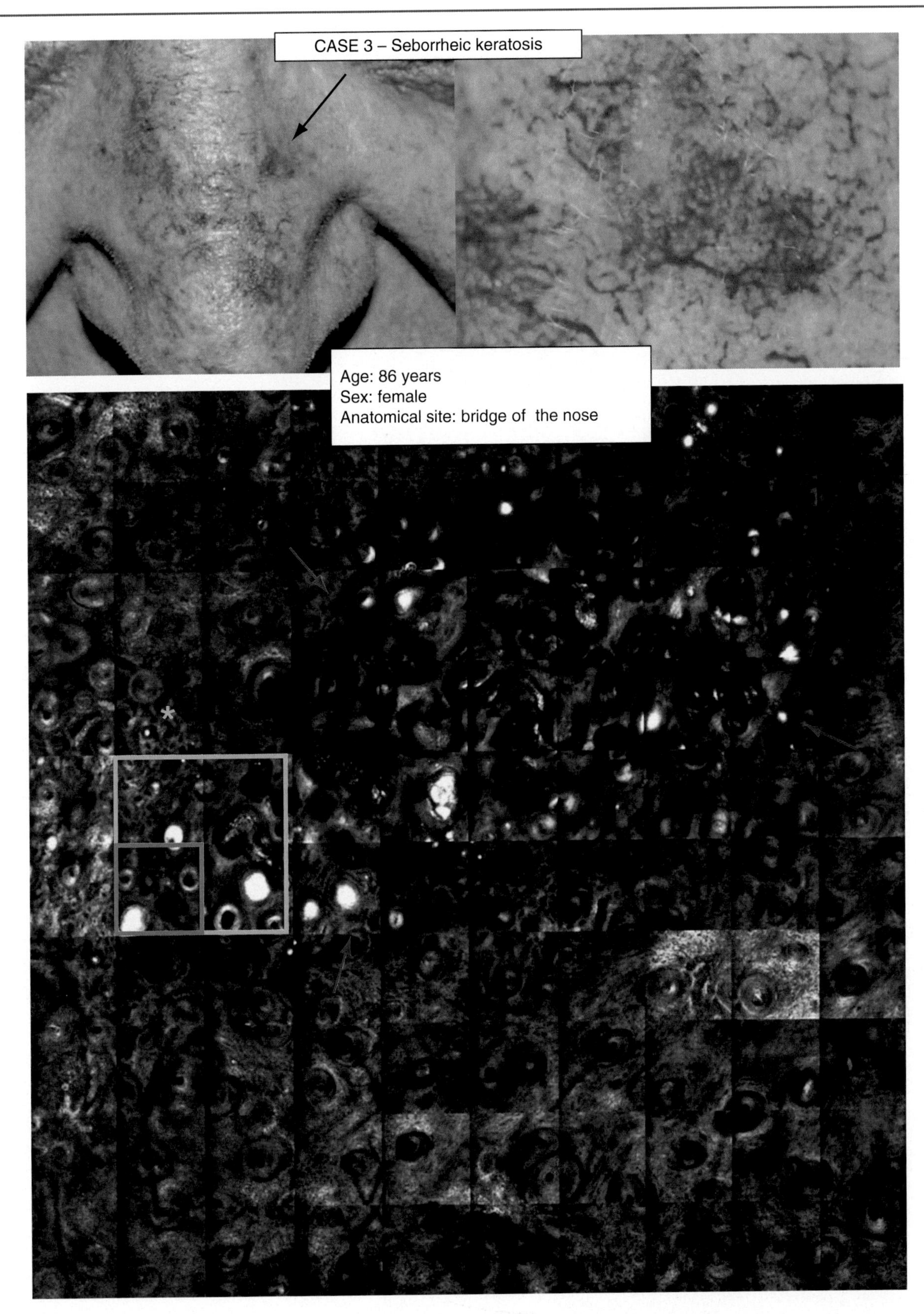

Fig. 20.3 RCM mosaic (5 × 5 mm) obtained at the level of the dermo-epidermal junction/upper dermis. A round to oval area displaying epidermal projections, keratin-filled invaginations and bright horn cysts is observed (*red arrows*). Multiple follicular openings (*red asterisk*) and focal cord-like rete ridges (*green asterisk*) are seen in the periphery

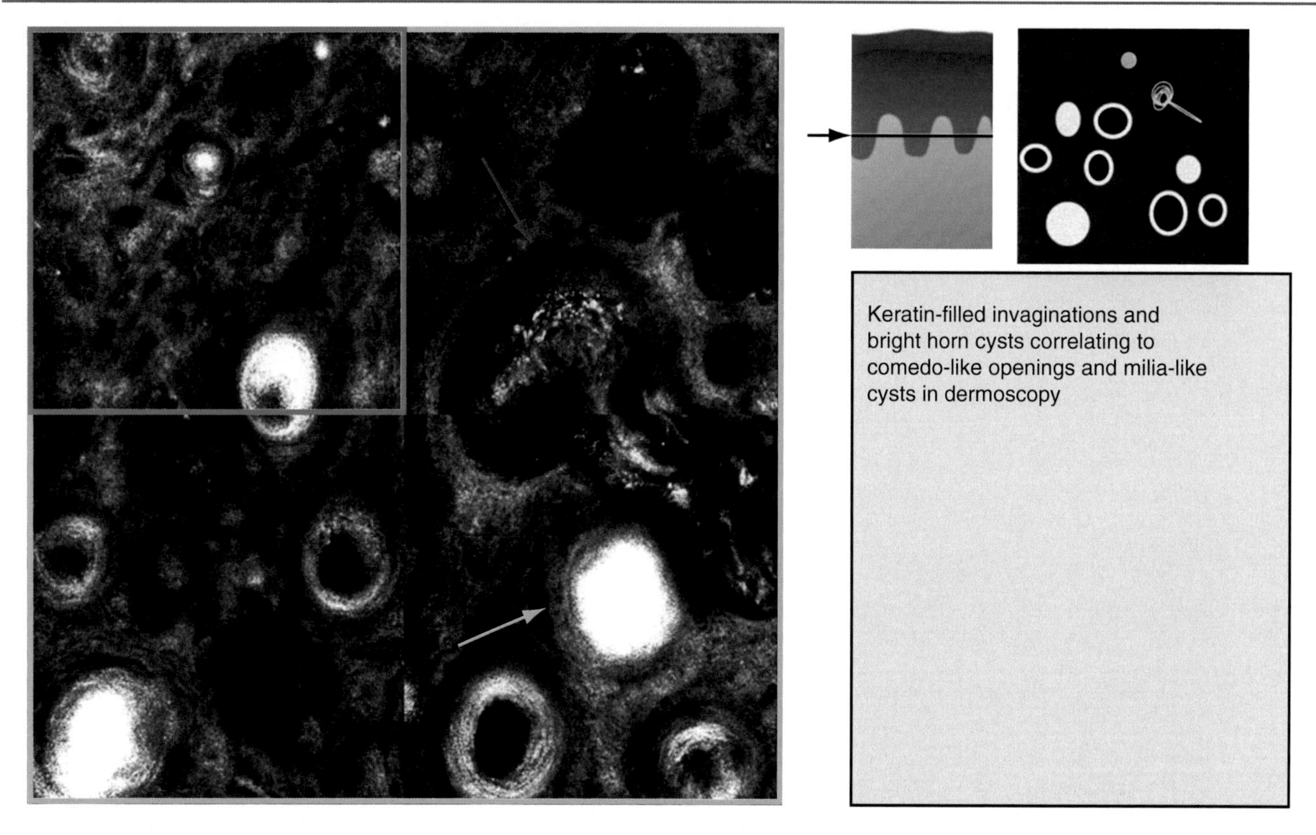

Fig. 20.3.1 RCM mosaic (1 × 1 mm) at the DEJ. Keratin-filled invaginations (*red arrow*) and bright reflecting horn cysts (*green arrow*) are seen. Cord-like rete ridges are observed in the periphery (*blue rectangle*)

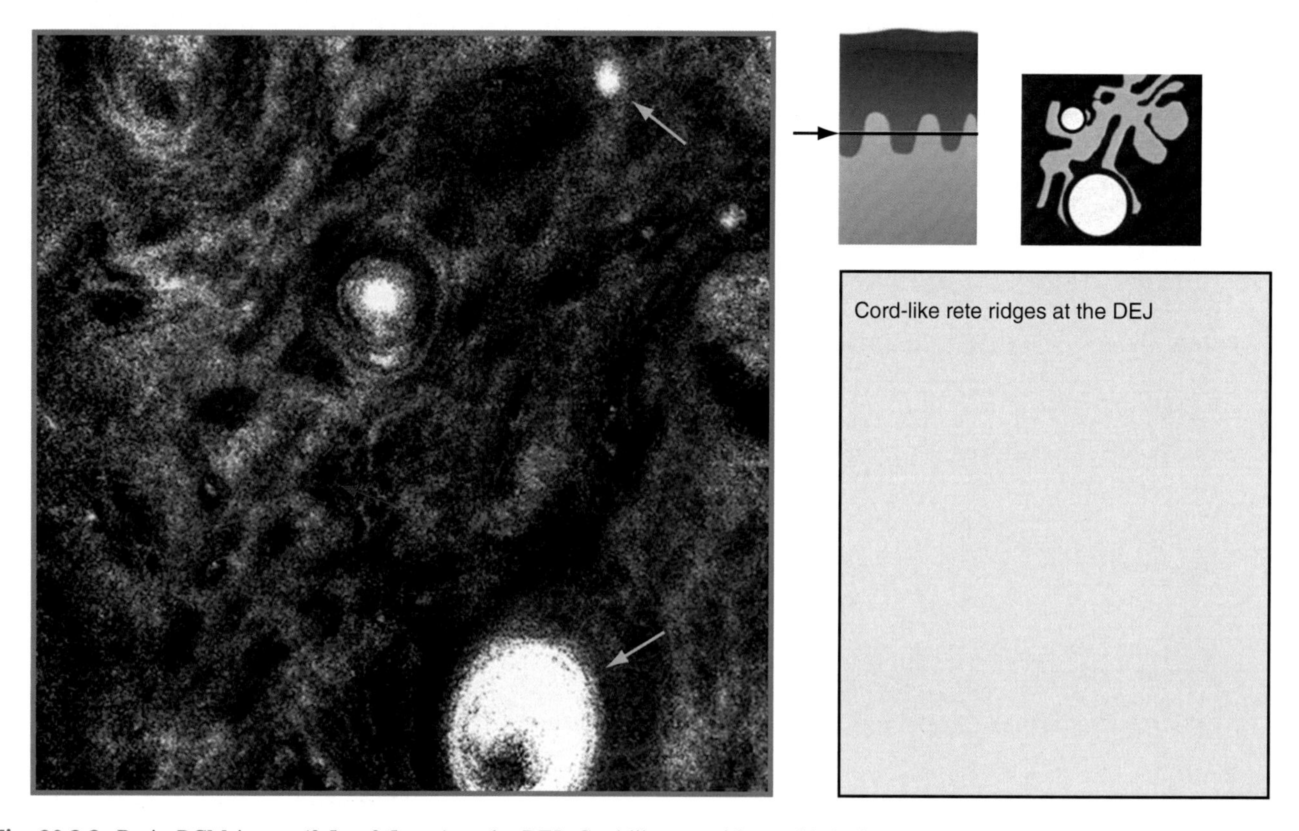

Fig. 20.3.2 Basic RCM image (0.5 × 0.5 mm) at the DEJ. Cord-like rete ridges with bulbous projections are observed in the periphery (*red arrow*). Bright reflecting horn cysts of variable size are seen (*green arrows*)

CASE 4 – Lichen planus-like keratosis
Age: 88 years
Sex: female
Anatomical Site: left temple

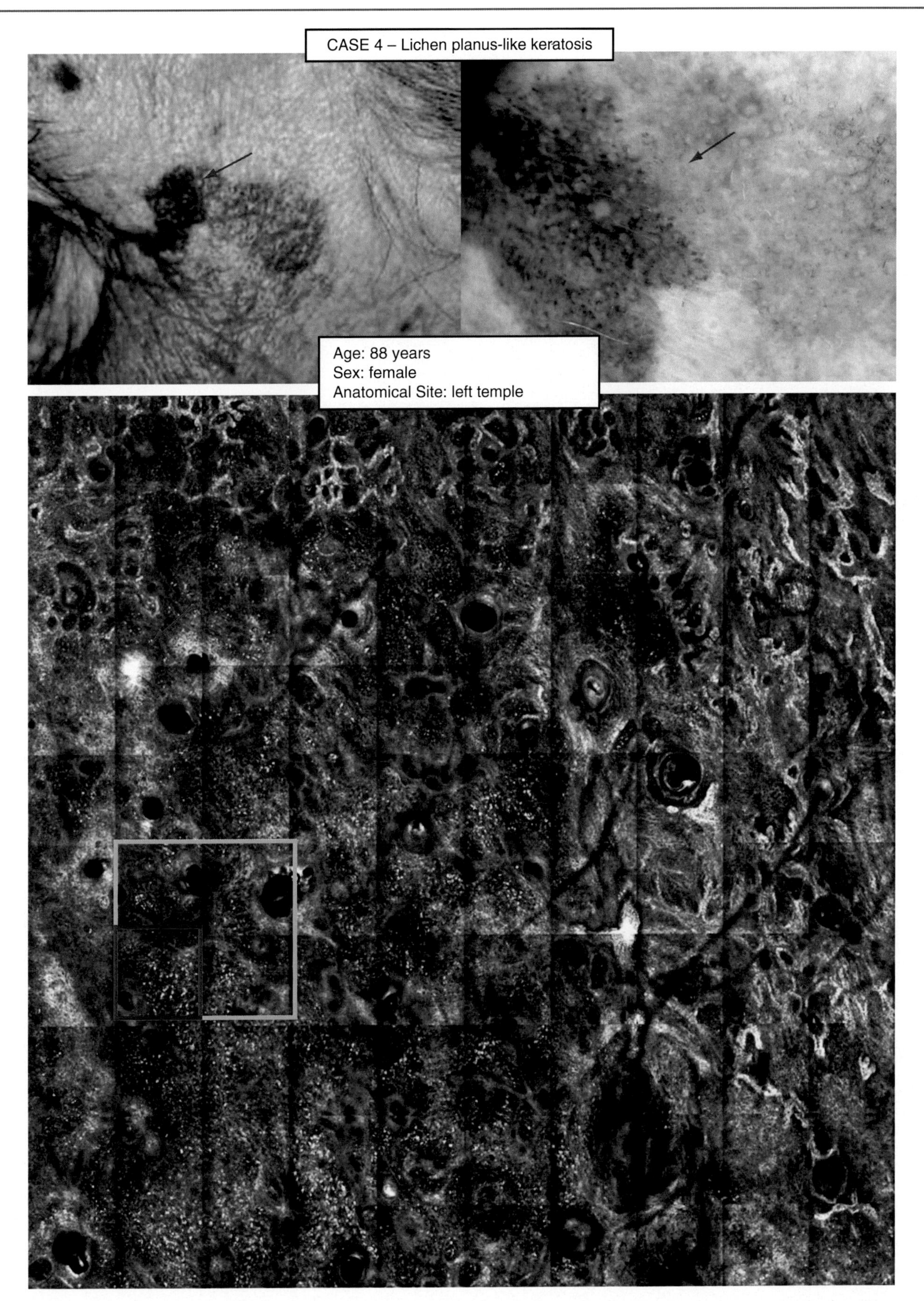

Fig. 20.4 RCM mosaic (5 × 5 mm) at the DEJ/upper dermis. Scattered and focally aggregated bright stellate spots and triangular cells (*rectangles*) are observed at upper dermis, correlating to an inflammatory infiltrate. Cord-like rete ridges (*asterisk*) and bright horn cysts are seen at the DEJ

Dermal inflammatory infiltrate composed of lymphocytes and melanophages

Fig. 20.4.1 RCM mosaic (1 × 1 mm) at the DEJ/upper dermis. Scattered small bright particles, correlating to lymphocytes and focally aggregated round to triangular cells, correlating to melanophages, are observed at upper dermis

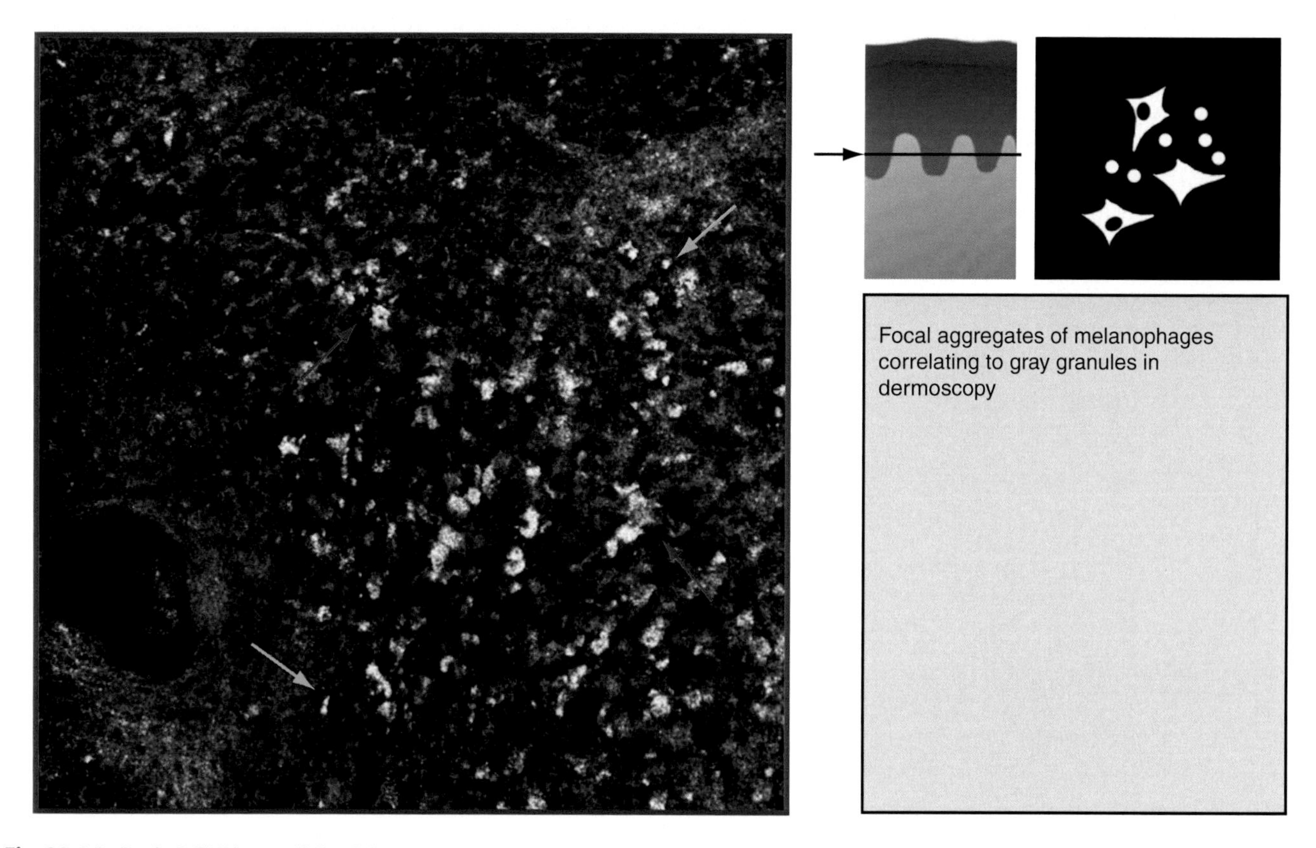

Fig. 20.4.2 Basic RCM image (0.5 × 0.5 mm) at the DEJ/upper dermis. Scattered and focally aggregated bright, round to triangular, non-nucleated cells, corresponding to melanophages are observed (*red arrows*). Bright stellate spots, correlating to lymphocytes, are additionally seen (*green arrows*)

Core Messages

- SL, SK and LPLK represent a spectrum of benign skin neoplasms with common clinical, dermoscopic, histopathologic and RCM features.
- Common RCM findings, such as a regular epidermal architecture, densely packed dermal papillae and/or cord-like rete ridges at the DEJ, are observed along with specific RCM features.
- The detection of key RCM features of SL, SK or LPLK in the absence of RCM findings suggestive of malignancy may enable a non-invasive diagnosis in clinically and dermoscopically equivocal cases.

References

1. Elgart GW (2001) Seborrheic keratoses, solar lentigines, and lichenoid keratoses. Dermatoscopic features and correlation to histology and clinical signs. Dermatol Clin 19(2):347–357
2. González S, Gill M, Halpern AC (2008) Reflectance confocal microscopy of cutaneous tumors. An atlas with clinical, dermoscopic and histological correlations. Informa Healthcare, London
3. Langley RGB, Burton E, Walsh N et al (2006) In vivo confocal scanning laser microscopy of benign lentigines: comparison to conventional histology and in vivo characteristics of lentigo maligna. J Am Acad Dermatol 55:88–97
4. Braun RP, Rabinovitz HS, Krischer J (2002) Dermoscopy of pigmented seborrheic keratosis: a morphological study. Arch Dermatol 138(12):1556–1560
5. Kopf AW, Rabinovitz H, Marghoob A, Braun RP, Wang S, Oliviero M, Polsky D (2006) "Fat fingers": a clue in the dermoscopic diagnosis of seborrheic keratoses. J Am Acad Dermatol 55(6):1089–1091
6. Laur WE, Posey RE, Waller JD (1981) Lichen planus-like keratosis. A clinicohistopathologic correlation. A clinicohistopathologic correlation. J Am Acad Dermatol 4(3):329–336
7. Bugatti L, Filosa G (2007) Dermoscopy of lichen planus-like keratosis: a model of inflammatory regression. J Eur Acad Dermatol Venereol 21(10):1392–1397

Basal Cell Carcinoma

21

Pantea Hashemi, Harold S. Rabinovitz,
Ashfaq A. Marghoob, and Alon Scope

21.1 In Vivo Confocal Reflectance Microscopy of Basal Cell Carcinoma

Basal cell carcinoma (BCC) is the most common human malignancy. In the last decades, there is an estimated increase in the incidence of BCC by 3–10% per annum [1]. The average lifetime risk for Caucasians to develop BCC is approximately 30% [2, 3]. BCC most commonly occurs in adults, especially in the elderly population [4], although it may rarely be seen in children in the context of genetic diseases such as Gorlin syndrome. The risk of development of BCC increases rapidly at age greater than 55 years [5].

Both constitutional and environmental factors contribute to the development of BCC. Sun exposure has been mainly implicated as having a causative role in the development of BCC since most patients are Caucasians with fair skin phenotypes and since BCC mostly arises on exposed, sun-damaged body sites [6, 7]. In addition, exposures to ionizing radiation, arsenic, coal tar derivatives and oral methoxsalen (psoralen), as well as immune system compromise can predispose individuals to the development of BCC [8, 9].

BCC is believed to arise from pluripotent progenitor basaloid keratinocytes [10]. The morphology of the neoplastic keratinocytes is similar to that seen in germinative buds at the undersurface of embryonic epidermis, from which the entire follicular-sebaceous unit arises. The keratin profile of the germinative cells of BCC is similar to that of the lower part of the hair follicle and distinct from the adjacent basal keratinocytes of surface epidermis [11].

Clinically, BCCs are slow-growing neoplasms that can infiltrate and invade adjacent tissues, rarely killing the patient because of direct extension into vital organs, such as the brain; cases of metastasis have been very rarely reported [12]. BCC has been classified, based on clinico-pathologic correlation, into five subtypes: nodular, superficial, morpheaform, infundibulocystic and fibroepithelial tumor of Pinkus [13]. Classic nodular BCC, the most common form, occurs most frequently on sun-exposed areas of the head and presents as a translucent pearly pink papule or nodule with a rolled border and telangiectasia, at times exhibiting central crusting or ulceration. Superficial BCC, the second most common subtype, manifests as a well-defined, circumscribed reddish plaque with slightly raised margins, frequently on the trunk, that clinically simulates Bowen's disease, nummular eczema, contact dermatitis or fungal infections. Morpheaform BCC, also known as sclerosing or infiltrative BCC, is a more aggressive but less common variant (roughly 1–5% of all BCCs) that appears as a white or yellow depressed scar-like plaque. Because morpheaform BCC is more difficult to detect clinically, it can result in local destruction of eyes, ears and nose [6, 14, 15]. Fibroepithelioma of Pinkus is a rare variant of BCC which clinically presents as a single or multiple well-defined red plaques and flesh-colored nodule without ulceration, mostly on the trunk. Different subtypes of BCC, particularly the nodular subtype, can appear pigmented [16] and, at times, can simulate melanoma [17].

On histopathology, most BCC subtypes show aggregates of atypical basaloid cells with peripheral palisading of nuclei, stroma with fibroplasia, and frequently clefts between the neoplastic aggregates and the stroma. Dendritic melanocytes can often be seen within the neoplastic aggregates, although only 25% of the aggregates contain melanin, and even fewer are clinically pigmented [18, 19].

Although many BCCs are clinically evident, the overall accuracy of dermatologists for the diagnosis of BCC was

P. Hashemi (✉)
Dermatology Service, Memorial Sloan-Kettering Cancer Center,
New York, NY, USA
e-mail: panteahashemi@gmail.com

H.S. Rabinovitz
Skin and Cancer Associates/ADM, Plantation, FL, USA
e-mail: harold@admcorp.com

A.A. Marghoob
Dermatology Service, Memorial Sloan-Kettering Cancer Center,
Suffolk, Hauppauge, NY, USA
e-mail: marghooa@mskcc.org

A. Scope
Department of Dermatology, Sheba Medical Center,
Tel Hashomer, Israel
e-mail: scopea1@gmail.com

R. Hofmann-Wellenhof et al. (eds.), *Reflectance Confocal Microscopy for Skin Diseases*,
DOI 10.1007/978-3-642-21997-9_21,

Table 21.1 RCM features found in BCC with their respective histopathologic correlates

RCM terms	Definition	Histopathologic correlate
Dark silhouettes	Hyporeflective areas at the level of DEJ or superficial dermis outlined by bright collagen bundles in the surrounding dermis	Aggregates of basaloid cells with peripheral palisading of nuclei in nonpigmented BCC
Bright tumor islands	Round to oval, cord-like or lobulated bright structures at the level of DEJ or superficial dermis, often well-demarcated by a surrounding dark cleft	Aggregates of basaloid cells with peripheral palisading of nuclei, mostly in pigmented BCC
Cleft-like dark spaces	Black areas, shaped like clefts/slits that separate the bright tumor islands from the surrounding dermis	Clefting or mucin surrounding the neoplastic aggregates
Dendritic cells	Bright delicate, dendritic structures within bright tumor islands or in the overlying epidermis	Dendritic melanocytes within neoplastic aggregates in pigmented BCC or Langerhans cells in the spinous layer of the overlying epidermis
Plump-bright cells	Oval to stellate cells with indistinct borders and without apparent nucleus in the dermis	Melanophages
Canalicular vessels	Dilated vessels coursing in the *en-face* plane of imaging	Telangiectatic blood vessels

reported to be around 70% [20]. To this end, dermoscopy can aid in the early recognition of BCC. Dermoscopic features seen in pigmented BCC include blue-gray ovoid nests, blue-gray globules, leaf-like structures and spoke wheel-like areas, in the absence of a pigment network [21]. Additional dermoscopic features including arborizing vessels, pink-white shiny areas and ulceration can also be seen in nonpigmented BCC [22]. However, diagnosis of BCC can be at times challenging even with dermoscopy, particularly in small nodular BCC on the face, in morpheaform BCC, and in some cases of superficial BCC hardly exhibiting any dermoscopic criteria.

Reflectance confocal microscopy (RCM) can augment dermoscopic diagnosis, allowing the clinician to diagnose BCC more confidently in real-time. Most RCM features of BCC come to view at the level of the superficial dermis or dermal-epidermal junction (DEJ) (fig 21.1, fig 21.2). In the mosaic images, akin to low-power magnification microscopy, bright tumor islands present as oval, polycyclic or elongated, cord-like structures often well defined from the surrounding dermis by cleft-like dark spaces (fig 21.3). Bright tumor islands are typically seen in pigmented BCCs (fig 21.3). The presence of tumor islands as hypo reflective areas ("dark silhouettes") that are darker than the surrounding dermis or basal epidermis are mostly seen in non pigmented BCCs (fig 21.1, 21.2, 21.4). Tumor silhouette is a new RCM criterion, particularly valuable in evaluation of nonpigmented BCCs in which bright tumor islands are often not seen on RCM. However, the dense stroma around the neoplastic aggregates creates a distinct imprint on mosaic images of dark silhouettes outlined by bright collagen bundles at the level of the superficial dermis [23] fig 21.1.1, fig 21.4.1. The bright tumor islands and the dark silhouettes seen on RCM correlate on histopathology with aggregates of basaloid cells with peripheral palisading of nuclei (Table 21.1). The cleft-like dark spaces around tumor islands is an interesting in vivo RCM observation, (fig 21.3.1) since the cleft seen around the neoplastic aggregates on histopathology is considered an artifact of tissue processing. The clefting on RCM probably corresponds to mucin surrounding the neoplastic aggregates.

In individual RCM images, akin to higher power microscopy, elongated nuclei can exhibit peripheral palisading within the tumor islands be discerned as exhibiting peripheral palisading of nuclei within the tumor islands. The adjacent dermal stroma contains plump-bright oval to stellate cells with indistinct borders compatible with melanophages, (fig 21.1.2) or small bright dots compatible with smaller inflammatory cells such as lymphocytes. Dilated blood vessels coursing in the *en-face* plane of imaging can be seen in real-time or video-mode RCM imaging, juxtaposed to the tumor islands (fig 21.1.1) [23–25]; these blood vessels often exhibit rolling of leukocytes (fig 21.4.2). At times, multiple bright dendritic structures and dendritic cells can be seen within the tumor islands (fig 21.2.2, fig 21.5.2); these dendritic cells within neoplastic aggregates of BCC have been shown by immunohistochemistry to be melanocytes [26]. Interestingly, concomitant dendritic cells in the overlying spinous layer of the epidermis have been shown to correlate with Langerhans cells [27]. Observation of the bright delicate, dendritic structures within the tumor nodules, in the absence of melanocytic features, can be a helpful clue in the diagnosis of challenging cases of BCC [28]. Elongated nuclei, polarization of nuclei ("streaming") and a pleomorphic overlying epidermis have also been previously described as features of BCC [24, 25].

Rishpon et al. analyzed a series of 50 histologically proven BCCs and found a set of reproducible RCM criteria for the diagnosis of BCC (manuscript in preparation). RCM mosaic images revealed bright tumor islands or dark silhouettes consistently in all lesions (100%), clefting between tumor islands and the surrounding stroma in 25 lesions (50%), dendritic structures and dendritic cells within or between the tumor islands in 20 (40%) and round non-nucleated cells in the dermis in 47 lesions (94%). Canalicular vessels coursing in the *en-face* plane of imaging were observed in 43/48 (89%) of cases during real-time imaging. Canalicular vessels correlate with the tortuous, arborizing telangiectatic vessels seen on dermoscopy. However, canallicular vessels on RCM can be seen even in lesions that did not show arborizing vessels on dermoscopy, suggesting a higher sensitivity of RCM for detecting vascular morphology.

To date, it is not possible to fully differentiate among the various histopathologic subtypes of BCC; by RCM however, some features may be helpful [24]. Nodular BCC is characterized on RCM by large bright tumor islands surrounded by dark non refractive cleft-like spaces and / or by large dark tumor silhouettes in the superficial dermis. Superficial BCC is mostly characterized on RCM by dark tumor silhouettes surrounded by the spinous layer of the epidermis that become apparent when imaging immediately below the basal epidermis. Morpheoform BCC is difficult to detect with RCM because the dark silhouettes tend to be small and thin and do not stand out sufficiently from the bright collagen in the surrounding dermis.

In summary, RCM is useful for the diagnosis of BCC and demonstrates reproducible features that correlate well with histopathologic criteria. Improvement in penetration depth, resolution, breadth of field of view and imaging speed, may further increase the utility of RCM for the diagnosis of BCC in routine clinical practice.

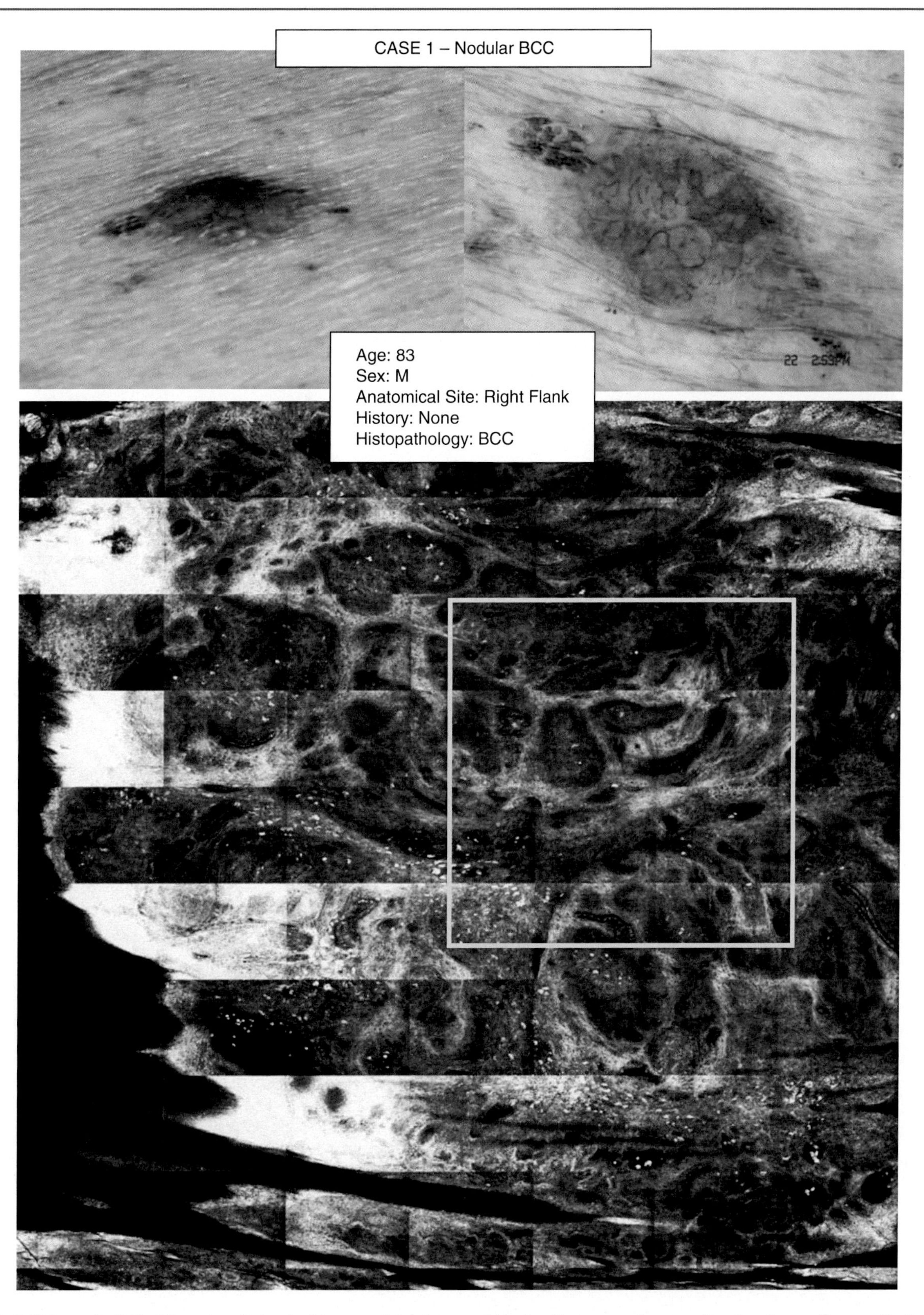

Fig. 21.1 RCM mosaic (3.5×4.5 mm) at the level of the superficial dermis reveals dark silhouettes of different sizes and shapes surrounded by bright collagen bundles. In addition, there are numerous bright dots both within the silhouettes and surrounding dermis as well as canalicular vessels (Published with kind permission of © Harold S. Rabinovitz 2012. All Rights Reserved)

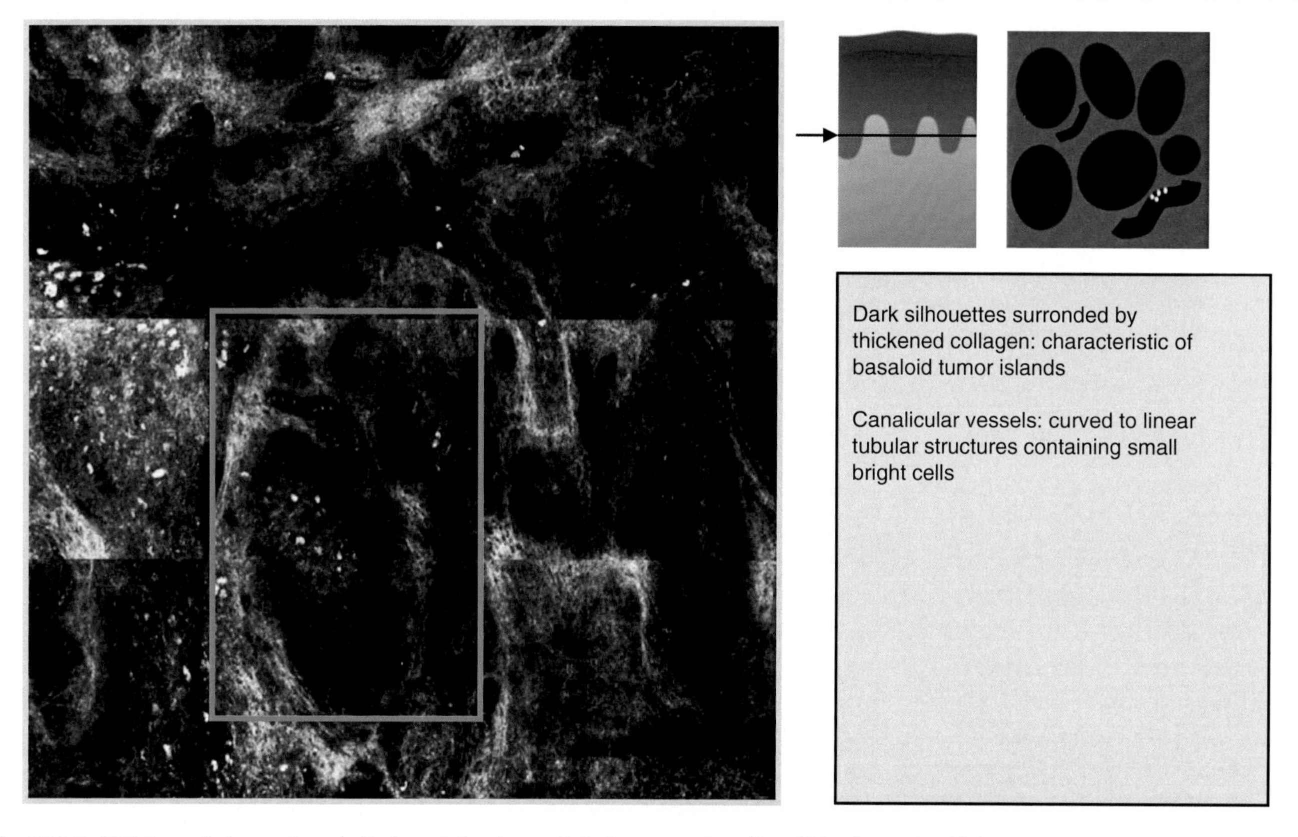

Fig. 21.1.1 RCM mosaic (approximately 2×2 mm) showing a relatively hypo-refractile area ("dark silhouette") that is surrounded by bright and thickened collagen bundles. Curved to linear tubular structures that contain a row of small bright structures can also be seen; these are canalicular vessels – dilated blood vessels which run parallel to the *en face* plane of confocal imaging and which harbor leukocytes that move during real-time imaging (Published with kind permission of © Harold S. Rabinovitz 2012. All Rights Reserved)

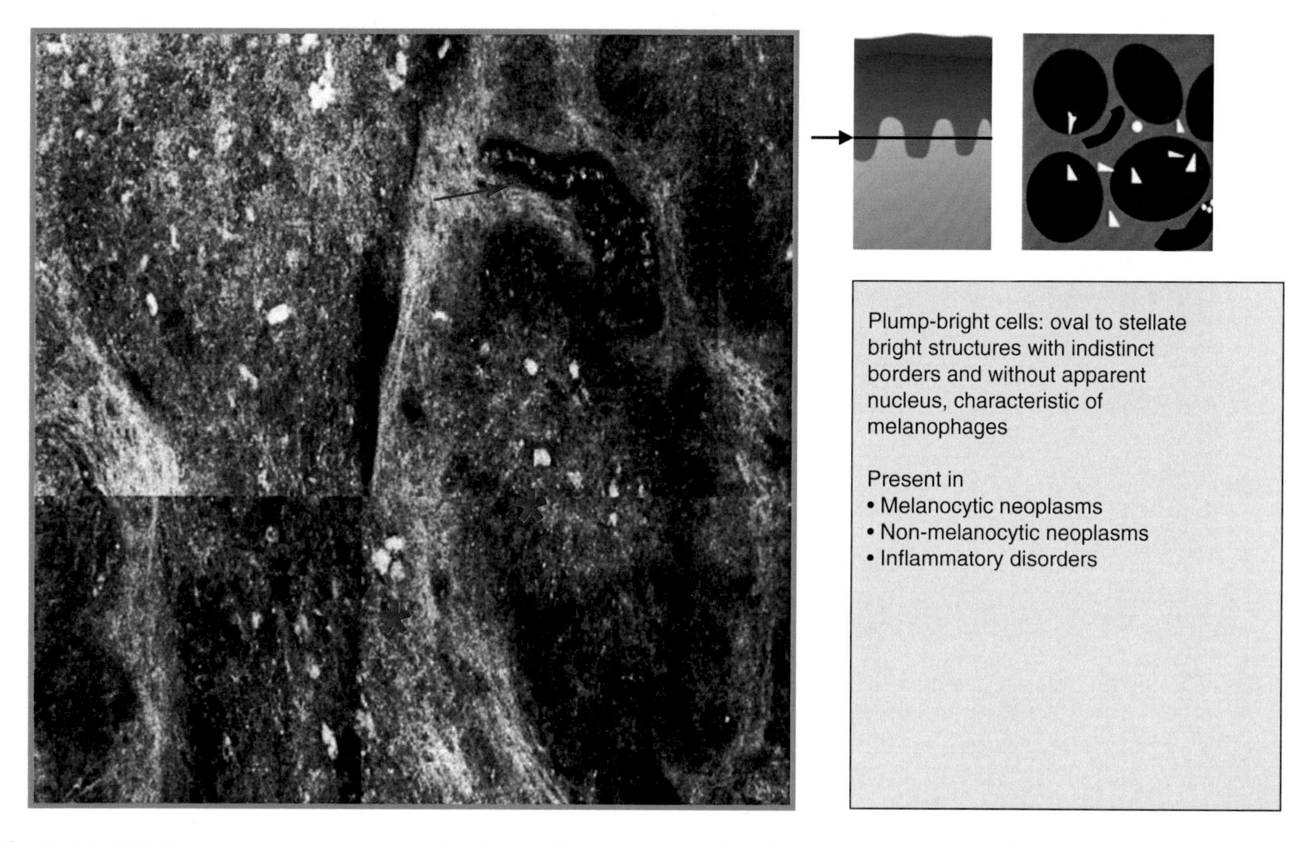

Fig. 21.1.2 RCM image (approximately 1×1 mm) at the superficial dermis level depicts plump-bright oval to stellate structures without apparent nuclei (*); these cells correlate with melanophages and are seen within tumor islands as well as in the surrounding dermis. Within the canalicular vessels are small bright cells which correlate with leukocytes (→) (Published with kind permission of © Harold S. Rabinovitz 2012. All Rights Reserved)

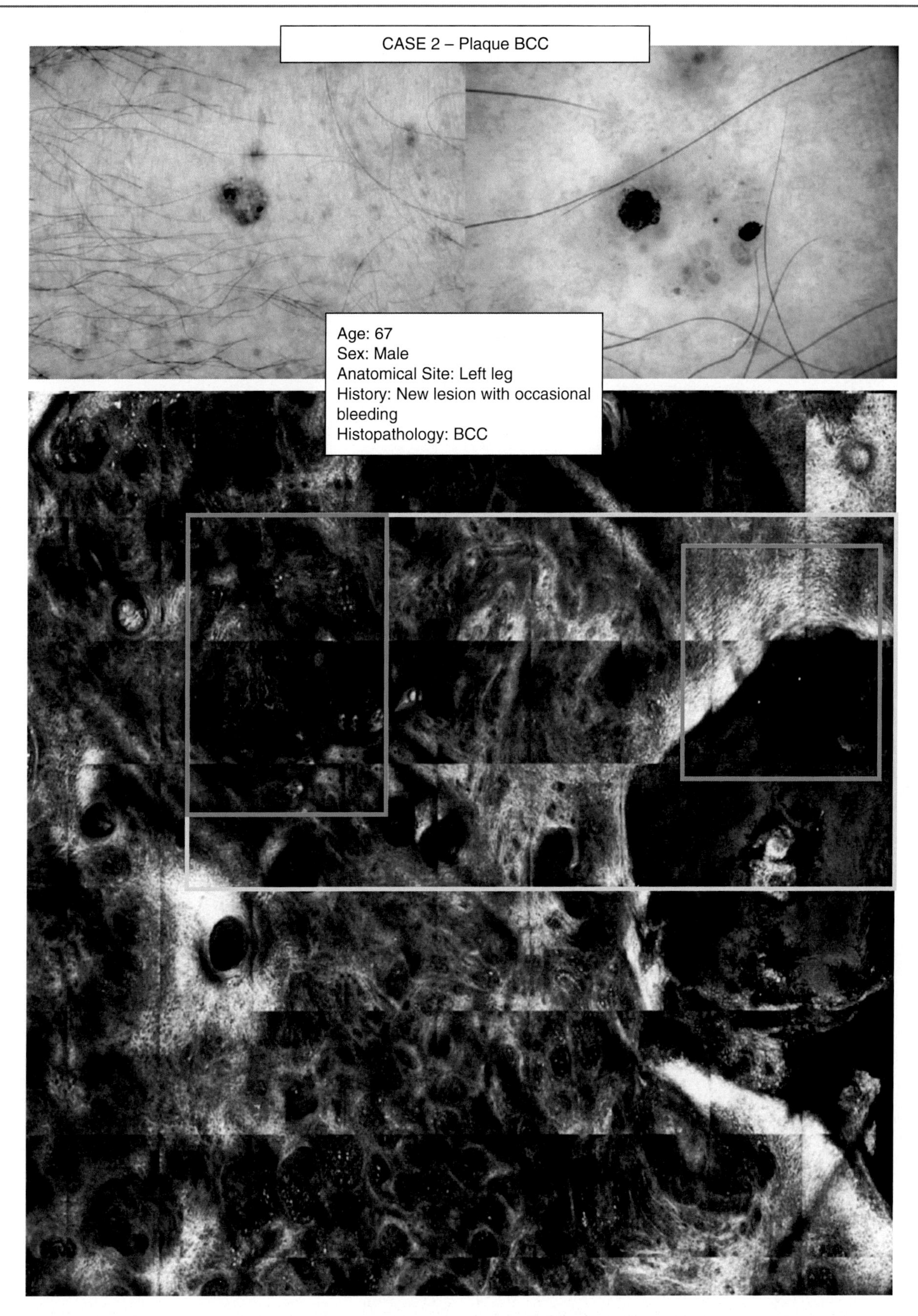

Fig. 21.2 RCM mosaic (4 × 4 mm) at the level of the dermal-epidermal junction shows lobulated dark silhouettes of different sizes and shapes. On the right hand side there is a dark oval area which corresponds to the ulceration that is seen on the clinical and dermoscopic images (Published with kind permission of © Harold S. Rabinovitz 2012. All Rights Reserved)

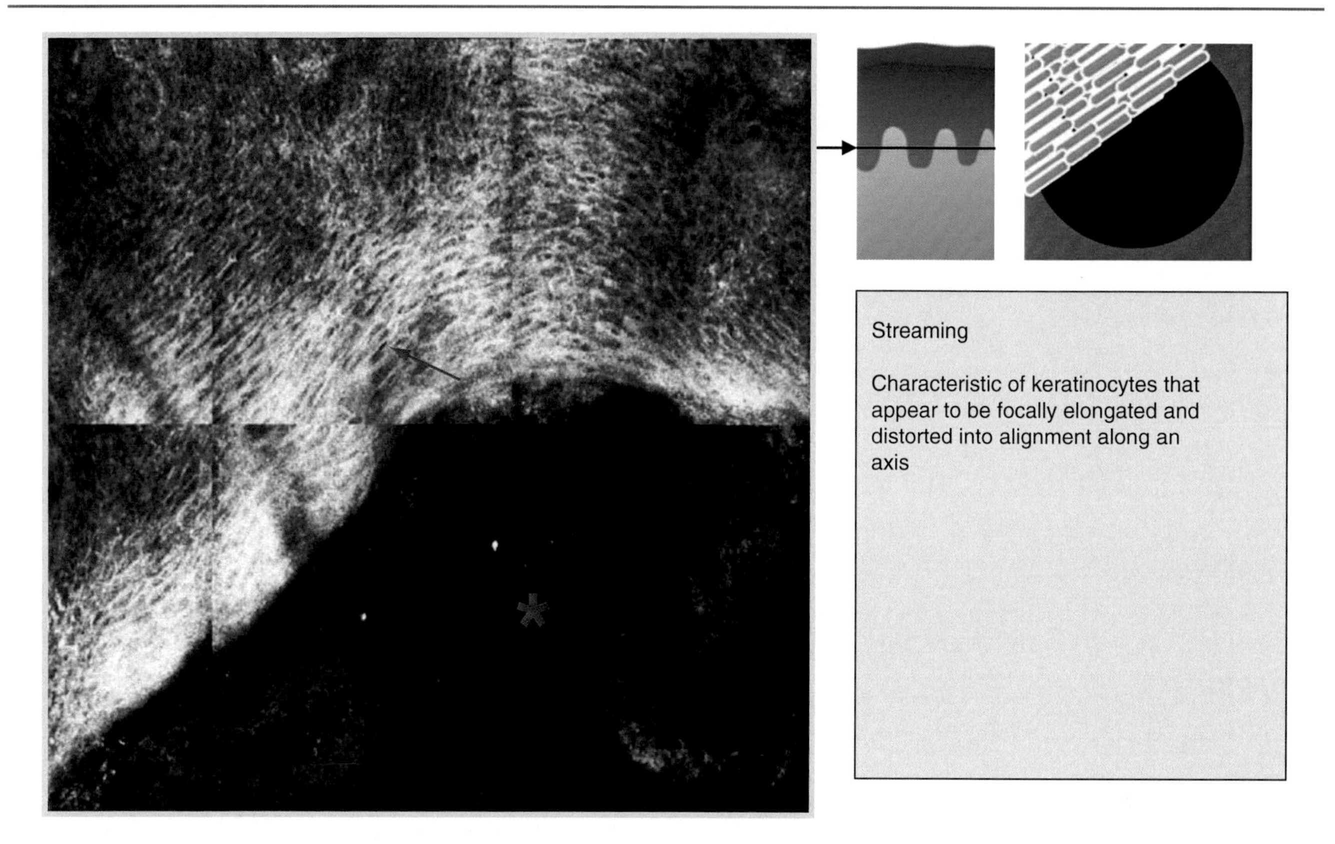

Fig. 21.2.1 RCM mosaic (approximately 2×2 mm) showing the dark oval area which corresponds to an ulceration (*). The refractive area above shows cells that appear to be focally elongated and distorted into alignment along an axis ("streaming") (→); these cells are spinous-layer keratinocytes (Published with kind permission of © Harold S. Rabinovitz 2012. All Rights Reserved)

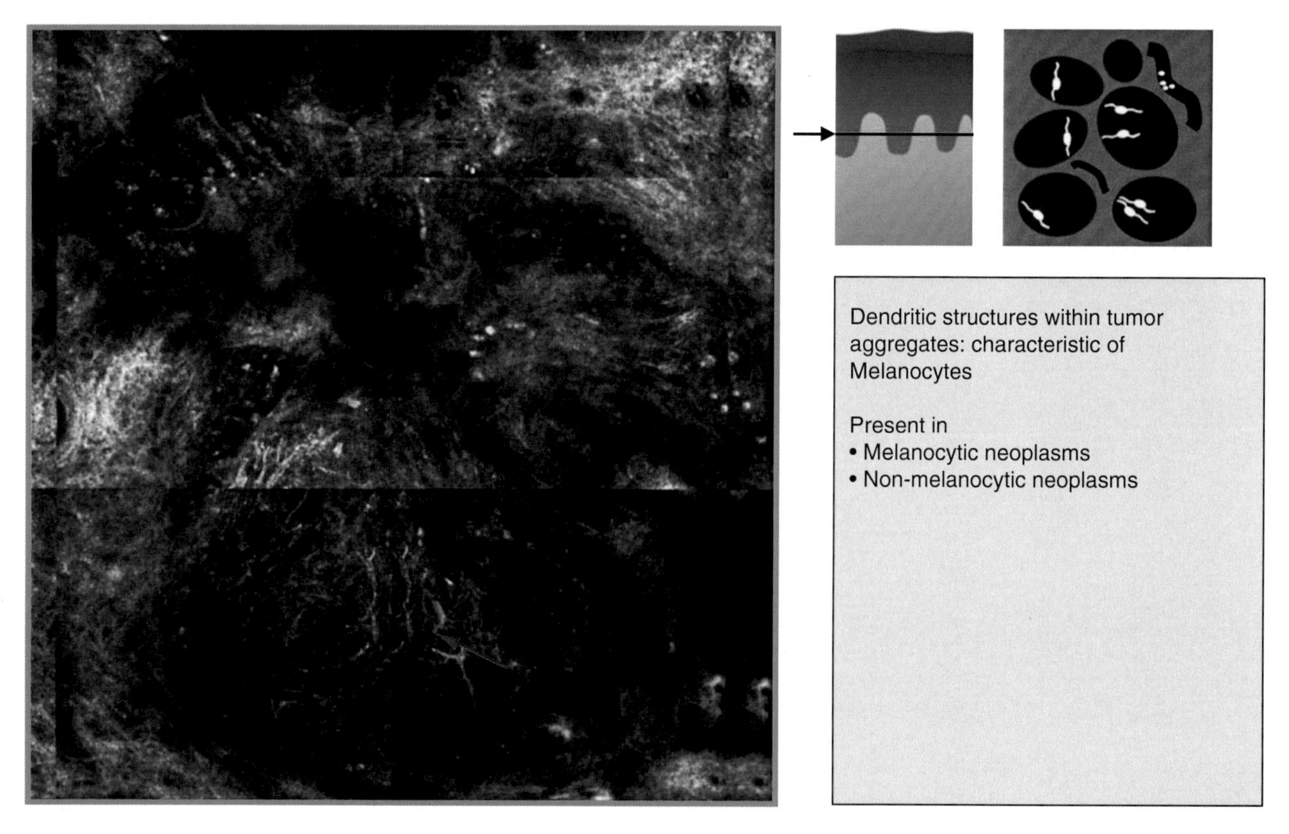

Fig. 21.2.2 RCM image (1×1 mm) at the DEJ depicts dendritic structures within a poorly defined tumor island (→); these dendritic structures correspond to melanocytes within neoplastic aggregates (Published with kind permission of © Harold S. Rabinovitz 2012. All Rights Reserved)

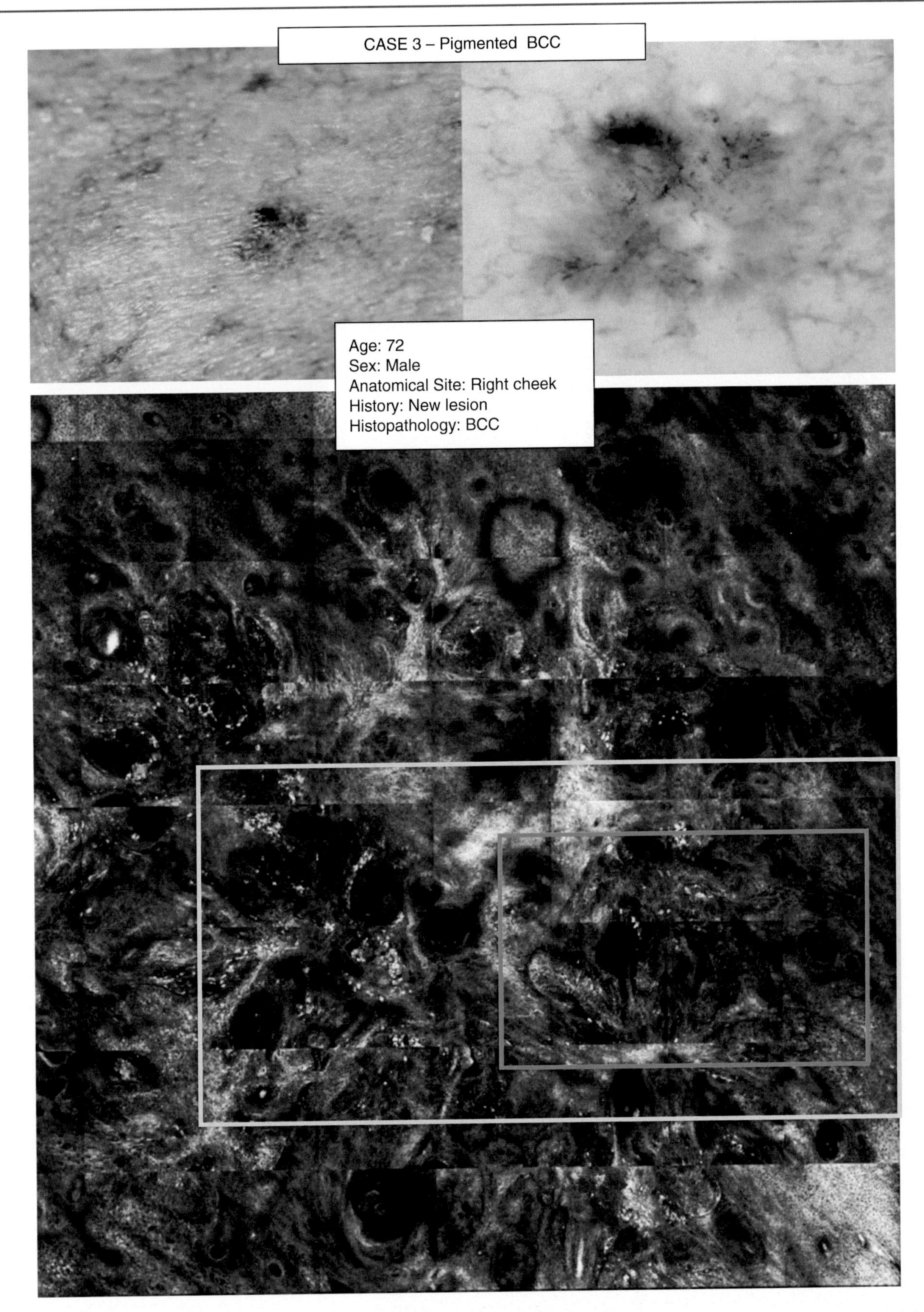

Fig. 21.3 RCM mosaic (4×4 mm) at the level of the superficial dermis reveals bright tumor islands, dark sillouettes and numerous bright spots (Published with kind permission of © Harold S. Rabinovitz 2012. All Rights Reserved)

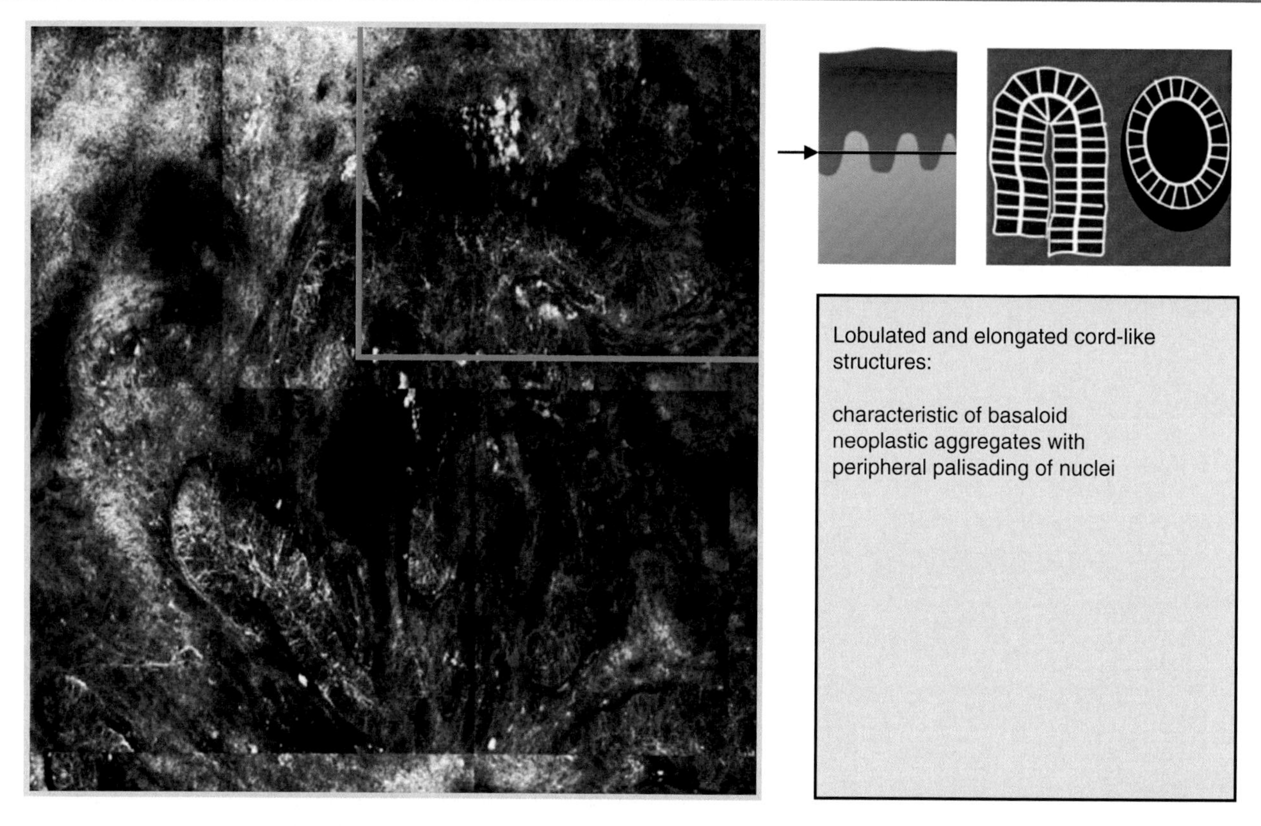

Fig. 21.3.1 RCM mosaic (approximately 1.5×1.5 mm) showing a bright tumor islands as elongated cord-like structures. These bright tumor islands harbor bright dendritic structures and are demarcated from the surrounding dermis by cleft-like dark spaces (Published with kind permission of © Harold S. Rabinovitz 2012. All Rights Reserved)

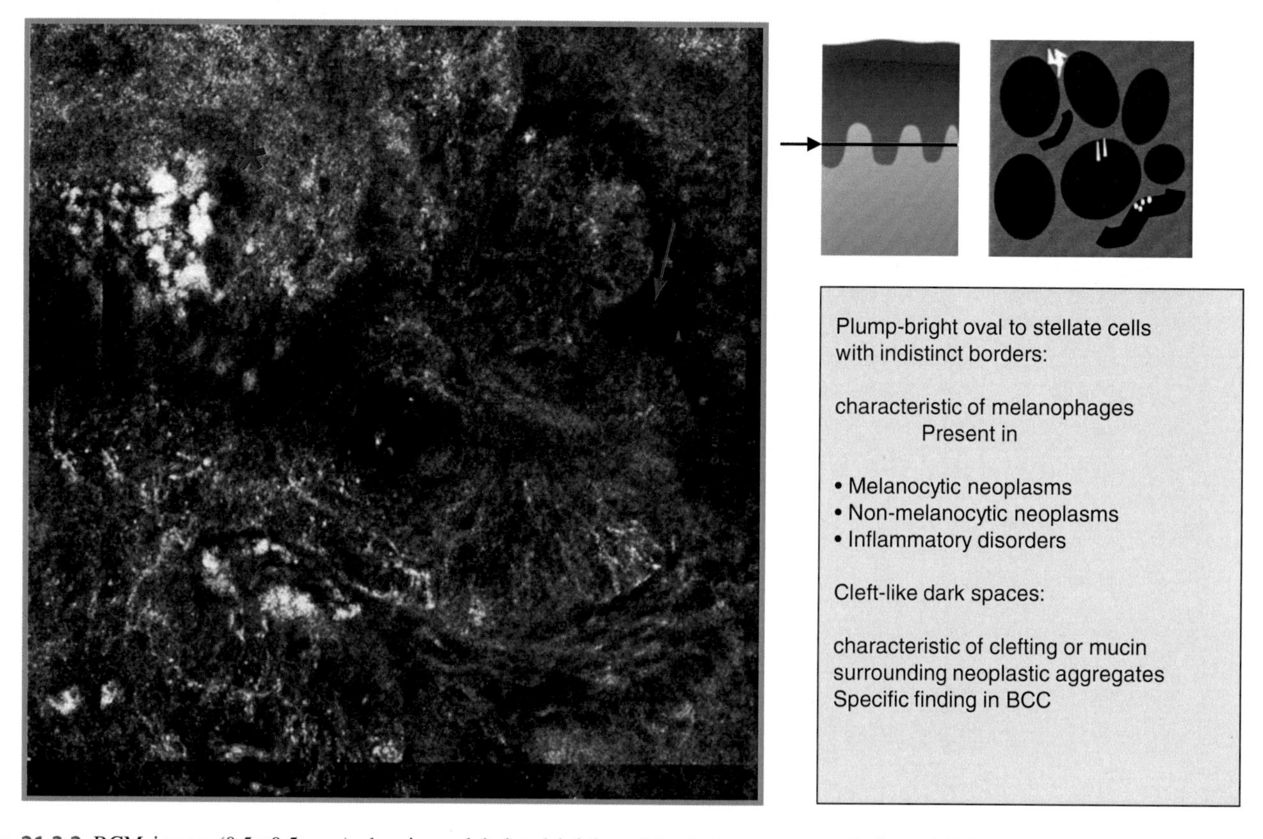

Fig. 21.3.2 RCM image (0.5×0.5 mm) showing a lobulated bright tumor island that is well demarcated by surrounding cleft-like dark spaces (→). Fine dendritic processes can be seen within the tumor island. An aggregate of plump-bright stellate structures, characteristic of melanophages, can also be seen (*) (Published with kind permission of © Harold S. Rabinovitz 2012. All Rights Reserved)

Case 4 – Plaque BCC
Age: 42
Sex: Male
Anatomical Site: Left side cheek
History: New lesion
Histopathology: BCC

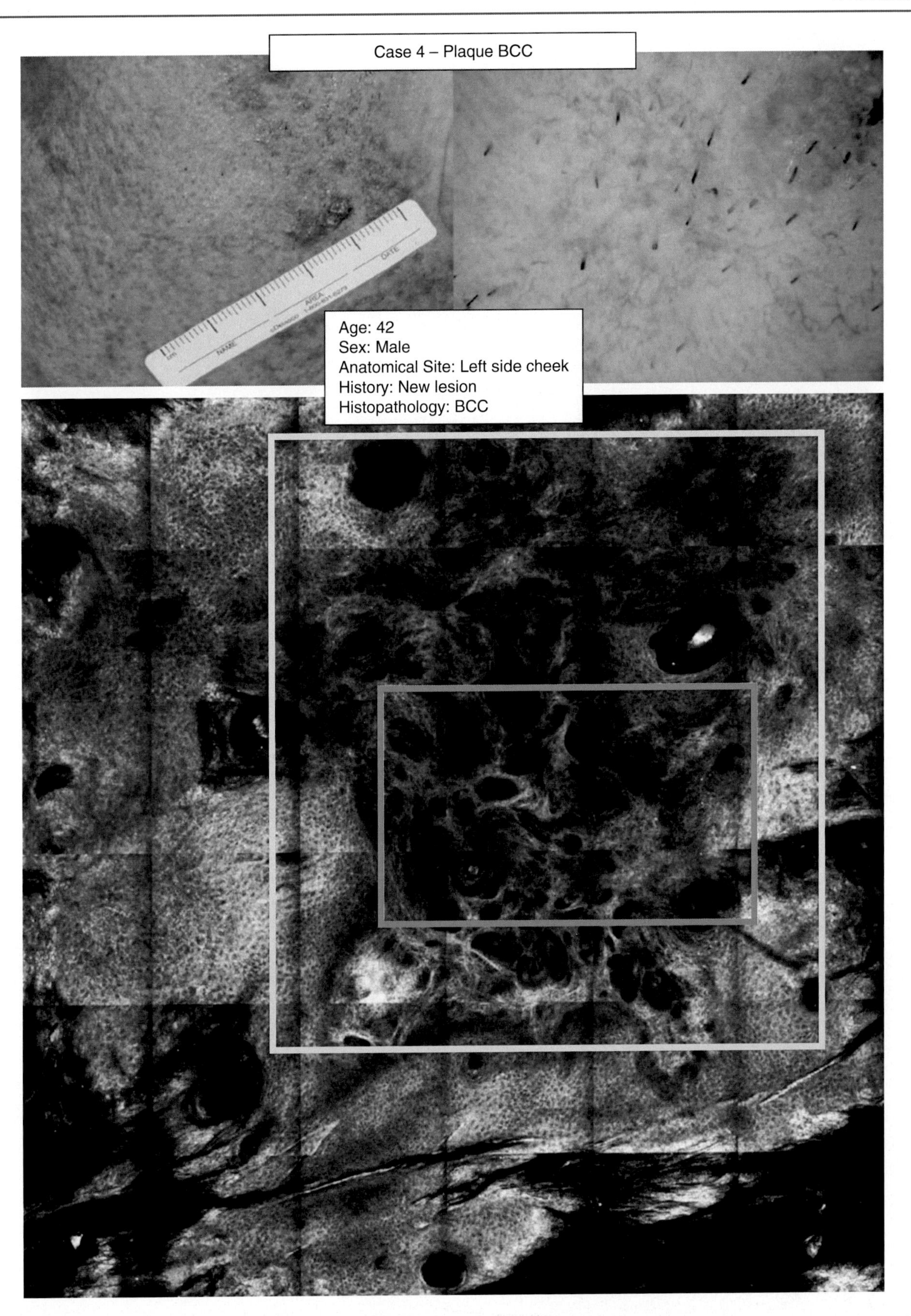

Fig. 21.4 RCM mosaic (3×3 mm) at the level of the dermal-epidermal junction reveals central dark silhouettes surrounded by thickened collagen. Surrounding this area is epidermis showing a honeycomb pattern of the spinous layer (Published with kind permission of © Harold S. Rabinovitz 2012. All Rights Reserved)

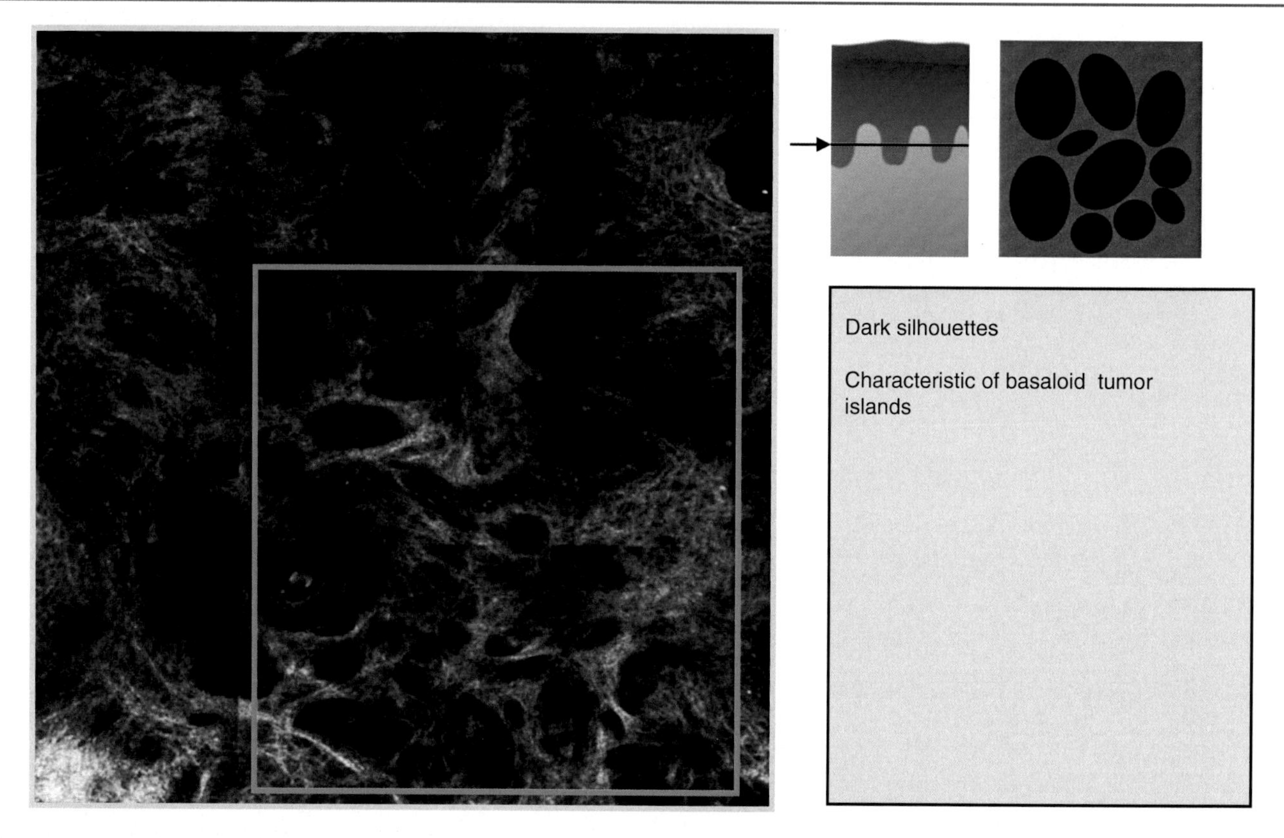

Fig. 21.4.1 RCM mosaic (approximately 2×2 mm) showing dark silhouettes surrounded by thickened collagen bundles; these dark silhouettes are characteristic of basaloid neoplastic aggregates in nonpigmented BCC (Published with kind permission of © Harold S. Rabinovitz 2012. All Rights Reserved)

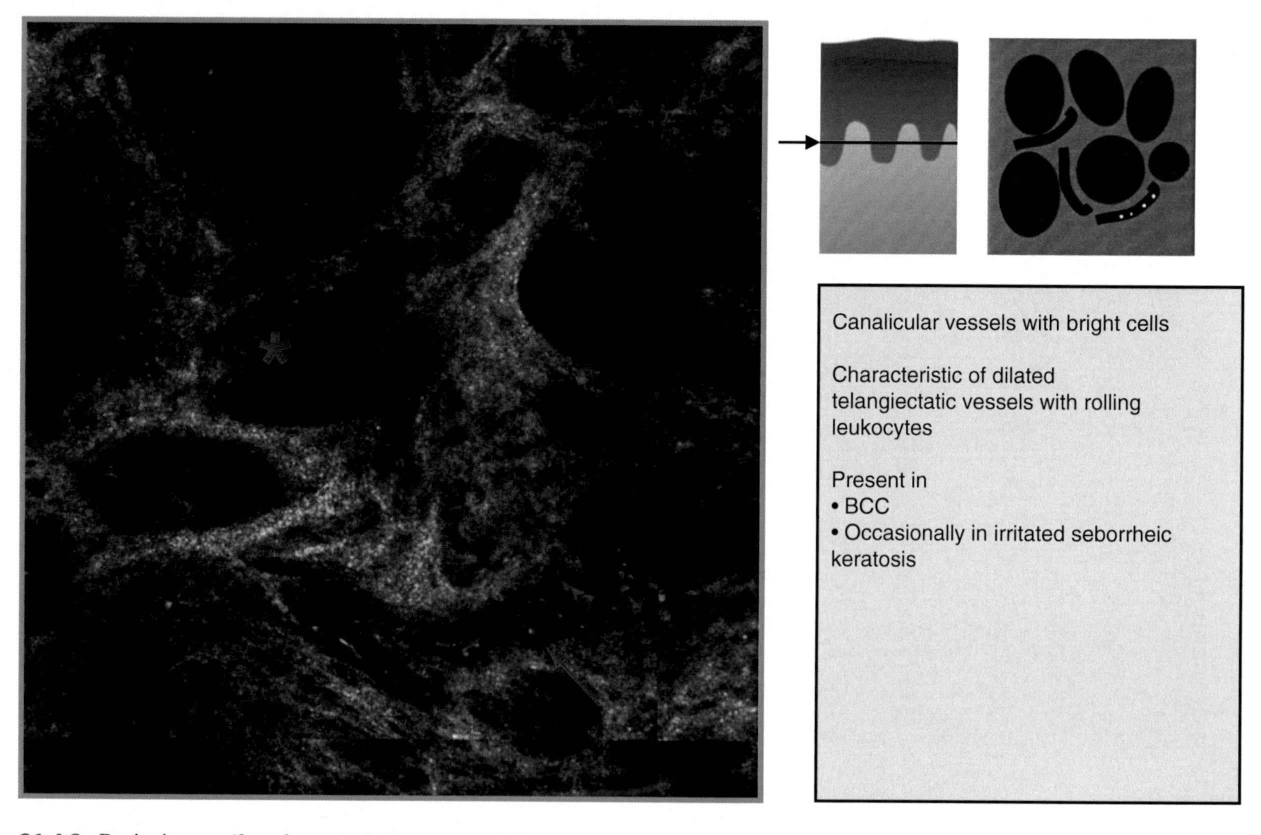

Fig. 21.4.2 Basic image (2 × 2 mm) depicts tumor islands surrounded by thickened collagen bundles (*). There are canalicular vessels with bright cells characteristic of dilated, telangiectatic vessels in the surrounding dermis (→) (Published with kind permission of © Harold S. Rabinovitz 2012. All Rights Reserved)

CASE 5 – Superficial BCC
Age: 81
Sex: Male
Anatomical Site: Left upper back
History: New lesion
Histopathology: BCC

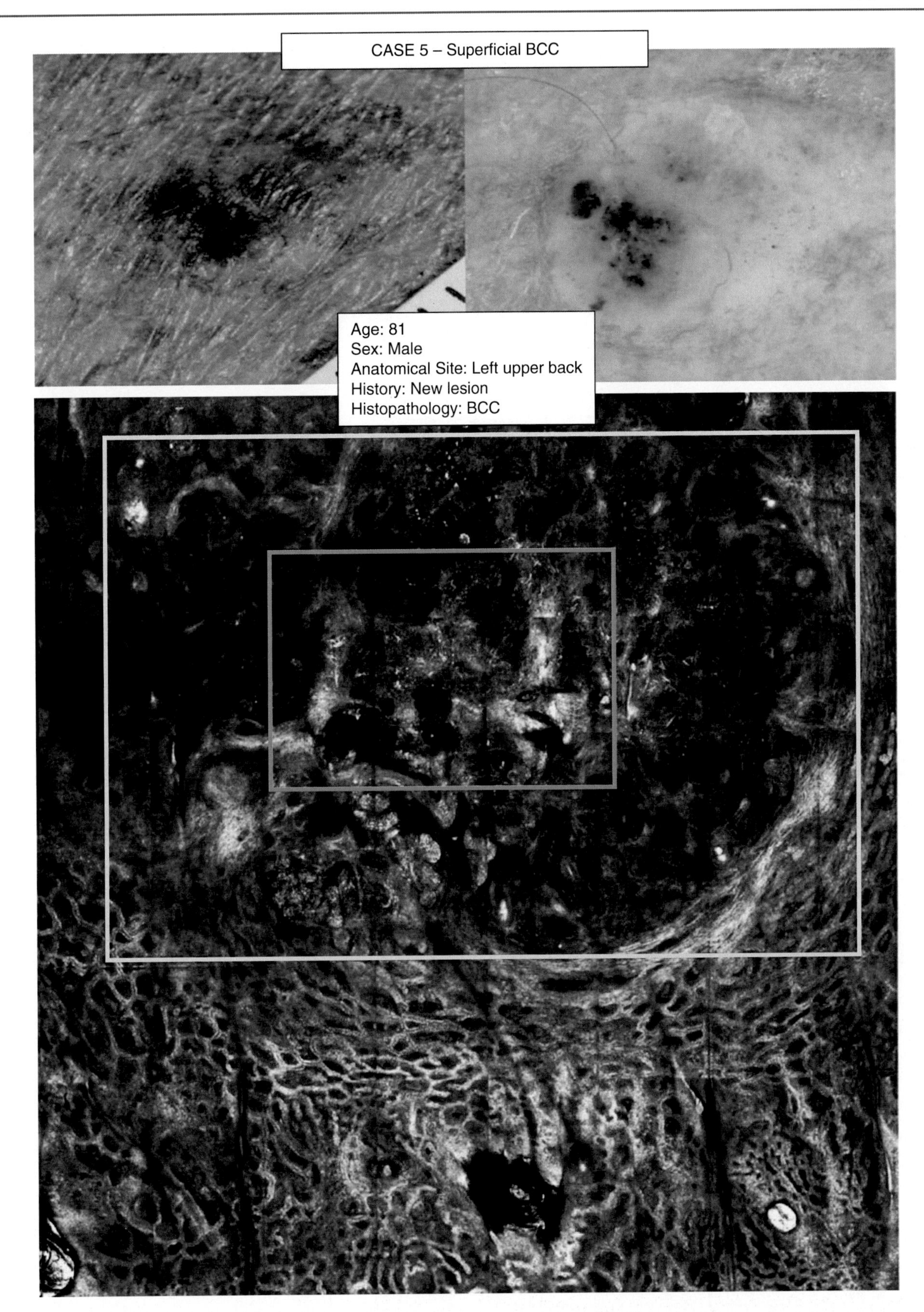

Fig. 21.5 RCM mosaic (4 × 4 mm) at the level of the superficial dermis reveals a complete replacement of the normal architecture by irregularly shaped lobulated bright tumor islands and dark silhouettes of different sizes and shapes. In addition, there are numerous bright spots. At the inferior portion are bright elongated connecting cords-like structures characteristic of solar lentigo (Published with kind permission of © Harold S. Rabinovitz 2012. All Rights Reserved)

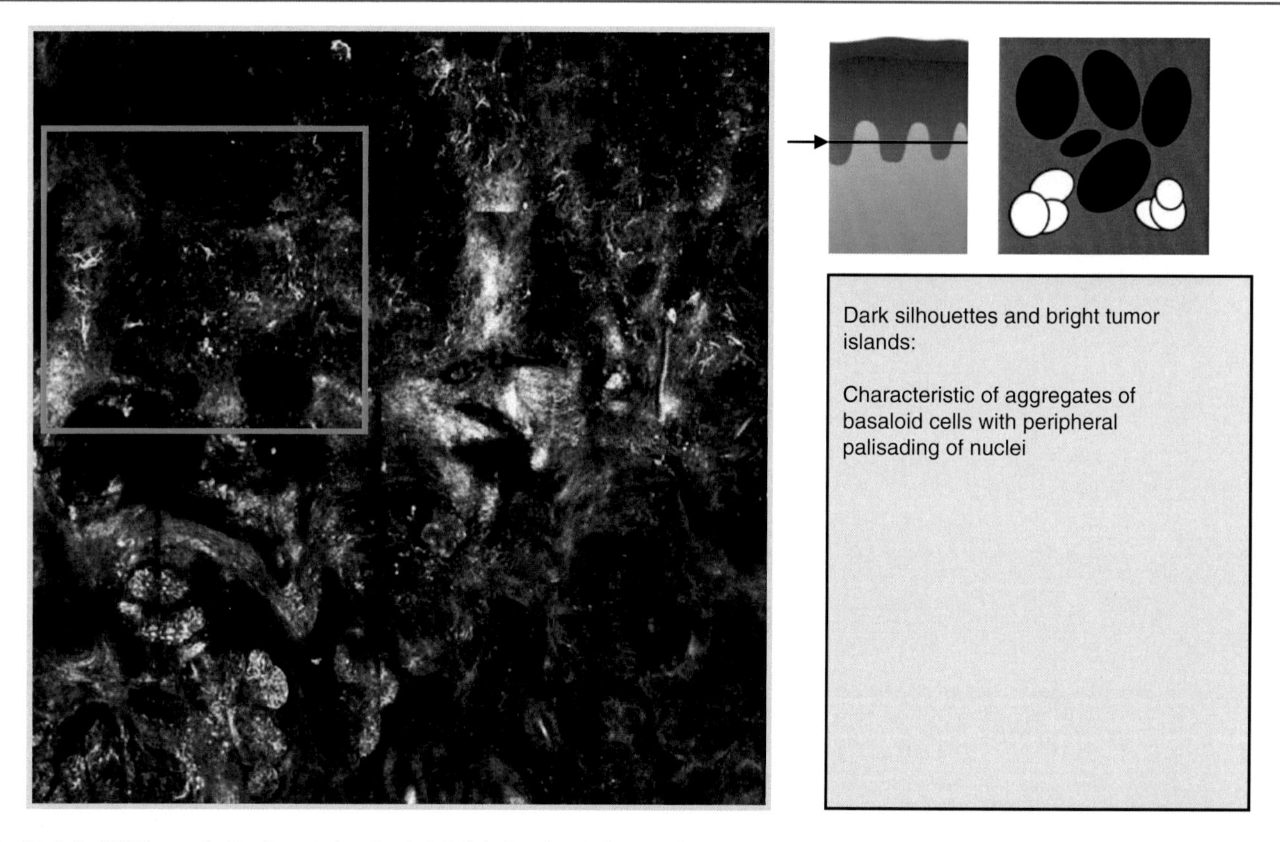

Fig. 21.5.1 RCM mosaic (2×2 mm) showing bright lobulated and elongated tumor islands that contain cells with dendritic processes (Published with kind permission of © Harold S. Rabinovitz 2012. All Rights Reserved)

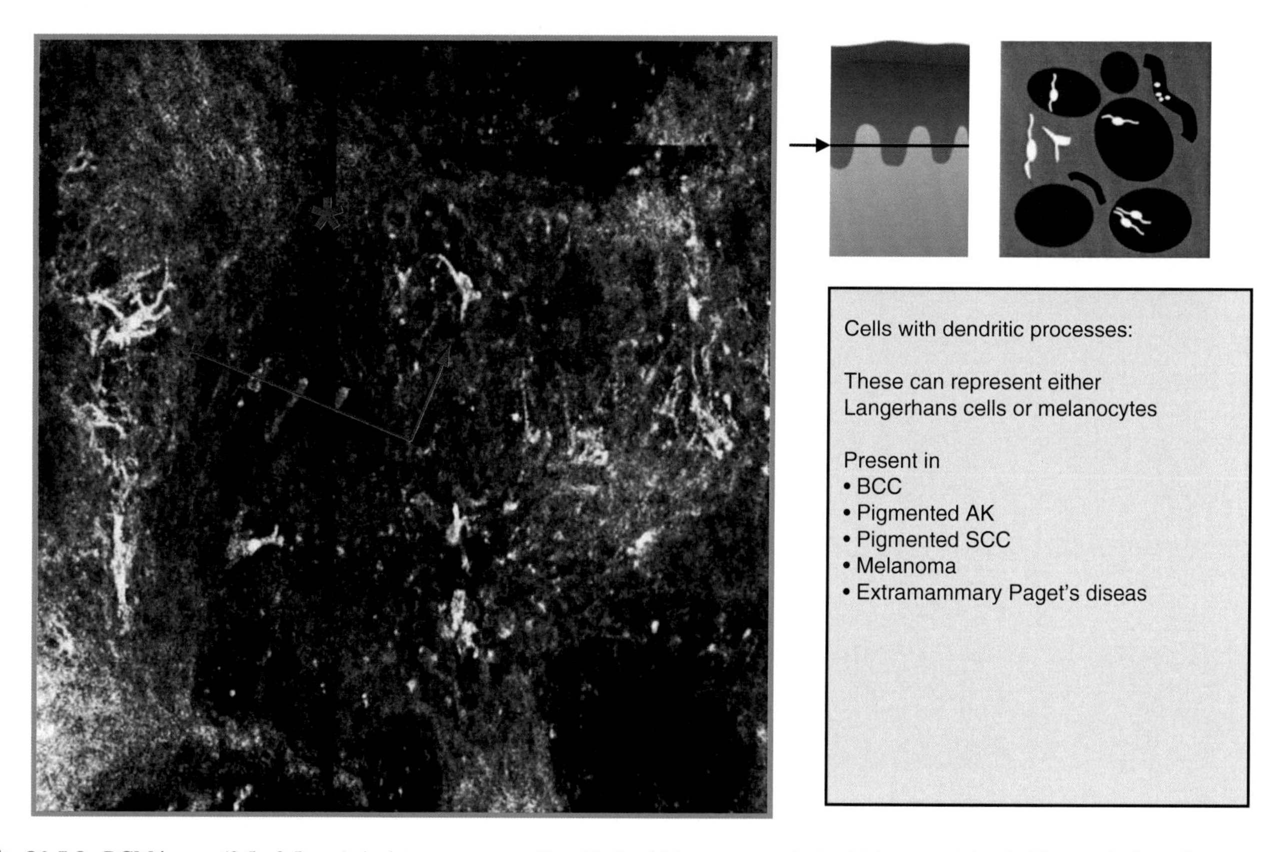

Fig. 21.5.2 RCM image (0.5×0.5 mm) depicts numerous cells with dendritic processes (→) within tumor islands (*), correlating with dendritic melanocytes within neoplastic aggregates of BCC (Published with kind permission of © Harold S. Rabinovitz 2012. All Rights Reserved)

Core Messages

- In RCM mosaic images, BCC is characterized by bright tumor islands well delineated from surrounding dermis by dark cleft-like spaces, or by dark silhouettes outlined by bright collagen bundles; the bright tumor islands and dark silhouettes correspond on histopathology to aggregates of neoplastic basaloid cells with peripheral palisading of nuclei.
- At higher magnification RCM, BCC shows elongated nuclei and at times bright dendritic structures within the tumor island, and a surrounding stroma that exhibits canalicular vessels coursing *en face* and plump-bright cells.

References

1. Christenson LJ, Borrowman TA, Vachon CM, Tollefson MM, Otley CC, Weaver AL, Roenigk RK (2005) Incidence of basal cell and squamous cell carcinomas in a population younger than 40 years. JAMA 294:681–690
2. Lear JT, Smith AG (1997) Basal cell carcinoma. Postgrad Med J 73:538–542
3. Roewert-Huber J, Lange-Asschenfeldt B, Stockfleth E, Kerl H (2007) Epidemiology and aetiology of basal cell carcinoma. Br J Dermatol 157(Suppl 2):47–51
4. Harris RB, Griffith K, Moon TE (2001) Trends in the incidence of nonmelanoma skin cancers in southeastern Arizona, 1985–1996. J Am Acad Dermatol 45:528–536
5. Dahl E, Aberg M, Rausing A, Rausing EL (1992) Basal cell carcinoma. An epidemiologic study in a defined population. Cancer 70:104–108
6. Goldberg LH (1996) Basal cell carcinoma. Lancet 347:663–667
7. Gallagher RP, Hill GB, Bajdik CD, Fincham S, Coldman AJ, McLean DI, Threlfall WJ (1995) Sunlight exposure, pigmentary factors, and risk of nonmelanocytic skin cancer. I. Basal cell carcinoma. Arch Dermatol 131:157–163
8. Rubin AI, Chen EH, Ratner D (2005) Basal-cell carcinoma. N Engl J Med 353:2262–2269
9. Nijsten TE, Stern RS (2003) The increased risk of skin cancer is persistent after discontinuation of psoralen+ultraviolet A: a cohort study. J Invest Dermatol 121:252–258
10. Crowson AN, Magro CM, Kadin ME, Stranc M (1996) Differential expression of the bcl-2 oncogene in human basal cell carcinoma. Hum Pathol 27:355–359
11. Shimizu N, Ito M, Tazawa T, Sato Y (1989) Immunohistochemical study on keratin expression in certain cutaneous epithelial neoplasms. Basal cell carcinoma, pilomatricoma, and seborrheic keratosis. Am J Dermatopathol 11:534–540
12. Ting PT, Kasper R, Arlette JP (2005) Metastatic basal cell carcinoma: report of two cases and literature review. J Cutan Med Surg 9:10–15
13. Bernard Ackerman, Helmut Kerl, Jorge Sanchez et al (2000) A clinical atlas of 101 common skin diseases: with histopathologic correlation. Ardor Scribbendi, 1st edn
14. Boyd AS (2004) Tumors of the epidermis. In: Branhill R (ed) CAeToD, 2nd edn. McGraw-Hill Co, New York, pp 575–634
15. Johnson TM, Tschen J, Ho C, Lowe L, Nelson BR (1994) Unusual basal cell carcinomas. Cutis 54:85–92
16. Maloney ME, Jones DB, Sexton FM (1992) Pigmented basal cell carcinoma: investigation of 70 cases. J Am Acad Dermatol 27: 74–78
17. Scope A, Mecca PS, Marghoob AA (2009) skINsight lessons in reflectance confocal microscopy: rapid diagnosis of pigmented basal cell carcinoma. Arch Dermatol 145:106–107
18. Carucci J, Leffell DJ (2003) Basal cell carcinoma. In: Freedberg IM, Eisen AZ, Wolff K et al (eds) Fitzpatrick's dermatology in general medicine. McGraw-Hill, New York, pp 747–754
19. Kirkham N (2002) Tumors and cysts of the epidermis. In: Elder DE, Elenitas R, Johnson BL et al (eds) Lever's histopathology of the skin. Lippincott Williams & Wilkins, Philadelphia, pp 836–849
20. Presser SE, Taylor JR (1987) Clinical diagnostic accuracy of basal cell carcinoma. J Am Acad Dermatol 16:988–990
21. Menzies SW, Westerhoff K, Rabinovitz H, Kopf AW, McCarthy WH, Katz B (2000) Surface microscopy of pigmented basal cell carcinoma. Arch Dermatol 136:1012–1016
22. Pan Y, Chamberlain AJ, Bailey M, Chong AH, Haskett M, Kelly JW (2008) Dermatoscopy aids in the diagnosis of the solitary red scaly patch or plaque-features distinguishing superficial basal cell carcinoma, intraepidermal carcinoma, and psoriasis. J Am Acad Dermatol 59:268–274
23. Braga JC, Scope A, Klaz I, Mecca P, Gonzalez S, Rabinovitz H, Marghoob AA (2009) The significance of reflectance confocal microscopy in the assessment of solitary pink skin lesions. J Am Acad Dermatol 61:230–241
24. Nori S, Rius-Diaz F, Cuevas J, Goldgeier M, Jaen P, Torres A, Gonzalez S (2004) Sensitivity and specificity of reflectance-mode confocal microscopy for in vivo diagnosis of basal cell carcinoma: a multicenter study. J Am Acad Dermatol 51:923–930
25. Gonzalez S, Tannous Z (2002) Real-time, in vivo confocal reflectance microscopy of basal cell carcinoma. J Am Acad Dermatol 47:869–874
26. Agero AL, Busam KJ, Benvenuto-Andrade C, Scope A, Gill M, Marghoob AA, Gonzalez S, Halpern AC (2006) Reflectance confocal microscopy of pigmented basal cell carcinoma. J Am Acad Dermatol 54:638–643
27. Segura S, Puig S, Carrera C, Palou J, Malvehy J (2007) Dendritic cells in pigmented basal cell carcinoma: a relevant finding by reflectance-mode confocal microscopy. Arch Dermatol 143: 883–886
28. Segura S, Puig S, Carrera C, Palou J, Malvehy J (2009) Development of a two-step method for the diagnosis of melanoma by reflectance confocal microscopy. J Am Acad Dermatol 61:216–229

22 Actinic Keratosis

Martina Ulrich and Susanne Astner

22.1 Introduction

The incidence of actinic keratoses (AK) is continuously rising worldwide and the most common risk factor is chronic UV exposure. Actinic keratoses have recently been classified as cutaneous squamous cell carcinoma (SCC) in situ [1, 2] and have the potential to develop into invasive squamous cell carcinoma. The risk for progression has been estimated around 10% [3]; however, much higher rates have been reported in immunosuppressed patients after organ transplantation [4]. In this regard early recognition and treatment of AK remains crucial. Clinically, AK present as erythematous to brown plaques with a scaly surface and rough palpation. Different grades of hyperkeratosis can be observed. In contrast to other epithelial malignancies, such as basal cell carcinoma, AK develop multiple in areas of chronic UV exposure. This has been referred to as actinic field cancerization [5]. The diagnosis of AK is usually based on clinical evaluation, but biopsies are routinely performed to rule out invasive squamous cell carcinoma or other skin diseases. The differential diagnosis is broad and includes among others porokeratoses, seborrheic keratoses, basal cell carcinoma or Bowen's disease. Dermoscopy has recently been applied for the diagnosis of AK, the classic features include the presence pink-to-red 'pseudonetwork' surrounding the hair follicles, scale, fine, linear-wavy vessels surrounding the hair follicles and keratotic plugs within the hair follicles. Altogether these criteria result in a "strawberry" appearance of the lesion [6]. However, hyperkeratotic scale often obscures other features and the sensitivity and specificity of these criteria have not yet been determined.

Histopathologically, AK are characterized by a proliferation of atypical keratinocytes, which starts at the basal cell layer and leads to architectural disarray with basal crowding of the keratinocytes. Mitoses and nuclear pleomorphism are commonly seen and parakeratosis alternating with orthokeratosis at the follicle ostia can be observed in the stratum corneum. Solar elastosis is present in the dermis as well as an inflammatory infiltrate of variable degree. The proliferation of atypical keratinocytes may involve the complete epidermis, in this regard AK have been classified into three different grades histopathologically. In grade I the proliferation of atypical keratinocytes is limited to the lower third of the epidermis, whereby in grade II the lower two thirds of the epidermis is involved and in grade III full thickness epidermal atypia is present [7].

22.2 RCM Features of AK

Characteristic RCM features of AK have been determined (Table 22.1), showing high sensitivity and specificity in two independent studies and good correlation to established histological criteria of AK [8, 9]. A recent study showed the reproducibility of these findings among the variable degrees of AK and SCC [10].

At the level of the stratum corneum superficial disruption with single detached keratinocytes seen as bright, polygonal cells of high reflectance can be observed (Fig. 22.1). Furthermore, nucleated cells with dark centre and sharp demarcation appear within highly reflective cells of the stratum corneum corresponding to parakeratosis (Fig. 22.1). On RCM mosaics a hyperkeratotic scale can often be observed, overlying the centre of the AK lesion and impairing the visualization of deeper lying structures (Fig. 22.2). Atypical honeycomb pattern and architectural disarray of variable degree are seen at the level of the stratum granulosum and stratum spinosum corresponding to different grades of keratinocyte dysplasia on histopathological exam (Fig. 22.1 and 22.2). On RCM atypical honeycomb pattern is characterized by variation of size and shape of keratinocytic nuclei and irregular cell borders. At the dermal layers solar elastosis can be visu-

M. Ulrich (✉) • S. Astner
Department of Dermatology and Venerology,
Charité University Medicine Berlin, Berlin, Germany
e-mail: martina.ulrich@charite.de; susanne.astner@charite.de

R. Hofmann-Wellenhof et al. (eds.), *Reflectance Confocal Microscopy for Skin Diseases*,
DOI 10.1007/978-3-642-21997-9_22,

Table 22.1 Patterns of actinic keratoses and their respective confocal microscopic correlates

Histologic features	RCM correlate	Differential diagnosis
Hyperkeratosis	superficial scale (RCM mosaics) single detached corneocytes (single images)	Warts, Seborrheic keratoses, Inflammatory skin diseases (e.g., psoriasis)
Parakeratosis	nucleated cells with dark centre and sharp demarcation at the level of the stratum corneum	Eczema (e.g., contact dermatitis), Psoriasis, Porokeratosis (at the borders/ cornoid lamella)
Proliferation of atypical keratinocytes	Atypical honeycomb pattern variation of size and shape of keratinocytic nuclei irregular cell borders architectural disruption/loss of normal epidermal stratification	Bowen's disease Malignant melanoma Basal cell carcinoma
Solar elastosis	Moderately refractive lace-like material adjacent to collagen bundles	Other epithelial malignancies Lentigo maligna melanoma Actinically damaged skin
Inflammatory infiltrate	Small highly refractile cells within the epidermal layers and the superficial dermis	Inflammatory skin diseases (e.g., eczema, psoriasis) Cutaneous T-cell lymphoma
Blood vessel dilatation	Round or oval dark spaces filled with moderately refractive small cells that show movement on in-vivo examination and correspond to erythrocytes	Inflammatory skin diseases other cutaneous tumours, but different morphology of blood vessels on RCM imaging – BCC: horizontally oriented branched and linear vessels – Seborrheic keratoses: looped vessels

alized, appearing as moderately refractive lace-like material adjacent to collagen bundles. Variable degree of inflammation seen as small, round cells of bright reflectance may also be observed (Fig. 22.1). Dilated blood vessels showing blood flow on in vivo examination are another common finding of AK. These blood vessels have been further characterized as round vessels traversing into the dermal papilla [10].

22.3 Subtypes of Actinic Keratoses

22.3.1 Pigmented AK

Pigmented AK represents an important differential diagnosis of pigmented macules and plaques of the face. The most important differential diagnosis includes lentigo maligna (LM), flat seborrheic keratoses and solar lentigo. Whereby (pigmented) AK and LM may both show atypical honeycomb pattern on RCM imaging; LM characteristically shows additional features such as non-edged papillae, pagetoid melanocytes in the epidermis, follicular distribution of atypical cells, atypical cells at the junction and nucleated cells in the dermis. In this regard, a score has been developed to simplify diagnosis of pigmented macules of the face [11]. Please refer to Chap. 16 & 20 for further details.

22.3.2 Hyperkeratotic AK

On clinical grounds hyperkeratotic AK are the one of the most important differential diagnosis of invasive squamous cell carcinoma. In this regard, improved diagnosis would be preferable. However, unfortunately hyperkeratosis limits the use of RCM as thick superficial scale interferes with the visualization of deeper epidermal-dermal structures due to its high refraction index. Several approaches are applicable to improve visualization in these cases including careful curettage of the scale or the use of topical keratolytic agents before evaluation. Curettage should only include the hyperkeratotic scale and not deeper layers to avoid artificial alterations and bleeding.

22.3.3 Actinic Cheilitis

Actinic cheilitis (AC) represents the equivalent of AK on the lip. In contrast to facial skin, the stratum corneum thickness on the lip is reduced often allowing better visualization of deeper structures than in AK at other body sites. The criteria of AC on RCM are similar to those of AK and include atypical honeycomb pattern at the level of the stratum granulosum and spinosum (Fig. 22.3), parakeratosis, single detached corneocytes in the stratum corneum as well as blood vessel dilatation and solar elastosis [12]. However, marked inflammatory infiltrate may be present in AC. Thus, impeding the correct diagnosis of AC and its differentiation from inflammatory lip conditions such as eczema or lichenoid dermatitis. In this regard, careful follow-up is recommended and biopsy has to be considered in cases that do not respond to therapy. A possible approach to lesions with marked inflammation on RCM imaging might be a short-term treatment with topical steroids followed by a second RCM evaluation.

CASE 1 – Actinic keratoses
Age: 68 years
Sex: Male
Anatomical Site: Scalp
History: rough lesion on the forehead for several months
*

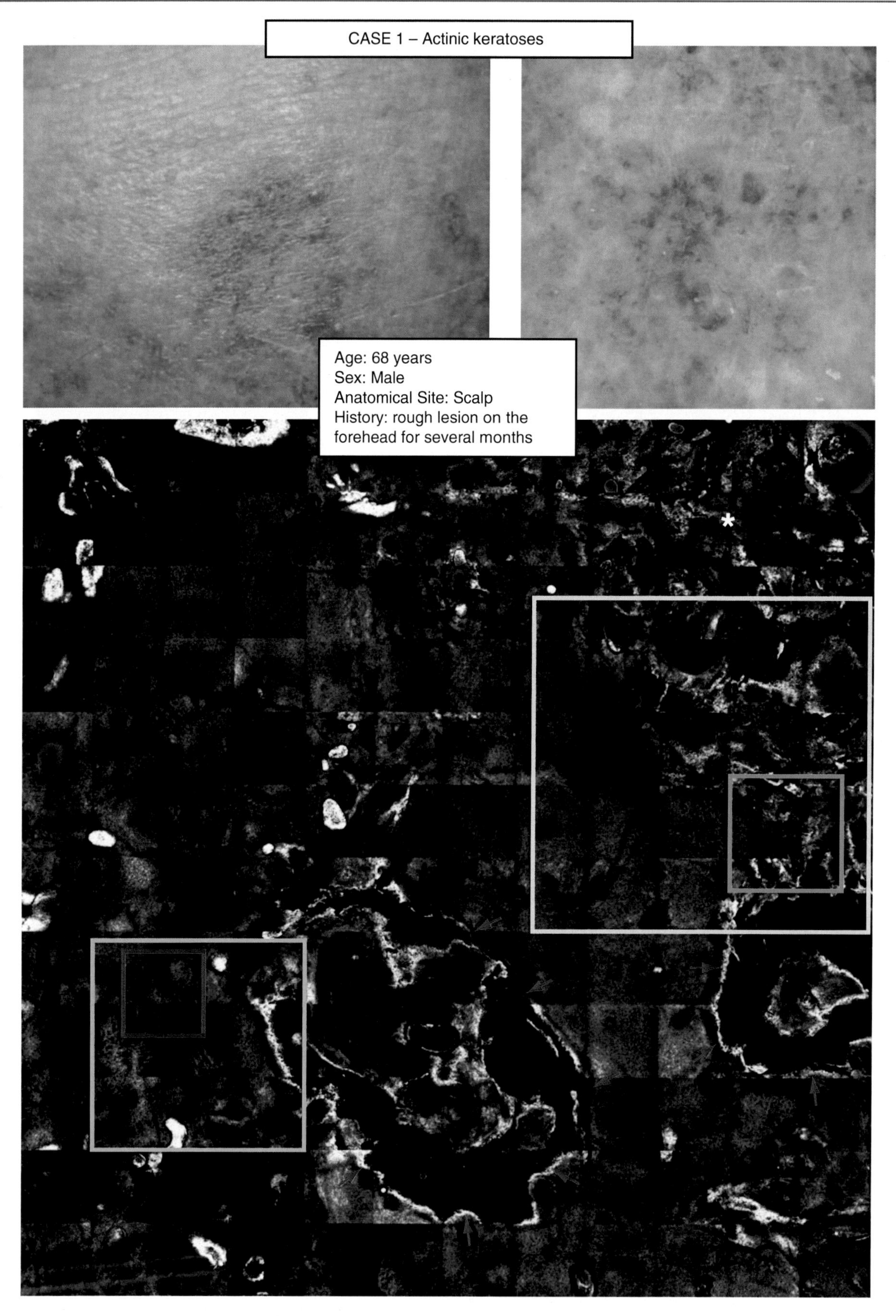

Fig. 22.1 RCM mosaic (6 × 6 mm) illustrating superficial disruption of the stratum corneum (*) and areas with hyperkeratotic superficial scale (→), partially interfering with the visualization of deeper epidermal and dermal structures

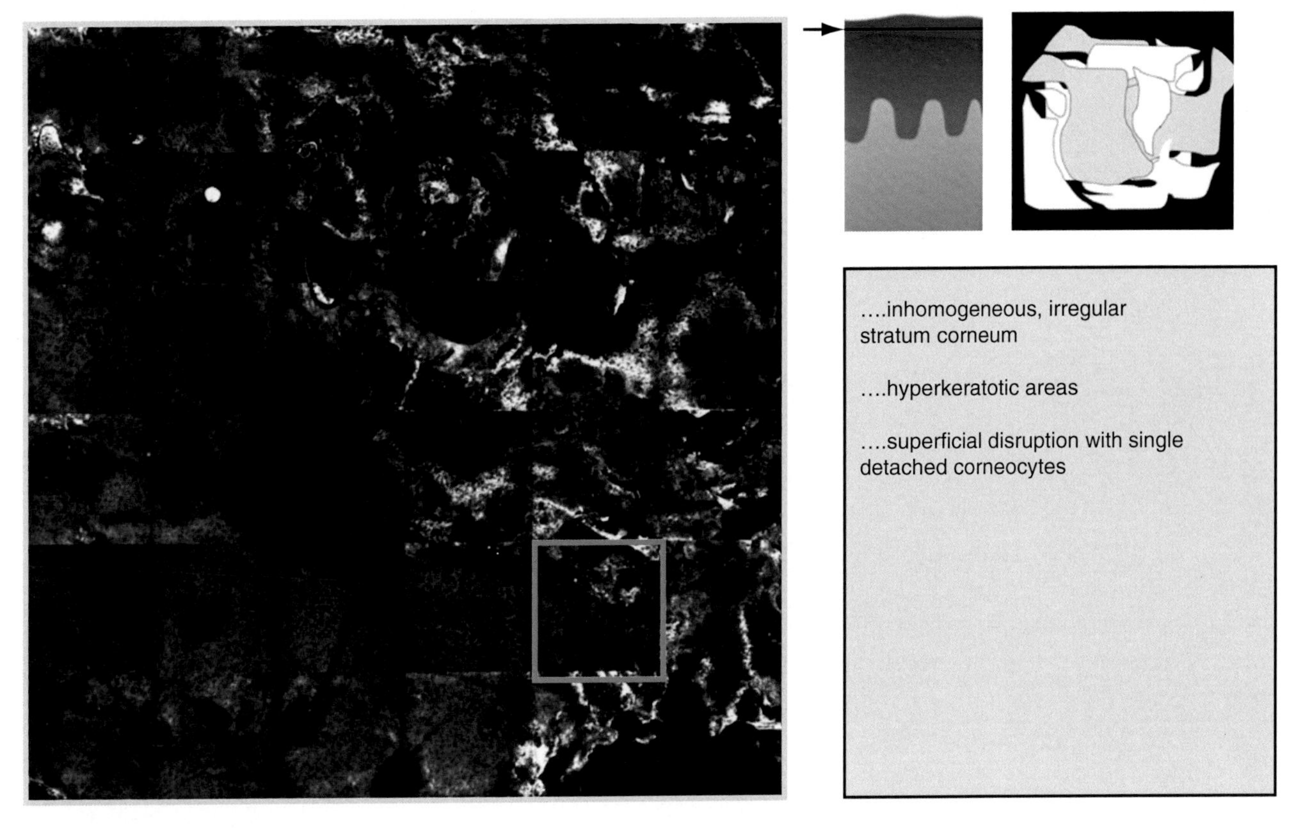

Fig. 22.1.1 RCM mosaic (3 × 3 mm) illustrating inhomogeneous appearance of the stratum corneum with hyperkeratotic areas

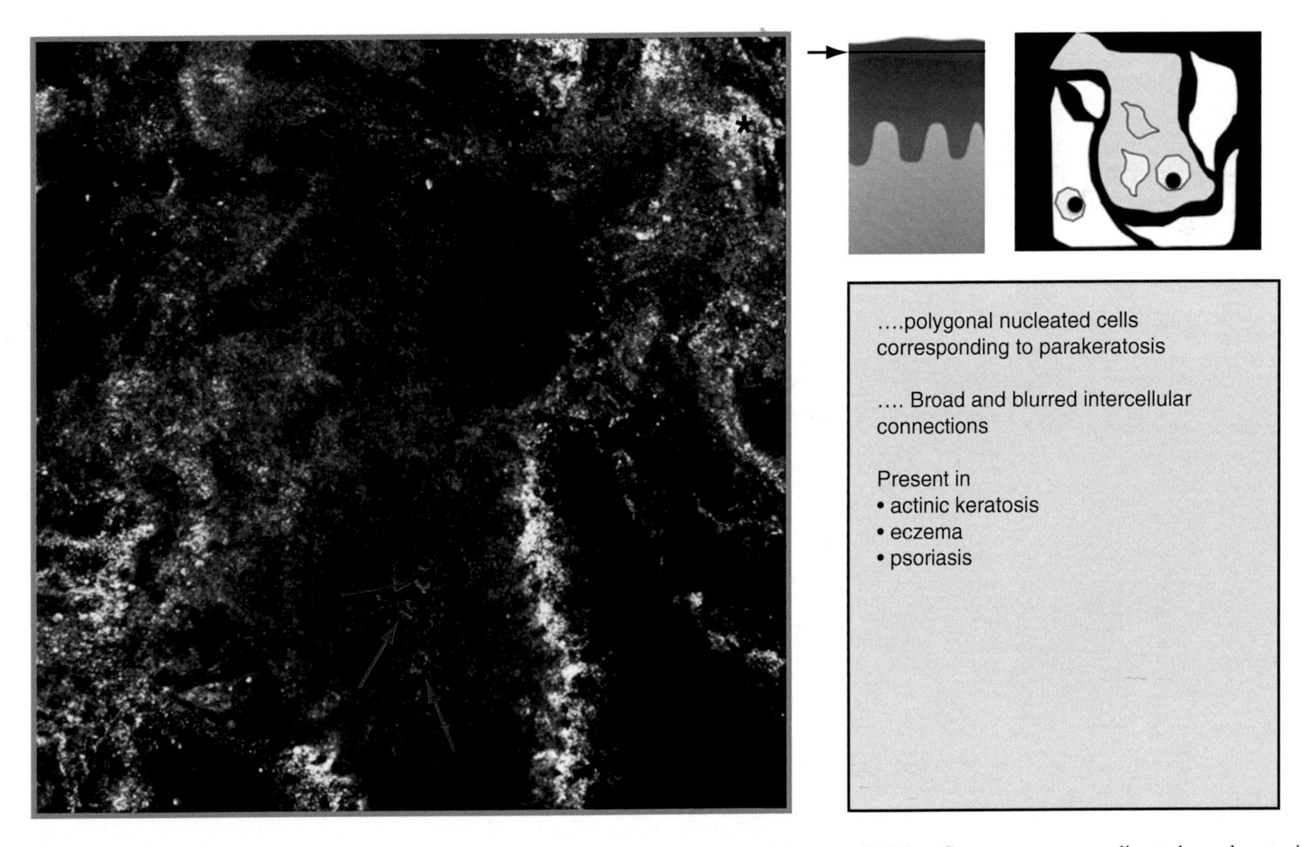

Fig. 22.1.2 Basic image (0.5 × 0.5 mm) obtained at the level of the stratum corneum with areas of bright reflectance corresponding to hyperkeratosis (*) and polygonal, nucleated cells corresponding to parakeratosis (→)

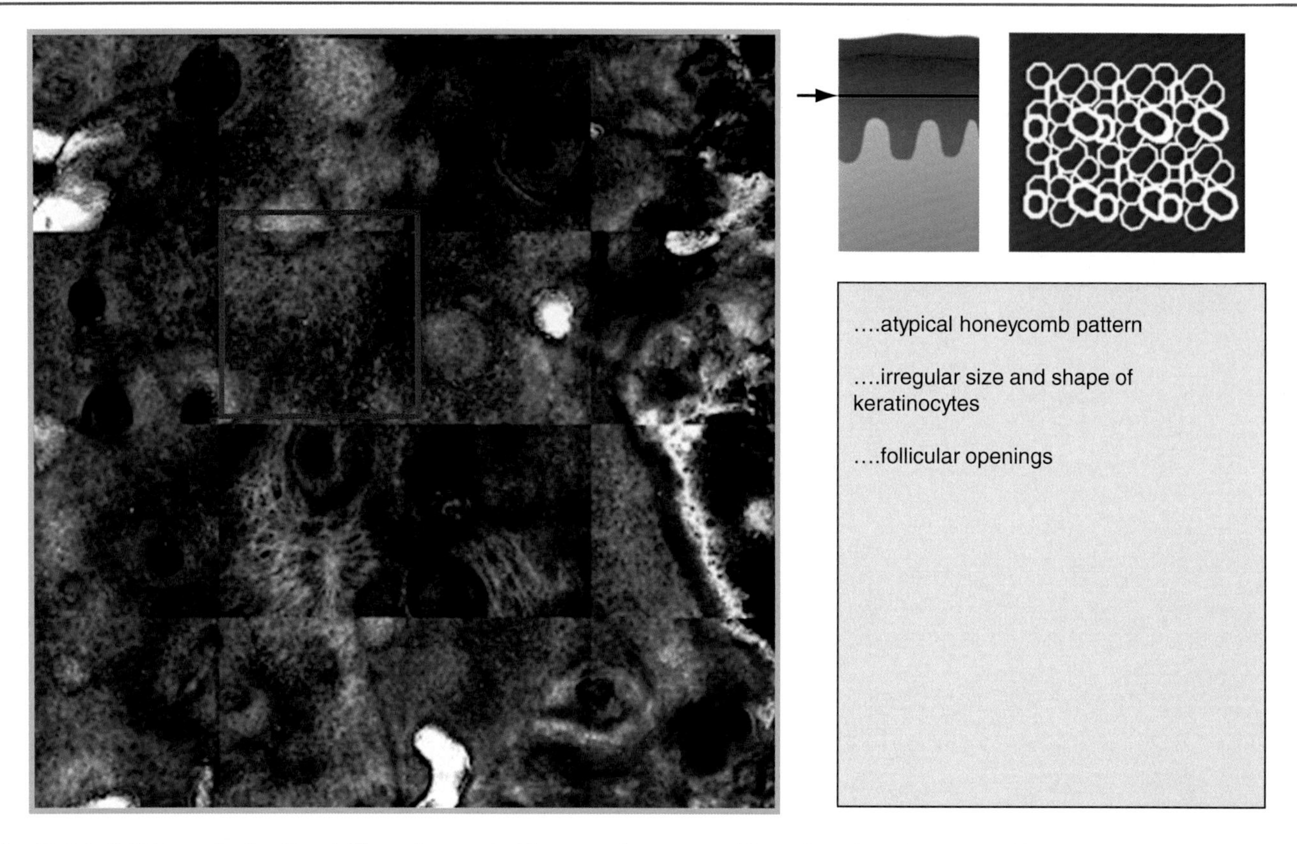

Fig. 22.1.3 RCM mosaic (2 × 2 mm) illustrating atypical honeycomb pattern and loss of regular epidermal architecture. Furthermore, enlarged follicular openings can be visualized

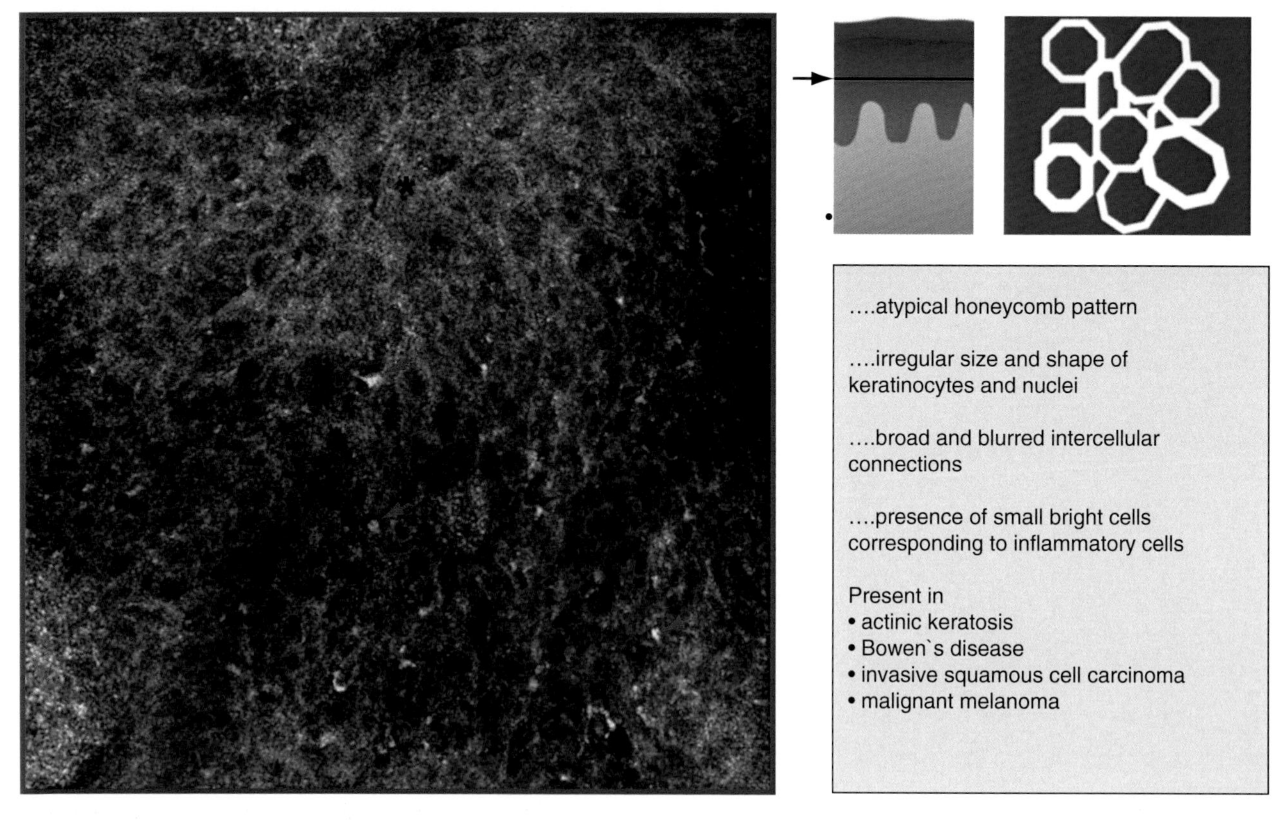

Fig. 22.1.4 Basic image (0.5 × 0.5 mm) at the level of the spinous-granular layer showing atypical honeycomb pattern with variation of cell size and shape. Broadened and blurred intercellular connections (*) at the upper part of the image. Furthermore, the presence of small bright round cells can be observed (→) corresponding to inflammatory cells

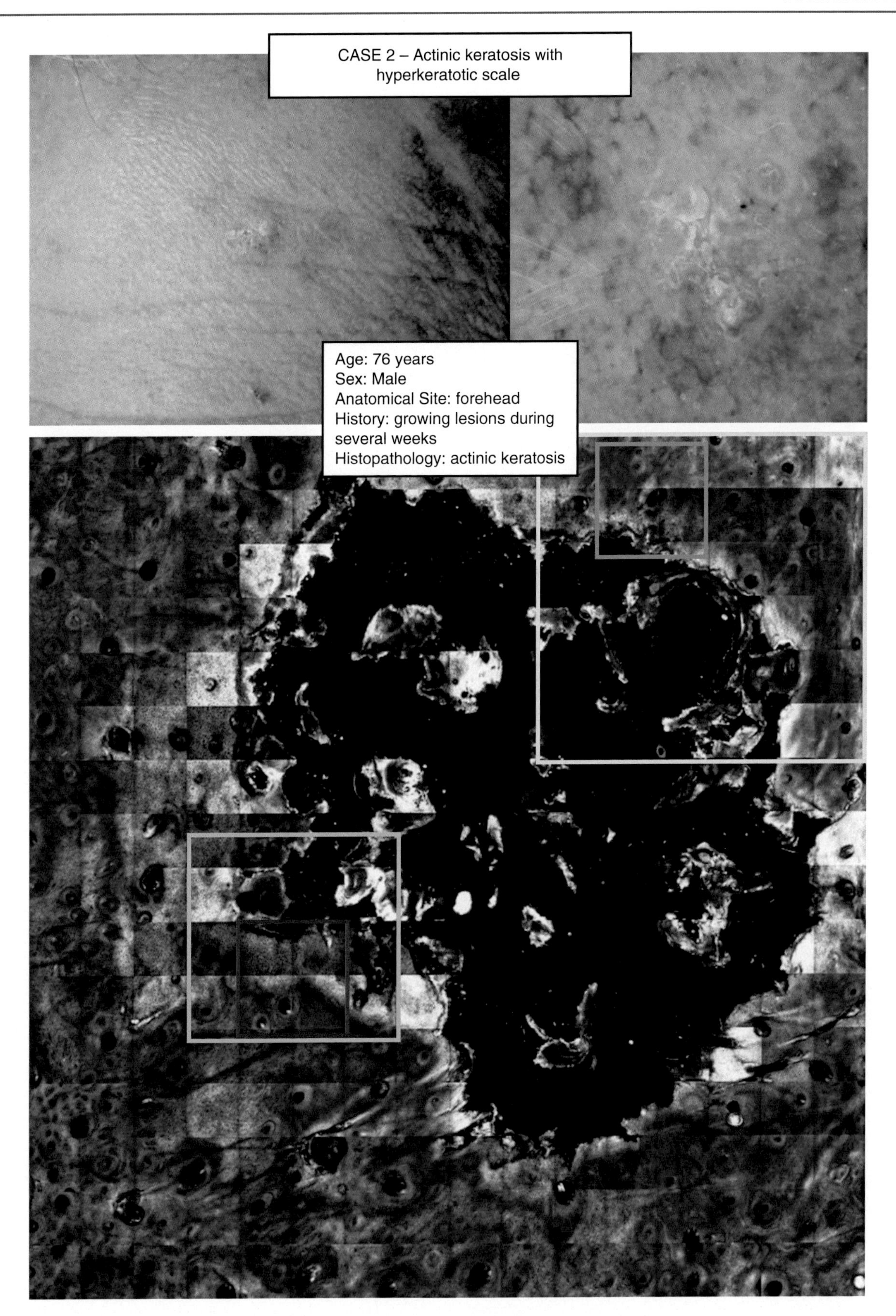

Fig. 22.2 RCM mosaic (8 × 8 mm) showing a dark area in the center of the lesion due to overlying superficial scale that interferes with visualization of deeper epidermal and dermal structures. Within this dark area irregular moderately to high refractive structures can be observed corresponding to hyper-and parakeratosis. At the border of the lesion visualization of the granular-spinous layer is possible

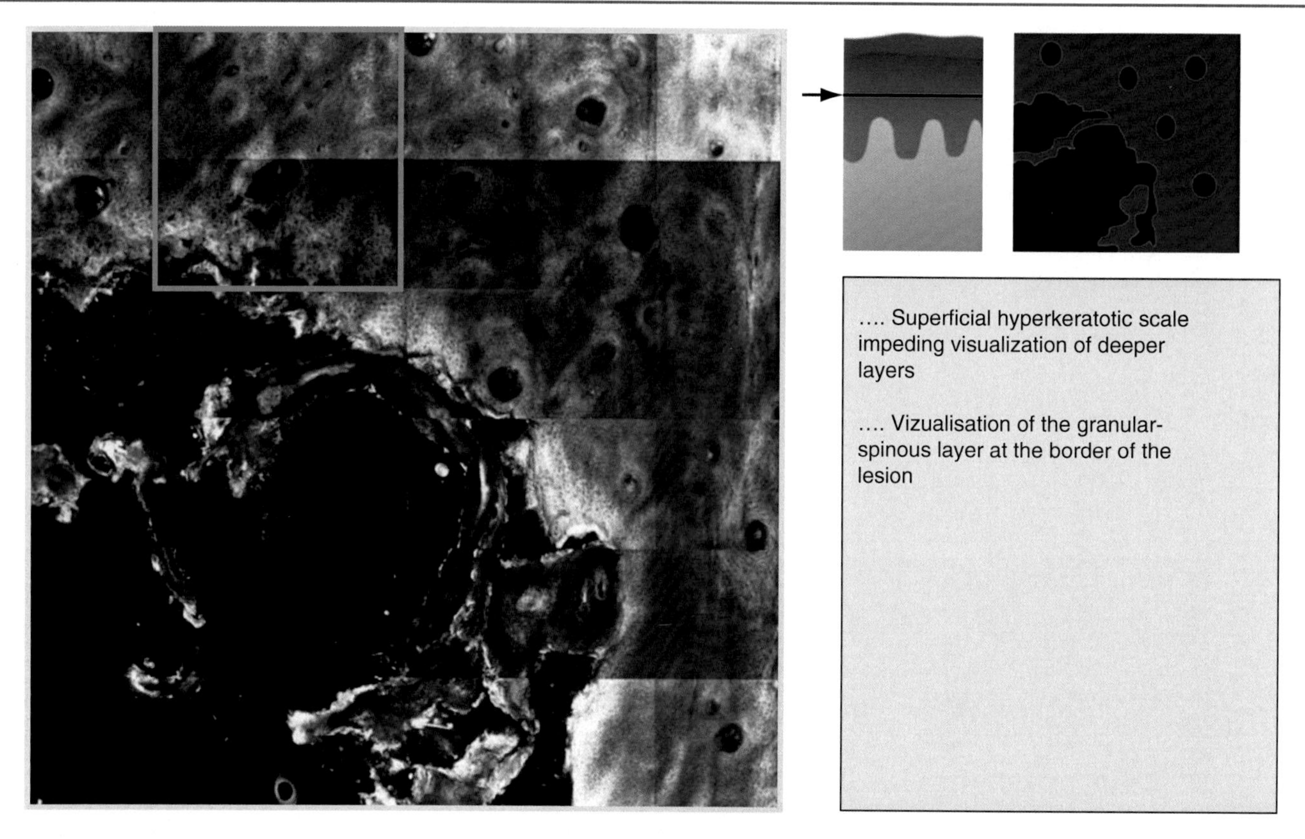

Fig. 22.2.1 RCM mosaic (3 × 3 mm) illustrating area of superficial scale at the left lower part of the lesion at which visualization of epidermal structures/cells is not possible. At the upper part of the lesion an area without overlying hyperkeratosis can be seen and detailed visualization of the granular-spinous layer is possible. Due to the presence of the scale, investigation of the central part of the lesion cannot be performed, invasive squamous cell carcinoma cannot be excluded

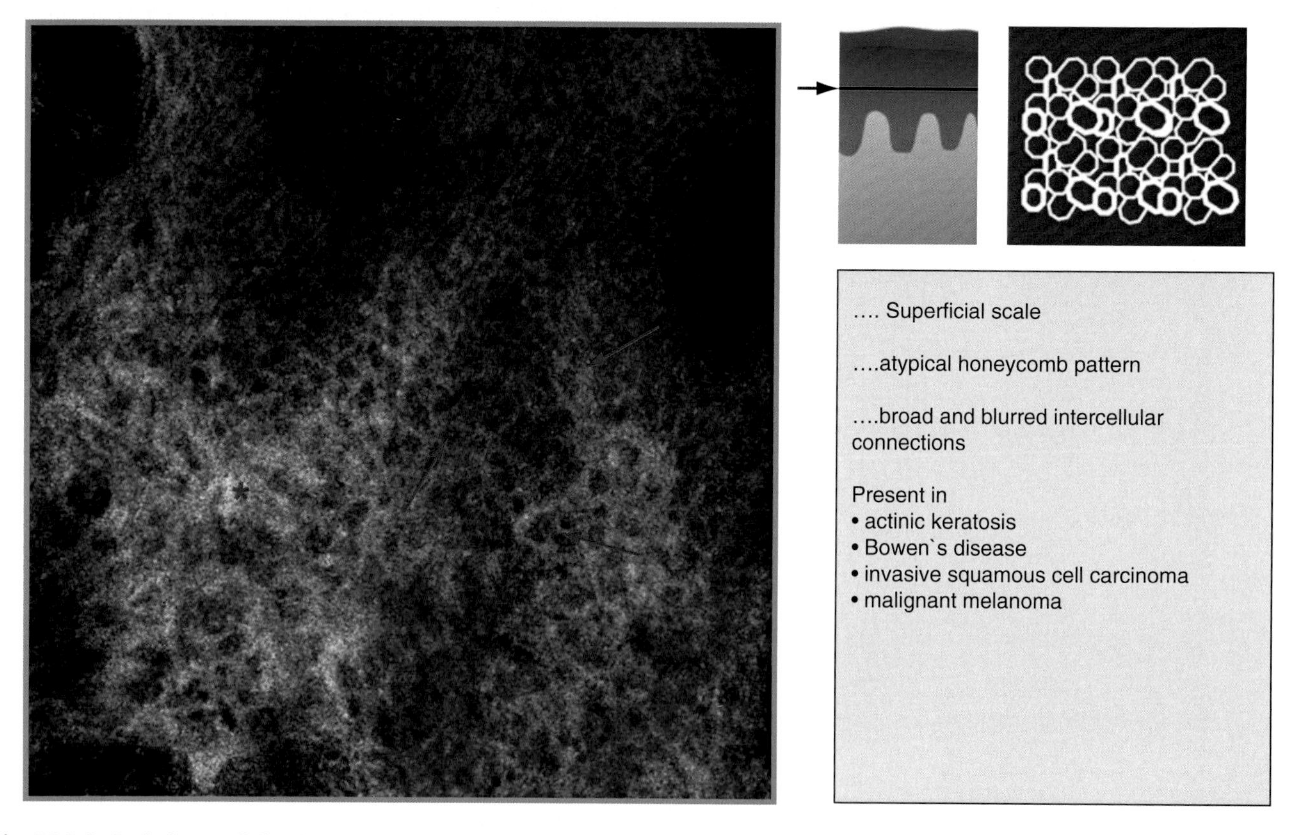

Fig. 22.2.2 Basic image (0.5 × 0.5 mm) obtained at the granular-spinous layer with broadened and blurred intercellular connections (*) and atypical honeycomb pattern showing variation of cell size and shape (→)

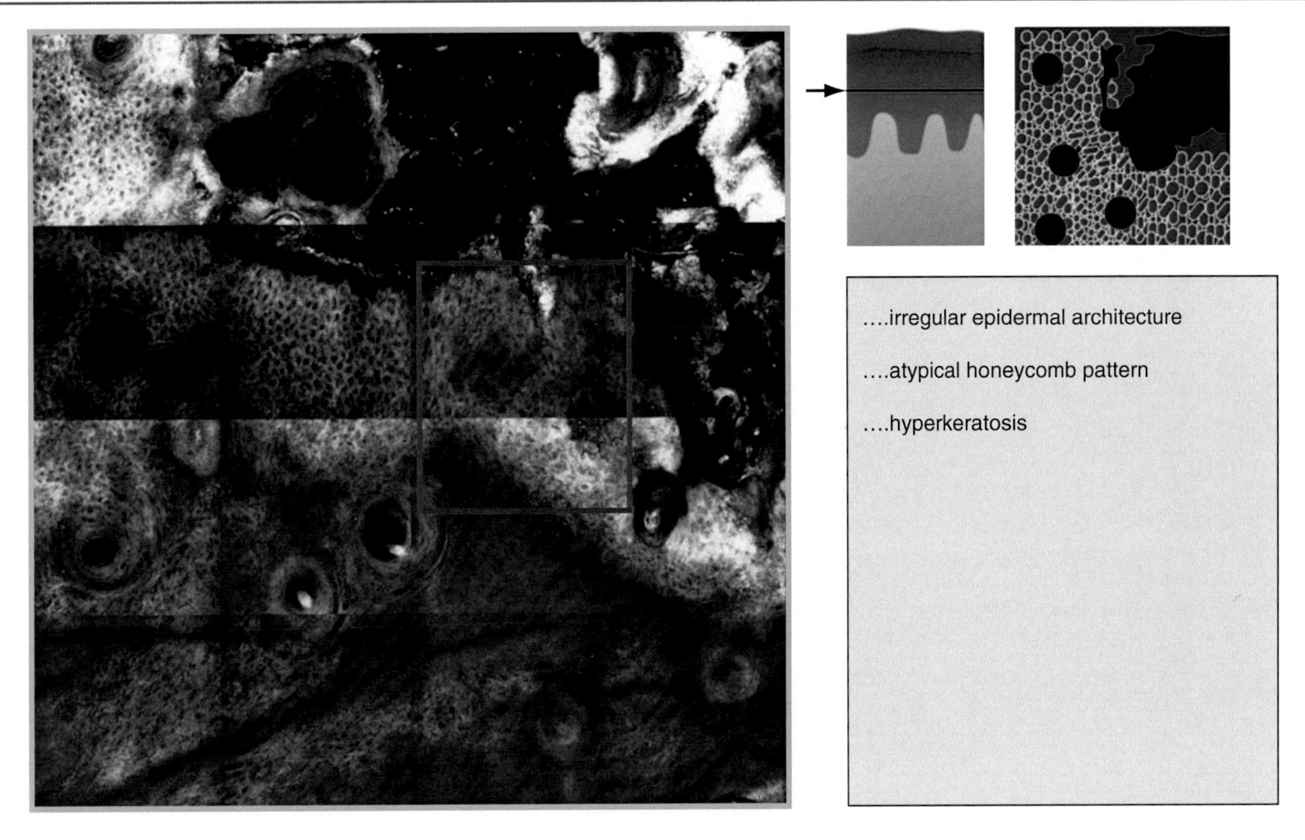

Fig. 22.2.3 RCM mosaic (2 × 2 mm) illustrating irregular architecture of the epidermis with atypical honeycomb pattern, hyperkeratotic areas and follicular openings

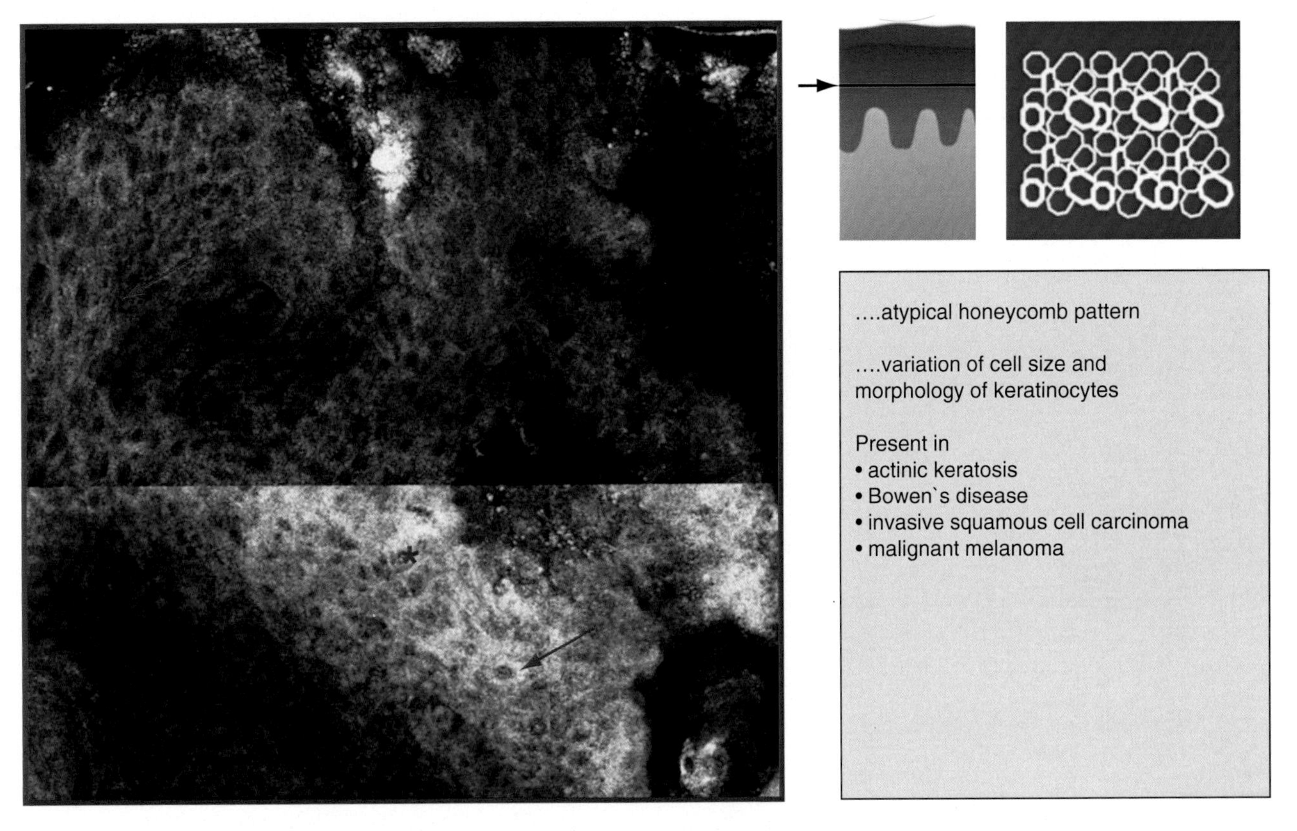

Fig. 22.2.4 Basic image (0.5 × 0.5 mm) illustrating atypical honeycomb pattern at the superficial parts of the epidermis with varying size and shape of the keratinocytes and nuclei (→). The intercellular connections are irregular and broadened (*)

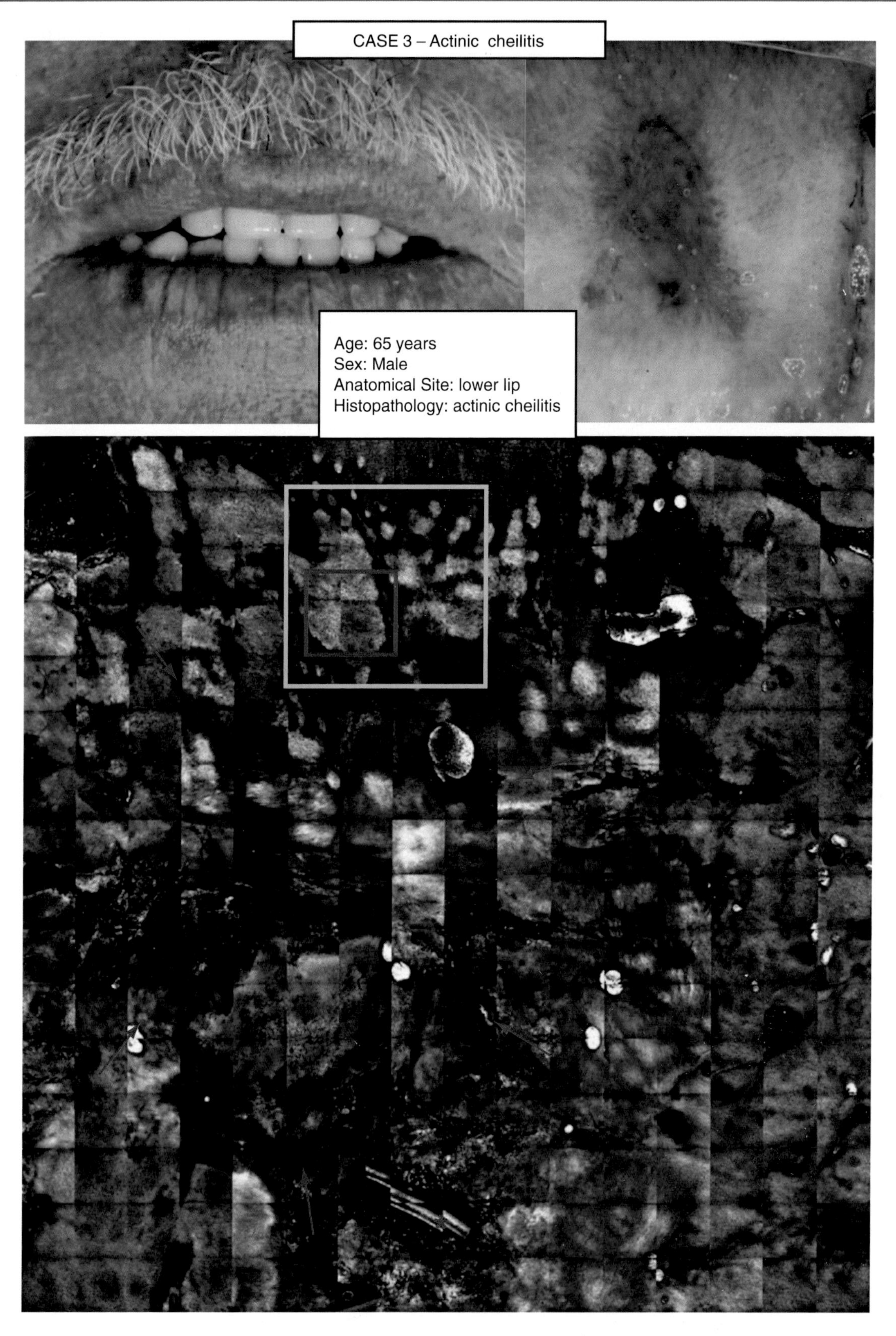

Fig. 22.3 RCM mosaic (8 × 8 mm) obtained at the level of the stratum spinosum illustrating epithelium of the vermillion border. The central part of the mosaic shows the erosive area (*red arrows*), whereas the lower part represents the surrounding normal skin where adnexal structures such as hairs (red star) can be visualized

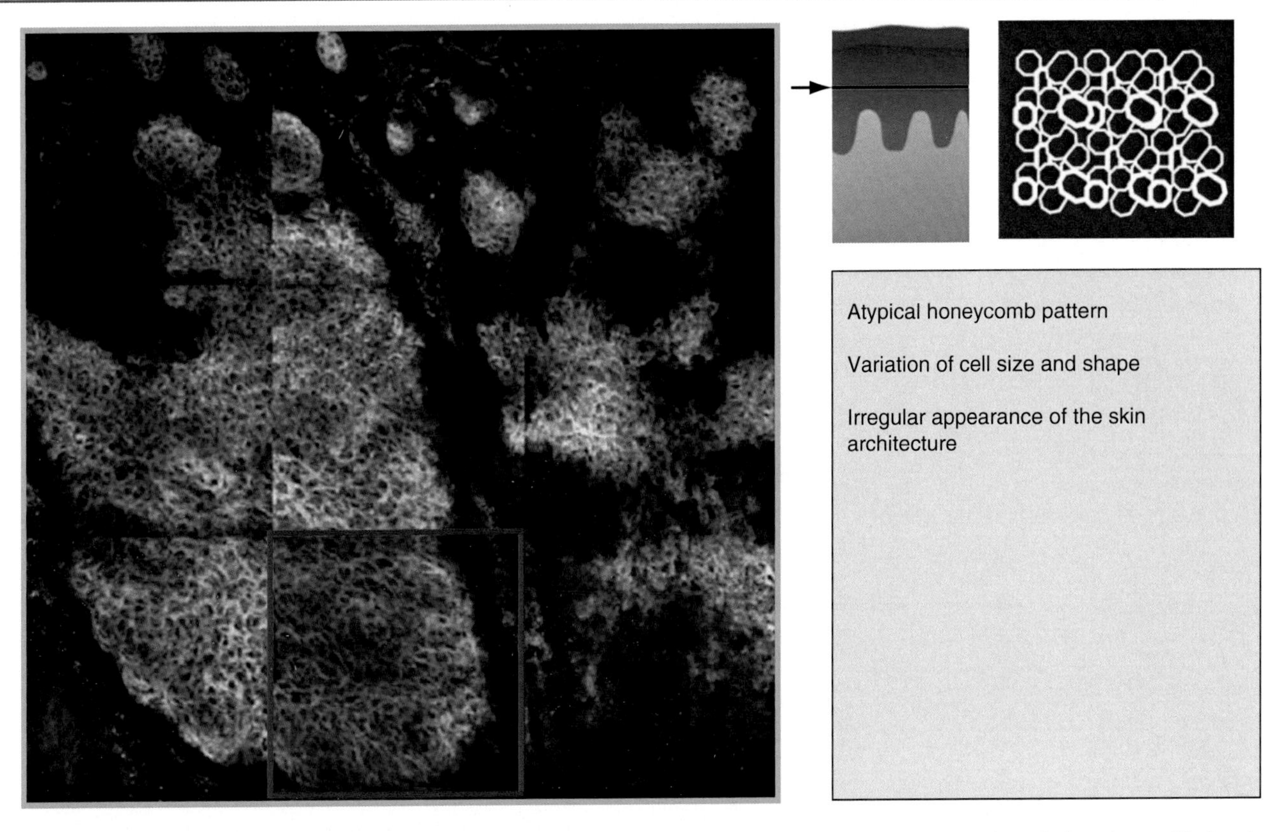

Fig. 22.3.1 RCM mosaic (1.5 × 1.5 mm) obtained at the level of the stratum spinosum showing atypical honeycomb pattern. The mosaic shows small "islands" of epithelium which is caused by superficial disruption with scaling and crusting and partly interferes with the visualization of deeper layers

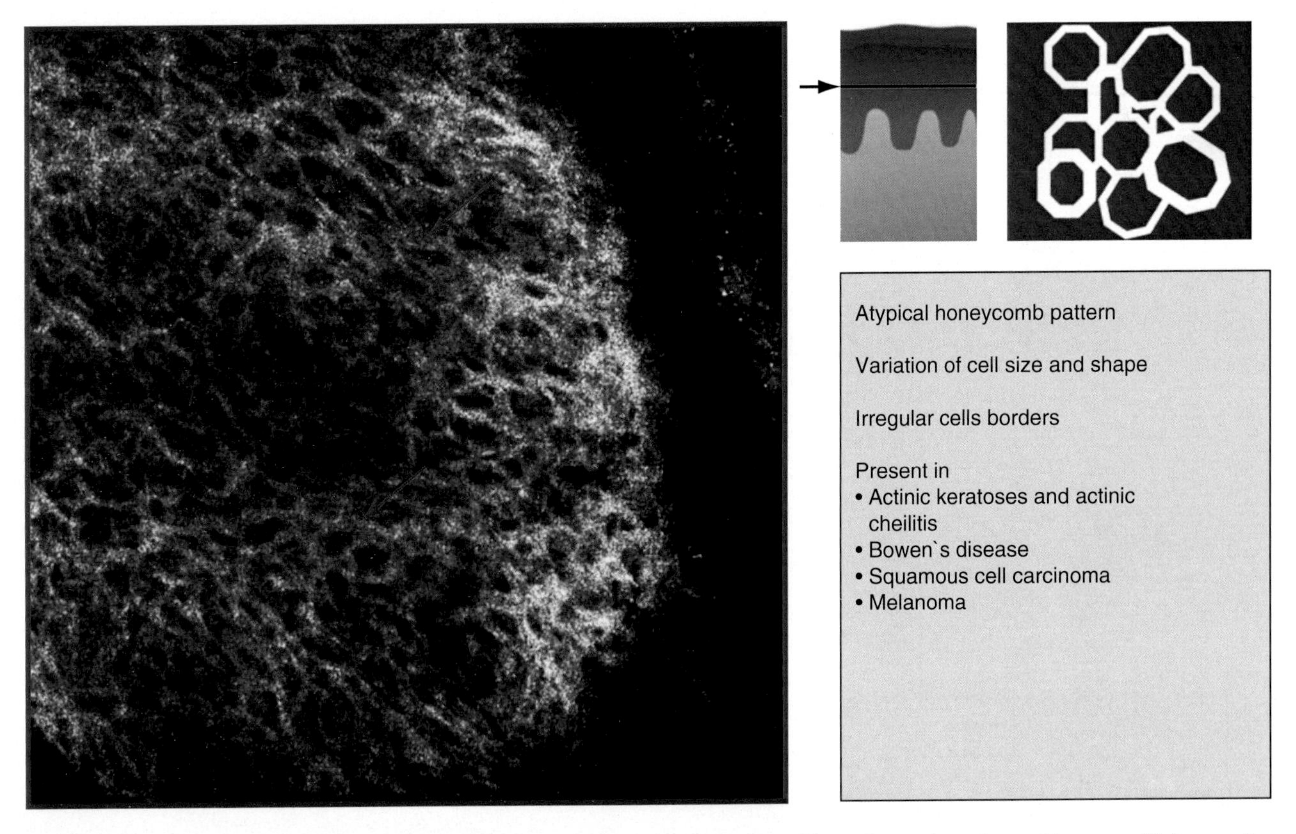

Fig. 22.3.2 Basic image (0.5 × 0.5 mm) obtained at the level of the stratum spinosum illustrating an irregular architecture with large cells and nuclei (*) that show great variation in size and morphology. In some areas intercellular borders are blurred and irregular (→)

Core Messages

- Actinic keratoses are characterized by the presence of atypical honeycomb pattern on RCM showing:
- Irregular size and shape of keratinocytes and nuclei.
- Irregular borders of keratinocytes.
- Alteration of the stratum corneum with single detached keratinocytes and superficial scale.
- Presence of polygonal, nucleated keratinocytes in the stratum corneum (parakeratoses).
- Loss of regular epidermal architecture resulting in disarranged epidermal pattern.
- Blood vessel dilatation with round to oval blood vessels traversing the dermal papilla.
- Solar elastosis characterized by moderately refractive lace-like material adjacent to collagen bundles.
- Absence of other RCM criteria (e.g., pagetoid melanocytic cells, non-edged papillae, elongated cells/nuclei with palisading) to distinguish non-pigmented AK from amelanotic melanoma or superficial basal cell carcinoma and pigmented AK from Lentigo maligna.

References

1. Ackerman AB (2003) Solar keratosis is squamous cell carcinoma. Arch Dermatol 139:1216–1217
2. Röwert-Huber J, Patel MJ, Forschner T, Ulrich C, Eberle J, Kerl H, Sterry W, Stockfleth E (2007) Actinic keratosis is an early in situ squamous cell carcinoma: a proposal for reclassification. Br J Dermatol 156(Suppl 3):8–12
3. Fuchs A, Marmur E (2007) The kinetics of skin cancer: progression of actinic keratosis to squamous cell carcinoma. Dermatol Surg 33(9):1099–1101
4. Euvrard S, Kanitakis J, Claudy A (2003) Skin cancers after organ transplantation. N Engl J Med 348(17):1681–1691
5. Braakhuis BJ, Tabor MP, Kummer JA, Leemans CR, Brakenhoff RH (2003) A genetic explanation of Slaughter's concept of field cancerization: evidence and clinical implications. Cancer Res 63(8):1727–1730
6. Zalaudek I, Giacomel J, Argenziano G, Hofmann-Wellenhof R, Micantonio T, Di Stefani A, Oliviero M, Rabinovitz H, Soyer HP, Peris K (2006) Dermoscopy of facial nonpigmented actinic keratosis. Br J Dermatol 155(5):951–956
7. Cockerell CJ (2000) Histopathology of incipient intraepidermal squamous cell carcinoma ("actinic keratosis"). J Am Acad Dermatol 42(1Pt 2):11–17
8. Ulrich M, Maltusch A, Rius-Diaz F, Röwert-Huber J, González S, Sterry W, Stockfleth E, Astner S (2008) Clinical applicability of in vivo reflectance confocal microscopy for the diagnosis of actinic keratoses. Dermatol Surg 34(5):610–619
9. Horn M, Gerger A, Ahlgrimm-Siess V, Weger W, Koller S, Kerl H, Samonigg H, Smolle J, Hofmann-Wellenhof R (2008) Discrimination of actinic keratoses from normal skin with reflectance mode confocal microscopy. Dermatol Surg 34(5):620–625
10. Rishpon A, Kim N, Scope A, Porges L, Oliviero MC, Braun RP, Marghoob AA, Fox CA, Rabinovitz HS (2009) Reflectance confocal microscopy criteria for squamous cell carcinomas and actinic keratoses. Arch Dermatol 145(7):766–772
11. Guitera P, Pellacani G, Crotty KA, Scolyer RA, Li LX, Bassoli S, Vinceti M, Rabinovitz H, Longo C, Menzies SW (2010) The impact of in vivo reflectance confocal microscopy on the diagnostic accuracy of lentigo maligna and equivocal pigmented and nonpigmented macules of the face. J Invest Dermatol 130(8):2080–2091
12. Ulrich M, González S, Lange-Asschenfeldt B, Roewert-Huber J, Sterry W, Stockfleth E, Astner S (2010) Non-invasive diagnosis and monitoring of actinic cheilitis with reflectance confocal microscopy. J Eur Acad Dermatol Venereol [Epub ahead of print]

Squamous Cell Carcinoma

23

Theresa Cao, Margaret Oliviero, and Harold S. Rabinovitz

23.1 Introduction

Cutaneous squamous cell carcinoma (SCC), one of the most common malignant neoplasms in fair-skinned individuals, classically presents as a pink to red scaly papule or plaque that at times can be difficult to distinguish clinically from other skin lesions, such as basal cell carcinomas, irritated seborrheic keratoses, lichen planus-like keratoses, or inflammatory skin diseases like psoriasis. Pigmented SCC clinically presents as a variegated brown papule or plaque with variable amounts of scale and can be confused with superficial spreading melanoma [1]. Dermoscopy can aid in the correct diagnosis when characteristic features of SCC such as vessels as dots or coiled (glomerular) vessels and a scaly surface are present; however, significant surface scale can obscure the vascular structures [2–5]. Pigmented SCCs are also diagnostically challenging as they may have clinical and dermoscopic features that are suggestive of a melanocytic neoplasm. The dermoscopic clues to pigmented Bowen's disease described by Cameron et al. include a linear arrangement of brown or gray dots and coiled vessels; however, some of the other reported features that have been observed that are described in the literature are atypical vascular structures, globules, and blotches of pigment [1, 3]. Pigmented SCCs are uncommon, however, comprising only 0.01–7% of all SCCs, with most cases occurring in oral and ocular mucosa rather than in skin [6]. Histopathologically, SCC is defined as a squamous epithelial neoplasm that demonstrates crowded, enlarged, and pleomorphic nuclei, dykeratosis, and parakeratosis [7]. In vivo reflectance confocal laser microscopy (RCM) features of SCC correlate well with histopathology; however, RCM has limitations of depth of penetration of the diode laser to the superficial reticular dermis, and depth of invasion may not be accurately determined due to limited visualization beyond the dermo-epidermal junction (DEJ), especially in lesions with significant surface scale or hyperplasia.

23.2 RCM Features

The key RCM features of SCC are presence of an atypical honeycomb or disarranged pattern of the spinous-granular (SG) layer, round nucleated cells at the SG layer, and round blood vessels traversing through the dermal papillae perpendicular to the skin surface [8]. Scale crust appears as brightly reflective amorphous islands on the surface of the skin, visualized on the mosaic image. Polygonal nucleated cells at the stratum corneum represent parakeratosis while round nucleated cells in the SG layer correspond to dyskeratotic cells (Figs. 23.2, 23.2.2, 23.2.4)[8]. Cells of irregular size and shape at the SG layer create an atypical honeycomb pattern, but if the honeycomb pattern is completely replaced by severe architectural disarray of the SG layer, the term disarranged epidermal pattern is used [8] (Fig. 23.1–23.1.3; 23.2–23.2.1; 23.3–23.3.1).

Pigmented SCC presents a diagnostic challenge on confocal microscopy as well because similarly to its dermoscopy, there are features that can cause confusion with a melanocytic neoplasm. Pigmented SCCs may show numerous dendrites, (Figs. 23.1.2; 23.3.1–23.3.2) which if misclassified as atypical dendritic melanocytes then would be interpreted as melanoma. Sometimes small edged papillae may also be visualized at the DEJ (Figs. 23.1.4; 23.3.3–23.3.4). The clue to making the correct diagnosis is scale crust, a markedly atypical honeycomb pattern or disarranged pattern at the SG layer, and presence of tightly coiled vessels in the dermal papillae, as is seen in non-pigmented SCC (Figs. 23.1.4; 23.2.3).

As actinic keratoses are considered by some as incipient SCC or to be part of a spectrum of keratinocyte neoplasia, they too show RCM features similar to those of SCC but with a milder, more focal atypical honeycomb pattern and fewer round vessels in the superficial dermis [8].

T. Cao (✉)
Dermatology Residency, Nova Southeastern University/Broward General Medical Center, Fort Lauderdale, FL, USA
e-mail: theresacao@gmail.com

M. Oliviero
Skin & Cancer Associates, Plantation, FL, USA

H.S. Rabinovitz
Skin & Cancer Associates, Plantation, FL, USA

University of Miami Miller School of Medicine, Miami, FL, USA

R. Hofmann-Wellenhof et al. (eds.), *Reflectance Confocal Microscopy for Skin Diseases*,
DOI 10.1007/978-3-642-21997-9_23, © Springer-Verlag Berlin Heidelberg 2012

SCC CASE 1
Age: 59
Sex: F
Anatomical Site: Right lower leg
History: None
Histopathology: SCC in situ

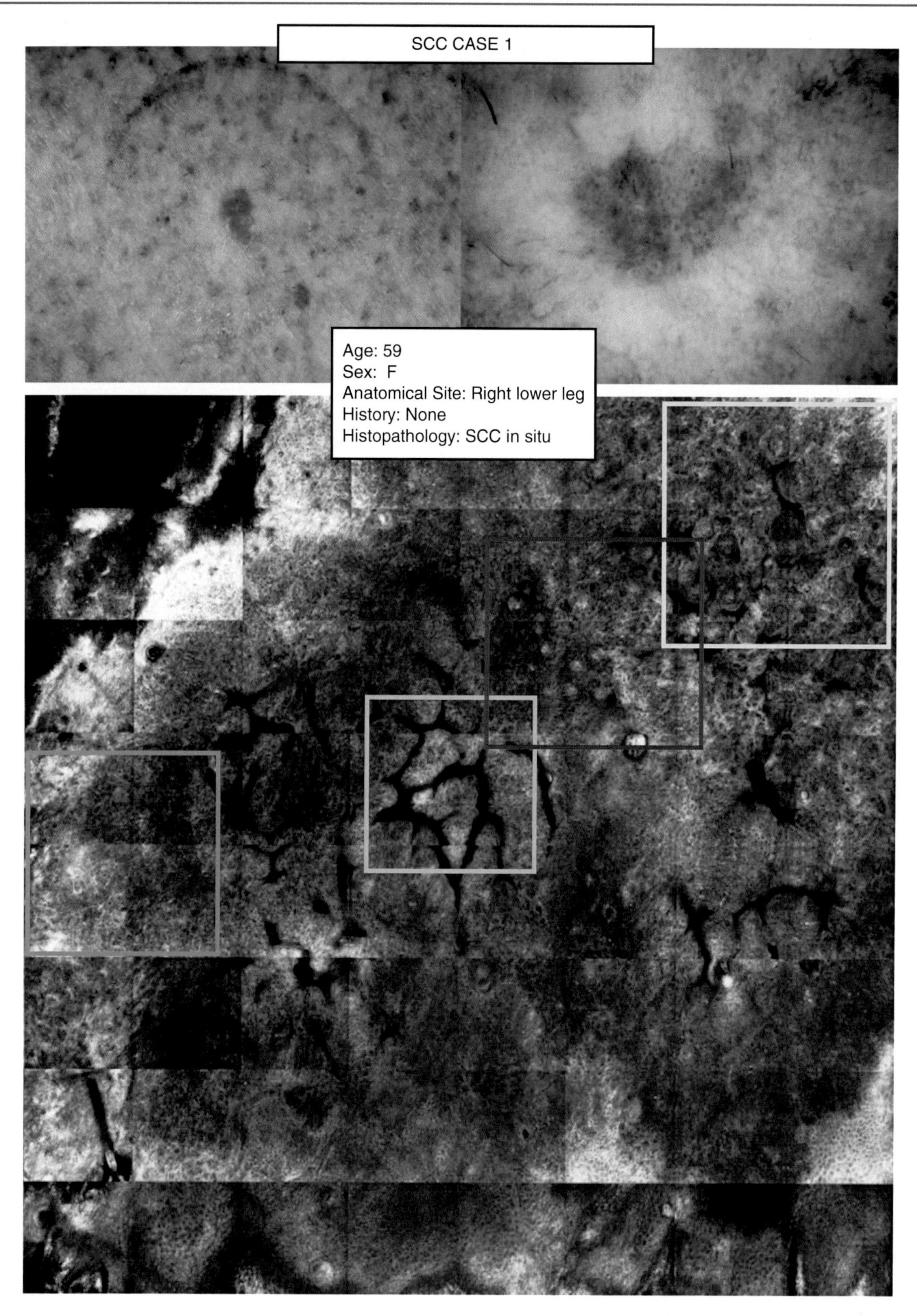

Fig. 23.1 RCM mosaic (4 × 4 mm) at the spiny granular layer shows an atypical honeycomb pattern with broadened and irregular keratinocyte outlines, areas of complete architectural disarray, i.e. a disarranged pattern, a few dendritic cells at the periphery, and small, round, bright spots. There are also surface changes of bulbous islands of keratinocytes separated by nonrefractile linear areas corresponding to ridges and fissures that were not appreciated on the dermoscopic image (Published with kind permission of © Harold S. Rabinovitz 2012. All Rights Reserved)

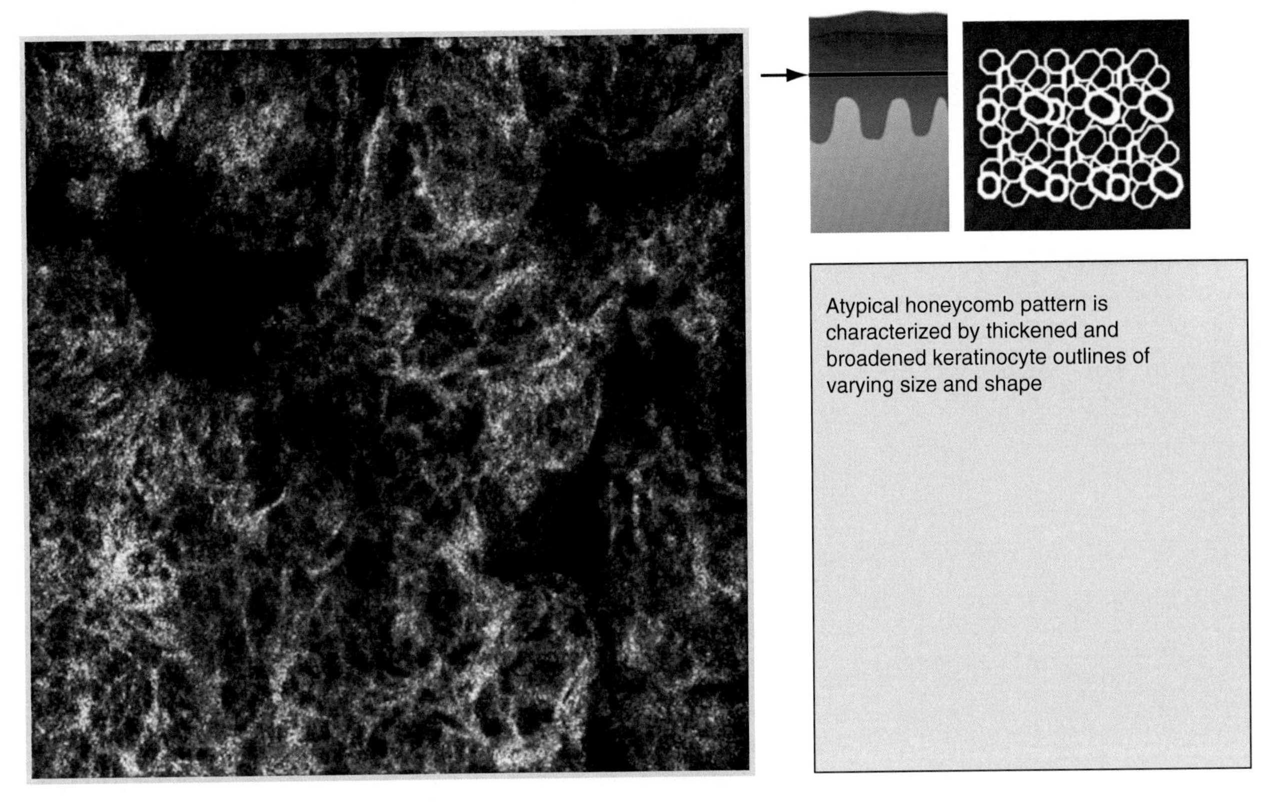

Fig. 23.1.1 Basic image (0.5 × 0.5 mm) at the spiny granular layer showing a disarranged epidermis with an atypical honeycomb pattern composed of distorted keratinocytes of varying size and shape (Published with kind permission of © Harold S. Rabinovitz 2012. All Rights Reserved)

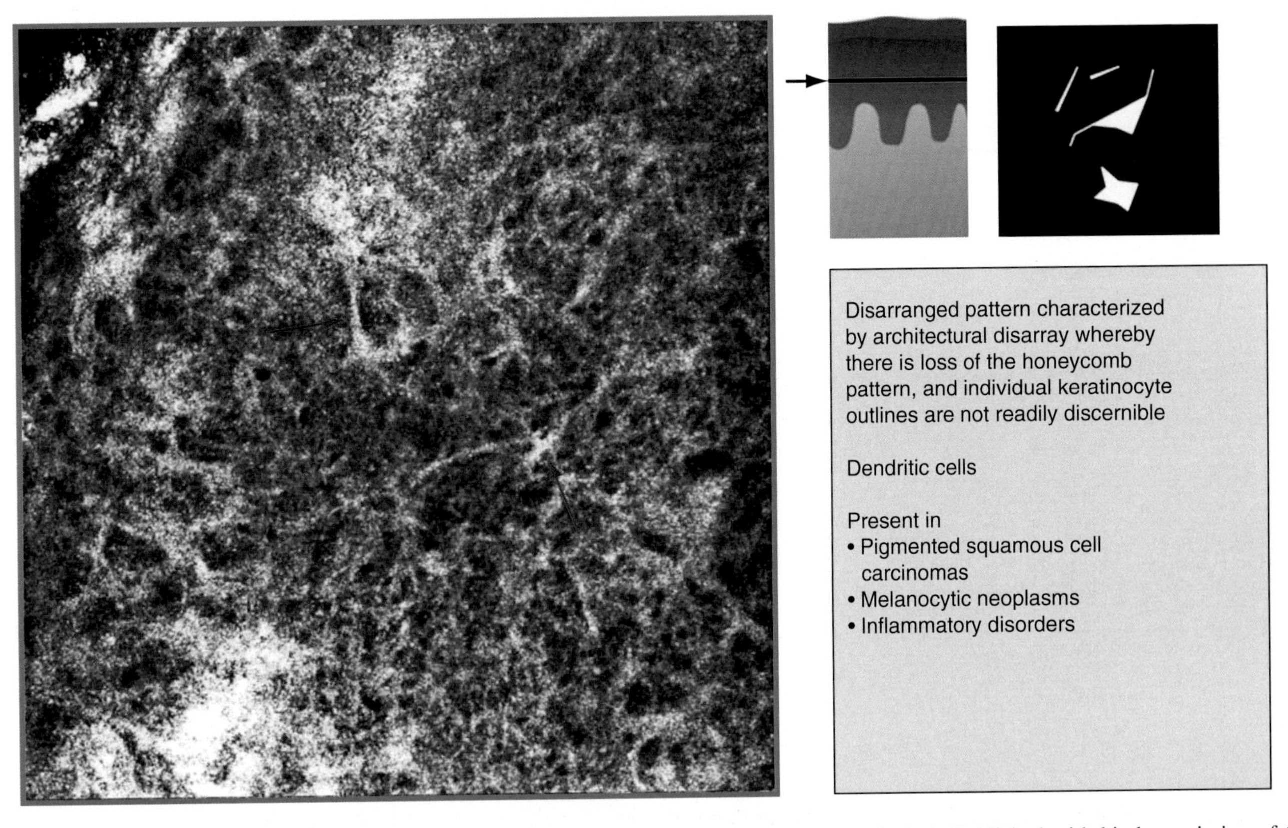

Fig. 23.1.2 Basic image (0.5 × 0.5 mm) shows a disarranged pattern and a few dendritic cells (→) (Published with kind permission of © Harold S. Rabinovitz 2012. All Rights Reserved)

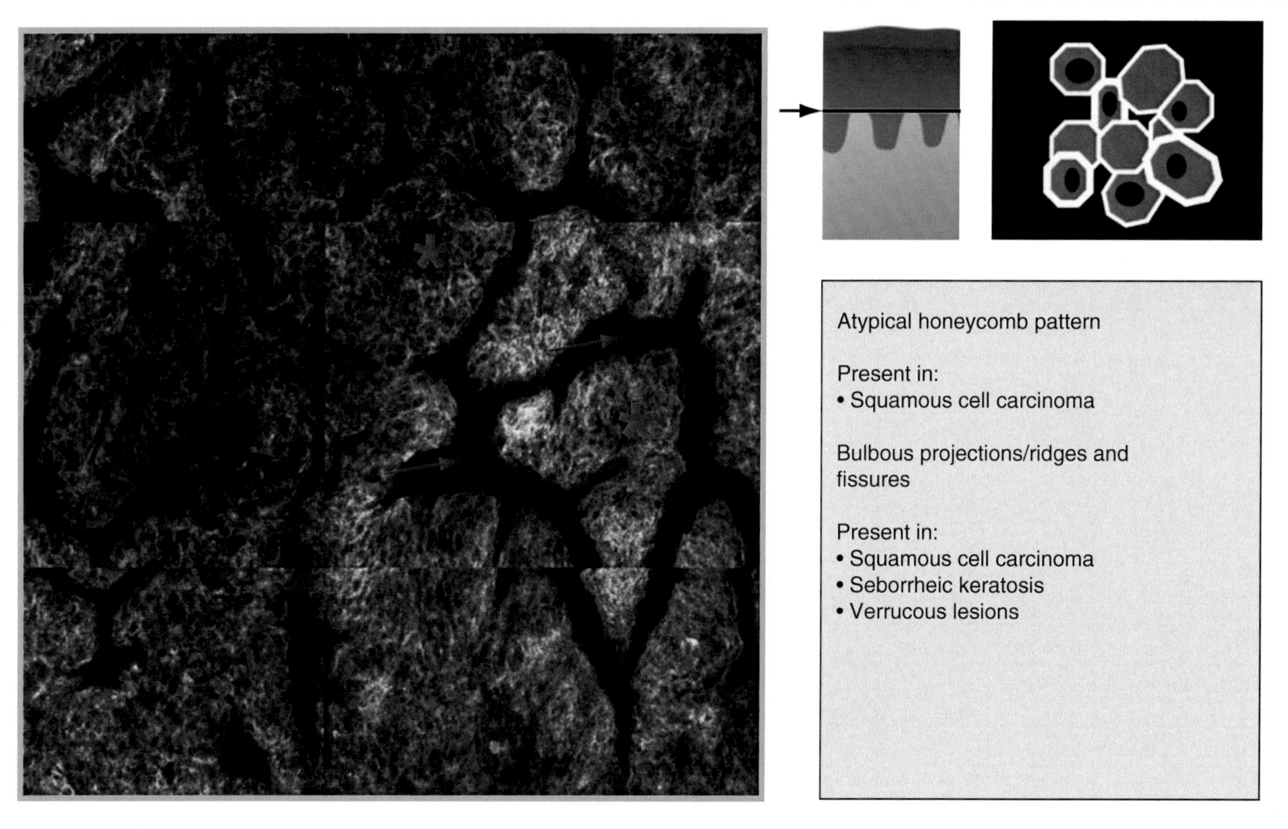

Fig. 23.1.3 RCM mosaic (1 × 1 mm) at the SG layer shows islands of atypical honeycomb pattern separated by linear nonrefractile areas corresponding to round, bulbous projections/linear ridges (*) and fissures (→), respectively. Similar surface changes of ridges and fissures without an atypical honeycomb pattern may be seen in seborrheic keratoses and verrucous lesions (Published with kind permission of © Harold S. Rabinovitz 2012. All Rights Reserved)

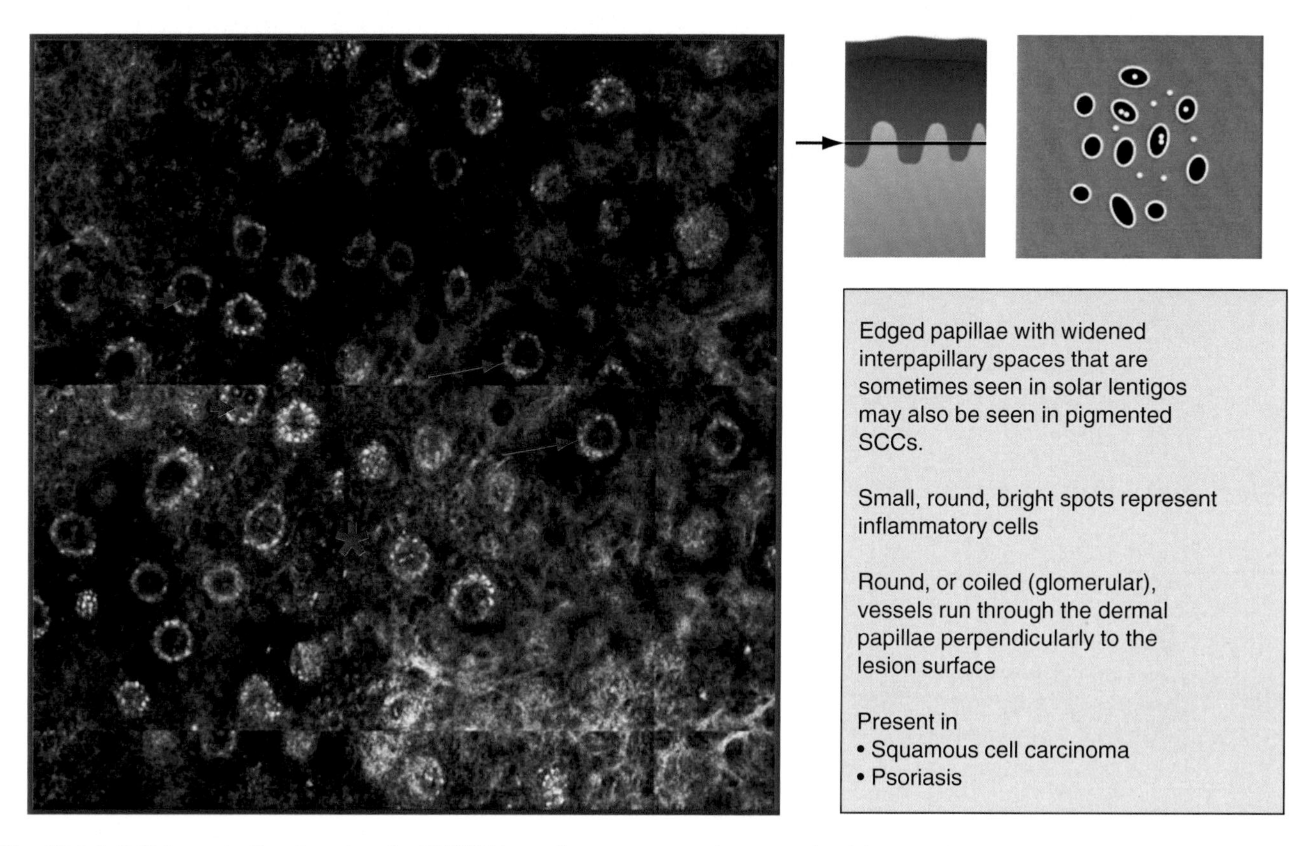

Fig. 23.1.4 RCM mosaic (2 × 2 mm) at the DEJ/SG layer shows an atypical honeycomb pattern focally and multiple small edged papillae (long →). Within some of the papillae are two adjacent small dark vessel lumina containing refractile blood vessels, representing a vessel coursing upward and downward through the papillae, giving a buttonhole appearance (short →) to the papillae. There are also some small, round, bright spots corresponding to inflammatory cells (*) (Published with kind permission of © Harold S. Rabinovitz 2012. All Rights Reserved)

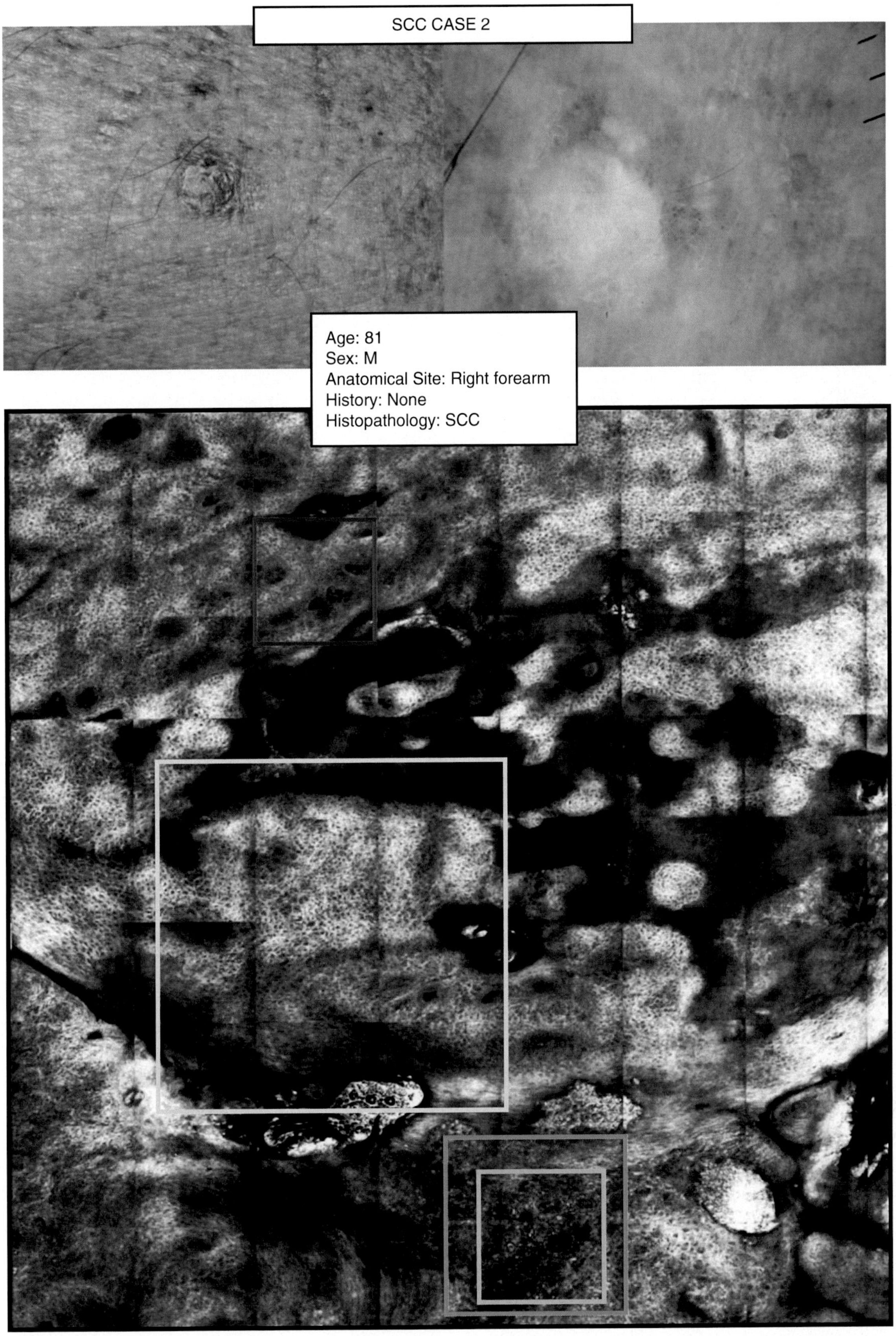

SCC CASE 2

Age: 81
Sex: M
Anatomical Site: Right forearm
History: None
Histopathology: SCC

Fig. 23.2 RCM mosaic (5 × 5 mm) at SG/DEJ shows an atypical honeycomb pattern with broadened keratinocyte outlines and cells of different size and shape. Large, round nucleated cells represent dyskeratotic cells, and multiple round, dark holes represent dermal papillae containing coiled vessels running perpendicularly to the lesion surface (Published with kind permission of © Harold S. Rabinovitz 2012. All Rights Reserved)

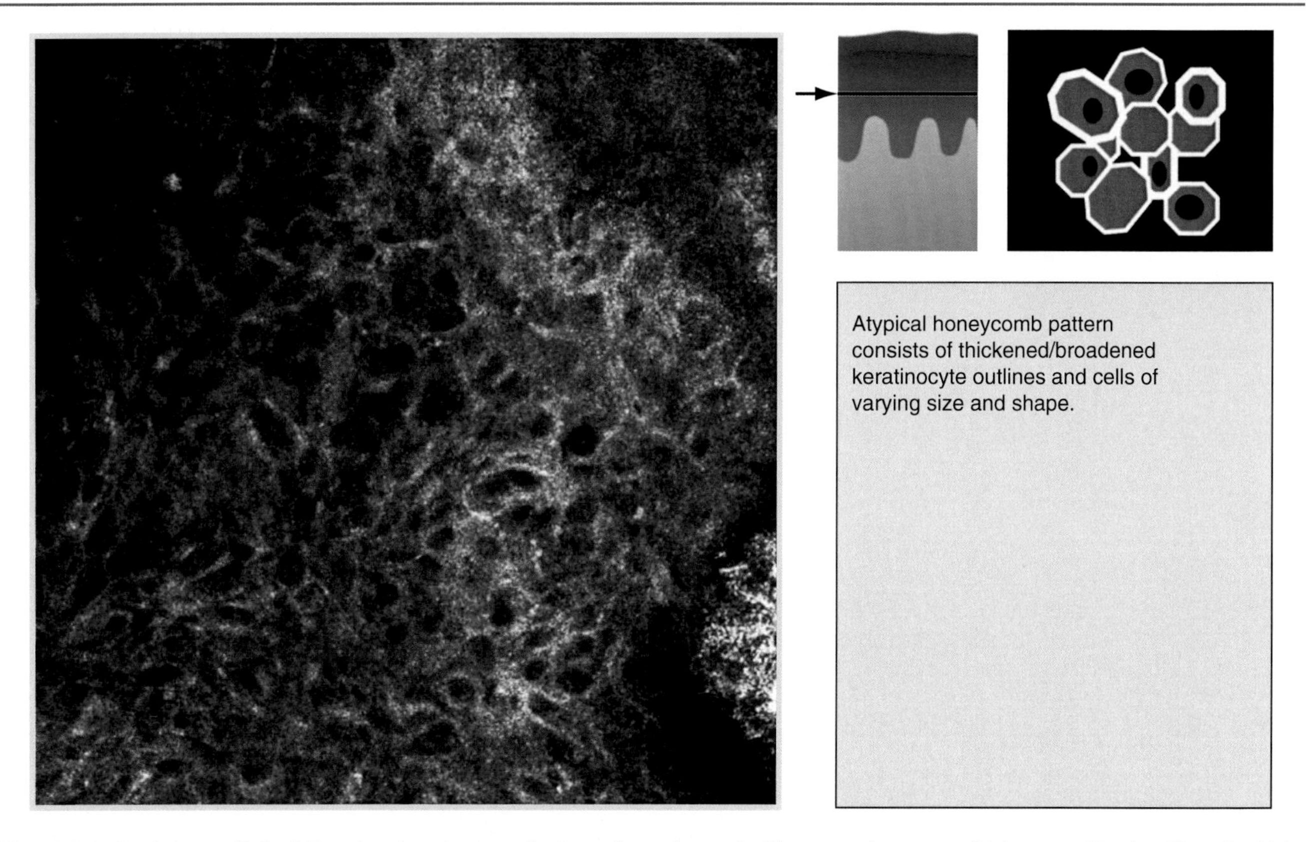

Fig. 23.2.1 Basic image (0.5 × 0.5 mm) at the spiny granular layer shows the atypical honeycomb pattern at higher magnification. Note the thickened/broadened keratinocyte outlines and pleomorphism (Published with kind permission of © Harold S. Rabinovitz 2012. All Rights Reserved)

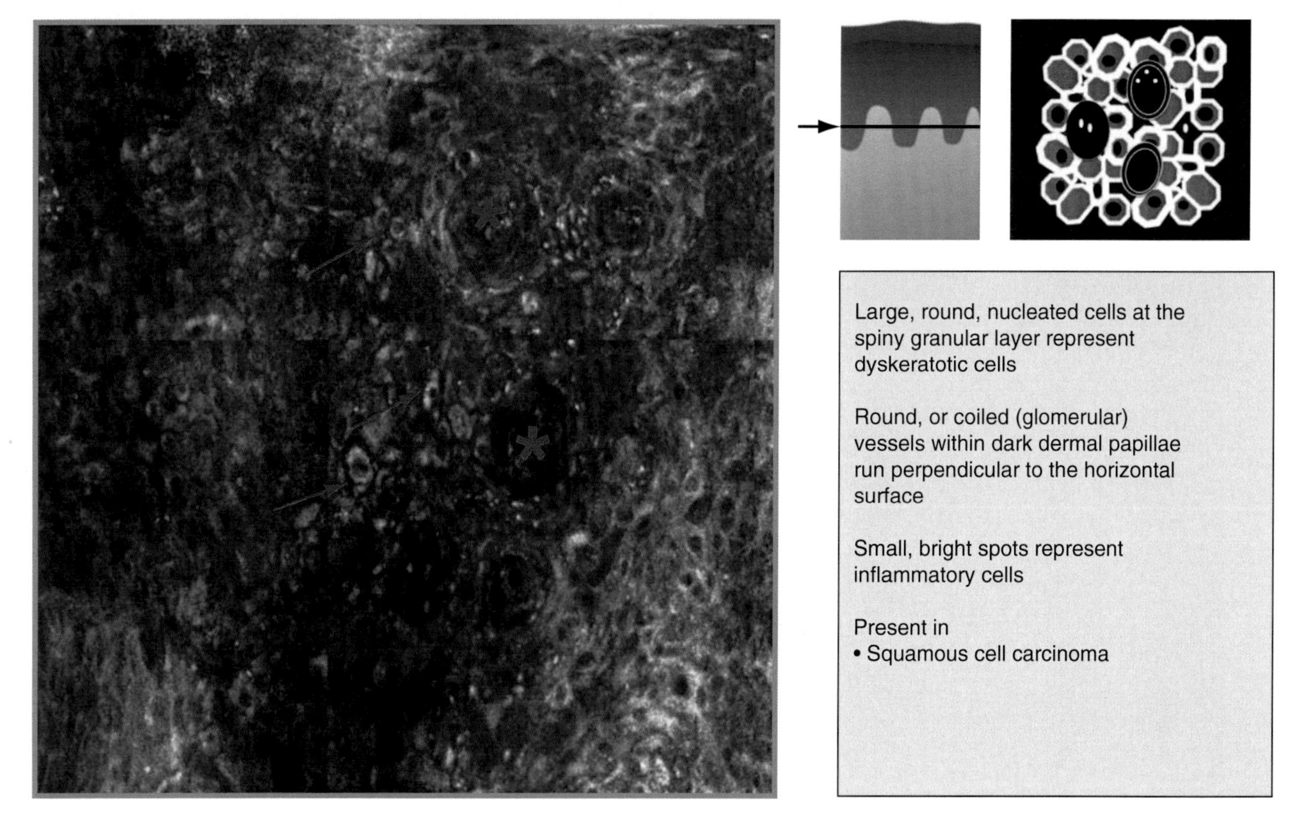

Fig. 23.2.2 RCM mosaic (2 × 2 mm) shows again atypical honeycomb pattern at the bottom right and a disarranged pattern in the remainder of the image with large, round, nucleated cells (→) suggestive of dyskeratotic keratinocytes, and round, coiled vessels traversing perpendicularly within dark dermal papillae (*). Scattered small, bright spots are also seen primarily around the dermal papillae (Published with kind permission of © Harold S. Rabinovitz 2012. All Rights Reserved)

Coiled (glomerular) vessels within dark dermal papillae run perpendicular to the horizontal surface

Fig. 23.2.3 Basic image (0.5 × 0.5 mm) at the papillary dermis shows the dark, round dermal papillae (*) which contain round, coiled vessels (→) that run perpendicularly to the horizontal plane of imaging (Published with kind permission of © Harold S. Rabinovitz 2012. All Rights Reserved)

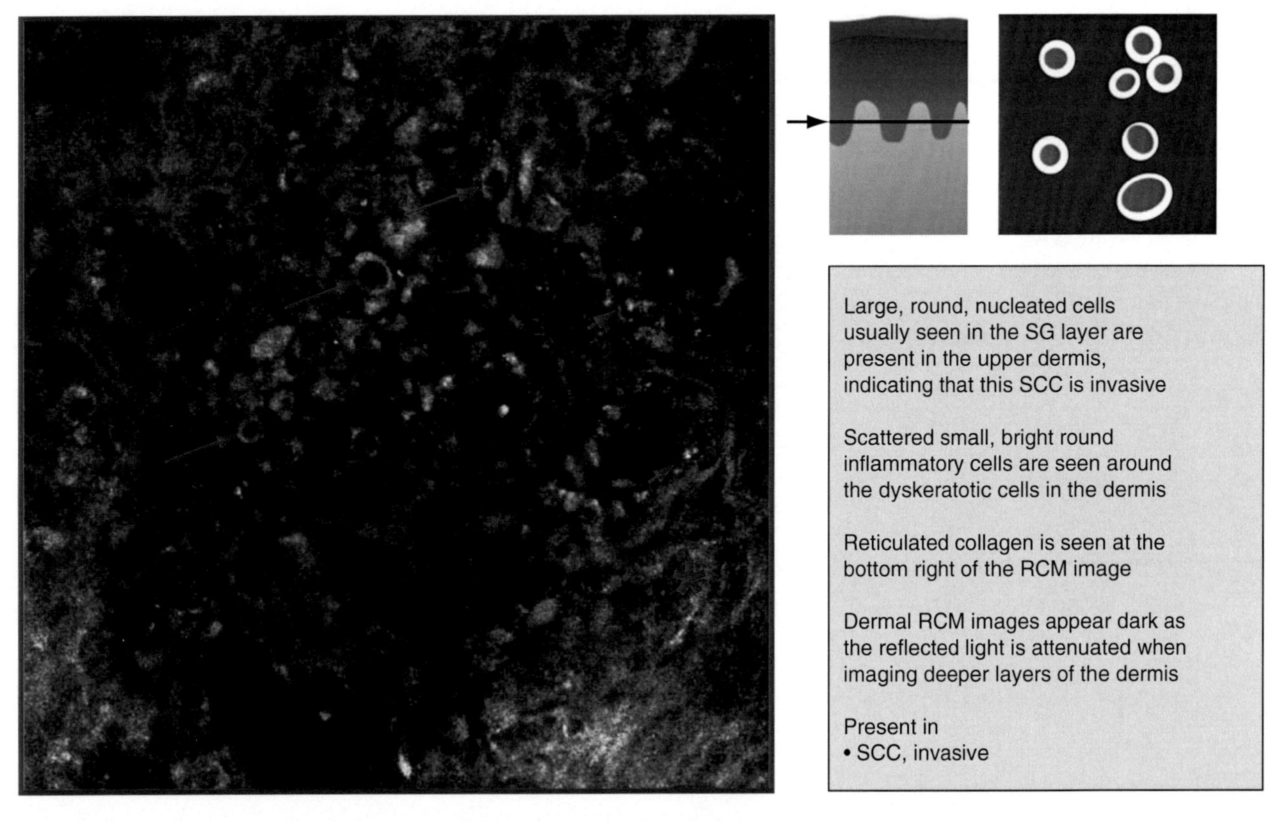

Fig. 23.2.4 Basic image (0.5 × 0.5 mm) of the upper dermis shows large, round, nucleated cells (long →) that are usually seen in the SG layer invading the dermis and surrounded by small, bright round inflammatory cells (short →) and reticulated collagen (*), indicating that the lesion is an invasive SCC (Published with kind permission of © Harold S. Rabinovitz 2012. All Rights Reserved)

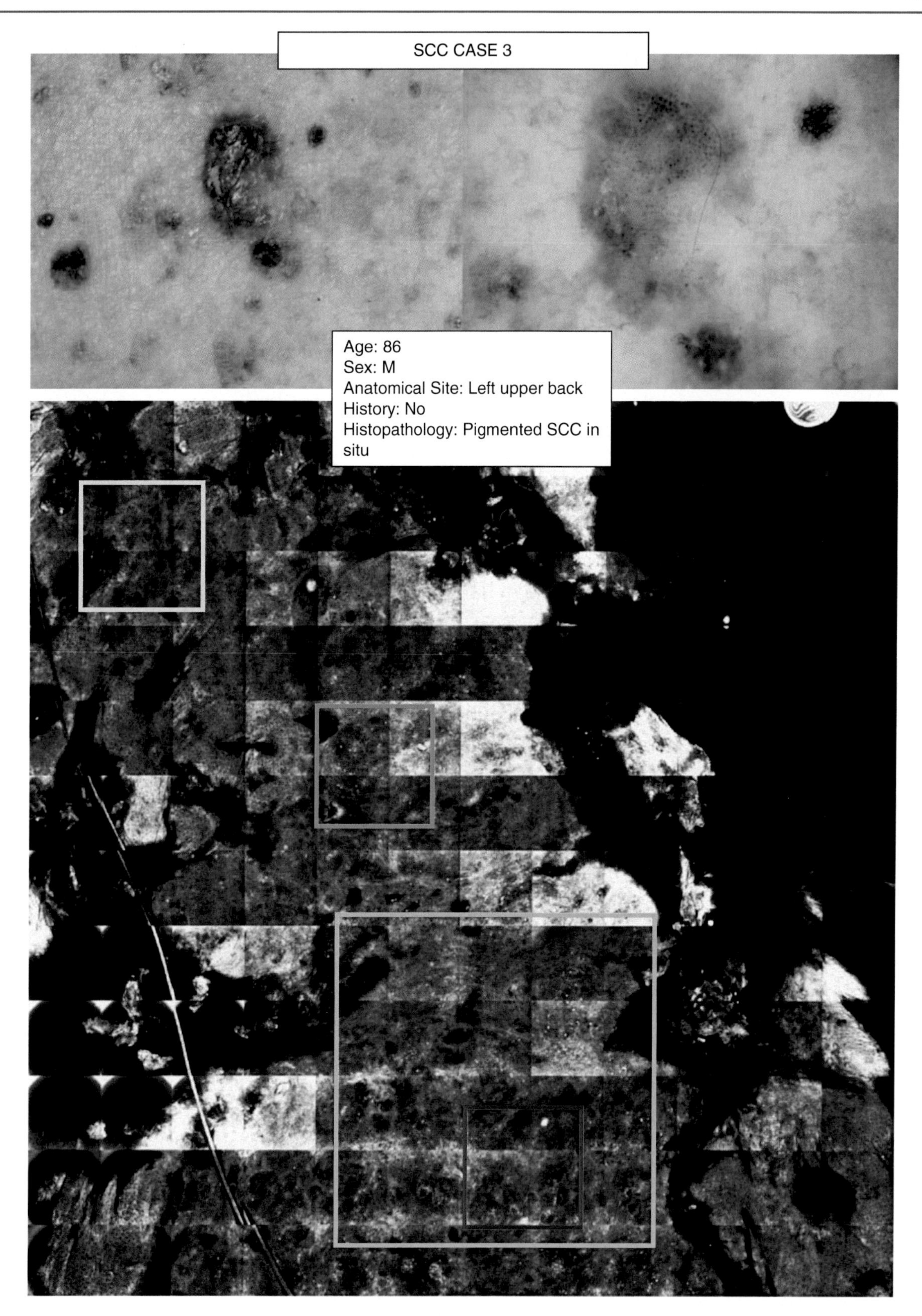

Fig. 23.3 RCM mosaic (6 × 6 mm) at the SG layer shows a disarranged honeycomb pattern with numerous round, bright and dendritic cells infiltrating the epidermis (Published with kind permission of © Harold S. Rabinovitz 2012. All Rights Reserved)

Disarranged honeycomb pattern occurs because of replacement of normal epidermis by pleomorphic, neoplastic keratinocytes

Numerous dendritic cells infiltrating the epidermis may represent melanocytes or Langerhan's cells

Scattered small, round bright spots represent inflammatory cells

Fig. 23.3.1 A higher magnification RCM mosaic (2 × 2 mm) of the SG layer at the top left of the lesion shows a disarranged honeycomb pattern with numerous bright dendritic cells (→) and small, bright round cells (*) infiltrating the epidermis (Published with kind permission of © Harold S. Rabinovitz 2012. All Rights Reserved)

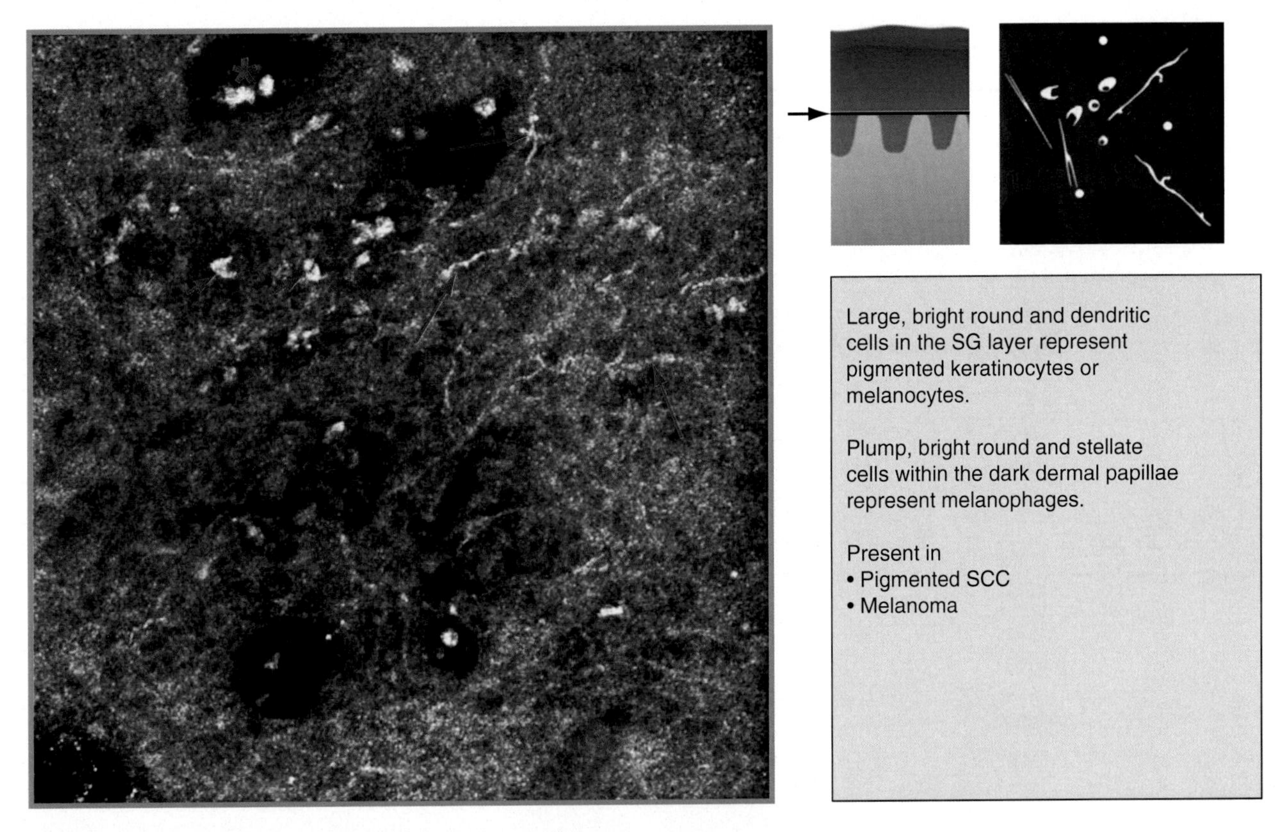

Fig. 23.3.2 Basic image (0.5 × 0.5 mm) of the SG layer shows bright round (short →) and dendritic cells (long →) representing pigmented keratinocytes and melanocytes infiltrating the epidermis, and bright round and stellate spots representing melanophages (*) within the dark dermal papillae (Published with kind permission of © Harold S. Rabinovitz 2012. All Rights Reserved)

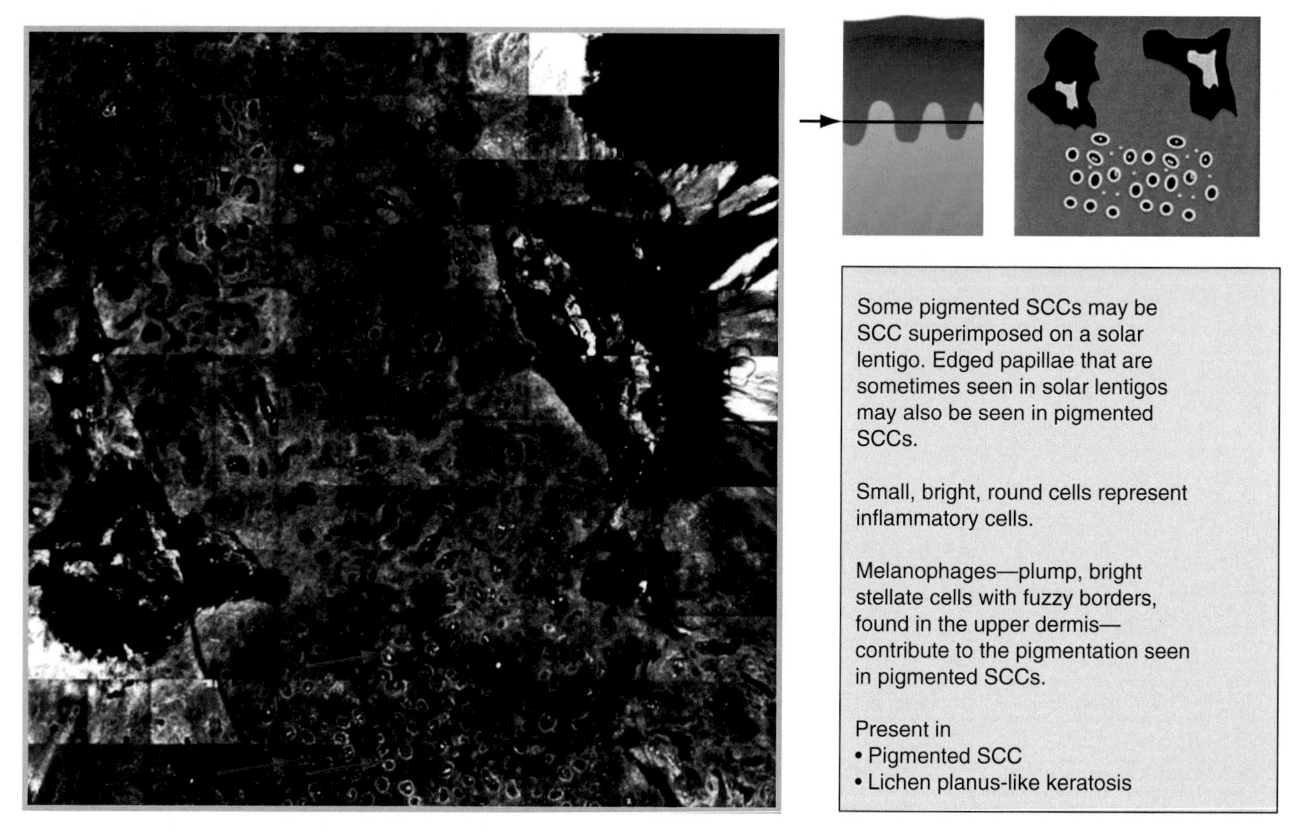

Fig. 23.3.3 RCM mosaic (6 × 6 mm) at the DEJ shows edged papillae (→), which correspond to bright rings of pigmented keratinocytes lining the dark dermal papillae. Elongated cords are seen at the left of the image. Small, round, bright cells at the upper left of the image represent inflammatory cells. Bright round to stellate spots within the dermal papillae correspond to melanophages. Both the pigmented keratinocytes and melanophages account for the brown color of the pigmented SCC (Published with kind permission of © Harold S. Rabinovitz 2012. All Rights Reserved)

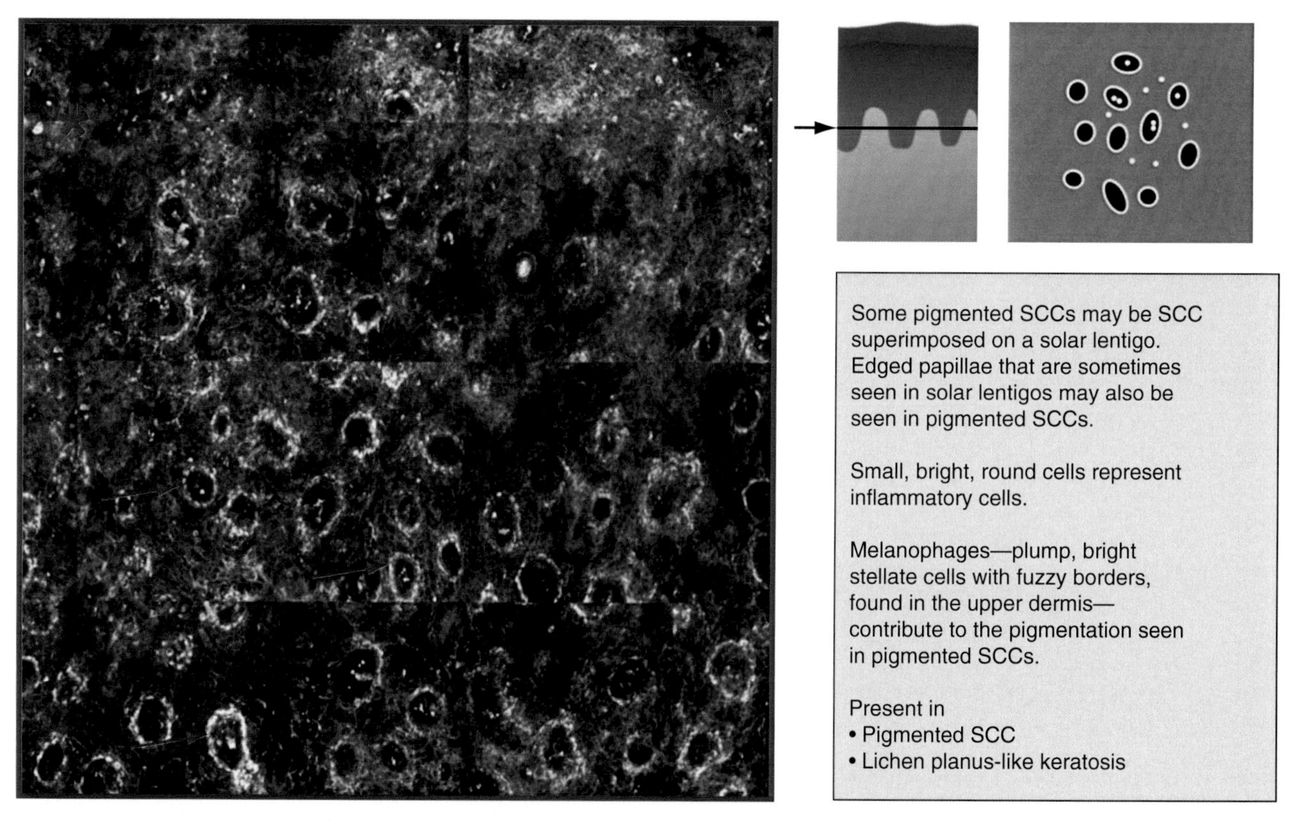

Fig. 23.3.4 A higher magnification RCM mosaic (2 × 2 mm) at the DEJ again shows edged papillae (→), which correspond to bright rings of pigmented keratinocytes lining the dark dermal papillae. Small, round, bright cells (*) corresponding to inflammatory cells are seen scattered between dermal papillae at the top of the image. Bright round to stellate spots within the dermal papillae correspond to melanophages. Small, thin dendritic structures surround some of the edged papillae (Published with kind permission of © Harold S. Rabinovitz 2012. All Rights Reserved)

Core Messages

- Scale crust and parakeratosis (large, round nucleated polygonal cells) at the stratum corneum.
- Atypical honeycomb pattern or disarranged pattern of the SG layer.
- Large, round nucleated cells at the SG layer.
- Round, coiled blood vessels traversing vertically through the dermal papillae.
- Dendritic cells in the SG layer and small edged papillae at the DEJ, as well as other features listed above, are found in pigmented SCC.

References

1. Cameron A, Rosendahl C, Tschandl P, Riedl E, Kittler H Dermatoscopy of pigmented Bowen's disease. J Am Acad Dermatol. 2010 Apr;62(4):597-604. Epub 2010 Jan 15.
2. Zalaudek I, Argenziano G, Leinweber B, Citarella L, Hofmann-Wellenhof R, Malvehy J, Puig S, Pizzichetta MA, Thomas L, Soyer HP, Kerl H (2004) Dermoscopy of Bowen's disease. Br J Dermatol 150:1112–1116
3. Bugatti L, Filosa G, De Angelis R (2004) Dermoscopic observation of Bowen's disease. JEADV 18:572–574
4. Pan Y, Chamberlain A, Bailey M, Chong A, Haskett M, Kelly J (2008) Dermatoscopy aids in the diagnosis of the solitary red scaly patch or plaque—features distinguishing superficial basal cell carcinoma, intraepidermal carcinoma, and psoriasis. J Am Acad Dermatol 59(2):268–274
5. Argenziano G, Zalaudek I, Corona R, Sera F, Cicale L, Petrillo G, Ruocco E, Hofmann-Wellenhof R, Soyer HP (2004) Vascular structures in skin tumors: a dermoscopy study. Arch Dermatol 140: 1485–1489
6. Satter EK (2007) Pigmented squamous cell carcinoma. Am J Dermatopathol 29(5):486–489
7. Ackerman AB, Mones JM (2006) Solar (actinic) keratosis is squamous cell carcinoma. Br J Dermatol 155:9–22
8. Rishpon A, Kim N, Scope A, Porges L, Oliviero M, Braun R, Marghoob A, Alessi-Fox C, Rabinovitz H (2009) Reflectance confocal microscopy criteria for squamous cell carcinomas and actinic keratoses. Arch Dermatol 145(7):766–772

24 Cutaneous Lymphoma

Regina Fink-Puches, Verena Ahlgrimm-Siess,
Edith Arzberger, and Rainer Hofmann-Wellenhof

24.1 Introduction

Primary cutaneous lymphomas (CLs) represent a heterogeneous group of skin neoplasms with a wide spectrum of clinical, histological and immunophenotypic features [1]. Primary CL arises in the skin, is restricted to the skin at the time of diagnosis and often remains confined to the skin for longer periods of time, whereas secondary CL represents infiltrates of a disseminated nodal or extranodal lymphoma in the skin.

The clinical presentation of cutaneous T-cell lymphoma (CTCL) is variable and depends on the subtype [2]. Mycosis fungoides (MF) represents the most common type of CTCL, accounting for about two-thirds of all CTCLs and for almost 50% of all primary CLs [3, 4].

The primary cutaneous CD30+ lymphoproliferative disorders, including lymphomatoid papulosis (LyP), are the second most common form of CTCL, accounting for approximately 30% of CTCLs [3].

Other types of CTCLs are very rare and primary cutaneous B-cell lymphomas (PCBCL) are less common than cutaneous T-cell lymphomas [5].

24.2 Mycosis Fungoides (MF)

Classical MF is clinically characterized by the progressive evolution of erythematous patches, plaques and tumors over years.

R. Fink-Puches (✉) • V. Ahlgrimm-Siess • E. Arzberger
Department of Dermatology, Medical University of Graz, Graz, Austria
e-mail: regina.fink@meduni-graz.at

R. Hofmann-Wellenhof
Department of Dermatology and Venerology, Medical University of Graz, Graz, Austria
e-mail: rainer.hofmann@medunigraz.at

24.2.1 Histopathologic and RCM Features

24.2.1.1 MF, Patch Type

In histopathology, early lesions of MF reveal a patchy lichenoid or band-like infiltrate in the upper dermis, mainly consisting of lymphocytes and histiocytes; small lymphocytes typically predominate over large atypical cells. The papillary dermis shows moderate to marked fibrosis. Epidermotropism of lymphocytes is usually observed; these atypical cells characteristically colonize the basal layer of the epidermis either in single units or in a linear configuration [6]. The lymphocytes are often surrounded by a clear halo but there is usually little or no spongiosis [7, 8]. The histopathological diagnosis of early MF may be extremely difficult, differentiation from inflammatory skin conditions may be impossible.

RCM: Architectural disarray of the epidermis with focal loss of the honeycomb pattern ("poorly visible" cell demarcations) is characteristically observed with RCM (Figs. 24.1, 24.1.1.1, and 24.1.1.2). In some cases ("spongiotic histopathological pattern"), bright and thickened intercellular demarcations, corresponding to mild spongiosis, are seen [9] (Fig. 24.1.1.2). Epidermotropic atypical lymphocytes, which vary in size, shape and reflectivity, may be visualized scattered among keratinocytes (Figs. 24.1, 24.1.1.1 and 24.1.1.2) A perivascular distribution of atypical lymphocytes and inflammatory cells within dermal papillae may lead to a loss of the typical ringed appearance of dermal papillae at the DEJ [9]. Deeper dermal structures are difficult to identify because of the limited penetration of light in RCM.

Altogether, RCM changes seen in early MF are discrete and often unspecific.

24.2.1.2 MF, Plaque Type

Plaques of MF are characterized by a dense band-like infiltrate within the upper dermis in histology. Epidermotropism is generally more pronounced than in the patches of MF. The presence of discrete intraepidermal clusters of lymphocytes

R. Hofmann-Wellenhof et al. (eds.), *Reflectance Confocal Microscopy for Skin Diseases*,
DOI 10.1007/978-3-642-21997-9_24, © Springer-Verlag Berlin Heidelberg 2012

(Pautrier's microabscesses) is a highly characteristic feature, which is commonly found at this stage [7].

RCM: The examination of plaques in mycosis fungoides characteristically reveals an infiltration of the epidermis by scattered atypical lymphocytes, which vary in size, shape and brightness. The cell size of these lymphocytes usually does not exceed the size of surrounding keratinocytes. Intraepidermal aggregates of atypical lymphocytes correspond to Pautrier's microabscesses seen in histopathology (Figs. 24.1, 24.1.2.1 and 24.1.2.2). A marked reactive architectural disarray of the epidermis is often associated. At the DEJ, a loss of the typical ringed appearance of dermal papillae is observed due to infiltration by atypical lymphocytes and inflammatory cells [10]. Loss of detail and contrast below the papillary dermis hinders the visualization of the dense dermal infiltrate of atypical lymphocytes seen in histopathology.

24.2.1.3 MF, Tumor Type

In histopathology, a dense nodular or diffuse infiltrate is typically found within the entire dermis, also involving the subcutaneous fat. A further increase in tumor cell number and size is seen compared to patch MF; variable proportions of small, medium-sized and large cerebriform cells as well as blast cells with prominent nuclei and intermediate forms are observed within the neoplastic infiltrate [6]. Large atypical lymphocytes are characteristically present in tumor type MF. Interestingly, epidermotropism of atypical lymphocytes may be absent.

RCM: Epidermotropic, atypical lymphocytes are also rarely seen with RCM in tumor type MF; large pleomorphic atypical lymphocytes may be occasionally detected [10]. A loss of the ringed appearance of the DEJ, reflecting infiltration of dermal papillae by atypical lymphocytes and inflammatory cells, may be observed [9]. Again, the deep nodular collections of atypical lymphocytes seen in histopathology are not visible with RCM due to the technical limitations of this method.

24.3 Folliculotropic MF

Folliculotropic MF is a variant of MF, which occurs mostly in adults. Grouped follicular papules, acneiform lesions, indurated plaques, and sometimes tumors may be clinically present; the head and neck area is usually the predominant location of the skin lesions. Folliculotropic MF exhibits a worse prognosis than common MF and thus requires more intensive treatment (3).

24.3.1 Histopathological and RCM Features

In histopathology, a prominent periadnexal dermal infiltrate with variable infiltration of the follicular epithelium is observed in addition to histopathologic findings of classic MF.

RCM: Single scattered atypical lymphocytes and consecutive architectural disarray of the remaining epidermis may be additionally found (Figs. 24.1, 24.1.1.1 and 24.1.1.2). The dermal lymphocytic infiltrate is predominately observed around adnexal openings and blood vessels (Figs. 24.2, 24.2.1, and 24.2.2). A periadnexal loss of the honeycomb pattern may be observed due to the neoplastic infiltrate (Figs. 24.2.2). A loss of the ringed appearance of dermal papillae at the DEJ may be also evident in folliculotropic MF (Figs. 24.2 and 24.2.1).

24.4 Sezary's Syndrome

Sezary's syndrome (SS), the leukemic variant of MF, is a rare disease. It is characterized by erythroderma, often marked exfoliation, edema and intense pruritus followed by lichenification. Lymphadenopathy, alopecia, onychodystrophy, and palmoplantar hyperkeratosis are other common findings in SS [11]. The prognosis is generally poor, with a median survival between 2 and 4 years.

24.4.1 Histopathological and RCM Features

The histological features of SS may be similar to those of MF. The cellular infiltrate is more often monotonous and epidermotropism is usually less marked than in MF or may be even absent; typical Pautrier's microabscesses, however, are occasionally observed. In up to one-third of biopsies from patients with otherwise classical SS the histologic picture may be nonspecific [3, 6].

RCM: A diffuse infiltration of atypical lymphocytes varying in size and shape may be found at epidermal layers as well as at the DEJ (Figs. 24.1.1.1 and 24.1.1.2). The normal honeycomb pattern of the epidermis and the typical ringed appearance of dermal papillae are focally lost (Figs. 24.3 and 24.3.1). Number and diameter of papillary blood vessels are typically increased (Fig. 24.3.2).

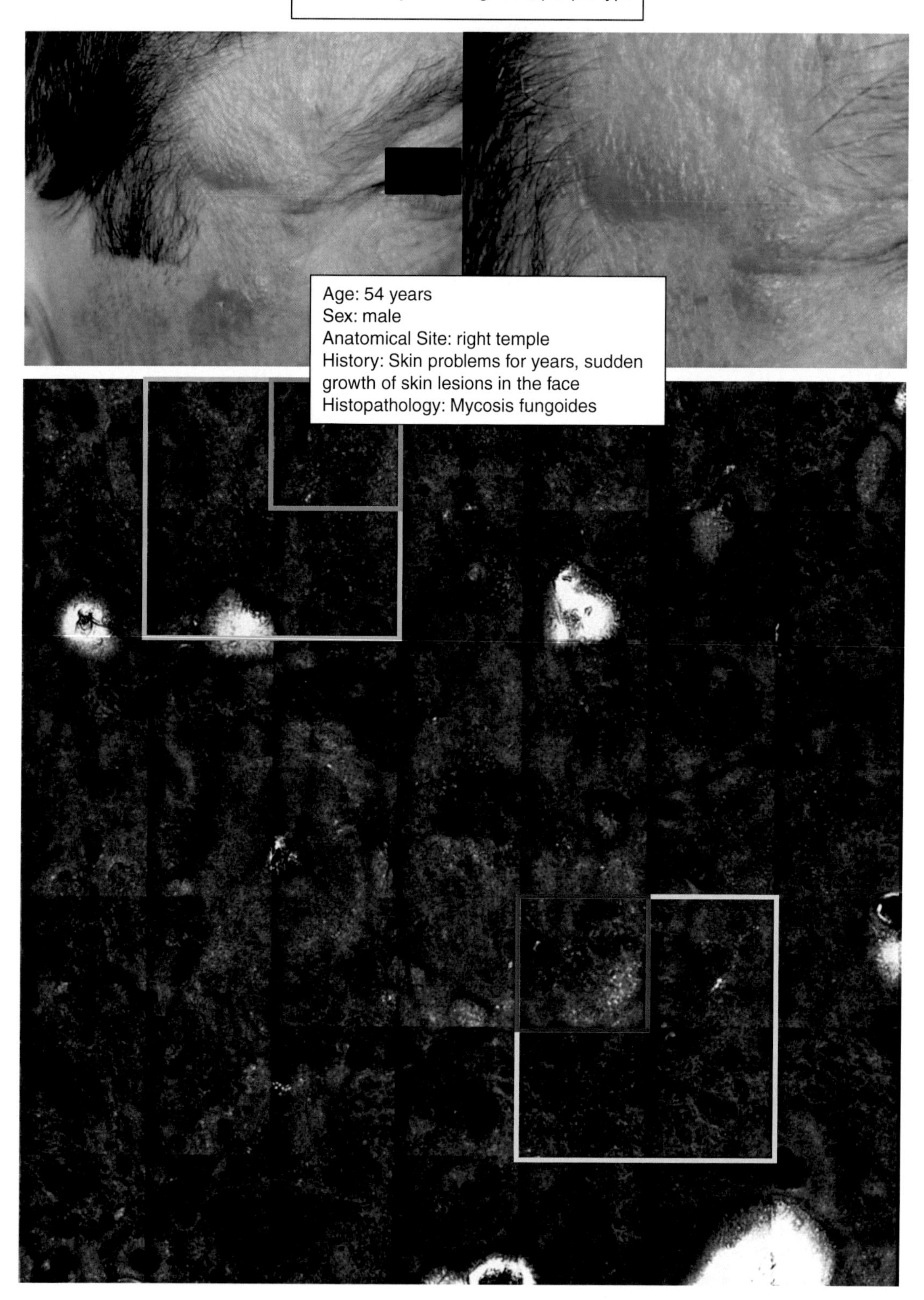

Fig. 24.1 RCM mosaic (3.5 × 3.5 mm) at the level of the DEJ reveals focal loss of the honeycomb-pattern and blurred intercellular connections due to focal scatter of atypical lymphocytes (*green/blue rectangles*). Intraepidermal aggregates of atypical cells are observed, corresponding to the Pautrier's microabscesses seen in histopathology. Marked reactive architectural disarray of the surrounding epidermis is associated (*yellow/red rectangles*)

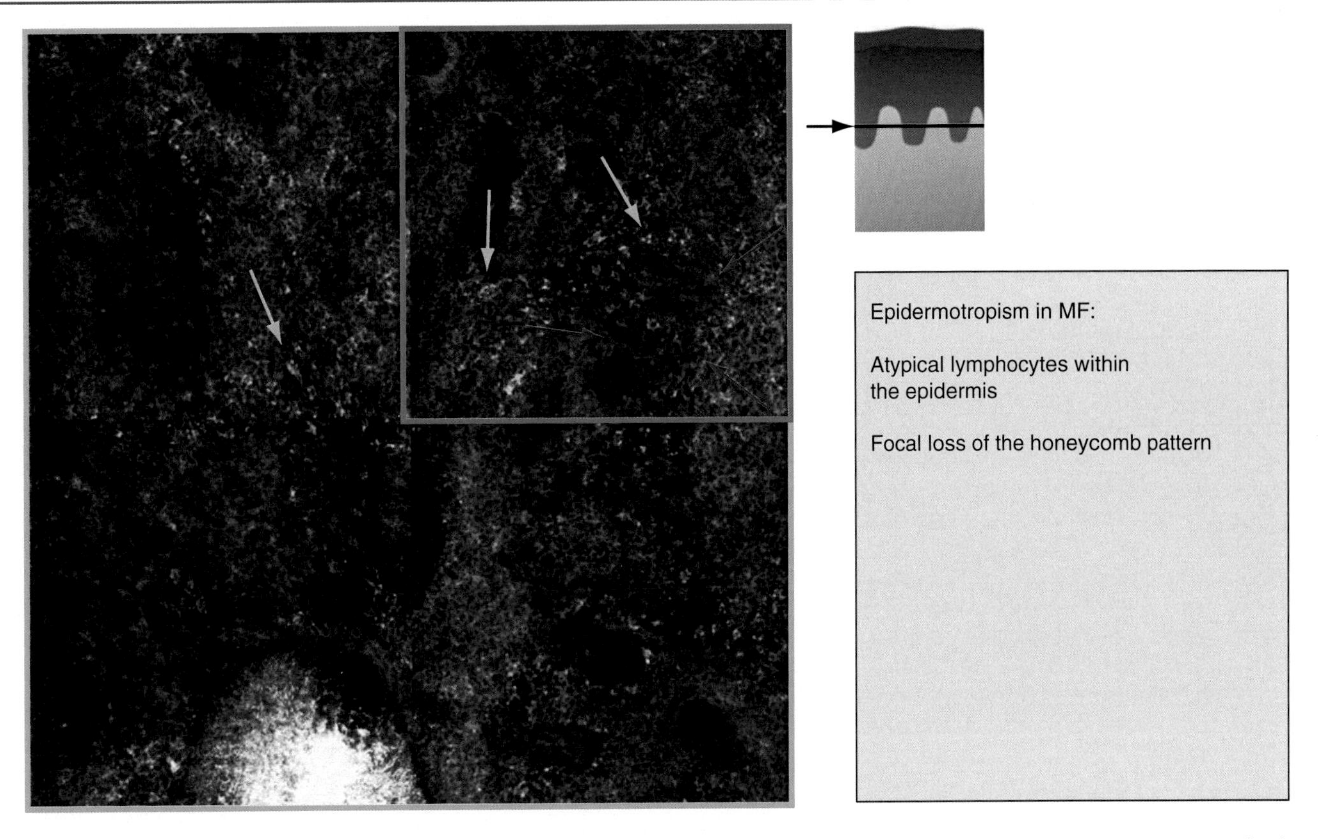

Fig. 24.1.1.1 RCM mosaic (1 × 1 mm) at the DEJ. Atypical lymphocytes scattered throughout the epidermis (*green arrows*) and consecutive loss of the honeycomb pattern are seen (*red arrows*)

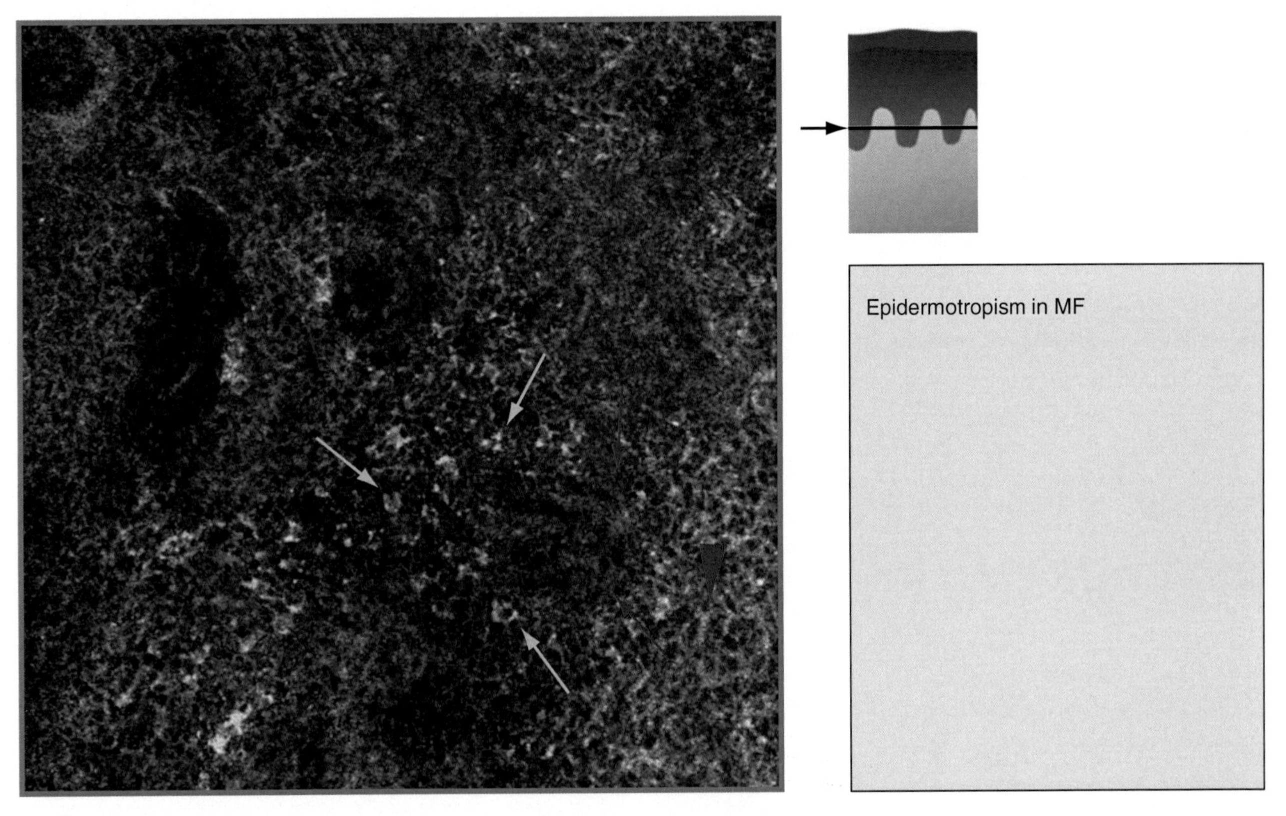

Fig. 24.1.1.2 Basic RCM image (0.5 × 0.5 mm) at the DEJ shows scattered atypical lymphocytes with marked variation of cell size, shape and reflectivity (*green arrows*). Cell size of lymphocytes does not exceed the size of surrounding keratinocytes. Blurred and thickened intercellular connections (*arrowhead*) and focal loss of the honeycomb pattern (*red arrows*) are seen

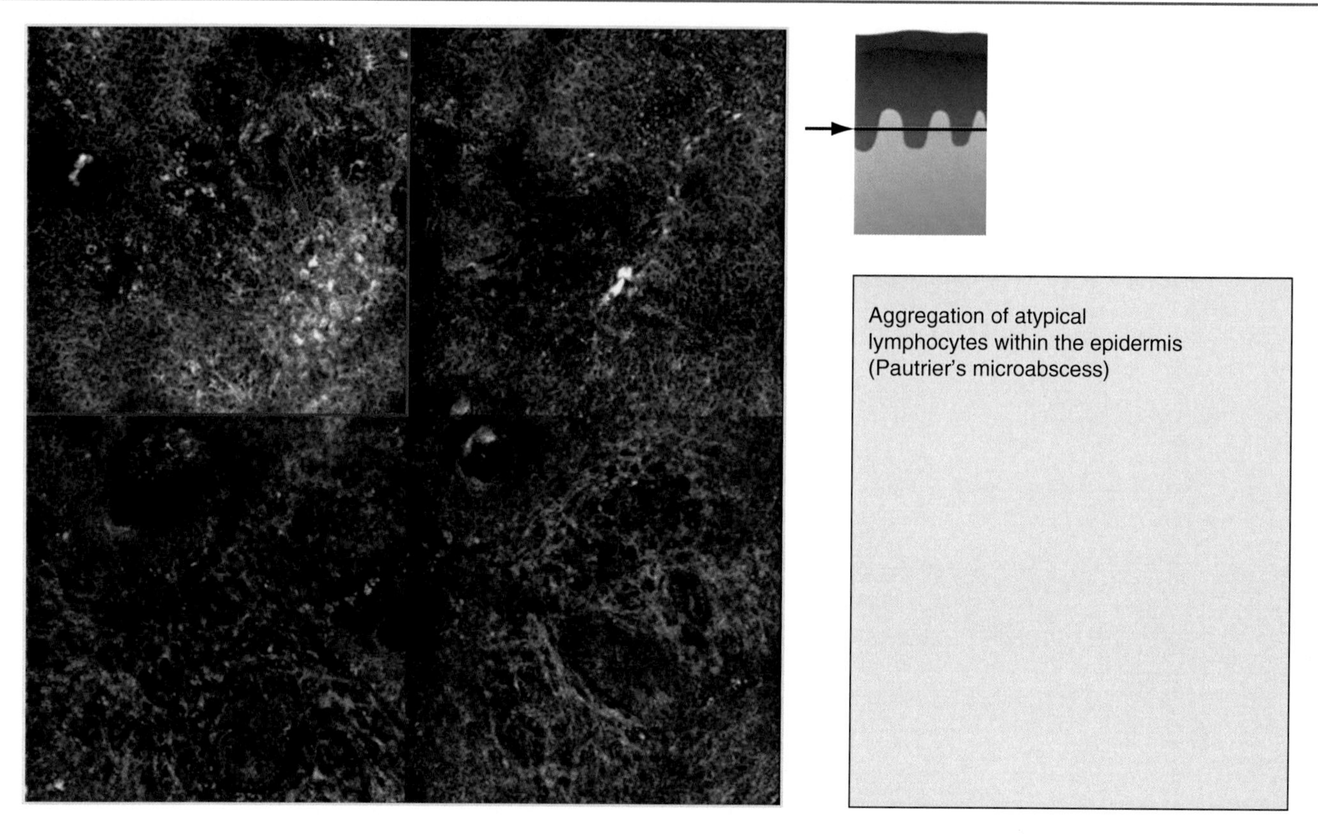

Fig. 24.1.2.1 RCM mosaic (1 × 1 mm) at the DEJ. Aggregation of atypical lymphocytes within the epidermis (Pautrier's microabscess) is observed (*red arrows*). Again, architectural disarray of the surrounding epidermis is evident

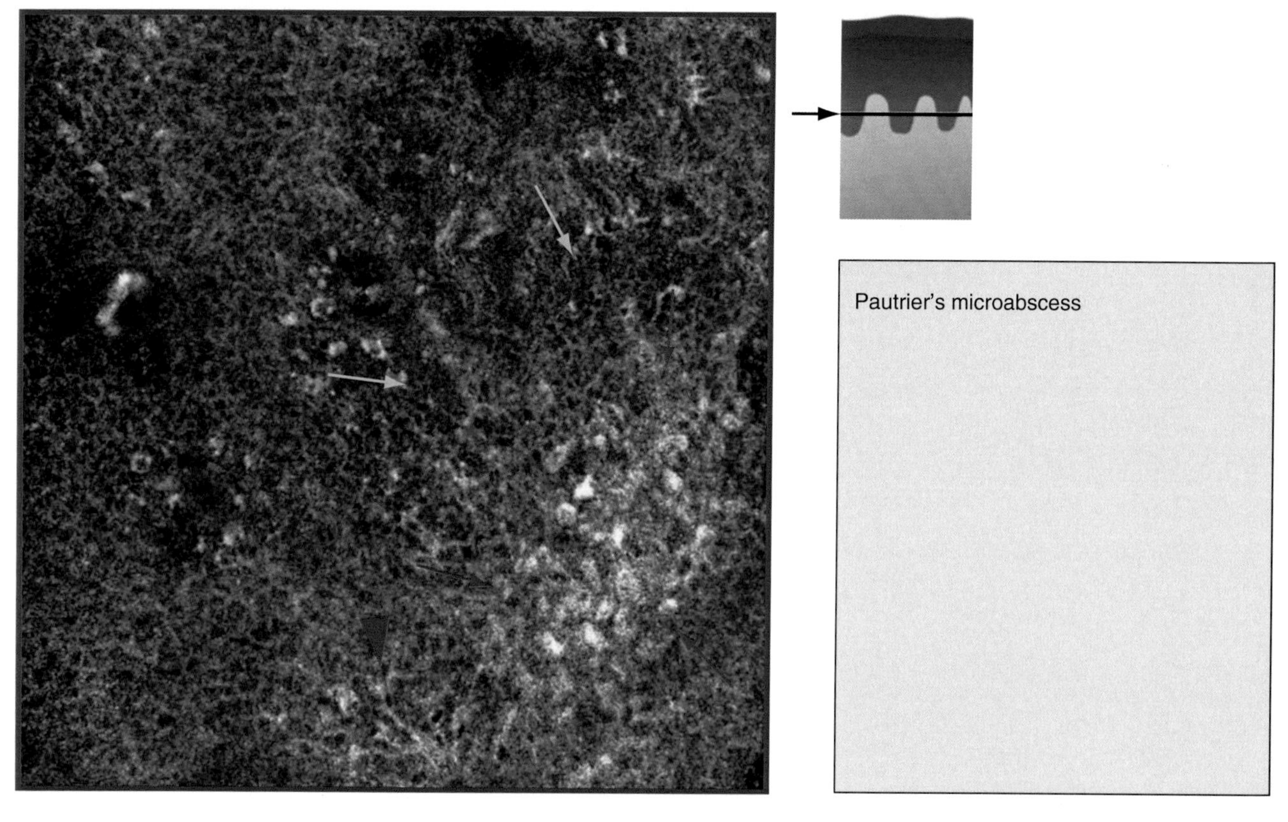

Fig. 24.1.2.2 Basic RCM image (0.5 × 0.5 mm) at the DEJ. Aggregated atypical lymphocytes, varying in size, shape and reflectivity are observed within the epidermis (*red arrows*). The surrounding epidermis shows blurred and thickened intercellular connections (*arrowhead*) and focal loss of the honeycomb pattern (*green arrows*)

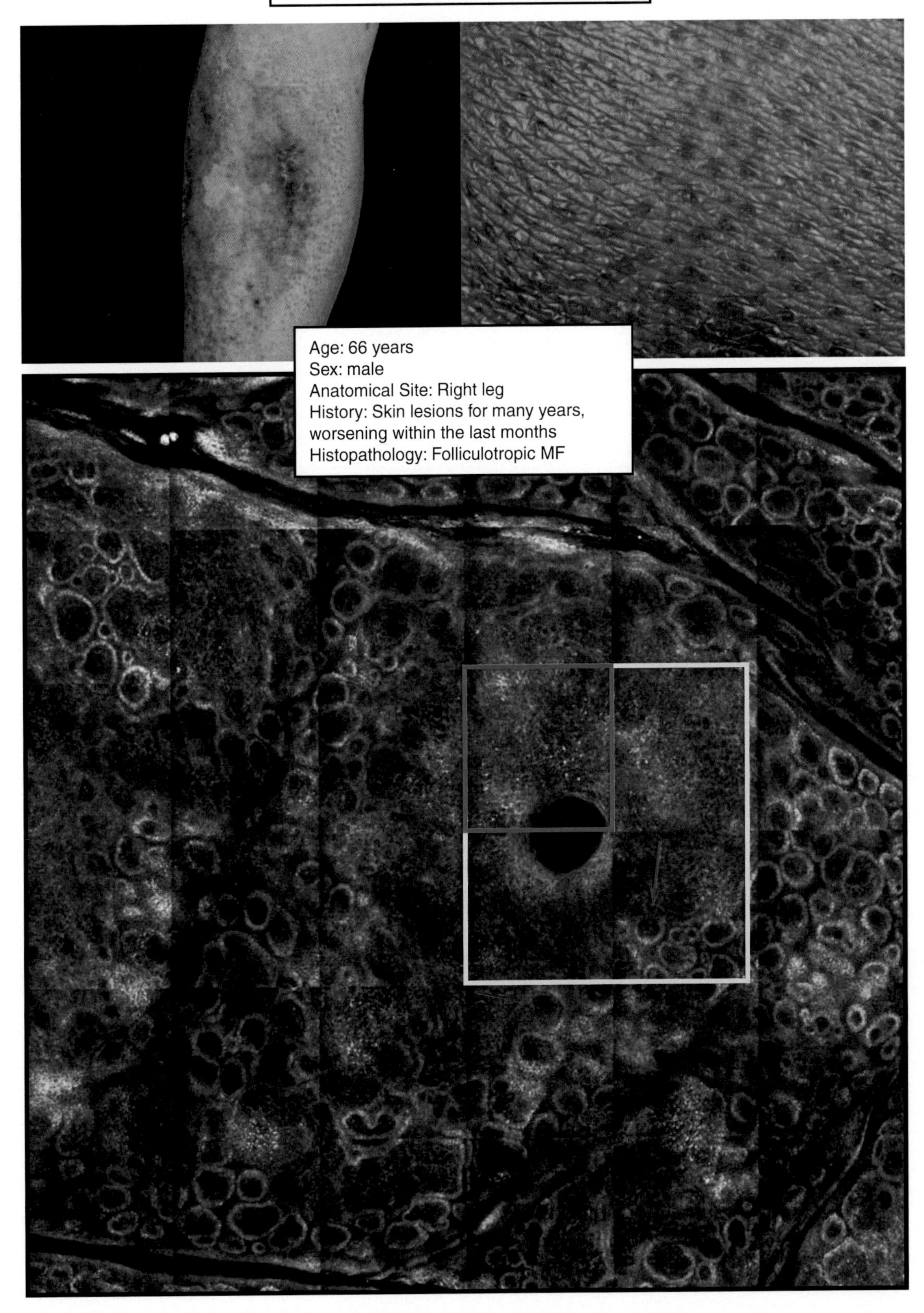

Fig. 24.2 RCM mosaic (3 × 3 mm) at the DEJ. At scanning magnification, RCM reveals a prominent dermal infiltration by small bright cells around an adnexal opening (*rectangles*). A focal loss of the ringed appearance of dermal papillae (*arrows*) is observed

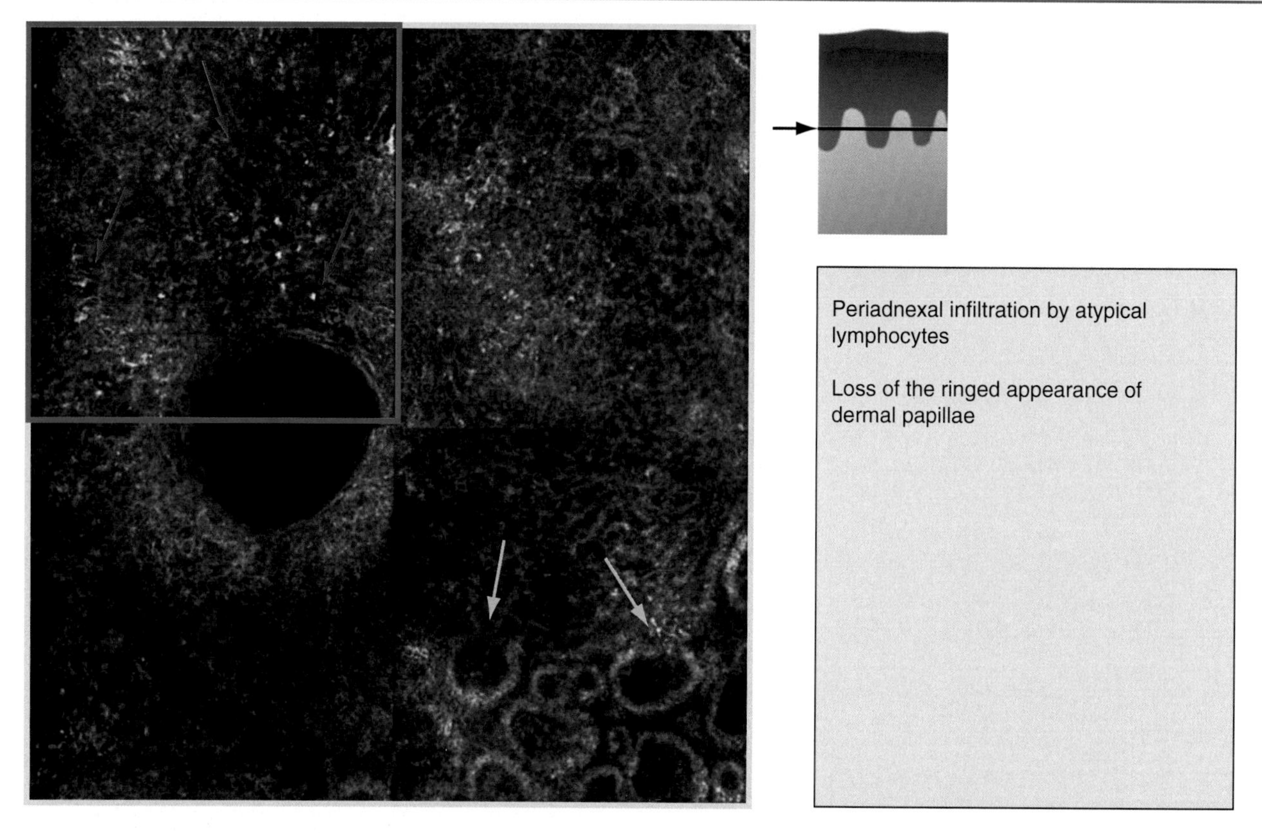

Fig. 24.2.1 RCM mosaic (1 × 1 mm) at the DEJ. Atypical lymphocytes (*red arrows*) are detected around an adnexal opening. The ringed appearance of dermal papillae is focally lost due to infiltration by atypical lymphocytes (*green arrows*)

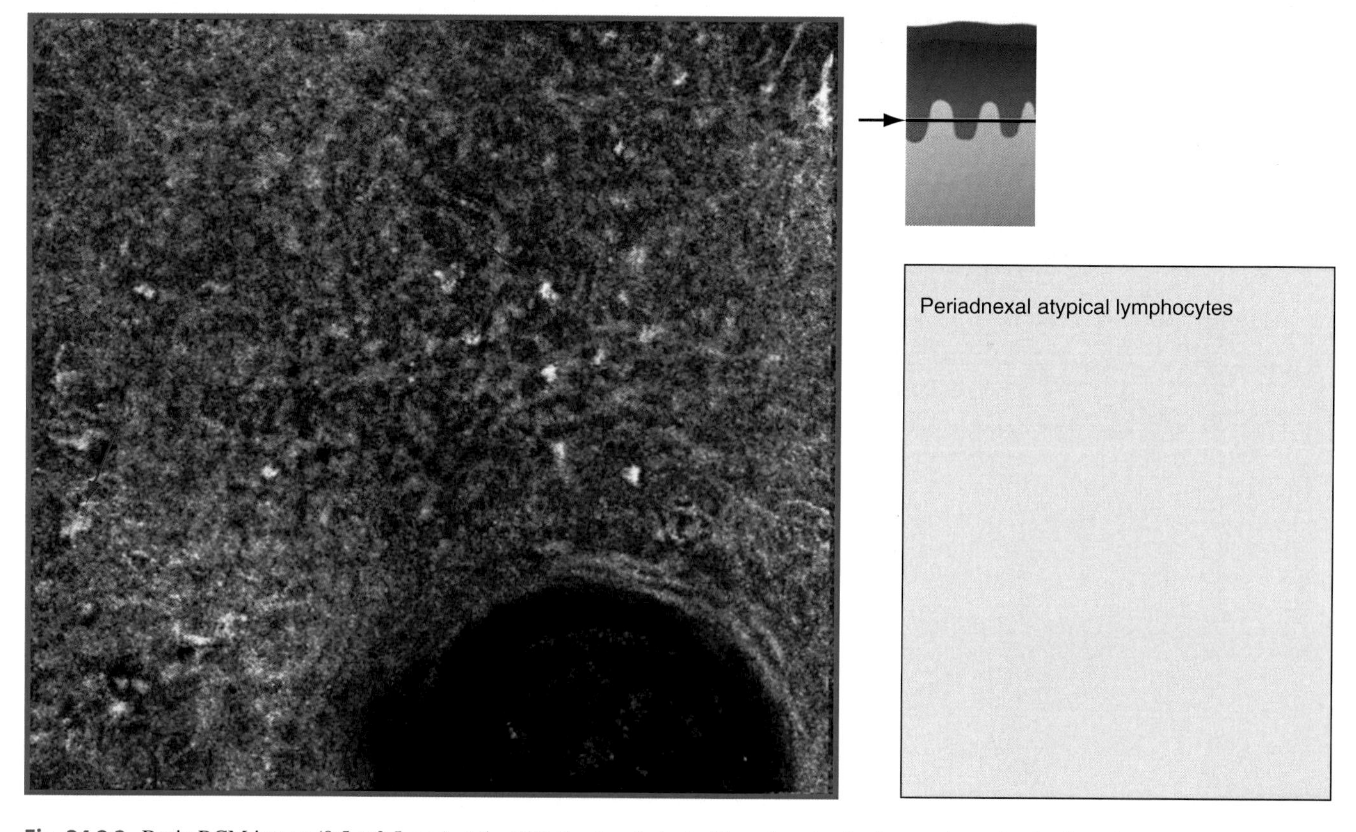

Fig. 24.2.2 Basic RCM image (0.5 × 0.5 mm) at the DEJ. Scattered atypical lymphocytes (*red arrows*) varying in size, shape and reflectivity are seen in the surrounding of an adnexal opening

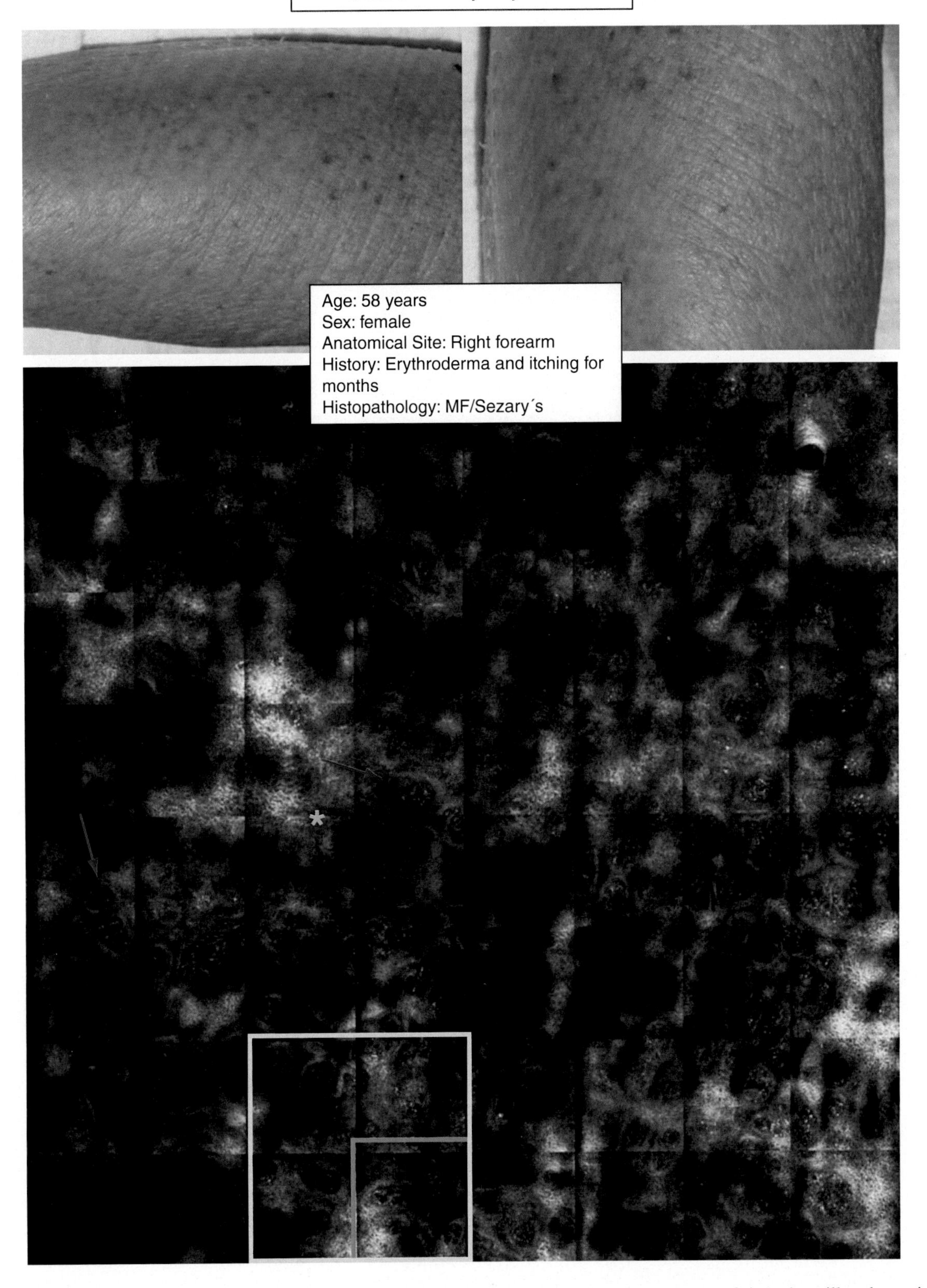

Fig. 24.3 RCM mosaic (4 × 4 mm) at the level of the DEJ reveals focal loss of the ringed appearance of dermal papillae due to infiltration by atypical cells (*arrows*). Reactive epidermal disarray with presence of blurred and thickened intercellular connections (*asterisk*) is seen

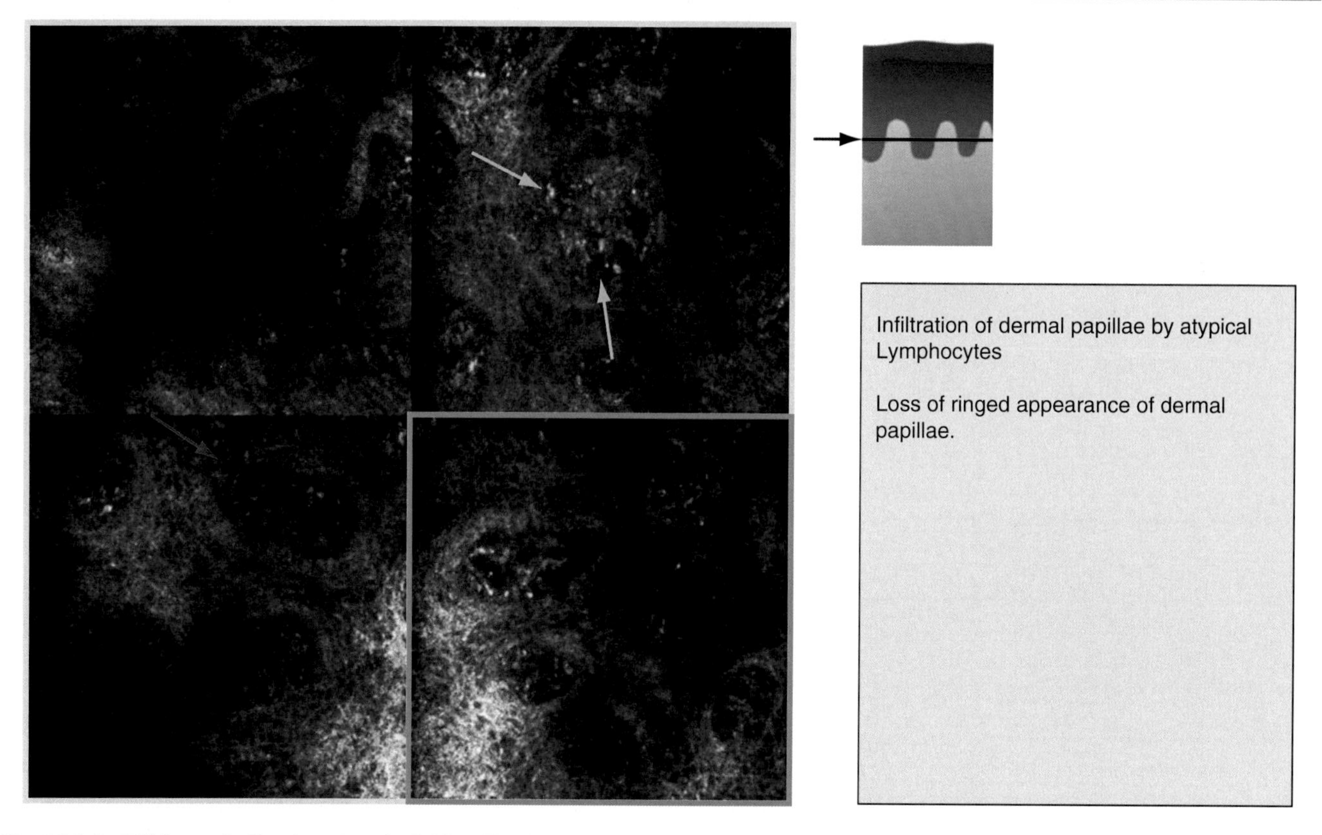

Fig. 24.3.1 RCM mosaic (1 × 1 mm) at the DEJ. Infiltration of dermal papillae by atypical lymphocytes (*green arrows*) and consecutive loss of the ringed appearance of dermal papillae (*red arrow*)

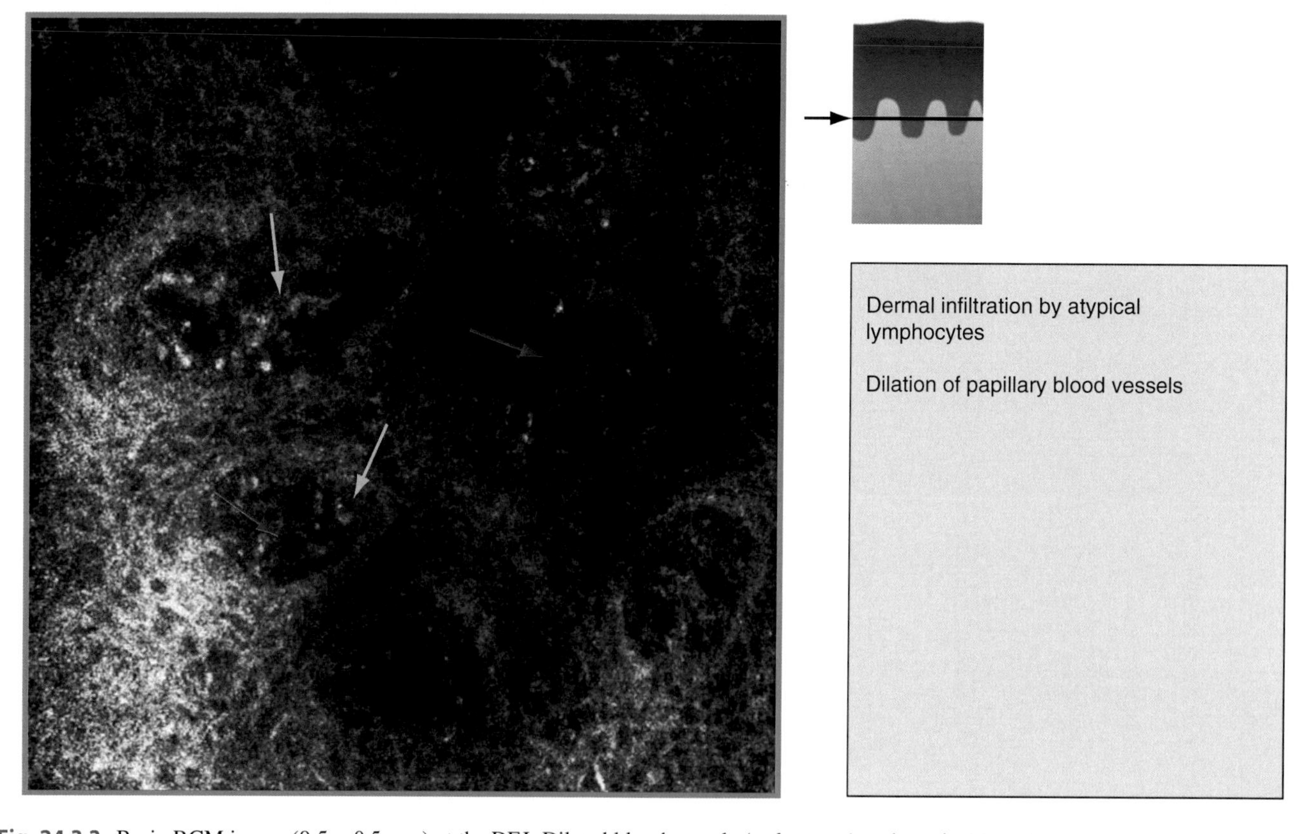

Fig. 24.3.2 Basic RCM image (0.5 × 0.5 mm) at the DEJ. Dilated blood vessels (*red arrows*) and atypical lymphocytes, varying in size, shape and reflectivity (*green arrows*) are observed within dermal papillae

24.5 Lymphomatoid Papulosis

Lymphomatoid papulosis (LyP), the most common form of primary cutaneous CD30+ lymphoproliferative disorders, generally occurs in adults but may also occur rarely in children. LyP is characterized by the presence of papular, papulonecrotic, and/or nodular skin lesions at various stages of development, which are predominantly located on the trunk and limbs.

24.5.1 Histopathologic and RCM Features

The histopathological appearance of LyP is extremely variable and, in part, correlates with the stage of development of the biopsied skin lesion. Three histologic subtypes of LyP (Types A, B, and C) have been described, which represent a spectrum with overlapping features. In LyP Type A, being the most common histologic variant and accounting for 75% of all LYP specimens, large, sometimes multinucleated (CD30+) lymphocytes are intermingled singly or in small clusters with numerous inflammatory cells. Epidermotropism is variable.

RCM: A focal loss of the honeycomb pattern and blurred intercellular connections may be observed at upper epidermal layers as well as around adnexal openings due to infiltration by inflammatory and neoplastic cells, which vary in size and shape (Figs. 24.4 and 24.4.1). The size of neoplastic cells does not exceed the size of surrounding keratinocytes. In some lesions of LyP, sharply demarcated polygonal areas filled with homogeneous material of low reflectivity, suggestive of epidermal necrosis, may be observed (Figs. 24.4, 24.4.1 and 24.4.2).

24.6 Primary Cutaneous B-Cell Lymphomas

Primary cutaneous B-cell lymphomas (PCBCL) represent a heterogeneous group of lymphoproliferative disorders characterized by clonal proliferation of neoplastic B-cells in the skin. The most important representatives are primary cutaneous follicle-center cell lymphoma, primary cutaneous marginal-zone lymphoma and primary cutaneous diffuse large B-cell lymphoma, leg type.

Cutaneous B-cell lymphomas usually present as well-circumscribed, red to purple papules, plaques or nodules on the trunk, head, or neck region or as rapidly growing red to purple tumors on the legs [12].

24.6.1 Histopathological and RCM Features

Histopathology of primary cutaneous B-cell lymphomas shows nodular to diffuse infiltrates of large nucleated atypical cells within the dermis, sometimes extending into the subcutaneous tissue, and sparing of the epidermis.

RCM: According to these histopathological features, RCM findings in primary cutaneous B-cell lymphomas are very discrete and unspecific. In some cases, a subtle inflammatory infiltrate around adnexal structures may be observed at the dermoepidermal junction and scanning of the papillary dermis may reveal aggregates of large nucleated atypical cells. Loss of detail and contrast below the papillary dermis hinders the visualization of the dense dermal infiltrates of atypical lymphocytes, the key feature of primary cutaneous B-cell lymphoma.

CASE 4 – Lymphomatoid papulosis
Age: 42 years
Sex: female
Anatomical Site: Right thigh
History: Recurrent papulonecrotic lesions for many years
Histopathology: Lymphomatoid papulosis

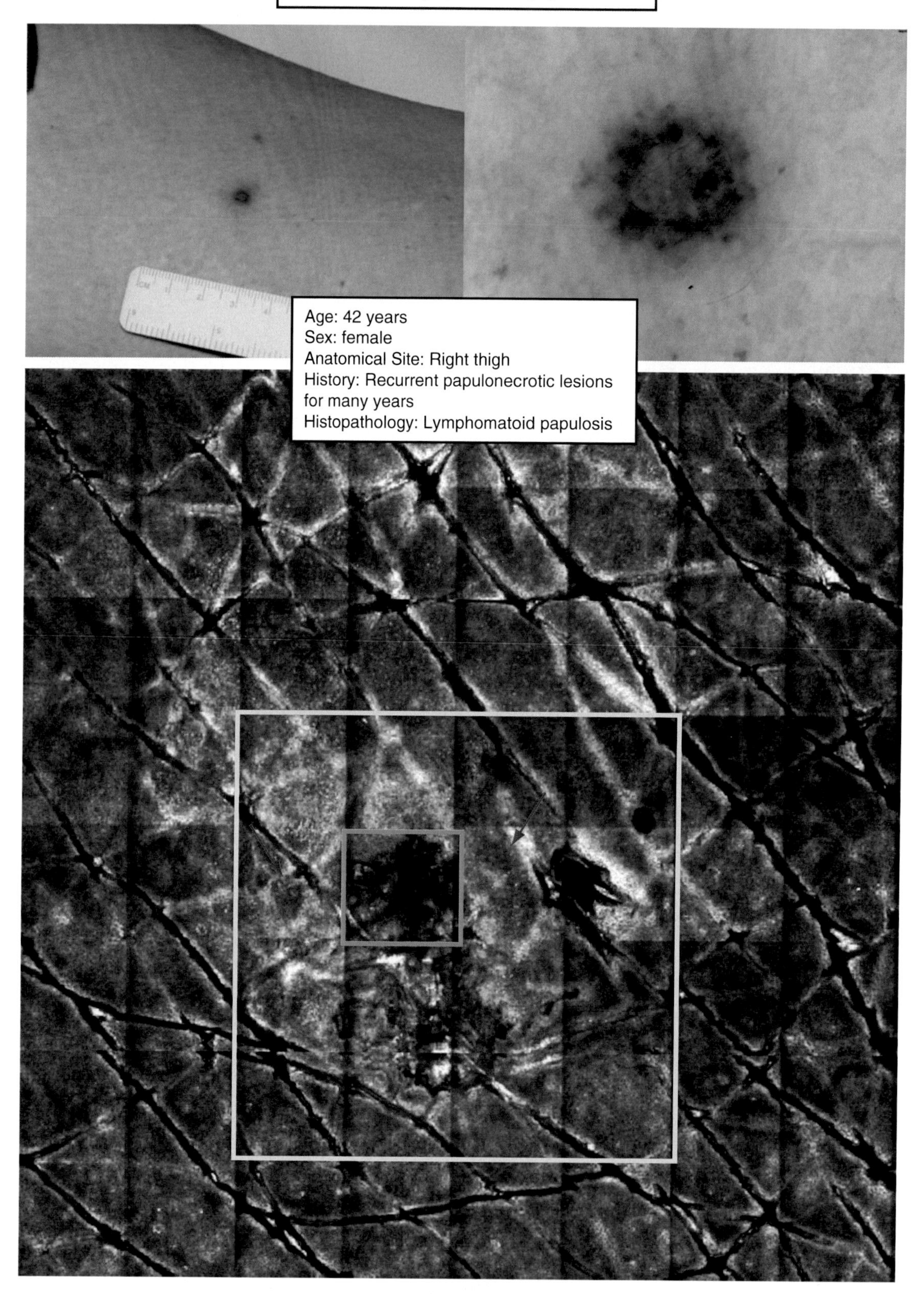

Fig. 24.4 RCM mosaic (4 × 4 mm) at upper epidermal layers reveals a sharply demarcated hyporeflective area with peripheral infiltration by atypical cells (*yellow rectangle*) and focal disarray of the honeycomb pattern (*arrow*) with blurred intercellular connection

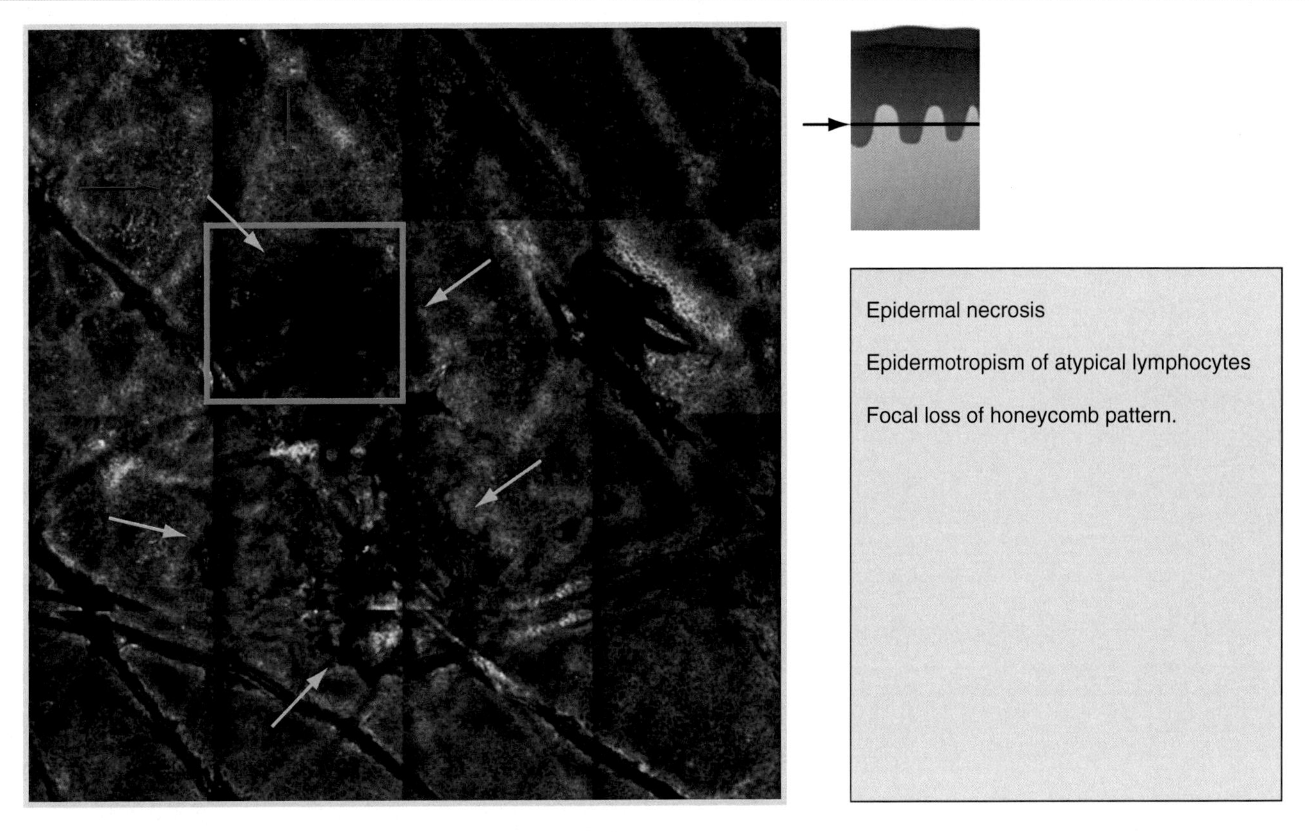

Fig. 24.4.1 RCM mosaic (2 × 2 mm) at upper epidermal layers. A sharply demarcated polygonal area filled with structureless homogeneous material, suggestive of epidermal necrosis, is shown (*green arrows*). Peripheral infiltration by atypical lymphocytes and focal loss of surrounding honeycomb pattern (*red arrows*) is visible

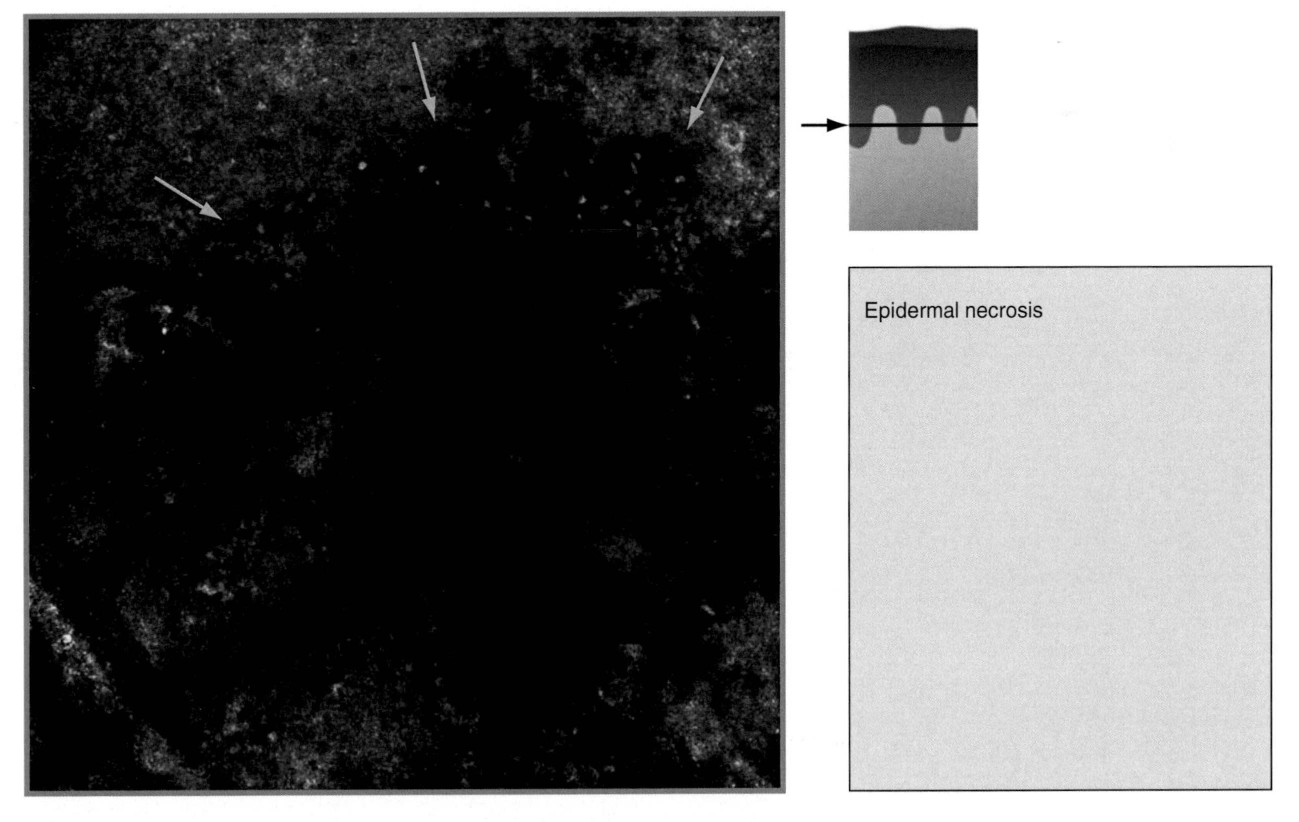

Fig. 24.4.2 Basic image (0.5 × 0.5 mm) at upper epidermal layers. A sharply demarcated polygonal area filled with structureless material, suggestive of epidermal necrosis, is visible (*green arrows*). Atypical lymphocytes and consecutive loss of the honeycomb pattern are observed in the surrounding epidermis (*red arrow*)

Core Messages

- RCM enables the visualization of some of the histopathologic features of CTCL, such as scattered epidermotropic lymphocytes, Pautrier´s microabscesses and infiltration of the upper dermis.
- The presence of intraepidermal clusters of small atypical lymphocytes, which vary in size, shape and reflectivity (Pautrier's microabscesses) is a highly characteristic RCM feature of MF and may lead to a correct diagnosis together with the clinical picture.
- RCM exhibits features similar to MF in MF-variants (folliculotropic MF, Sezary's Syndrome) and other CTCLs (Lymphomatoid papulosis).
- Cutaneous B-cell lymphomas present only unspecific or discrete RCM features, since histopathologic key features are missed due to limited penetration of light.

References

1. Burg G, Kempf W (2005) Cutaneous lymphomas, 1st edn. Taylor & Francis, New York
2. Foss F, Whittaker S (2006) Past, present and future developments in cutaneous T-cell lymphomas (CTCL). Semin Oncol 33(suppl 3):S1–S2
3. Willemze R, Elaine S, Jaffe ES, Burg G et al (2005) WHO-EORTC classification for cutaneous lymphomas. Blood 105:3768–3785
4. Fink-Puches R, Zenahlik P, Bäck B et al (2002) Primary cutaneous lymphomas: applicability of current classification schemes (European Organization for Research and Treatment of Cancer, World Health Organization) based on clinicopathologic features observed in a large group of patients. Blood 99:800–805
5. Prince HM, Yap LM, Blum R et al (2003) Primary cutaneous B-cell lymphomas. Clin Exp Dermatol 28:8–12
6. Cerroni L, Kerl H, Gatter K (2009) An illustrated guide to skin lymphoma, 3rd edn. Blackwell Science, Oxford
7. Weedon D, Strutton G (2002) Skin Pathology, 2nd edn. Churchill Livingstone, Elsevier Science, Edinburgh, pp 1105–1111
8. Nickoloff BJ (1988) Light microscopic assessment of 100 patients with patch/plaque-stage mycosis fungoides. Am J Dermatopathol 10:469–477
9. Agero AL, Gill M, Ardigo M et al (2007) In vivo reflectance confocal microscopy of mycosis fungoides: a preliminary study. J Am Acad Dermatol 57:435–441
10. Koller S, Gerger A, Ahlgrimm-Siess V et al (2009) In vivo reflectance confocal microscopy of erythematosquamous skin diseases. Exp Dermatol 18:536–540
11. Wieselthier JS, Koh HK (1990) Sezary syndrome: diagnosis, prognosis and critical review of treatment options. J Am Acad Dermatol 22:381–401
12. Willemze R, Kerl H, Sterry W et al (1997) EORTC classification for primary cutaneous lymphomas: a proposal from the Cutaneous Lymphoma Study Group of the European Organization for Research and Treatment of Cancer. Blood 90:354–371

25 Potpourri of Nonmelanocytic Skin Lesions

Elvira Moscarella, Iris Zalaudek, Gerardo Ferrara, Caterina Catricalà, and Giuseppe Argenziano

25.1 Introduction

Differential diagnosis of melanoma includes not only melanocytic nevi, but also a series of non-melanocytic, benign and malignant, pigmented and nonpigmented skin tumors. Under routine conditions it is not a rare event facing common lesions that show unusual morphologic features or, on the other hand, uncommon skin tumors that exhibit peculiar clinical and dermoscopic characteristics. In this setting RCM can be a reliable tool for improving the confidence of the clinician when dealing with such difficult-to-interpret lesions. We present a series of lesions that can be encountered in a clinical setting of patients with pigmented and non-pigmented skin tumors. For some of these lesions (ink-spot lentigo and dermatofibroma) RCM features have been already described by clinical studies including series of cases [1, 2]. Other lesions here described (lichen planus-like keratosis, angiokeratoma, pyogenic granuloma, sebaceous adenoma, and eccrine poroma) have only been presented as single cases [3–5], and for those lesions further studies are needed to better define clear and reproducible criteria for their recognition under RCM.

E. Moscarella (✉) • C. Catricalà
Department of Oncological Dermatology, Istituto Dermatologico San Gallicano, Rome, Italy
e-mail: elvira.moscarella@gmail.com

I. Zalaudek
Department of Dermatology, Medical University of Graz, Graz, Austria
e-mail: iris.zalaudek@gmail.com

G. Ferrara
Pathological Anatomy Department, Ospedale G. Rummo, Benevento, Italy
e-mail: gerardo.ferrara@libero.it

G. Argenziano
Dermatology Unit, ASMN Hospital, Reggio Emilia, Italy
e-mail: g.argenziano@gmail.com

R. Hofmann-Wellenhof et al. (eds.), *Reflectance Confocal Microscopy for Skin Diseases*,
DOI 10.1007/978-3-642-21997-9_25, © Springer-Verlag Berlin Heidelberg 2012

25.2 Ink-Spot Lentigo

Reticulated black solar lentigo, usually called ink-spot lentigo, is often typified clinically by irregular shape and black color resembling an ink-spot. These lesions occur in patients of Celtic ancestry, and are usually located on sun-exposed areas [6]. The most common presentation includes a single ink-spot lentigo among an extensive number of solar lentigines on the back or shoulders of a fair skin individual. Ink-spot lentigines can initially suggest melanoma because of their dark color and irregular shape; however, further investigation with dermoscopy reveals the characteristic features of these benign lesions, namely, a black broken-up network with or without intermingled bluish melanophages. Histopathologic examination reveals a 'skip' hyperpigmentation of the basal layer, with or without extension of the melanin throughout all levels of the epidermis. Melanocytes are not increased in number, uniform and small in size, and melanophages are usually present in the dermis. By RCM the lesion is characterized by a regular architecture and edged papillae are visible at dermo-epidermal junction. At the surface of the lesion, hyper refractile, small, roundish cells are detected; they appear crowded, with a so-called carpet-like distribution. Differentiation with melanoma can be made confidently by observing the cytological morphology and the lesion architecture. Cells in an ink-spot lentigo are roundish, small and homogeneous as compared to melanoma cells, and the epidermal architecture is not affected at all (Fig. 25.1).

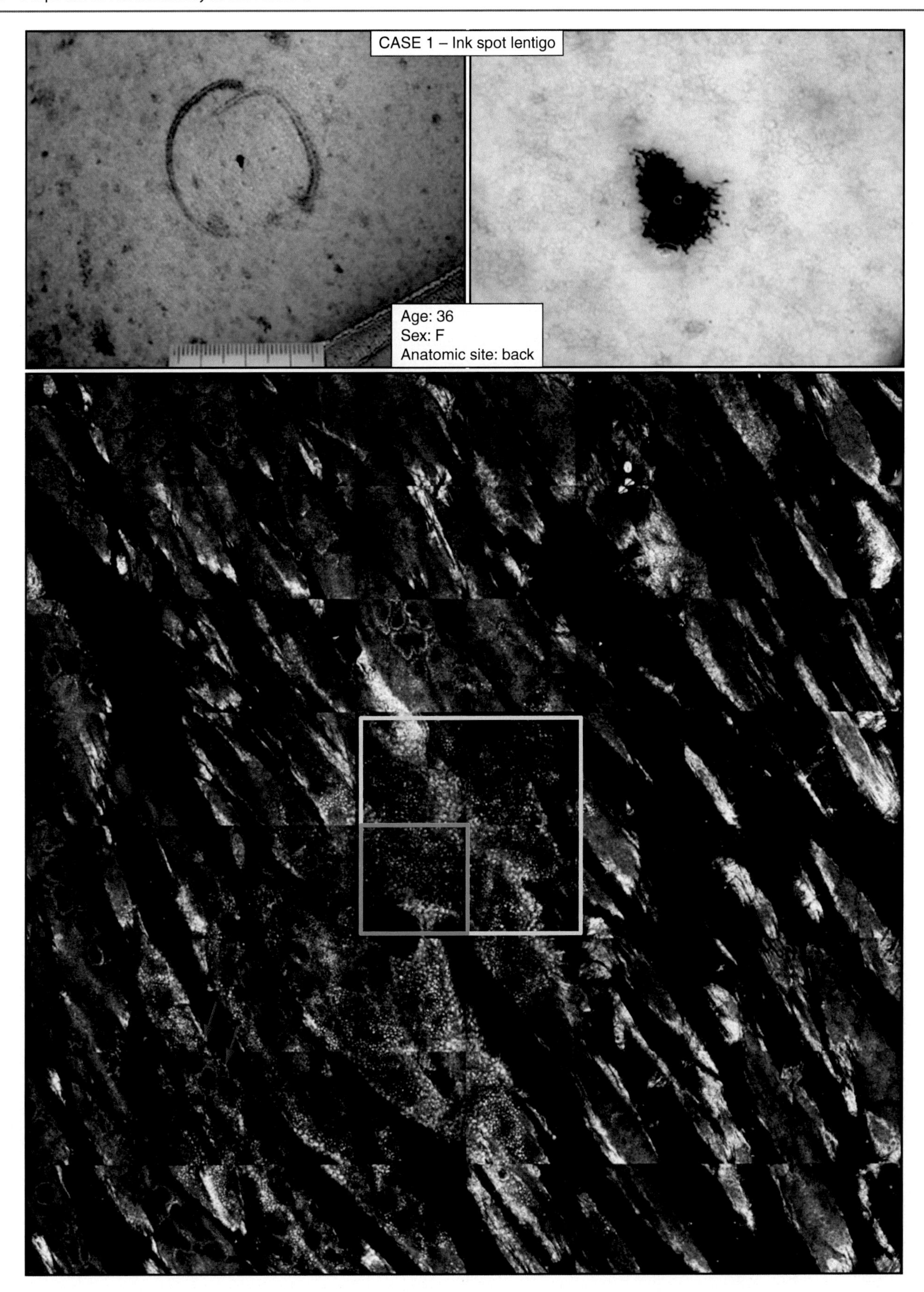

Fig. 25.1 RCM mosaic of the lesion at DEJ that shows the presence of edged papillae at the periphery of the lesion (→), the central portion appears crowded of highly pigmented cells

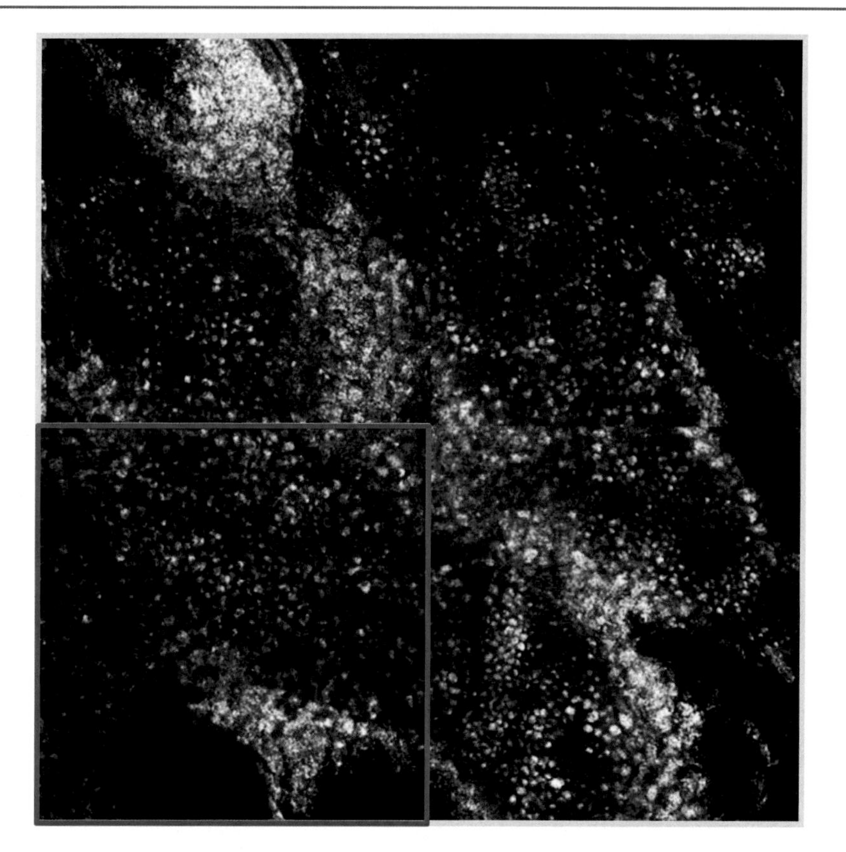

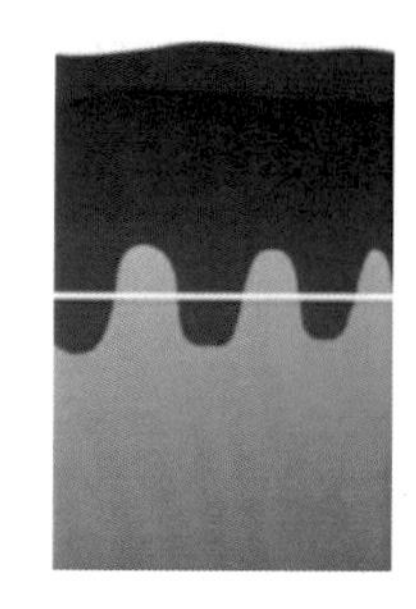

Fig. 25.1.1 RCM mosaic at the center of the lesion, small, roundish, highly refractile cells are present in carpet-like distribution

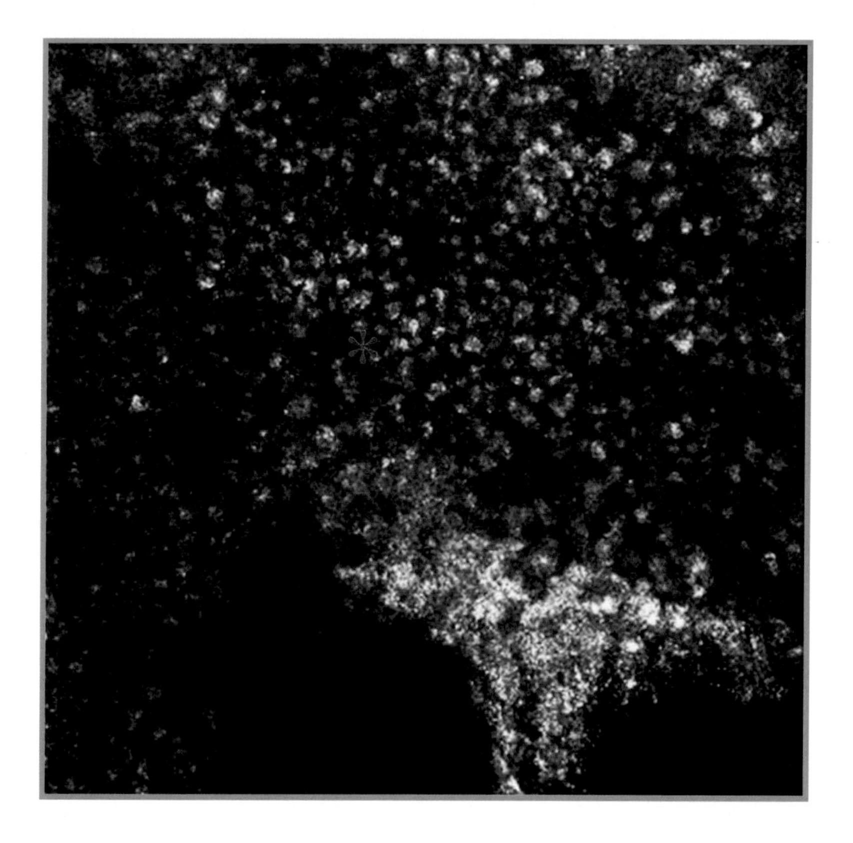

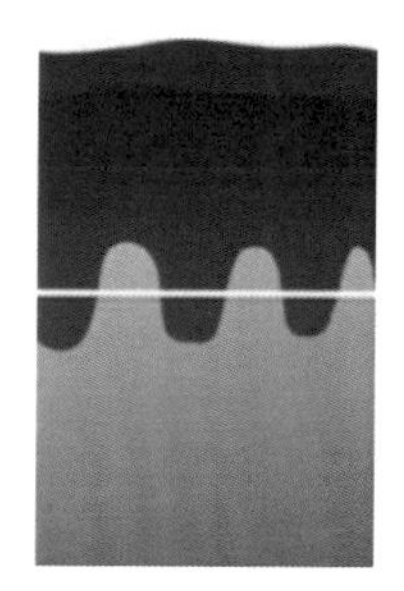

Fig. 25.1.2 A carpet of pigmented keratinocytes, no atypical melanocytes are detected

25.3 Lichen Planus-Like Keratosis

Lichen planus-like keratosis (LPLK) is defined as a solar lentigo or a seborrheic keratosis that is undergoing regression [7, 8]. Clinically, it is a solitary lesion that predominantly occurs on the face and sun-exposed areas of the trunk and upper extremities of adult and elderly patients. Early LPLK is usually a pink to red papule; as it progresses the papule may become darker and violaceous. In late LPLK the lesion may evolve into a hyperpigmented macule. The most consistent histopathologic features observed in LPLK are represented by a lichenoid lymphocytic infiltrate, often in a 'patchy' distribution that obscures the dermo-epidermal junction, by hyperkeratosis with focal parakeratosis and variable hypergranulosis and acanthosis. Remnants of either a seborrheic keratosis or an actinic keratosis can be detected. Eosinophils and plasma cells are sometimes present in the lichenoid infiltrate.

On dermoscopy we can recognize two main patterns associated with LPLK, namely, the localized granular pattern and the diffused granular pattern, both characterized by the presence of brownish-gray, reddish-brown, bluish-gray or whitish-gray coarse granules. However, on dermoscopy, some cases of LPLK may represent a dermoscopic pitfall, being difficult to differentiate from other pigmented lesions, such as lentigo maligna or regressive melanoma [9, 10]. RCM features of LPLK are represented by abundant presence of plump bright cells (melanophages) in the upper dermis, together with inflammatory cells, recognizable as bright spots and small bright cells. Of importance is the recognition of remnants of cords, indicating the preexisting solar lentigo or seborrheic keratosis, and the presence of edged papillae at the dermo-epidermal junction with no architectural disarray. In the upper layers a preserved honeycombed or cobblestone pattern is visible, with absence of atypical cells and pagetoid infiltration. As for dermoscopy, also with RCM, the absence of features reminiscent of a regressed benign lesion does not allow a precise diagnosis. In those cases, in which only an inflammatory infiltrate is present and no signs of the preexisting lesion can be detected, the histopathologic examination should always be performed (Fig. 25.2).

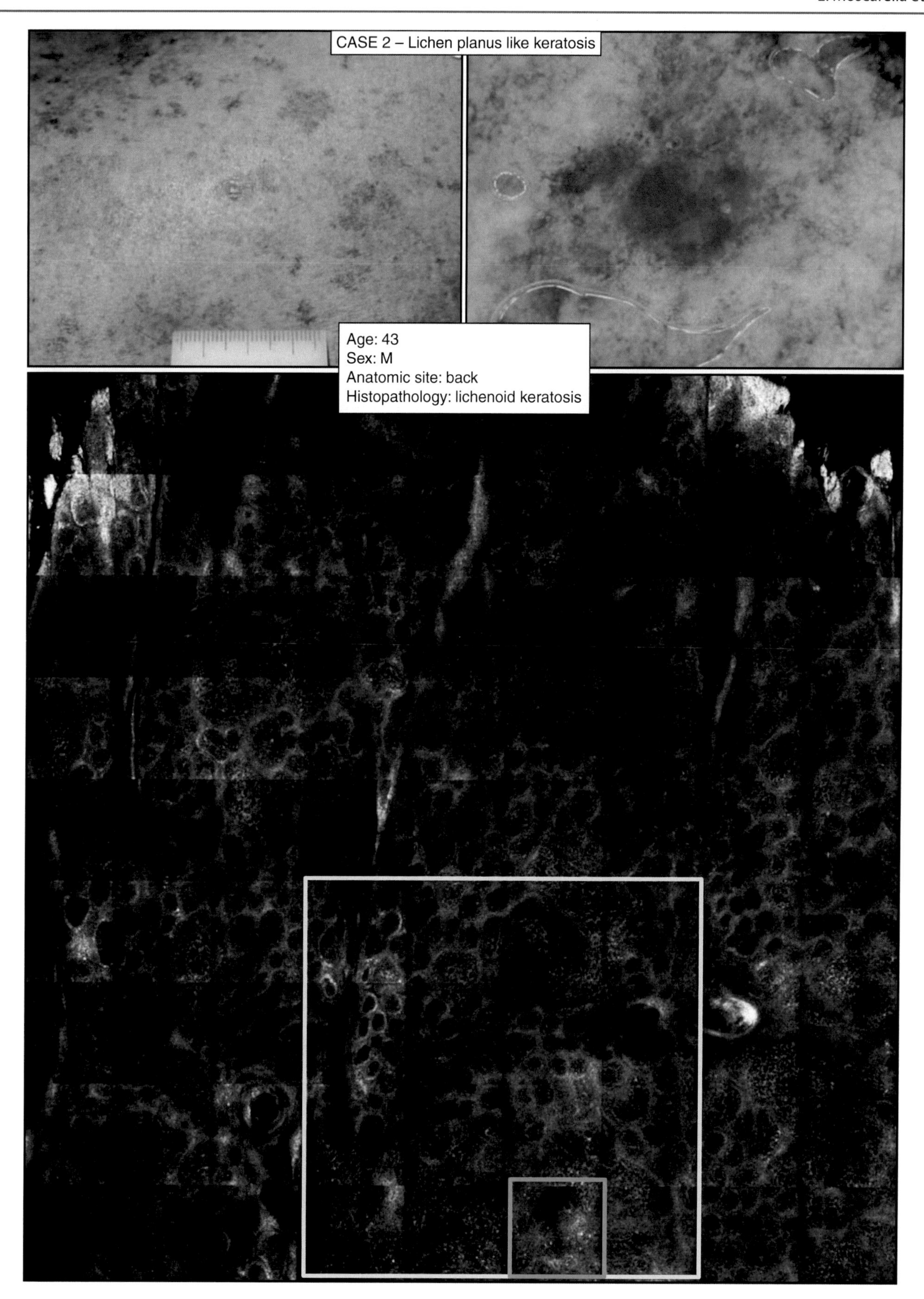

Fig. 25.2 RCM mosaic just above dermal epidermal junction, showing an abundant inflammatory infiltrate, with prevalence of melanophages. Remnants of cords may be detected

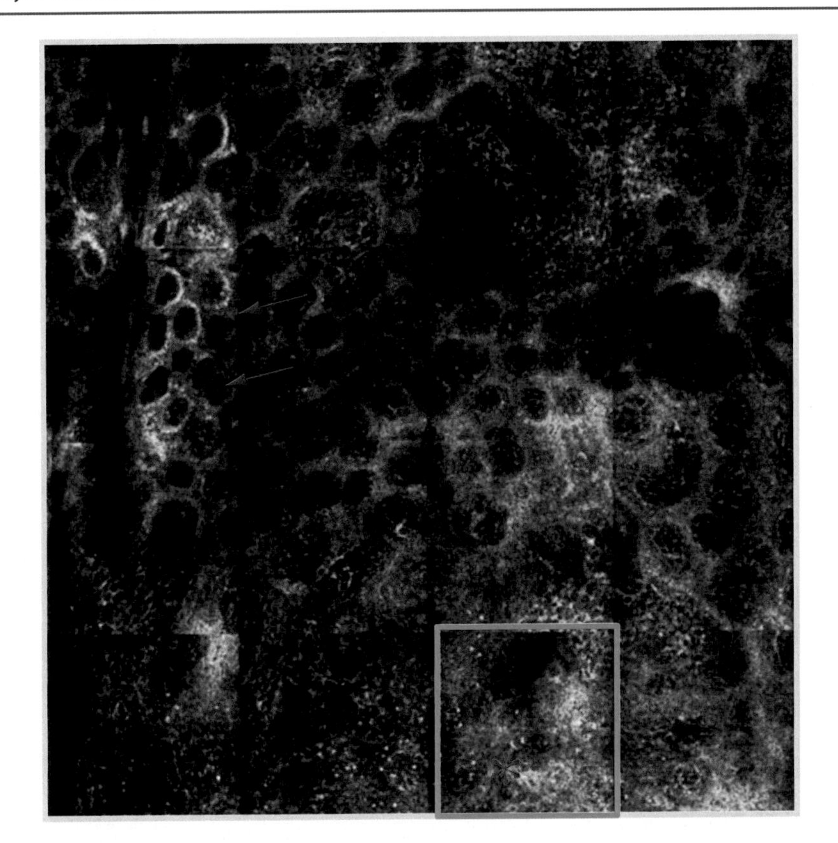
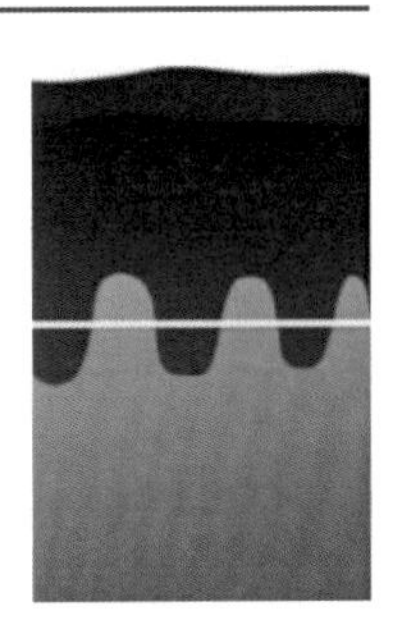

Fig. 25.2.1 RCM mosaic showing dermal papillae rimmed by bright, monomorphic cells (→)

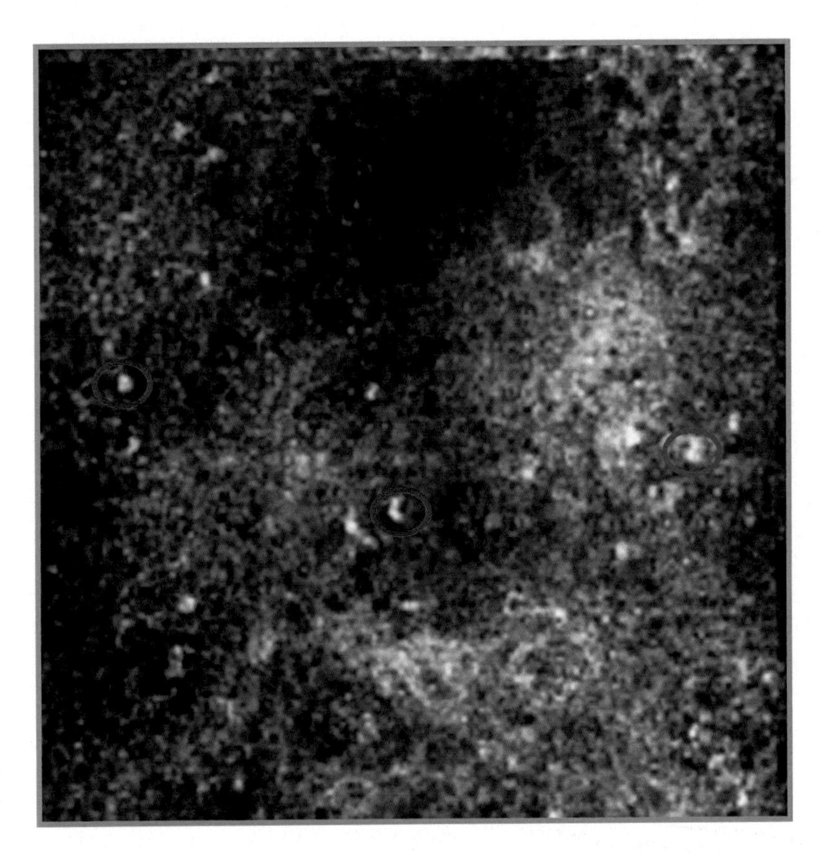
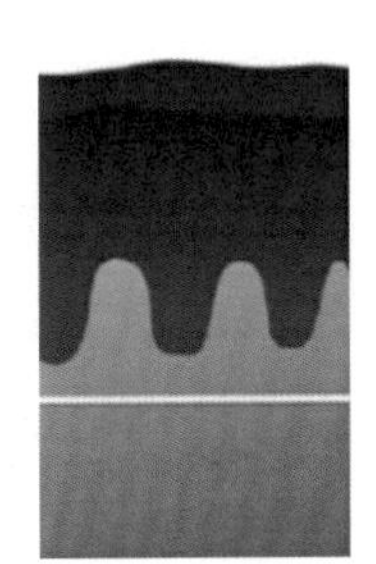

Fig. 25.2.2 Basic image at upper dermis level, showing melanophages, as plump bright cells (*red circle*), some of them showing nuclei (*blue circle*)

25.4 Angiokeratoma

During in vivo imaging, blood flow into capillary vessels can be easily appreciated, therefore, the documentation of vascular components in melanocytic and non melanocytic skin tumors has been an important aspect of the microscopic evaluation, including dilatation, elongation, tortuosity, and apparent neovascularization. Recently, RCM features of different vascular skin tumors have been described [4]. In a previous report a benign angioma was described under RCM, which revealed a greater number of tortuous and dilated capillary loops in the upper dermal layer [11]. In the routine practice it is not uncommon that vascular benign tumors may be confounded with melanoma. That is especially the case of angiokeratoma and pyogenic granuloma.

Angiokeratomas clinically present as elevated, warty, dark red to purple, slightly compressible papules, small nodules or plaques. The lesions often have irregular borders and black pigmentation, which is mostly attributable to superficial hemorrhage or associated hemosiderin pigment deposition in the dermis. Angiokeratomas exhibit an exophytic profile, with numerous ectatic thin-walled vascular channels that expand the papillary dermis. The epidermis is variably hyperplastic and hyperkeratotic. Thrombosis of these vessels is common and is responsible for the clinical mimicry of melanoma. The overlying epidermis encompasses the vascular spaces, and displays variable degrees of acanthosis and hyperkeratosis.

On dermoscopy angiokeratomas usually display dark red, to blue or black lacunae. When hyperkeratosis is present, it appears as a white-yellow hue over the lacunae.

RCM mosaic image nicely correlate with dermoscopy, showing numerous dilated spaces, large in diameter, correlating with dermoscopic lacunes, and corresponding to ectatic vascular lumina below the DEJ. The epidermis is thickened and shows a regular honeycombed pattern (Fig. 25.3).

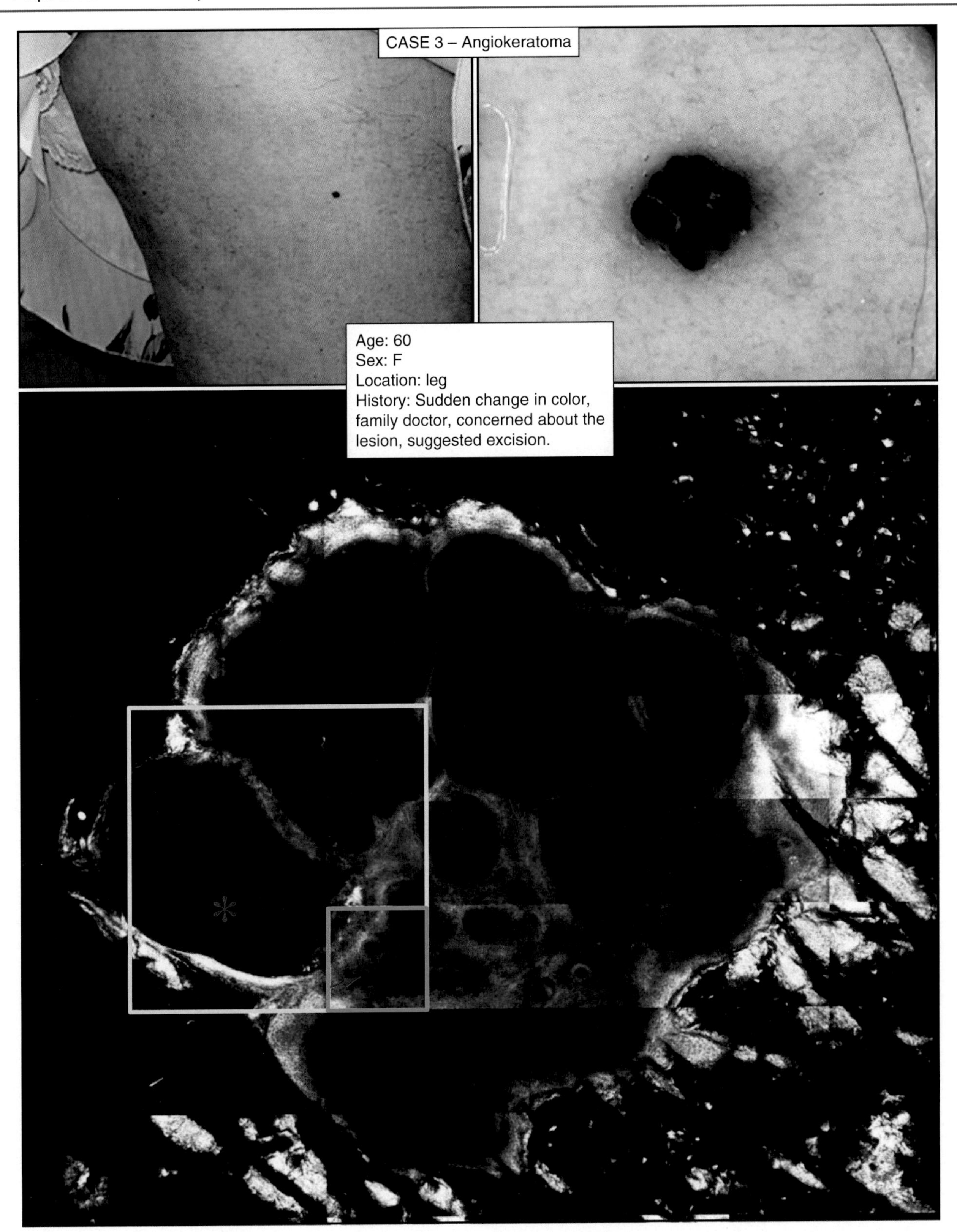

Fig. 25.3 RCM mosaic showing numerous lumina, as dark dilated spaces, large in diameter (*), that correlate with dermoscopic lacunes. They appear filled with hyporefractile cells (erythrocytes). Epidermis shows a regular honeycombed pattern, no atypical cells can be visualized (→)

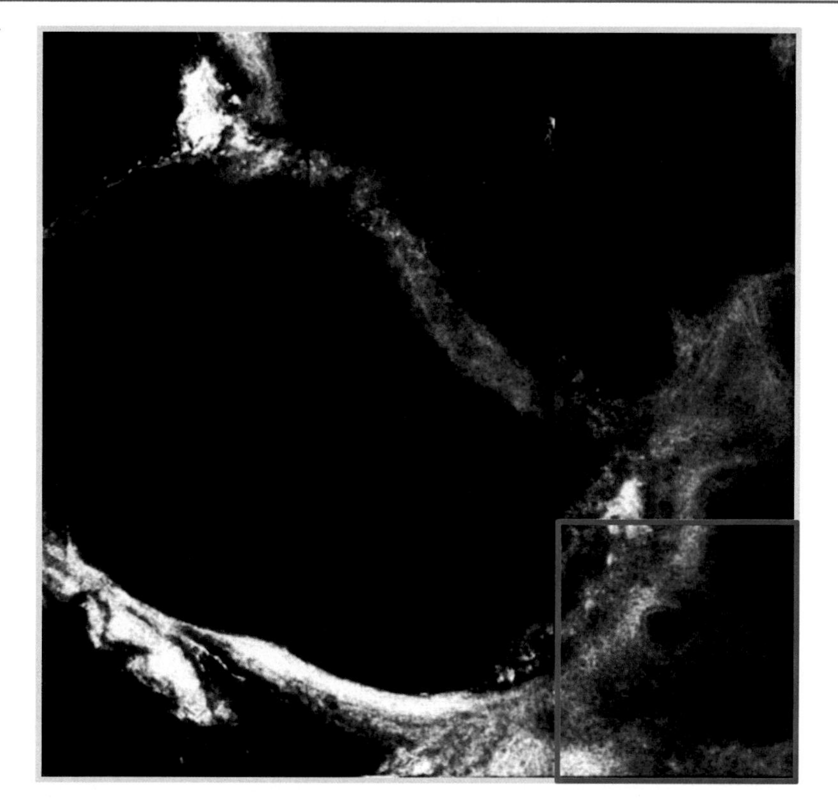
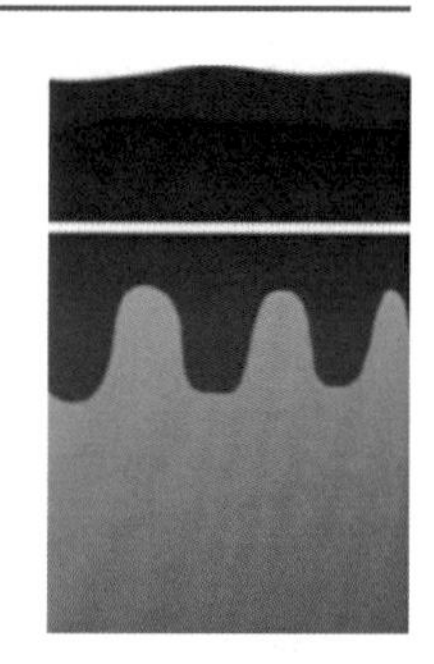

Fig. 25.3.1 RCM mosaic of a dark lacunae, filled by low refractile cells (erythrocytes)

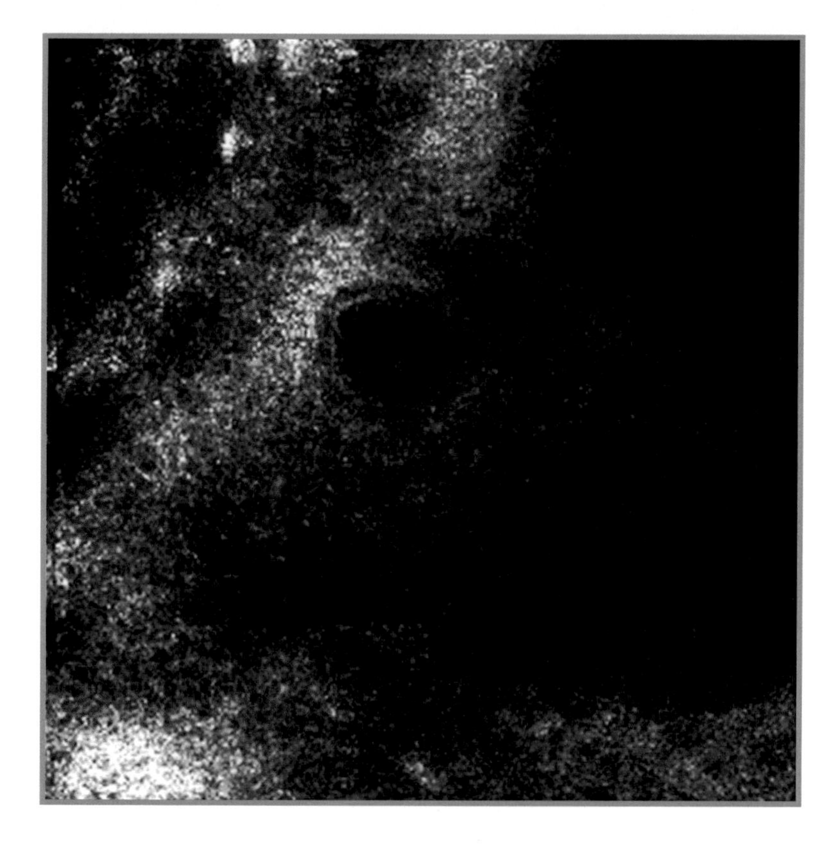
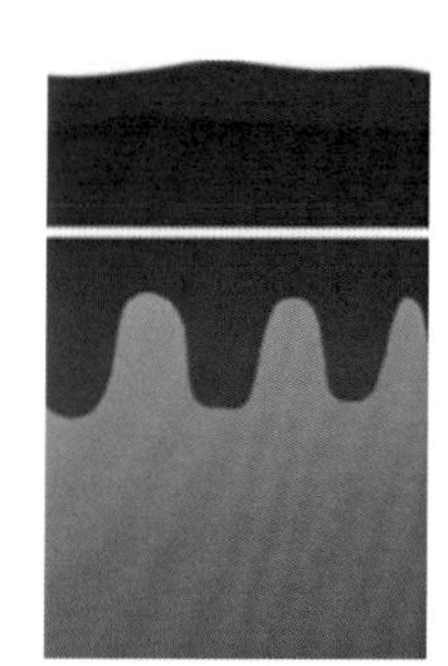

Fig. 25.3.2 Basic image showing preserved epidermal pattern

25.5 Pyogenic Granuloma

Pyogenic granuloma is a benign, acquired, vascular lesion of the skin and mucous membranes [12]. It usually presents as a solitary, rapidly growing, papule or nodule that bleeds easily after minor trauma. It occurs most often on the fingers, face, lips and oral mucous membranes, but can occur on any body site. In most cases, patient history and clinical appearance provide adequate information to make a correct diagnosis, however, Spitz nevi and amelanotic melanoma may be clinically and dermoscopically confused with pyogenic granuloma. Because some clinicians tend to remove these lesions with non-surgical treatments, such as liquid nitrogen or electrodessication, it is important to make a reliable preoperative diagnosis. If there is no possibility to be sure about the diagnosis, histopathologic examination of these lesions is strictly recommended because of its differential diagnosis with malignant tumors. RCM features of pyogenic granuloma have not been reliably described yet; however confocal examination seems to be useful in correctly diagnosing these lesions, because it immediately highlights the vascular nature of this tumor [4]. Histopathologically, a typical exophytic pyogenic granuloma shows close to the surface a proliferation of blood capillaries with a lobular pattern set in an edematous and/or sclerotic matrix. An epidermal collarette is usually present, causing in some cases slight pedunculation of the lesion. A dermal mixed inflammatory infiltrate is a common finding. Older pyogenic granulomas tend to be more organized with fibrous septa intersecting the lesion and producing a lobular pattern. Dermoscopy features have been described, the most common features being reddish homogeneous areas, white collaret, 'white rail' lines that intersect the lesion, and ulceration [13]. RCM mosaic of the lesion reveals a well circumscribed lesion, surrounded by a white halo that correlates with the dermoscopic white collaret. Spinous keratinocytes are arranged in a honeycombed pattern, with a great number, elongation, and density of dermal capillaries at lower levels, arranged as bright canalicular structures within roundish or oval lobules. In vivo imaging allows visualization of lymphocyte rolling (Fig. 25.4).

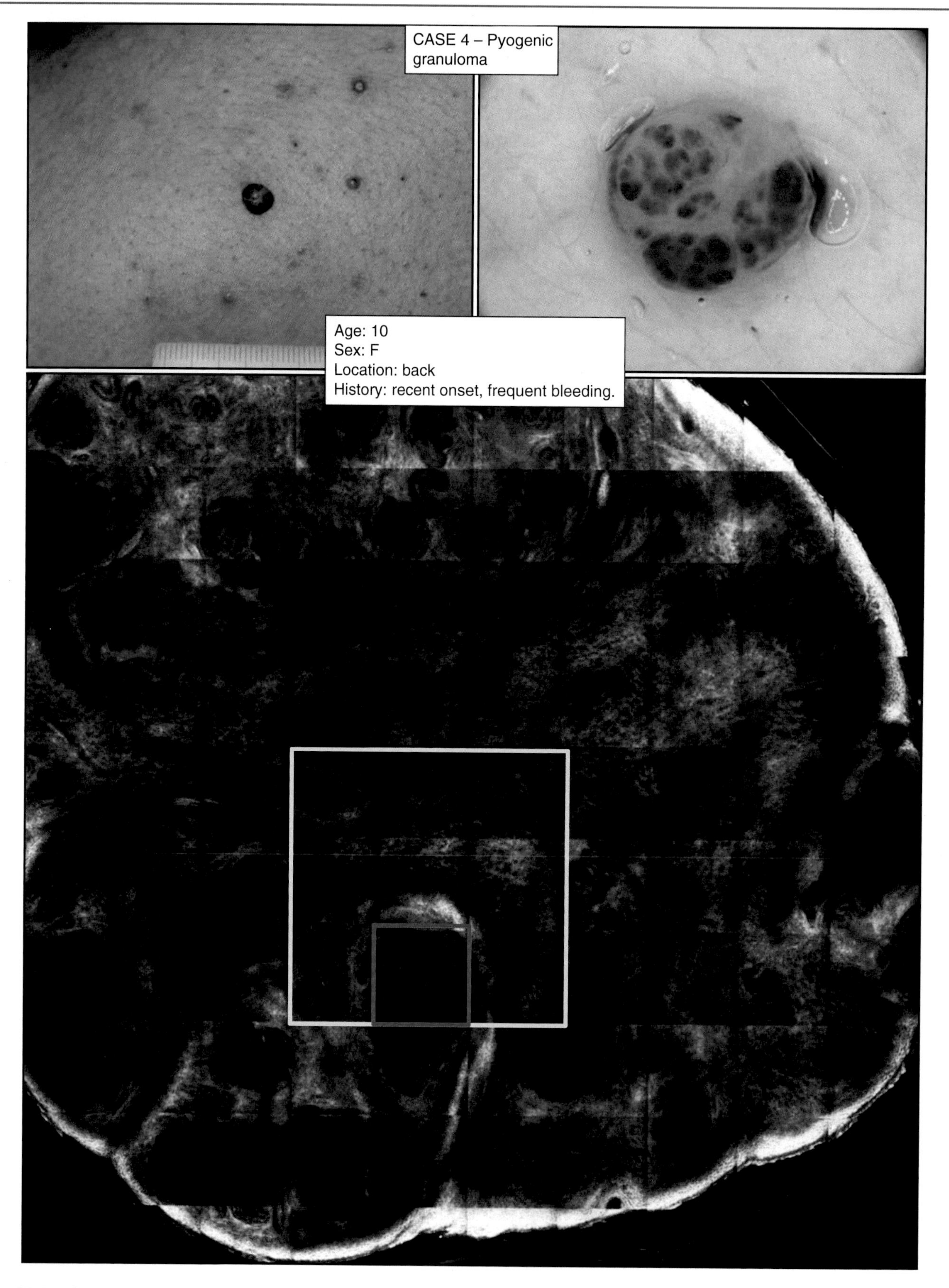

Fig. 25.4 RCM mosaic at dermal epidermal level shows well-circumscribed lesion, surrounded by a white collaret. Dermal capillaries, arranged as bright canalicular structures within roundish to oval lobules, appear in great number and density

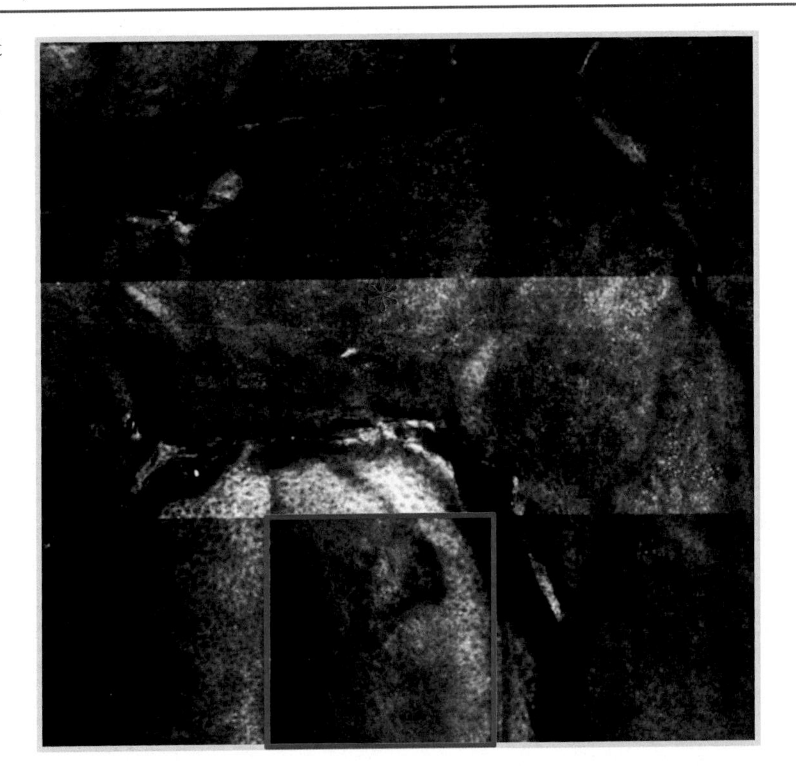
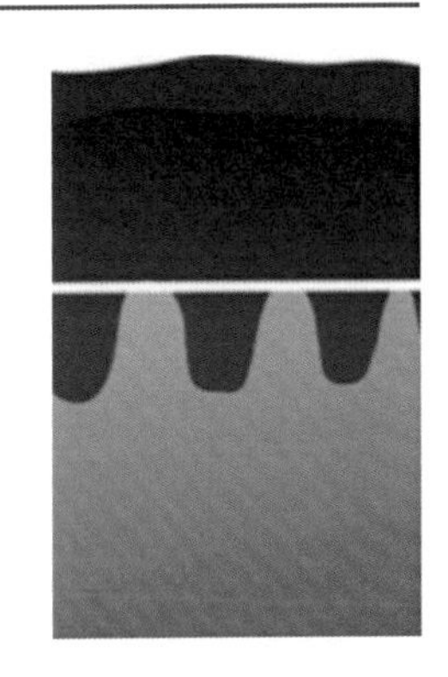

Fig. 25.4.1 Mosaic image at spinous layer showing a regular honeycombed pattern with no atypical cells (*)

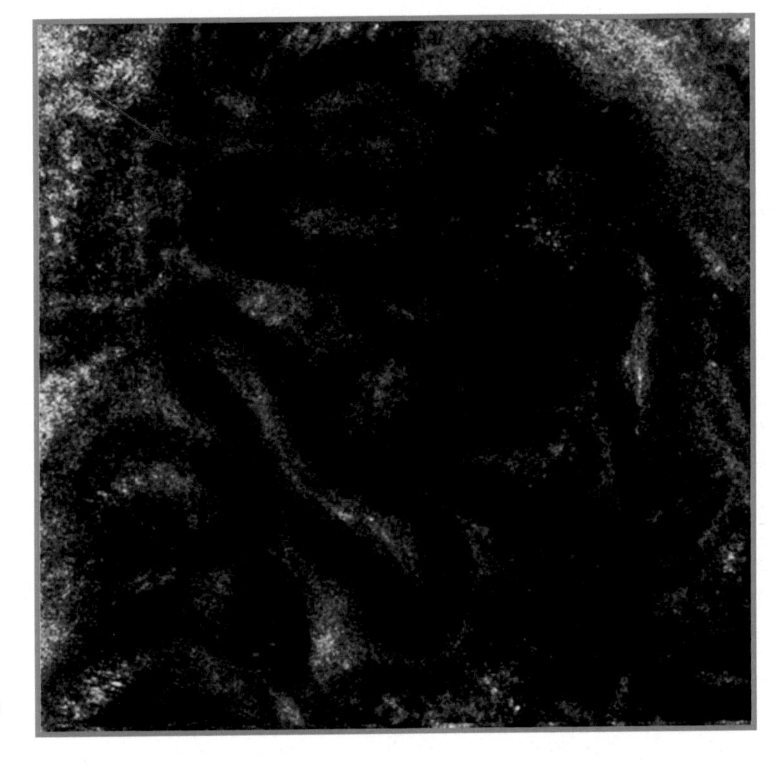
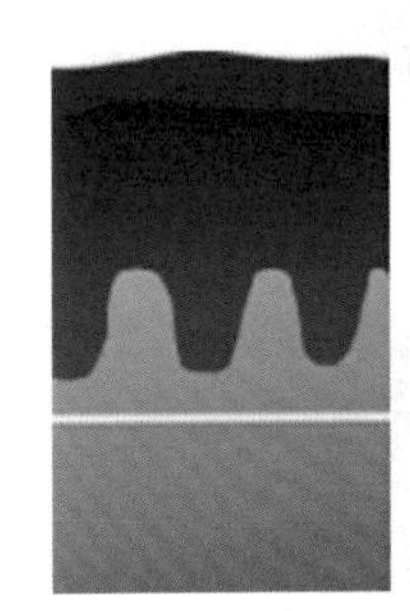

Fig. 25.4.2 Canalicular structures in dermis (→)

25.6 Dermatofibroma

Dermatofibroma (DF) is a common cutaneous nodule of unknown etiology that frequently develops on the extremities (mostly the lower legs) and is usually asymptomatic, although pruritus and tenderness are not uncommon [14]. DF is usually easy to diagnose clinically because of a firm fibrous consistency and surface dimpling on compression. Sometimes it can show atypical clinical presentations, simulating atypical melanocytic lesions, or it undergoes excision for its symptomatic presentation. A number of well-described, histopathologic subtypes of dermatofibroma have been described. The overlying epidermis is usually acanthotic. Pseudoepitheliomatous hyperplasia, basaloid proliferation, and hyperpigmentation of the basal layer may be noted. The bulk of the tumor is within the mid dermis where no capsule is present and the periphery of the lesion blends with the surrounding tissue. Fascicles of spindle cells with variable collagen deposition are characteristic. Xanthomization and hemorrhage are variably present as well. At the periphery, the spindle cells typically wrap around normal collagen bundles. Occasionally, melanocytes have been reported to be interspersed amongst the spindle cells. Numerous small blood vessels may also be present. Typically, dermoscopy of a DF shows a faint network or pseudonetwork surrounding a pale amorphous, scar-like area [15]. Sometimes the central white area shows white lines and brown holes. RCM features of DF have been described [16], namely, a normal honeycombed or cobblestone pattern, and an increased density of bright dermal papillary rings. In the dermis, collagen bundles are brighter and thicker than those seen in normal skin; they can be seen as reticulated bundles within dermal papillae, but also as elongated bundles between the papillae. Occasionally, dilated blood vessels can be observed in the center or at the periphery of the lesion. When the lesion is clinically hypopigmented, or in fair skin types, bright papillary rings, that usually represent an important criteria for diagnosis, are not commonly seen. In atypical cases, such RCM features, together with the absence of criteria for melanocytic lesion, can support the differential diagnosis with melanoma (Fig. 25.5).

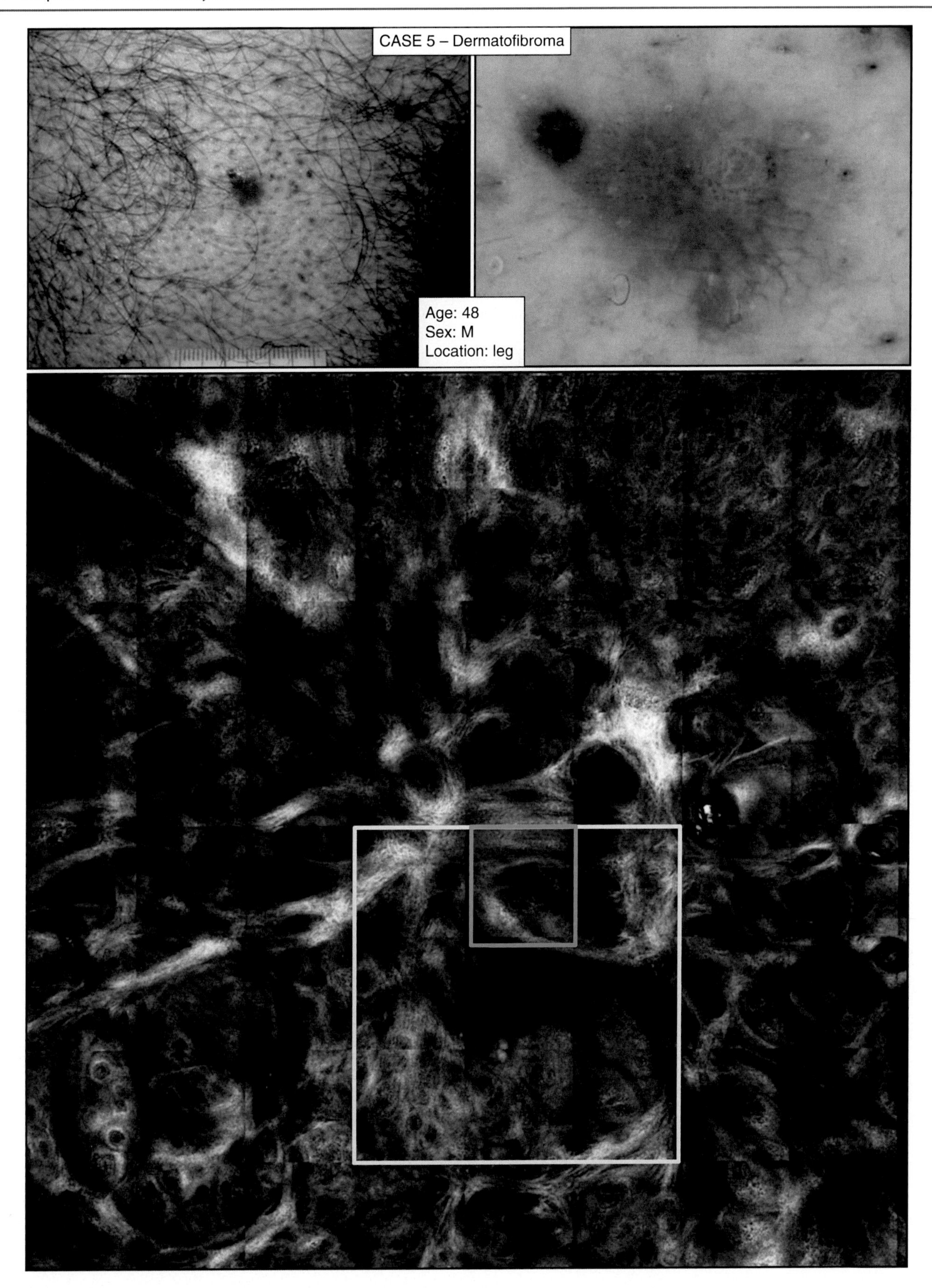

Fig. 25.5 RCM mosaic at the dermal level, showing hyper refractile, elongated, collagen bundles, that appear increased in number and size

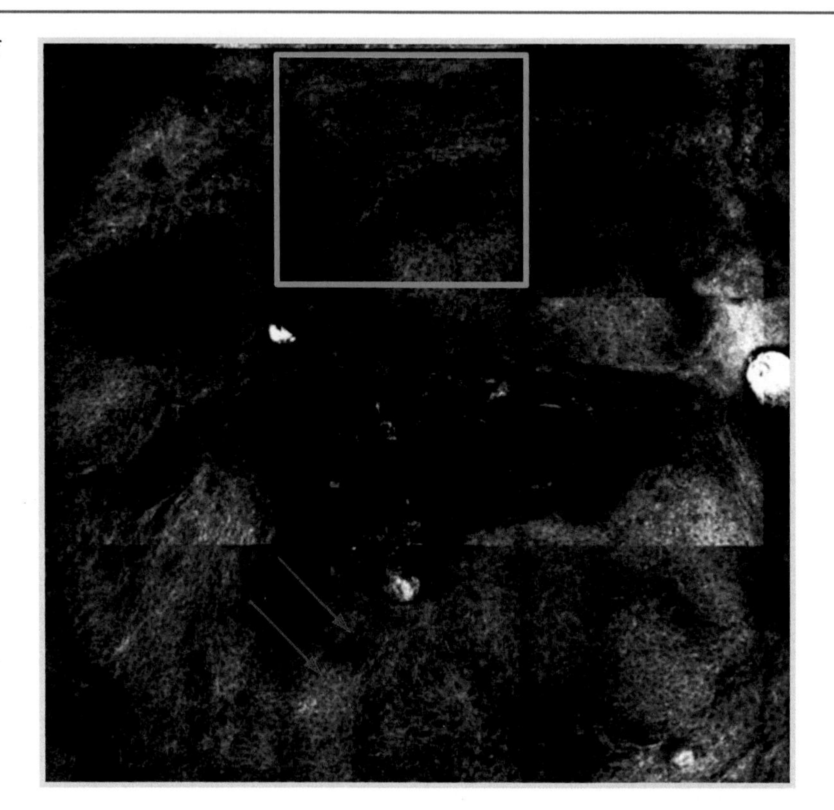

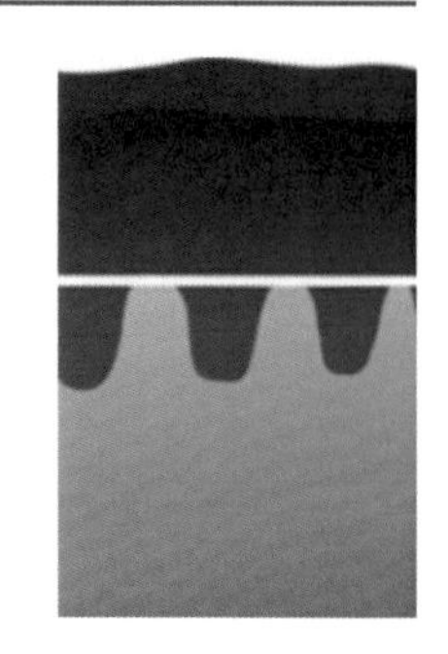

Fig. 25.5.1 RCM mosaic of the spinous layer, a typical honeycombed pattern characterizes the lesion (→)

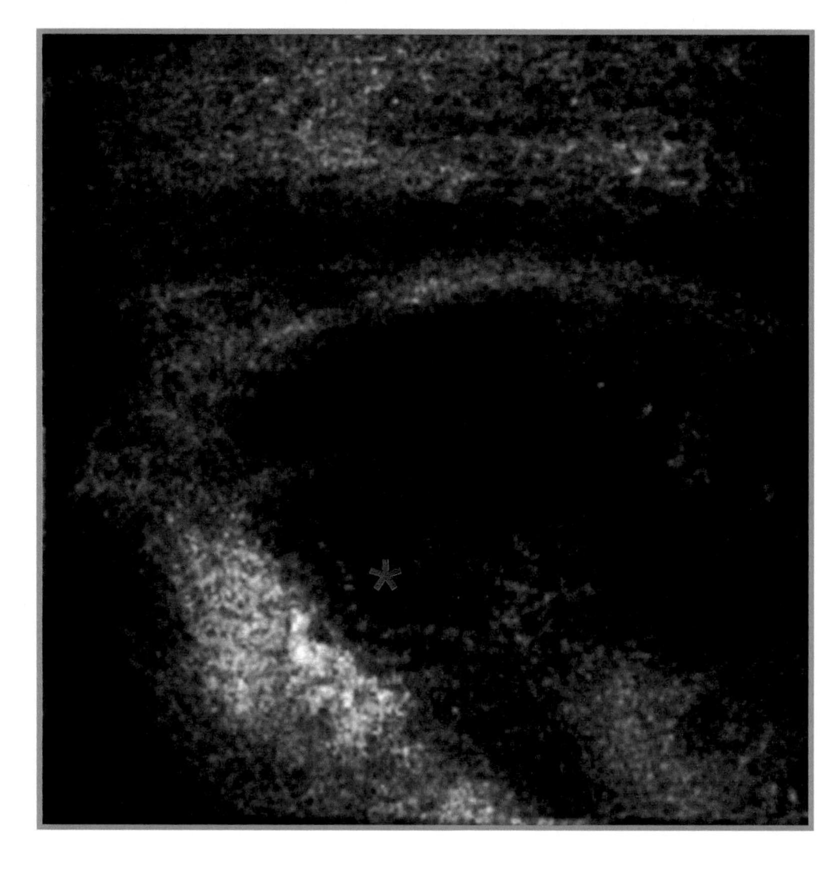

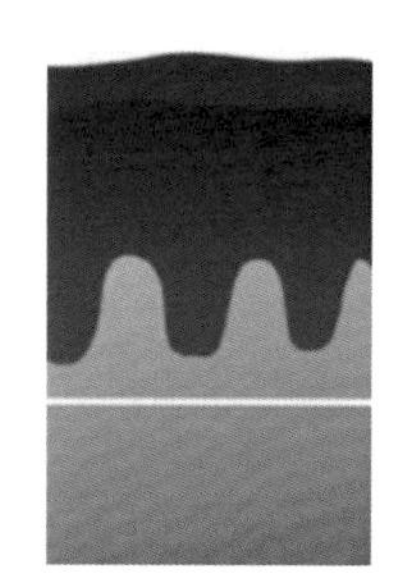

Fig. 25.5.2 Dilated vessels seen in superficial dermis (*)

25.7 Sebaceous Adenoma

Sebaceous adenoma (SA) typically presents as a solitary yellow nodule on the face or scalp. When SA are numerous, they could be associated with the Muir-Torre syndrome [17]. SA are benign cutaneous adnexal neoplasms that do not have a potential for aggressive growth or metastasis. However, local recurrence is occasionally encountered following incomplete removal of the tumor. When multiple SA are associated with the Muir-Torre syndrome, visceral carcinomas, including adenocarcinomas of the colon, stomach, duodenum, hematologic system, genitourinary tract, endometrium, and larynx (in decreasing order of frequency) may also be present. Clinically, it presents as a yellowish or pinkish papule or nodule, usually located on the face or scalp. The preoperative clinical impression is usually that of a basal cell carcinoma. On dermoscopy it may resemble a sebaceous hyperplasia, but with less prominent vessels. Sebaceous hyperplasia are characterized on dermoscopy by the presence of crown vessels, distributed around a central yellow-white globular structure. In SA this "crown" distribution appears less evident [18]. Histopathologically, the tumor is multilobulated with frequent connection to the epidermis. At low-power view, sebaceous adenoma is sharply demarcated from the surrounding tissue, with a proliferation of variously sized sebaceous lobules consisting of central, larger, mature sebaceous cells (sebocytes), peripheral, smaller, undifferentiated, germinative basaloid cells, and transitional cells. As already mentioned, the main clinical and dermoscopic differential diagnosis is with basal cell carcinoma. As RCM features of BCC are nowadays well known, the differential diagnosis by RCM can be simply made by the absence of features reminding to BCC. However, some peculiar RCM features of sebaceous adenoma can be also noted. The tumor shows similar features to those already described for sebaceous hyperplasia. The RCM mosaic reveals a well-circumscribed lesion, characterized by the presence of multiple sebaceous ducts that appear as dark, lobulated spaces on the lesion surface. Sebaceous lobules can also be detected, with round cells showing brightly refractile, speckled cytoplasm and central round, dark nuclei (Fig. 25.6).

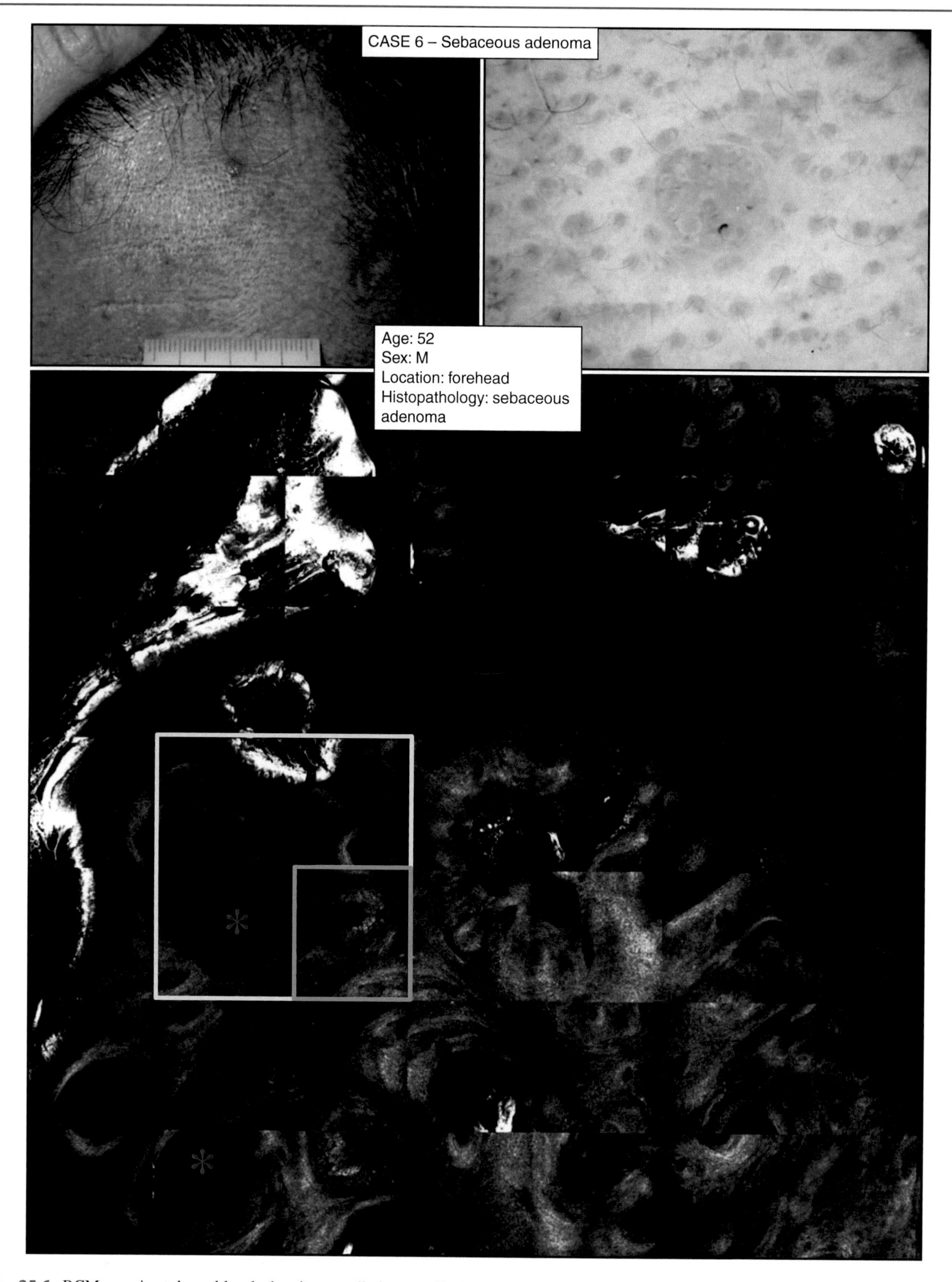

Fig. 25.6 RCM mosaic at dermal level, showing a well-circumscribed lesions, characterized by the presence of multiple sebaceous ducts (*) as dark, lobulated spaces on the lesion surface

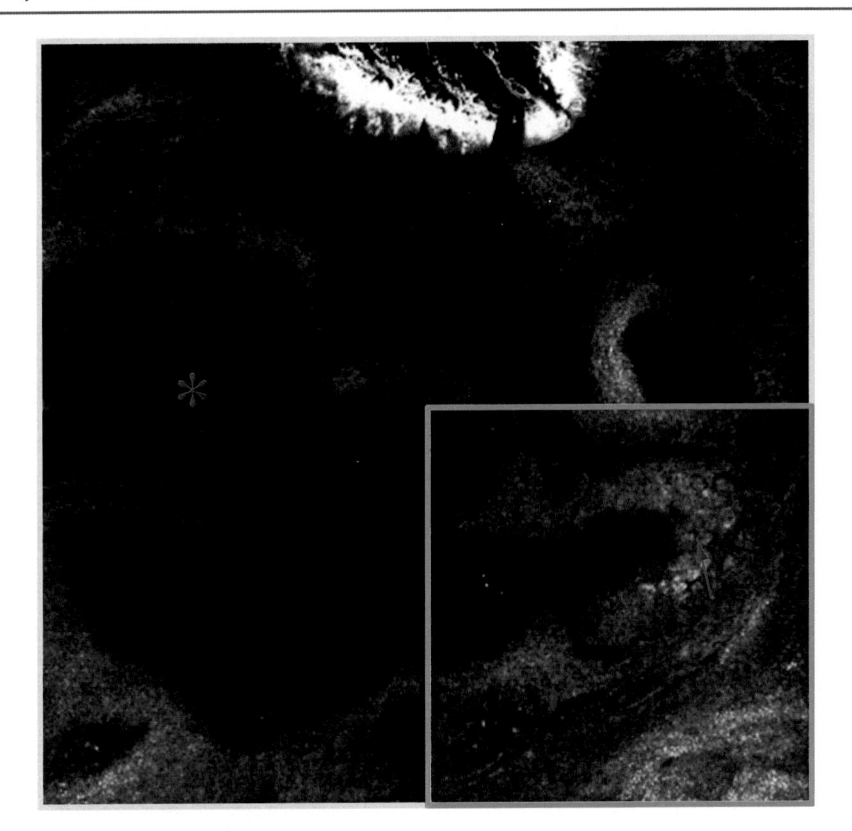

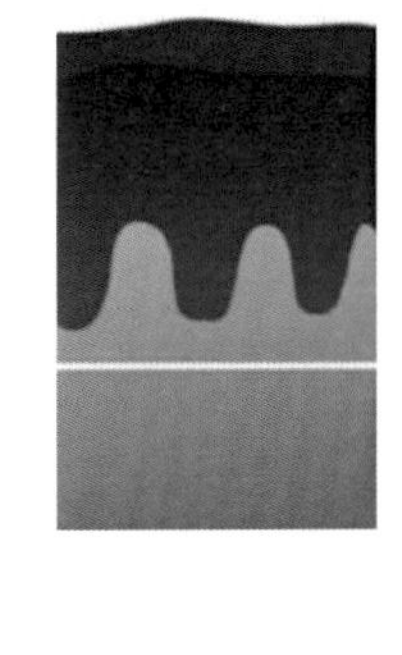

Fig. 25.6.1 RCM image at dermal level, showing a sebaceous duct (*), and a sebaceous lobule (→)

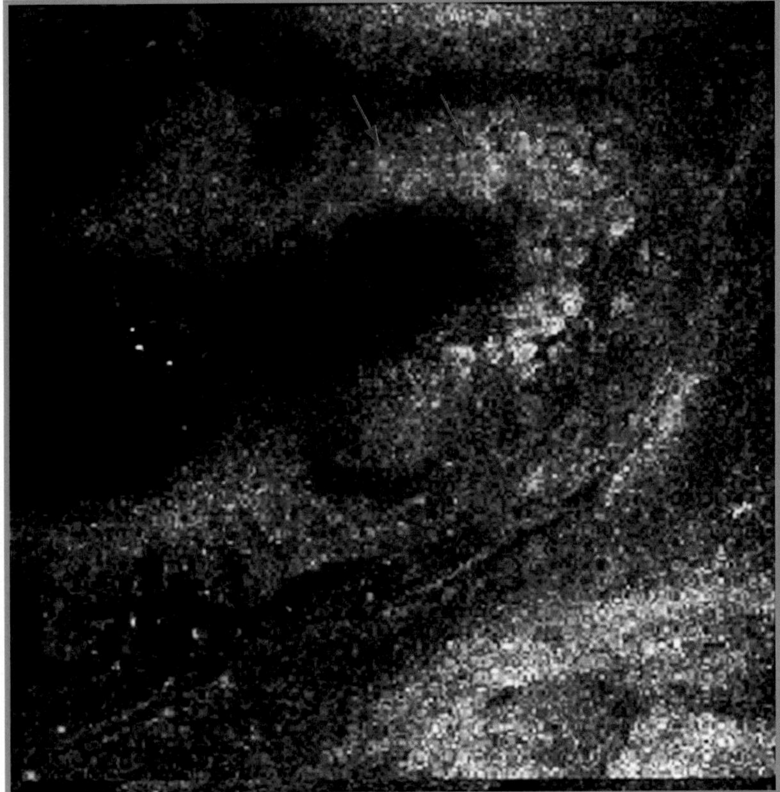

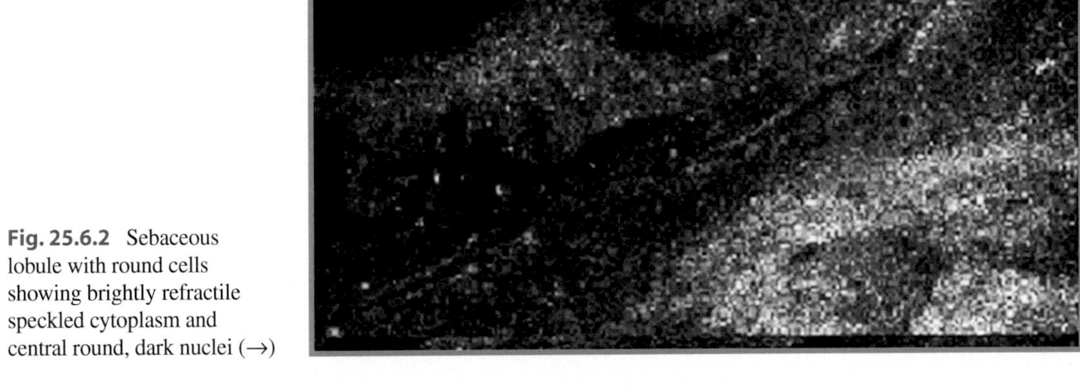

Fig. 25.6.2 Sebaceous lobule with round cells showing brightly refractile speckled cytoplasm and central round, dark nuclei (→)

25.8 Eccrine Poroma

Eccrine poroma (EP) is a tumor of the sweat gland that occurs commonly in adults on the soles, but it can develop also on the palms, trunk and in the head-neck regions [19]. Clinically, the tumor appears slightly pedunculated and has a normal or erythematous color and a firm consistency. The surface is usually smooth and often lobulated. However, many clinical presentation have been described, and the tumor can also present pigmentation. This variable clinical presentation gives reason of the difficulty in making a reliable differential diagnosis with many other skin tumors, including basal cell carcinoma and melanoma. Dermoscopic features of EP have been previously described, leading to the conclusion that both pigmented and amelanotic EP may be clinically and dermoscopically indistinguishable from melanoma and non-melanoma skin cancers [20]. RCM can help differentiating this tumor from other malignancies. Features of the pigmented variant have been described and correlated with histopathologic findings of the tumor [21]. Histopathologically, the tumor is composed by broad bands of epithelial cells which are typically intermediate in size between basilar and malpighian keratinocytes. The borders between the tumor and the epidermis are usually easy to recognize. Areas of ductal differentiation are seen as tubules lined by a dense eosinophilic cuticle. These lesions have a variable downward proliferation: cases of so-called 'dermal duct tumor' show loss of connection with the epidermis. Not uncommonly, the stroma is highly vascular.

RCM shows a well demarcated border between the tumor and the surrounding keratinocytes, with the tumoral cells organized in an atypical honeycombed pattern compared to the surrounding epithelial cells. Tumoral bands are surrounded by an abundant stroma, and an increased vascularization is detected, as well. Confocal images also reveal the presence of non refractile dark round spaces, which correspond to area of ductal differentiation within the tumor [21]. Together with these specific features, the absence of criteria for basal cell carcinoma and for melanocytic lesions can lead to the final diagnosis (Fig. 25.7).

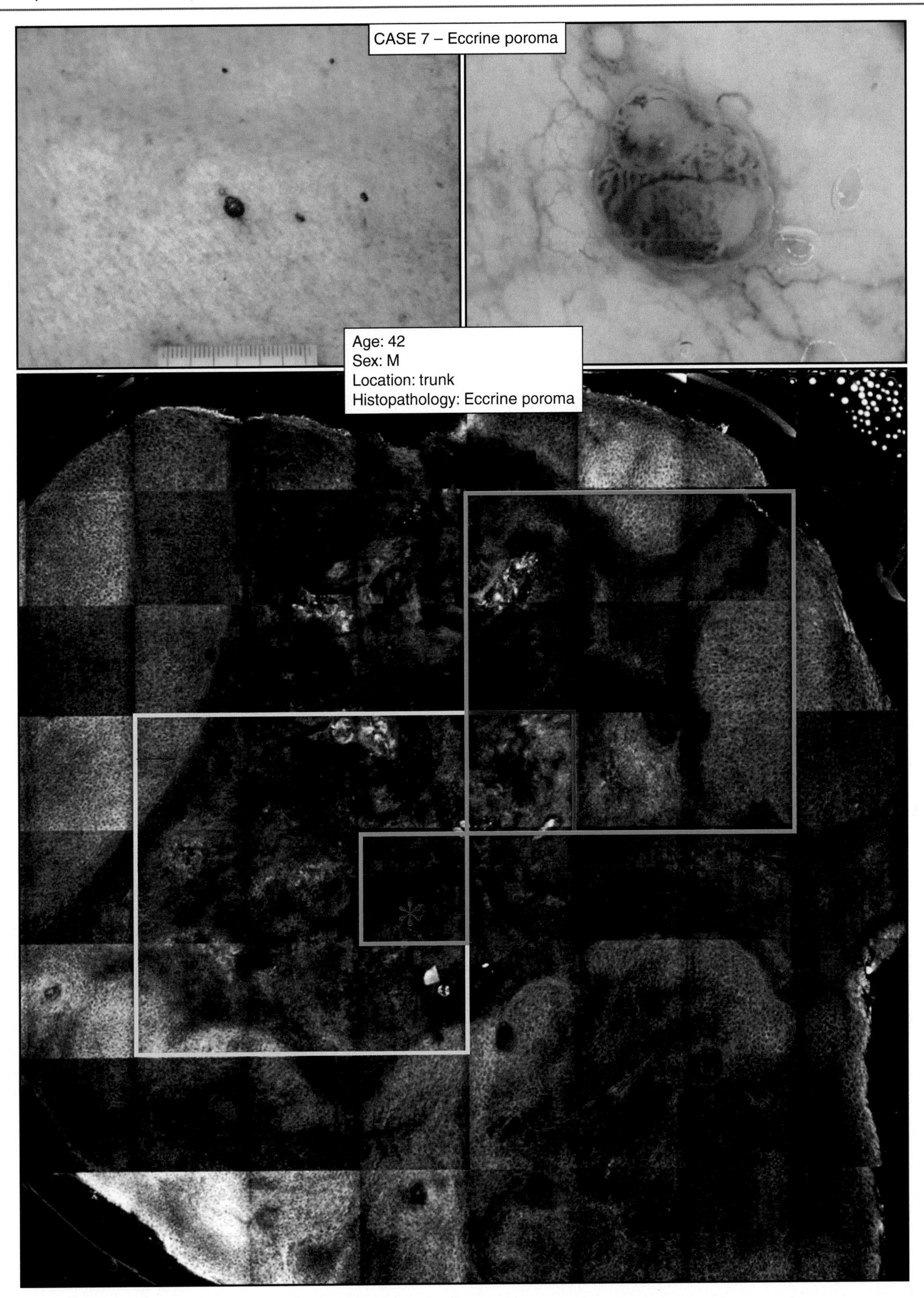

Fig. 25.7 RCM mosaic at deep spinous layer, showing a well-demarcated border between the tumor and surrounding epithelium, with the tumoral cells (*) organized in a disarranged honeycombed pattern compared to the surrounding epithelial cells (→)

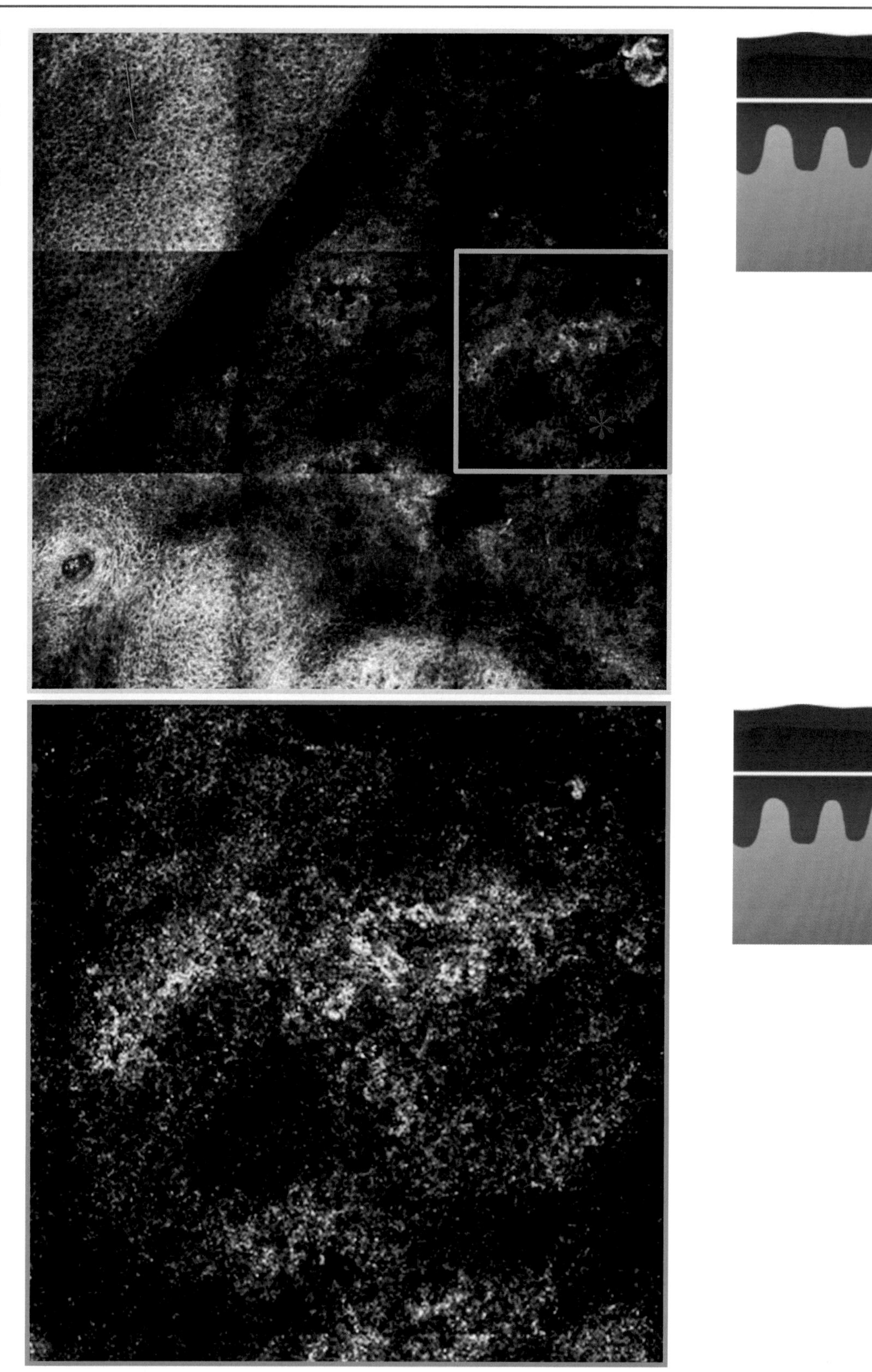

Fig. 25.7.1–25.7.2 Tumoral cells (*) are organized in an atypical honeycombed pattern, keratinocytes contour are differently refractile, compared to the surrounding epithelial cells (→) organized in a regular honeycombing

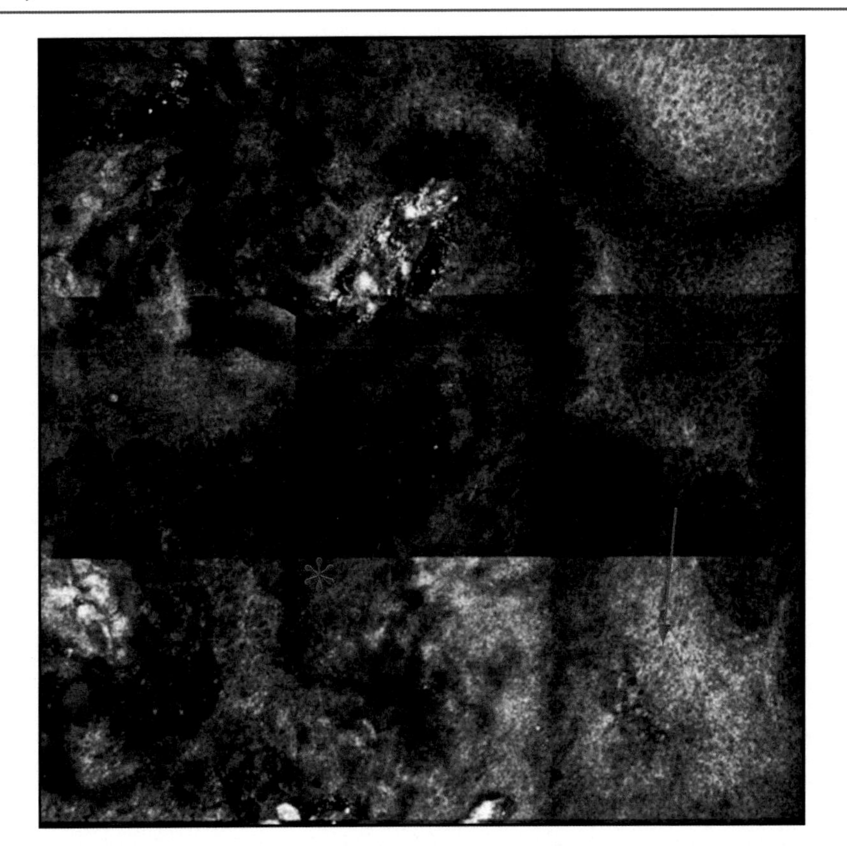

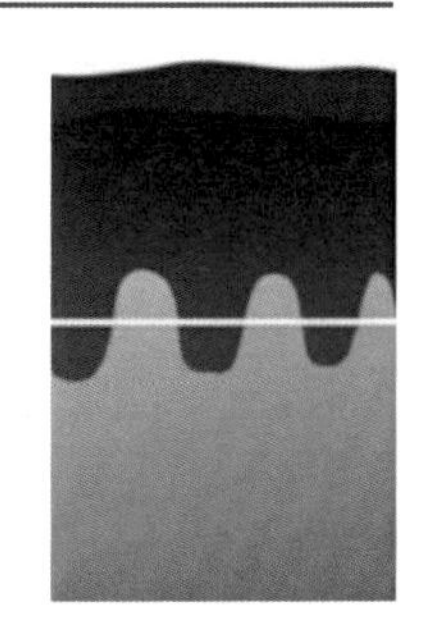

Fig. 25.7.3 Tumoral bands (→) are surrounded by abundant stroma (*), and an increased vascularization is detected

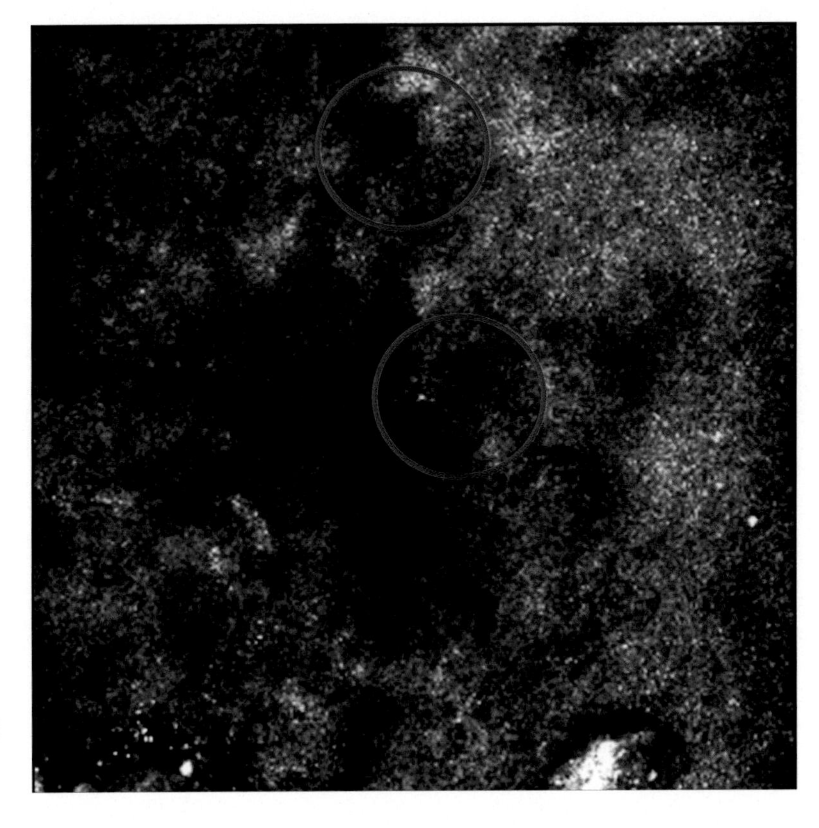

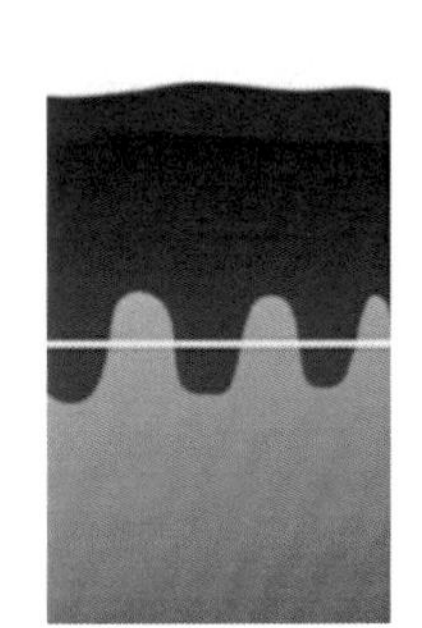

Fig. 25.7.4 Presence of nonrefractile dark round spaces (O), which correspond to area of ductal differentiation within the tumor

References

1. Langley RG, Burton E, Walsh N, Propperova I, Murray SJ (2006) In vivo confocal scanning laser microscopy of benign lentigines: comparison to conventional histology and in vivo characteristics of lentigo maligna. J Am Acad Dermatol 55:88–97
2. Scope A, Ardigo M, Marghoob AA (2008) Correlation of dermoscopic globule-like structures of dermatofibroma using reflectance confocal microscopy. Dermatology 216:81–82
3. Guitera P, Li LX, Scolyer RA, Menzies SW (2010) Morphologic features of melanophages under in vivo reflectance confocal microscopy. Arch Dermatol 146:492–498
4. Astner S, González S, Cuevas J, Röwert-Huber J, Sterry W, Stockfleth E, Ulrich M (2010) Preliminary evaluation of benign vascular lesions using in vivo reflectance confocal microscopy. Dermatol Surg 36:1099–1110
5. Tachihara R, Choi C, Langley RG, Anderson RR, González S (2002) In vivo confocal imaging of pigmented eccrine poroma. Dermatology 204:185–189
6. Bolognia JL (1992) Reticulated black solar lentigo ('ink spot' lentigo). Arch Dermatol 128:934–940
7. Lumpkin LR, Helwig EB (1966) Solitary lichen planus. Arch Dermatol 93:54–55
8. Shapiro L, Ackerman AB (1966) Solitary lichen planus-like keratosis. Dermatologica 132:386–392
9. Zaballos P, Blázquez S, Puig S, Salsench E, Rodero J, Vives JM, Malvehy J (2007) Dermoscopic pattern of intermediate stage in seborrhoeic keratosis regressing to lichenoid keratosis: report of 24 cases. Br J Dermatol 157:266–272
10. Bugatti L, Filosa G (2007) Dermoscopy of lichen planus-like keratosis: a model of inflammatory regression. J Eur Acad Dermatol Venereol 21:1392–1397
11. Aghassi D, Anderson RR, Gonzalez S (2000) Time-sequence histologic imaging of laser-treated cherry angiomas with in vivo confocal microscopy. J Am Acad Dermatol 43:37–41
12. Mooney MA, Janninger CK (1995) Pyogenic granuloma. Cutis 55:133–136
13. Zaballos P, Llambrich A, Cuéllar F, Puig S, Malvehy J (2006) Dermoscopic findings in pyogenic granuloma. Br J Dermatol 154:1108–1111
14. Chen TC, Kuo T, Chan HL (2000) Dermatofibroma is a clonal proliferative disease. J Cutan Pathol 27(1):36–39
15. Puig S, Romero D, Zaballos P, Malvehy J (2005) Dermoscopy of dermatofibroma. Arch Dermatol 141:122
16. Scope A, Ardigo M, Marghoob AA (2008) Correlation of dermoscopic globule-like structures of dermatofibroma using reflectance confocal microscopy. Dermatology 216:81–82
17. Eisen DB, Michael DJ (2009) Sebaceous lesions and their associated syndromes: part I. J Am Acad Dermatol 61:549–560
18. Kim NH, Zell DS, Kolm I, Oliviero M, Rabinovitz HS (2008) The dermoscopic differential diagnosis of yellow lobularlike structures. Arch Dermatol 144:962
19. Pinkus H, Rogin JR, Goldman P (1956) Eccrine poroma, tumors exhibiting features of the epidermal sweat duct unit. Arch Dermatol 74:511–521
20. Nicolino R, Zalaudek I, Ferrara G, Annese P, Giorgio CM, Moscarella E, Sgambato A, Argenziano G (2007) Dermoscopy of eccrine poroma. Dermatology 215(2):160–163
21. Tachihara R, Choi C, Langley RG, Anderson RR, Gonzalez S (2002) In vivo confocal imaging of pigmented eccrine poroma. Dermatology 204:185–189

Part VII

Inflammatory Skin Diseases

26 The Semiology and Patterns of Inflammatory Skin Conditions

Marco Ardigò and Marina Agozzino

26.1 Introduction

Histopathological contribution to the clinical diagnosis of inflammatory skin diseases can be conditioned by the complication in obtaining skin samples from patients that are generally scared from pain and scars deriving from biopsies. Moreover, histopathological diagnosis can be difficult because of inadequate biopsies (too superficial, too little, in the wrong lesion stage) or unsatisfactory pathology report, especially when the histopathological examination lack the support of exhaustive and detailed clinical information. A concrete contribution to minimize the problems can derive from the application of RCM for evaluation of inflammatory skin processes. In particular, its and axial resolution and its noninvasive and easy clinical application represent the goals for a large diffusion of this relatively new technology not only for diagnosis and management of skin cancers but also for inflammatory skin diseases.

RCM gives the clinician the possibility of a real time and non invasive "virtual" punch biopsy ranging from 2 to 8 mm in dimension. In this way it is possible to obtain a collection of microscopical changes and consequential, immediate "clinical-confocal" correlation [2, 3]. Therefore, RCM works as a "clinical tool" able to increase the sensibility and sensitivity of the dermatologist interpretation of skin inflammation integrating real time clinical and microscopical features [4]. Furthermore, RCM can help the clinician with the biopsy site selection throughout the identification of the lesion and its exact area in which main microscopical criteria are visible and more present.

As reported in literature, RCM of inflammatory skin diseases does not only have advantages, but is also restricted by some limitations: first of all, the "in-vivo" application of RCM to the sample avoids the fixation artefacts usually present in optical histology [1]; second, because of its non invasiveness, the procedure can be repeated as desired in more than one and in different areas of the same lesion during the same confocal section; third, the en-face approach to tissue allows for visualization of larger fields of epidermal epithelium as well as of the dermo-epidermal junction and the upper dermis (inducing the reader to rebuilt a new microscopical approach to the skin layers with re-definition of criteria) [2, 3]. On the other side, limits are related to the lack of resolution in deepness, the impossibility to discriminate different sub-type of leukocytes, the new horizontal approach (that makes more difficult to directly translate the criteria assumed from optical microscopy to confocal microscopy) and black and white "stained" images.

For a correct application of RCM to inflammatory skin diseases it is necessary to first of all get experience with confocal features of normal skin; second develop knowledge about differences existing in different normal skin sites, ages, and races; third, confocalists need to become confident with single microscopical criteria (as spongiosis, interface changes, papillomatosis, etc.) visualization at RCM.

The last step is to re-built specific microscopical patterns (i.e. the application of the "pattern method" commonly used in optical microscopy) taking advantages of the new RCM horizontally oriented, in vivo, approach.

26.1.1 The Pattern Method

On the basis of the commonly used microscopical classification of inflammatory skin diseases for optical microscopy [5], it is easily possible to identify four main groups of inflammatory skin disorders with RCM characterized by common main criteria: (1) Spongiotic dermatitis (i.e. allergic and irritant contact dermatitis), (2) hyperkeratotic diseases (i.e. psoriasis, seborrheic dermatitis), (3) diseases with interface involvement (i.e. lupus erythematosus, lichen planus and its variant, dermatomyositis, morphea, etc.),

M. Ardigò (✉) • M. Agozzino
San Gallicano Dermatological Institute,
Rome, Italy
e-mail: ardigo@ifo.it; marinaagozzino@gmail.com

R. Hofmann-Wellenhof et al. (eds.), *Reflectance Confocal Microscopy for Skin Diseases*,
DOI 10.1007/978-3-642-21997-9_26, © Springer-Verlag Berlin Heidelberg 2012

Table 26.1 The pattern analysis method

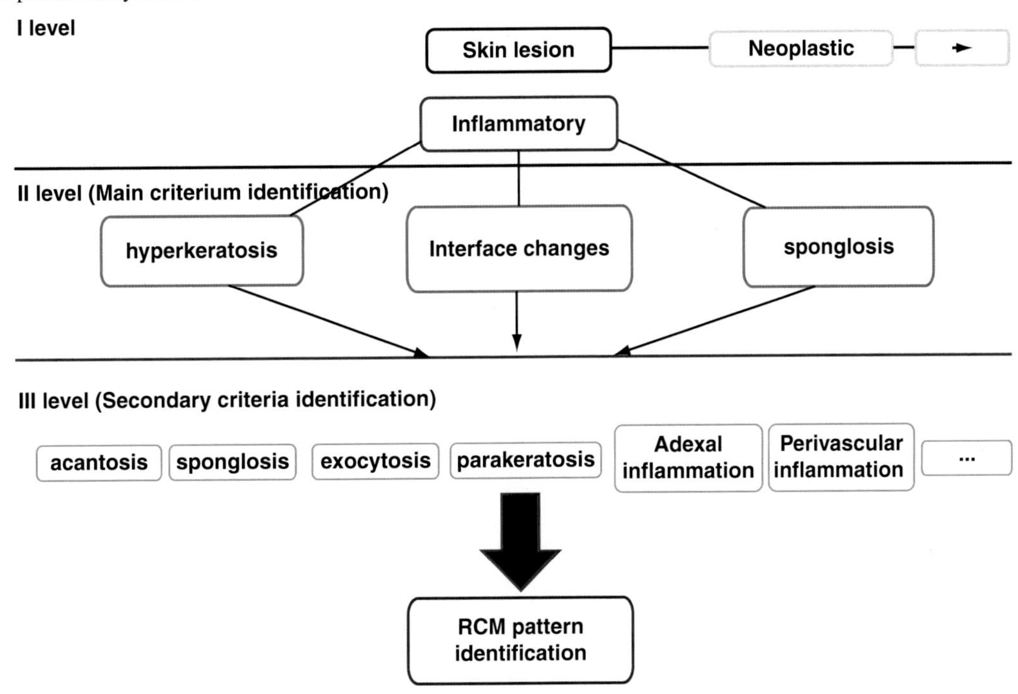

(4) pigmentary nontumoral skin disorders (i.e. vitiligo, melasma and postinflammatory pigmentation) [6–13].

RCM has been already demonstrated to be able to identify all of these main inflammatory microscopical features with high grade of correspondence and correlation to optical histology (i.e. spongiosis, interface changes, acanthosis, hyperkeratosis, alteration of pigmentation distribution and amount) [6–13]. RCM let the reader to collocate the skin disorder in the majority of the cases in one of the four previous mentioned groups. Moreover, looking for secondary RCM microscopical features (i.e. exocytosis of inflammatory cells in the epidermis or in the adnexal epithelium, perivascular inflammation, papillomatosis, dilated vessels, etc.) it is possible, in most of the cases, to support the clinical diagnosis avoiding or strongly reducing the use of skin biopsies. The specificity and sensitivity of the pattern method is increased proportionally to the number of confocal criteria that are typical for the entity considered (Table 26.1).

The en-face, in vivo approach to skin microscopy provided by RCM allows for easier detection of the main diagnostic microscopical features present in the pathological process if they are located in the upper skin [2, 3]. Moreover, the larger fields of epidermis seen with RCM as compared to optical histology and from the in vivo examination rules out the artefact deriving from tissue fixation and processing [1, 9, 11]. On the contrary, some other criteria are missing such as involvement of the deeper dermis because of the lack of image resolution in the deeper skin layers. For all of these reasons, new collections of criteria, located in the upper skin and more simply visible with the horizontal, in vivo approach are required for an effective RCM examination of skin inflammation.

26.2 RCM Criteria for Inflammatory Skin Diseases

The possibility of the application of the "pattern method" (that needs the collection of useful, repeatable, microscopical criteria) throughout the identification of "main" as well as "secondary" microscopical features represents the backbone of the RCM application for diagnosis of inflammatory skin diseases (Table 26.2).

26.2.1 Main Criteria

As already described in the introduction, the four main criteria, respectively defining the four main groups of inflammatory skin diseases, are (1) spongiosis (spongiotic disorders), (2) corneum and epidermal thickening (hyperkeraotic/acanthotic dermatosis) (3) interface changes (interface dermatosis), (4) amount and location of pigment and melanocytes activity (pigmentary disorders).

1. *Spongiosis*: Darker area relative to the surrounding epithelium of the stratum spinosum with intercellular spaces between the keratinocytes being larger than normal; this feature is generally associated with the presence of round-to-polygonal, mildly refractive cells (exoctosis). This feature can range from few, diffuse bright elements infiltration of the epidermis with irregular dark areas, trough the tendency to aggregation of the bright cellular elements in the contest of better defined, darker areas, to the presence of clear-cut, dark, round to poly-lobated areas fulfilled by bright inflammatory cells at the level of the epidermis corresponding to vesicles [6–9].

Table 26.2 Histological criteria vs the RCM correspondence

Histo criterium	RCM definition
1. Parakeratosis	Highly refractile, nucleated polygonal structures at the level of the stratum corneum
2. Hyperkeratosis	Stacked images captured starting from the top of the stratum corneum and progressing deeper in 5 μm-step to the first cellulated epidermal layer for a total thickness > of 20–40 μm (depending on anatomical site)
3. Hypo/hyper-granulosis	Reduction or increase of layers and field of cells with bright granules in the center of the nucleus, located immediately below the stratum corneum
4. Disarrayed epidermis	Loss of the normal honeycomb-like architecture of the epidermis at the level of the stratum spinosum
5. Spongiosis	Darker area relative to the surrounding epithelium of the stratum spinosum with intercellular spaces between keratinocytes larger than normal; this features is generally associated with the presence of round-to-polygonal, mildly refractive cells (exoctosis)
6. Exocytosis	Single or aggregates of round-to-polygonal, mildly refractive cells at the level of the stratum spinosum
7. Vescicle	Dark, round to poly-lobated areas fulfilled by bright inflammatory cells at the level of the epidermis
8. Acanthosis	Stacked images captured starting at the first nucleated epidermal layer and progressing deeper in 5 μm-steps until reaching the DEJ for a total thickness > of 60-90 microns (depending on anatomical site)
9. Papillomatosis	(evaluated using *Viva Block™* software and *Vertical Viva Stack™* software imaging) increase number and density of DP at the DEJ as well as elongation of the interpapillary epidermal crests associated to enlarged DP > of 80 μm in diameter
10. Non edged dermal papillae	Absence of the bright papillary rims at the DEJ
11. Interface changes	Focused to diffuse round-to-polygonal, mildly refractive cells at the level of the dermoepidermal junction, as singles or clusters, associated with total or partial obliteration of the ring-like structures around the dermal papillae
12. Dilated vessels	Prominent round or linear dark canalicular structures within the dermal papillae
13. New born vessels	Thin or imperceptible walled, linear or serpingenous small canalicular structures containing flowing of single white and red blood cells disposed in "Indian" line
14. Dermal inflammation	Single, aggregates or diffuse round-to-polygonal, mildly refractive cells at dermal level
15. Perivascular inflammation	Round-to-polygonal, mildly refractive cells around the dermal vessels
16. Melanophages	Polygonal, bright structures larger than inflammatory cells and sometimes dendritic in the dermis
17. Periadnexal inflammation	Round-to-polygonal, mildly refractive cells around and inside the adnexal epithelium
18. Dilated infundibular structure	Black round or oval lumina, ranging in diameter from 140 to 190 μm (in comparison with normal adnexal infundibula ranging from 45 to 80 μm) in the dermis or enlarged canalicular structure cut tangentially by RCm section
19. Follicular Hyperkeratosis	Highly refractive material inside the adnexa infundibulum
20. Thick dermal fibers	Thicker and increased dermal fibers

2. *Stratum corneum and epidermal thickening*: Evaluated, respectively, using the Viva Stack software analysis. In particular, epidermal acanthosis can be evaluated by the number of single frames needed to move from the first cellulated layer of the epidermis to the DEJ (fixed step size = for example 5 μm) that reveals the epidermal thickness for a total thickness > of 60–90 (depending on anatomical site). Differently, hyperkeratosis can be measured counting stack images needed to move from the top of the stratum corneum and progressing deeper in 5 μm-steps to the first cellulated epidermal layer for a total thickness > of 20–40 μm (depending on anatomical site) [11].
3. *Interface changes*: Round-to-polygonal, mildly refractive cellular structures located at the level of the dermoepidermal junction, as singles or clusters, present focally or in quite all the field of tissue evaluated and associated with total or partial obliteration of the ring-like structures around the dermal papillae [9].
4. *Melanocyte activity and quantification*: at the level of the DEJ, the reduction or disappearance of the brightness of the papillary rims corresponds to melanocyte suffering (i.e. in interface dermatitis) or absence (i.e. in vitiligo). Involvement of pigmentation can be also seen at the DEJ as well as at lower levels of the stratum spinosum as absence or reduction of brightness of keratinocytes corresponding to defective or absent melanin distribution from melanocytes to keratinocytes. On the contrary, increased melanocyte activity can be evaluated by the presence of an increased amount of bright keratinocytes at the level of the epidermis (bight cobblestone pattern) as well as increased brightness of papillary rims [10, 13].

26.2.2 Secondary Criteria

The next step necessary for the interpretation of RCM of inflammatory cutaneous processes is represented by the assumption of the secondary pathological criteria that can be seen in the different skin layers reachable with RCM.

26.2.2.1 Stratum Corneum

a. *Parakeratosis*: presence of highly refractile, round to polygonal and/or sometimes polylobulated structures consistent with parakeratosis and/or neutrophils at the level of the stratum corneum [11, 12].
b. *Disrupted corneocytes*: single, but generally multiple and in sheets, discrete, large (larger than normal keratinocytes) homogeneously mildly bright cellular structures, with no visible nucleus, composing totally of partially the stratum corneum [7, 8].

26.2.2.2 Stratum Granulosum/Spinosum

a. *Epidermal atrophy*: Evaluated using the Viva Stack software analysis by the number of single frames needed to move from the first cellulated layer of the epidermis to the DEJ (fixed step size = example 5 μm) that revealed an epidermal thickness < of 60–90 (depending on anatomical site).
b. *Hypo/hypergranulosis*: Reduction or increase of layers and field of cells, distributed in a honeycomb-like pattern, larger than normal keratinocytes and with bright granules in the center of the dark nucleus, located immediately below the stratum corneum [11].
c. *Disarrayed epidermis*: Loss of the normal honeycomb-like architecture of the epidermis at the level of the stratum granulosum/spinosum [6].
d. *Necrotic keratinocytes*: Mildly bright, polygonal structures that are larger than the surrounding keratinocytes and that seems to be leaned on the epithelium and located at the level of the stratum spinosum [6].
e. *Exocytosis*: Single or aggregates of round-to-polygonal, mildly refractive cells at the level of the stratum spinosum [6–9].
f. *Papillomatosis*: Evaluated using also *Viva Block™* software, junctional dermal papillae detectable in upper epidermal layers, increase number and density of DP at the DEJ as well as thin interpapillary epidermal spaces associated to enlarged DP > of 80 μm in diameter [11].
g. *Bright cobblestone*: plump, bright keratinocytes above the DEJ [13].

26.2.2.3 Dermo-Epidermal Junction

a. *Nonrimmed papillae*: Absence of the bright papillary rims at the DEJ with identifiable papillae [9].
b. *Nonedged papillae*: Incomplete, irregular or absent papillary rims with no identifiable papillae [10].
c. *Dilated dermal papillae*: Dermal papillae with increased diameter.

26.2.2.4 Upper Dermis

a. *Dilated vessels*: Prominent round to oval black areas delimited by thin mildly bright lines visible within the dermal papillae, at the level of the DEJ, or, at the level of the upper dermis, as enlarged canalicular structures, delimited by mildly bright parallel lines and cut tangentially by RCM section. Both the features are characterized by white and red blood cells flowing inside the black lumen [9, 11].
b. *New-born vessels*: Thin or imperceptible walled, linear or serpingenous small structures containing flowing of single white and red blood cells disposed in "indian line" [14].
c. *Dermal inflammation*: Single, aggregated or diffuse round-to-polygonal, mildly refractive cells at the dermal level [9, 11].
d. *Perivascular inflammation*: Round-to-polygonal, mildly refractive cells around the dermal vessels [9].
e. *Melanophages*: Polygonal, bright cellular structure larger than inflammatory cells, but less big than neoplastic/activated melanocytes when presenting short dendrites, located at the level of the dermis and generally located close to blood vessels [9, 13].

26.2.2.5 Adnexal Involvement

a. *Adnexal inflammation*: Round-to-polygonal, mildly refractive cells around and involving the adnexal epithelium, and visible between keratinocytes [9].
b. *Dilated infundibular structures*: Black round or oval lumina, ranging in diameter from 140 to 190 μm (in comparison with normal adnexal infundibula ranging from 45 to 80 μm) [9].
c. *Infundibular hyperkeratosis*: Highly refractive material visible inside the adnexal infundibulum [9].
d. *Dermal sclerosis*: Thick and increased number of dermal fibers [9, 14].

26.3 RCM Patterns

The pattern analysis method in confocal microscopy does not differ procedurally from the one used for optical histology; the difference existing for RCM make it necessary to newly describe the already known criteria using new methods. New specific criteria, when possible, can be also considered for a specific diagnosis in order to compensate the limits of RCM. In summary, first of all, the reader needs to identify the main feature assigning one of the 4 main groups to the lesion under evaluation; the second step is represented by collection of one or more "secondary" criteria that are found in the different skin layers and are needed in order to make the confocal examination as much specific as possible. Better if the secondary criteria are in collection with the concept that the more there are the more specific is the diagnosis. The last step is represented by the correlation of the confocal microscopical pattern obtained by RCM observation to the pre-proposed clinical diagnosis checking the effective coherence of the data obtained obtaining a confocal-clinical correlation.

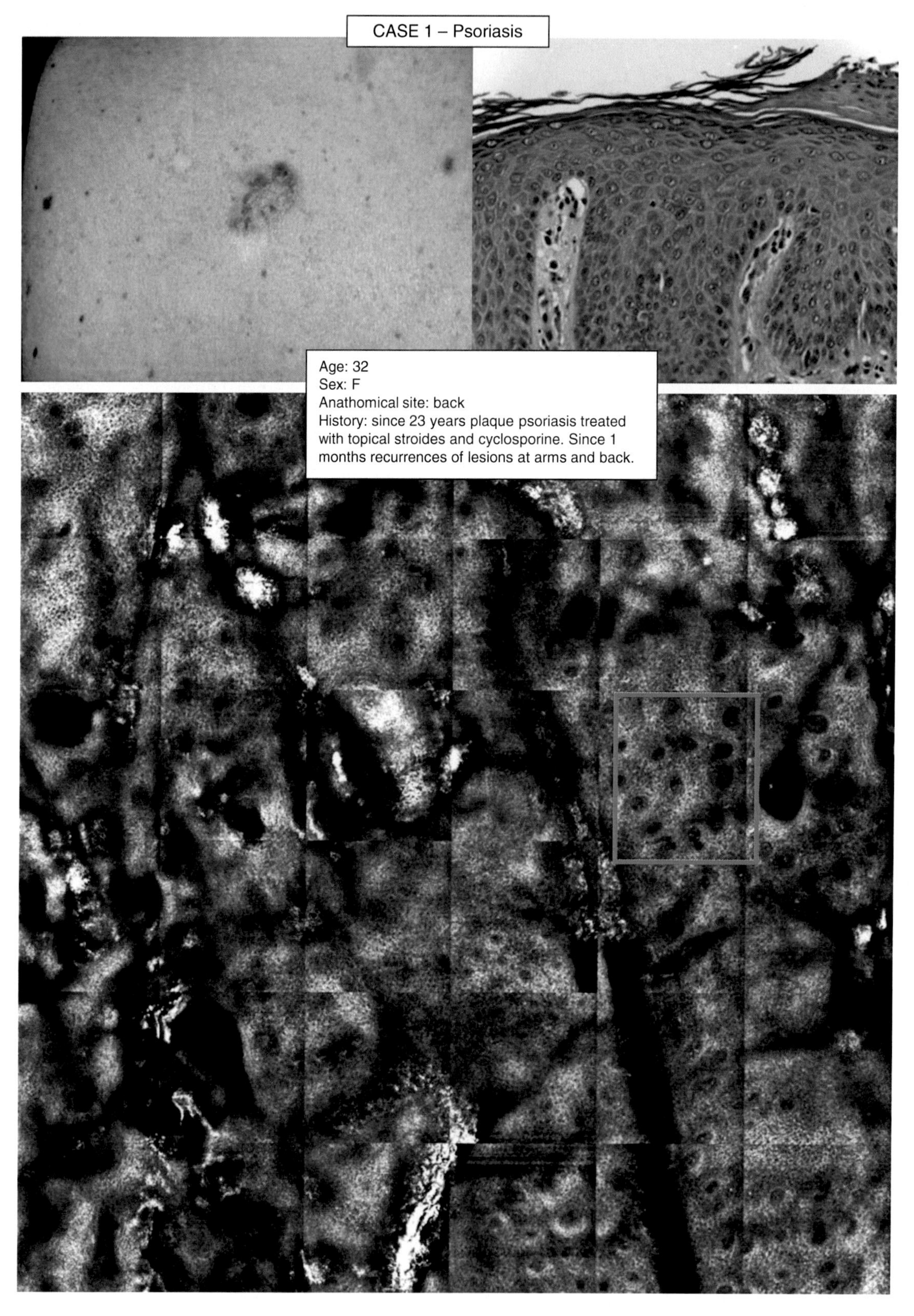

Fig. 26.1 RCM mosaic (3 × 3 mm) taken at the level of the stratum spinosum. The dermal papillae increased in density, irregularly distributed, and already visible in the superficial layers which is a sign of elongation of the rete ridges (papillomatosis)

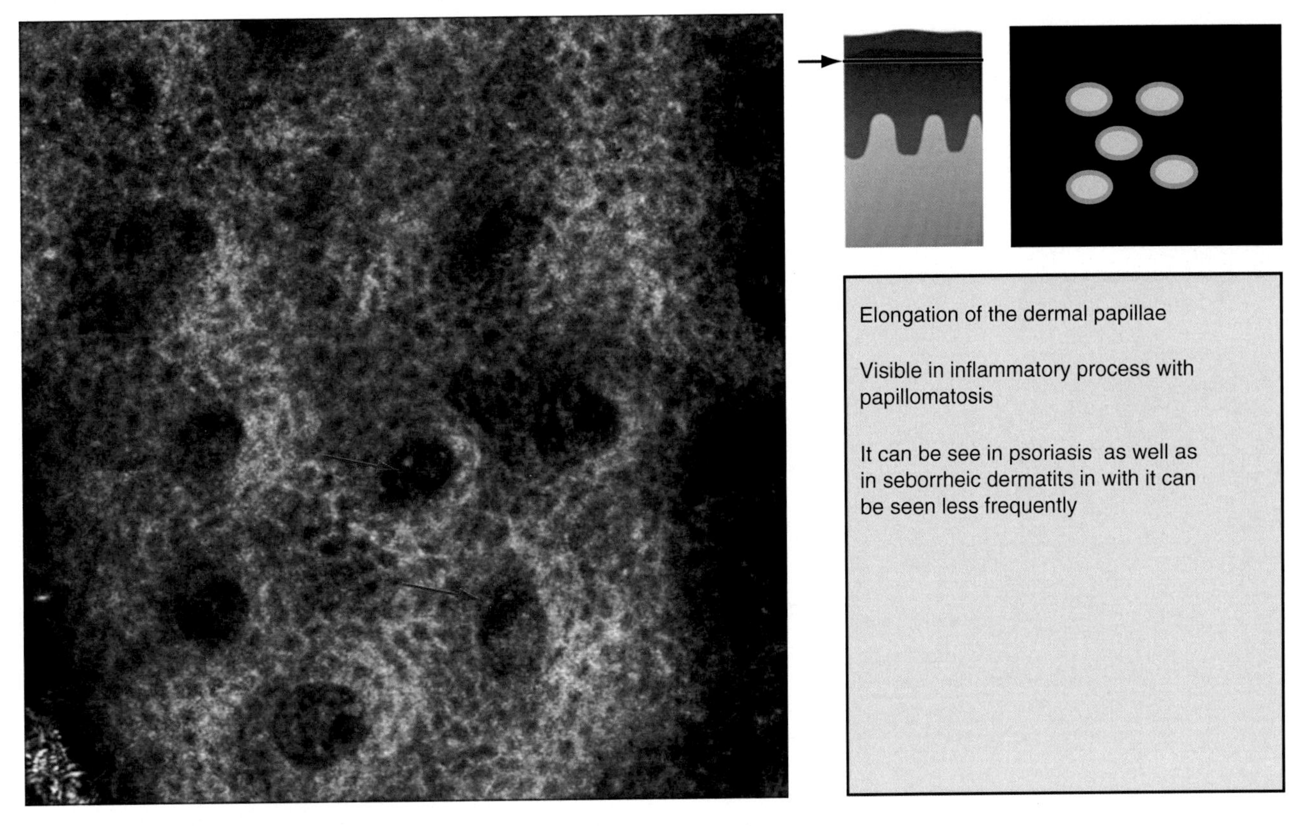

Fig. 26.1.1 Basic image (0.5 × 0.5 mm) at the level of the spinous layer. The presence of the dermal papillae is visible in the upper layers because of papillomatosis inducing elongation of the rete ridges. Dilated vessels are visible inside the papillae (→) corresponding to vessels filling the elongated papillae. Normal epidermal structures with honeycombed features (*)

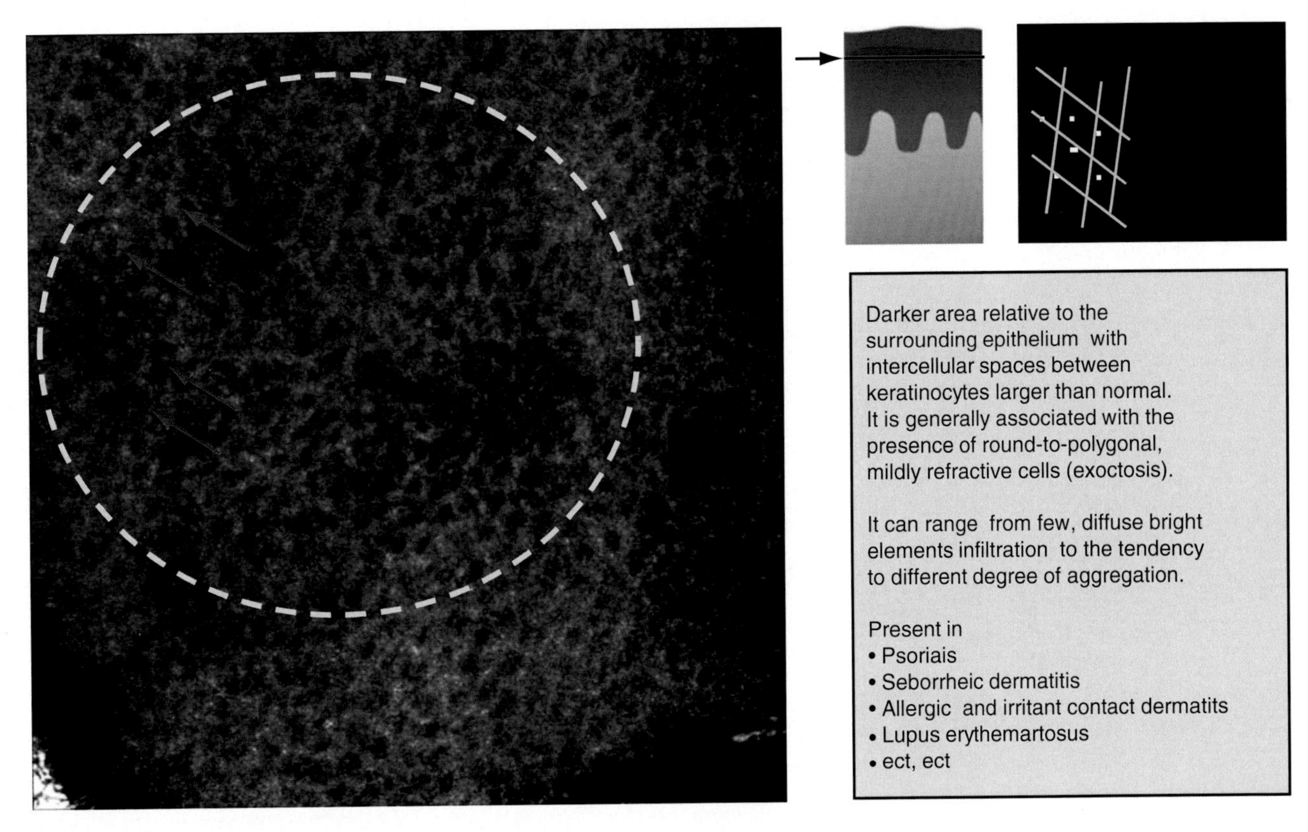

Fig. 26.2 Basic image (0.5 × 0.5 mm) shows a relatively darker area compared to the surrounding epithelium (*yellow circle*) at the level of the stratum spinosum with intercellular spaces between keratinocytes larger than normal associated with the presence of round mildly refractive cells between keratinocytes (exocytosis)

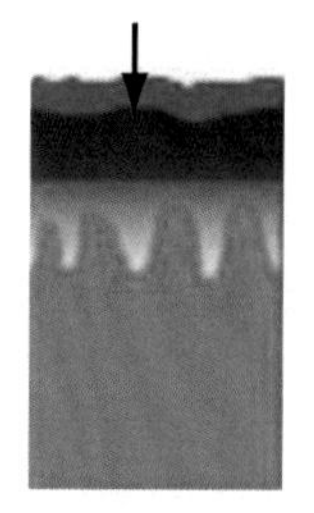

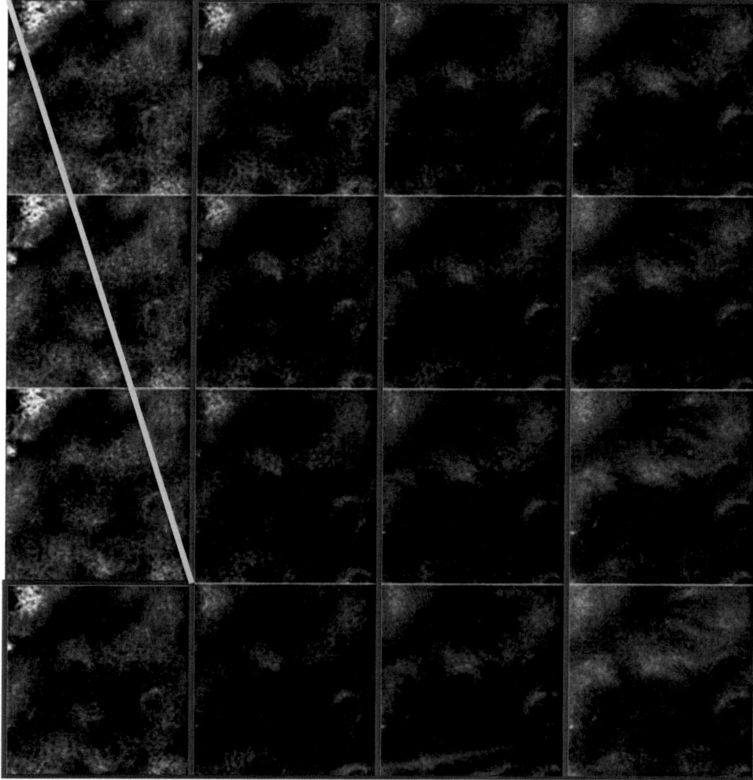

Fig. 26.3.1 and 26.3.2 VivaStack 5 μm step starting from the top of the squamous layer going deep to the first cellulated layer in order to define the thickness of the stratum corneum (hyperkeratosis) as 5 × 5 μm = 25 μm (*yellow boxes*). The same procedure is used to define acanthosis starting from the first cellulated layer to the papillary dermis as 25 × 5 μm = 125 μm (*red boxes*)

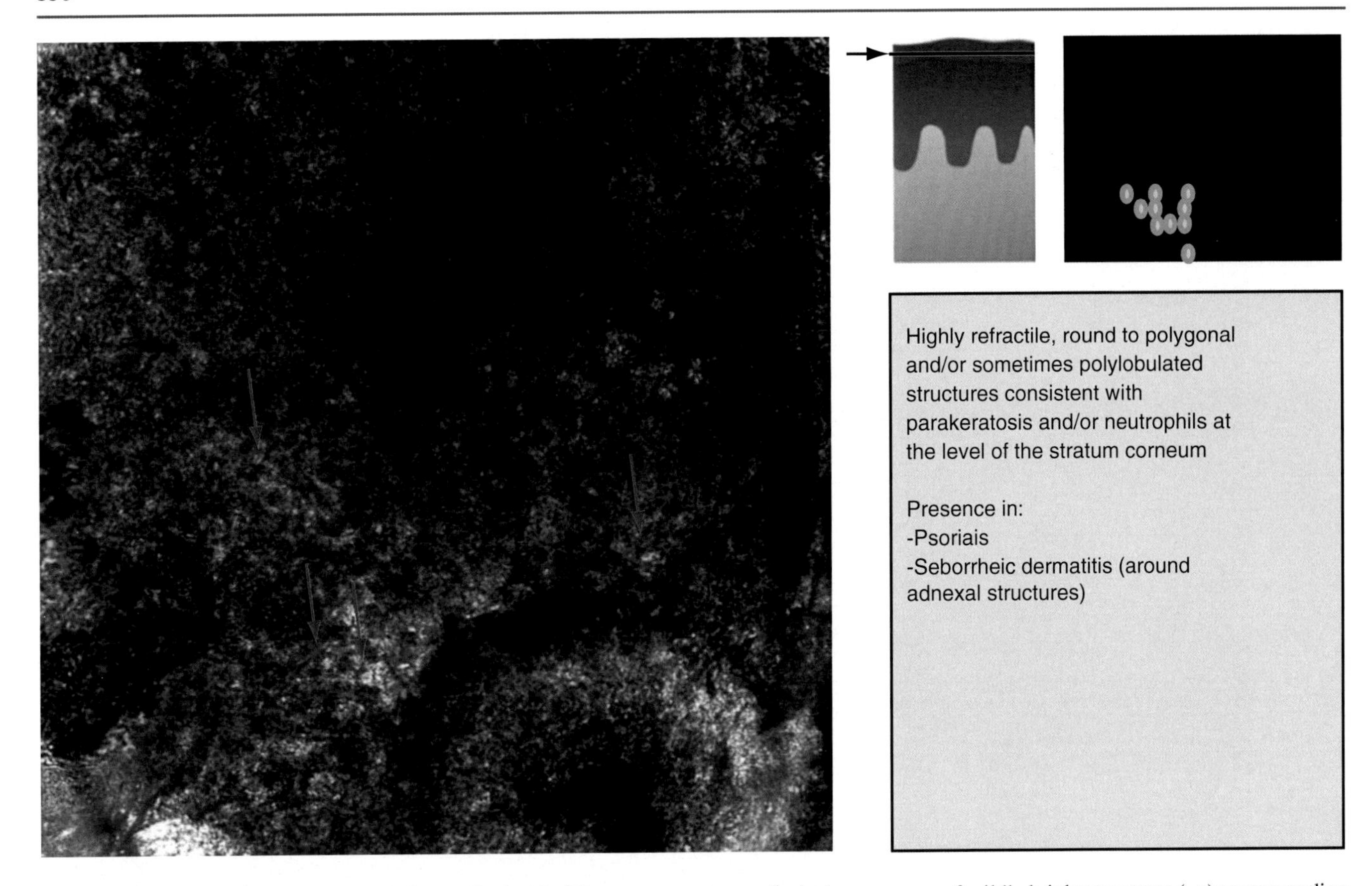

Fig. 26.4 Basic image (0.5 × 0.5 mm) taken at the level of the stratum corneum disclosing presence of mildly bright structures (→) corresponding to parakeratotic keratinocytes

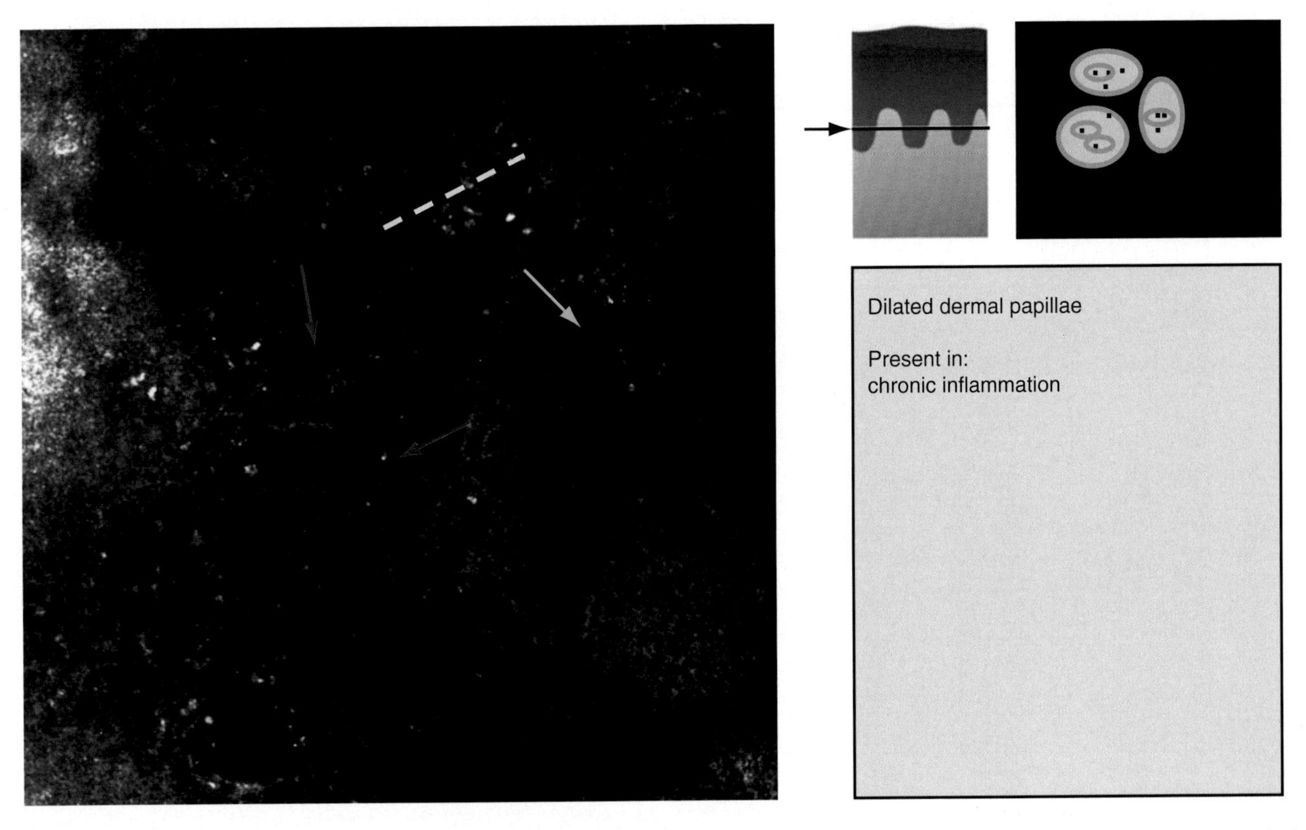

Fig. 26.5 Basic image (0.5 x 0.5 mm) showing dilated dermal papilae (yellow-line). Inside dermal papillae, dilated vessels are seen as black, round to polylobulated structures (*green* →). Interpapillary septa are thinner in comparison with normal

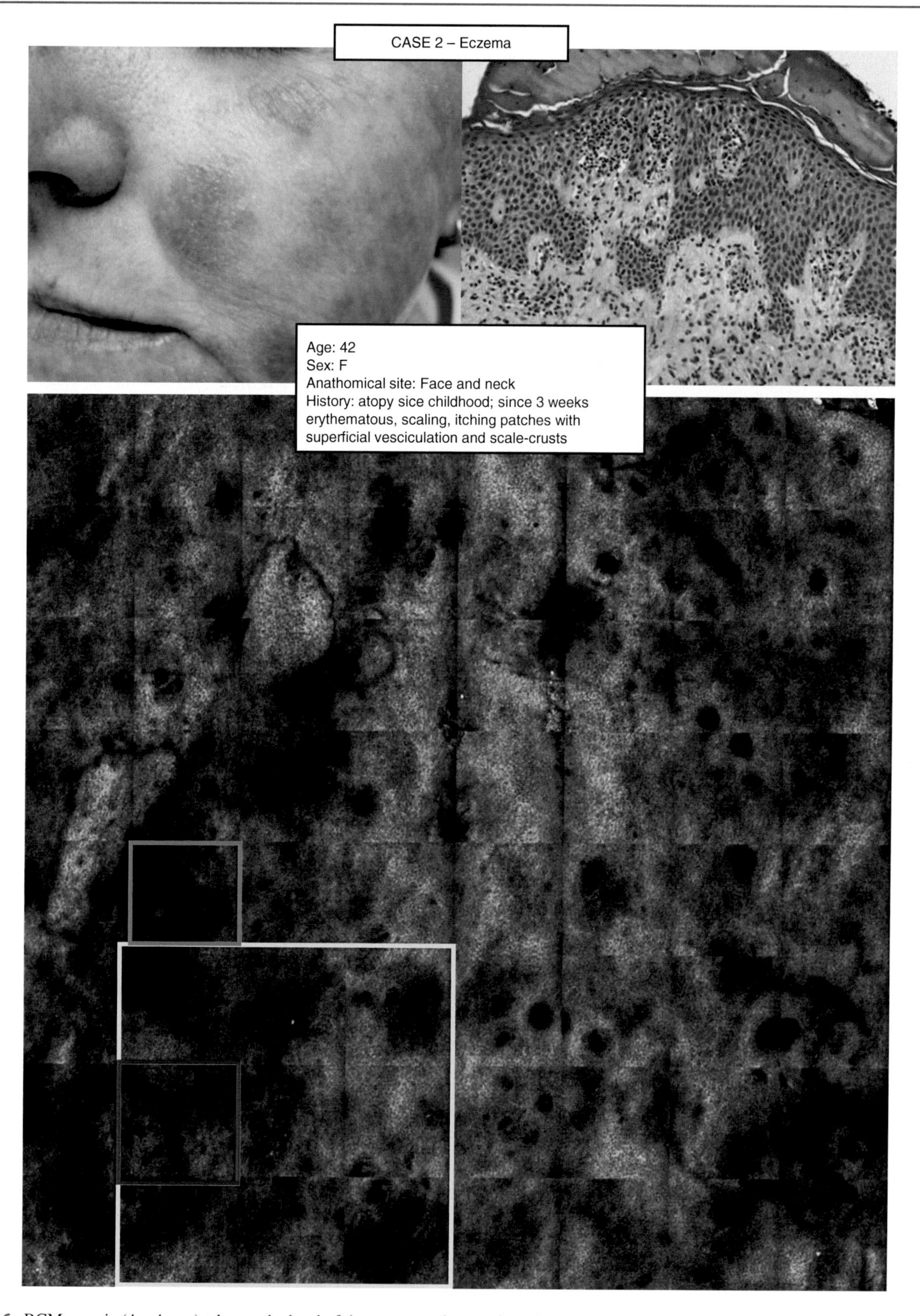

Fig. 26.6 RCM mosaic (4 × 4 mm) taken at the level of the stratum spinosum just above the dermo-epidermal junction discloses the presence of papillae filled by dilated vessels and inflammatory cells

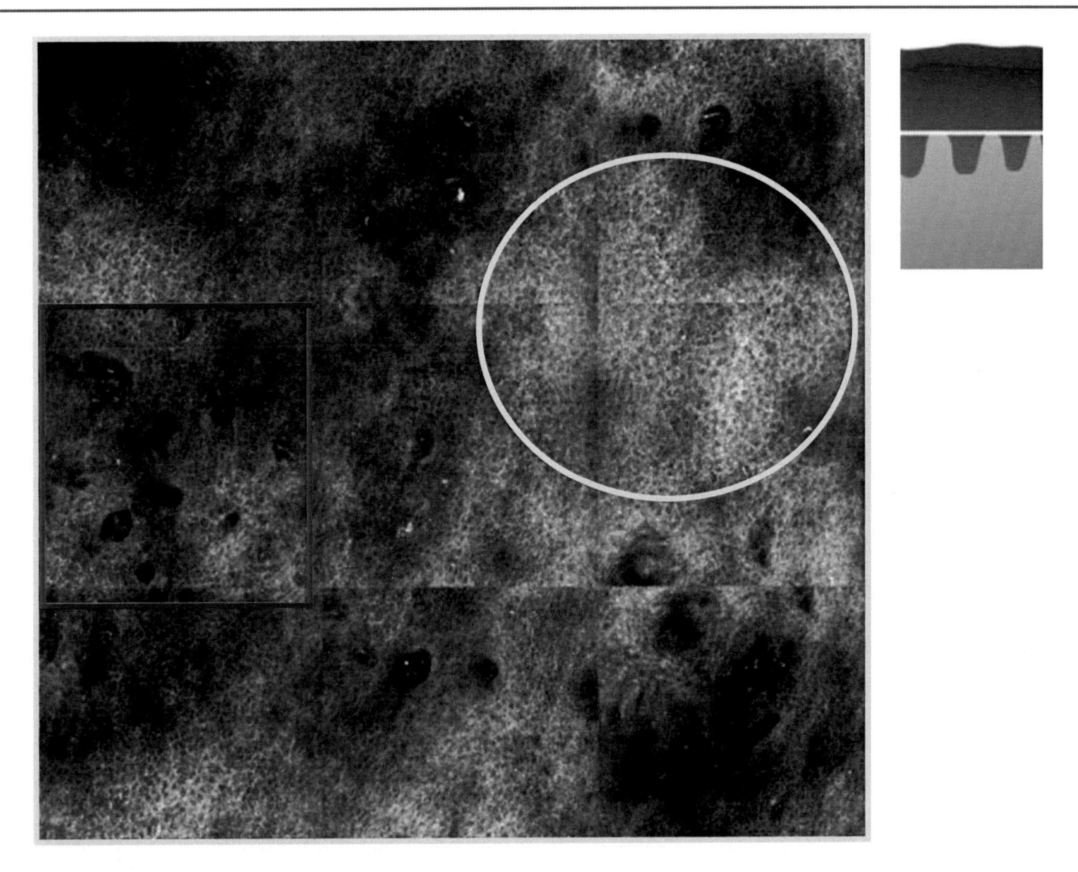

Fig. 26.6.1 RCM mosaic (1.5 × 1.5 mm) at the level of the spinous layer, above the DEJ. Dermal papillae are irregularly visible at this level (*red box*). The epidermal epithelium shows focal normal honeycombed structure (*yellow circle*)

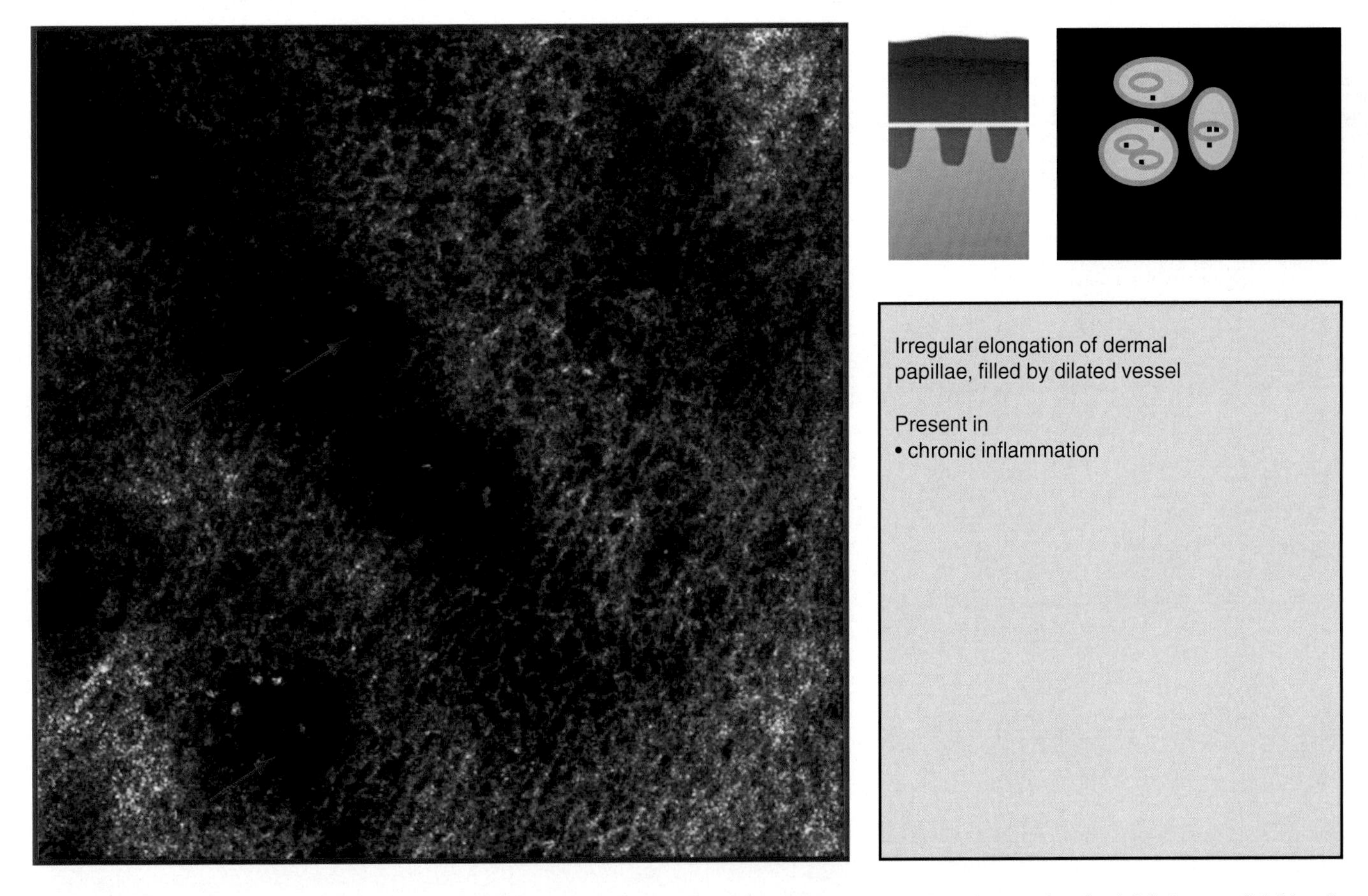

Fig. 26.6.2 Basic image (0.5 × 0.5 mm) as particular of the previous block. Elongated dermal papillae (that are already visible in superficial level) contains dilated vessels and inflammatory cells that are seen as bright round to polygonal structures (→)

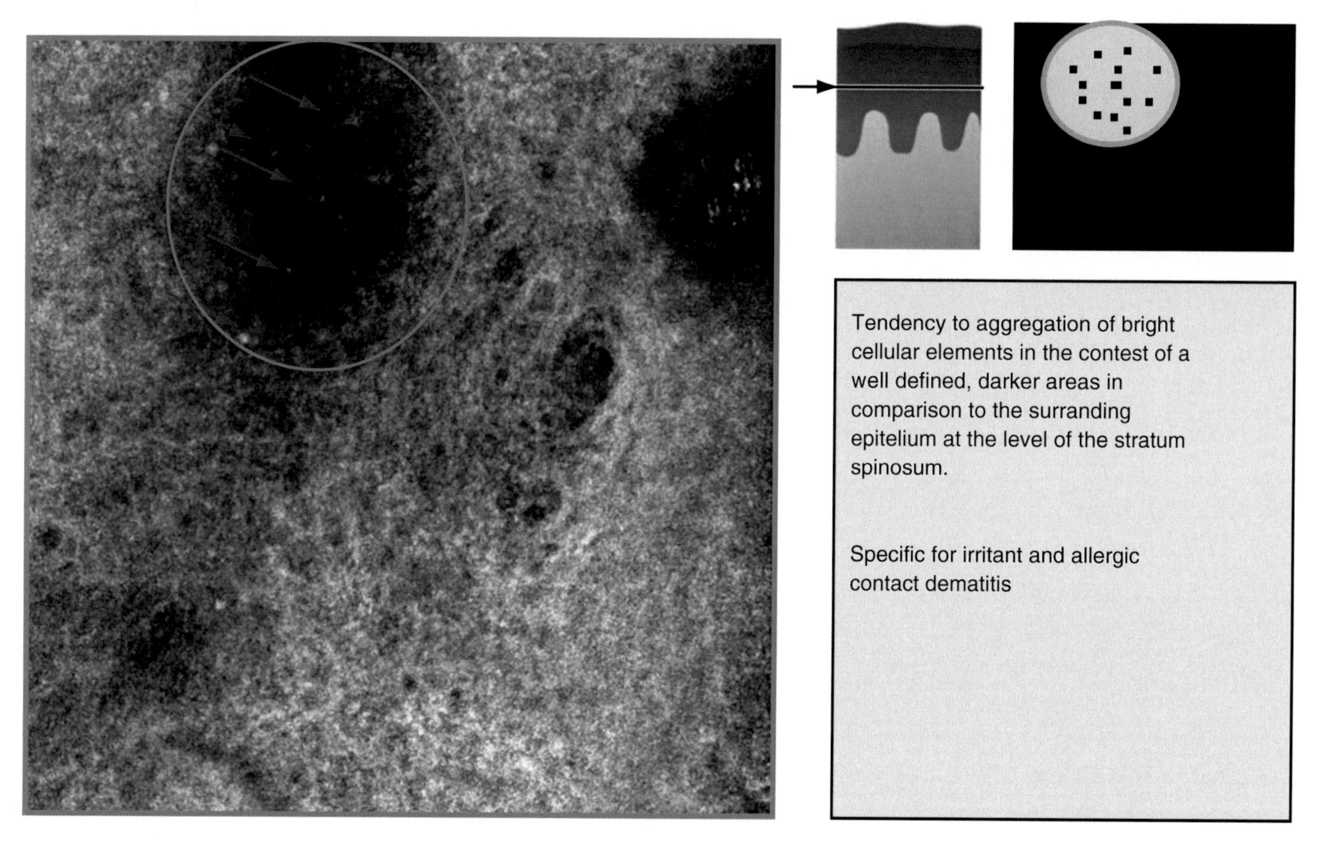

Fig. 26.6.3 Basic image (0.5 × 0.5 mm) showing spongiotic vesicle visible as well defined dark areas filed by mildly bright cellular structures corresponding to inflammatory cells

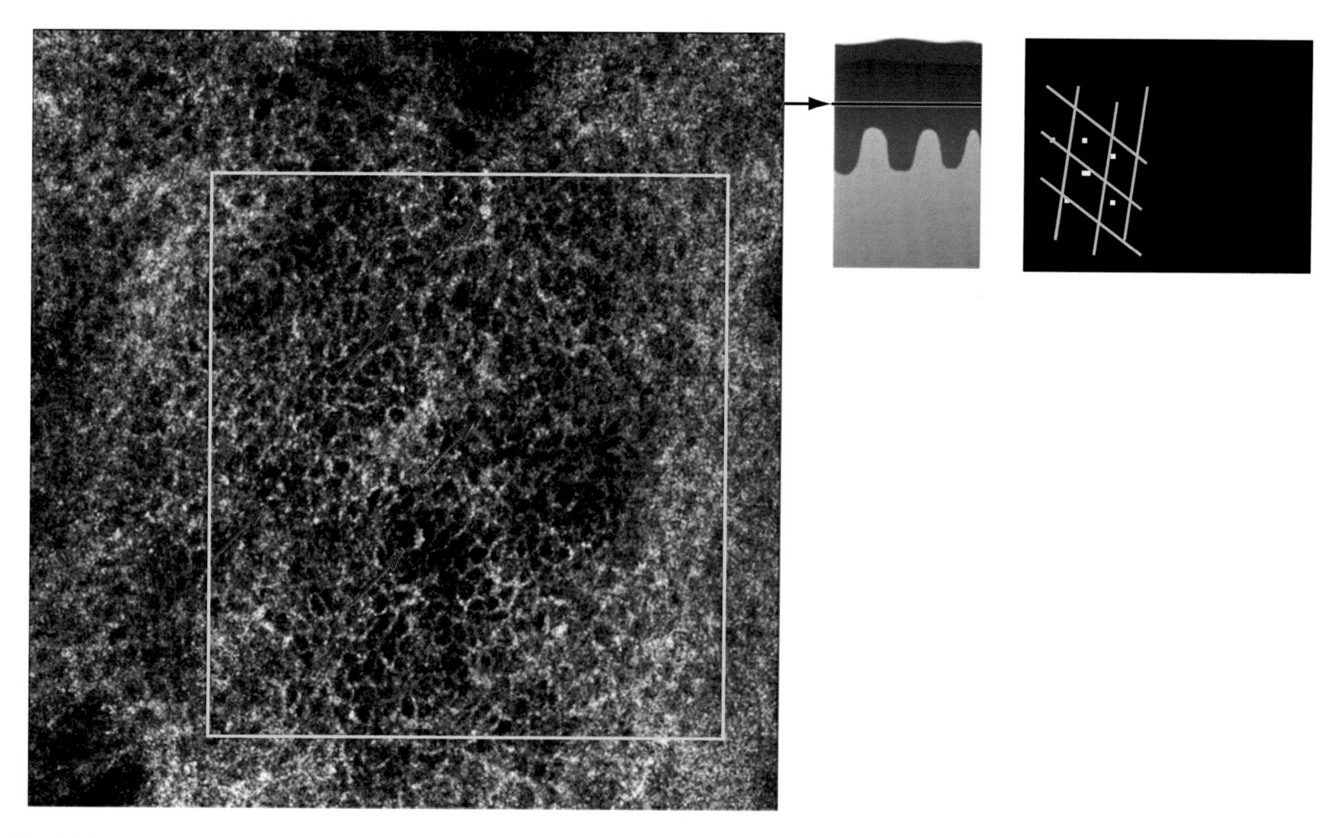

Fig. 26.7 Basic image (0.5 × 0.5 mm) at the level of the stratum spinosum that discloses the presence of darker area relative to the surrounding epithelium with intercellular spaces between keratinocytes larger than normal (*yellow box*) and associated with the presence of round-to-polygonal, mildly refractive cells (exocytosis) (→)

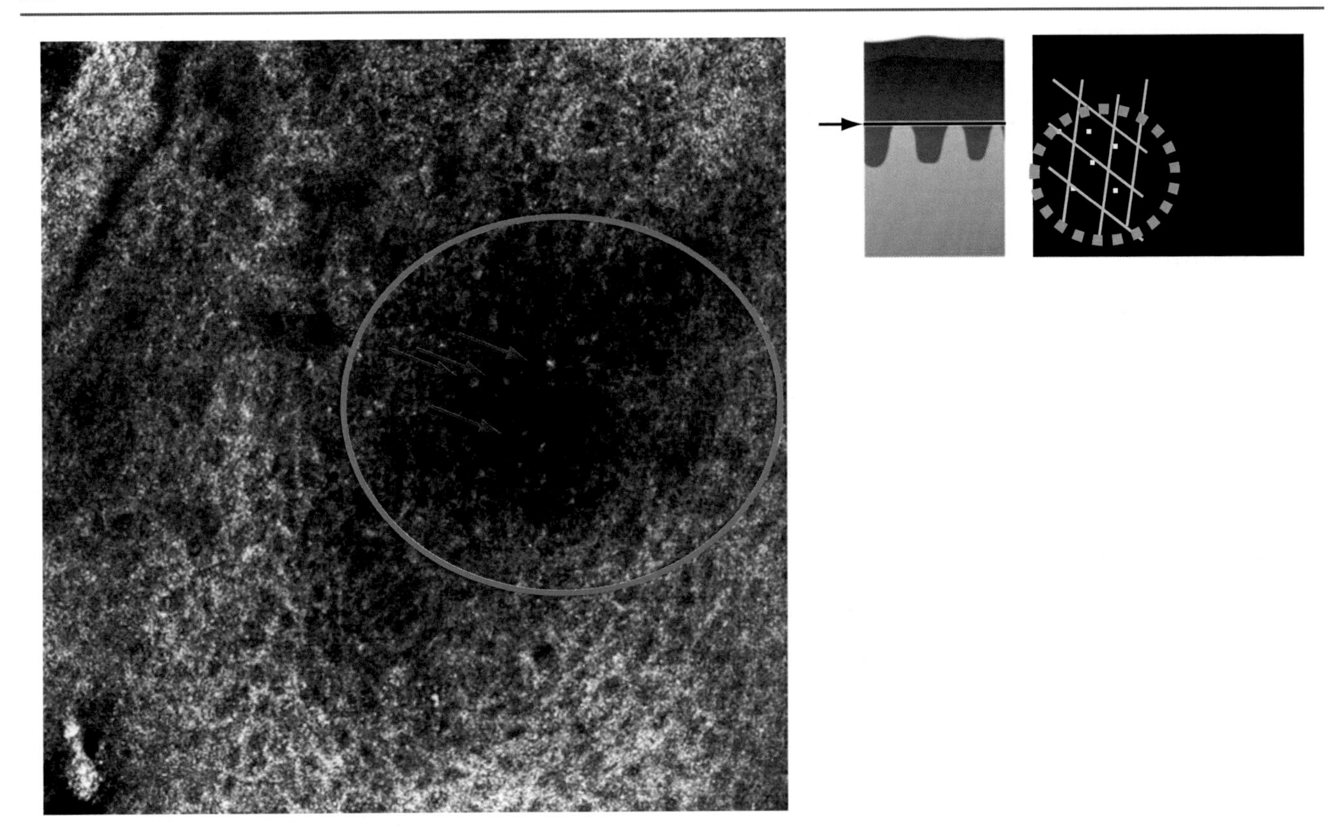

Fig. 26.8 Basic image (0.5 × 0.5 mm) incipient spongiosis forming vesicle at the level of the spinous layer

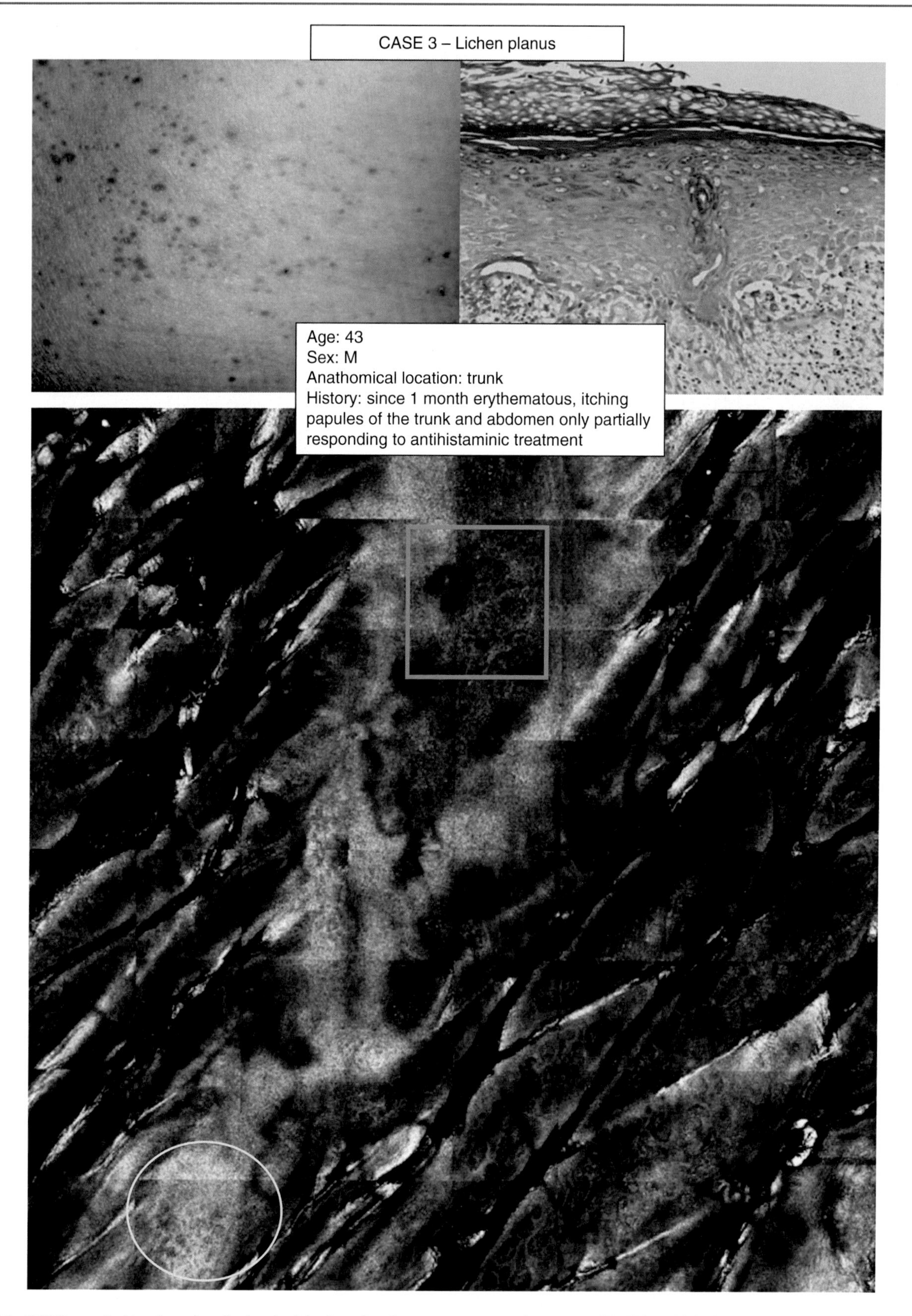

Fig. 26.9 RCM mosaic (4 × 4 mm) at the level of the interface between stratum spinosum and DEJ in which disarrayed epidermis (*yellow circle*) and bright inflammatory cells obscuring the DEJ are visible (*blue square*)

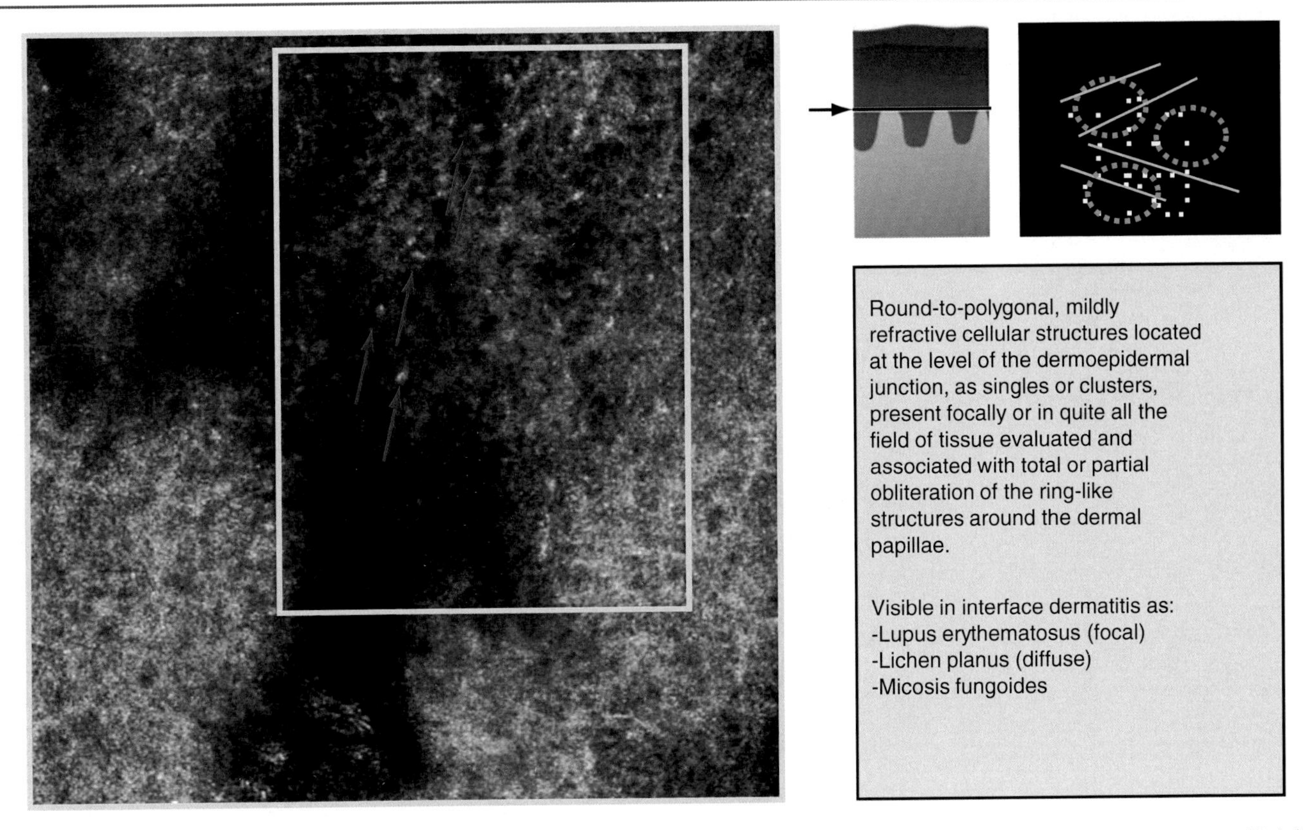

Fig. 26.10 Basic image (0.5 × 0.5 mm) at the interface between stratum spinosum and the DEJ in which the presence of aggregates of bright round to polygonal cellular structures (→) obscuring the papillary rims are visible

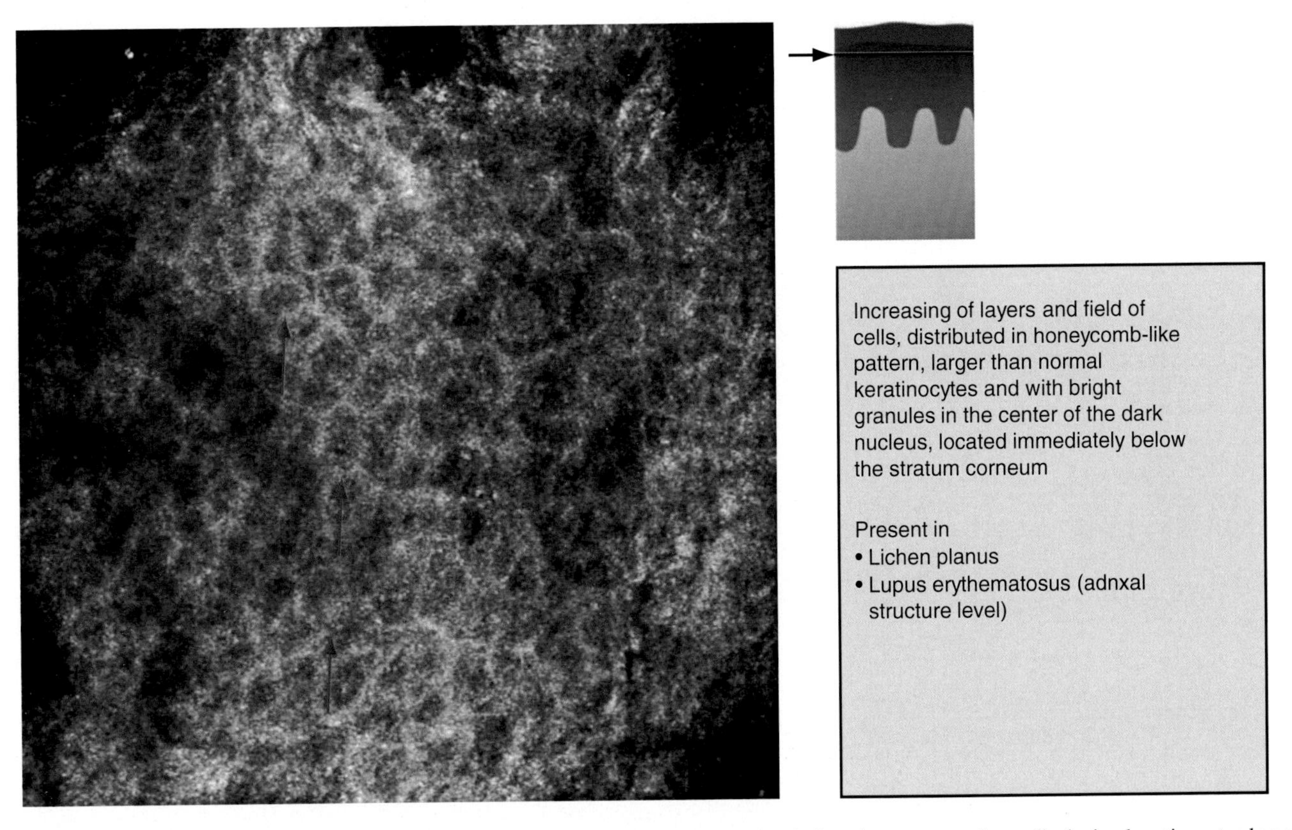

Fig. 26.11 Basic image (0.5 × 0.5 mm) taken at the level of the first cellulated layer just below the squamous layer disclosing keratinocytes larger than the usually seen in spinous later and characterized by bright granules and corresponding to hypergranulosis (→)

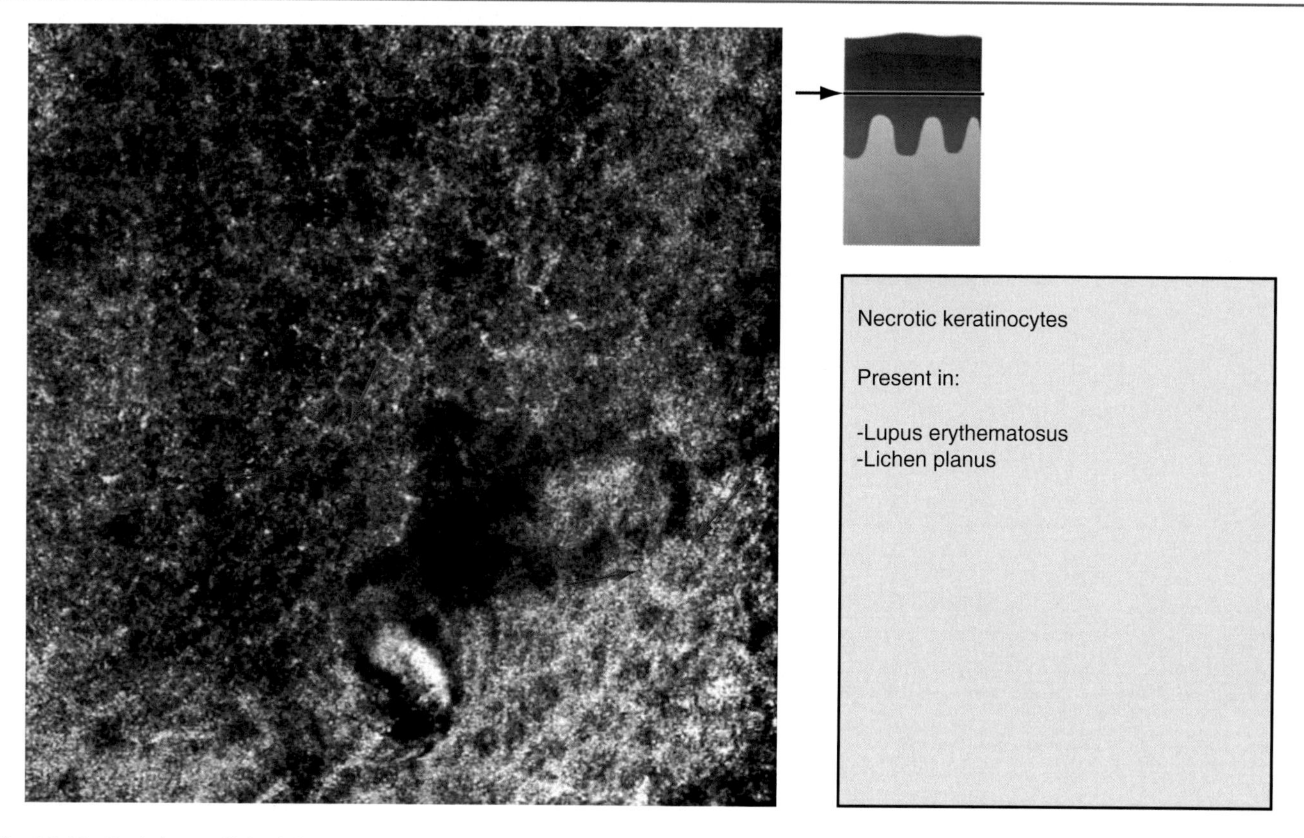

Fig. 26.12 Basic image (0.5 × 0.5 mm) at the level of the spinous layer showing disarray of the normal honeycomb pattern of the epidermis and mildly bright, polygonal structures larger than surrounding keratinocytes and that seems to be leaned on the epithelium corresponding to necrotic keratinocytes (→)

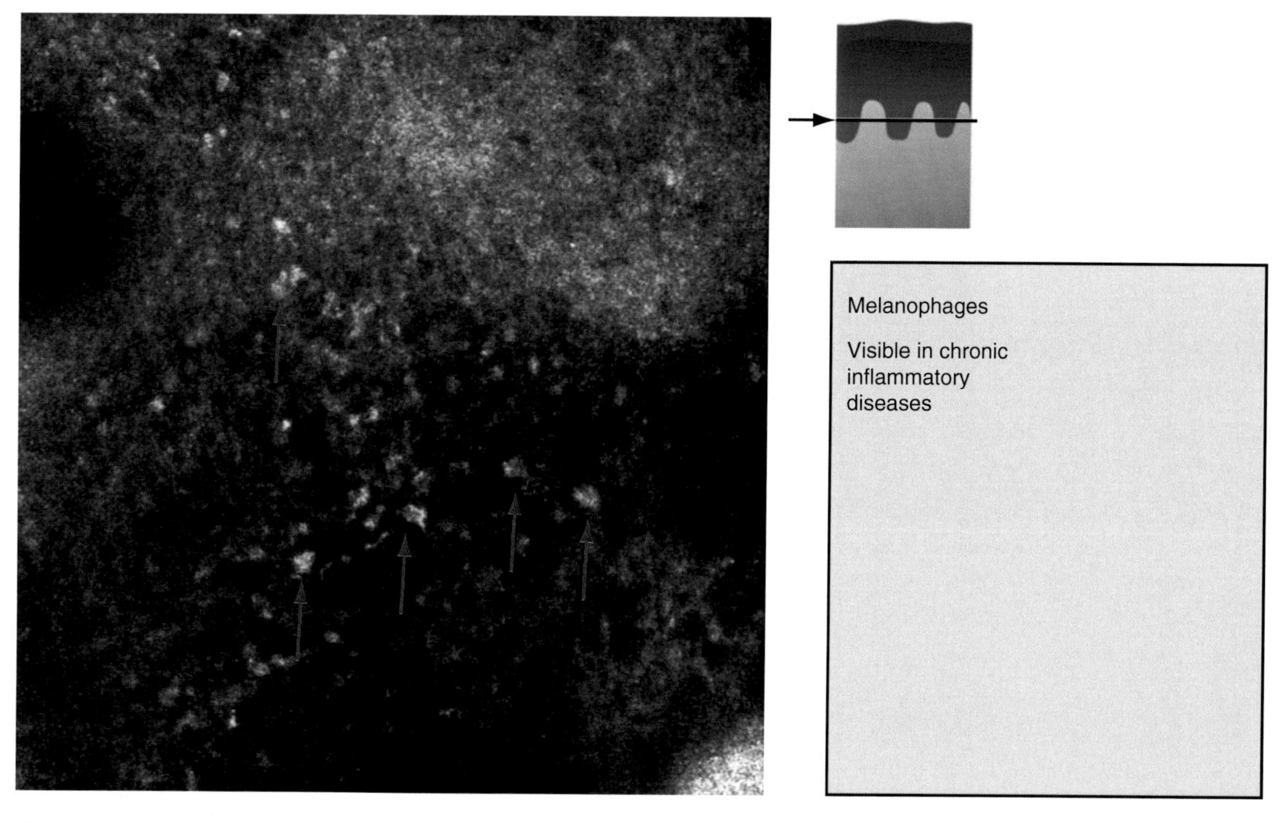

Fig. 26.13 Basic image (0.5 × 0.5 mm) showing polygonal, bright cellular structure larger than inflammatory cells, but less big than neoplastic/activated melanocytes when presenting short dendrites, located at the level of the dermis and generally located close to blood vessels corresponding to melanophages (→)

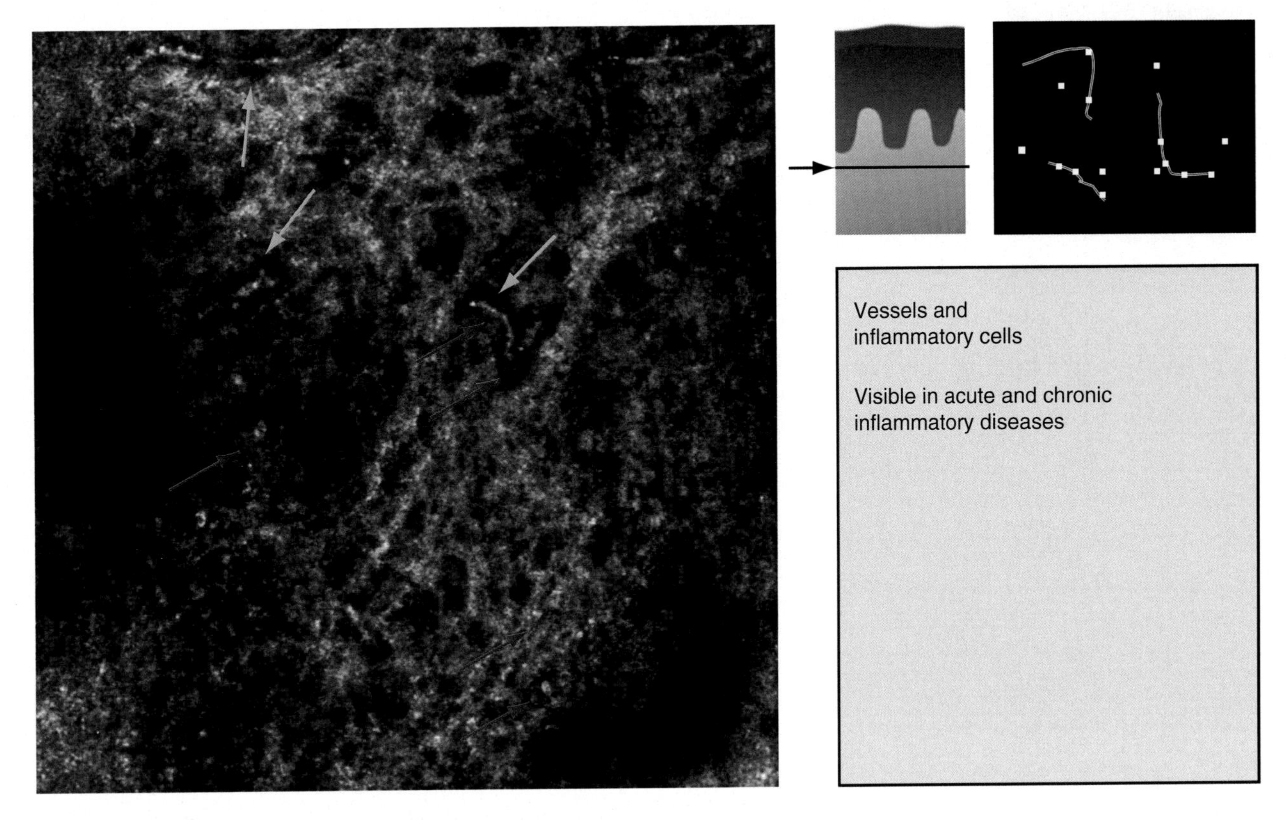

Fig. 26.14 Basic image (0.5 × 0.5 mm) at the level of the superficial dermis disclosing prominent, linear to serpiginous, canalicular black areas delimited by thin mildly bright lines visible in the dermal stroma (*green* →). Presence of bright cells flowing inside the black lumen and outside between dermal fibers (*red* →)

Core Messages

- RCM is a clinical tool that when integrated by clinical presentation and history is effective in evaluation and management of inflammatory skin diseases.
- A strong and solid correlation between the four main and the several secondary RCM microscopical features and optical microscopy has already been demonstrated.
- The confocal reader needs to use the microscopical pattern method (collection of single microscopical criteria) for identification and management of inflammatory skin diseases.

References

1. Elenitsas R, Nousari CH, Seykora JT (2005) Laboratory methods. In: Elder DE, Elenitzas R, Johnson BL, Murphy GF (eds) Lever's histopathology of the skin, 9th edn. Lippincott Williams & Wilkins, Philadelphia, pp 59–60
2. Gonzalez S, Rajadhyaksha M, Gonzalez-Serva A, White WM, Anderson RR (1999) Confocal reflectance imaging of folliculitis in vivo: correlation with routine histology. J Cutan Pathol 26(4): 201–205
3. Rajadhyaksha M, Gonzalez S, Zavislan JM, Anderson RR, Webb RH (1999) In vivo confocal scanning laser microscopy of human skin II: advances in instrumentation and comparison with histology. J Invest Dermatol 113(3):293–303
4. Rajadhyaksha M (1999) Confocal reflectance microscopy: diagnosis of skin cancer without biopsy? In: Frontiers of Engineering. Washington, DC: National Academies Press, pp 24–33
5. Bernard Ackerman A, Chongchitnant N, Sanchez J, Guo Y, Bennin B (2007) Histologic diagnosis of inflammatory skin diseases: an algorithmic method based on pattern analysis, 3rd edn. Ardor Scribendi, New York
6. Gonzalez S, Gonzalez E, White WM, Rajadhyaksha M, Anderson RR (1999) Allergic contact dermatitis: correlation of in vivo confocal imaging to routine histology. J Am Acad Dermatol 40(5 Pt 1): 708–713
7. Swindells K, Burnett N, Rius-Diaz F, Gonzalez E, Mihm MC, Gonzalez S (2004) Reflectance confocal microscopy may differentiate acute allergic and irritant contact dermatitis in vivo. J Am Acad Dermatol 50(2):220–228
8. Astner S, Gonzalez S, Gonzalez E (2006) Noninvasive evaluation of allergic and irritant contact dermatitis by in vivo reflectance confocal microscopy. Dermatitis 17(4):182–191
9. Ardigo M, Maliszewski I, Cota C, Scope A, Sacerdoti G, Gonzalez S et al (2007) Preliminary evaluation of in vivo reflectance confocal microscopy features of discoid lupus erythematosus. Br J Dermatol 156(6):1196–1203
10. Ardigo M, Malizewsky I, Dell'Anna ML, Berardesca E, Picardo M (2007) Preliminary evaluation of vitiligo using reflectance confocal microscopy. J Eur Acad Dermatol Venereol 21:1344–1350
11. Ardigo M, Cota C, Berardesca E, González S (2009) Concordance between in vivo reflectance confocal microscopy and histology in

the evaluation of plaque psoriasis. J Eur Acad Dermatol Venereol 23:660–667

12. González S, Rajadhyaksha M, Rubinstein G, Anderson RR (1999) Characterization of psoriasis in vivo by reflectance confocal microscopy. J Med 30:337–356
13. Ardigo M, Cameli N, Berardesca E, Gonzalez S. Characterization and evaluation of pigment distribution and response to therapy in melasma using in vivoreflectance confocal microscopy: a preliminary study. J Eur Acad Dermatol Venereol. 2010;24(11):1296-1303
14. Grazziotin TC, Cota C, Buffon RB, Araújo Pinto L, Latini A, Ardigò M (2010) Preliminary evaluation of in vivo reflectance confocal microscopy features of Kaposi's sarcoma. Dermatology 220:346–354

Hyperkeratotic Dermatitis

27

Marina Agozzino, Elvira Moscarella, Silvana Trincone, and Marco Ardigò

27.1 Introduction

The definition of hyperkeratotic skin diseases is referred to inflammatory skin disorders, clinically characterized by scaling and erythema, and microscopically showing variable thickening of the stratum corneum and epidermis (acanthosis) associated with variable degree of inflammation involving epidermis and dermis. Hyperkeratosis can be orthokeratotic as well as with parakeratosis; acanthosis can be regular, generally associated with papillomatosis (i.e. in psoriasis) or irregularly distributed and with different degree of epidermal thickening. Papillomatosis, histopathologically, is seen as elongation of the rete ridges, dilated dermal papillae and normal epidermal structures. The main hyperkeratotic skin diseases, in terms of frequency and social impact, are plaque psoriasis and seborrheic dermatitis.

27.1.1 Psoriasis and Seborrheic Dermatitis

Psoriasis is an inflammatory skin disease, with an estimated prevalence of 0.6–4.8% worldwide [1, 2]. This disease is characterized by polymorphic clinical presentations ranging from the typical plaques to the pustules, and to the erytroderma. Its pathogenesis is based on a genetic background involving T-cells and interleukin patterns [3] The typical plaque psoriasis, appears as hyperkeratotic plaques or papules, that are pink-salmon colored, well demarked and with notable hyperkeratotic scales which are whitish-silver in color. Lesions could have different shapes, from round to annular to oval and may be located all over the body [4, 5]. It has been reported that some triggering factors could rouse psoriasis, and these are: alcohol consumption, smoking, trauma, endocrine diseases, infections, stressful life events and the exposure to some drugs [2, 6–11]. Histopathologically, psoriasis is characterized by the presence of hyperkeratosis with parakeratosis, reduction of the granular layer and acanthosis. Papillomatosis is generally present as elongation of dermal papillae that are commonly filled by dilated vessels. At optical histology, spongiosis is mild or generally absent and epidermal and dermal inflammation is seen in variable degree according to the clinical inflammation.

Seborrheic dermatitis is a chronic, relapsing inflammatory skin condition [12]. This dermatitis prefers areas rich in sebaceous glands (face, scalp, sternal area, interscapular region). Clinically it is characterized by scaly, smooth and poorly defined erythematous patches, and there are many variations in extent and morphologic characteristics according to the area of the skin involved. Itching is moderate. Seborrheic dermatitis is one of the most frequent skin disorders (2–5% of population). Most common age of onset is between 20 and 50 years, but an infantile form which usually involves the scalp, the face, and the diaper area is also frequent [13]. Persons infected with the human immunodeficiency virus (HIV) express a more severe form. Malassezia furfur plays an important role in the pathogenesis of this dermatitis. Seborrheic dermatitis has been reported to be trigged by stress, but no controlled data are available. The diagnosis is correlated to the history and clinical examination. Differential diagnosis is with psoriasis, atopic dermatitis, and, in children, tinea capitis. The histopathologic picture of seborrheic dermatitis can be described to be halfway between psoriasis and chronic dermatitis. The epidermis shows slight to moderate acanthosis and spongiosis [14].

27.2 RCM Features of Hyperkeratotic Skin Disorders

Clinical diagnosis of plaque psoriasis and seborrheic dermatitis is only rarely difficult. In the cases in which both the entities are present on the same patient, usually sebo-psoriasis, which is a middle-entity both clinically and histopathologically, is

M. Agozzino (✉) • E. Moscarella • S. Trincone • M. Ardigò
San Gallicano Dermatological Institute, Rome, Italy
e-mail: marinaagozzino@gmail.com;
elvira.moscarella@gmail.com; ardigo@ifo.it

R. Hofmann-Wellenhof et al. (eds.), *Reflectance Confocal Microscopy for Skin Diseases*,
DOI 10.1007/978-3-642-21997-9_27, © Springer-Verlag Berlin Heidelberg 2012

diagnosed. The possibility of a non-invasive, real time, microscopical discrimination of the two entities from other inflammatory diseases such as chronic eczema, pytiriasis rosea, etc., will let the clinician better select the treatment and consequently, enable follow-up of the therapeutical response. In particular it has been already demonstrated in the literature that the identification of the main diagnostic microscopical features characterizing plaque psoriasis is easily possible using RCM [15, 16]. RCM examination of plaque psoriasis demonstrates different degrees of changes that are analyzed considering the different skin layers in the following paragraphs.

Stratum corneum: exhibits focal highly refractile, round to polygonal or sometimes polylobulated structures consistent with parakeratosis and/or neutrophils. Stack images captured starting from the top of the stratum corneum and progressing deeper in 3 to 5 μm-steps to the first cellulated epidermal layer for a total thickness > of 20–40 μm (depending on anatomical site) show increased thickness of the stratum corneum.

Epidermis: in normal skin, the granular compartment consists of layers of cells with bright granules located in the middle of the nucleus and located immediately below the stratum corneum. This compartment is absent or reduced in mostly of the psoriatic lesions. Acanthosis of the epidermis, is constantly, variable, present and can be evaluated using Viva Stack software analysis, starting from the upper part of the epidermis immediately below of the stratum corneum to the DEJ and considering the entire thickness of the cell layers. A variable degree of increased epidermal thickening can be observed in all the lesions with thickness ranging from 100 to 300 μm, compared to 60–90 μm in normal skin. En face honeycomb-like appearance of the stratum spinosum is observed in association with the acanthosis. Frequently, the honeycombed pattern can be seen as darker than the surrounding skin (not affected by the psoriasis). In these areas, the presence of round-to-polygonal, mildly refractive cells associated with the darker epidermal areas can be observed corresponding to exocytosis events of inflammatory cells associated with epidermal spongiosis. Viva Block software can be used to obtain mosaics of images (2–8 × 2–8 mm) at the level of the dermo-epidermal junction. These mosaics are useful for the evaluation of papillomatosis that is seen as the presence of grouped, multiple, dilated DP, filled with prominent blood vessels, separated by thinner interpapillary rete ridges and visible above the DEJ in the upper layers of the stratum spinosum. The dermal papillae can range from 100 to 250 μm; the diameter of the DP seems to be proportional to the depth of the acanthotic inter-papillary epidermal ridges. This enlargement of the dermal papillae was evident when compared to the control group, in which the diameter of the DP was <80 μm.

Dermo-epidermal junction: at this level, nonrimmed papillae, showing just a shadow of this structure, are seen in high percentage of the lesions, but not in the normal skin of the same patients.

Upper dermis: in the upper dermis, the dermal papillae are filled with prominent blood vessels that are readly visible above the dermo-epidermal junction at the level of the stratum spinosum. Examination using video reveals prominent dark canalicular structures, round or linear, filling the papillary dermis throughout the DP rings in all the lesions corresponding to dilated blood vessels in the papillary dermis. In most of the cases, there is presence of round-to-polygonal, mildly refractive cells around the dilated vessels in papillary dermis that corresponds to perivascular inflammatory cell infiltration [15].

Please note that all the RCM features visible in plaque psoriasis have been demonstrated to have a high degree of correlation between the observed RCM features and the histological findings [15, 16]. In a study published in literature, RCM successfully identified presence of parakeratosis, reduction or absence of the granular layer, papillomatosis and acanthosis with normal honeycomb pattern of epidermis and dilated vessels in the upper dermis in >90% of the cases. However, presence of a hyperkeratotic stratum corneum was evidenced only in 70% of the lesions probably because of the RCM examination of plaque psoriasis needs the application of keratolytic agents prior to imaging to minimize light scattering due to the scales. However, the thickness of the stratum corneum ranged from 25 μm to a maximum of 150 μm compared to the control group, which ranged from 20 μm (flexural face of arms) to a maximum of 40 μm (back) [15]. Different degrees of spongiosis were also detected in 72% of the lesions examined with RCM, which was less frequently reported by conventional histopathology (44%, strongly suggesting that tissue coarctation by processing and fixation often masks the presence of spongiosis). The non rimmed dermal papillae evident at the level of the dermo-epidermal junction are similar to the one reported in vitiligo supporting the hypothesis that inhibition of melanogenesis and/or increased melanocyte apoptosis induced by elevated TNF-alpha in PP lesions can be responsible of this feature [15].

In contrast to plaque psoriasis, in seborrheic dermatitis the stratum corneum shows at Vivastack examination, hyperkeratosis that is generally associated with only sparse parakeratosis typically more visible in peri-adnexal areas as a clue for seborrheic dermatitis. Moreover, the RCM examination shows thickening of the epidermis (acantho-

Table 27.1 Summary of the main RCM features of psoriasis and seborrheic dermatitis and the differences existing between the entities

Plaque psoriasis	Seborrheic dermatitis
Thickening of the stratum corneum	Thickening of the stratum corneum
Parakeratosis	Focal and prevalently periadnexal parakeratosis
Reduced or absent granular layer	Reduced or absent granular layer
Thickening of the epidermis	Thickening of the epidermis
Honeycombed epidermis	Honeycombed epidermis
Slight to moderate spongiosis	More prominent spongiosis
Papillomatosis	Irregularly distributed papillomatosis
Dilated vessels visible in DP vertically oriented to the epidermis	Dilated vessels seen in the upper dermis horizontally oriented to the epidermis
Few or absence of inflammatory cells in the upper dermis	Inflammatory cells in the upper dermis

sis) in association with papillomatosis that is seen less regularly distributed than in plaque psoriasis. The main RCM difference existing between plaque psoriasis and seborrheic dermatitis is represented by the presence of much more inflammation in the epidermis (seen as more prominent spongiosis). In seborrheic dermatitis, the blood vessels are commonly dilated, but generally visible horizontally oriented to the epidermis and not vertically oriented and filling the papillae as in plaque psoriasis (Table 27.1). Dermal inflammation is much more represented in seborrheic dermatitis visible as more represented inflammatory cells in upper dermis. In conclusion RCM features of seborrheic dermatitis are in common with plaque psoriasis but visible in different distribution and amount.

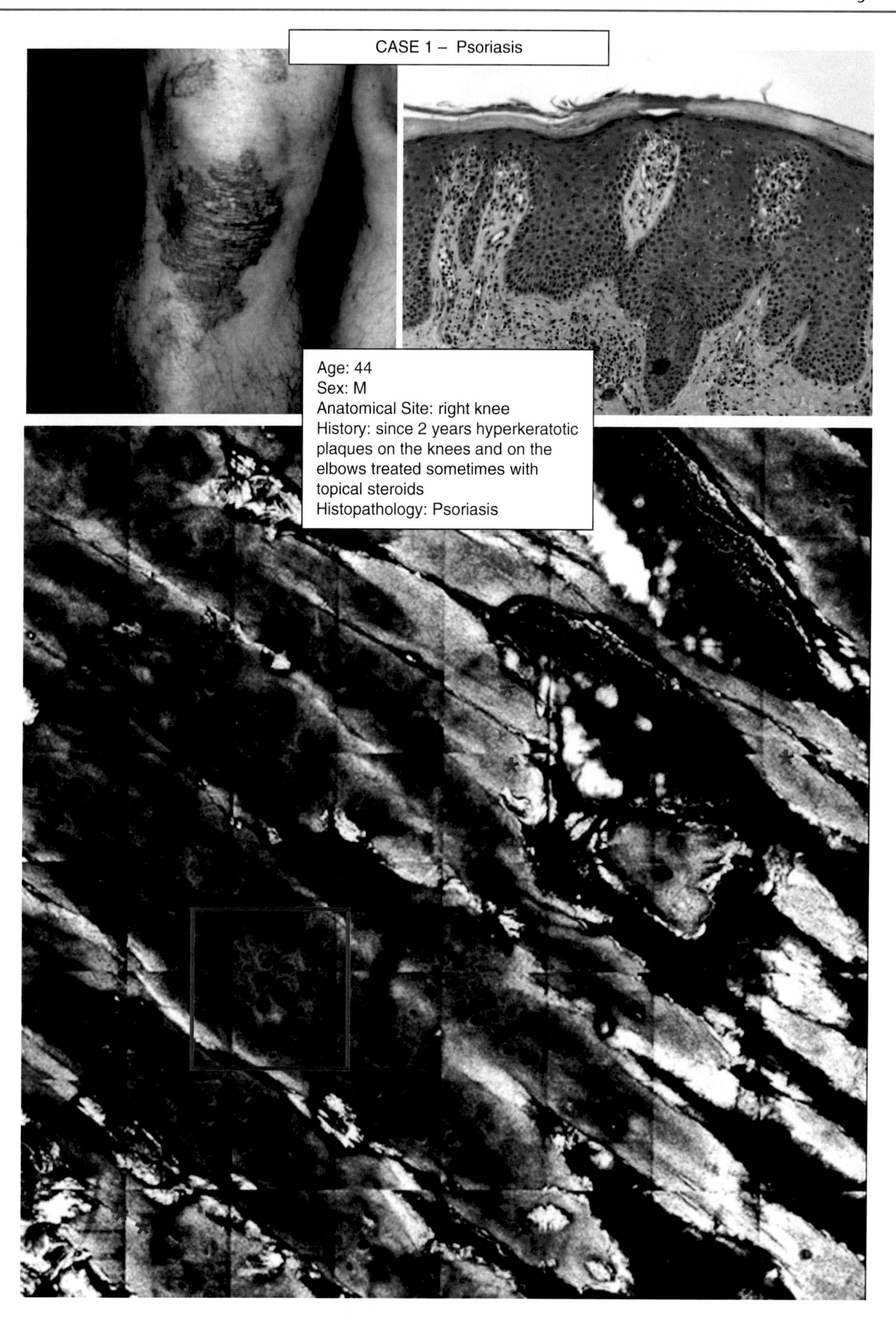

Fig. 27.1 RCM mosaic (3 × 3 mm) taken prevalently at the level of the stratum spinosum. Areas of the squamous layer are also visible (*). The papillae increased in density, irregularly distributed, and are already visible in superficial layers as sign of elongation of the rete ridges (papillomatosis)

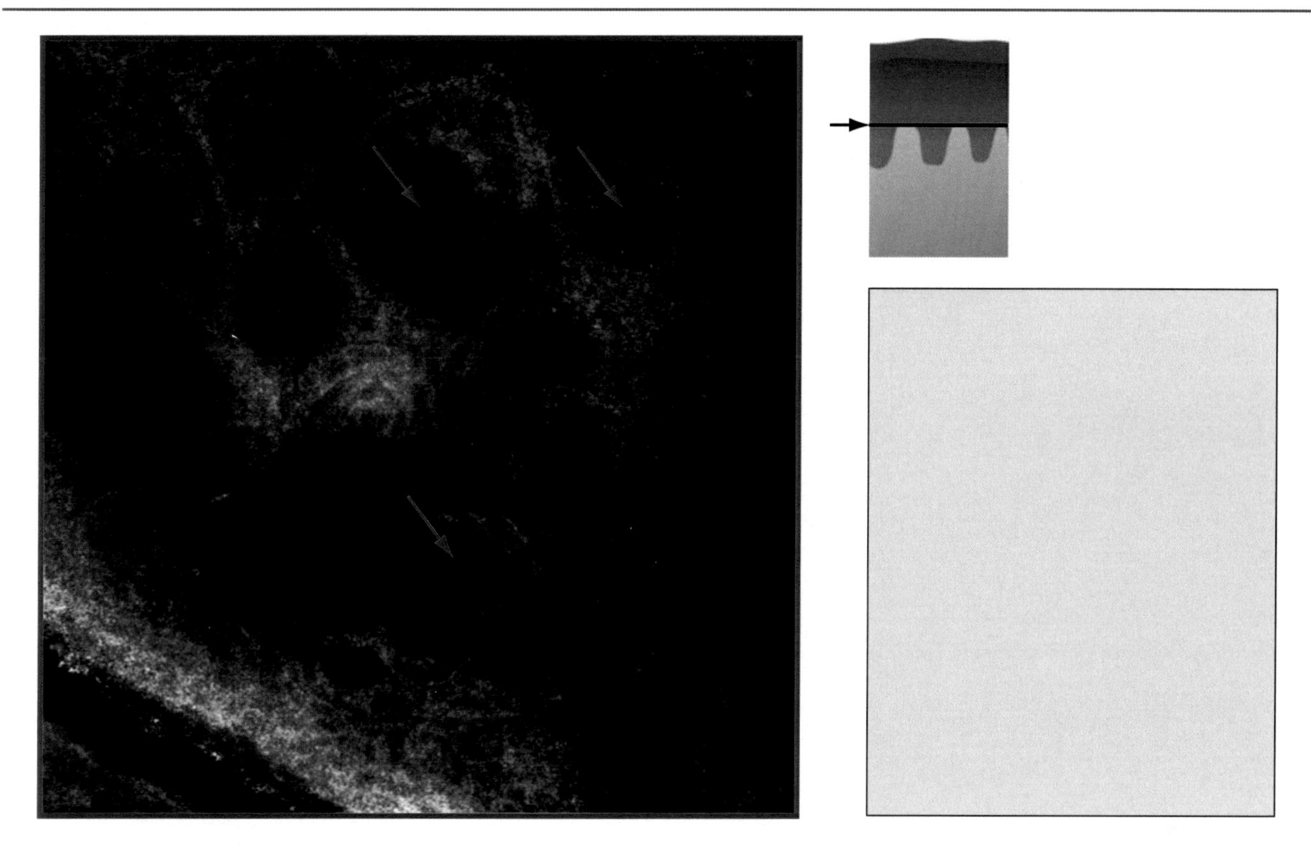

Fig. 27.1.1 Basic image (0.5 × 0.5 mm) as particular of the previous block at the level of the spinous layer. Presence of dermal papillae is visible in the upper layers because of papillomatosis inducing elongation of the rete ridges. Dilated vessels are visible inside the papillae (→) corresponding to vessels filling the elongated papillae

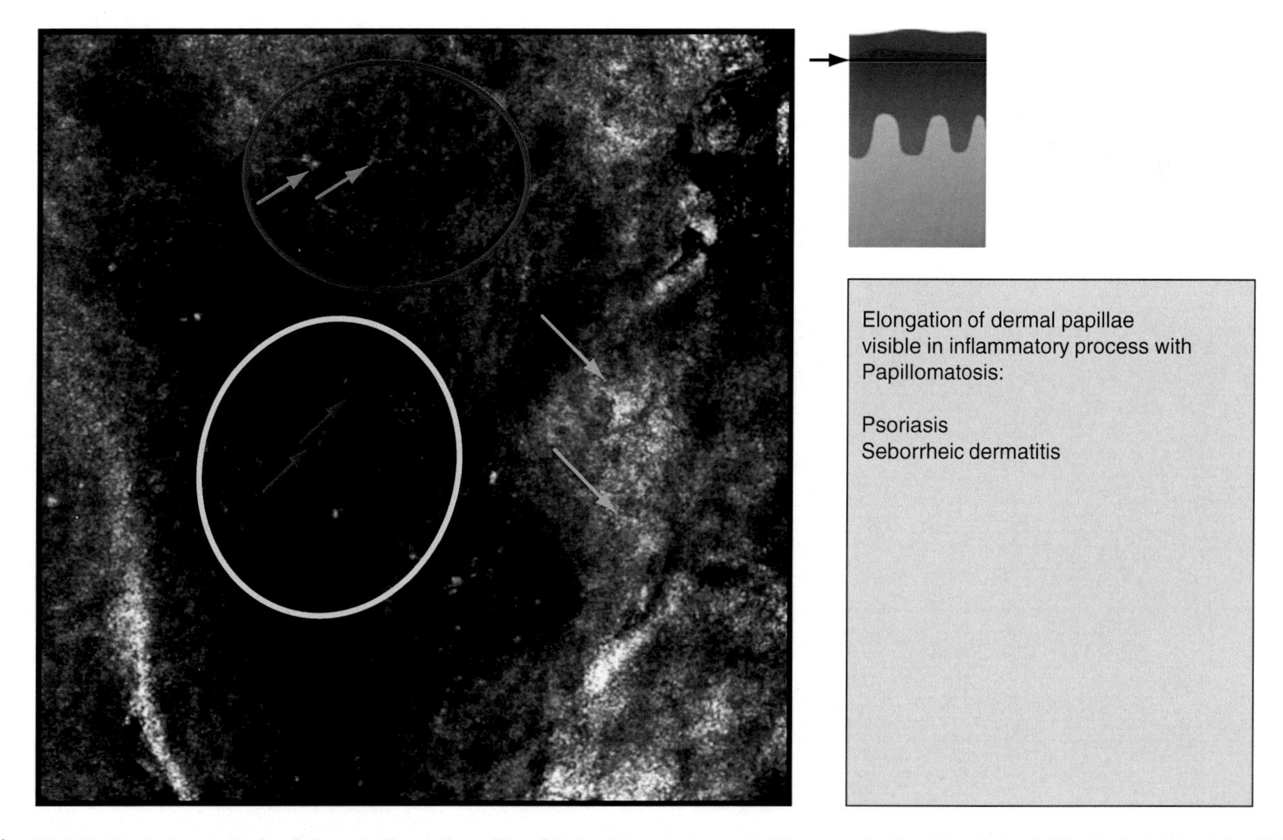

Fig. 27.1.2 Basic image (0.5 × 0.5 mm). Dermal papillae filled with dilated vessels (*red* →) are already visible just below the first cellular layer of the epidermis (*yellow circle*). Parakeratosis is also displayed (*green* →). Honeycombed epidermis is visible (*red circle*) with mildly bright round cellular structures between keratinocytes corresponding to exocytosis of inflammatory cells (*blue* →)

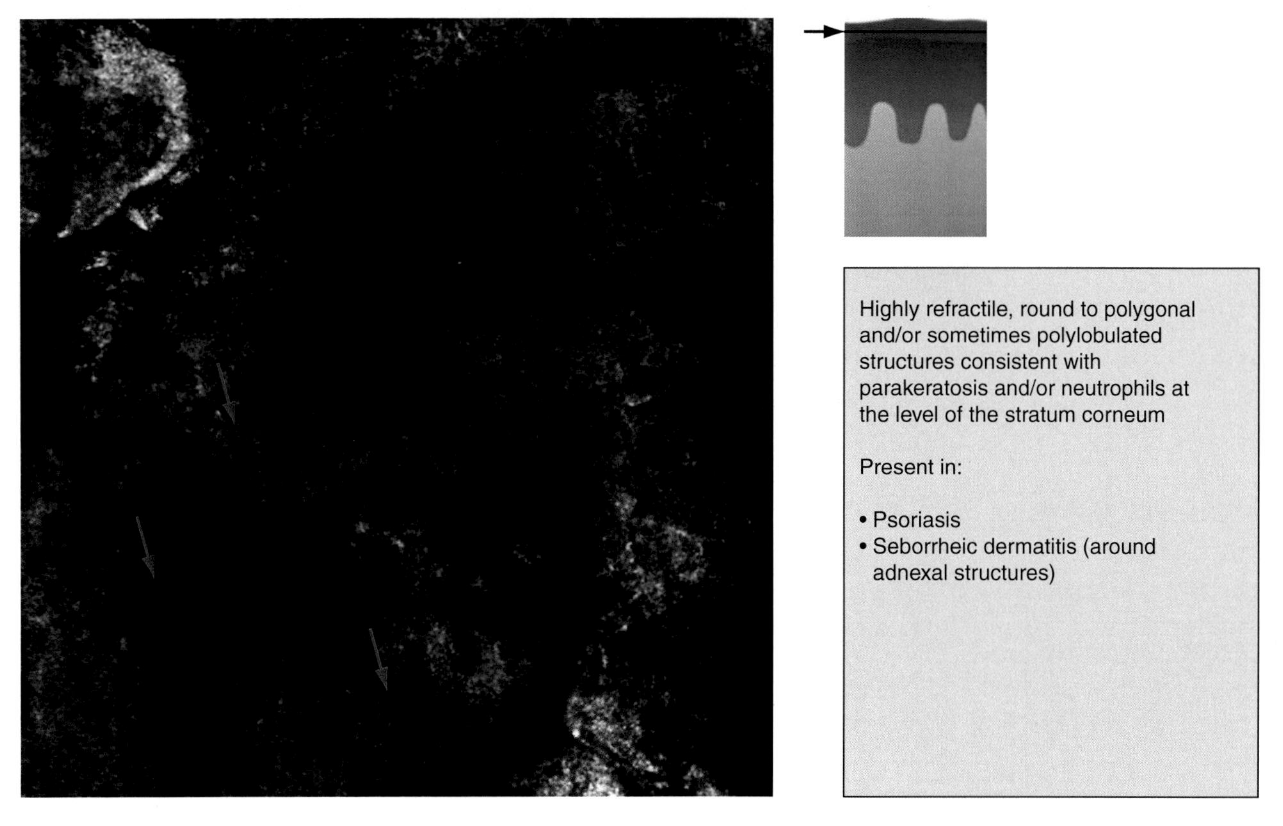

Fig. 27.1.3 Basic image (0.5 × 0.5 mm) taken at the level of the stratum corneum disclosing presence of mildly bright structures (→) corresponding to parakeratotic keratinocytes

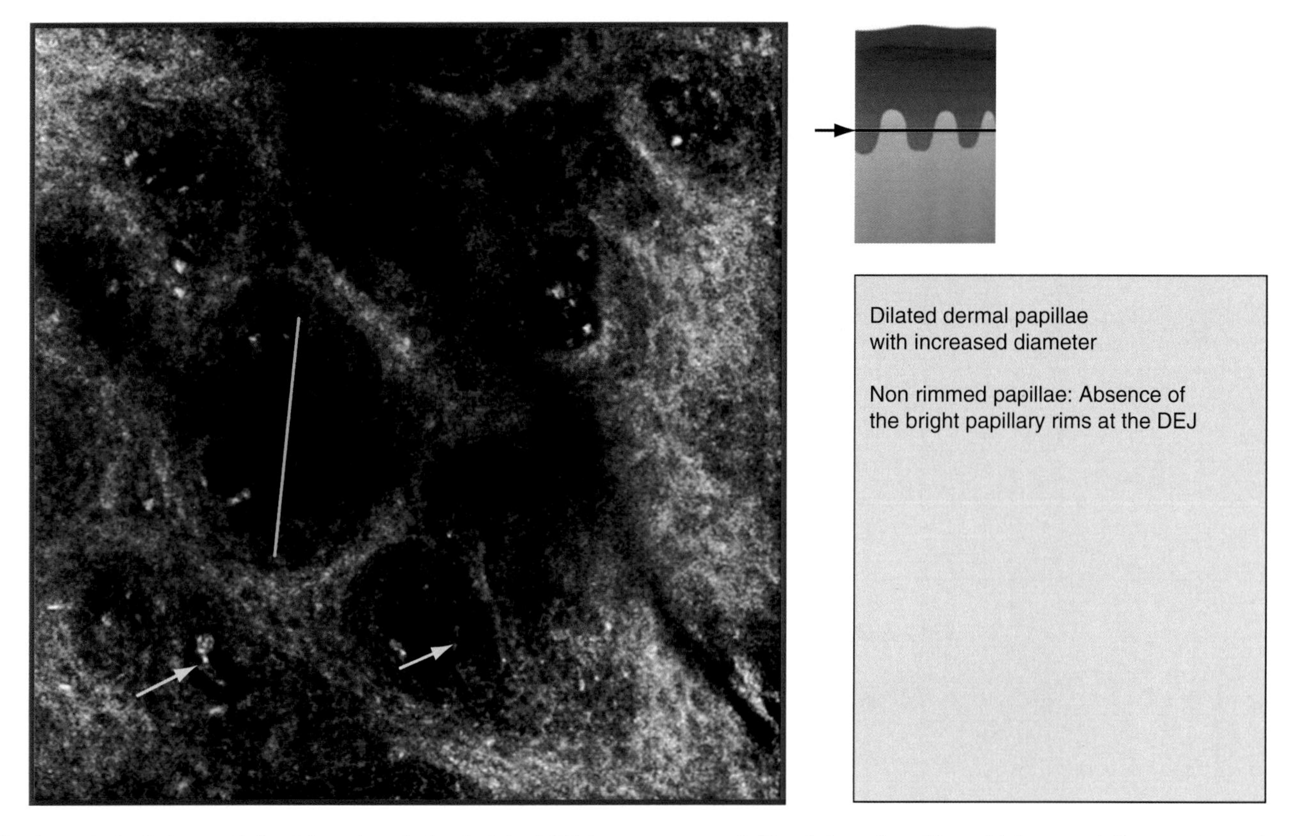

Fig. 27.1.4 Basic image (0.5 × 0.5 mm) at the level of the DEJ shows presence of dilated dermal papillae with increased diameter (*green line*). Inside the papillae dilated vessels are visible as black round to polylobated structures and are separated by thinner septa (*yellow* →)

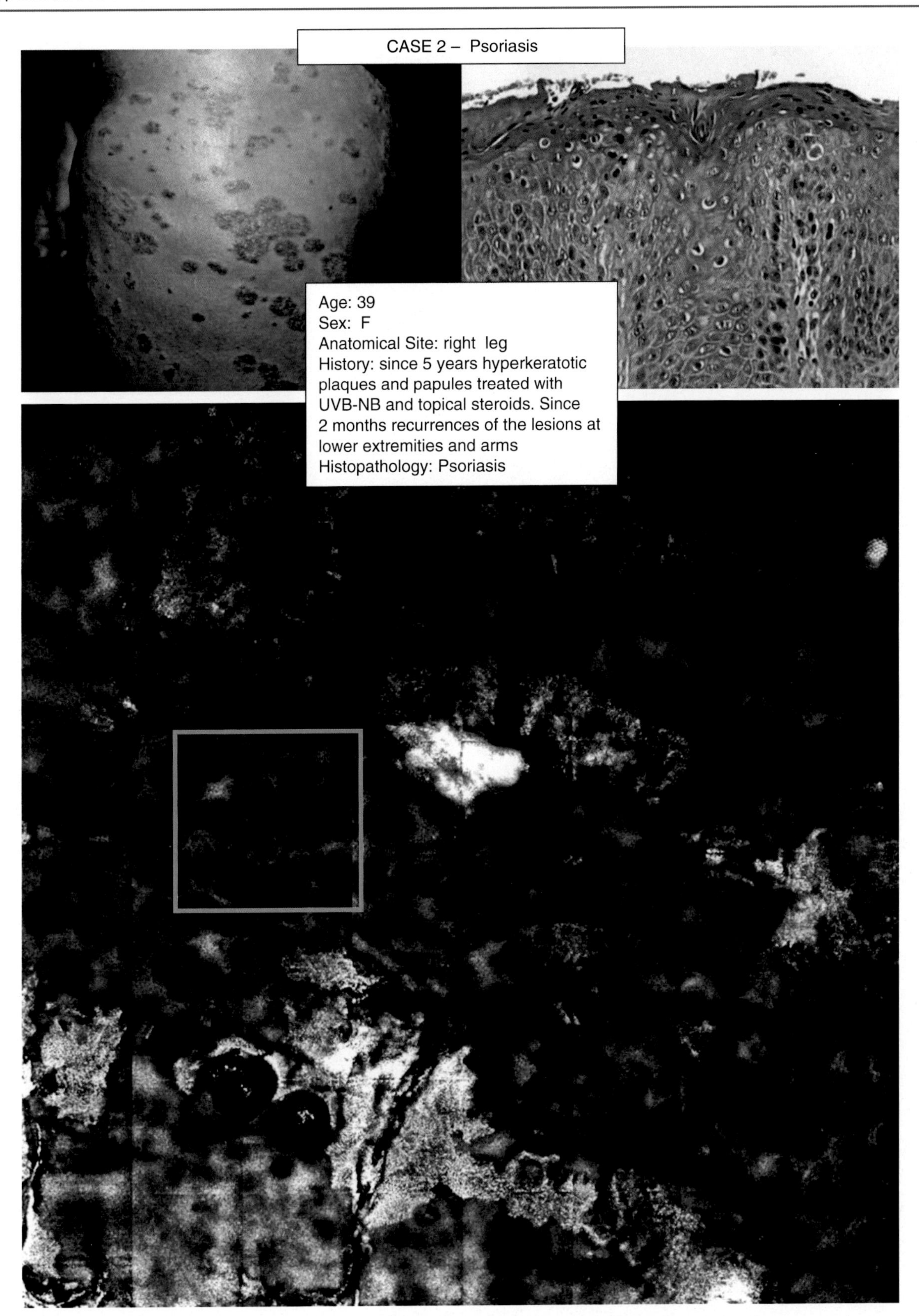

Fig. 27.2 RCM Viva Block mosaic (3×3 mm) taken at the level of the DEJ reveals multiple dermal papillae increased in density and diameter that are separated by thin interpapillary epidermal septa as sign of papillomatosis

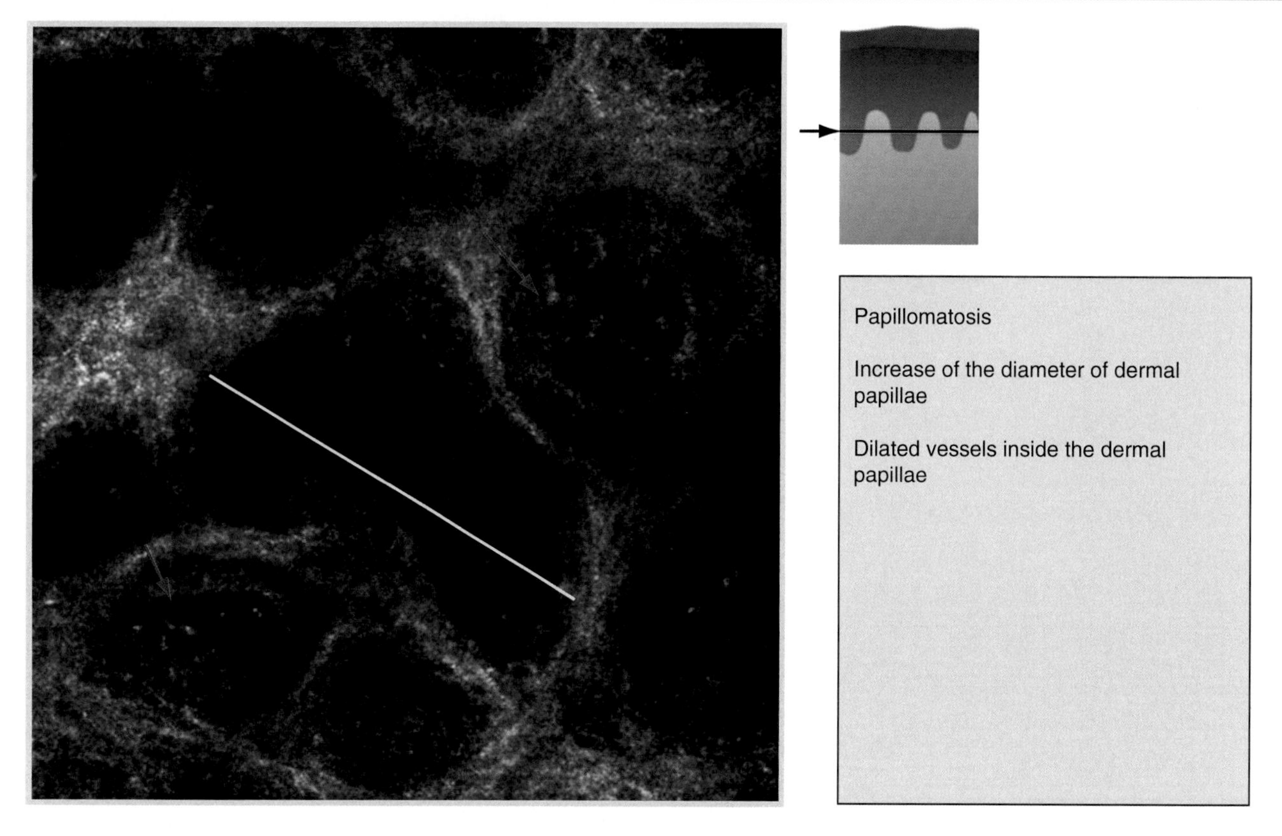

Fig. 27.2.1 Basic image (0.5 × 0.5 mm) as focus of the previous block. At the dermo-epidermal junction presence of papillomatosis with an increased diameter of the dermal papillae (DP) (~150 μm) (*yellow line*). The DP are separated by a thin epithelial septum, filled with prominent round or linear dark canalicular structures inside the dermal papillae, which correspond to dilated vessels →

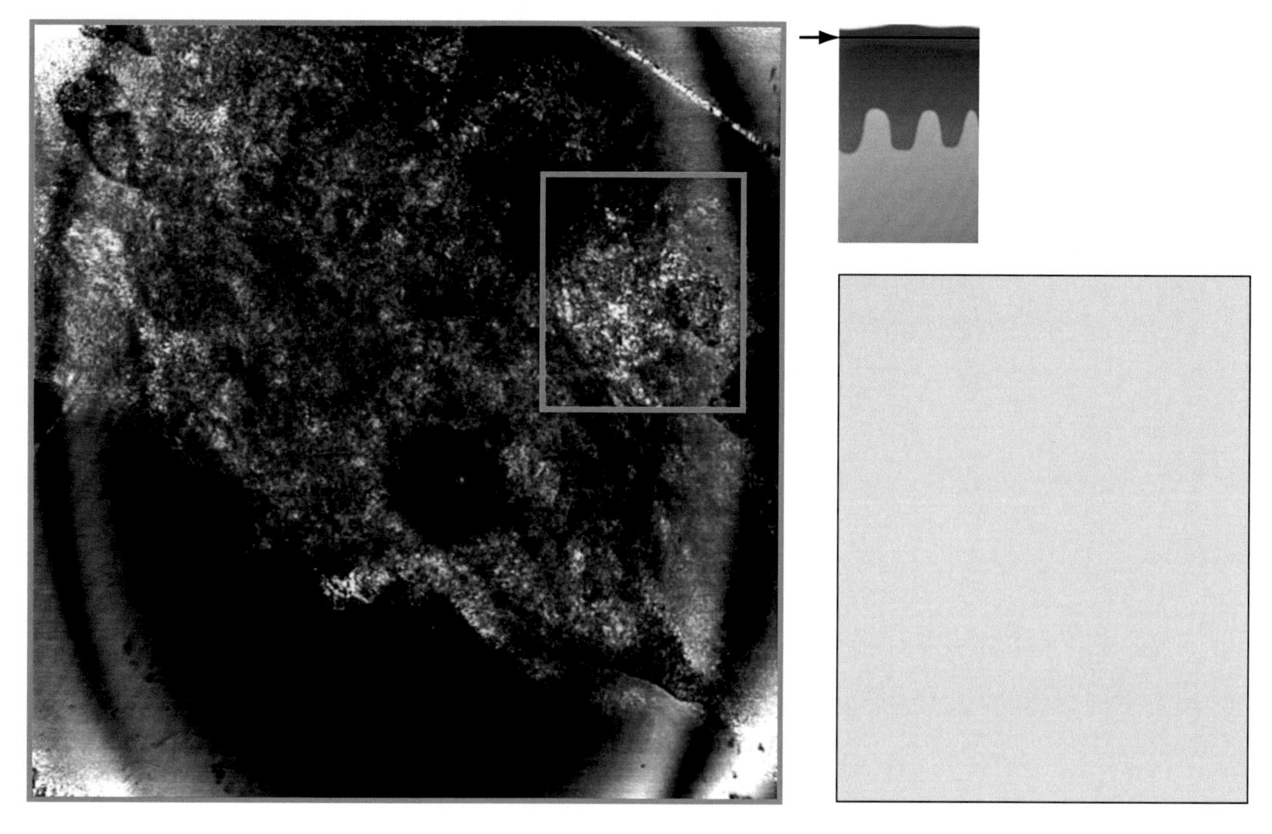

Fig. 27.2.2 RCM single frame (0.5 × 0.5 mm) taken at the level of the stratum corneum exhibits focal highly refractile, round to polygonal structures consistent with parakeratosis or aggregates of neutrophils

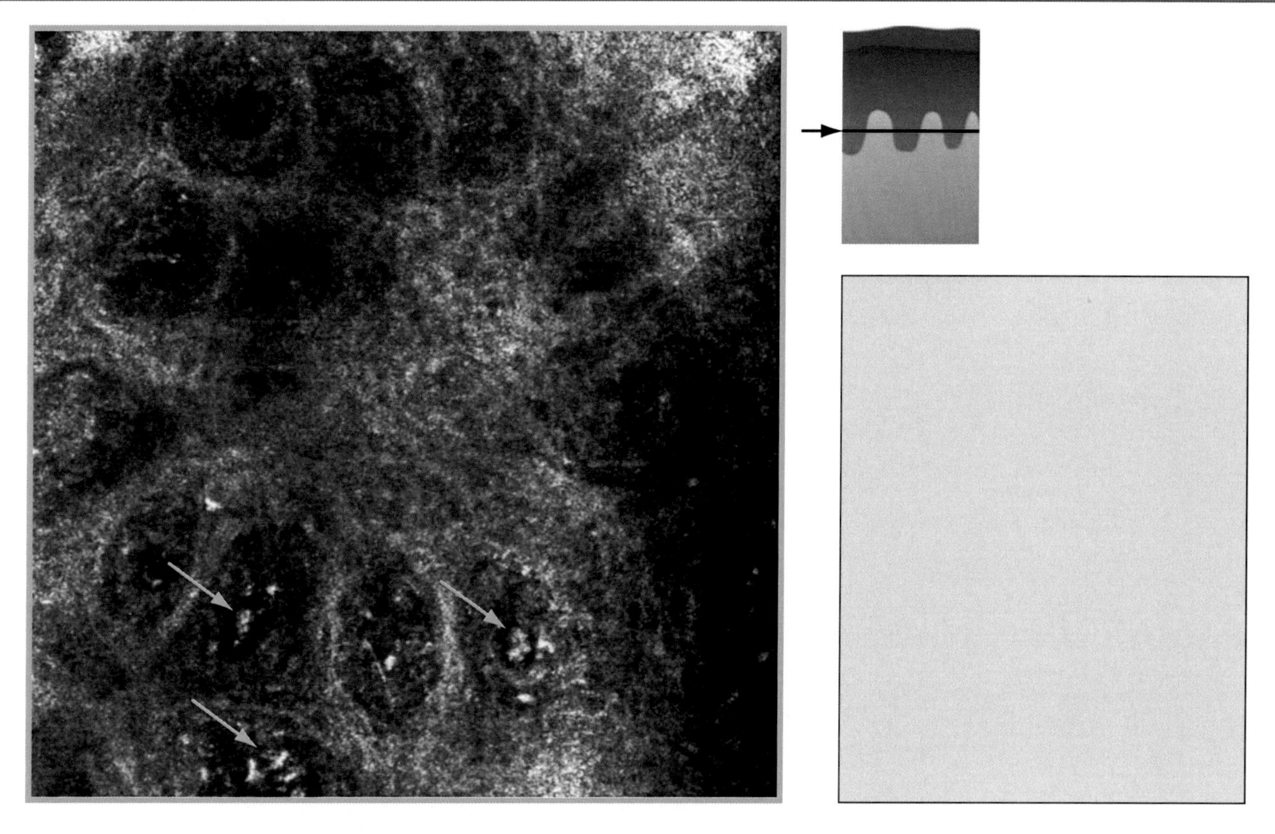

Fig. 27.2.3 Basic image (0.5 × 0.5 mm) at the level of DEJ show the presence of dilated dermal papillae filled by dilated vessels surrounded and filled by bright cellular structures corresponding to intravascular white blood cells and perivascular inflammation (*green* →)

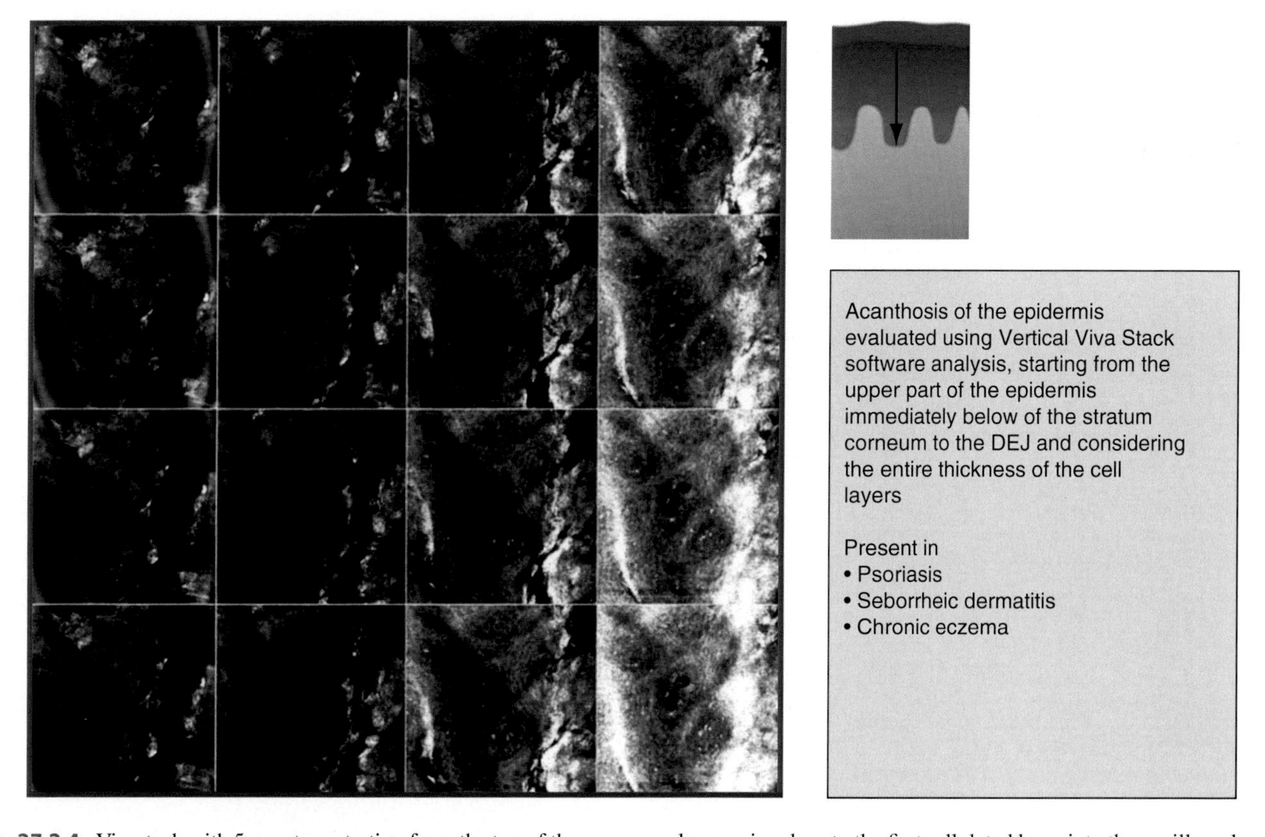

Fig. 27.2.4 Vivastack with 5 μm steps starting from the top of the squamous layer going deep to the first cellulated layer into the papillary dermis (acanthosis) as 16 × 5 μm = 80 μm. Acanthosis definition > of 60–90 μm, depending on anatomical site

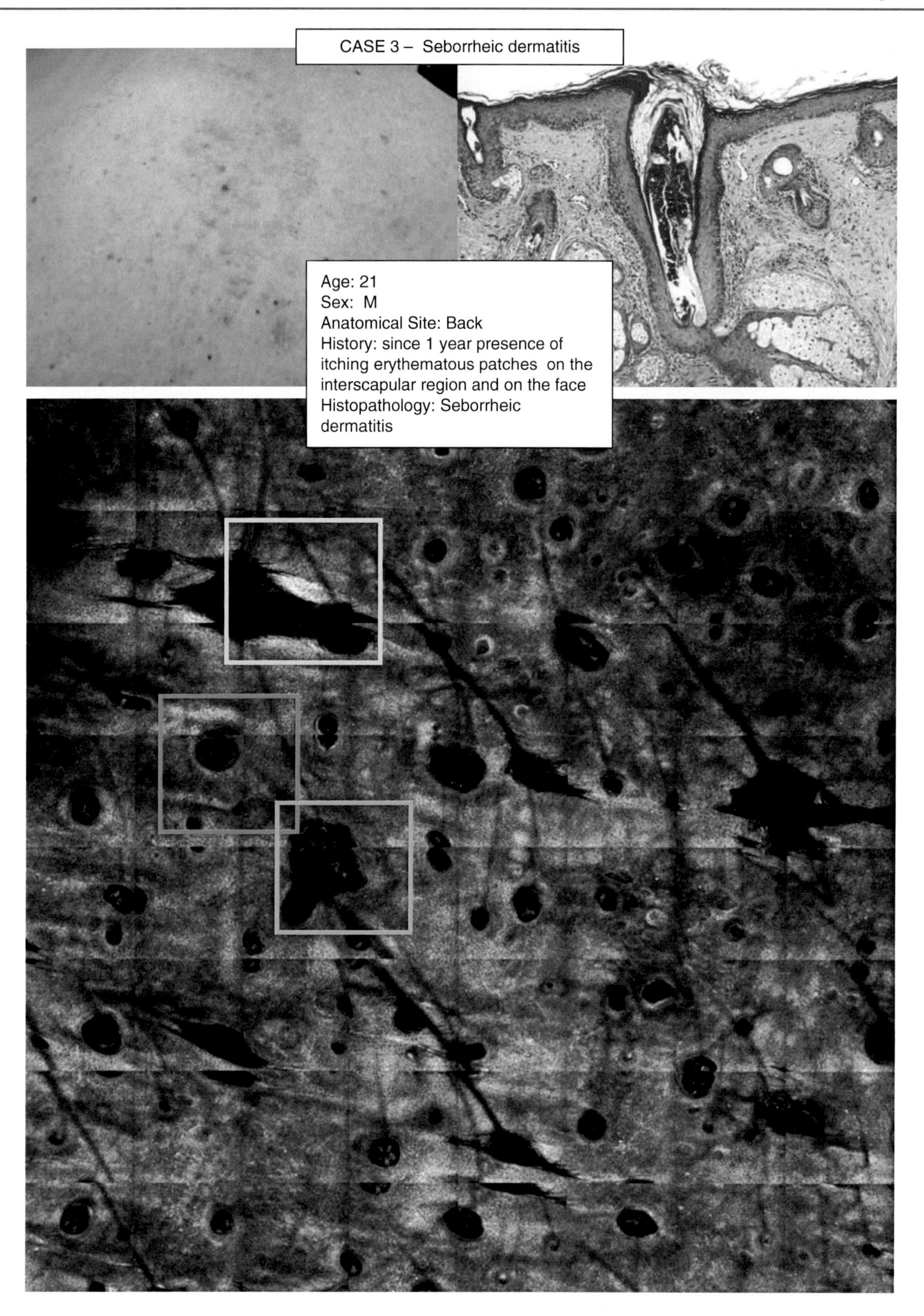

Fig. 27.3 RCM mosaic (3 × 3 mm) at the level of the spinosus layer disclosing parakeratosis (yellow square), epidermal infiltration of inflammatory cells around adnexal follicle (blue square) and around sebaceous gland (green square).

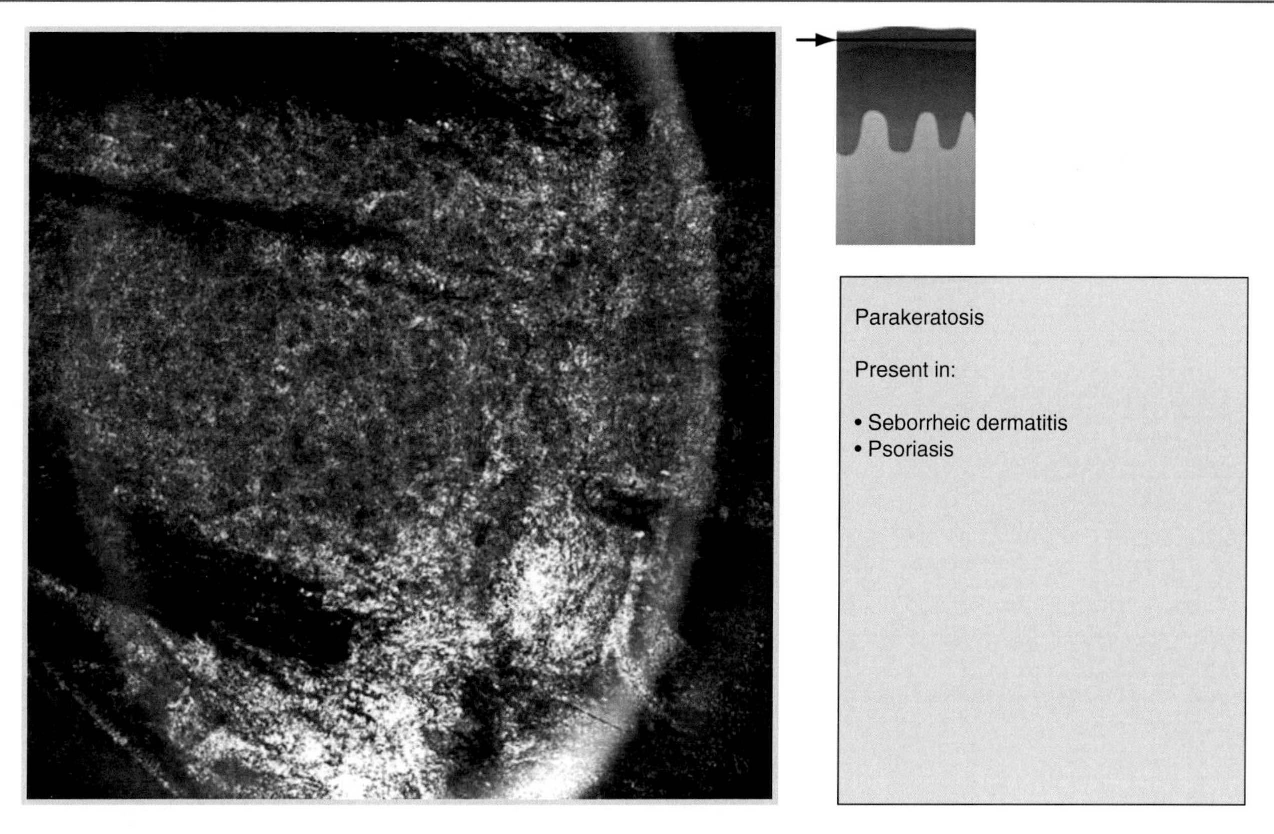

Fig. 27.3.1 RCM single frame (0.5× 0.5 mm) taken at the top of stratum corneum exhibits focal highly refractile, round to polygonal structures consistent with parakeratosis and/or neutrophils

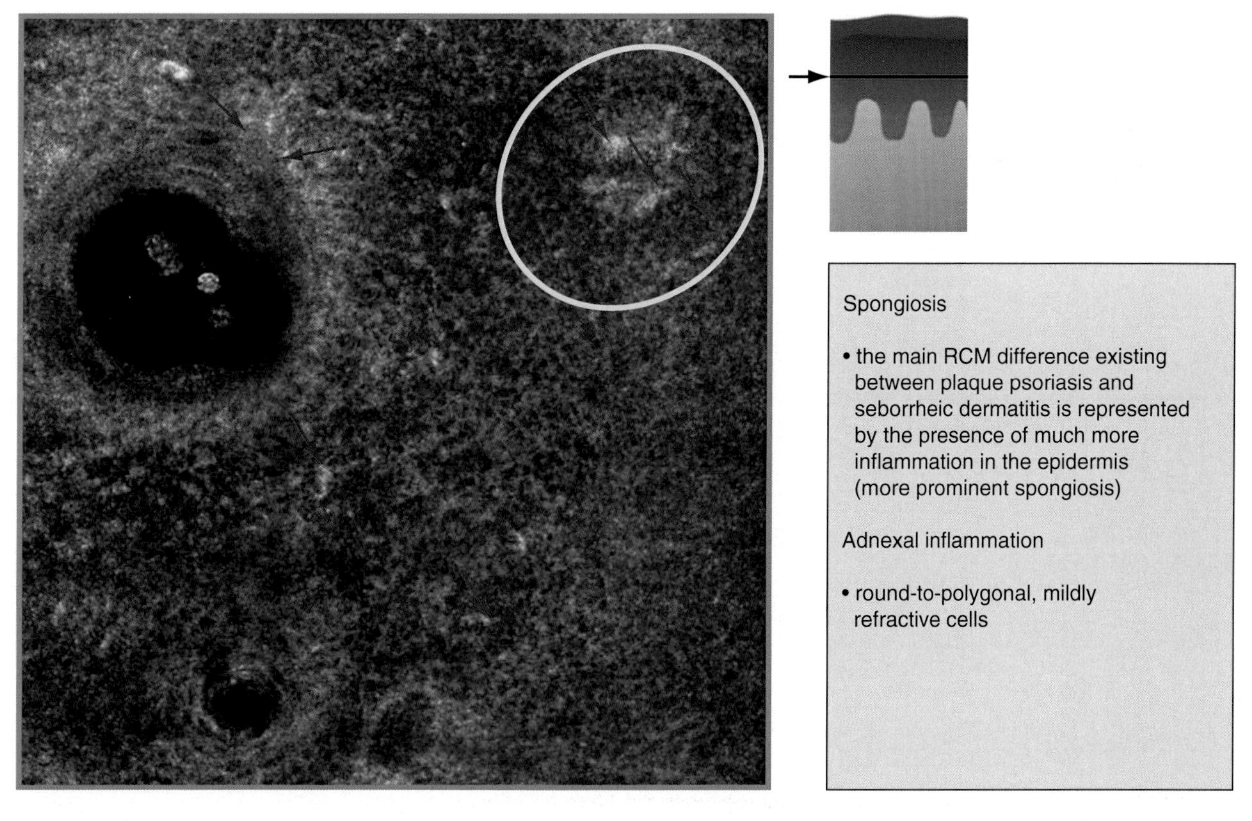

Fig. 27.3.2 Basic image (0.5 × 0.5 mm) as a particular of the previous block. Epidermal infiltration of inflammatory cells that are seen as bright round to polygonal structures (*red* →) in the contest of darker areas (spongiosis) (*yellow circle*). Adnexal inflammation: round-to-polygonal, mildly refractive cells around and involving the adnexal epithelium (*red* →)

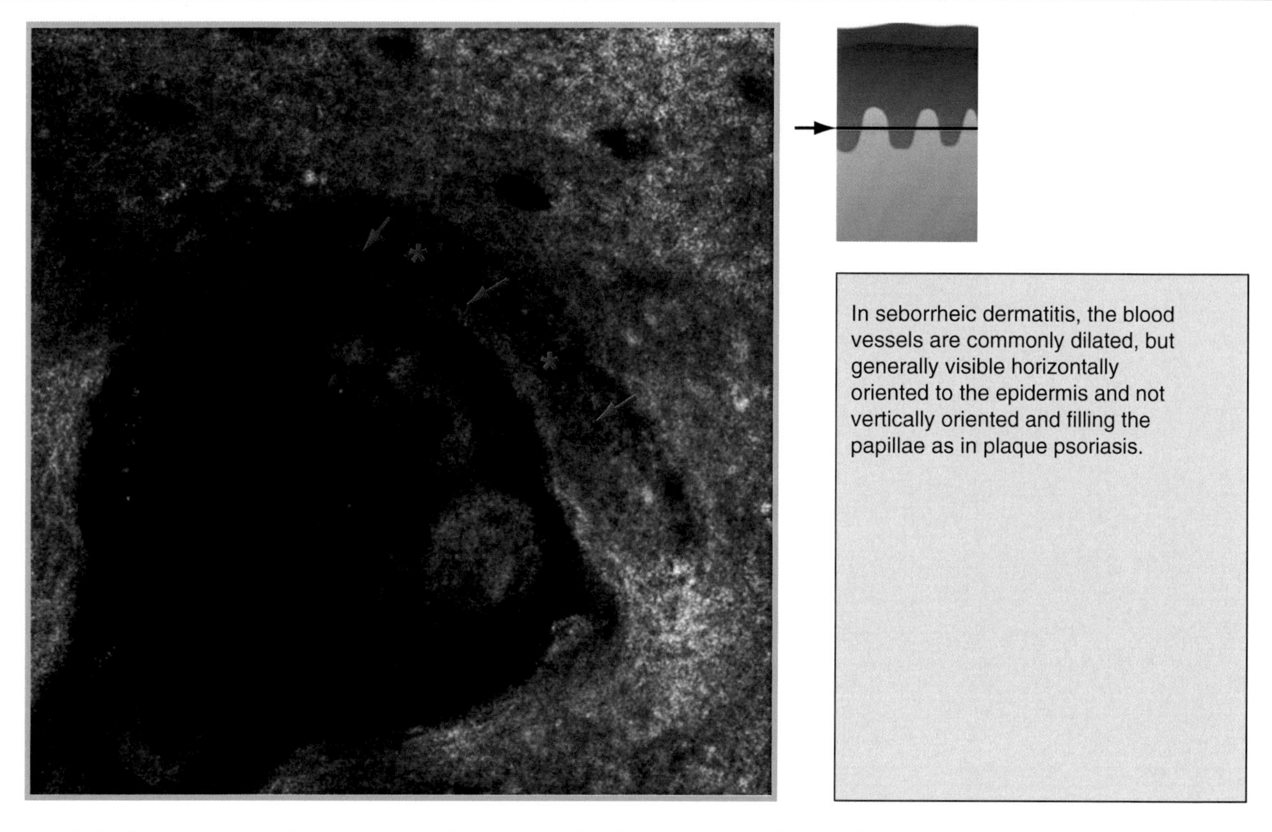

Fig. 27.3.3 Basic image (0.5 × 0.5 mm) as a particular of the previous block. Presence of dilated blood vessel around sebaceous gland. Vessels are visible as dark canalicular structures horizontally oriented to the epidermis (*), filled by moving bright cells corresponding to white blood cells (→)

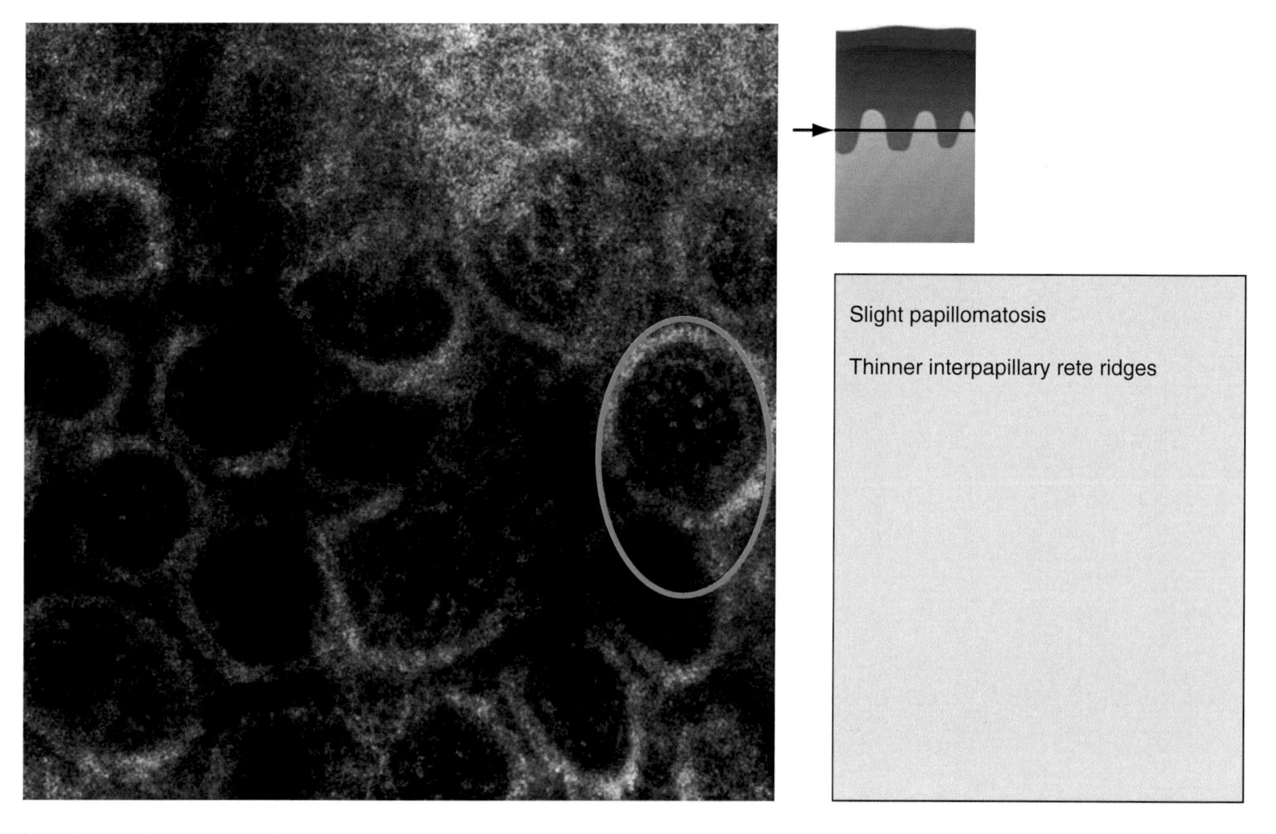

Fig. 27.3.4 Basic image (0.5 × 0.5 mm) presence of grouped, multiple, dilated rimmed dermal papillae, filled with prominent blood vessels (blue circle), separated by thinner interpapillary rete ridges (*) as sign of papillomatosis

Core Messages

- Hyperkeratotic skin diseases can be differentiated from the other inflammatory skin diseases using RCM.
- Vivastack examination is able to estimate the thickness of the stratum corneum and epidermis disclosing hyperkeratosis and acanthosis.
- RCM discloses the presence of parakeratosis, reduction or absence of the granular layer, papillomatosis and acanthosis with normal honeycomb pattern of epidermis and dilated vessels in the upper dermis in >90% of the cases.
- RCM examination of hyperkeratotic disorders needs the application of keratolytic agents prior to imaging to minimize light scattering due to the scales.
- Seborrheic dermatitis differs from plaque psoriasis prevalently in the location of parakeratosis in peridnexal areas, presence of much more spongiosis and presence of more sings of dermal inflammation characterized by dilated vessels horizontally oriented to the epidermis.

References

1. Raychaudhuri SP, Farber EM (2001) The prevalence of psoriasis in the world. J Eur Acad Dermatol Venereol 15:16–17
2. Naldi L (2004) Epidemiology of psoriasis. Curr Drug Targets Inflamm Allergy 3:121–128
3. Gudjonsson JE, Johnston A, Sigmundsdottir H, Valdimarsson H (2004) Immunopathogenic mechanisms in psoriasis. Clin Expo Immunol 135:1–8
4. De Berker D (2002) Diagnosis and management of nail psoriasis. Dermatol Ther 15:165–172
5. Gregoriou S, Kalogeromitros D, Kosionis N, Gkouvi A, Rigopoulos D (2008) Treatment options for nail psoriasis. Expert Rev Dermatol 3(3):339–344
6. Brauchli YB, Jick SS, Curtin F, Meier CR (2008) Association between beta-blockers, other antihypertensive drugs and psoriasis: population-based case-control study. Br J Dermatol 158(6):1299–1307
7. Tagami H (1997) Triggering factors. Clin Dermatol 15:677–685
8. Tsankov N, Kazandjieva J, Drenovska K (1998) Drugs in exacerbation and provocation of psoriasis. Clin Dermatol 16:333–351
9. Abel EA, DiCicco LM, Orenberg EK et al (1986) Drugs in exacerbation of psoriasis. J Am Acad Dermatol 15:1007–1022
10. Naldi L, Chatenoud L, Linder D et al (2005) Cigarette smoking, body mass index, and stressful life events as risk factors for psoriasis: results from an Italian case-control study. J Invest Dermatol 125:61–67
11. Naldi L, Parazzini F, Peli L et al (1996) Dietary factors and the risk of psoriasis Results of an Italian case-control study. Br J Dermatol 134:101–106
12. Hay JR, Graham-Brown RA (1997) Dandruff and seborrhoeic dermatitis: causes and management. Clin Exp Dermatol 22:3–6
13. Foley P, Zuo Y, Plunkett A, Merlin K, Marks R (2003) The frequency of common skin conditions in preschool-aged children in Australia: seborrheic dermatitis and pityriasis capitis (cradle cap). Arch Dermatol 139:318–322
14. Elder D et al. Lever's Histopathology of the skin, 9th edition 184–187
15. Ardigo M, Cota C, Berardesca E, González S (2009) Concordance between in vivo reflectance confocal microscopy and histology in the evaluation of plaque psoriasis. J Eur Acad Dermatol Venereol 23:660–667
16. González S, Rajadhyaksha M, Rubinstein G, Anderson RR (1999) Characterization of psoriasis in vivo by reflectance confocal microscopy. J Med 30:337–356

Spongiotic Dermatitis

28

Susanne Astner and Martina Ulrich

28.1 Introduction

Cutaneous inflammation is frequently observed as a primary or secondary phenomenon with a variety of endogenous, infectious or reactive skin processes and may occur in the epidermis, dermis or subcutaneous tissue. Clinically, the appearance of erythema, edema, vesicle, pustule or plaque formation may be observed, resulting in a characteristic morphology that often facilitates the clinical differential diagnosis. While the patterns of inflammation vary widely within the clinical spectrum of dermatological diseases, spongiotic dermatitis is among the most frequently observed [1–3]. Spongiotic dermatitis may run an acute, subacute or chronic course and is the key histopathologic feature of contact dermatitis, eczema, including nummular and dyshidrotic eczema and others such as atopic dermatitis, photoallergic reactions or drug eruptions [3]. Among them, acute contact dermatitis is a disease of particularly high prevalence and significant socioeconomic impact. Based on their heterogeneous etiology, allergic and irritant contact dermatitis (ACD and ICD respectively) may be differentiated [4–7]. Yet, while some clinical aspects, histological or immunological features may help in their distinction, the exact differentiation of ACD and ICD is not easily accomplished [5–7].

On histopathological evaluation, mild contact dermatitis is characterized by the presence of inter- or intracellular edema, an elongation of the intercellular bridges and a discrete inflammatory infiltrate. Early in the disease, the infiltrate consist of neutrophils, whereby these are more common in irritant contact dermatitis than in allergic contact dermatitis where eosinophils are frequently observed. With subacute and chronic disease, reactive hyperproliferation, parakeratosis and intraepidermal necrosis may be appreciated depending on the subtype of spongiform reaction pattern [3, 5].

Reflectance confocal microscopy (RCM).has previously been used for evaluation of acute contact dermatitis, as an example of spongiotic dermatitis [8]. Initial studies were performed by comparing RCM features of ACD and ICD to respective findings of routine histology, whereby corresponding features were detected [9]. Further investigations were performed to study the kinetic evolution of ICD and ACD over time, thereby gaining new insights into the dynamic and morphology of contact dermatitis [10]. All RCM evaluations were based on features previously described by routine histology [5, 7, 11].

28.2 General RCM Features of Spongiotic Dermatitis

The main feature of spongiotic dermatitis on RCM is the presence of intra- or intracellular spongiosis [9]. This corresponds to increased intercellular brightness due to inter-, or intracellular fluid accumulation, whereby the regular honeycombed morphology of the upper epidermal layers appears accentuated [8–10]. Another feature frequently observed is vesicle formation, which – either focal or widespread in extent – is seen on RCM as well-demarcated, dark hollow spaces between granular and spinous keratinocytes. Often small round, weakly refractile cells may be seen in the centre of vesicles and microvesicles, these may correspond to apoptotic keratinocytes or inflammatory cells [9]. Lastly, exocytosis is regularly associated with spongiotic dermatitis, whereby the inflammatory cells are seen on RCM as bright, round highly refractile structures of about 8–10 μm, interspersed between keratinocytes. Inflammatory cells may also be observed to various extents in perifollicular, perivascular or interstitial dermal distribution [8–10] (Table 28.1).

S. Astner (✉) • M. Ulrich
Department of Dermatology and Venereology,
Charité University Medicine Berlin,
Berlin, Germany
e-mail: susanne.astner@charite.de; martina.ulrich@charite.de

R. Hofmann-Wellenhof et al. (eds.), *Reflectance Confocal Microscopy for Skin Diseases*,
DOI 10.1007/978-3-642-21997-9_28, © Springer-Verlag Berlin Heidelberg 2012

Table 28.1 The relevant features for diagnosis of ACD and ICD respectively

RCM feature	ACD	ICD	Differential diagnoses
Superficial disruption/ detached corneocytes	+/–	+++	For example, actinic keratoses, dry skin, chronic eczema
Parakeratosis	+/–	+++	For example, actinic keratoses, DSAP, psoriasis
Spongiosis[a]	+++	+++	Concomitant spongiosis with other inflammatory/proliferative/infectious dermatoses
Vesicle formation[a]	+++	+++	For example, other forms of eczematous dermatoses, fungal disease, Mycosis fungoides
Exocytosis	++–+++	++–+++	Concomitant spongiosis with inflammatory/proliferative/infectious dermatoses
Necrosis[a]	+	+++	Burns, photothermal reaction, e.g. following PDT
Blood vessel dilatation	+[b]	+[b]	Any inflammatory, neoplastic or benign proliferative process
Superficial dermal inflammatory infiltrate	+–++	+–++[b]	Inflammatory dermatoses, autoimmune skin disorders
Increased epidermal thickness	+/–	+++	Psoriasis, regenerative hyperplasia, acanthosis

Left column indicates RCM feature, based on those previously described by RCM and established by H&E. Middle columns indicate the presence or absence of individual features, following a semiquantitative scoring (+/– rare, + mild, ++ moderate, +++ severe); right column indicates selected differential diagnoses to consider

[a]At the level of the granular and/or spinous layer respectively

[b]If optical penetration permits

28.3 RCM Features of Allergic Contact Dermatitis (Fig. 28.1)

The hallmark of acute ACD is seen on RCM by the presence of mild-moderate or marked spongiosis, depending somewhat on the severity of the clinical reaction [9]. Vesicle formation may be microfocal, diffuse or widespread within the epidermal compartment, thereby disrupting the architecture of the granular and spinous layer. Considering standardized readings of patch tests at 48 and 72 h, RCM may visualize inflammatory cells within the epidermal, dermal and perivascular compartment either in aggregates or as single cells [9, 10]. The dermal compartment is characterized by the presence of dilated blood vessels, seen as accentuated canalicular structures that exhibit blood flow on in vivo examination. Lymphocyte rolling may be observed, whereby lymphocytes may be distinguished from erythrocytes only by their somewhat larger diameter, and the tendency of marginalization within the blood flow [12]. Another, quantitative, aspect is the assessment of epidermal thickness, which – if measured in vivo – is comparable to that of normal skin, ranging from 45 to 55 μm [10]. Overall, the kinetic evolution of ACD follows characteristic dynamics and may persist up to 14 days following the induction of ACD by allergen exposure, with the exception of selected allergens with delayed onset or very mild forms of CD. Only later in the course, in subacute or chronic CD does epidermal hyperproliferation become a factor, corresponding to a mild increase in epidermal thickness and superficial disruption of the stratum corneum [10].

28.4 RCM Features of Irritant Contact Dermatitis (Fig. 28.2)

Considering distinguishing characteristics to ACD, ICD reactions exhibit a pronounced superficial disruption early on after the exposure to contact irritants, a finding that is generally absent in early ACD [9, 10]. Upon RCM evaluation, parakeratotic changes are seen as highly refractile, polygonal cells at the level of the stratum corneum, with a central dark or bright nucleus. The latter has been explained by direct corrosive effects of experimental irritants such as SLS, which may ultimately alter the refractility of the retained nuclei [9, 13]. In addition, individual corneocytes may appear as detached highly refractile polygonal cells which correspond clinically to subtle desquamation, reflecting the loss of SC-cohesiveness in response to contact irritants. Another characteristic feature of ICD is the regenerative hyperproliferation which may also be documented quantitatively by RCM in vivo [10]. Following serial measurements within the Z-axis, an increase of epidermal thickness may be quantified, being as large as two-fold compared to normal skin, or – in that regard – compared to sites exposed to contact allergens. Mean epidermal thickness values show a rapid increase after irritant exposure, followed by a delayed recovery over a period of 9–14 days. Another parameter more commonly seen in ICD reactions is the presence of intraepidermal necrosis. The latter is seen as circumscribed dark space with *irregular* borders, with detached keratinocytes at the periphery and may be a direct effect of cutaneous irritants [10]. It has been shown that ICD and ACD also differ in aspects of kinetic evolution such that ICD reactions have a more rapid onset and show a faster recovery compared to ACD. In addition, two consecutive studies have shown that RCM may detect and differentiate contact dermatitis in skin of color, where the interpretation of erythema is more difficult [14, 15]. When comparing individual susceptibility to ICD, the results of these studies indicated that Caucasians may have a lower irritancy threshold compared to African-Americans. At the same time, it was demonstrated that RCM may aid in the detection of subclinical reactions, where clinical features are absent or subtle, thereby verifying clinical readings of patch tests [15].

28.5 Discussion

Presently, patch testing represents the gold standard for confirmation of contact dermatitis, however its reproducibility has been questioned and challenged [2]. The virtue of RCM is the ability to study tissue in vivo, thus enabling sequential evaluations of dynamic processes and disease evolution over time. Following initial correlative clinical trials it was possible to define specific RCM features of ICD and ACD [9, 16]. Based on these findings it was suggested that RCM may aid in the differentiation of ACD and ICD [8, 9]. Yet RCM also creates new insights into the pathophysiologic mechanisms of evolving inflammatory processes [10, 17, 18]. While the visualization of features in the dermal layer may be limited by epidermal thickness or overlying inflammatory and disruptive changes, their absence may not always reflect the actual pathomorphology. Hence the interpretation of RCM findings must occur in a clinical-pathological context, by integrating selected RCM parameters into a diagnostic algorithm. Thereby, RCM observations may be utilized for confirmation, and enhancement, of equivocal patch test reactions [19].

CASE 1 – Allergic contact dermatitis

Age: 31
Sex: F
Anatomical site: Right forearm
History: Allergic contact dermatitis
Patch test: Allergic contact dermatitis

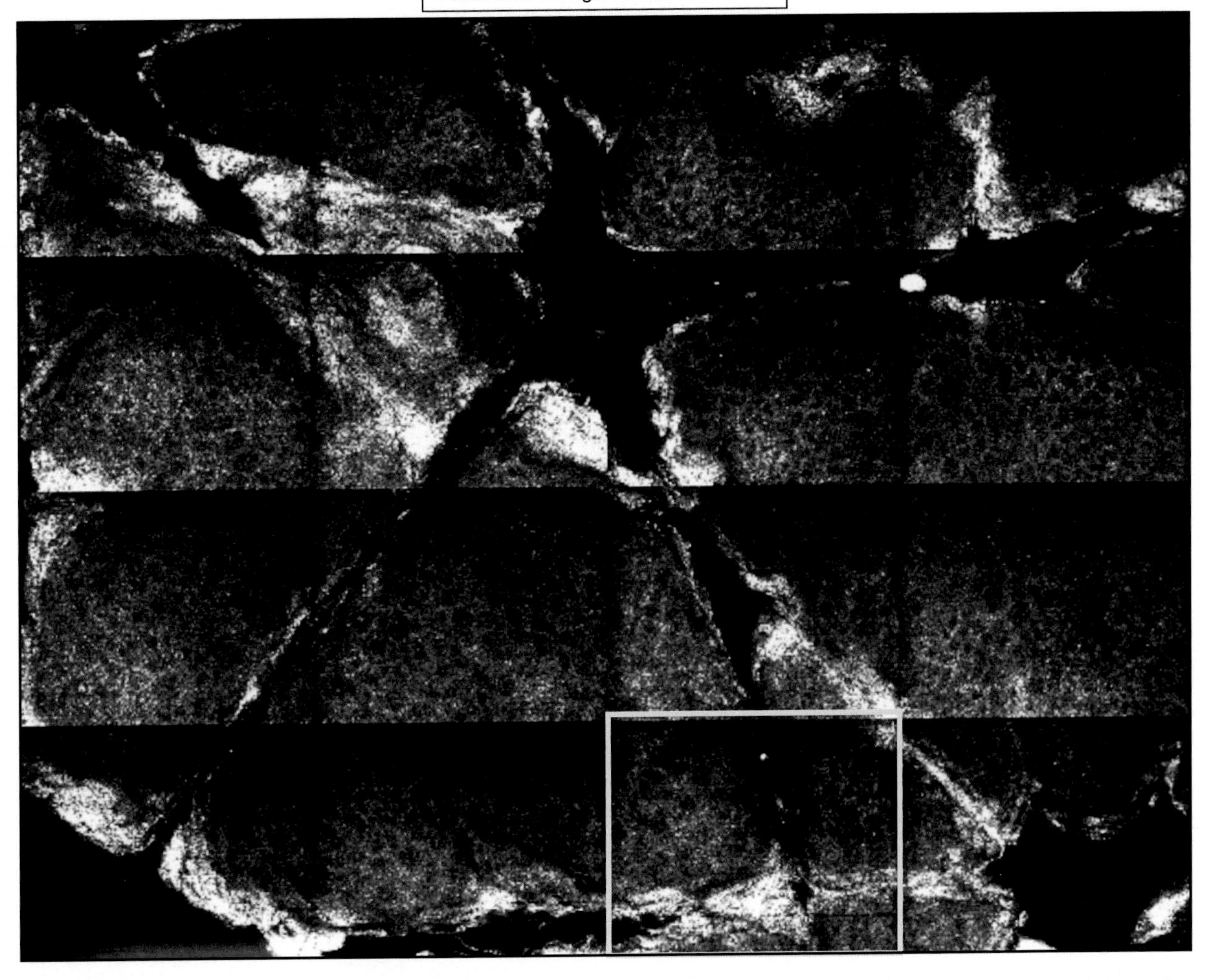

Fig. 28.1 RCM mosaic (1 × 0.8 mm) at the level of the granular layer reveals an increased brightness of the intercellular spaces, corresponding to moderate spongiosis. Epidermal architecture appears with an accentuated honeycombed pattern, with no atypia, yet focal loss of clear cell to cell demarcation

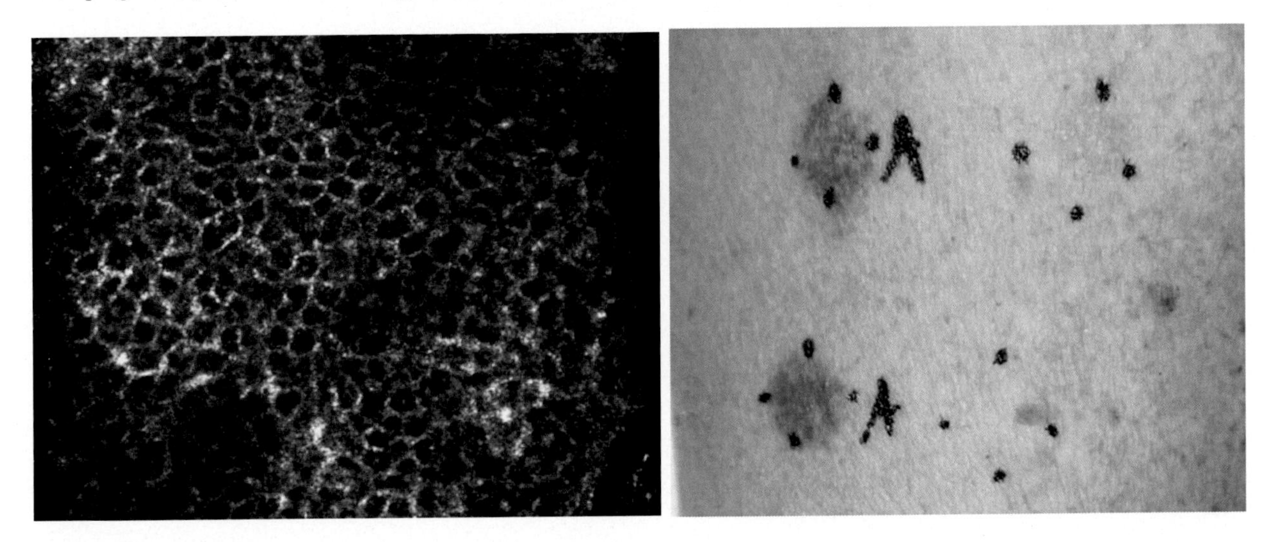

CASE 1 – Allergic contact dermatitis

Age: 31
Sex: F
Anatomical site: Right forearm
History: Allergic contact dermatitis
Patch test: Allergic contact dermatitis

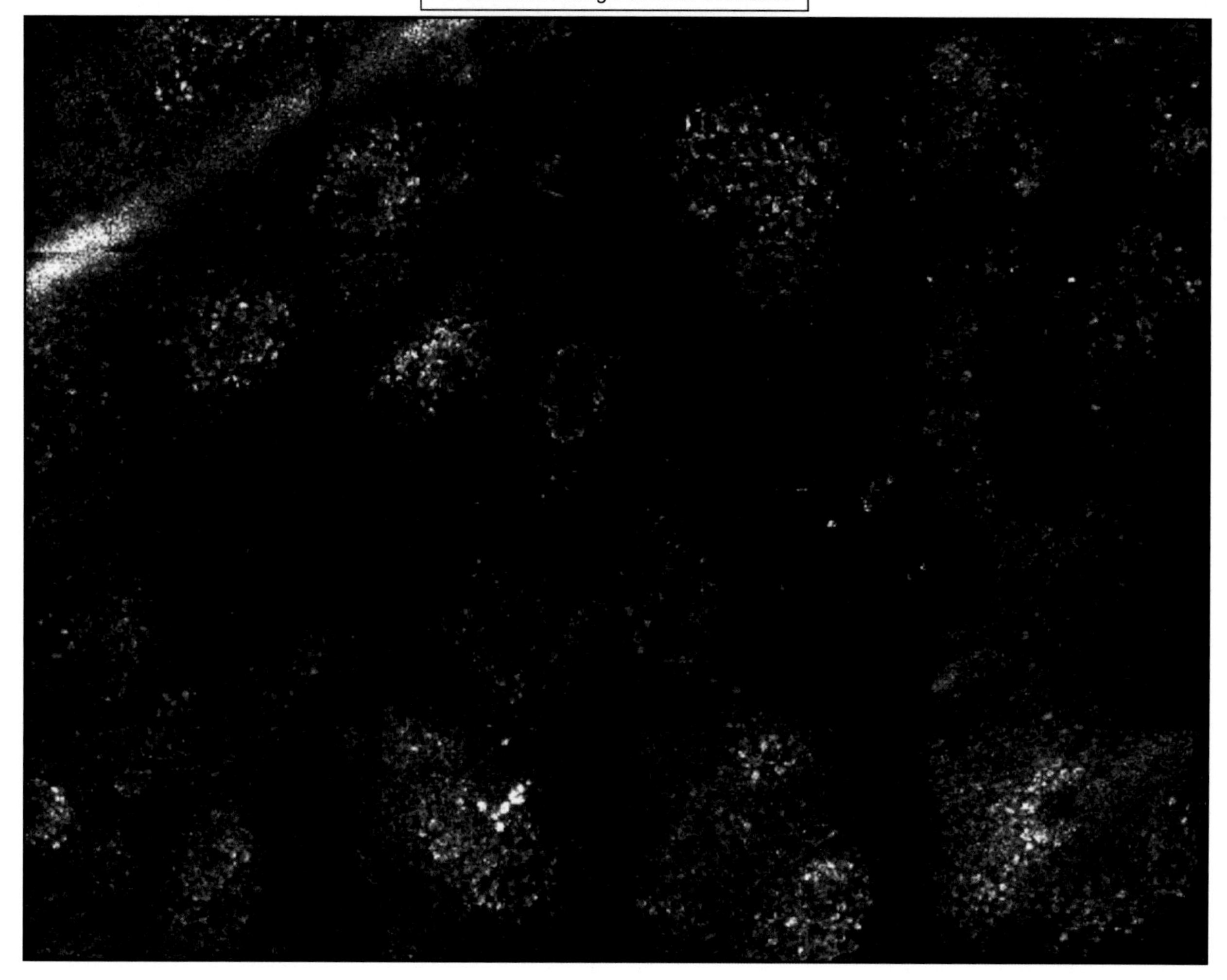

Fig. 28.1.2 Representative clinical image illustrating experimental allergen exposure (A) using routine patch tests resulting in the development of ACD with erythema, edema and microvesicle formation

Fig. 28.1.1 RCM mosaic (1 x 0,8 mm) at the level of the stratum corneum reveals a severely disrupted corneal layer with presence of parakeratosis and detached corneocytes. Figure 28.2.1 Illustrating detail of parakeratotic corneocytes, seen as bright polygonal cells with either bright (dashed square, left side) or dark central nuclei (dashed square right side). Clinical image with experimental allergen (A) and irritant (I) exposure, using 3 % SLS in aqueous solution.

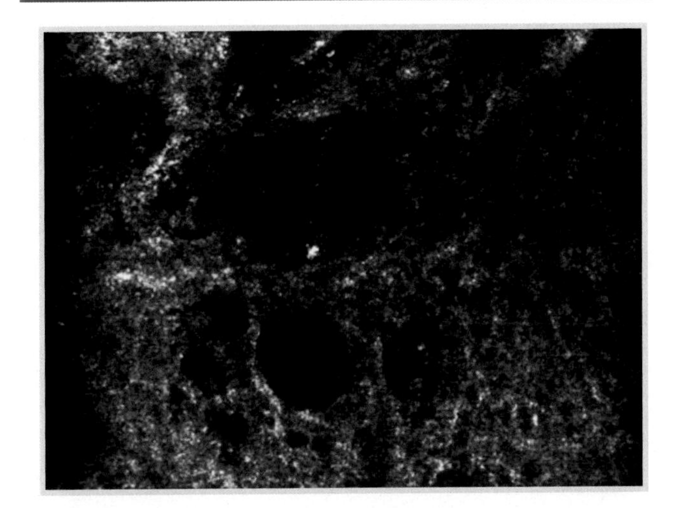

Fig. 28.1.3 RCM image (250 × 200 μm) obtained at the level of the granular layer, illustrating epidermal vesicle formation seen as round to oval dark space with good demarcation, contrasting surrounding spongiotic keratinocytes. Vesicle formation may be microfocal, focal, unilocular or multifocal; often multichambered microvesicles may be appreciated, seen as dark interconnected spaces with fine, membrane-like, intersecting vessel walls

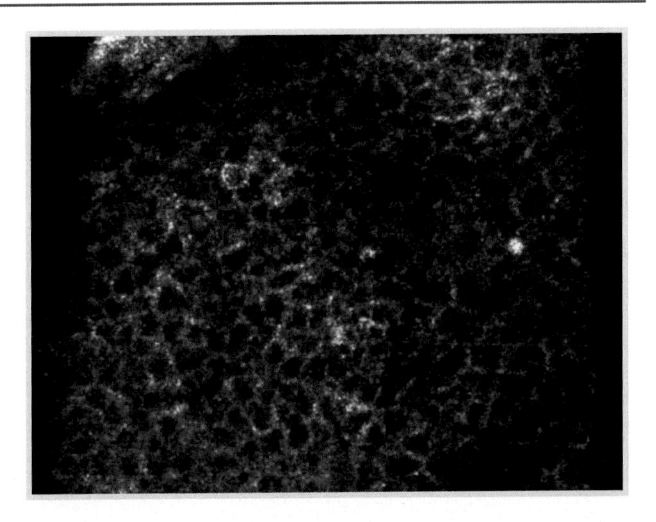

Fig. 28.1.4 RCM image (250 × 200 μm) obtained at the level of the granular layer, illustrating RCM features of exocytosis. Small, round to oval bright cells are seen interspersed between granular or spinous keratinocytes. Attention must be paid to the differentiation of pigmented basal cells, which may be based on either/and size/location/arrangement. In addition, inflammatory cells may be located at the level of the dermal layer, whereby small aggregates of round to oval bright cells may be seen in a perivascular or interstitial distribution.

CASE 2 – Irritant contact dermatitis

Age: 28
Sex: F
Anatomical site: Right forearm
History: Irritant contact dermatitis
Patch test: Irritant contact dermatitis

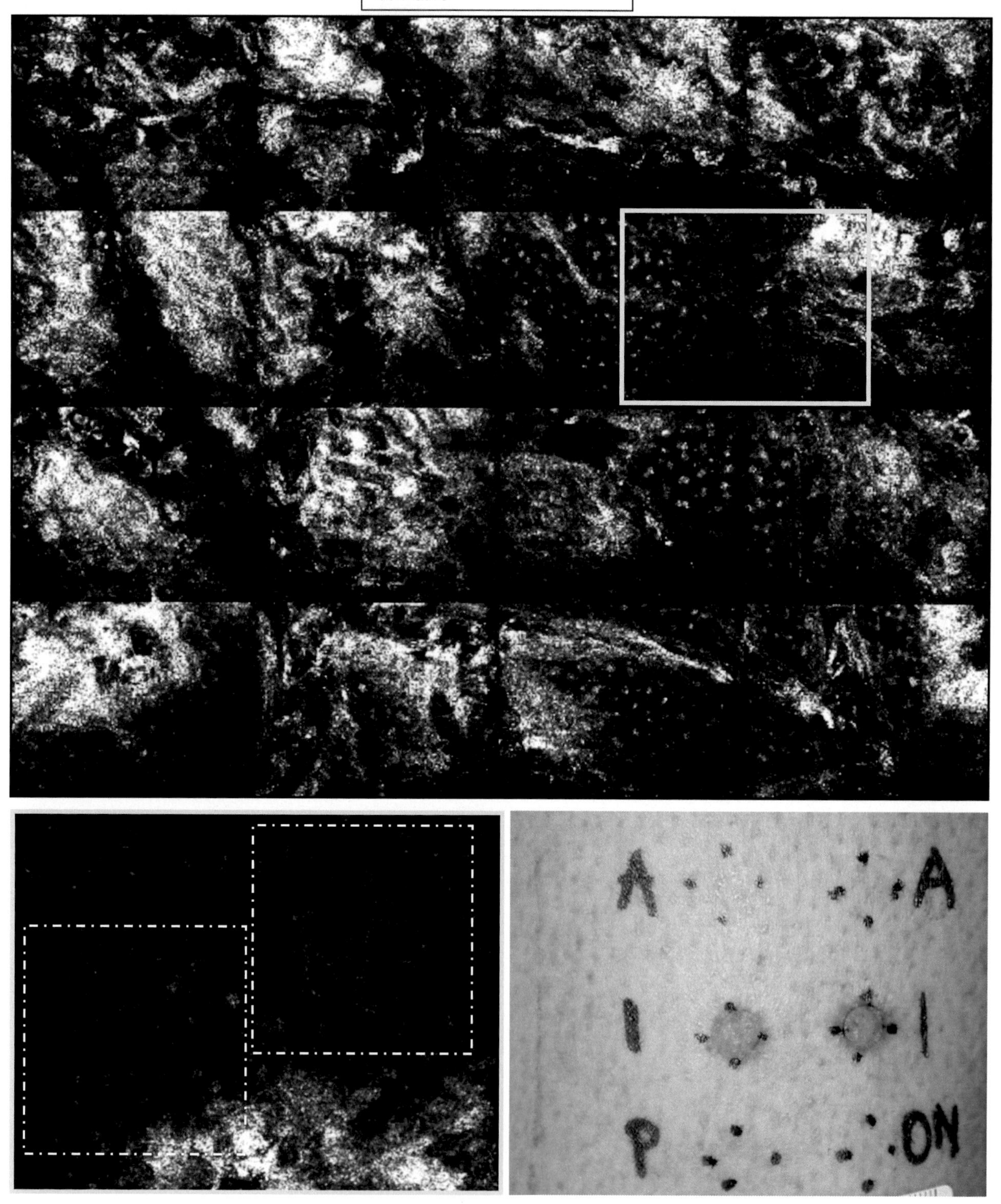

Figs. 28.2 and 28.2.1 RCM mosaic (1 x 0,8mm) at the level of the Stratum corneum reveals a severely disrupted corneal layer with presence of parakeratoses and detached corneocytes. Figure 28.2.1 Illustrating detail of parakeratotic coreneocytes, seen as bright polygonal cells with either bright or dark nuclei in the center (dashed white squares). Clinical image with experimental allergen (A) and irritant (I) exposure, using 3 % SLS in aqueous solution

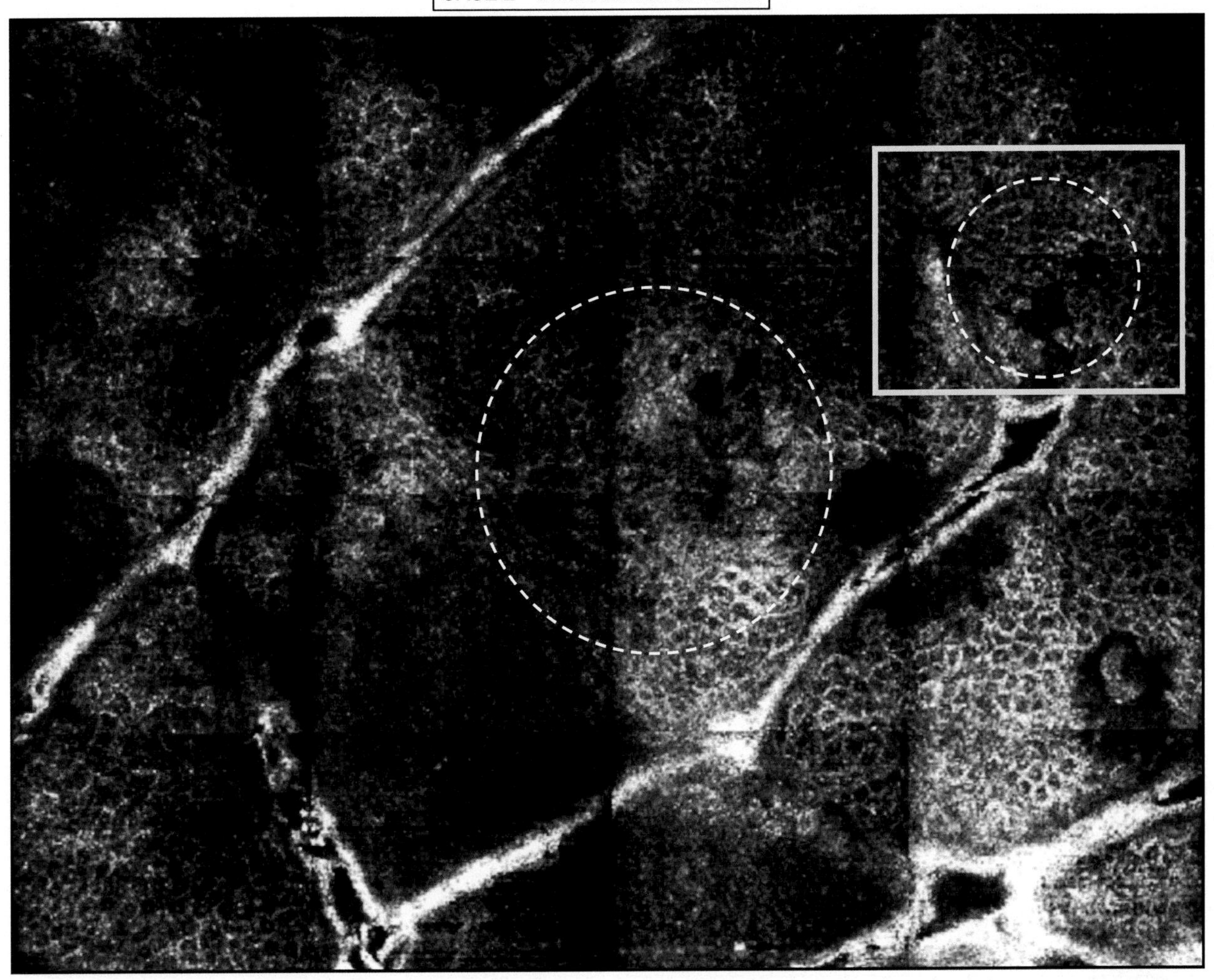

Fig. 28.2.2 RCM mosaic (1 × 0.800 mm) obtained at the level of the stratum granulosum reveals areas of necrosis corresponding to dark spaces with irregular demarcation and pronounced disruption of the epidermal architecture. Surrounding keratinocytes reveal the presence of spongiosis, seen as increased brightness of intercellular spaces, accentuating the honeycombed pattern of the granular layer. The overall architecture appears somewhat preserved by the visualization of skin folds and creases

Fig. 28.2.3 RCM image (250 × 200 μm) obtained at the level of the upper granular layer illustrating an area of circumscribed necrosis, seen as dark space with irregular configuration (*white dashed circle*). Contrasting the mechanism of vesicle formation, intraepidermal necrosis is disrupting the overall architecture by direct corrosive or chemical effects on keratinocytes

Core Messages

RCM permits the detection of epidermal spongiosis, vesicle formation and exocytosis.

The detection of selected features such as spongiosis or exocytosis alone is unspecific, and a broad differential diagnosis must be considered in a clinical-pathological context.

RCM enables the differentiation of irritant and allergic contact dermatitis based on morphologic and kinetic features.

RCM permits monitoring of dynamic inflammatory processes over time.

RCM evaluation may facilitate the detection of subclinical reactions.

References

1. Proposed National Strategy for the Prevention of Leading Work-Related Diseases and Injuries, Part 2. Washington, DC, Association of Schools of Public Health and National Institutes for Occupational Safety and Health, 1988, pp 65–95
2. Rietschel RL, Fowler JF, Fisher AA (2001) Fisher's contact dermatitis, 5th edn. Lippincott Williams & Wilkins, Baltimore
3. Gupta K (2008) Deciphering spongiotic dermatitides. Indian J Dermatol Venereol Leprol 74:523–526
4. Enk AH, Katz SI (1992) Early molecular events in the induction phase of contact sensitivity. Proc Natl Acad Sci USA 89:1398
5. Dvorak HF, Mihm MC, Dvorak AM et al (1974) Morphology of delayed type hypersensitivity reactions in man I: quantitative description of the inflammatory response. Lab Invest 31:111–130
6. Brasch J, Burgard J, Sterry W (1992) Common pathogenetic pathways in allergic and irritant contact dermatitis. J Invest Dermatol 98:166–170
7. Scheynius A, Fischer T (1986) Phenotypic difference between allergic and irritant patch test reactions in man. Contact Dermatitis 14:297–302
8. González S, González E, White WM, Rajadhyaksha M, Anderson RR (1999) Allergic contact dermatitis: correlation of in vivo confocal imaging to routine histology. J Am Acad Dermatol 40(5 Pt 1): 708–713
9. Swindells K, Burnett N, Rius-Diaz F et al (2004) Reflectance confocal microscopy may differentiate acute allergic and irritant contact dermatitis in vivo. J Am Acad Dermatol 50:220–228
10. Astner S, Gonzalez E, Cheung AC, Rius-Diaz F, Mihm MC, Doukas A, González S (2005) The kinetics of allergic and irritant contact dermatitis in vivo – a non-invasive evaluation. J Invest Dermatol 124:351–359
11. Scheynius A, Fischer T, Forsum U, Klareskog L (1984) Phenotypic characterization in situ of inflammatory cells in allergic and irritant contact dermatitis in man. Clin Exp Immunol 55:81–90
12. González S, Sackstein R, Anderson RR, Rajadhyaksha M (2001) Real-time evidence of in vivo leukocyte trafficking in human skin by reflectance confocal microscopy. J Invest Dermatol 117(2): 384–386
13. Fraschini A, Pellicciari C, Biggiogera M, Manfredi Romanini MG (1981) The effect of different fixatives on chromatin: cytochemical and ultrastructural approaches. Histochem J 13:763–769
14. Hicks S, Swindells KJ, Middelkamp-Hup MA, Sifakis MA, Gonzalez E, González S (2003) Confocal histopathology of irritant contact dermatitis in vivo and the impact of skin color (African-American versus Caucasian). J Am Acad Dermatol 48: 727–734
15. Astner S, Burnett N, Cheung AC, Rius- Díaz F, Doukas AG, González S, González E (2006) The impact of skin color on the susceptibility to irritant contact dermatitis: a non-invasive evaluation. J Am Acad Dermatol 54:458–465
16. Astner S, González S, Gonzalez E (2006) Non-Invasive evaluation of Allergic and Irritant Contact Dermatitis by in-vivo reflectance confocal microscopy. Dermatitis 17(4):182–191
17. González S, Rajadhyaksha M, Gonzalez-Serva A, White WM, Anderson RR (1999) Confocal reflectance imaging of folliculitis in vivo: correlation with routine histology. J Cutan Pathol 26(4): 201–205
18. González S, Rajadhyaksha M, Rubinstein G, Anderson RR (1999) Characterization of psoriasis in vivo by reflectance confocal microscopy. J Med 30:337–356
19. Astner S, Gonzalez E, Cheung AC, Rius-Diaz F, González S (2005) Pilot study on the sensitivity and specificity of in-vivo reflectance confocal microscopy in the diagnosis of allergic contact dermatitis. J Am Acad Dermatol 53(6):986–992

Interface Dermatitis

29

Elvira Moscarella, Marina Agozzino, Claudia Cavallotti, and Marco Ardigò

29.1 Introduction

The term interface dermatitis refers to those skin dermatoses in which an inflammatory process involves prevalently the dermo-epidermal junction, with injury and even necrosis of the basal cell keratinocytes. These dermatitis can be characterized further as being either vacuolar or showing lichenoid changes [1]. The most common interface dermatitis are characterized by prevalent lymphocytic interface infiltrate and are represented by two wide categories: cell-poor interface dermatitis, when only a sparse and focal infiltrate of inflammatory cells is present along the dermo-epidermal junction (erythema multiformis; autoimmune connective tissue disease, particularly systemic lupus erythematosus, dermatomyositis, and mixed connective tissue disease; graft-versus-host disease (GVHD); morbiliform viral exanthema; and some drug reactions), or cell rich, which typically occurs as a heavy band-like infiltrate that obscures the basal layers of the epidermis (lichen planus, lichenoid hypersensitivity reactions of drug or contact-based etiology, lichenoid reactions in the setting of hepatobiliary disease, secondary syphilis, and autoimmune CTD) [2].

Following we introduce the two most common skin inflammatory entities in which the interface changes represent the main macroscopic feature as emblematic for interface dermatitis: lupus erythematosus and lichen planus (and their variants) evaluated with RCM.

29.1.1 Lupus Erythematosus

Cutaneous lupus erythematosus is an autoimmune skin disorder. Clinically, it can be divided schematically in two different sub-types, sub-acute cutaneous (SCLE), and discoid lupus erythematosus (DLE), but histopathologically no significant differences exist in the different sub-types. A variant presenting involvement of the subcutis, but without interface changes, i.e. lupus panniculitis exists. The systemic variant of lupus erythematosus (SLE) is a more serious disease based on involvement by B-cells immunity, of the connective tissue and blood vessels. It is characterized by many clinical manifestations: fever (90%), skin manifestation (85%), arthritis, diseases involving the central nervous system, kidneys, heart, and lungs. Skin involvement can be also present in SLE showing discoid lesions or malar rush. Patients with SCLE express photodistributed, annular, papulosquamous eruptions accompanied by extracutaneous manifestations that, if present, are mild in nature, such as microhematuria or arthralgia [2]. DLE presents only a cutaneous expression with one or more plaques in photodistributed areas. Regarding the histopathologic features in lupus erythematosus we can find a heavier superficial and deep perivascular and periappendageal lymphocytic infiltrate, basement membrane zone thickening, keratotic follicular plugging, and variable acanthosis and atrophy. Atrophy is variable but it is usually present in lesions of SLE and SCLE [3, 4].

29.1.2 Lichen Planus

Lichen planus is a chronic or acute inflammatory dermatitis involving skin or mucosa. It manifests as violaceous, itchy, flat-topped, polygonal papules covered by a reticulated surface scale termed "*Wickham Striae*". The most frequent localization of the lesions is on the volar aspect of the forearms and other flexural surfaces of acral parts, but lesions may be widespread. This pathology is rare in childhood and most frequently affects adults between thirty and seventy years. Variants of lichen planus include the atrophic form (*lichen planus actinicus*), hypertrophic lichen planus, bullous lichen planus, and linear lichen planus. Scarring alopecia may be seen in association with lichen planus; this is termed *lichen*

E. Moscarella (✉) • M. Agozzino • C. Cavallotti • M. Ardigò
San Gallicano Dermatological Institute,
Rome, Italy
e-mail: elvira.moscarella@gmail.com;
marinaagozzino@alice.it; ardigo@ifo.it

R. Hofmann-Wellenhof et al. (eds.), *Reflectance Confocal Microscopy for Skin Diseases*,
DOI 10.1007/978-3-642-21997-9_29,

planopilaris. Regarding the histopathologic features we can find compact orthohypokeratosis overlying an epidermis that shows wedge-shaped thickening of the granular cell layer and a "sawtooth" pattern of acanthosis is prototypic for lichen planus. A dense, bandlike lymphocytic infiltrate obscures the dermoepidermal junction; in our lexicon, this is the defining feature of a lichenoid dermatitis [2]. Lichen follicularis represents a variant of lichen planus involving focally the hair follicle with hair loss and histologically characterized by a sort of "jumping" involvement of the skin with respect of the interadnexal epidermis; another variant of lichen, as previously reported, is called lichen planopilaris and is characterized by the involvement of both epidermis and adnexal structures. In this last variant, some or all the inflammatory papules are follicular and it is often characterized by scarring alopecia of the scalp, but not elsewhere [5].

29.2 RCM Features of Lichenoid Dermatitis

For both the entities, skin lupus and lichen planus, several experiences with the use of RCM have been already collected [6]. The data obtained disclosed that RCM is useful for interface dermatitis identification as a main feature of this group of entities. In particular, RCM demonstrated to be able to show, with high grade of correspondence with optical microscopy, the interface involvement as the presence of inflammatory cells infiltrate disposed in sheets or focally obscuring the DEJ. Using RCM on affected skin, all the different skin layers can be evaluated disclosing microscopical changes in common with the different interface dermatitis or differently specific, as the presence of inflammatory cells at the level of the epidermis seen as round to polygonal bright structures in the context of variable degree of spongiosis (see chapter on semeiology), the loss of the normal honeycombed-like architecture of the epidermis, or the presence of necrotic keratinocytes (possible in lupus and really common and specific for lichen planus in which are named Civatte Bodies) seen as mildly bright, polygonal structures larger than surrounding keratinocytes and that seem to be leaned on the epithelium. In all the interface dermatitis, looking at the level of the DEJ, the main and distinctive criteria is represented by the presence of the inflammatory involvement of the epidermis at the level of the dermo-epidermal interface; in particular, the papillary rims, usually visible in normal skin, are obscured by the presence of a sparse to a diffuse inflammatory cells infiltrate disposed in sheets or focally involving the junction. In particular, a diffuse involvement of the junction is more typical for lichen planus than lupus erythematosus in which the DEJ involvement is typically focal. Moreover, in lupus, presence of inflammatory infiltrate of the adnexal epithelium can be seen in most of the cases as round-to-polygonal, mildly refractile cells around and inside the adnexal epithelium between keratinocytes and generally associated with dilated adnexal ostia (larger than 80–100 μm) and accumulation of highly refractile material in the lumen corresponding to hyperkeratotic infundibula. At the level of the upper dermis, dilated vessels, diffused and aggregates of inflammatory cells can be seen associated with thickening of stroma fibers. The last feature is more commonly seen in long standing lupus [6]. Differently, the involvement of the adnexal structure in lichen is generally seen in the case of lichen planus pilaris or lichen follicularis, but less visible in the case of lichen planus.

In conclusion, in spite of the possibility to easily discriminate an interface dermatitis from other groups of inflammatory skin disorders, it is more difficult to identify the sub-type of interface dermatitis (lupus vs lichen) because of the few and little microscopical differences existing.

The point is that RCM is a clinical tool, thus the identification of the microscopical changes in real time have to be used in association with the clinical aspect of the lesion examined in order to contribute to the diagnosis and differential diagnosis. The clinical differentiation between lupus and lichen represents a problem in a very small number of cases, while the possibility to discriminate a spongiotic or a hyperkeratotic diseases from an interface dermatitis, in real time and non invasively, is desired and helpful in daily clinical practice.

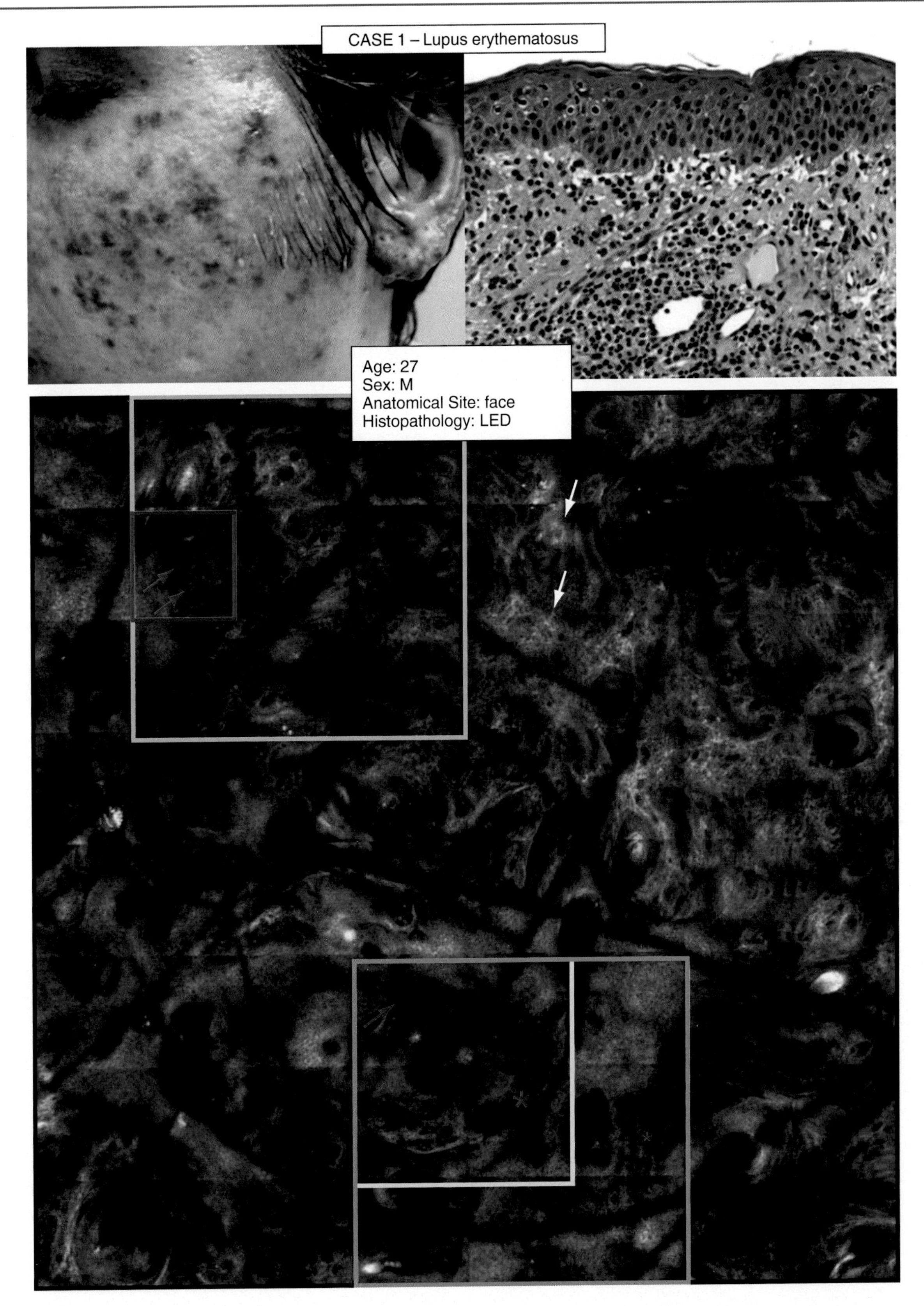

Fig. 29.1 RCM mosaic image (4 × 4) at the level of the upper dermis showing the presence of peri-adnexal epithelium inflammatory infiltrate (*red arrows*), seen as round-to-polygonal, mildly refractile cells around and inside the adnexal epithelium between keratinocytes. Dilated vessels diffused (*red asterisk*) and aggregates of inflammatory cells can be seen associated with thickening of stroma fibers (*white arrows*)

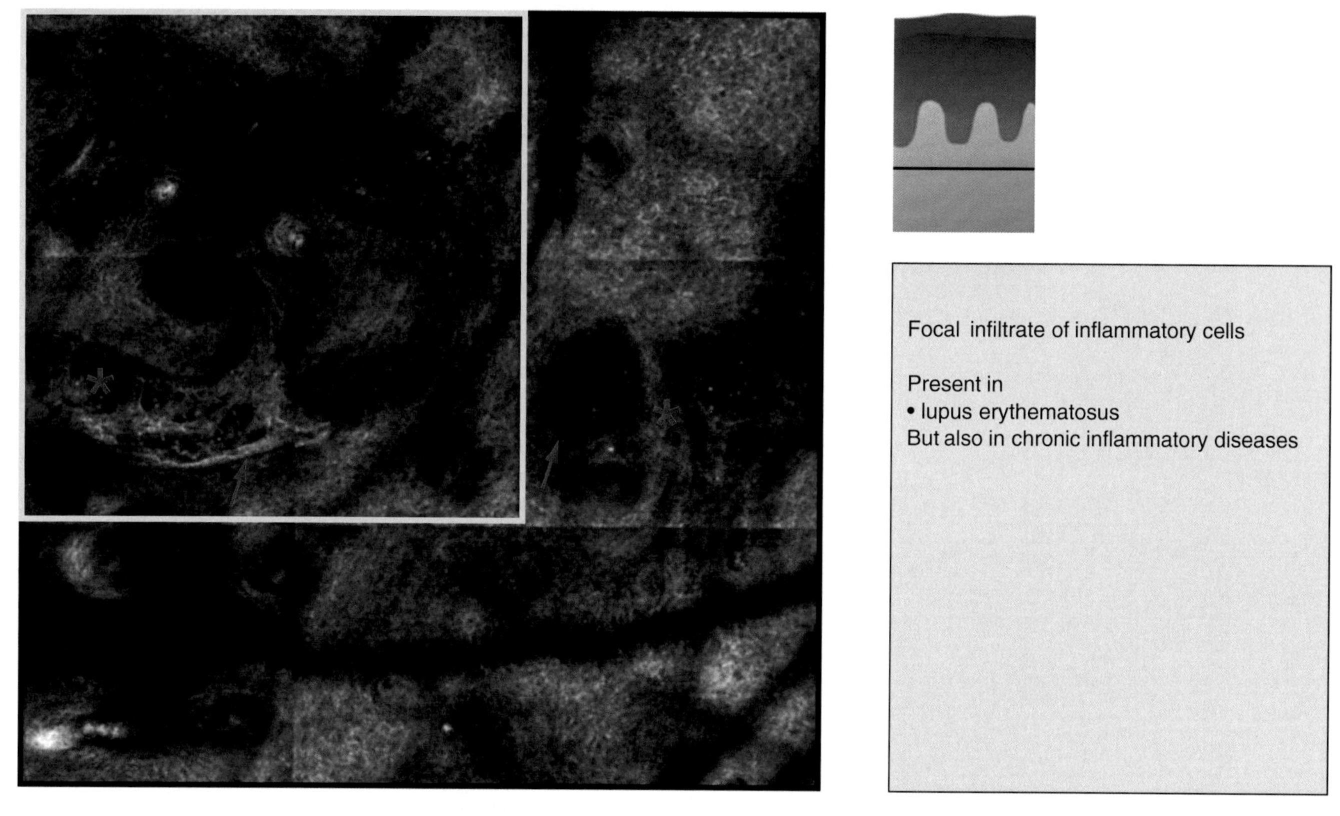

Fig. 29.1.1 RCM mosaic (1.5 × 1.5) showing dilated vessels (*red asterisks*) with perivascular infiltrate of inflammatory cells (*arrows*)

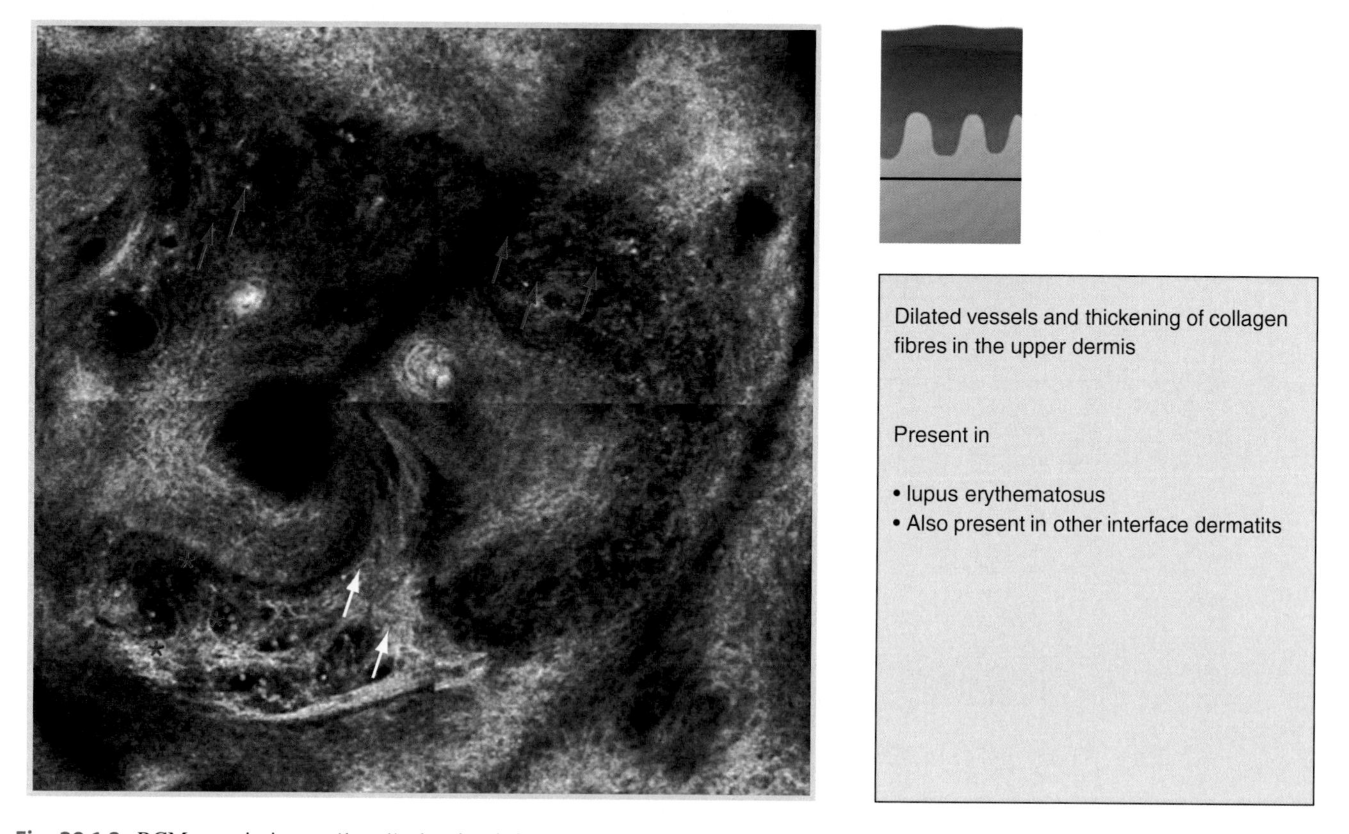

Fig. 29.1.2 RCM mosaic image (1 × 1) showing inflammatory cells (*red arrows*) in the superficial dermis, dilated vessels (*asterisks*) and thickening of collagen fibers (*white arrows*)

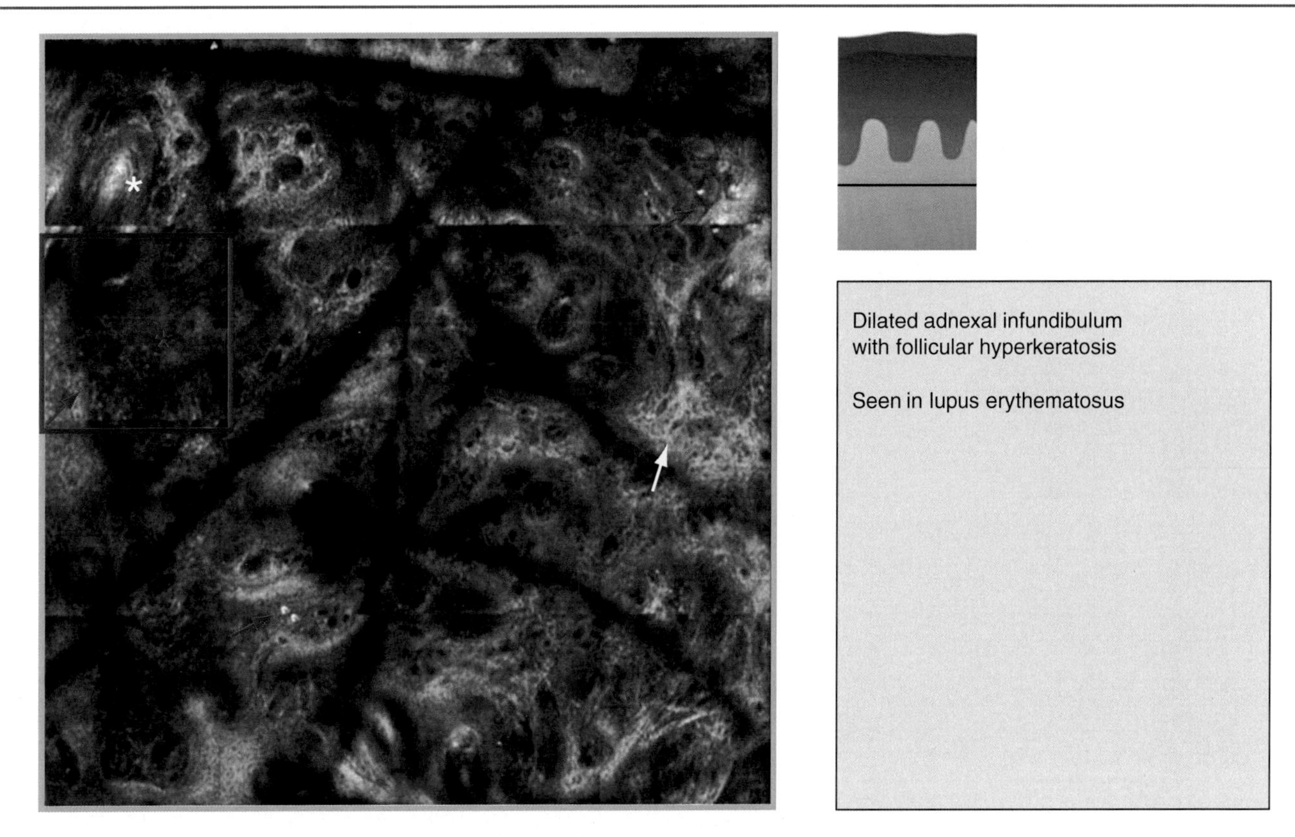

Fig. 29.1.3 RCM mosaic image (2 × 2) at the level of the upper dermis showing dilated adnexal infundibulum with follicular hyperkeratosis (*white asterisk*), periadnexal inflammatory cell infiltrate and sparse melanophages (*red arrows*) throughout degenerated collagen bundles (*white arrow*)

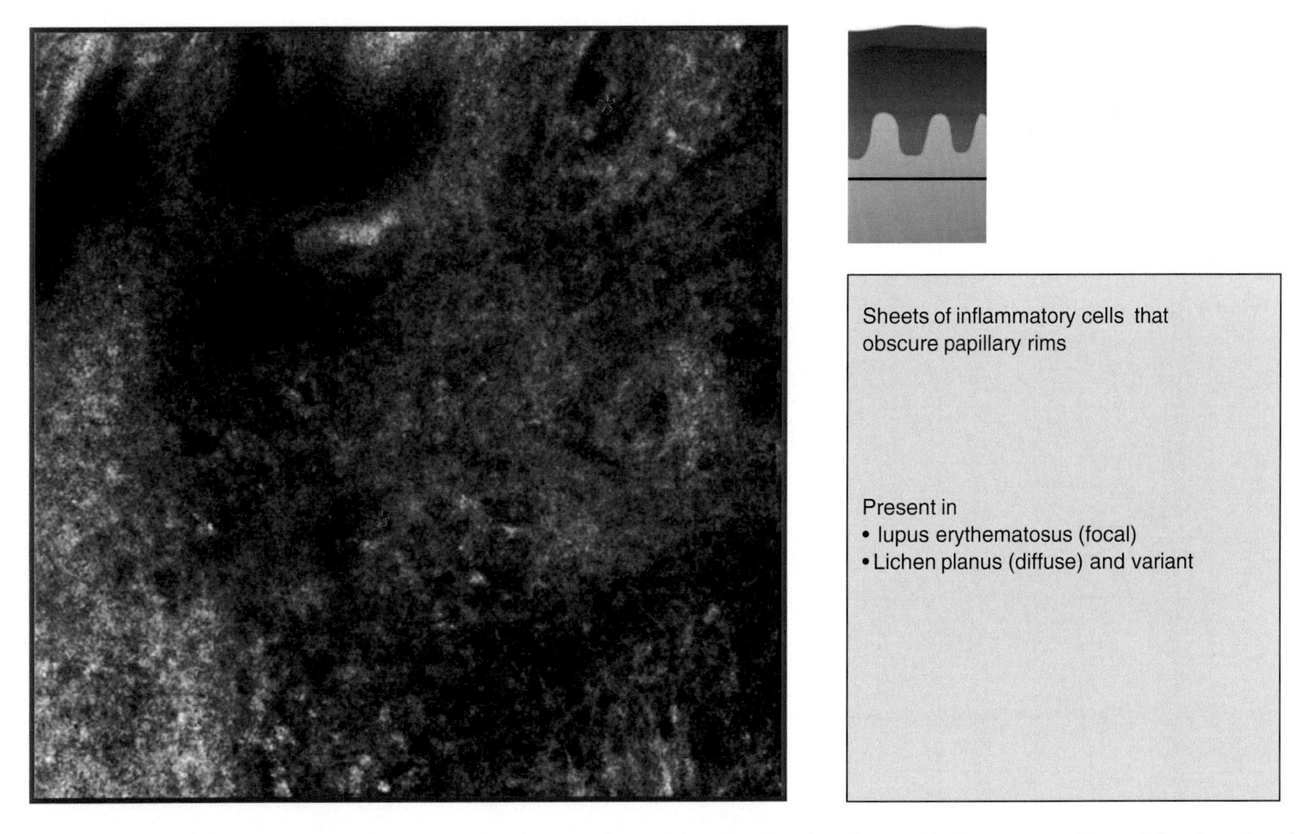

Fig. 29.1.4 RCM image (0.5 × 0.5) at the level of the dermal epidermal junction showing sheets of inflammatory cells partially obscuring the dermal-epidermal junction

CASE 2 – Lichen planus
Age: 73
Sex: F
Anatomical Site: leg

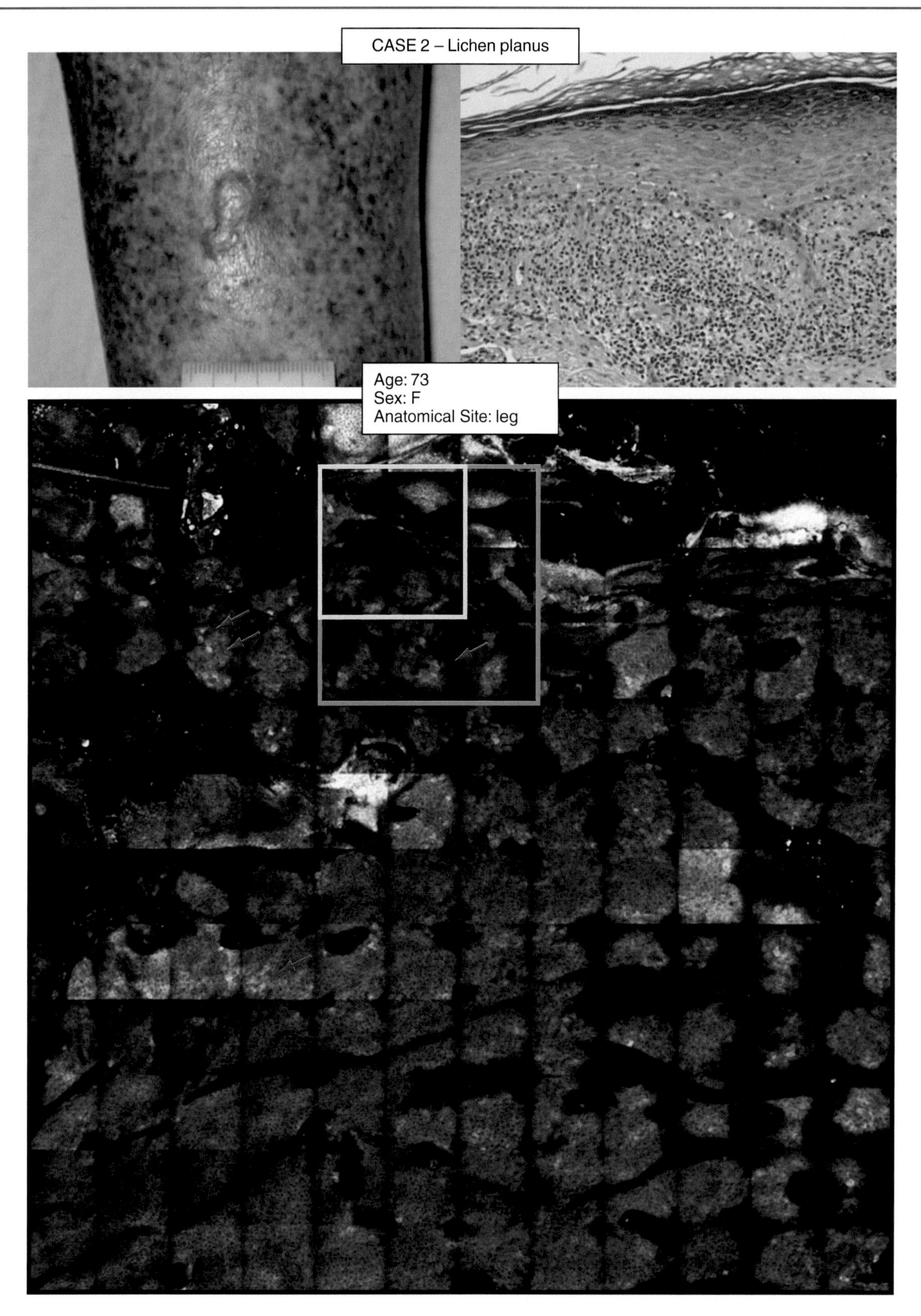

Fig. 29.2 RCM mosaic image (6 × 6) at the level of the spinous layer, showing the loss of the normal honeycombed-like architecture of the epidermis, and the presence of necrotic keratinocytes (*arrows*) seen as mildly bright, polygonal structures larger than surrounding keratinocytes and that seem to be leaned on the epithelium

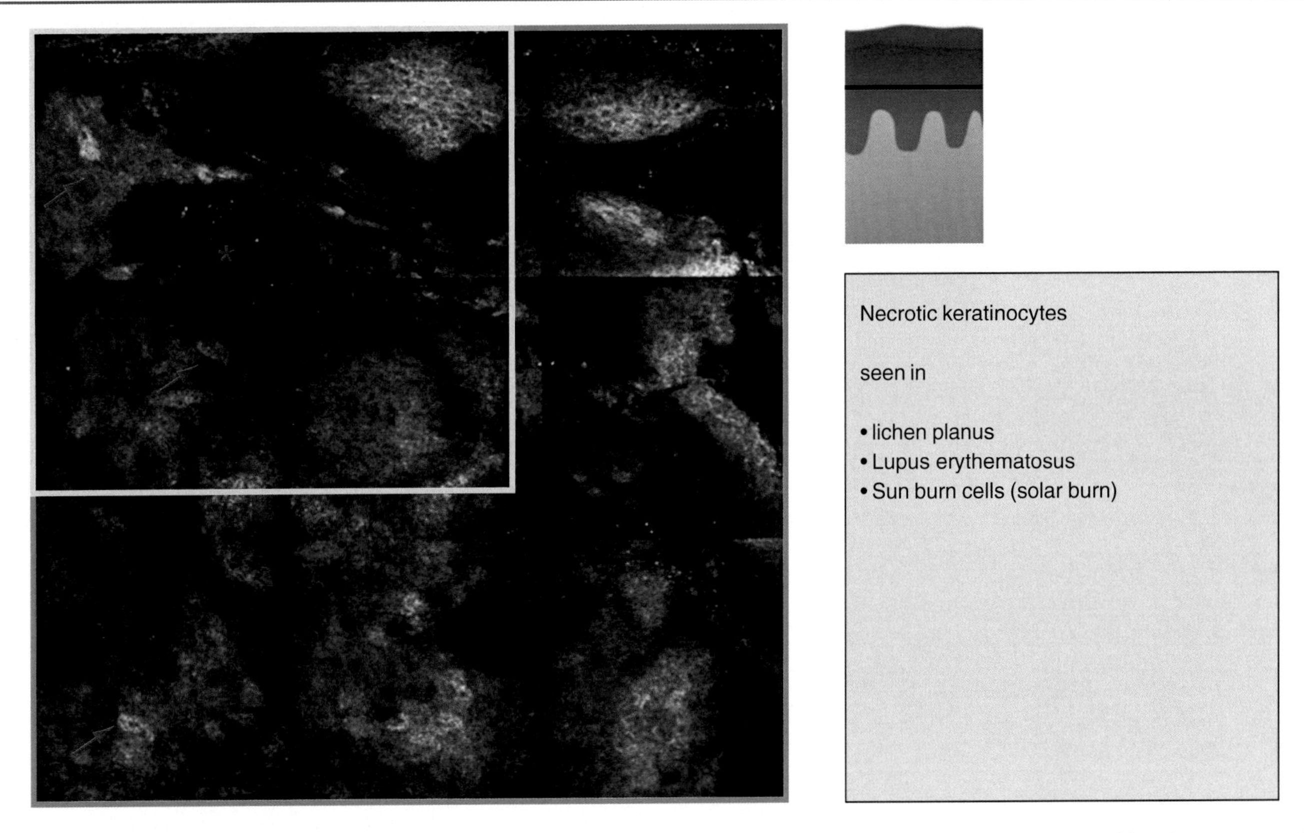

Fig. 29.2.1 RCM mosaic image (1.5 × 1.5) at the level of spinous layer that shows inflammatory cells at the level of the epidermis seen as round to polygonal bright structures in the context of spongiosis (*asterisk*) and a plenty of necrotic keratinocytes (*red arrows*)

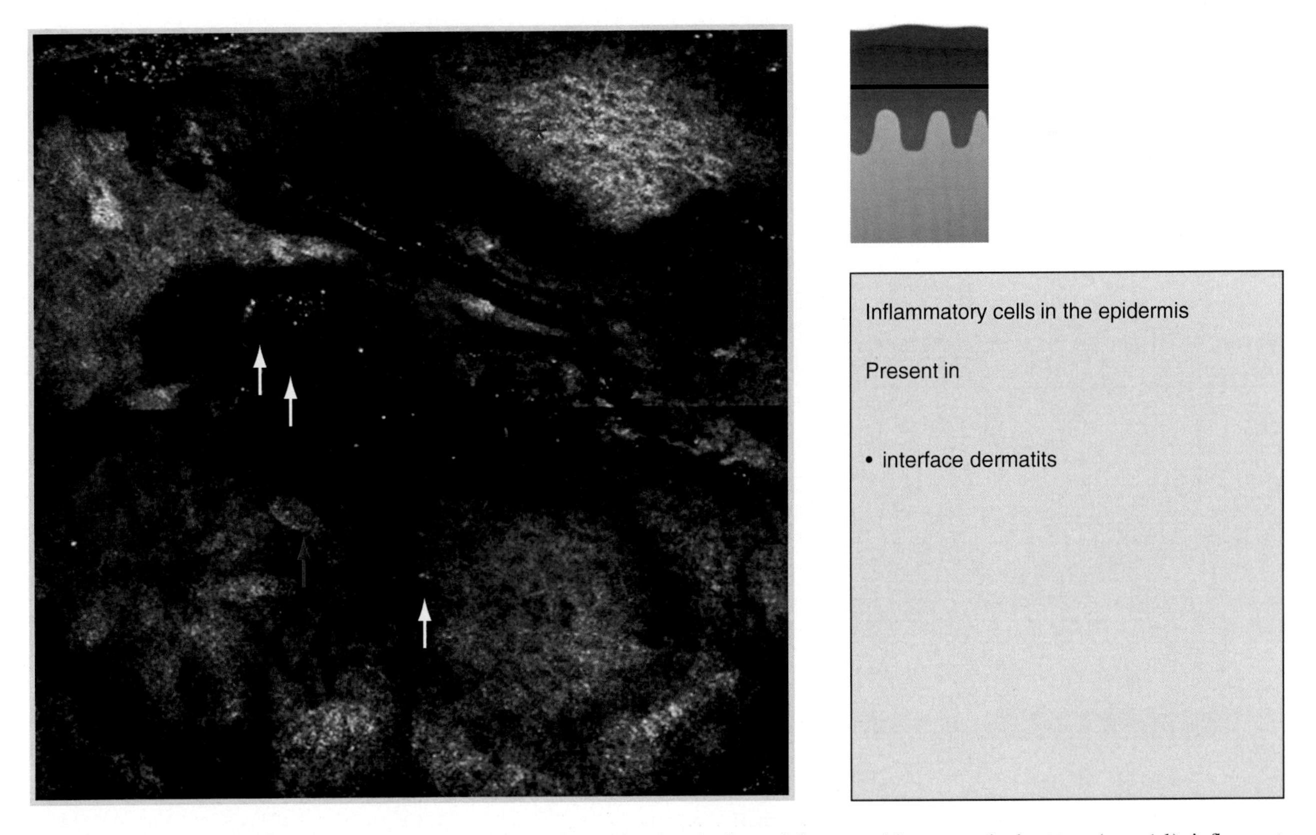

Fig. 29.2.2 RCM mosaic (1 × 1) at the level of the spinous layer showing the loss of the normal honeycombed pattern (*asterisk*), inflammatory cells (*white arrows*) both as single cells in the epidermis and in the area of spongiosis, and necrotic keratinocytes (*red arrow*)

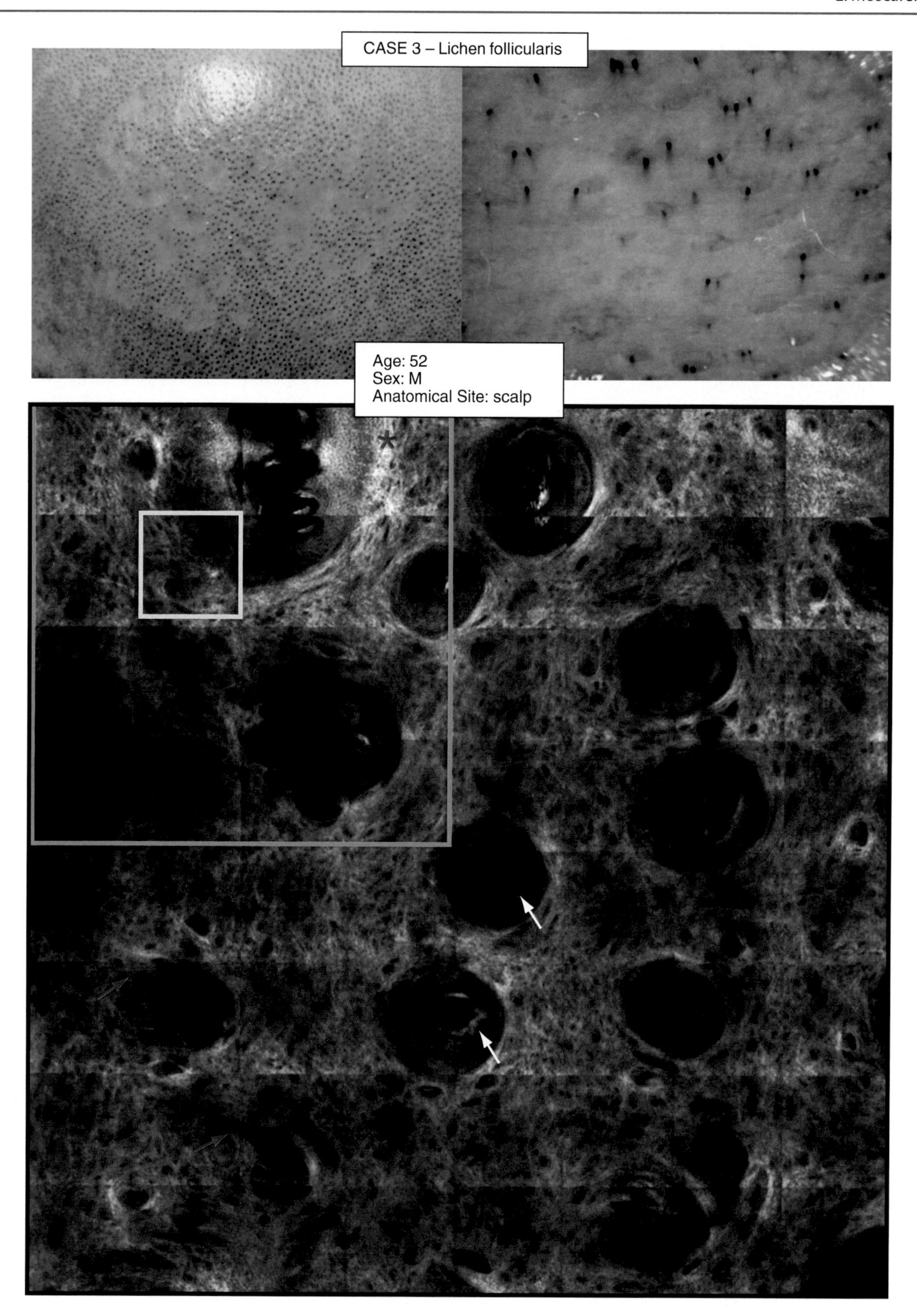

Fig. 29.3 RCM mosaic image (4 × 4) of a scalp at the level of the upper dermis. Follicular openings appear irregularly affected by the inflammatory infiltrate. Features of scarring alopecia can be visualized (*red arrow*), together with healthy follicles (*white arrows*). The presence of a perifollicular inflammatory infiltrate makes the follicular epithelium poorly distinguishable from the surrounding stroma (*red asterisk*)

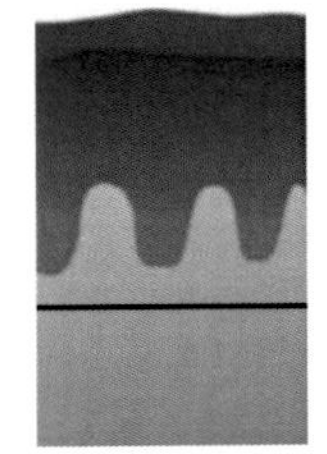

Perifollicular inflammatory infiltrate

Present in

- lichen follicularis and lichen planus pilaris
- lupus erythematosus

Fig. 29.3.1 RCM mosaic (2 × 2) at the level of the upper dermis showing ill-defined borders of the follicular epithelium, hair follicle is surrounded by dilated vessels and thickening of collagen bundles (*white arrow*)

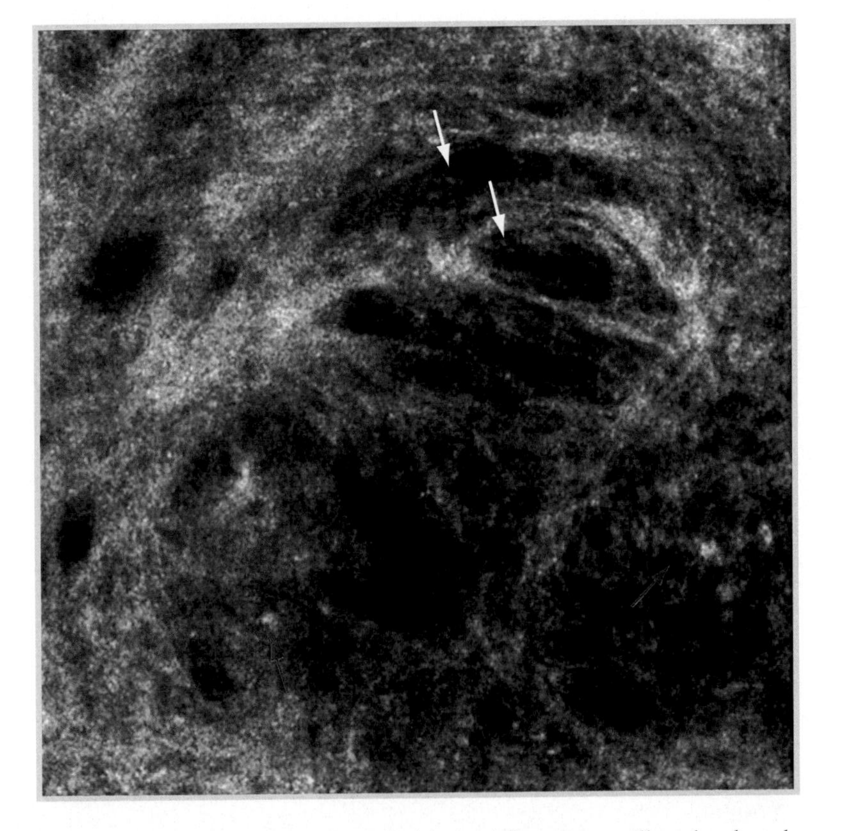

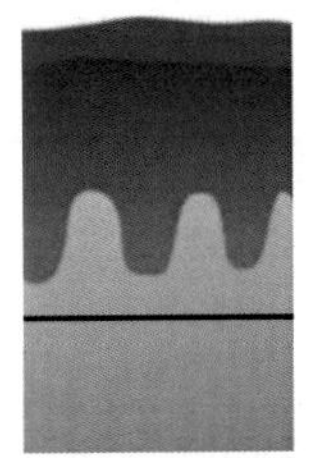

Perifollicular inflammatory infiltrate

Present in

- lichen follicularis and lichen planus pilaris
- lupus erythematosus

Fig. 29.3.2 RCM basic image (0.5 × 0.5) showing inflammatory cells and melanophages as roundish, bright cells within follicular epithelium, (*red arrows*) and dilated vessels (*white arrow*)

Table 29.1 Differences and common features of lupus and lichen planus

Lupus erythematosus	Lichen planus
1. Hypergranulosis	Hypergranulosis
2. Dilated, hyperkeratotic infundibula	Normal infundibula
3. Acanthosis to epidermal atrophy	Acanthosis to epidermal atrophy
4. Necrotic keratinocytes	Necrotic keratinocytes
5. Inflammatory cells in the epidermis	Inflammatory cells in the epidermis
6. Spongiosis	Moderate spongiosis
7. Interface changes 8. (focal)	Interface changes (diffuse)
9. Dilated vessels	Dilated vessels
10. Dermal inflammation	Dermal inflammation
11. Dermal sclerosis	Sparse dermal sclerosis

Core Messages

- The interface change is one of the main feature visible on RCM as the papillary rims, usually visible in normal skin, are obscured by the presence of a sparse to a diffuse inflammatory cells infiltrate disposed in sheets or focally involving the junction.
- Discrimination of lupus from lichen derives from the identification of the distribution of interface changes (focal in lupus and diffuse in lichen), and collection of secondary criteria.
- RCM can be useful both for diagnosis and differential diagnosis as well as for the treatment follow-up.

References

1. Hussein M-RA, Aboulhagag NM, Atta HS, Atta SM (2008) Evaluation of the profile of the immune cell infiltrate in lichen planus, discoid lupus erythematosus, and chronic dermatitis. Pathology 40(7):682–693
2. Crowson AN, Magro CM, Mihm MC (2008) Interface dermatitis. Arch Pathol Lab Med 132(4):652–666
3. Crowson AN, Magro CM (2001) The cutaneous pathology of lupus erythematosus: a review. J Cutan Pathol 28:1–23
4. Magro CM, Crowson AN, Harrist TJ (1996) The use of antibody to C5b-9 in the subclassification of lupus erythematosus. Br J Dermatol 134:855–862
5. Cainelli T, Giannetti A, Rebora A. Manuale di Dermatologia Medica e Chirurgica. McGraw-Hill
6. Ardigò M, Maliszewski I, Cota C, Scope A, Sacerdoti G, Gonzalez S, Berardesca E (2007) Preliminary evaluation of in vivo reflectance confocal microscopy features of Discoid lupus erythematosus. Br J Dermatol 156:1196–1203

Pigmentary Skin Disorders

30

Marina Agozzino, Elvira Moscarella,
and Marco Ardigò

30.1 Introduction

Acquired pigmentary skin disorders are common and therapeutically problematic skin diseases involving the skin of every age subjects. They are clinically classified in two main groups: hyperpigmented and hypopigmented disorders.

Acquired hyperpigmentations are characterized by the development of pigmented macules, generally involving the skin of sun-exposed areas, generally the face, with the tendency to confluence in larger areas of the skin. Microscopically the pigment can be confined in the epidermis (brown macules) or in the dermis (grey/blue macules), or can involve the two skin layers (brown to blue macules); the identification of its prevalent localization influences significantly the treatment selection [1]. The two most common hyperpigmetary conditions are melasma/chloasma and post-inflammatory pigmentation.

On the other side, the most common skin disorder characterized by the development of white skin macules, due to the reduction or disappearing of melanocytes from the dermo-epidermal junction, is vitiligo. The effective possibility to evaluate both the absence or reduction of melanocytes at the level of the DEJ as well as the increased pigmentation of keratinocytes, melanocytes activity, and increased amount of melanophages in the dermis has been already demonstrated with success in literature.

The clinical diagnosis of pigmentary disorders is generally sufficient; in some of the cases, skin biopsy can be useful, but avoided by the patient and not possible to be used routinely in the therapeutical follow-up. RCM have been also demonstrated to be powerful in the follow-up and patients management giving the possibility of a fine modulation of the treatment and reducing side effects and monitoring the response to treatment [2, 3].

30.2 Vitiligo and Its RCM Presentation

Vitiligo is a chronic disease characterized by circumscribed hypomelanotic maculae usually localized on face, dorsa of hands, genital areas, wrists, knees, with tendency to the diffusion all over the body. The occurrence of vitiligo is estimated to be approximately 1% in the U.S. and range from 0.5 to 2% worldwide [1, 4]. The average of age of onset is between the ages of 10 and 30 years but vitiligo can begin at any age. The prevalence seems to be the same in male and female, but is possible to observe an increased prevalence in patients affected by thyroid diseases and mellitus diabetes. This pathology is characterized by the disappearing of melanocytes and melanin from the epidermis and dermo-epidermal junction in involved skin. Three pathogenetic hypothesis have been postulated: according to the autoimmunitary theory the melanocytes are destroyed by activated lymphocytes; the neurogen hypothesis establishes that melanocytes destruction is due to the interaction between melanocytes and neurological cells; the auto destructive theory supposes that, during the normal melanin biosynthesis, some toxic substances destroy the melanocytes interacting with these [1, 5].

Vitiligo can be divided into four variations referred to as generalized, localized or segmental, universal and acrofacial (lip-tip) [4, 5]. This disease can be spread by reactive isomorphism or Koebner phenomenon, i.e. the induction of depigmentation after a local trauma.

30.2.1 RCM Features

RCM used on vitiligo lesional and non lesional skin provides, non invasively, microscopical informations useful for disease

M. Agozzino (✉) • E. Moscarella • M. Ardigò
San Gallicano Dermatological Institute, Rome, Italy
e-mail: marinaagozzino@gmail.com;
elvira.moscarella@gmail.com; ardigo@ifo.it

R. Hofmann-Wellenhof et al. (eds.), *Reflectance Confocal Microscopy for Skin Diseases*,
DOI 10.1007/978-3-642-21997-9_30, © Springer-Verlag Berlin Heidelberg 2012

management. In RCM, the en-face visualization of the skin layers of normal skin, melanin presents a higher reflectance index (1.7) in comparison with the total skin (1.4); therefore, melanocytes and pigmented keratinocytes are seen as bright structures on a dark background. Differently, vitiligo lesions show disappearance of the normal brightness at dermo-epidermal junction level with remnant of a "shadow" of the pre-existing papillary ring. Moreover, bright keratinocytes, seen in normal skin above the DEJ in higher phototypes, are generally absent in vitiligo lesions. The disappearance of brightness (i.e. pigment) at the dermo-epidermal junction level or above fits perfectly with the progressive loss of melanocytes and the reduction of epidermal pigmentation previously demonstrated with histopathology and histochemistry. Interestingly, non lesional skin of vitiligo patients shows an abnormal distribution pattern of brightness (i.e. pigment) at the dermo-epidermal junction. The characteristic ring structures are hardly recognizable, bright structures are incompletely distributed around the dermal papillae providing "half-ring" features or resembling "scalloped border-like" features. It has been speculated that these changes could derive from an initial and progressive disappearing of melanocytes or a congenital defective melanocyte distribution [2].

After UVB-narrow band treatment repigmented areas show a variable number of activated melanocytes located at the dermo-epidermal junction. Activated melanocytic cells can be seen as bipolar or stellate dendritic structures usually located around adnexal structures [2].

To note, decreased amount of pigment and melanocytes activity, generally associated with clinical and microscopical signs of inflammation, are typical of some inflammatory conditions like pityriasis, exitus of eczema etc., clinically characterized by whitening of the skin and have to be considered in differential diagnosis with vitiligo. In those cases, RCM let the confocalist to make an immediate differential diagnosis throughout the demonstration of persistence of pigmented keratinocytes and melanocytes at the DEJ (normal papillary rims) associated with bright, round, little structures in the epidermis, around dilated vessels and diffuse in the upper dermis as signs of inflammation.

30.3 Melasma/Chloasma and Postinflammatory Pigmentation and Their RCM Presentation

Melasma/chloasma is an acquired condition presenting hyperpigmented macules; usually it is localized on the sun-exposed skin of the face. This disease typically occurs in young women during the fertile age, being related to pregnancy or oral contraceptive pills use; in similar cases it can be related to endocrine disorders or hepatic diseases [4]. Oestrogen and progesterone seems to be involved in determine this pathology. Melasma/chloasma can be localized on the cheeks, forehead, nose, upper lip and chin and generally it is present with symmetrical localization. The macules are dark or clear brown with irregular borders. In many cases this condition may resolve after oral contraceptive interruption or few months after delivery; sometimes it could persist. A low percentage of affected individuals (10%) are men, particularly Latin American and Asians [5]. Effective treatment of melasma/chloasma are local combination of hydroquinone (2%) and tretinoin 0.025% or hydroquinone and glycolic acid, laser (erbium YAG, Q switched neodymium YAG, Q switched Ruby laser, Q switched Alexandrite and CO2 laser) and intense pulsed light (IPL) [6–9]. Sunscreen blocking UVA and UVB light should be used systematically in order to reduce the melanocytes activation and consequent pigment deposition [5].

30.3.1 RCM Features

Differently from the Wood light classification, that consider the melasma classifiable in three sub-groups (Epidermal type, Dermal type and Mixed type), RCM of melasma/chlosma lesions shows the presence of pigment located variable amount, but constantly involving all the three different skin layers (mixed type only):

- The epidermis, with increased number of bright keratinocytes (bright cobblestone pattern) that can be visible focally or in large aggregated in the normal honeycombed-like structure of the epidermis.
- The dermo-epidermal junction, with increased rimming around the dermal papillae or around adnexal epithelium that substitute the junctional rimming visible in other anatomical sites.
- The dermis, with presence of different number of melanophages, as polygonal bright structures, larger than inflammatory cells and smaller than neoplastic melanocytes when presenting dendritic feature.

Generally the pigment deposition involves prevalently the epidermis and the dermo-epidermal junction, but the presence of pigment in the dermis is constantly seen; recently, presence of bright pin-point elements that can correspond to "free" melanosomes in the upper dermis that have been lost from junctional defective or injured melanocytes [3].

Post-inflammatory pigmentations may occur at any site of previous existing acute or chronic inflammatory processes. Frequent causes of hyperpigmentations include: discoid lupus, sarcoid, chemical irritation, burns, lichen planus, irritant or allergic cutaneous dermatitis, acne, and many other cutaneous diseases or trauma [4]. It could be an esthetical problem especially for the patients with IV and V phototype [4]. The hyperpigmentation can appear as irregular macules generally of grey color (because the pigment is generally in deep dermis), but can be also brown in the early stage in which the epidermal component is more represented. Usually the lesions are asymptomatic and may occur in any cutaneous district. The epidermal component post-inflammatory hyperpigmentation has a good result with local hydroquinone [9] treatment. In some cases the macules resolve spontaneously, but this process usually takes long time. Otherwise the dermal hyper pigmentation may be permanent and does not respond to any treatment.

30.3.2 RCM Features

Differently from melasma/chloasma, RCM of post-inflammatory pigmentation is characterized by a typical distribution of pigment prevalently at the dermo-epidermal junction with the evidence of strongly bright rims associated with a variable involvement of the epidermis that is characterized by evident increased brightness of keratinocytes of the spinosum in early stage of the pigmentation, but by a less commonly seen bright cobblestone pattern than in melasma. Typically, no or closely absent bright melanophages in the upper dermis are seen in the postinflammatory pigmentation pattern of distribution of pigment. The last, does not fit with the histopathological description of the postinflammatory pigmentation in which melanophages has been described involving the deeper part of the papillary dermis and/or in reticular dermis [3]. The explanation of it can be related to the limit of penetration of the RCM in the skin tissue, but let the definition of the two pattern of distribution of pigment in melasma vs postinflammatory inflammation.

CASE 1 – Melasma
Age: 43
Sex: F
Anatomical Site: Face
History: since 4 years
hyperpigmented macules on the
skin of the face after pregnancy

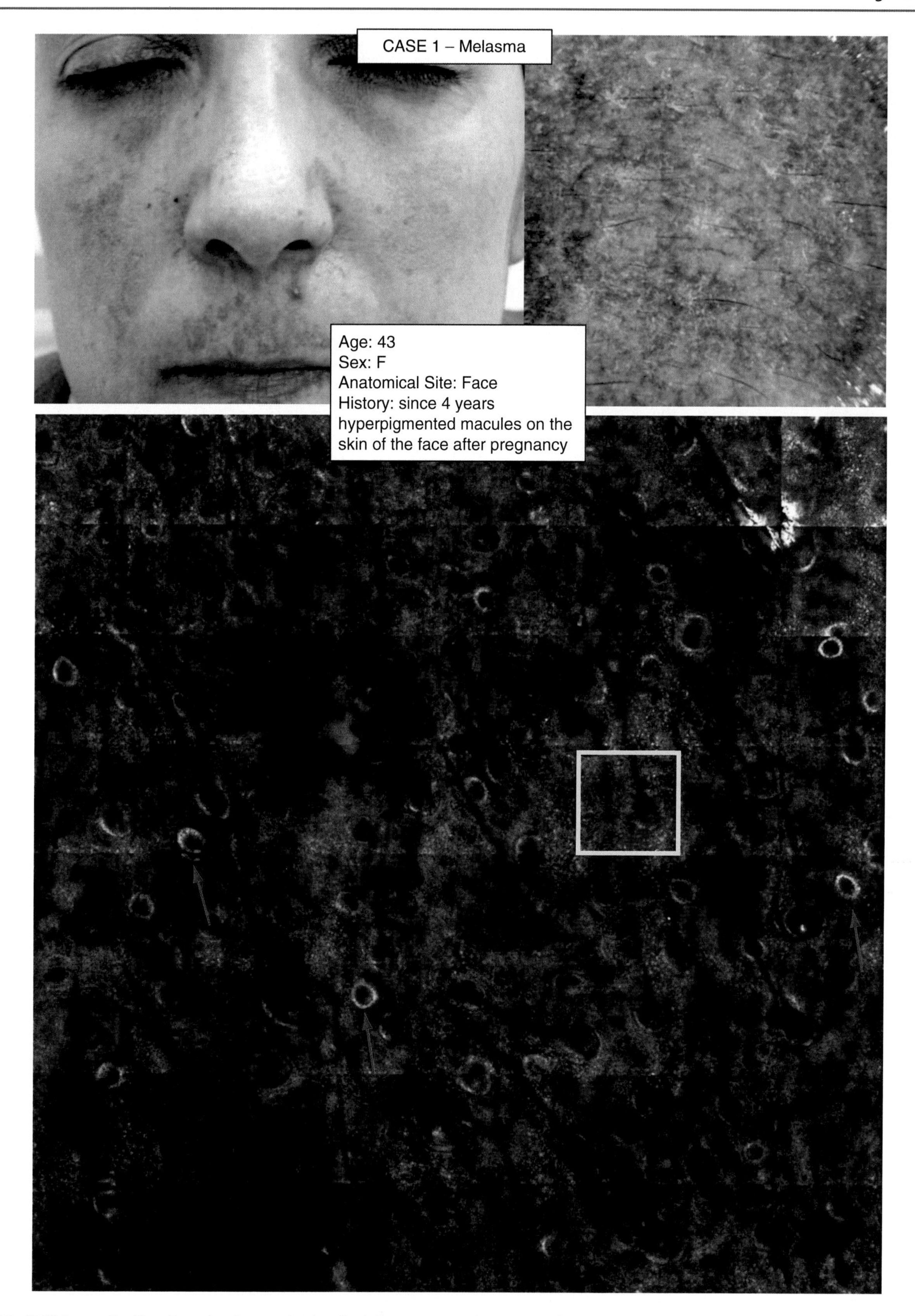

Fig. 30.1 RCM mosaic (4 × 4 mm) taken at the level of the stratum spinosum. Evidence of bright keratinocytes (*yellow square*) and focal periadnexal brightness (→) corresponding respectively to pigmented keratinocytes and increased pigmentation at the DEJ

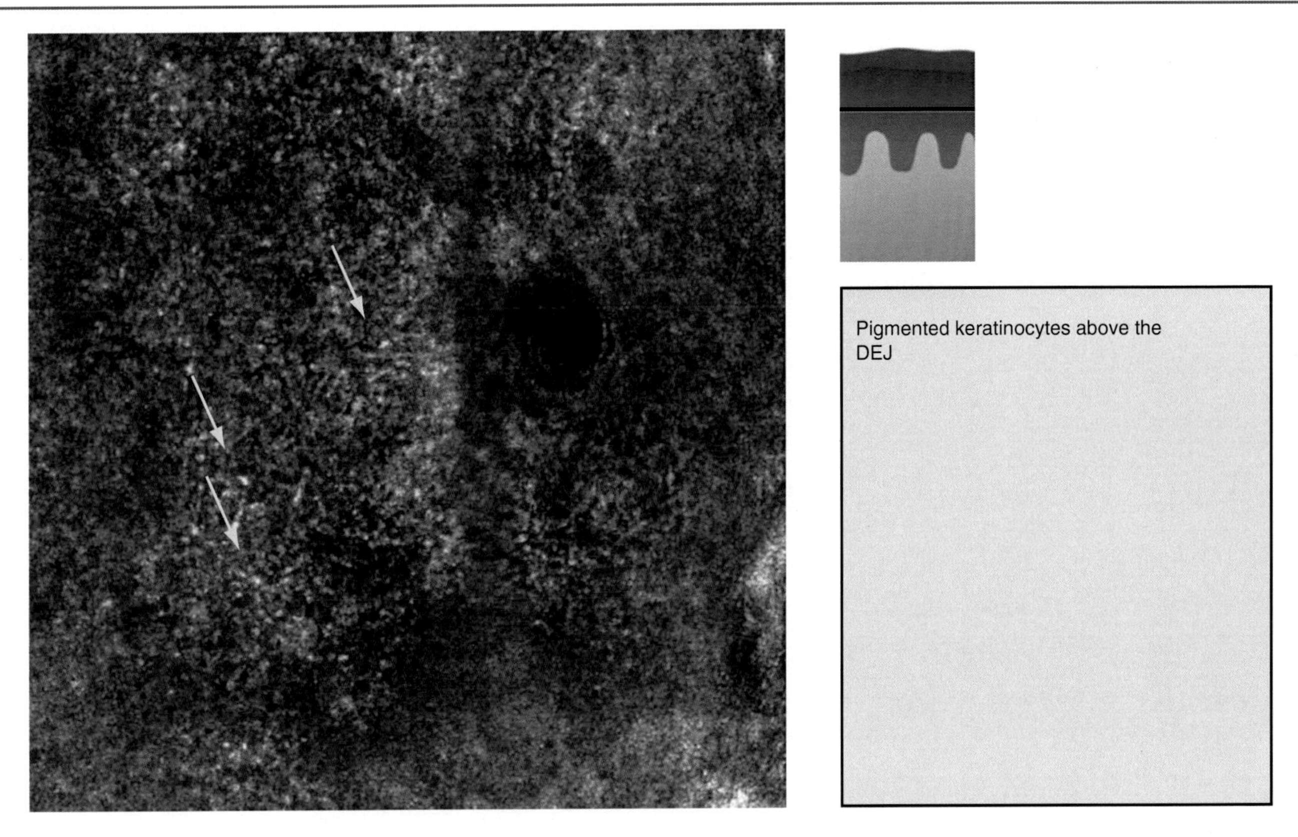

Fig. 30.1.1 Basic image (0.5 × 0.5 mm) as particular of the previous block at the level of the stratum spinosum. Presence of bright keratinocytes (→)

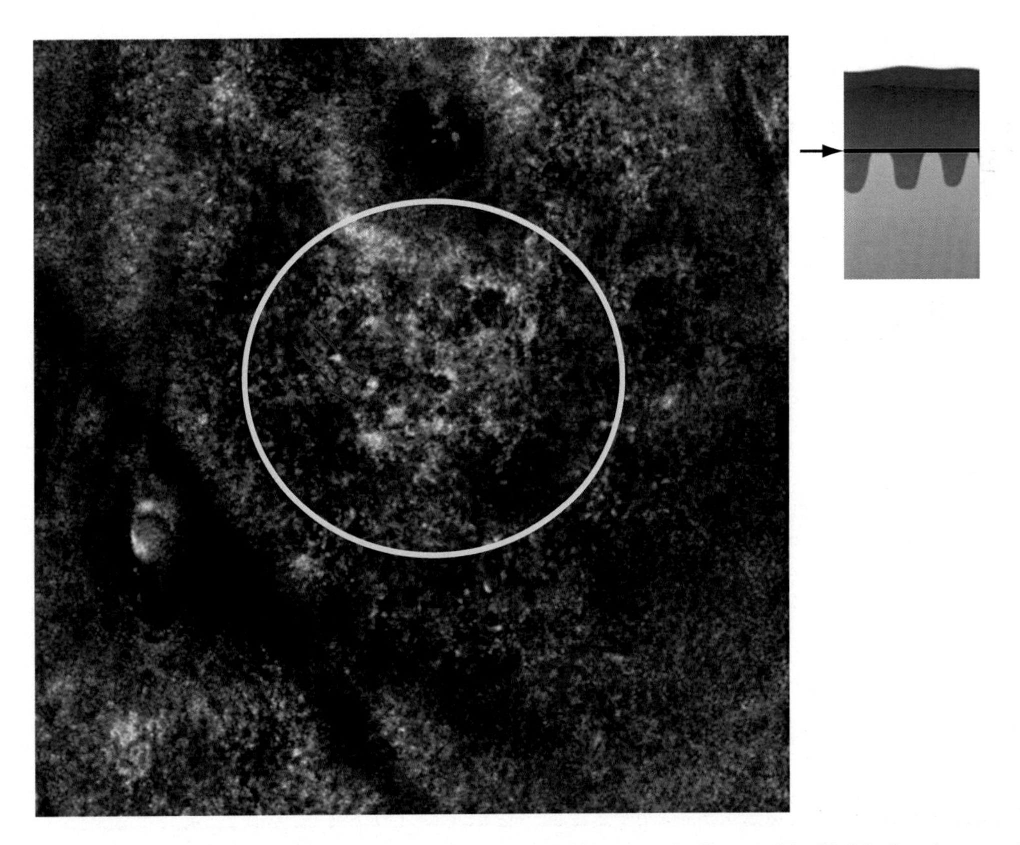

Fig. 30.2 Basic image (0.5 × 0.5 mm) at the supra-papillary plate, evidence of aggregate (*yellow circle*) of bright keratinocytes (→)

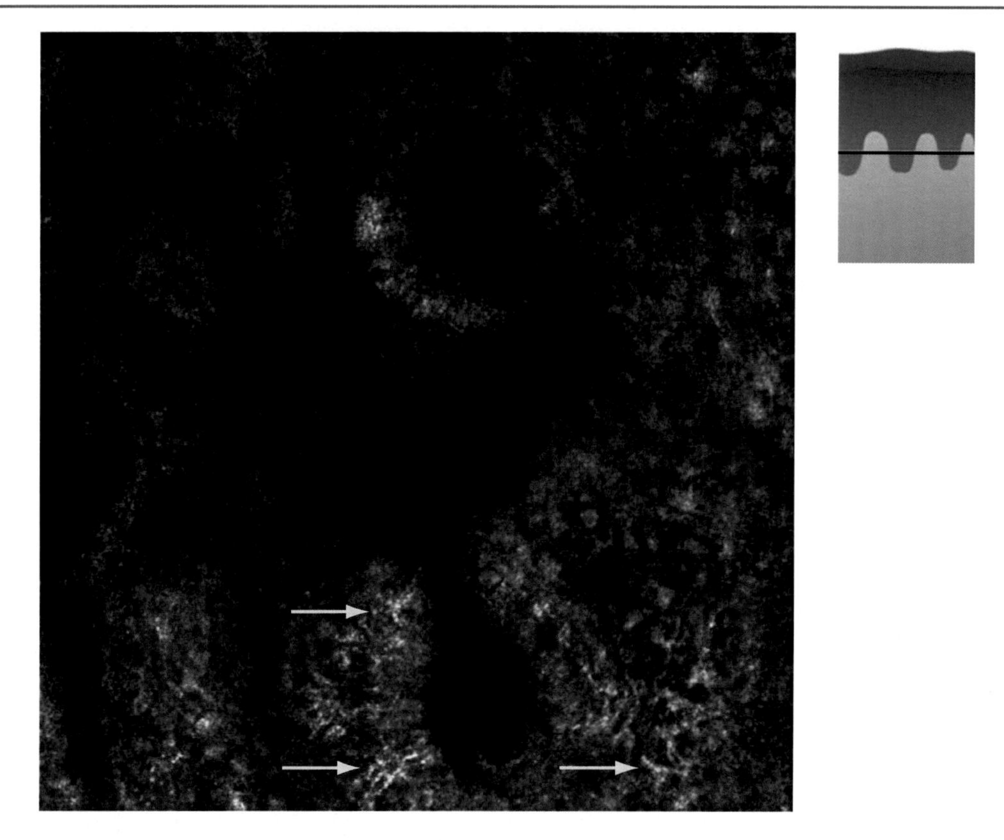

Fig. 30.3 RCM mosaic (0.5 × 0.5 mm) at the DEJ with increased rimming around the adnexal epithelium that substitute the junctional rimming on the face. To note the bright dendritic structures partially composing the rim that could correspond to activated melanocytes

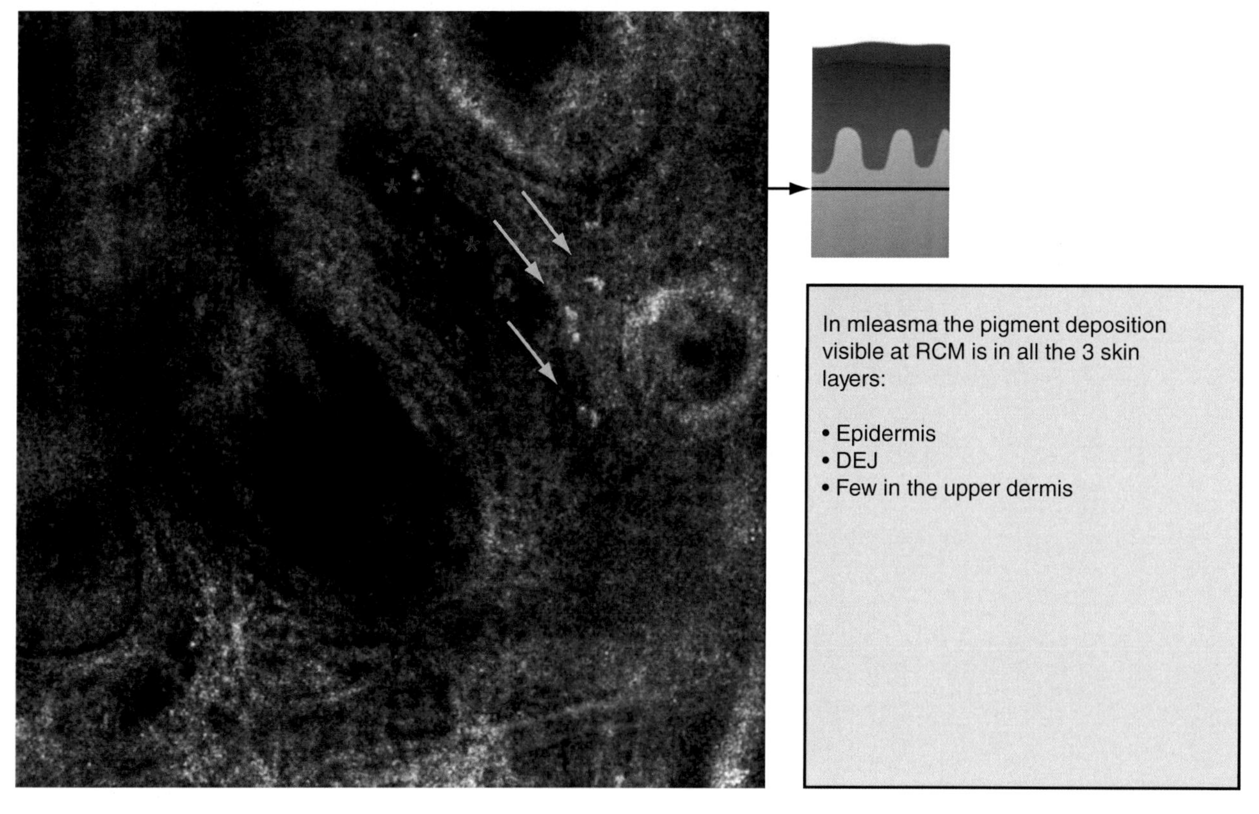

Fig. 30.4 Basic image (0.5 × 0.5 mm) presence of polygonal, bright cellular structure larger than inflammatory cells (→) corresponding to melanophages, located at the level of the dermis and located close to a blood vessel (*)

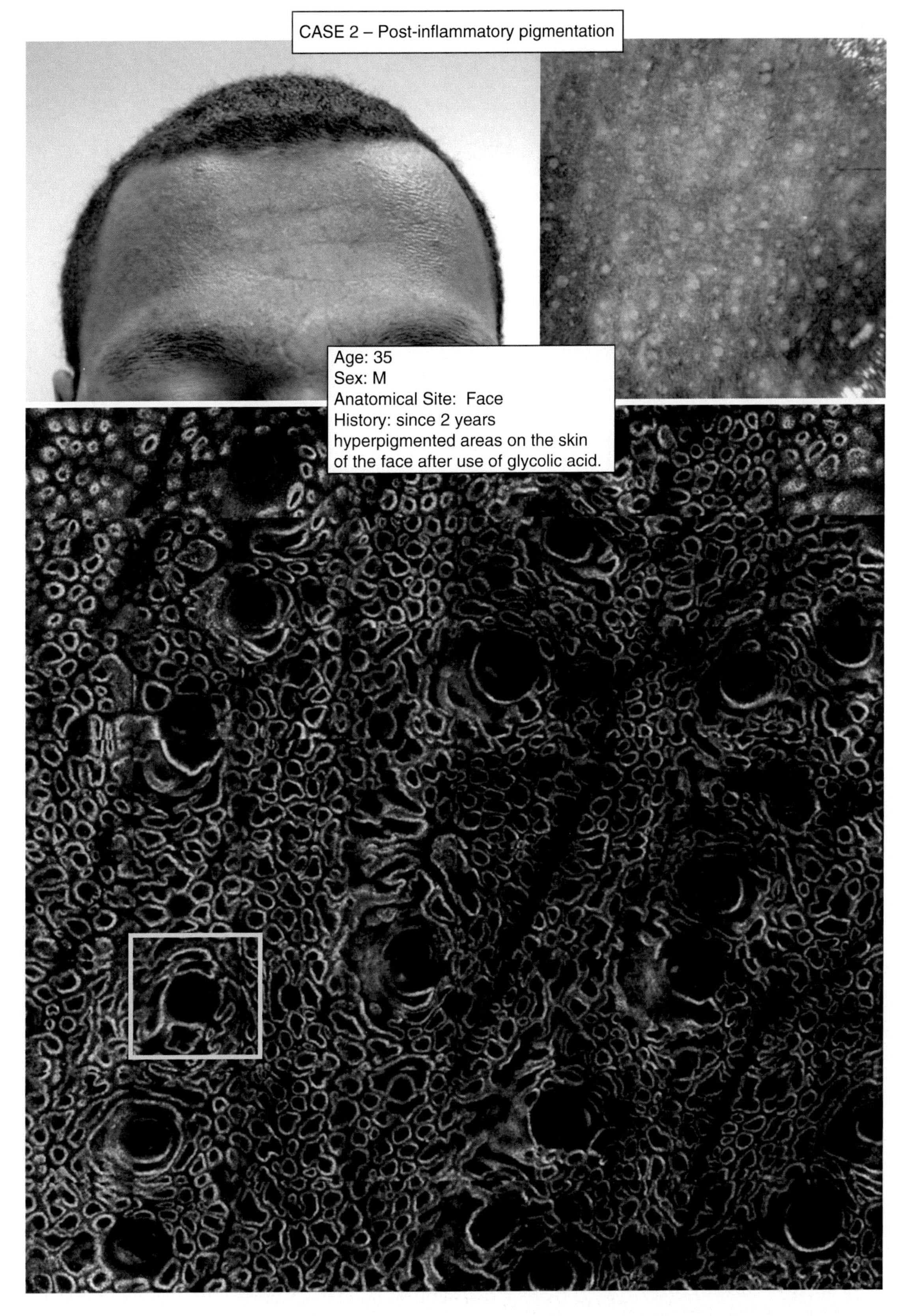

Fig. 30.5 RCM mosaic (3 × 3 mm) at the DEJ. Evidence of strongly bright rims around dermal papillae and adnexal structures

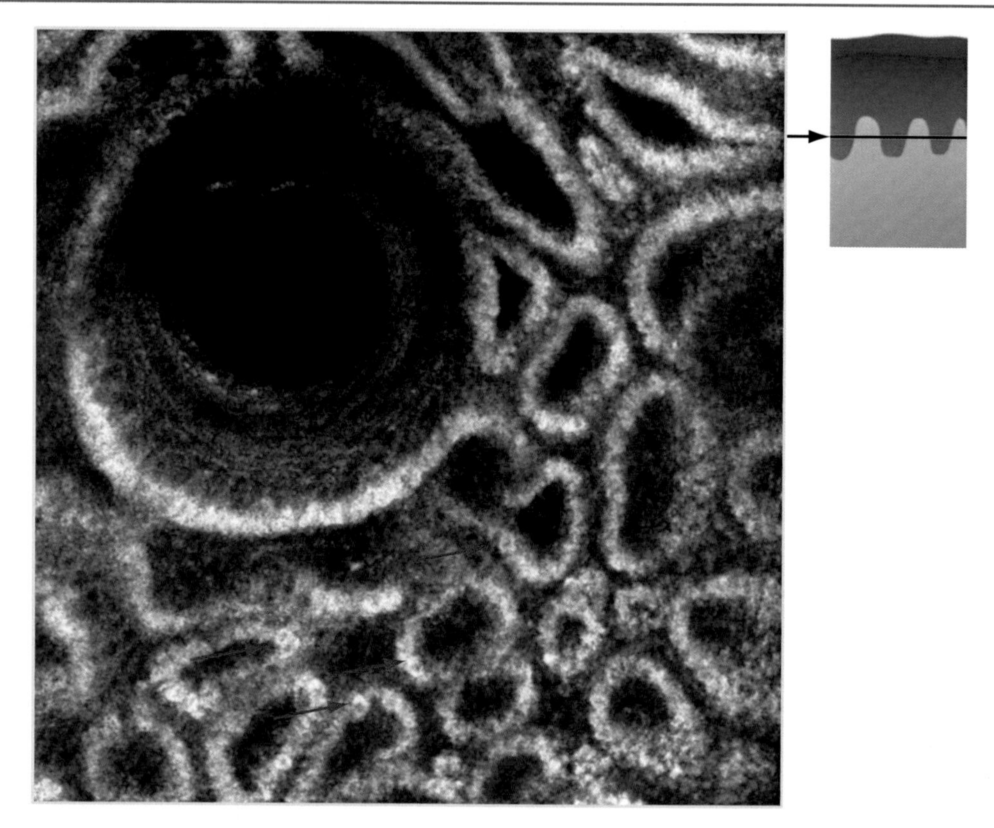

Fig. 30.5.1 Basic image (0.5 × 0.5 mm) as a particular of a previous block. Presence of strongly brightness of basal cells of the adnexal epithelium. To note the appearance of cells with bright cytoplasm and dark nuclei (→) at the DEJ and the circular arrangement of basilar keratinocytes around dermal papillae

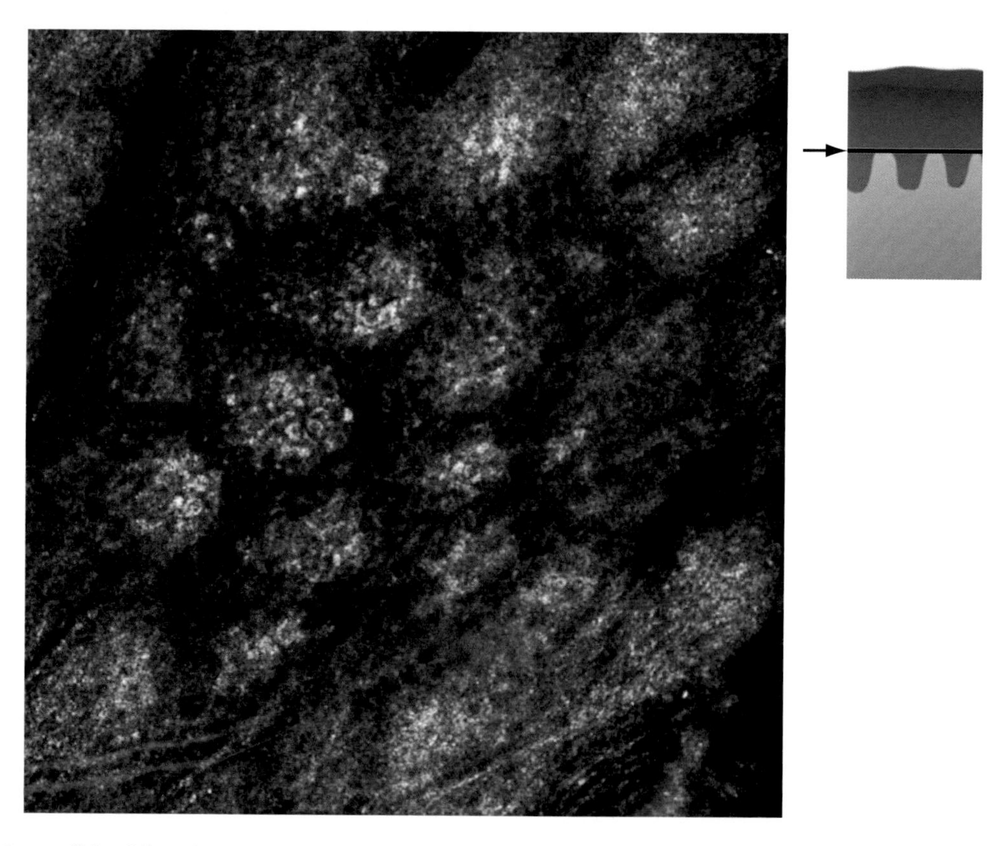

Fig. 30.6 Basic image (0.5 × 0.5 mm) suprapapillary plate evidence of bright cobblestone pattern

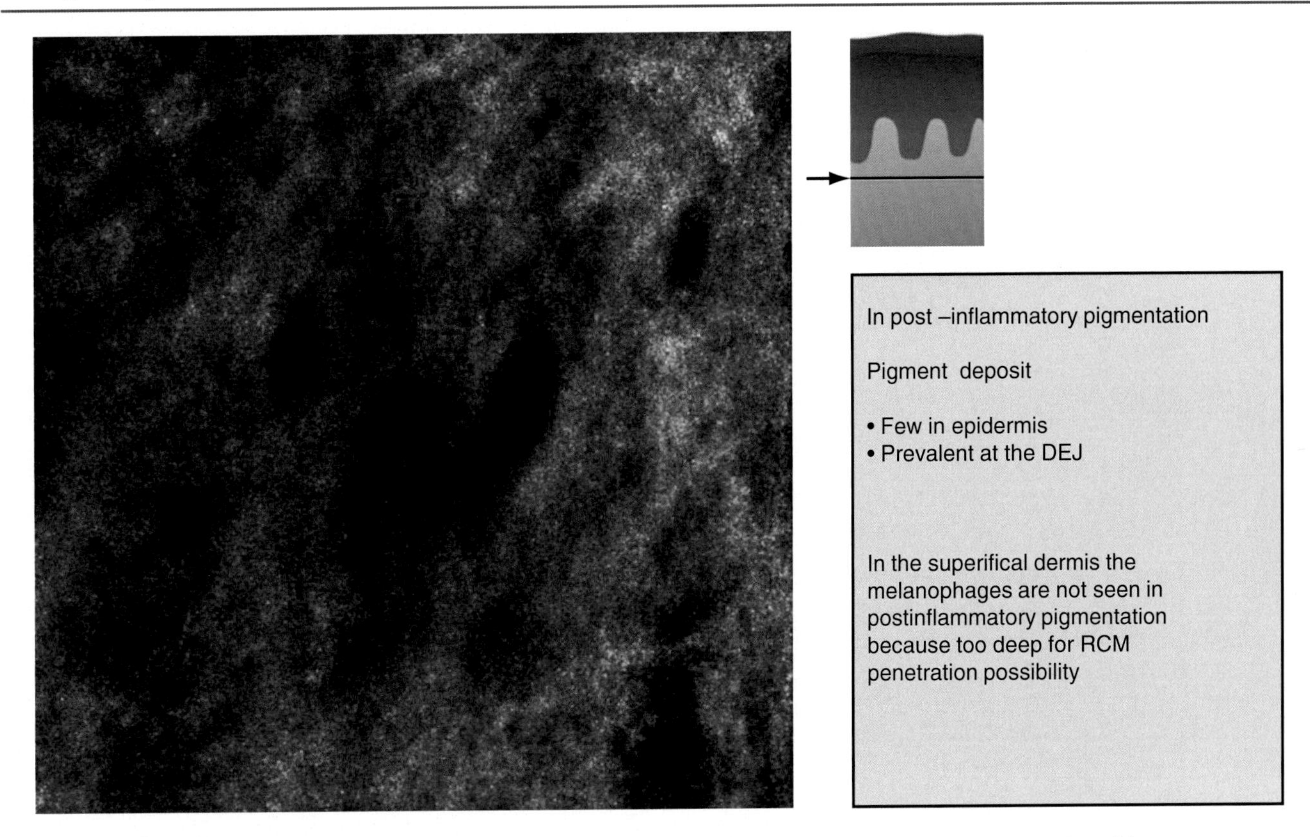

Fig. 30.7 Basic image (0.5 × 0.5 mm) taken at the level of the superficial dermis disclosing the absence of pigment deposition

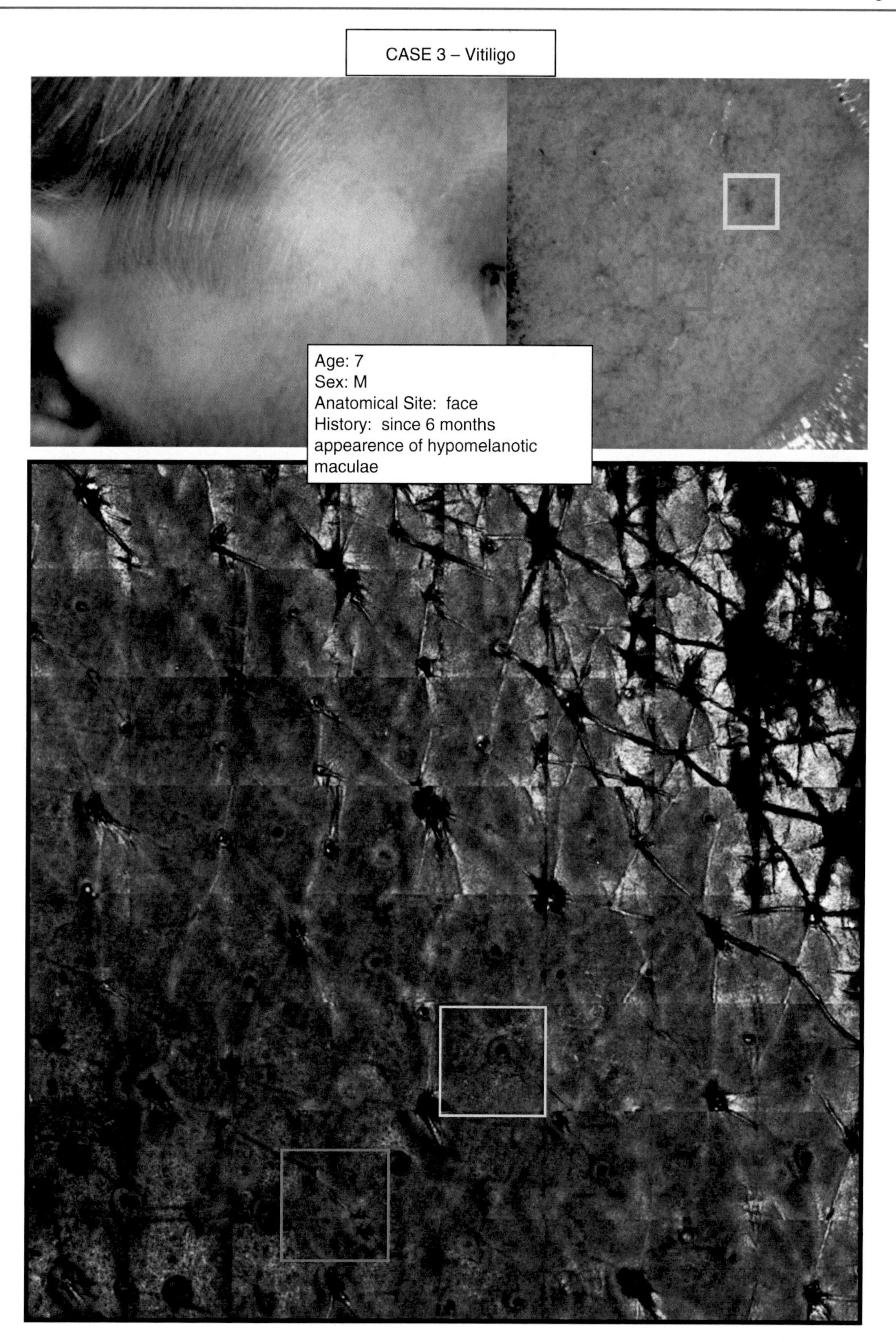

Fig. 30.8 RCM mosaic (4 × 4 mm) at the level of the stratum spinosum absence of epidermal pigmentation. Particular of repigmented area (*yellow box*) with presence of dendritic bright structures around adnexal epithelium

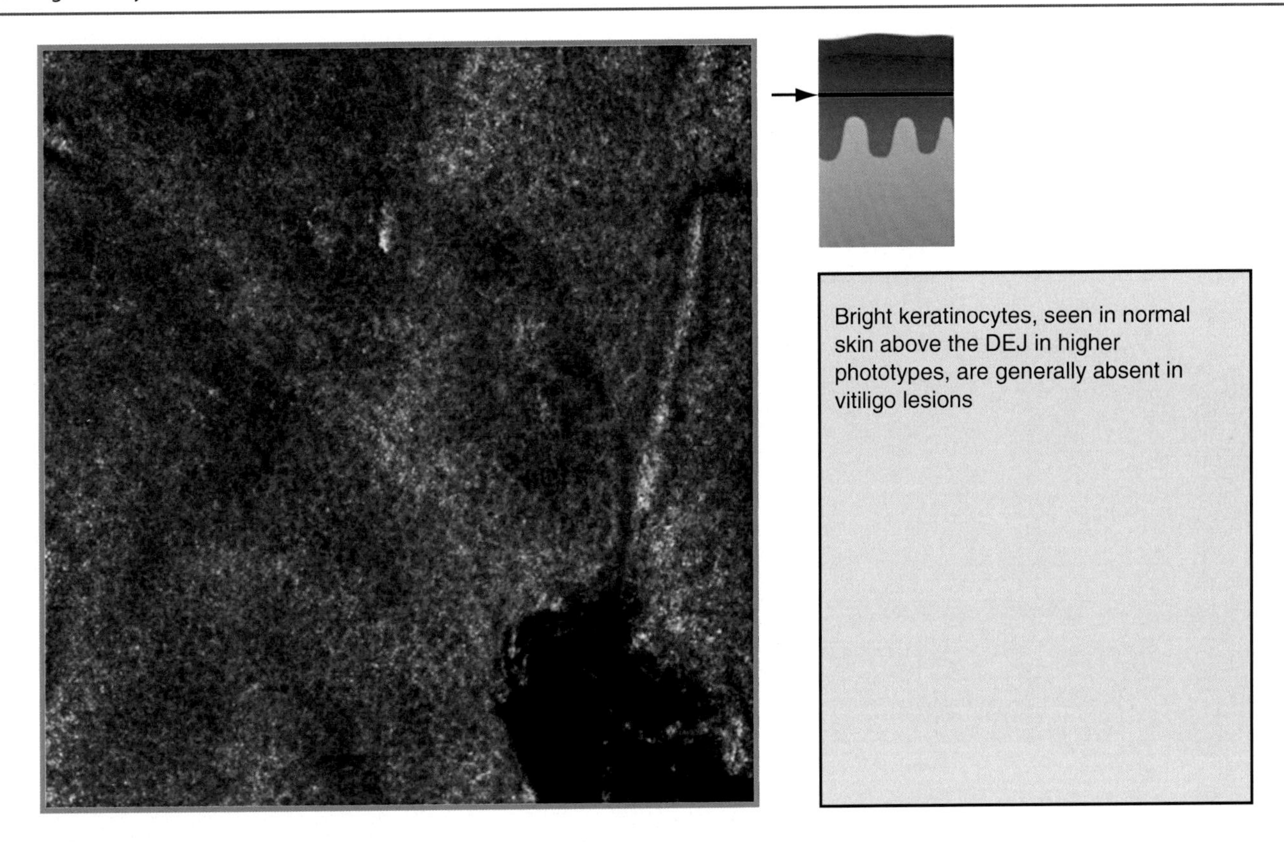

Fig. 30.8.1 Basic image (0.5 × 0.5 mm) normal honeycombed epidermis

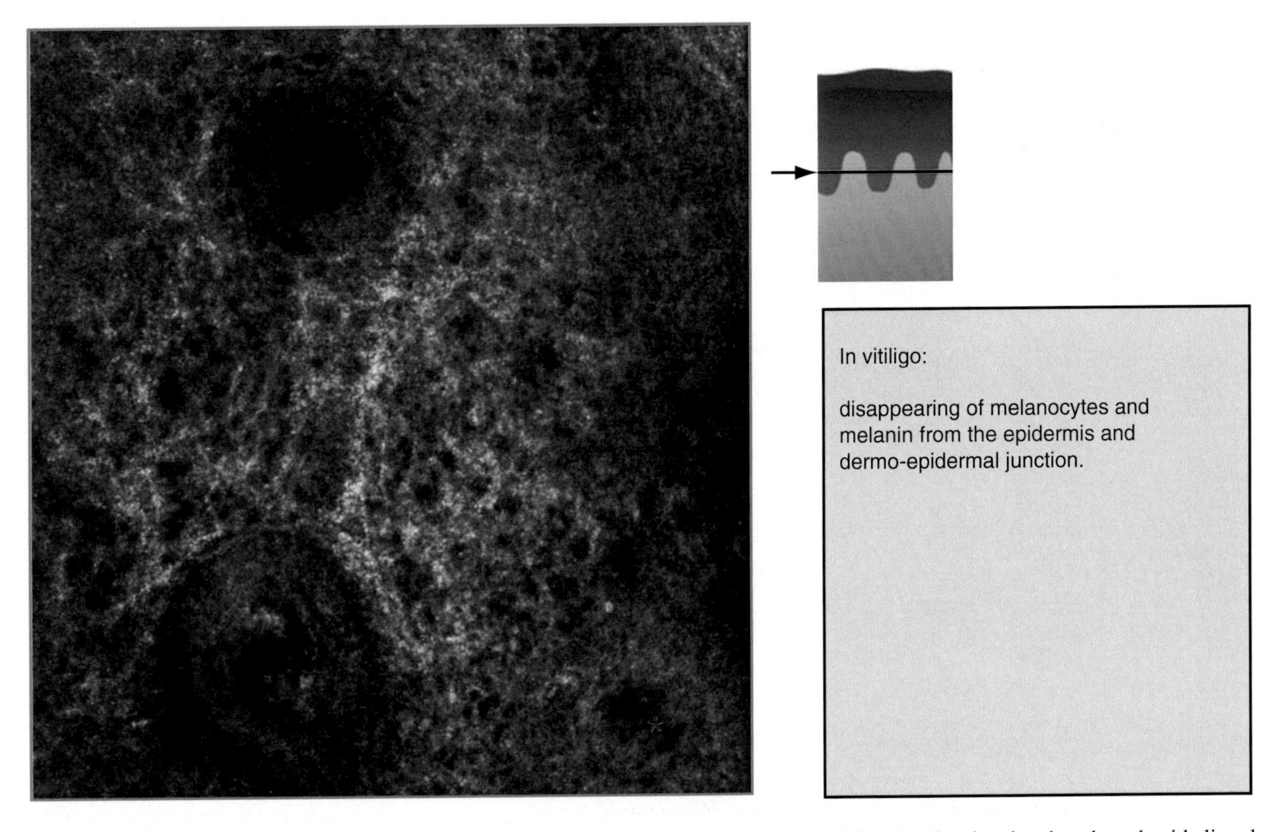

Fig. 30.8.2 Basic image (0.5 × 0.5 mm) absence of the normal brightness at derrmo-epidermal junction level and at the adnexal epithelium basal layer with remnant of a "shadow" of the pre-existing papillary ring (*)

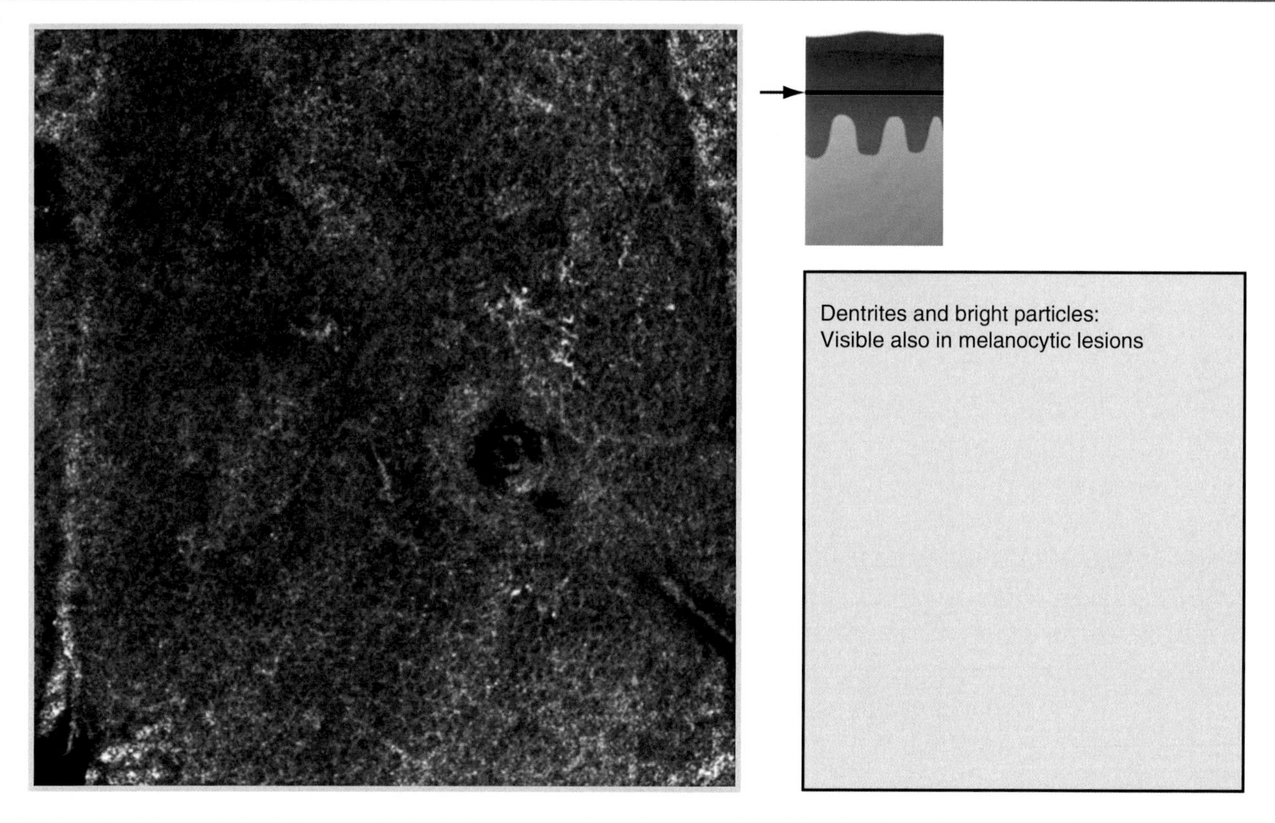

Fig. 30.8.3 Basic image (0.5 × 0.5 mm) at the level of the spinous layer. Presence of dendrites, bright particles and dendritic cells around adnexal structure

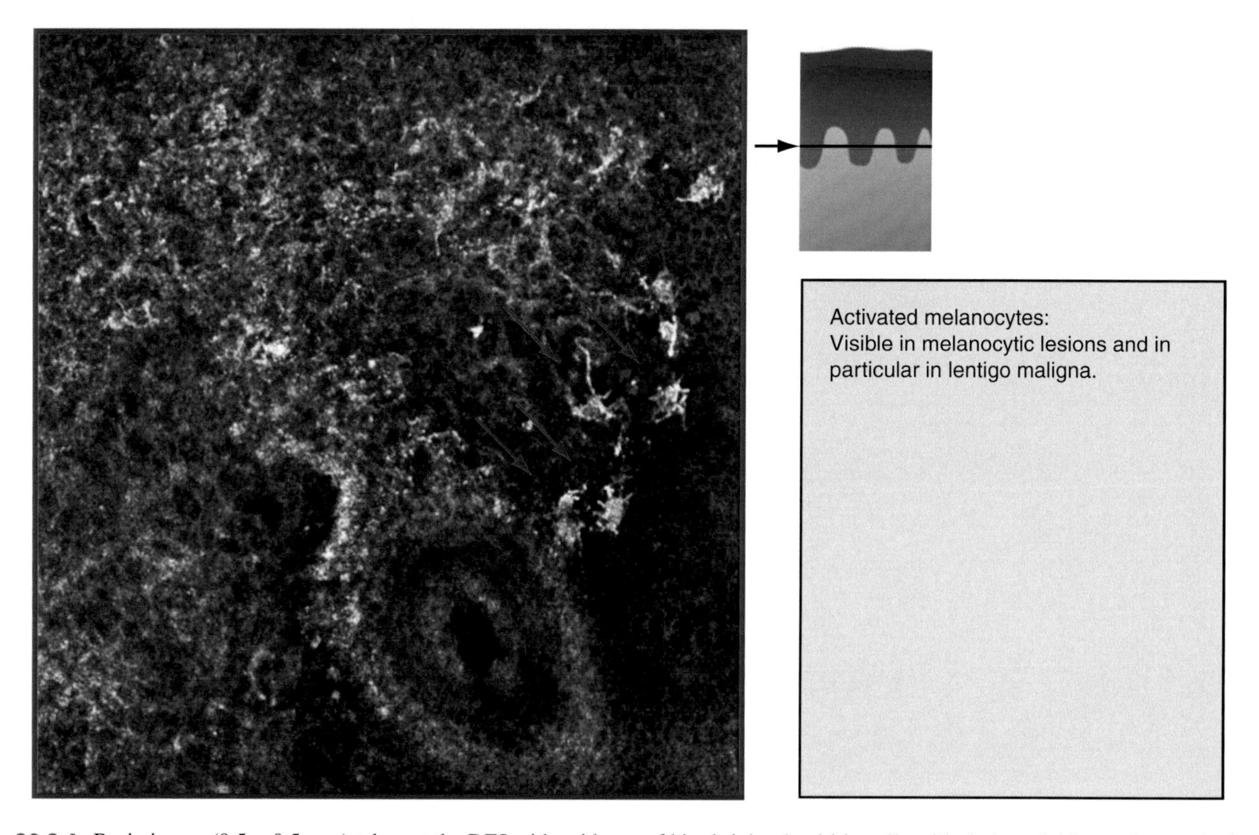

Fig. 30.8.4 Basic image (0.5 × 0.5 mm) taken at the DEJ with evidence of big, bright, dendritic cells with dark nuclei located around adnexal structures (→) corresponding to activated melanocytes

Core Messages

- Vitiligo is characterized by no brightness of epidermal keratinocytes as well as non rimmed papillae.
- No signs of inflammation are seen in vitiligo differently than in other ipopigmentary skin diseases.
- The pigmented skin of vitiligo patients shows abnormal pigment distribution at the DEJ.
- Melasma shows at RCM deposition of pigment in all three skin layers (mixed type).
- Melasma can be differentiated from postinflammatory pigmentation using RCM because showing different pattern of pigment distribution (postinflammatory pigmentation RCM patternis: prevalent at the DEJ and variable in the epidermis).
- RCM let the confocalist manage the pigmentary disorder treatment management.

References

1. Taieb A, Picardo M (2007) The definition and assessment of vitiligo: a consensus report of the Vitiligo European Task Force. Pigment Cell Res 20:27–35
2. Ardigo M, Malizewsky I, Dell'anna ML et al (2007) Preliminary evaluation of vitiligo using in vivo reflectance confocal microscopy. J Eur Acad Dermatol Venereol 21:1344–1350
3. Ardigo M, Cameli N, Berardesca E, Gonzalez S (2010) Characterization and evaluation of pigment distribution and response to therapy in melasma using in vivo reflectance confocal microscopy: a preliminary study. J Eur Acad Dermatol Venereol 24(11):1296–1303
4. Rose PT (2009) Pigmentary disorders. Med Clin N Am 93:1225–1239
5. Nim NY, Pandya AG (1998) Pigmentary diseases, office dermatology part I. Med Clin North Am 82:1185–1207
6. Nanda S, Grover C, Reddy BS et al (2004) Efficacy of hydroquinone 2% versus tretinoin 0,025% as adjunct topical agents for chemical peeling in patients with melasma. Dermat Surg 30:385–388
7. Perez MI (2005) The stepwise approach to the treatment of melasma. Cutis 75:217–222
8. Grimes PE, Callender V (2006) Tazarotene cream for postinflammatory hyperpigmentation and acne vulgaris in darker skin; a double-blind, randomised, vehicle-controlled study. Cutis 77:45–50
9. Grimes PE (2004) Microscponge formulation of hydroquinone 4% and retinol 0.15% in the treatment of melasma and postinflammmatory hyperpigmentation. Cutis 74(6):362–368

Part VIII

Monitoring of Skin Lesions and Therapy Control

31 Follow-up of Nevi

Rainer Hofmann-Wellenhof, Edith Arzberger,
Josef Smolle, and Verena Ahlgrimm-Siess

31.1 Introduction

RCM offers the unique opportunity to noninvasively monitor cytomorphologic changes in skin lesions in vivo over a longitudinal period of time. The value of RCM for monitoring and follow-up of melanocytic skin tumors has already been shown for lentigo maligna undergoing novel, noninvasive treatment modalities [1, 2]. In this context, RCM may be used for noninvasive diagnosis and evaluation of treatment effects as well as for long-term follow-up. There have been recent attempts to assess the value of RCM for monitoring of clinically and dermoscopically equivocal nevi in patients at high risk for cutaneous melanoma. The examination of dynamic changes in the life of nevi represents another innovative research focus.

31.2 Follow-up of Atypical Nevi

The most effective approach to improve the prognosis of cutaneous melanoma is early recognition and excision. Digital dermoscopic monitoring of equivocal nevi aims to facilitate the early detection of melanoma in patients with dysplastic mole syndrome by visualizing morphologic changes over time [3]. Most atypical nevi that are followed are stable; approximately only 5% show changes in size or architecture. Of these, only 11% are found to be melanoma [4]. Although the malignant/benign ratio in excised melanocytic skin lesions has already enhanced since the adoption of dermoscopy in routine melanoma screening, there is still scope for enhancement [5]. RCM has the potential to rigorously improve the management of patients with dysplastic mole syndrome; on the one hand, the cytomorphologic examination of clinically and dermoscopically equivocal melanocytic lesions may allow for an immediate, noninvasive differentiation of nevi from melanoma and may render follow-up visits unnecessary. On the other hand, RCM may help elucidating the benign origin of morphologic changes in nevi, which are due to normal evolution, sun exposure or irritation and may further reduce the number of unnecessary excisions (Fig. 31.1). Nevi that show signs of atypia in both imaging methods, that are not distinctive of melanoma, may be followed with RCM to detect dynamic morphologic changes suggestive of melanoma. The value of RCM as adjunct to routine dermoscopy melanoma screening has already been shown in the literature; RCM improved the specificity for the diagnosis of melanoma from 32% to 68%. The combination of both techniques allowed a significant improvement in the diagnostic sensitivity (98%) [6, 7].

31.3 Insights into Nevogenesis

Previous studies attempting to explain the evolution of nevi were based on the histopathologic evaluation of excised nevi or were dermoscopy-based observational studies [8–12]. Dynamic cytomorphologic changes in the life of nevi could therefore never be visualized and correlated with corresponding dermoscopic structures. In the daily routine, these nevi are frequently excised to rule out malignancy; clinical and dermoscopic aspects are often equivocal and patients commonly report changes in lesion size, elevation or color. RCM enables for the first time a dynamic, noninvasive dermatoscopic-histopathologic correlation in evolving nevi (Fig. 31.3). These observations may provide new insights into nevogenesis and may allow for a noninvasive differentiation of equivocal evolving nevi from melanoma in the future [13].

R. Hofmann-Wellenhof (✉) • E. Arzberger • V. Ahlgrimm-Siess
Department of Dermatology and Venerology,
Medical University of Graz, Graz, Austria
e-mail: rainer.hofmann@medunigraz.at

J. Smolle
Rectorate of the Medical University of Graz,
Graz, Austria

R. Hofmann-Wellenhof et al. (eds.), *Reflectance Confocal Microscopy for Skin Diseases*,
DOI 10.1007/978-3-642-21997-9_31, © Springer-Verlag Berlin Heidelberg 2012

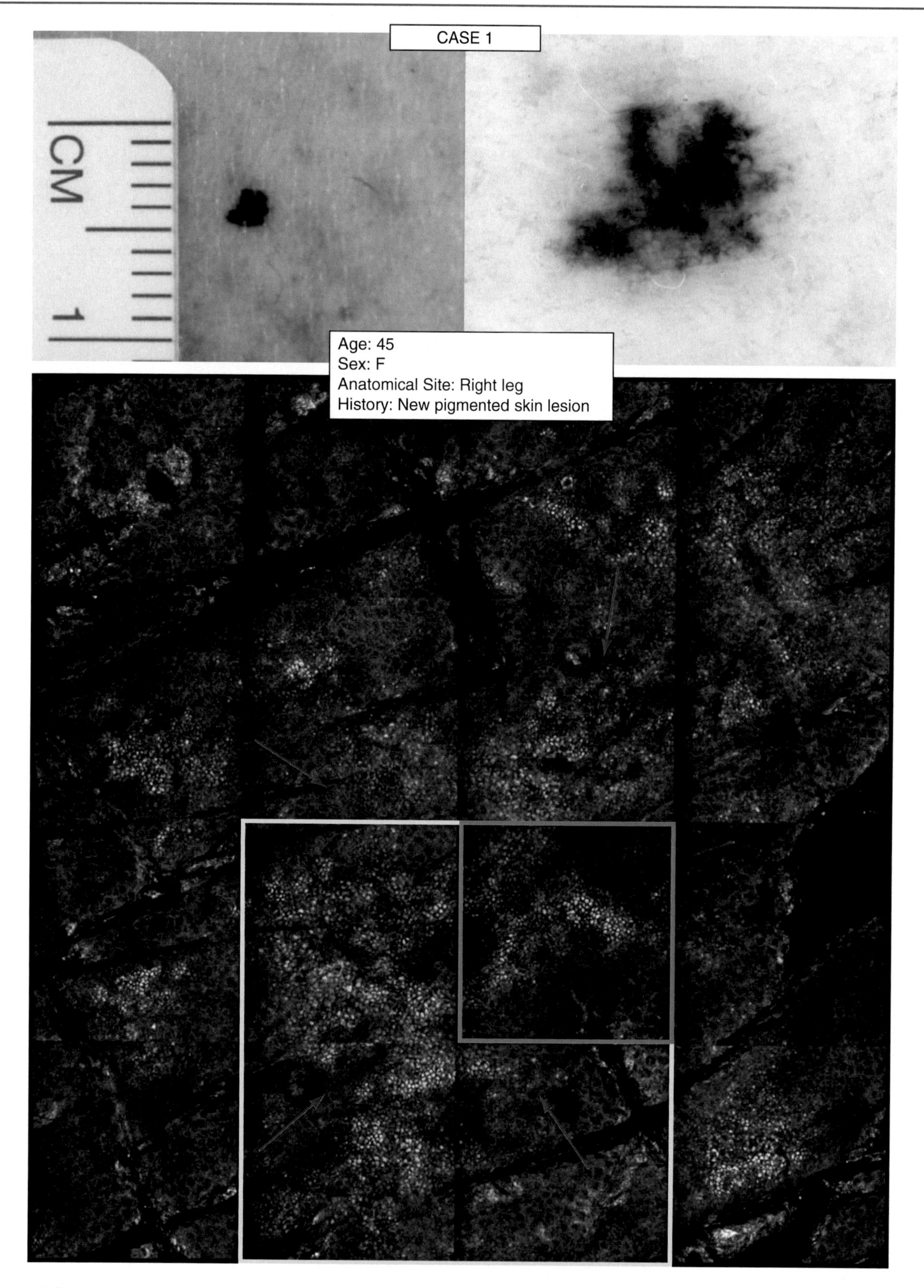

Fig. 31.1 RCM mosaic (2 × 2 mm) at the level of the upper epidermis reveals a peripheral typical honeycomb pattern and aggregated monomorphous, bright cells in the center (*arrows*)

Upper epidermis:

Typical cobblestone pattern adjacent to typical honeycomb pattern

Fig. 31.1.1 RCM mosaic (1 × 1 mm) at the upper epidermis. At higher magnification, areas with typical honeycomb pattern (*asterisk*) are observed adjacent to areas with aggregated, pigmented keratinocytes (cobblestone pattern; *arrows*)

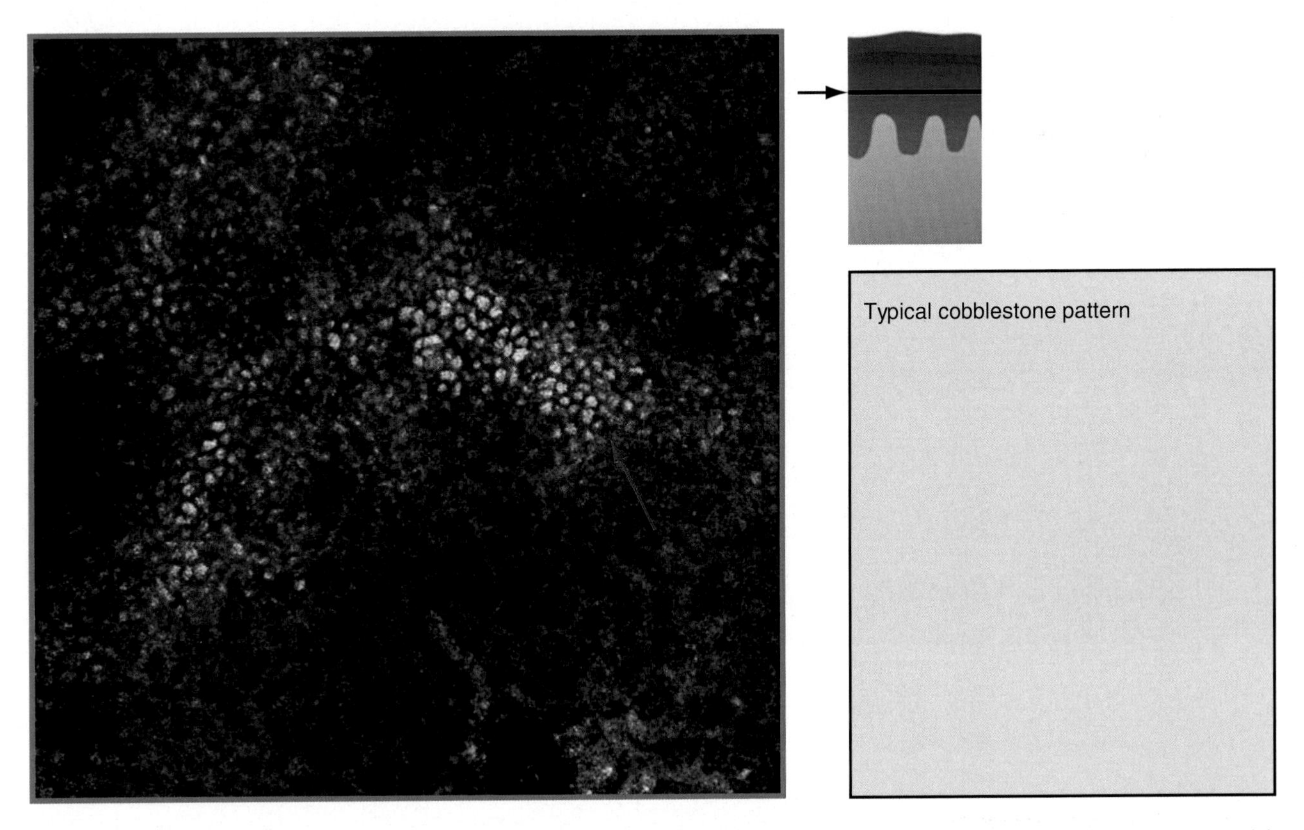

Fig. 31.1.2 Single RCM image (0.5 × 0.5 mm) at the upper epidermis. Monomorphous pigmented keratinocytes (*arrow*), whose nuclei are obscured by the bright melanin are aggregated back-to-back forming a typical cobblestone pattern

CASE 1

Age: 45
Sex: F
Anatomical Site: Right leg
History: New pigmented skin lesion

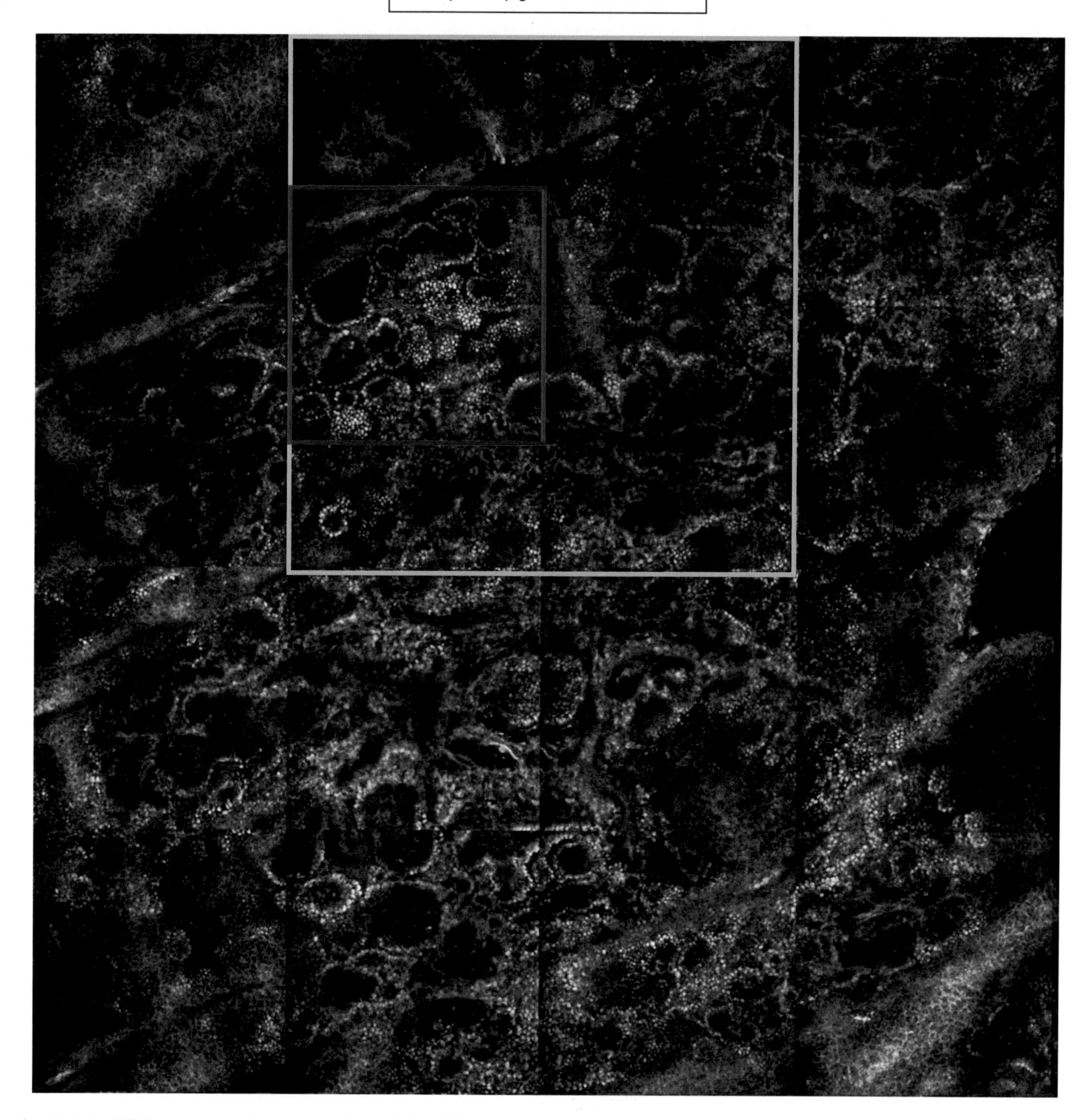

Fig. 31.1.3 RCM mosaic (4 × 4 mm) at the level of the DEJ reveals a so-called ringed pattern composed of edged dermal papillae (*arrow*)

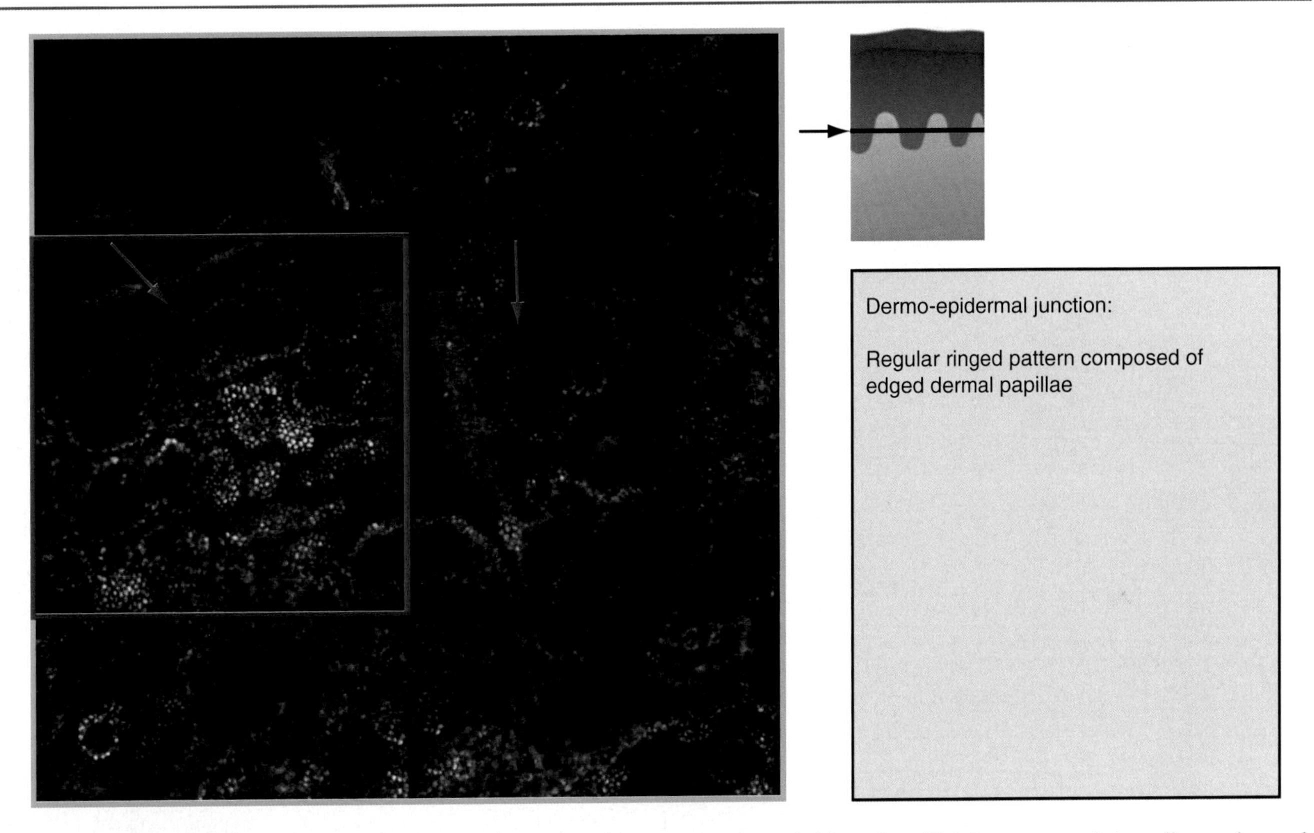

Fig. 31.1.4 RCM mosaic (1 × 1 mm) at the DEJ. Numerous dermal papillae surrounded by a rim of bright monomorphous cells are observed, forming a regular ringed pattern (*arrows*)

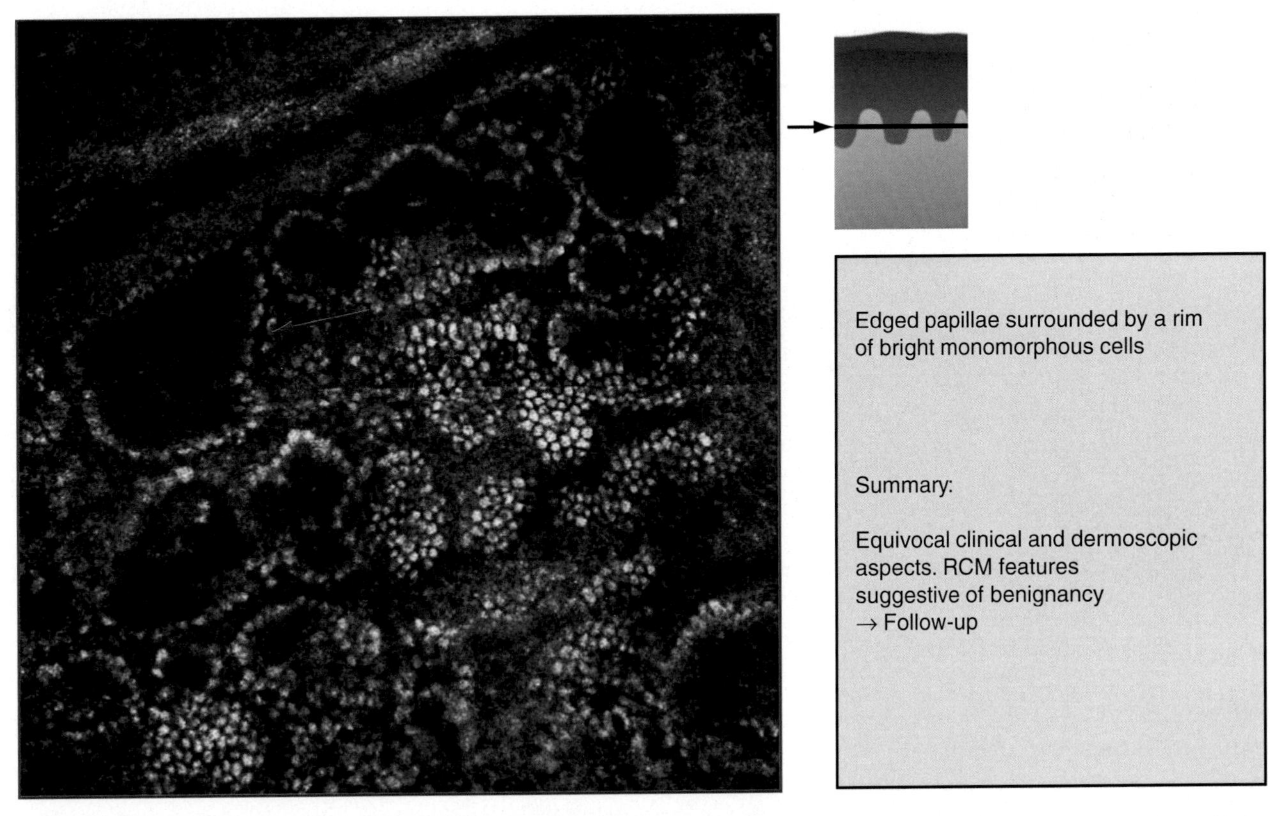

Fig. 31.1.5 Basic RCM image (0.5 × 0.5 mm) at the DEJ. Densely packed dermal papillae surrounded by a rim of bright, monomorphous cells, correlating to pigmented keratinocytes and melanocytes (*arrow*). Disk-like bright cell aggregates are seen when RCM sections higher, at the level of the suprapapillary plates (*asterisk*)

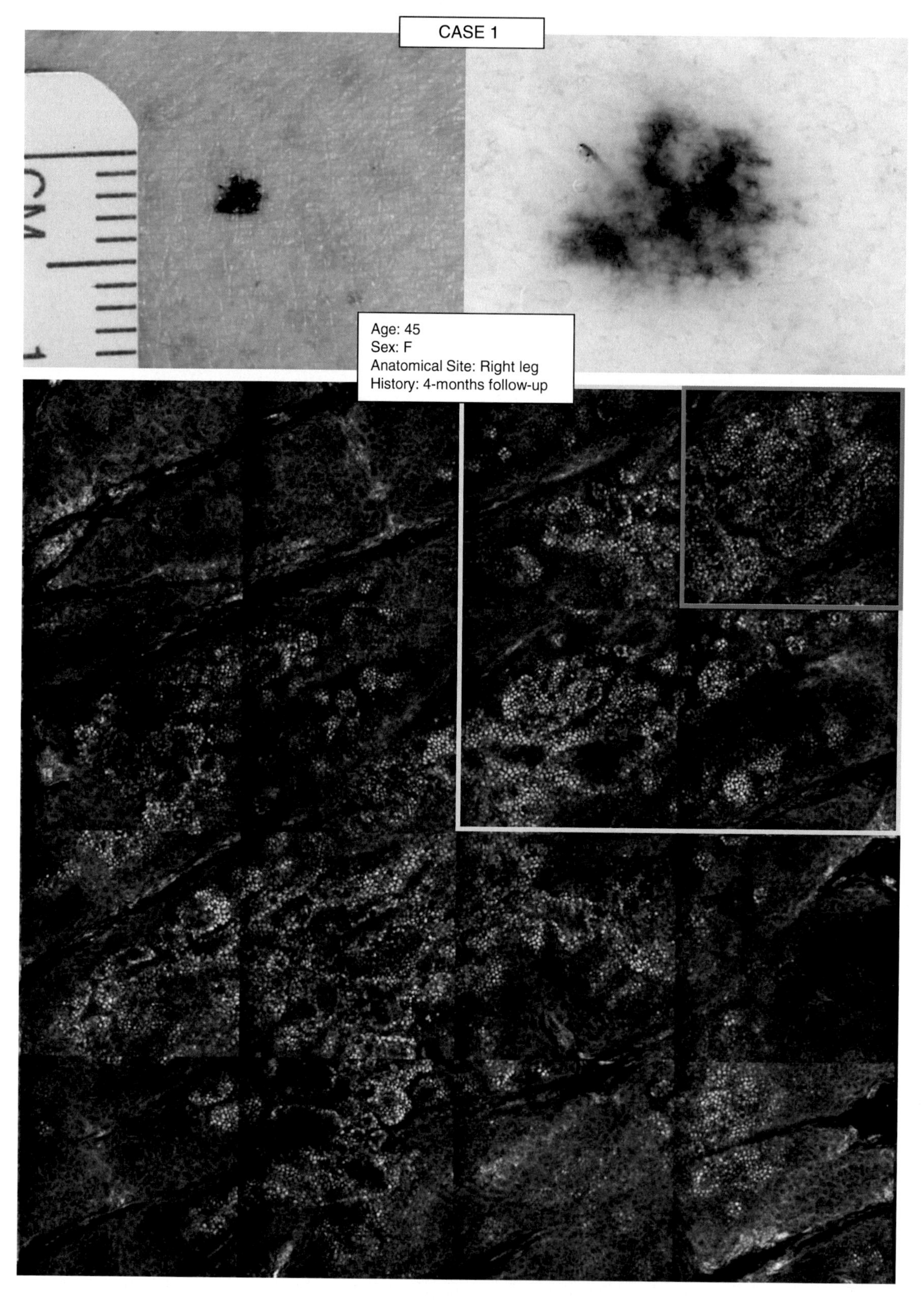

Fig. 31.2 Same lesion as in Fig. 31.1 after 4-months follow-up. RCM mosaic (2 × 2 mm) at the level of the epidermis. A typical peripheral honeycomb pattern is observed in the lesion periphery, the lesion center displays aggregated monomorphous, bright cells

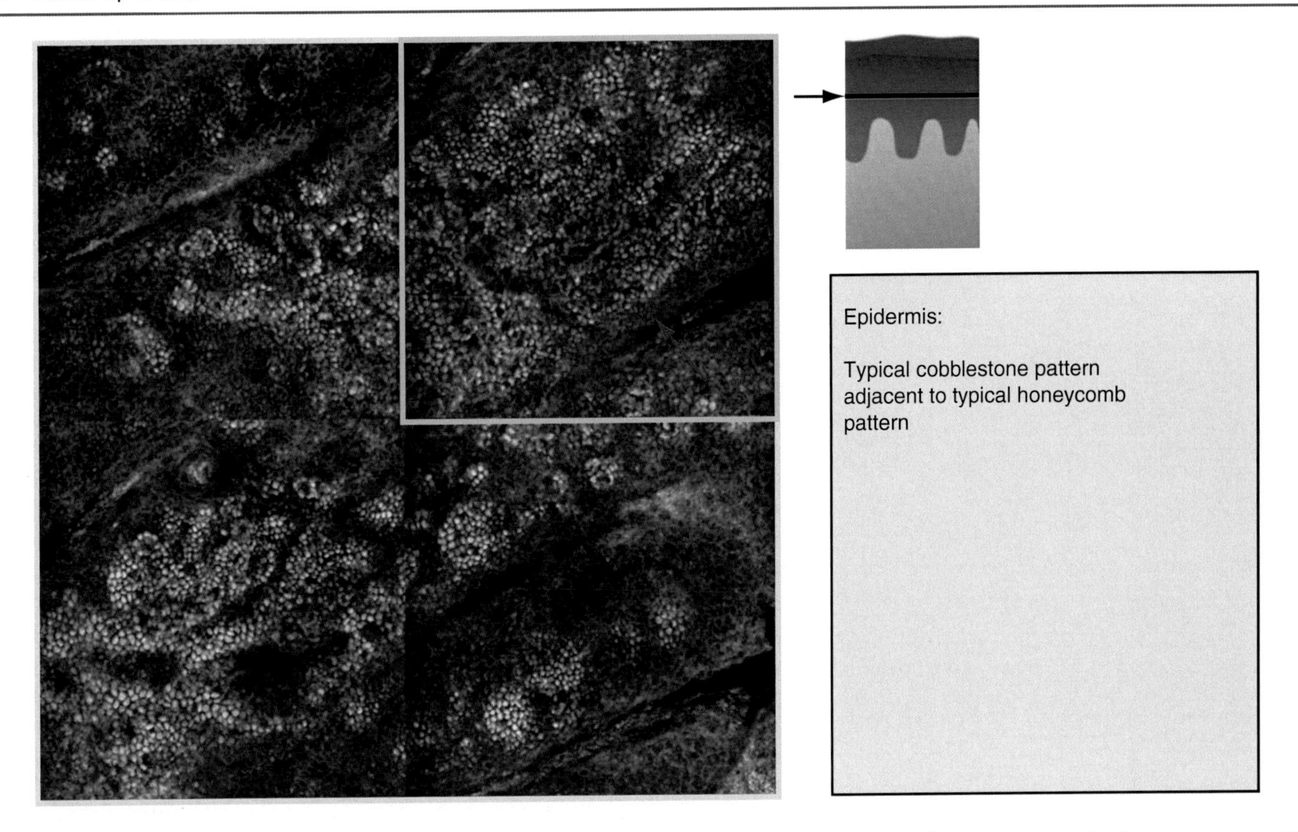

Fig. 31.2.1 RCM mosaic (1 × 1 mm) at the level of the epidermis shows areas with typical honeycomb pattern (*asterisk*) adjacent to areas with so-called cobblestone pattern (*arrow*)

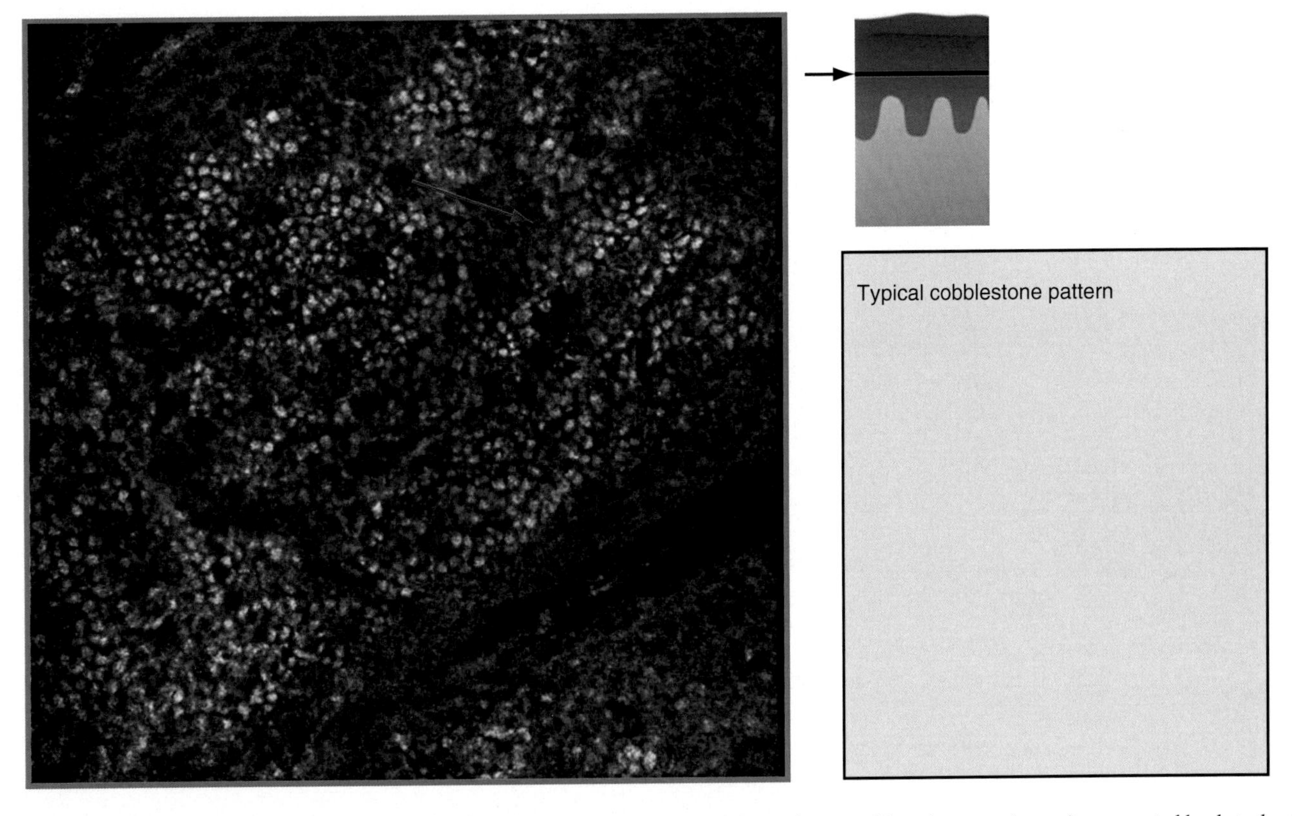

Fig. 31.2.2 Single RCM image (0.5 × 0.5 mm) at the epidermis shows monomorphous pigmented keratinocytes (*arrow*) aggregated back-to-back (typical cobblestone pattern)

CASE 1

Age: 45
Sex: F
Anatomical Site: Right leg
History: 4-months follow-up

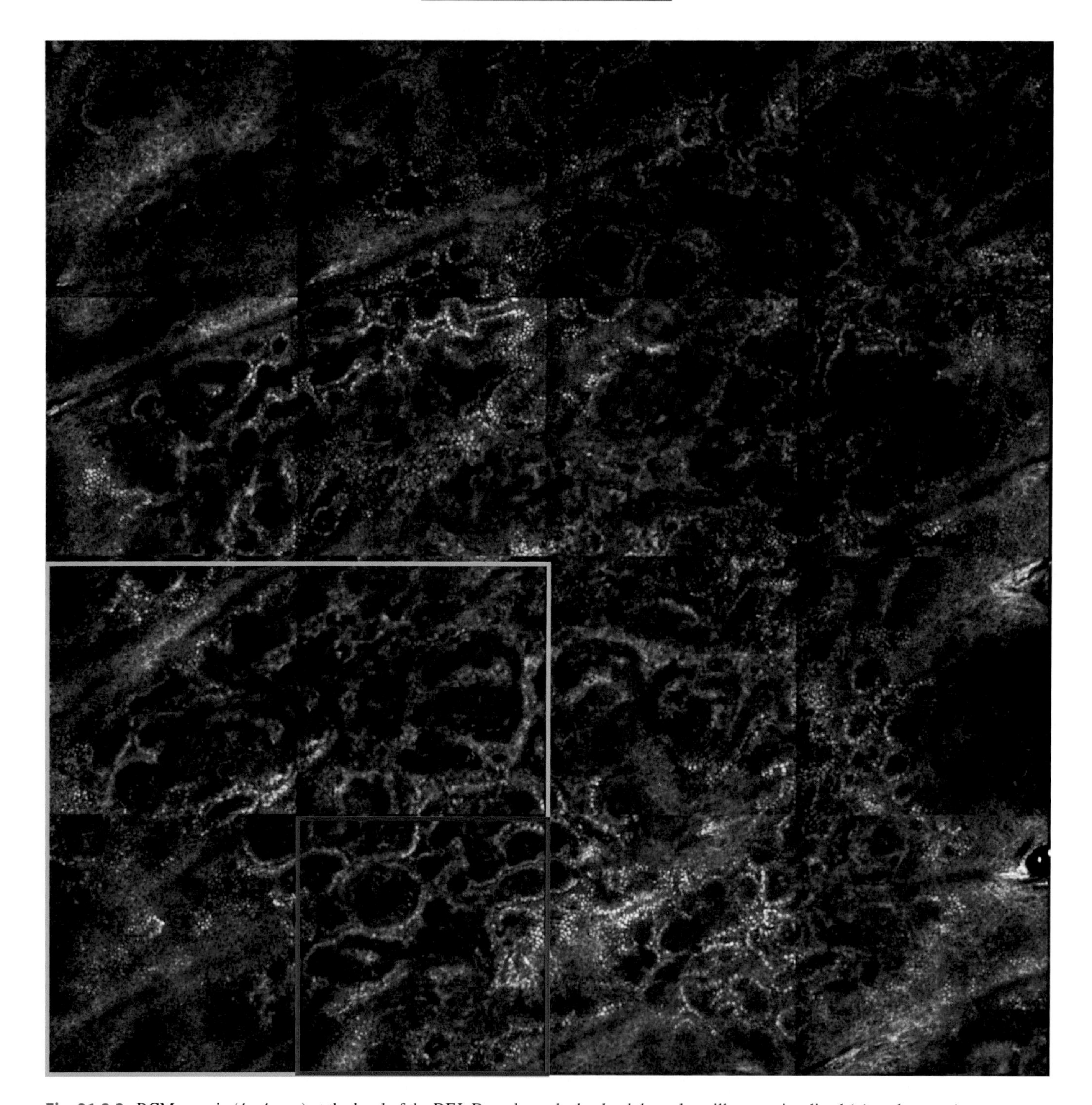

Fig. 31.2.3 RCM mosaic (4×4 mm) at the level of the DEJ. Densely packed, edged dermal papillae are visualized (*ringed pattern*)

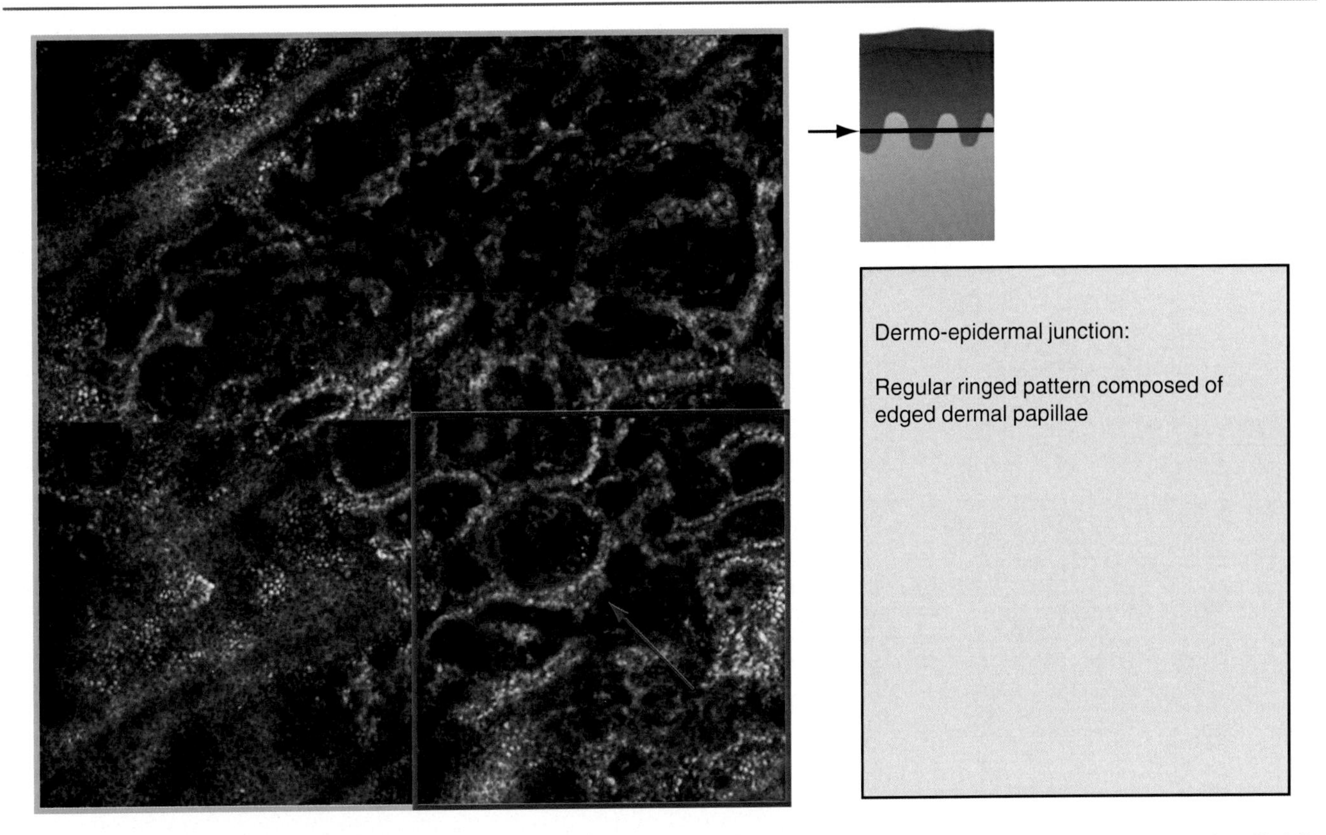

Fig. 31.2.4 RCM mosaic (1 × 1 mm) at the DEJ. A regular ringed pattern composed of numerous dermal papillae surrounded by a rim of bright monomorphous cells, correlating to pigmented keratinocytes and melanocytes is observed (*arrow*)

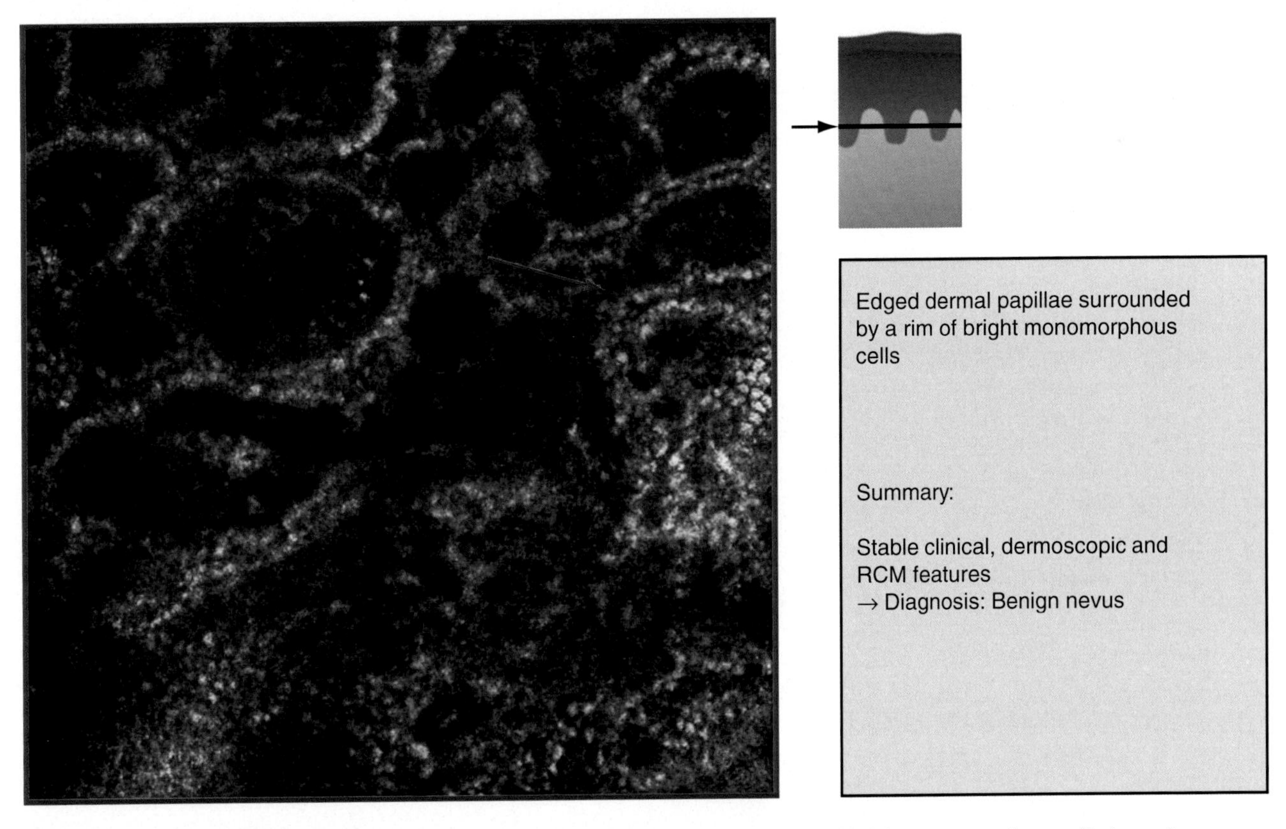

Fig. 31.2.5 Basic RCM image (0.5 × 0.5 mm) at the DEJ reveals edged papillae with a rim of bright, monomorphous cells (*arrow*)

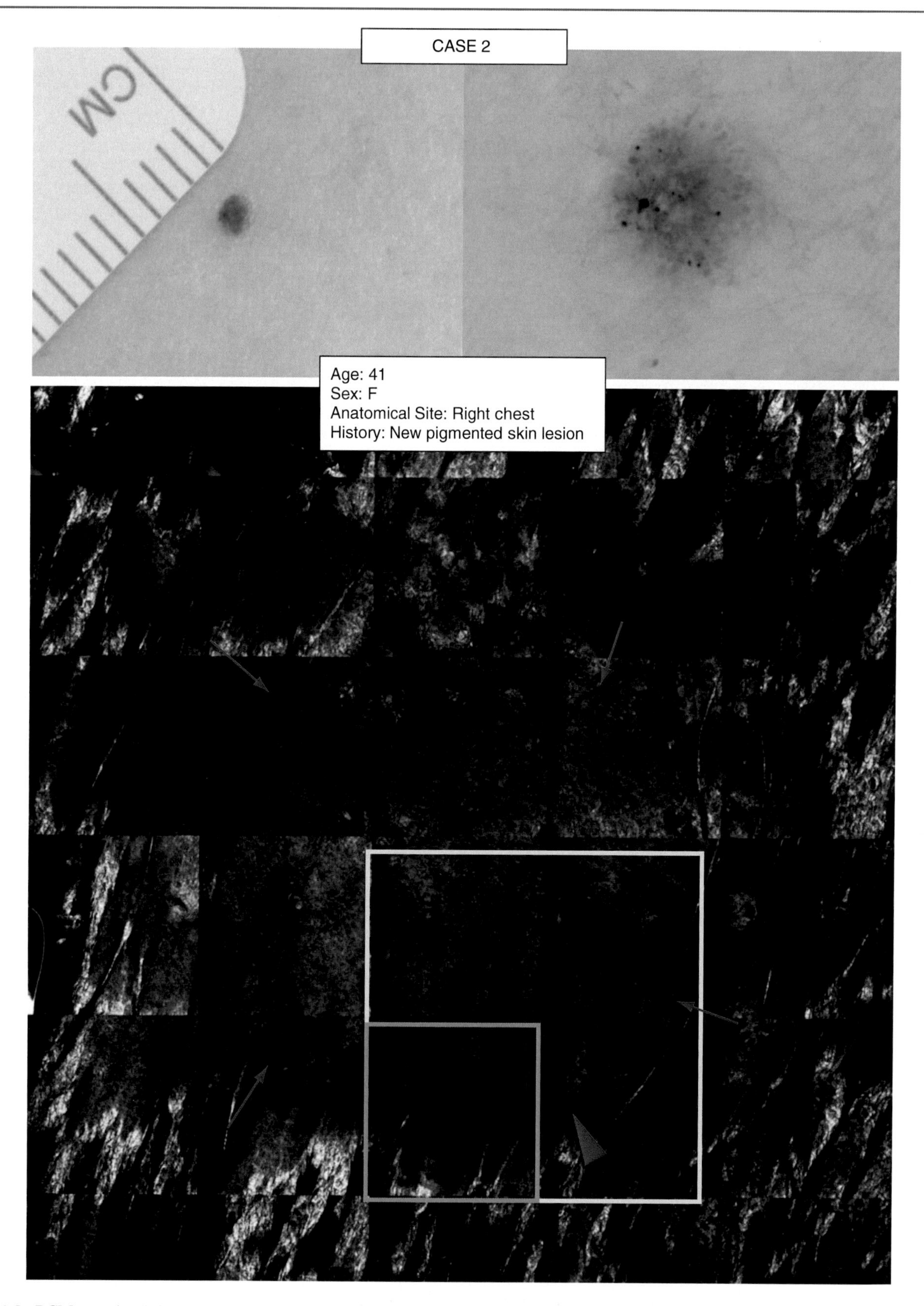

Fig. 31.3 RCM mosaic (4.5×4.5 mm) at the level of the upper epidermis shows an area with broadened honeycomb pattern (*arrows*) and a peripheral rim of reflective, round to oval structures (*arrowhead*)

Upper epidermis:

Broadened honeycomb pattern

Peripheral rim of reflective, round to oval structures

Fig. 31.3.1 RCM mosaic (1 × 1 mm) at the upper epidermis. At this resolution, a regular honeycomb pattern with enlarged holes and thickened lines of the meshwork (broadened honeycomb pattern) is observed in the lesion center (*arrows*). Reflective, round to oval structures, correlating to the tips of junctional melanocytic nests, are observed in the lesion periphery (*arrowhead*)

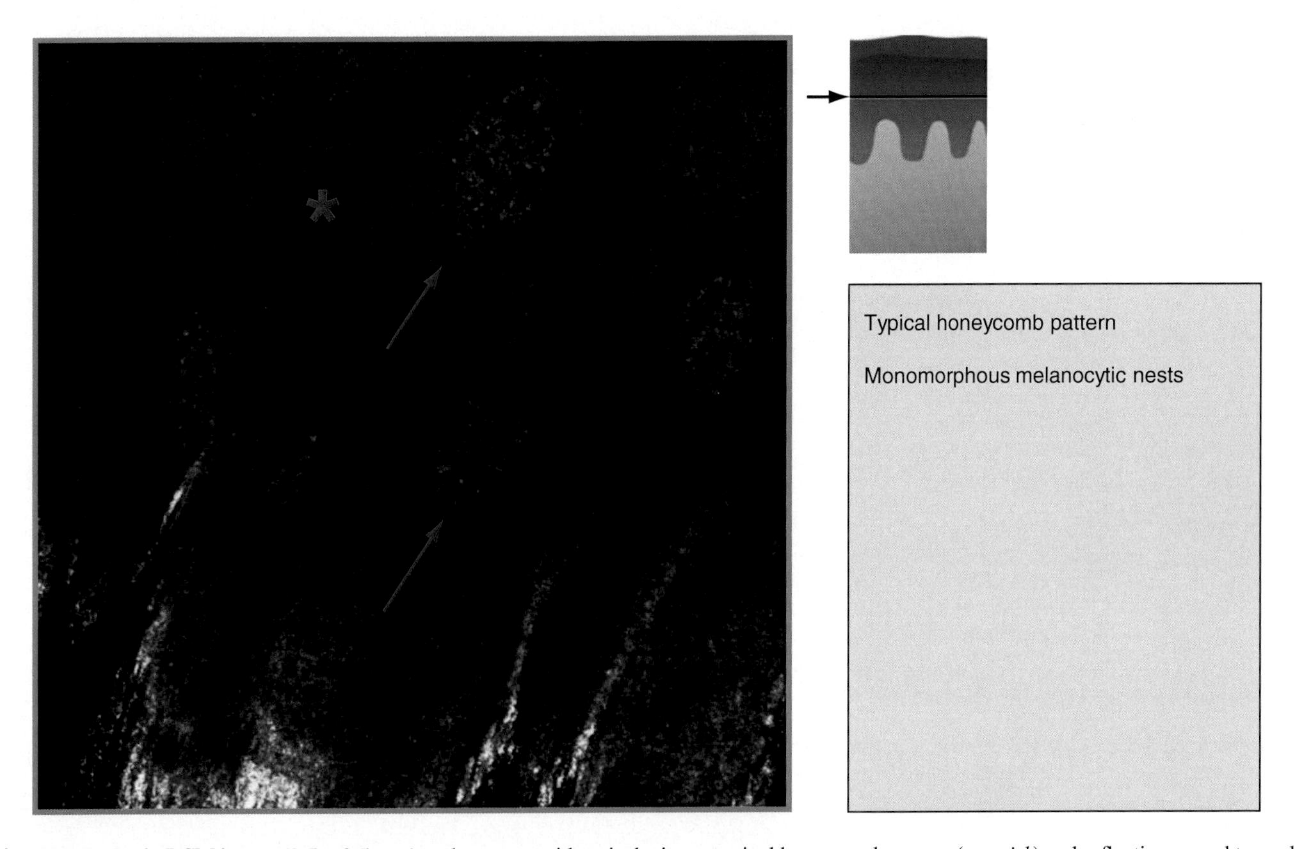

Fig. 31.3.2 Basic RCM image (0.5 × 0.5 mm) at the upper epidermis depicts a typical honeycomb pattern (*asterisk*) and reflective, round to oval, dense melanocytic nests (*arrows*). Distinct cellular outlines of melanocytes are not detectable within individual nests

CASE 2

Age: 41
Sex: F
Anatomical Site: Right chest
History: New pigmented skin lesion

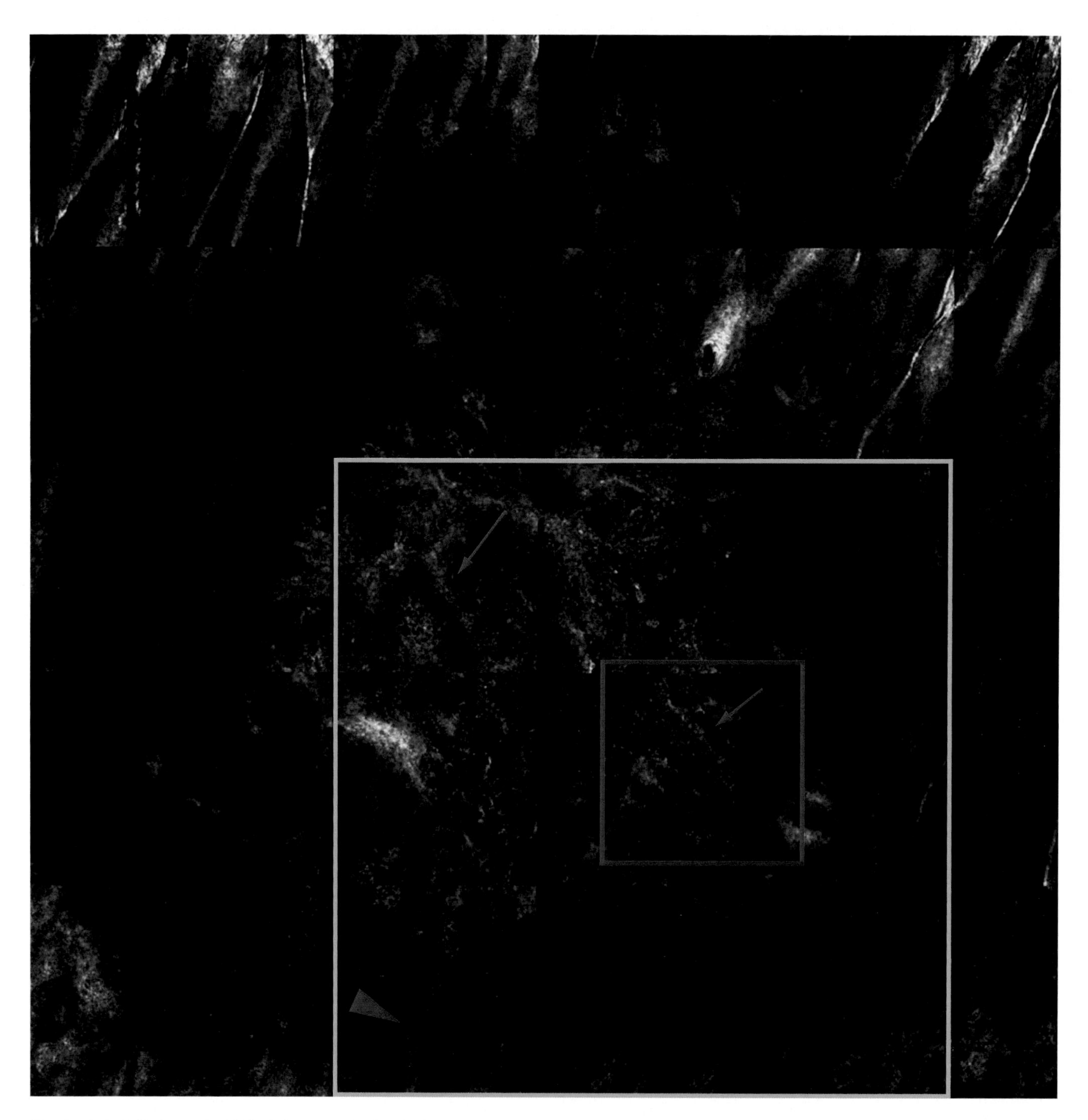

Fig. 31.3.3 RCM mosaic (4.5 × 4.5 mm) at the level of the DEJ reveals reflective, tubular structures in the lesion center (*arrows*) and reflective, round to oval structures in the lesion periphery (*arrowhead*), correlating to junctional melanocytic nests

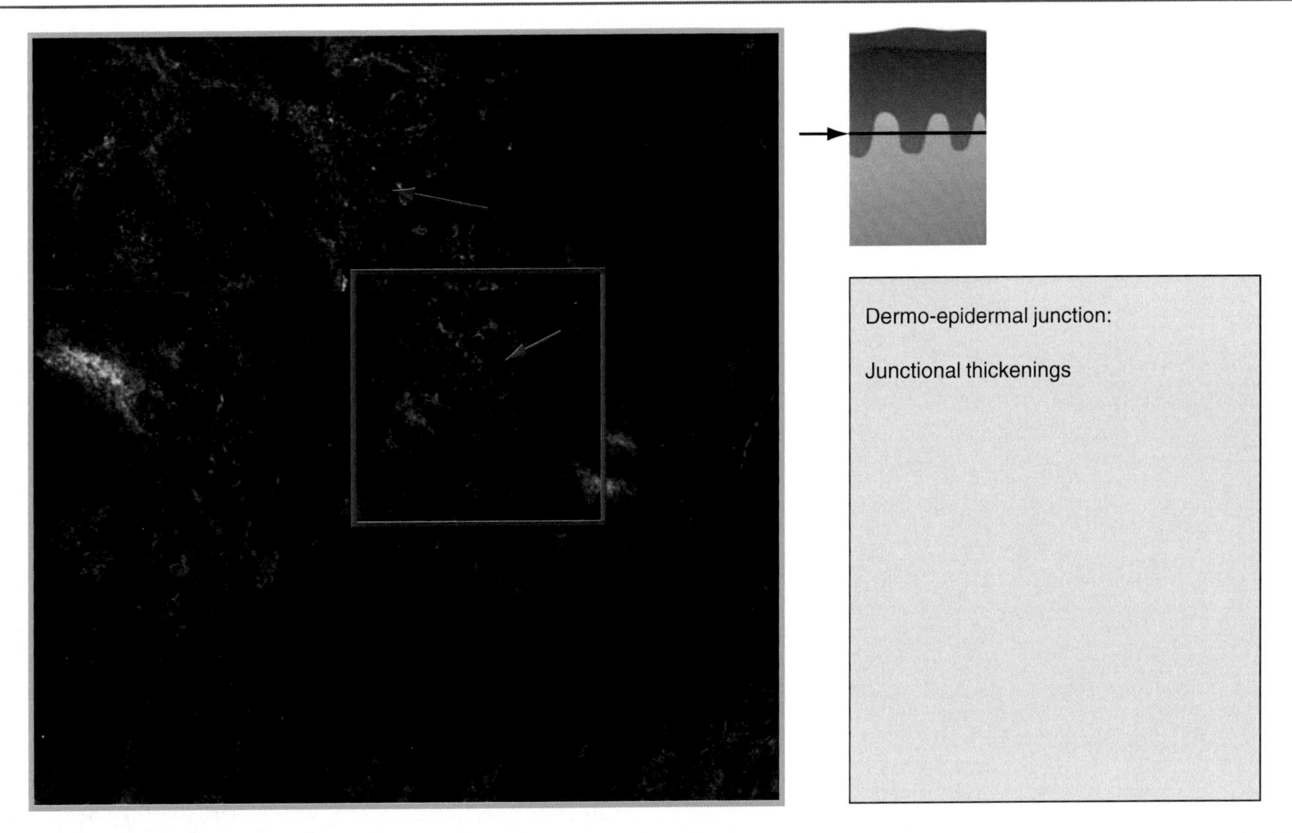

Fig. 31.3.4 RCM mosaic (1.5 × 1.5 mm) at the DEJ. Reflective, tubular melanocytic nests that expand the interpapillary spaces are visualized in the lesion center (*arrows*)

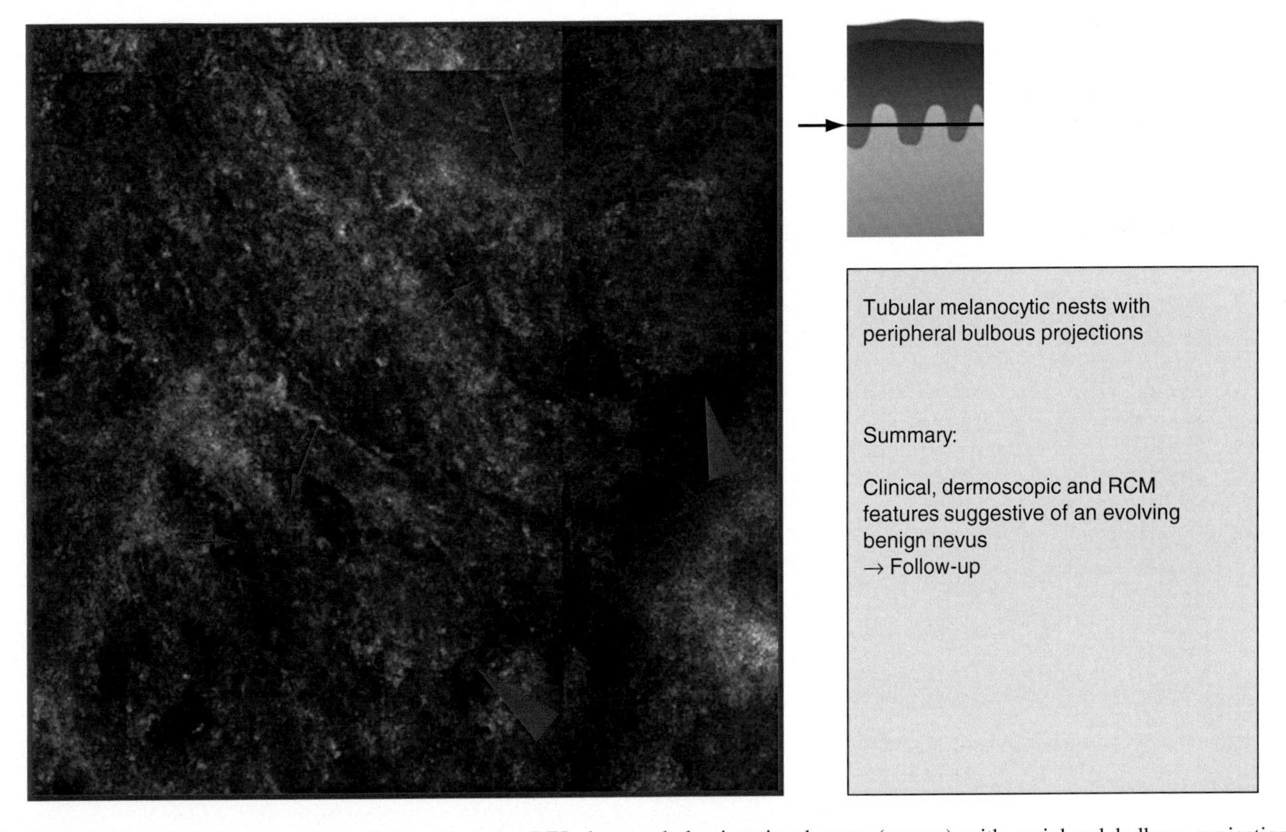

Fig. 31.3.5 Basic RCM image (0.5 × 0.5 mm) at the DEJ shows tubular junctional nests (*arrows*) with peripheral bulbous projections (*arrowheads*)

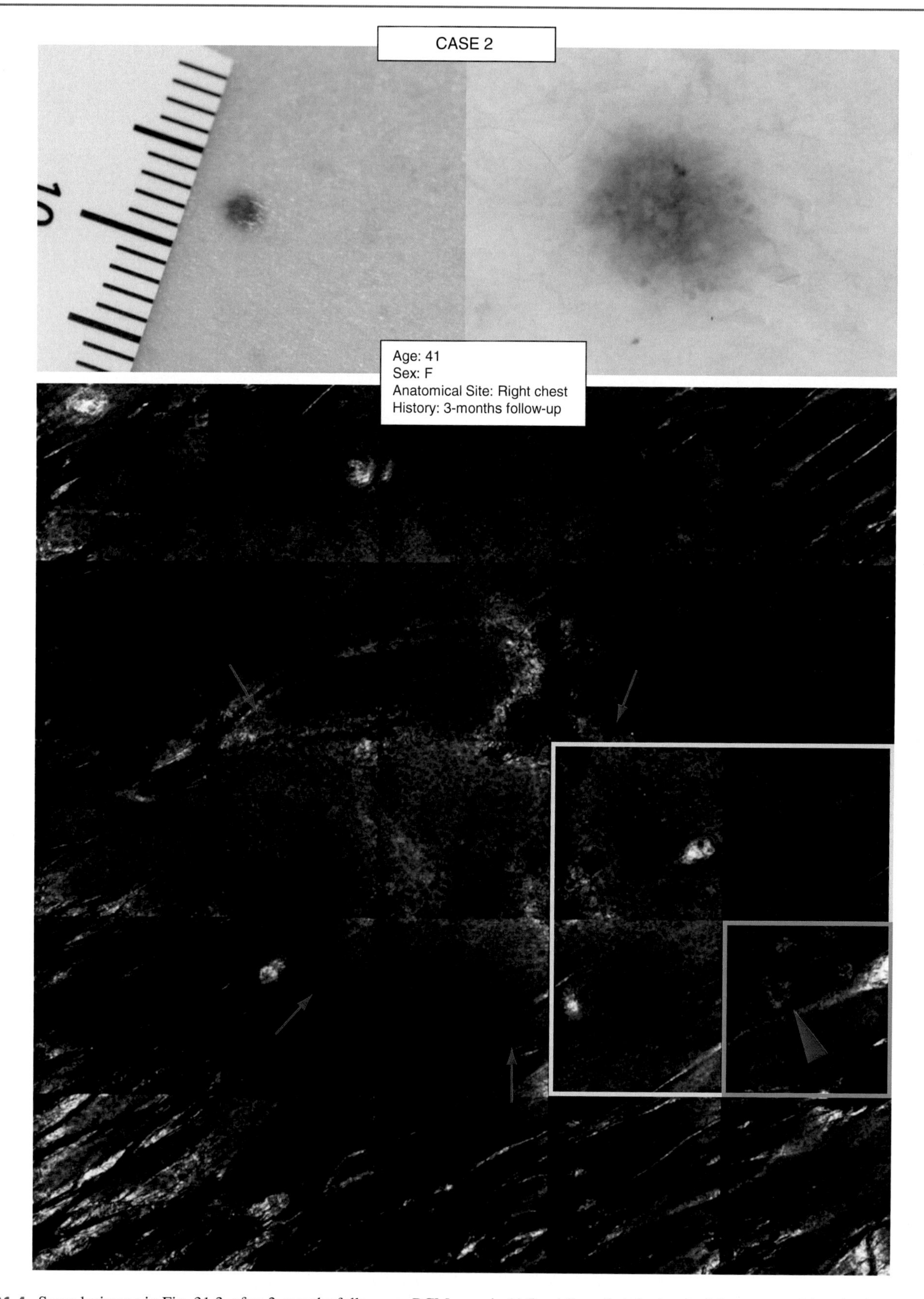

Fig. 31.4 Same lesion as in Fig. 31.3, after 3-months follow-up. RCM mosaic (4.5 × 4.5 mm) at the level of the upper epidermis shows a broadened honeycomb pattern in the center (*arrows*) and peripheral reflective, round to oval structures (*arrowhead*)

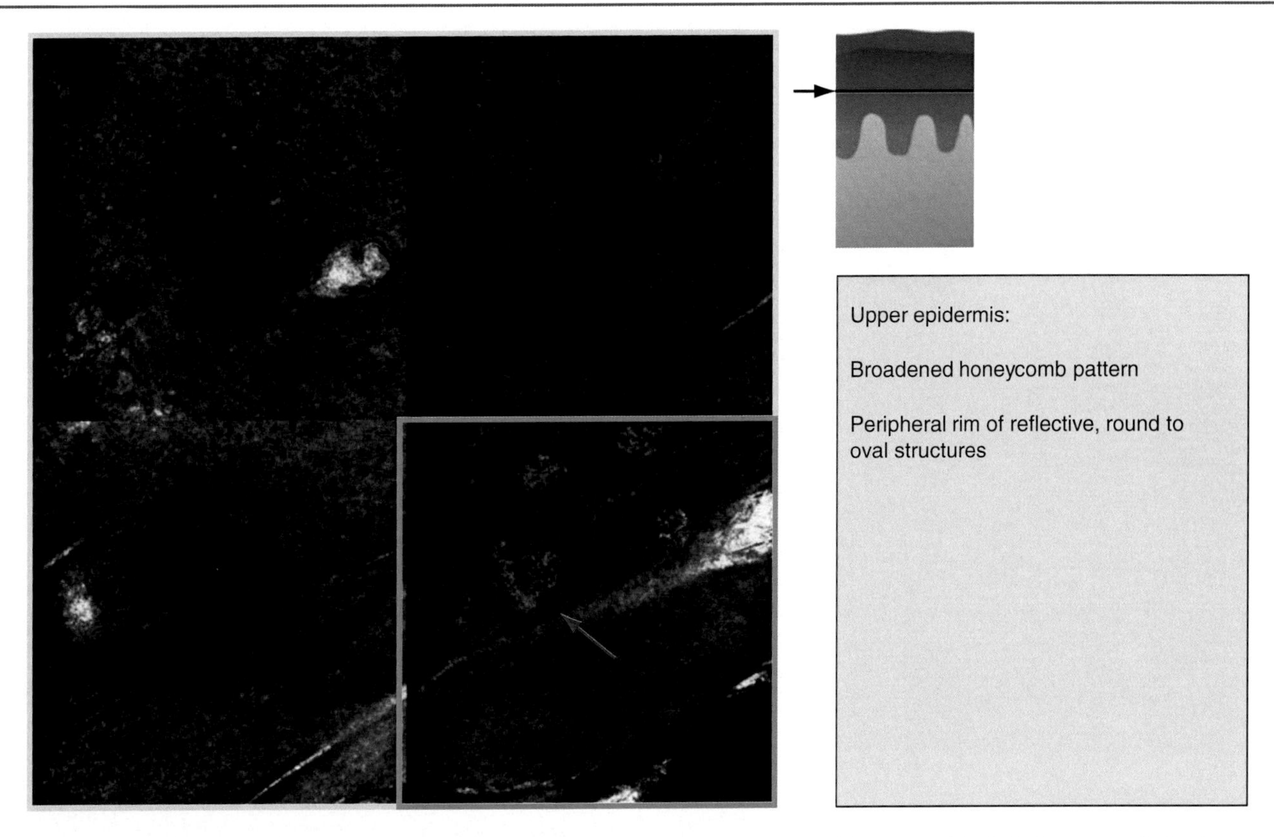

Fig. 31.4.1 RCM mosaic (1 × 1 mm) at the upper epidermis. A slightly broadened honeycomb is observed in the lesion center. Reflective, round to oval melanocytic nests are observed in the lesion periphery (*arrow*)

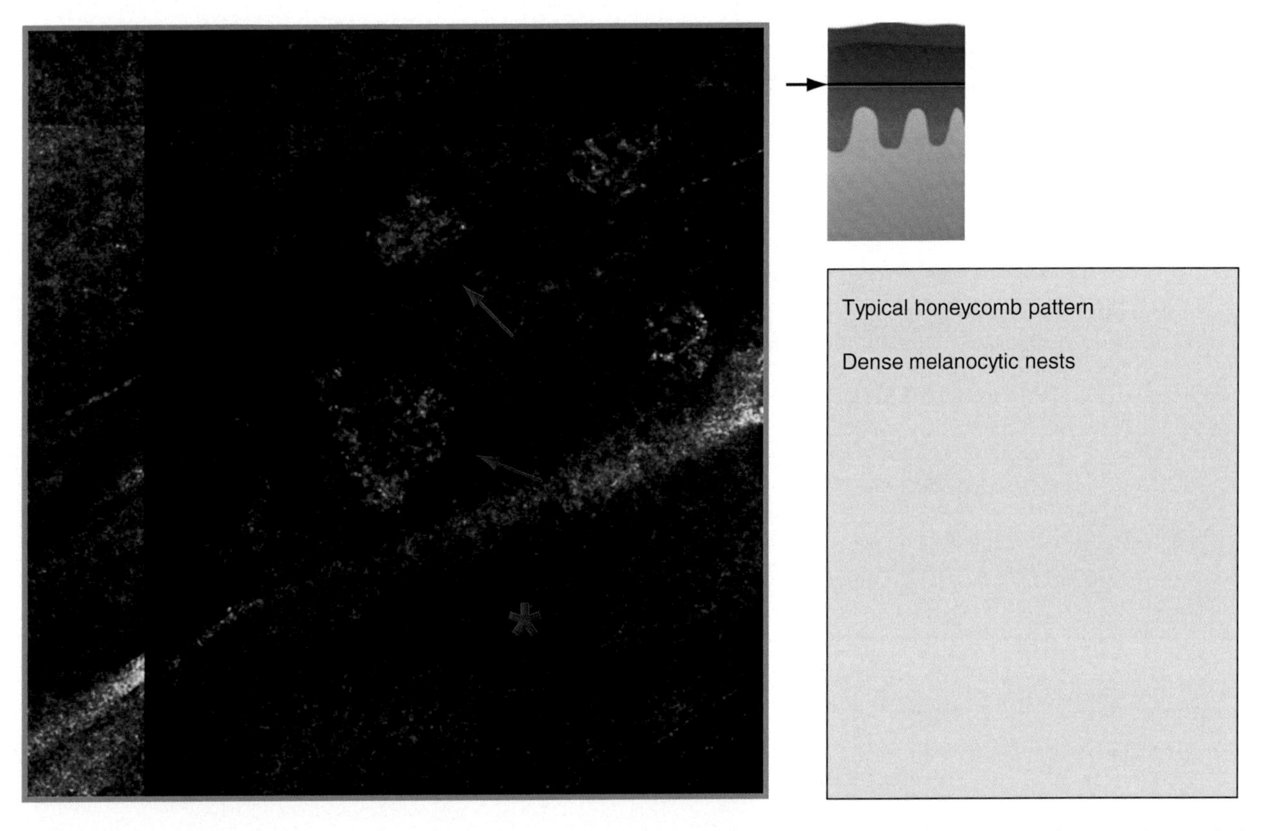

Fig. 31.4.2 Basic RCM image (0.5 × 0.5 mm) at the DEJ reveals a typical honeycomb pattern (*asterisk*) and reflective, round to oval, dense melanocytic nests (*arrows*)

CASE 2

Age: 41
Sex: F
Anatomical Site: Right chest
History: 3-months follow-up

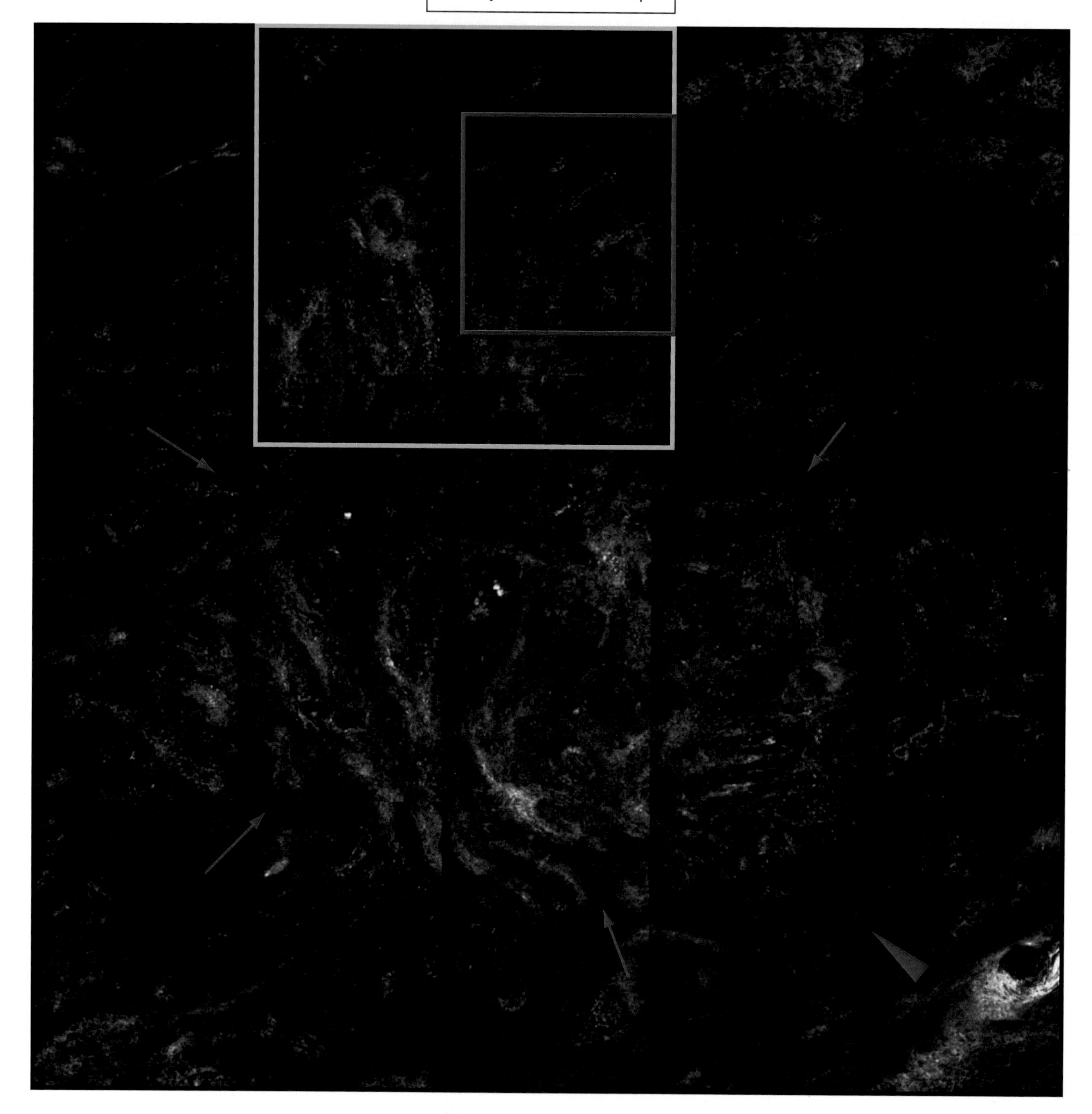

Fig. 31.4.3 RCM mosaic (4.5 × 4.5 mm) at the level of the DEJ. An area displaying central reflective tubular structures (*arrows*) and focal reflective, round to oval structures in the periphery (*arrowhead*) is observed, correlating to junctional melanocytic nests

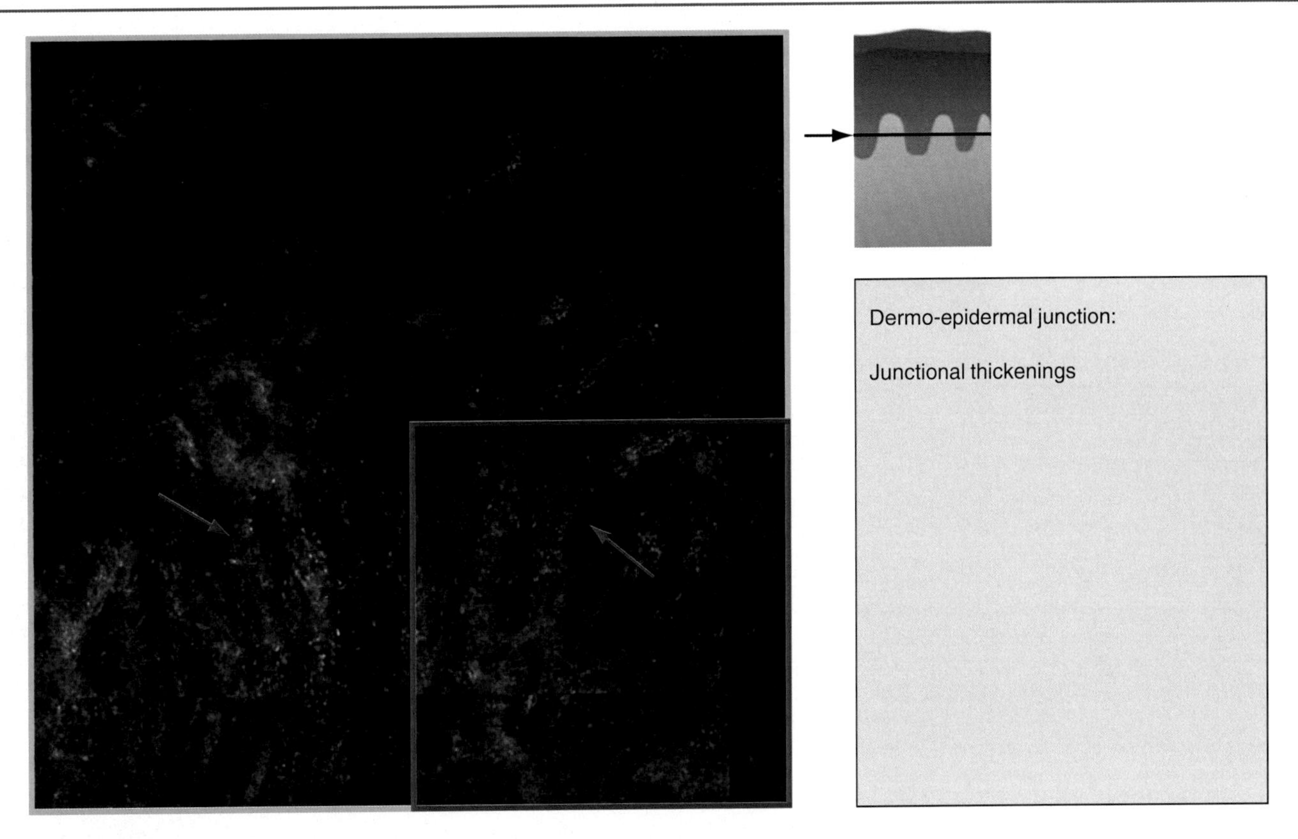

Fig. 31.4.4 RCM mosaic (1 × 1 mm) at the DEJ shows reflective, tubular melanocytic nests (*arrows*)

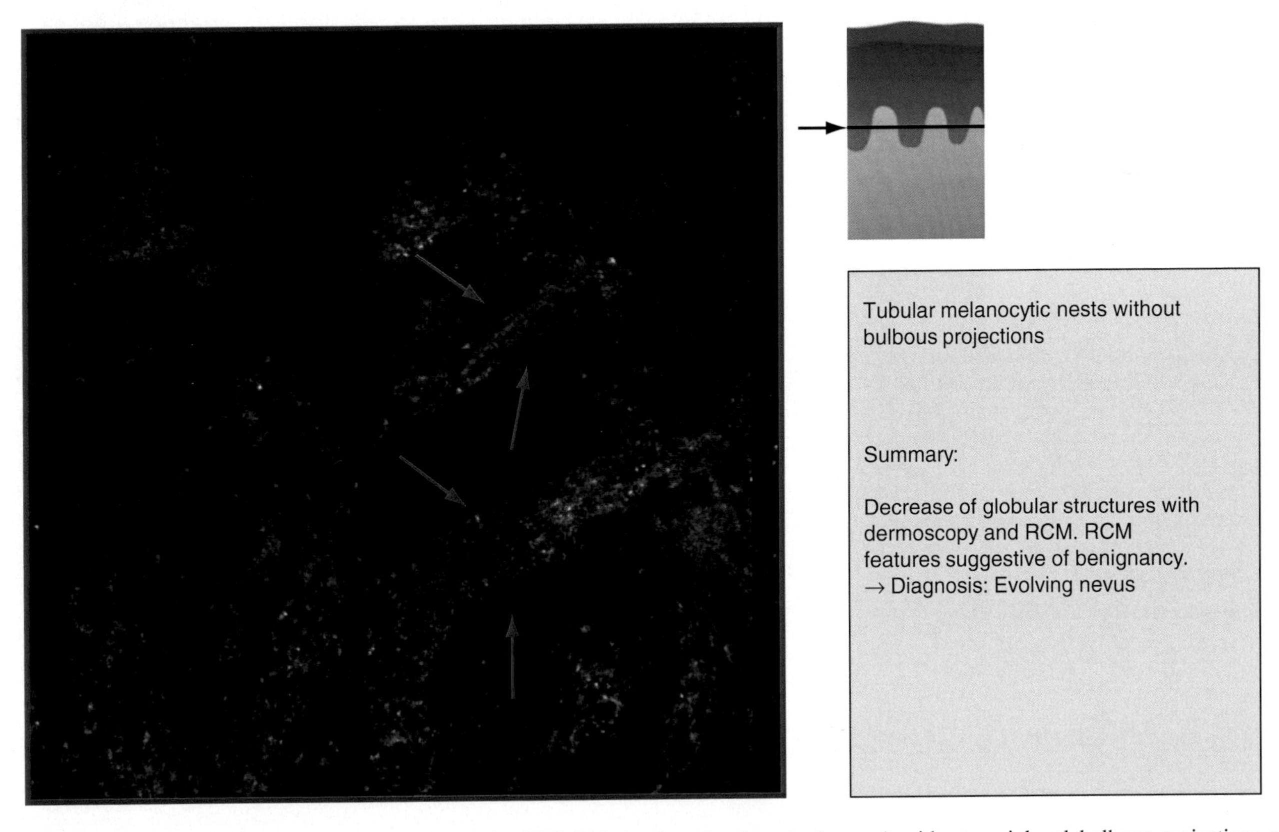

Fig. 31.4.5 Basic RCM image (0.5 × 0.5 mm) at the DEJ. Tubular junctional nests (*arrows*) without peripheral bulbous projections are visualized

References

1. Nadiminti H, Scope A, Marghoob A, Busam K, Nehal KS (2010) Use of reflectance confocal microscopy to monitor response of Lentigo maligna to nonsurgical treatment. Derm Surg 36(2):177–184
2. Naylor MF, Crowson N, Kuwahra R, Teague K, Garcia C, Mackinnis C, Haque R, Odom C, Jankey C, Cornelison RL (2003 Nov) Treatment of lentigo maligna with topical imiquimod. Br J Dermatol 149(Suppl 66):66–70
3. Haenssle HA, Krueger U, Vente C, Thoms KM, Bertsch HP, Zutt M, Rosenberger A, Neumann C, Emmert S (2006) Results from an observational trial: digital epiluminescence microscopy follow-up of atypical nevi increases the sensitivity and the chance of success of conventional dermoscopy in detecting melanoma. J Invest Dermatol 126(5):980–985
4. Menzies SW, Gutenev A, Avramidis M, Batrac A, McCarthy WH (2001 Dec) Short-term digital surface microscopic monitoring of atypical or changing melanocytic lesions. Arch Dermatol 137(12): 1583–1589
5. Carli P, De Giorgi V, Crocetti E, Mannone F, Massi D, Chiarugi A, Giannotti B (2004) Improvement of malignant/benign ratio in excised melanocytic lesions in the 'dermoscopy era': a retrospective study 1997–2001. Br J Dermatol 150(4):687–692
6. Langley RG, Walsh N, Sutherland AE, Propperova I, Delaney L, Morris SF, Gallant C (2007) The diagnostic accuracy of in vivo confocal scanning laser microscopy compared to dermoscopy of benign and malignant melanocytic lesions: a prospective study. Dermatology 215(4):365–372
7. Guitera P, Pellacani G, Longo C, Seidenari S, Avramidis M, Menzies SW (2009) In vivo reflectance confocal microscopy enhances secondary evaluation of melanocytic lesions. J Invest Dermatol 129(1): 131–138
8. Unna PG (1893) Nevi and nevocarcinome. Berl Klin Wochenschr 30:14–16
9. Masson P (1951) My conception of cellular nevi. Cancer 4:9–38
10. Cramer SF (1984) The histogenesis of acquired melanocytic nevi: based on a new concept of melanocytic differentiation. Am J Dermatopathol 6(Suppl):289–298
11. Kittler H, Seltenheim M, Dawid M, Pehamberger H, Wolff K, Binder M (2000) Frequency and characteristics of enlarging common melanocytic nevi. Arch Dermatol 136:316–320
12. Zalaudek I, Grinschgl S, Argenziano G, Marghoob AA, Blum A, Richtig E et al (2006) Age-related prevalence of dermoscopy patterns in acquired melanocytic nevi. Br J Dermatol 154:299–304
13. Pellacani G, Scope A, Ferrari B, Pupelli G, Bassoli S, Longo C, Cesinaro AM, Argenziano G, Hofmann-Wellenhof R, Malvehy J, Marghoob AA, Puig S, Seidenari S, Soyer HP, Zalaudek I (2009) New insights into nevogenesis: in vivo characterization and follow-up of melanocytic nevi by reflectance confocal microscopy. J Am Acad Dermatol 61(6):1001–1013

32 Monitoring of Nonsurgical Treatment of Skin Tumors

Martina Ulrich and Verena Ahlgrimm-Siess

32.1 Introduction

In the past decade, a variety of novel, noninvasive treatment modalities have been introduced for the therapeutic management of skin tumors. The ability to treat skin cancer without surgery prompted the search for new, noninvasive diagnostic techniques. Reflectance confocal microscopy (RCM) allows the in vivo assessment of skin and has been used as an adjunct technique in the diagnosis of various skin diseases with a focus on skin tumors. RCM enables repeated investigation of the same skin lesion over a longitudinal period of time without any tissue alterations, thus representing an ideal tool for diagnosis and follow-up of skin tumors undergoing nonsurgical treatment. In this regard, RCM may be used for the assessment of treatment efficacy as well as for the investigation of treatment effects including necrosis, apoptosis or inflammation. RCM offers some great advantages to patients as the noninvasive examination is painless and does not cause any scarring. Histopathological examination, however, still represents the current diagnostic gold standard and should be performed in all cases that cannot be classified with certainty by RCM.

32.2 Monitoring of Nonmelanoma Skin Cancer

32.2.1 Basal Cell Carcinoma

Diagnostic confocal criteria of basal cell carcinoma (BCC) have been well established within the past years; tumor islands sharply demarcated from the surrounding fibrotic dermis by dark cleft-like spaces, dilated and tortuous linear blood vessels that run parallel to the horizontal plane and elongated keratinocytes oriented along the same axis ("streaming") above tumor islands have been described as key RCM features of BCC [1, 2]. These well-defined criteria allow the distinction of BCC from normal skin with high sensitivity and specificity and serve as a basis for evaluating treatment response to noninvasive therapies.

A study examining the efficacy of Imiquimod as an adjunct treatment following to Moh`s micrographic surgery showed a high concordance between RCM and histology as well as a higher positive predictive value in the assessment of treatment response when RCM was used together with clinical assessment [3]. Another study evaluated the efficacy of cryotherapy for superficial BCC, showing that early cell necrosis at basal layer and within the superficial dermis 5 h after application of liquid nitrogen indicated effective cryotherapy [4]. In this regard, RCM may allow the immediate evaluation of treatment efficacy after cryotherapy and may indicate if a second cryotherapy session is needed (Table 32.1).

32.2.2 Actinic Keratoses

The diagnosis of actinic keratoses (AK) with RCM is based on the detection of an atypical honeycomb pattern with loss of the regular epidermal architecture and presence of an irregular and thickened stratum corneum. A high sensitivity and specificity of key RCM features of AK and a high interobserver agreement on RCM diagnosis has been shown [5, 6].

A recent study evaluated the applicability of RCM for monitoring treatment efficacy of Imiquimod in AK, showing that RCM was able to visualize the inflammatory response induced by Imiquimod in clinically visible as well as in subclinical lesions within an actinically damaged field [7]. RCM offered in vivo insights into immune-modulatory effects of Imiquimod by visualizing appearance of inflammatory cells, especially Langerhans cells, followed by apoptosis of atypical keratinocytes. At 4-week follow-up, disappearance of

M. Ulrich (✉)
Department of Dermatology and Venerology, Charité University Medicine Berlin, Berlin, Germany
e-mail: martina.ulrich@charite.de

V. Ahlgrimm-Siess
Department of Dermatology and Venerology, Medical University of Graz, Graz, Austria
e-mail: verena.ahlgrimm@medunigraz.at

R. Hofmann-Wellenhof et al. (eds.), *Reflectance Confocal Microscopy for Skin Diseases*,
DOI 10.1007/978-3-642-21997-9_32, © Springer-Verlag Berlin Heidelberg 2012

keratinocyte atypia and appearance of a regular epidermal architecture and a typical honeycomb pattern could be observed in the majority of patients by RCM. In some of the patients, RCM enabled the detection of residual disease after treatment. RCM may also be used for monitoring of other non invasive treatment modalities for AK such as PDT or hyaluronic acid (Figs. 32.1 and 32.2).

32.3 Monitoring of Melanocytic Lesions

32.3.1 Lentigo Maligna

The clinical diagnosis of Lentigo maligna is often challenging on the background of chronically sun-damaged skin and the detection of tumor margins may be hindered by the presence of ill-defined or amelanotic borders, which are commonly observed. RCM may be a helpful adjunct tool in diagnosis and noninvasive margin mapping; a confluence of mainly dendritic atypical melanocytes along a flattened dermo-epidermal junction and a descent of atypical melanocytes along adnexal structures have been shown to be characteristic confocal features of Lentigo maligna [8].

Although surgical excision including Moh's micrographic surgery represents the treatment of choice, nonsurgical treatments such as Imiquimod [13], radiation and cryotherapy have been alternatively used in particular cases [9–11]. RCM enabled not only the delineation of lateral tumor margins, but also monitoring of the inflammatory response and proof of tumor clearance after cessation of therapy. The dendritic appearance of Langerhans cells, however, represents a potential pitfall in the evaluation of treatment efficacy of Imiquimod in Lentigo maligna, as these cells may resemble residual dendritic melanocytes. According to our own experience and cases reported in the literature, these activated Langerhans cells completely disappear within 1 to 3 months after end of treatment.

32.4 Monitoring of Nonneoplastic Skin Lesions

The ability to visualize dynamic skin processes by RCM implicates a broad spectrum of potential applications not only in neoplastic, but also in inflammatory skin conditions and in monitoring of cosmetic procedures. A recent study evaluated the treatment of melasma with pyruvic acid and hydroquinone in 15 patients. In this preliminary study, RCM was able to provide precise information on the location and extent of pigment deposits and to assess treatment efficacy over time [12].

Table 32.1 Summary of clinical studies evaluating treatment response by RCM

Tumor type	Study	Results
Basal cell carcinoma	Torres et al. [3]	Evaluation of efficacy of Imiquimod in adjunct to Moh's micrographic surgery by RCM; a high concordance between RCM and histology and a higher positive predictive value than with clinical assessment alone was shown
	Ahlgrimm-Siess et al. [4]	RCM was able to assess the efficacy of cryotherapy immediately after therapy and to indicate the necessity for further treatment, such as a second cryotherapy session, when early necrosis within the dermis was absent
Actinic keratoses	Ulrich et al. [7]	RCM is able to visualize inflammatory response induced by Imiquimod in clinically visible as well as in subclinical lesions and allows the assessment of tumor clearance or detection of residual disease after treatment
Lentigo maligna	Nadiminti et al. [9–11]	RCM allows the assessment of treatment efficacy of various noninvasive treatment modalities in Lentigo maligna, including cryotherapy and Imiquimod
Melasma	Ardigo et al. [12]	RCM allows the evaluation of pigment distribution in melasma and monitoring of treatment effects over time

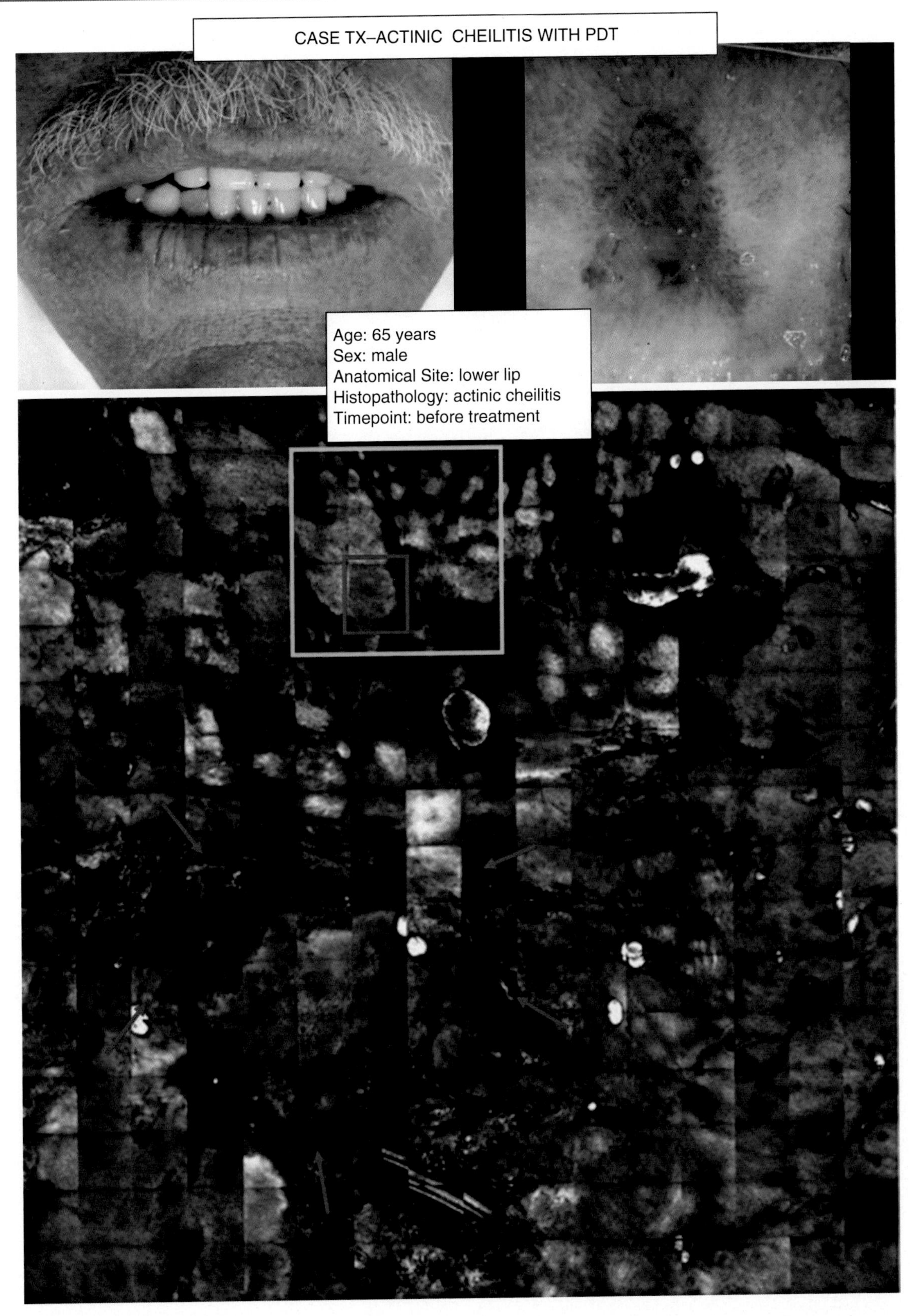

Fig. 32.1 RCM mosaic (8 × 8 mm) obtained at the level of the stratum spinosum illustrating epithelium of the vermillion border. The central part of the mosaic (*red arrows*) is showing the erosive area, whereas the lower part represents the surrounding normal skin where adnexal structures such as hairs (red star) can be visualized

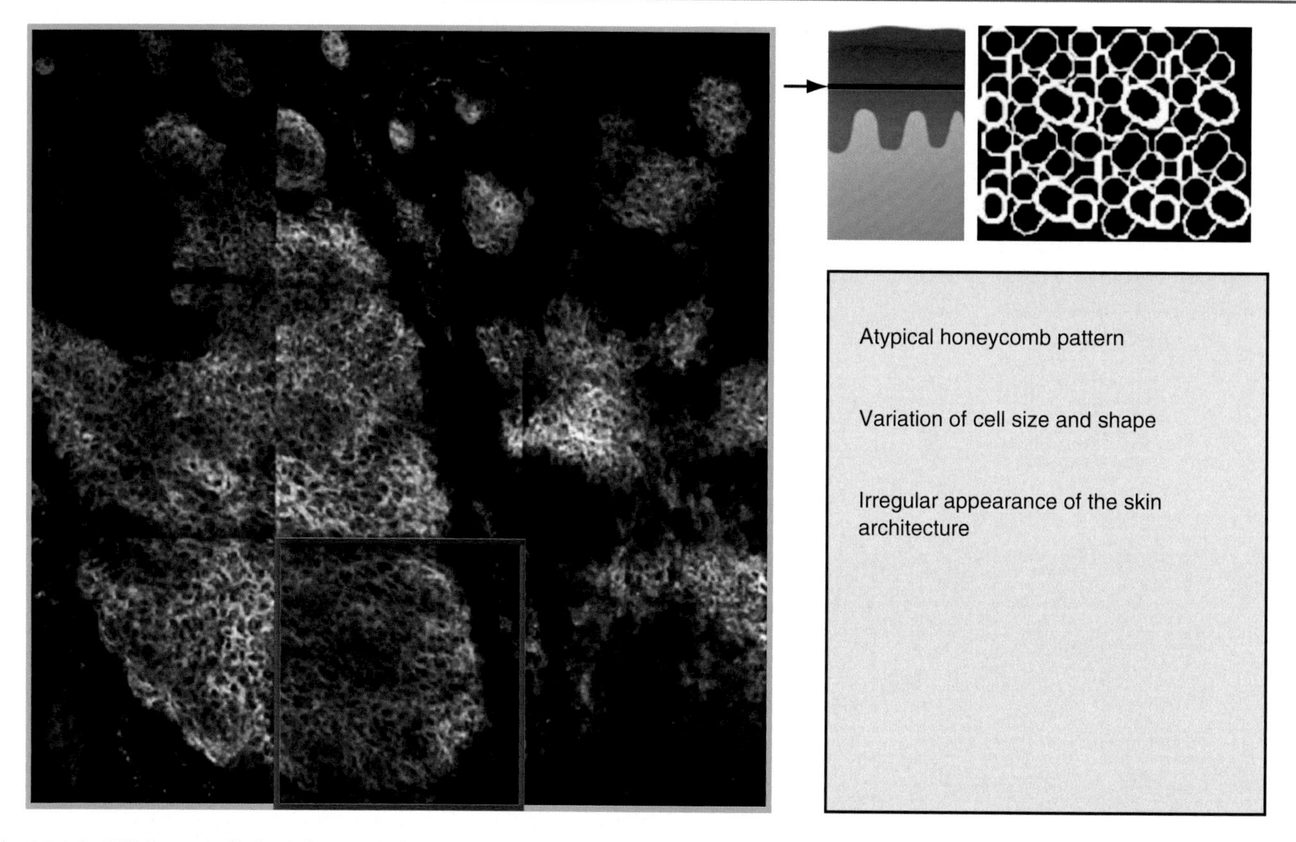

Fig. 32.1.1 RCM mosaic (1.5 × 1.5 mm) obtained at the level of the stratum spinosum showing atypical honeycomb pattern. The mosaic shows small "islands" of epithelium which is caused by superficial disruption with scaling and crusting and partly interferes with the visualization of deeper layers

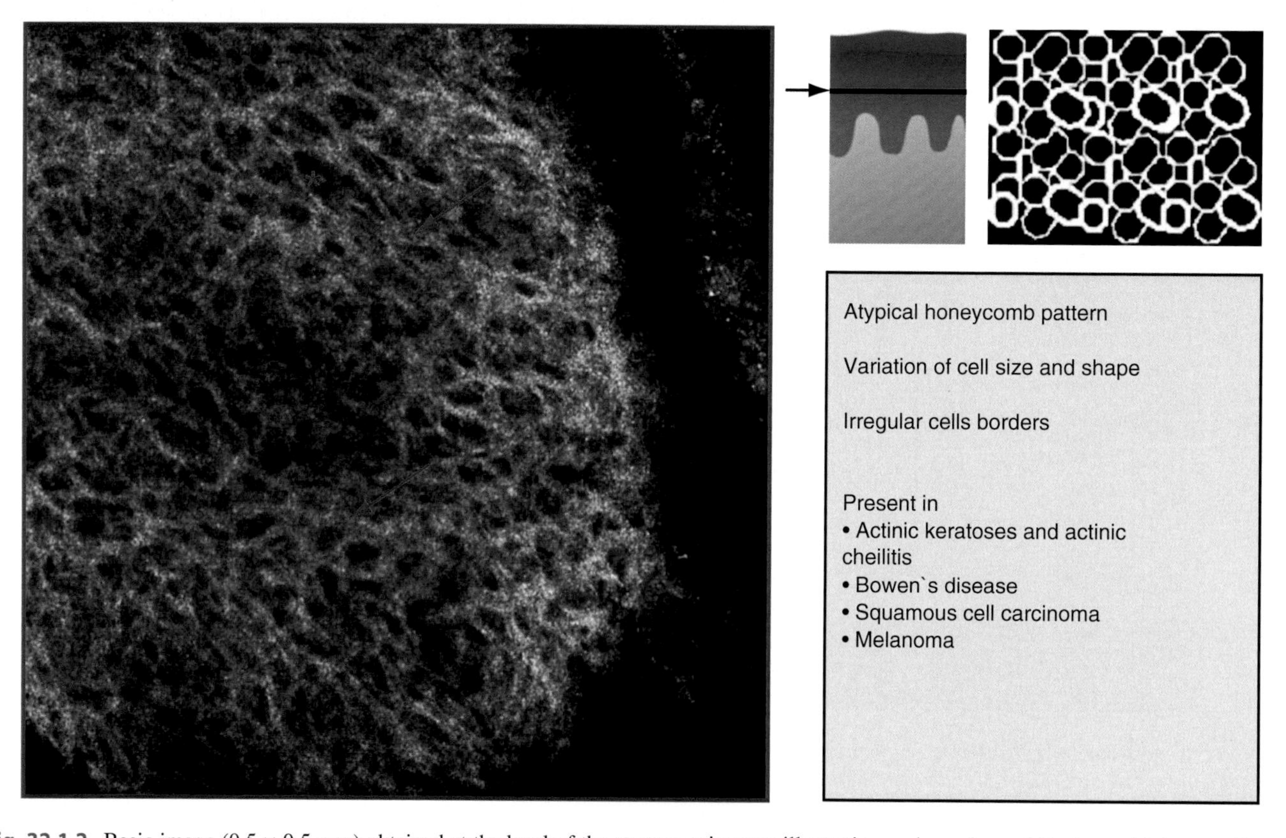

Fig. 32.1.2 Basic image (0.5 × 0.5 mm) obtained at the level of the stratum spinosum illustrating an irregular architecture with large cells and nuclei (*) that show great variation in size and morphology. In some areas intercellular borders are blurred and irregular (→)

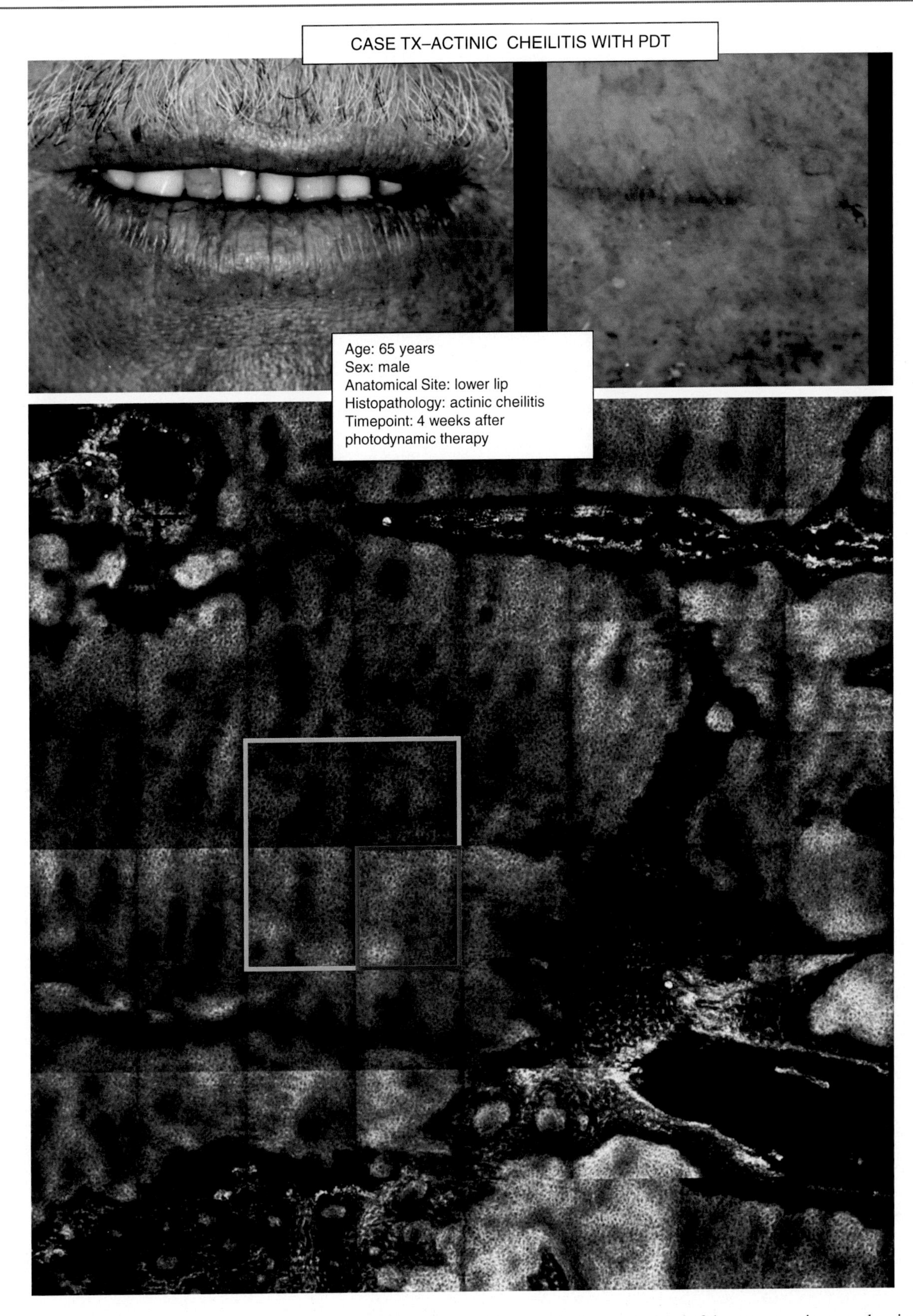

Fig. 32.1.3 RCM mosaic (4 × 4 mm) of the same lesion 4 weeks after PDT. Images obtained at the level of the stratum spinosum showing regular architecture with large epidermal islands, separated by normal skin folds (*)

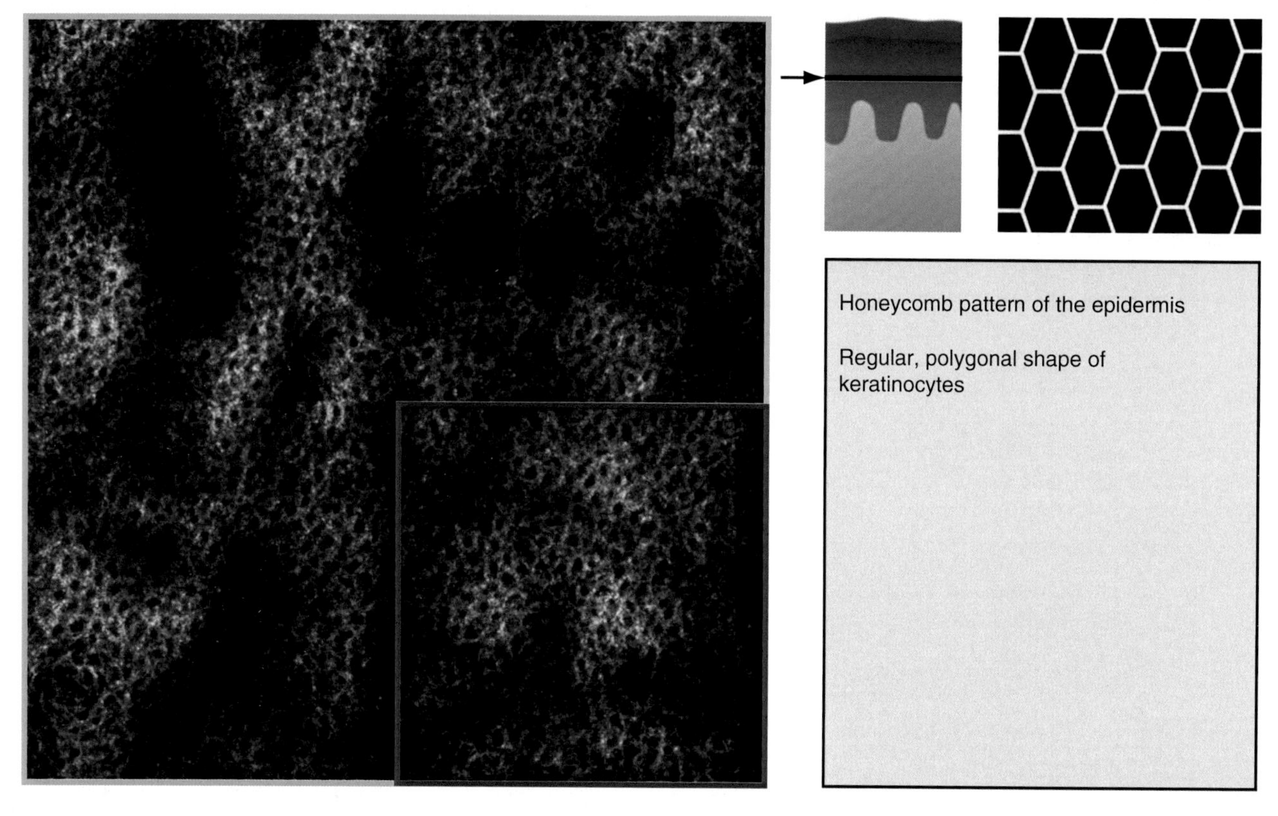

Fig. 32.1.4 RCM mosaic (1 × 1 mm) obtained at the level of the stratum spinosum showing typical honeycomb appearance of the epidermis. Cells show homogeneous size, shape and arrangement indicating clearance of actinic cheilitis and re-arrangement of normal honeycomb appearance

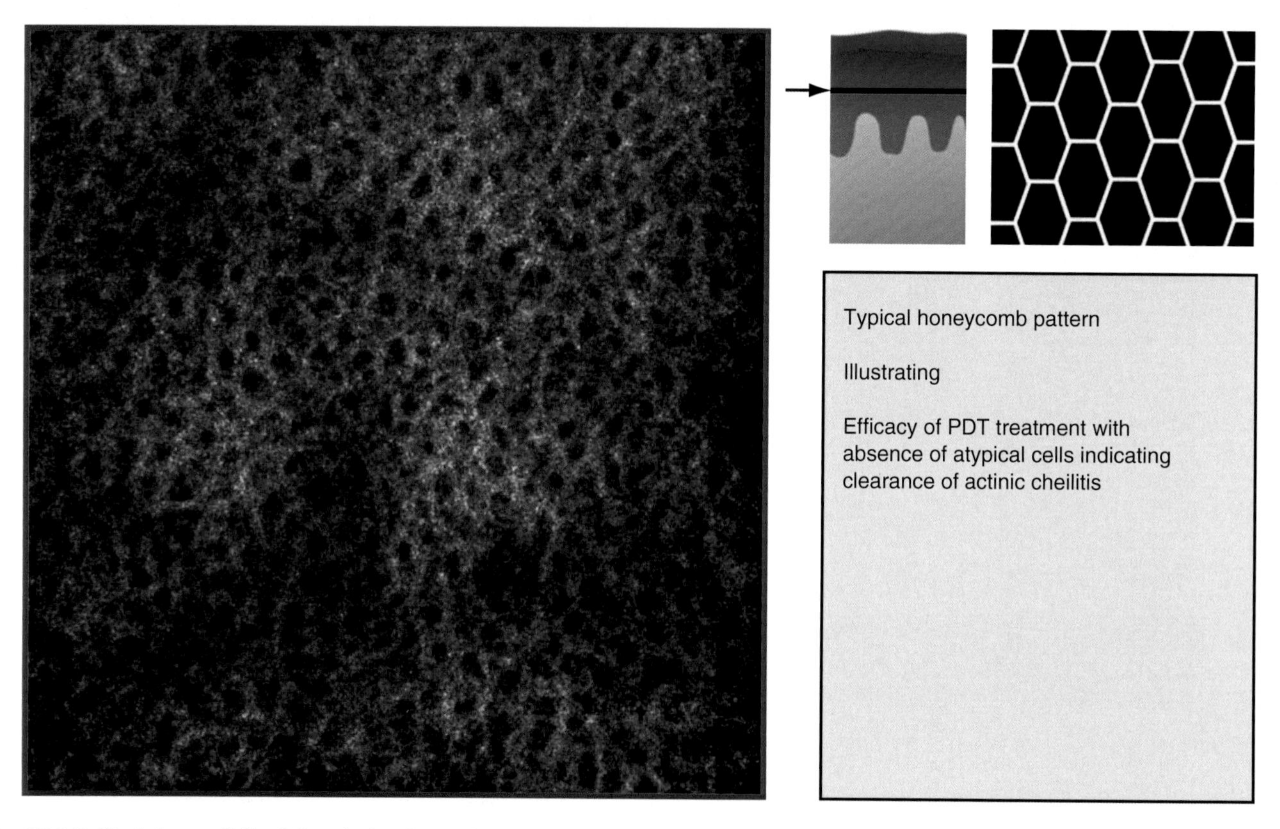

Fig. 32.1.5 Basic image (0.5 × 0.5 mm) showing typical honeycomb pattern

CASE AK_TX –ACTINIC KERATOSES (3% DICLOFENAC)
Age: 72 years
Sex: male
Anatomical Site: right cheek
Diagnosis: Actinic keratosis
Timepoint: before treatment:

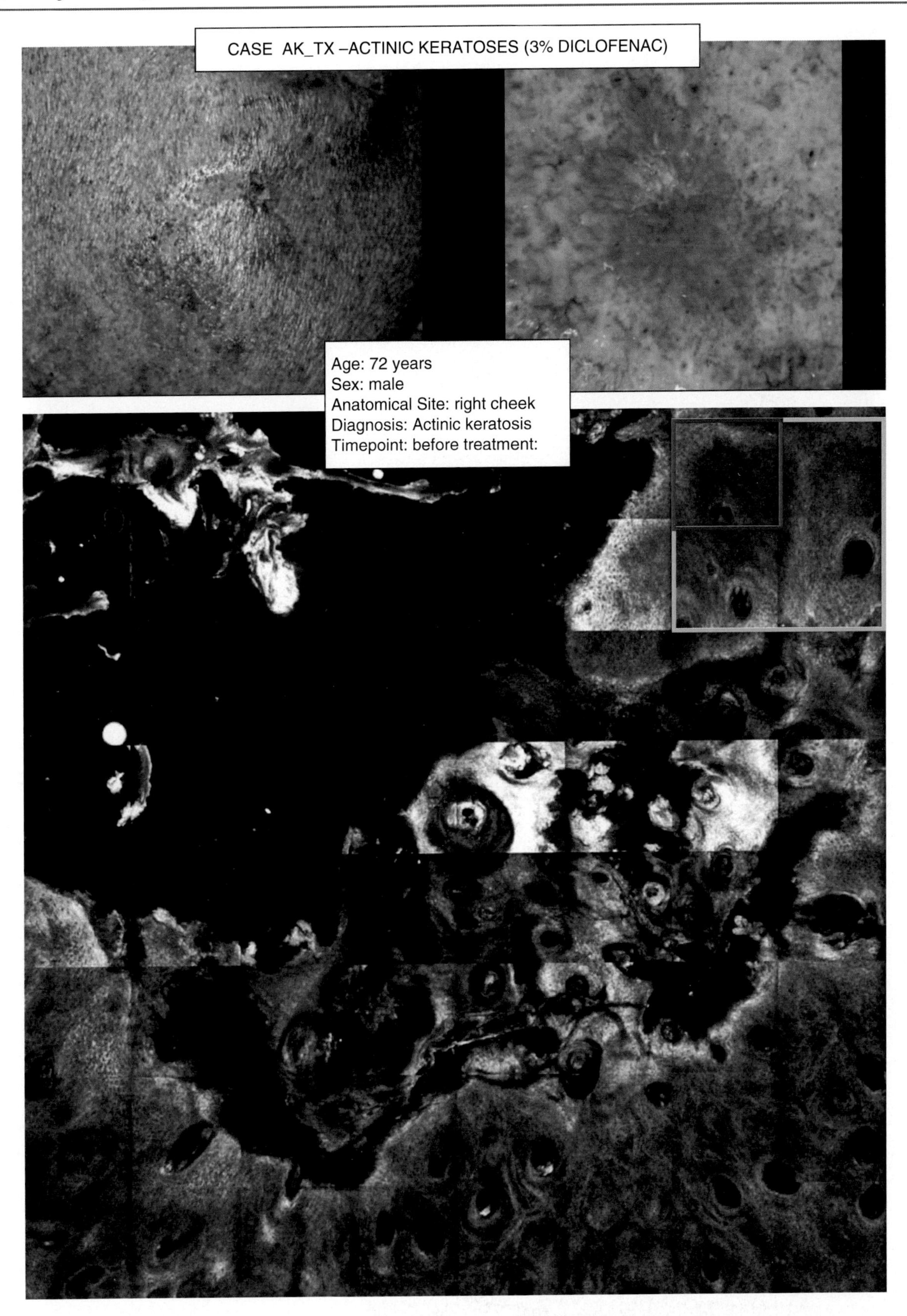

Fig. 32.2 RCM mosaic (4 × 4 mm) of an actinic keratoses on the right cheek illustrating irregular morphology of the epidermis. Dark areas in the center of the lesions are due to hyperkeratosis which causes reflection of the light and does impede the visualization of deeper layers

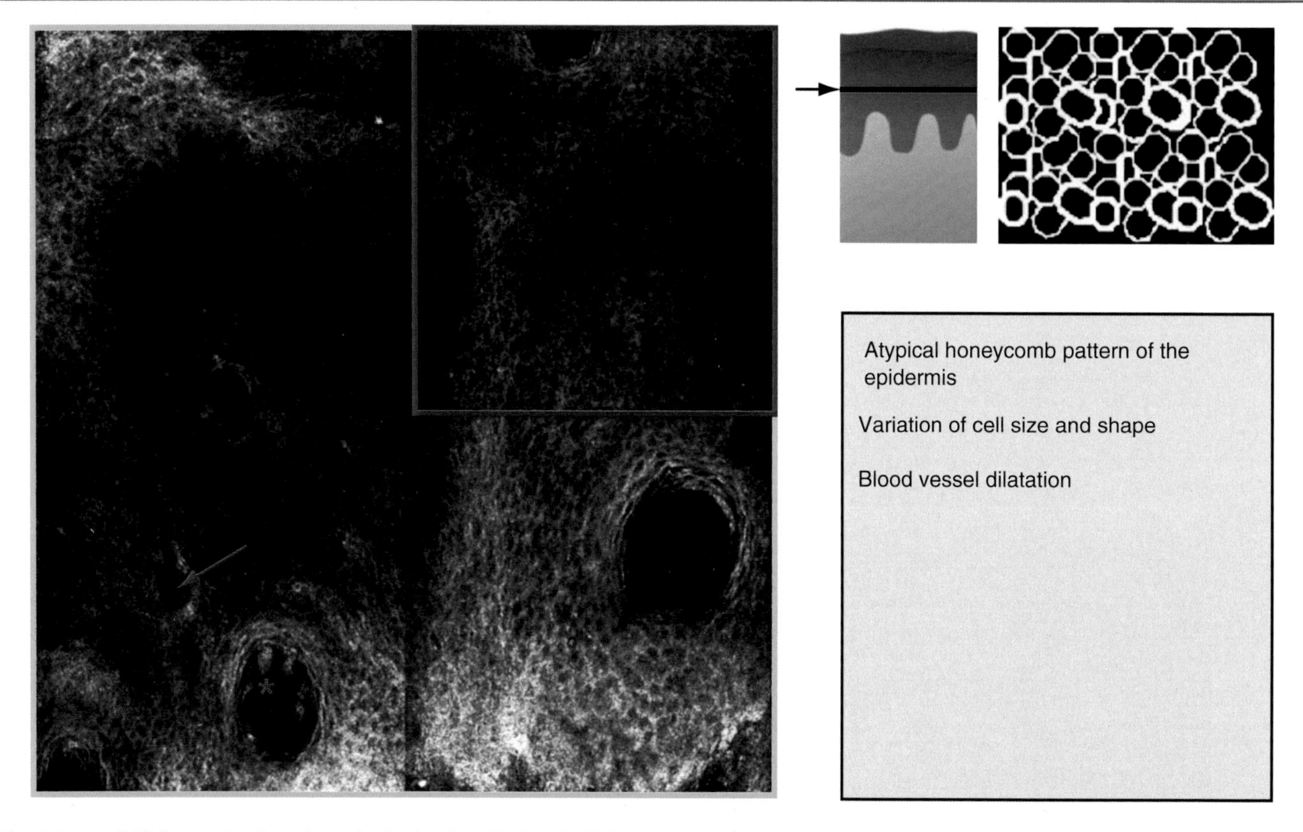

Fig. 32.2.1 RCM mosaic (1 × 1 mm) obtained at the level of the stratum spinosum and the DEJ illustrating atypical honeycomb pattern with cells that vary in size and shape. Slight blood vessel dilatation of the capillaries within the dermal papillae (*red arrow* →). A demodex mite can also be observed (*), a finding not specific for AK that can often be observed in facial skin

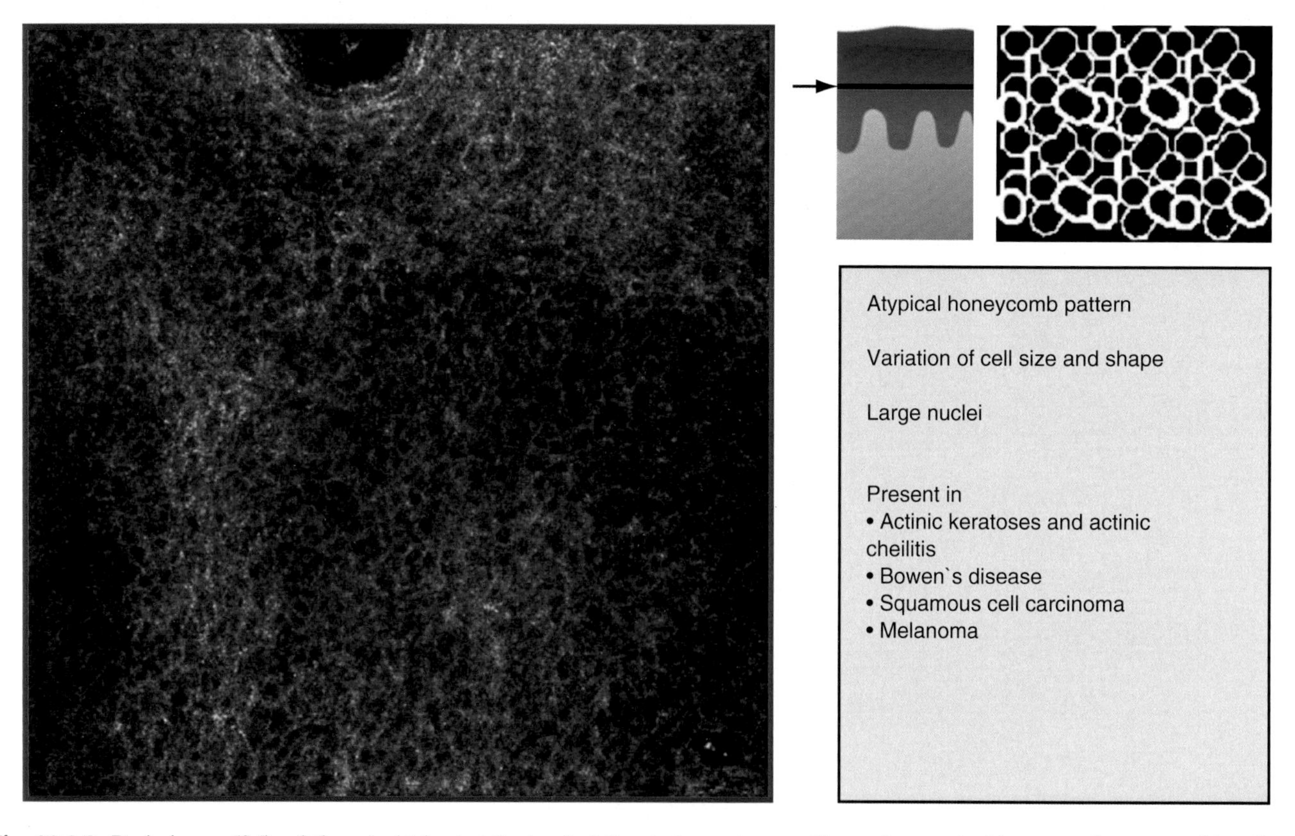

Fig. 32.2.2 Basic image (0.5 × 0.5 mm) obtained at the level of the stratum spinosum illustrating atypical honeycomb pattern with cells of different size and shape

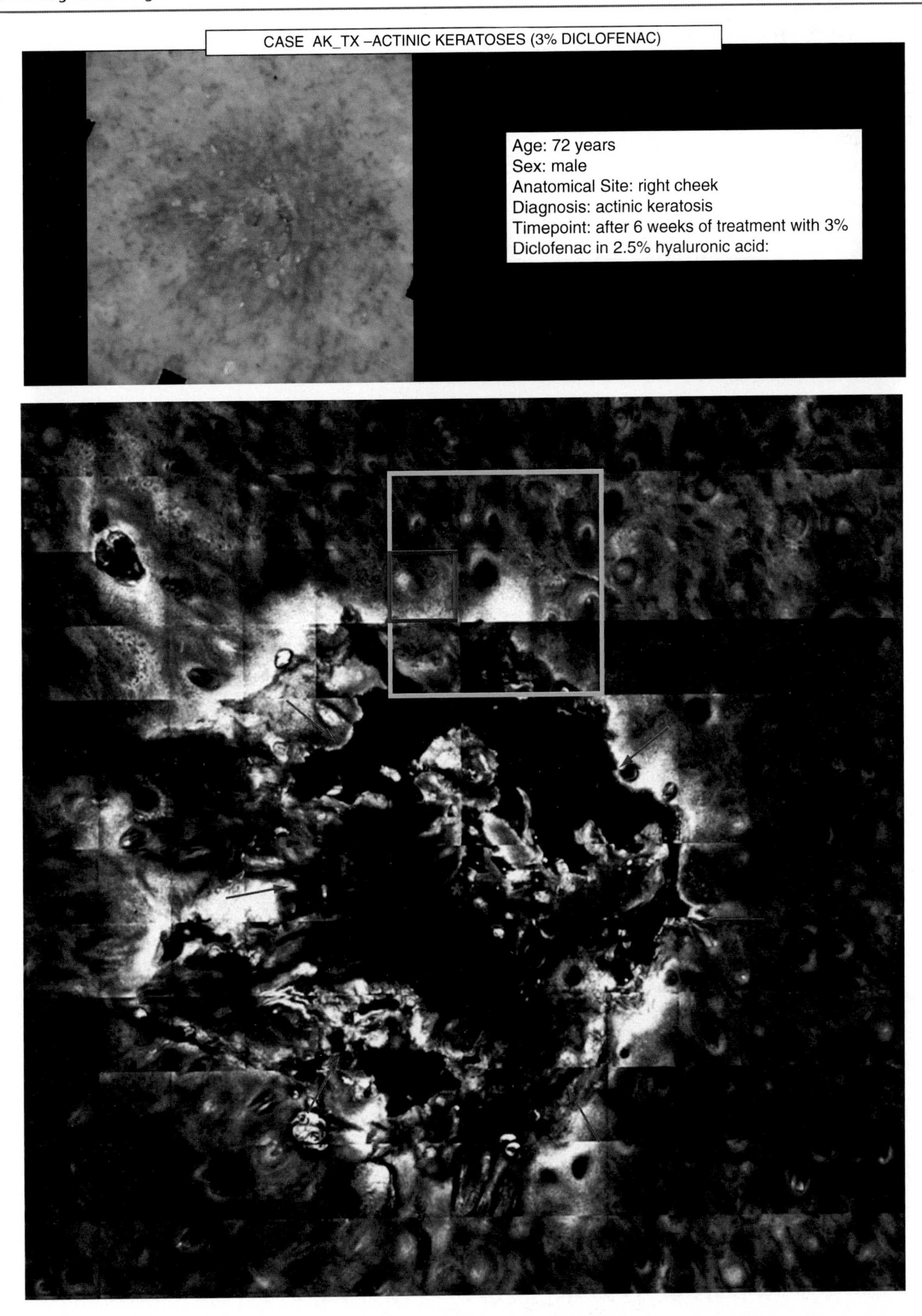

Fig. 32.2.3 RCM mosaic (6 × 6 mm) of the same lesion after 6 week treatment with 3% Diclofenac in hyaluronic acid illustrating remaining hyperkeratotic scale in the center of the lesion (*), showing irregular borders and sharp demarcation (*red arrows* →)from nonhyperkeratotic areas of the lesion

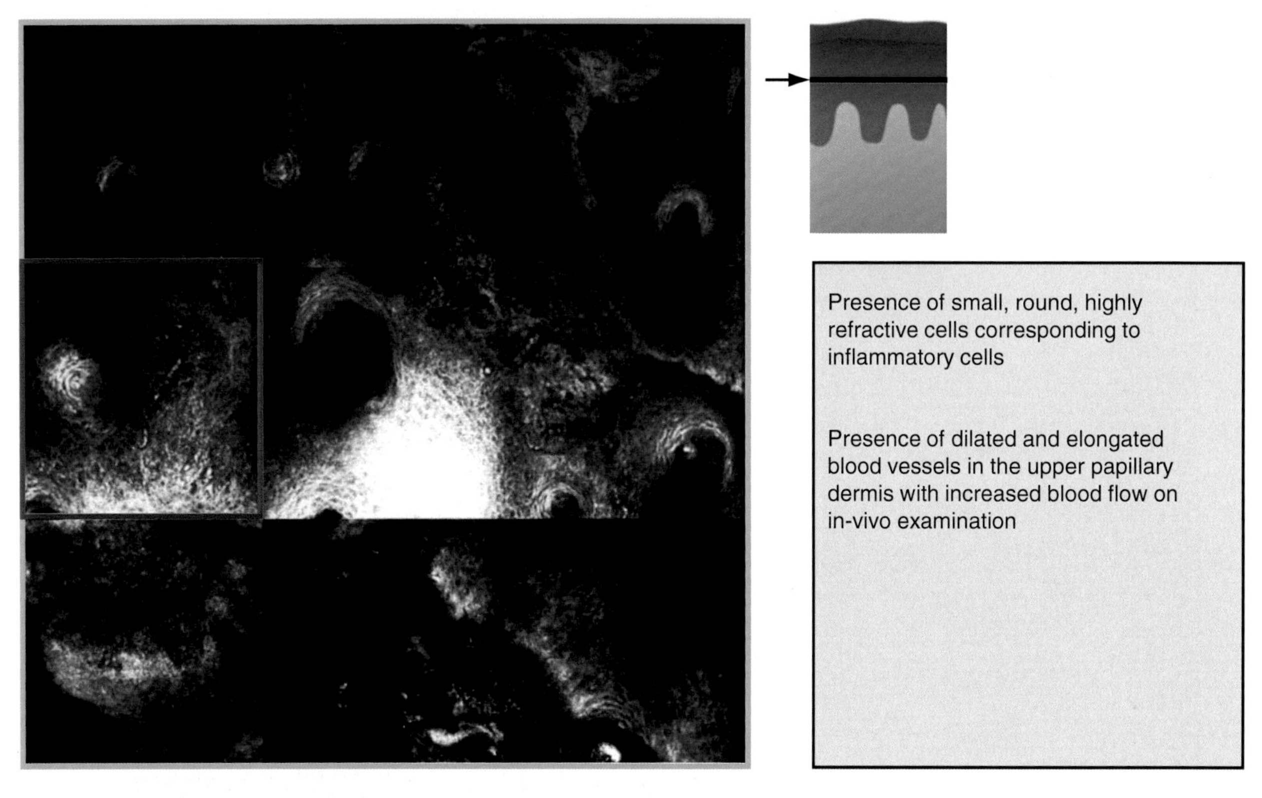

Fig. 32.2.4 RCM mosaic (1.5 × 1.5 mm) obtained at the DEJ illustrating inflammatory response induced by 3% Diclofenac in 2.5% hyaluronic acid

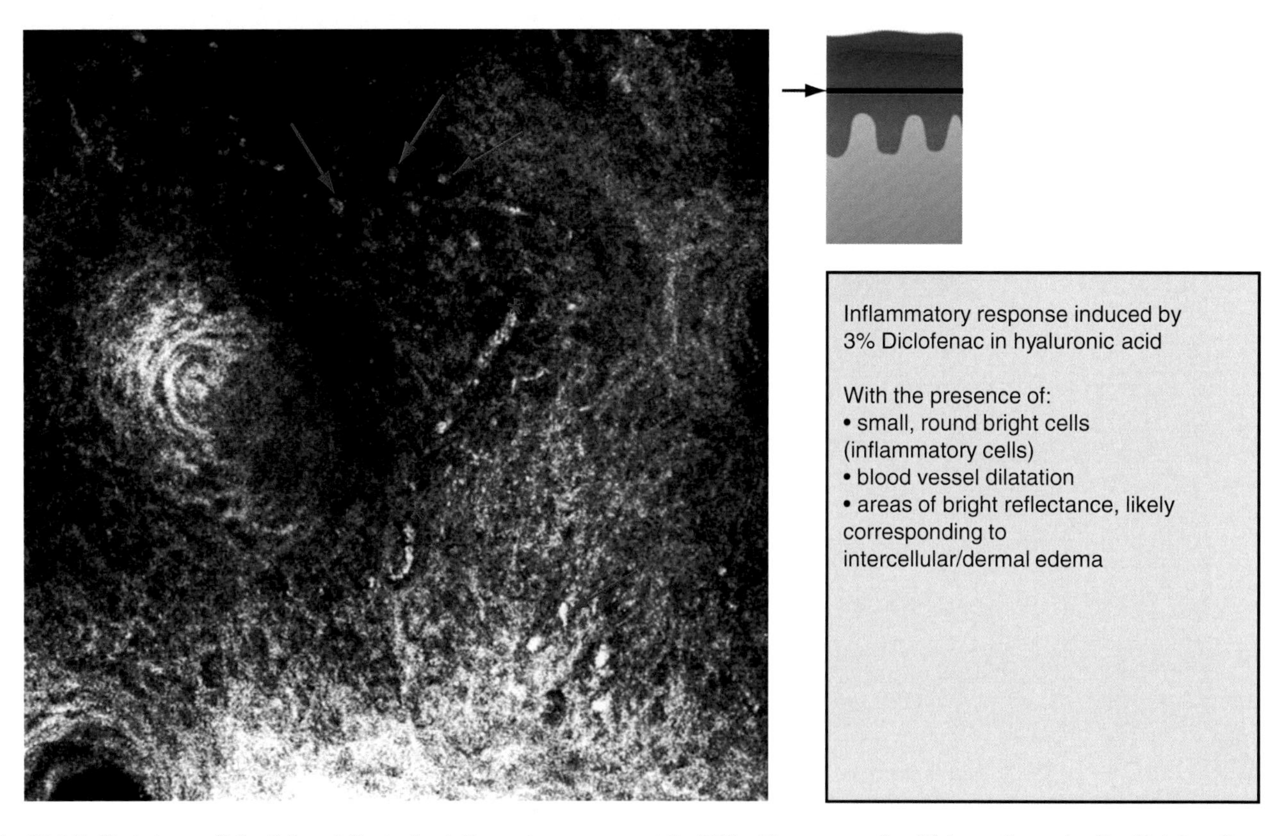

Fig. 32.2.5 Basic image (0.5 × 0.5 mm) illustrating inflammatory response at the DEJ with presence of multiple small round cells of bright reflectance in a perifollicular and perivascular distribution (→). Furthermore, dilated and elongated blood vessels (*) are present in the upper papillary dermis

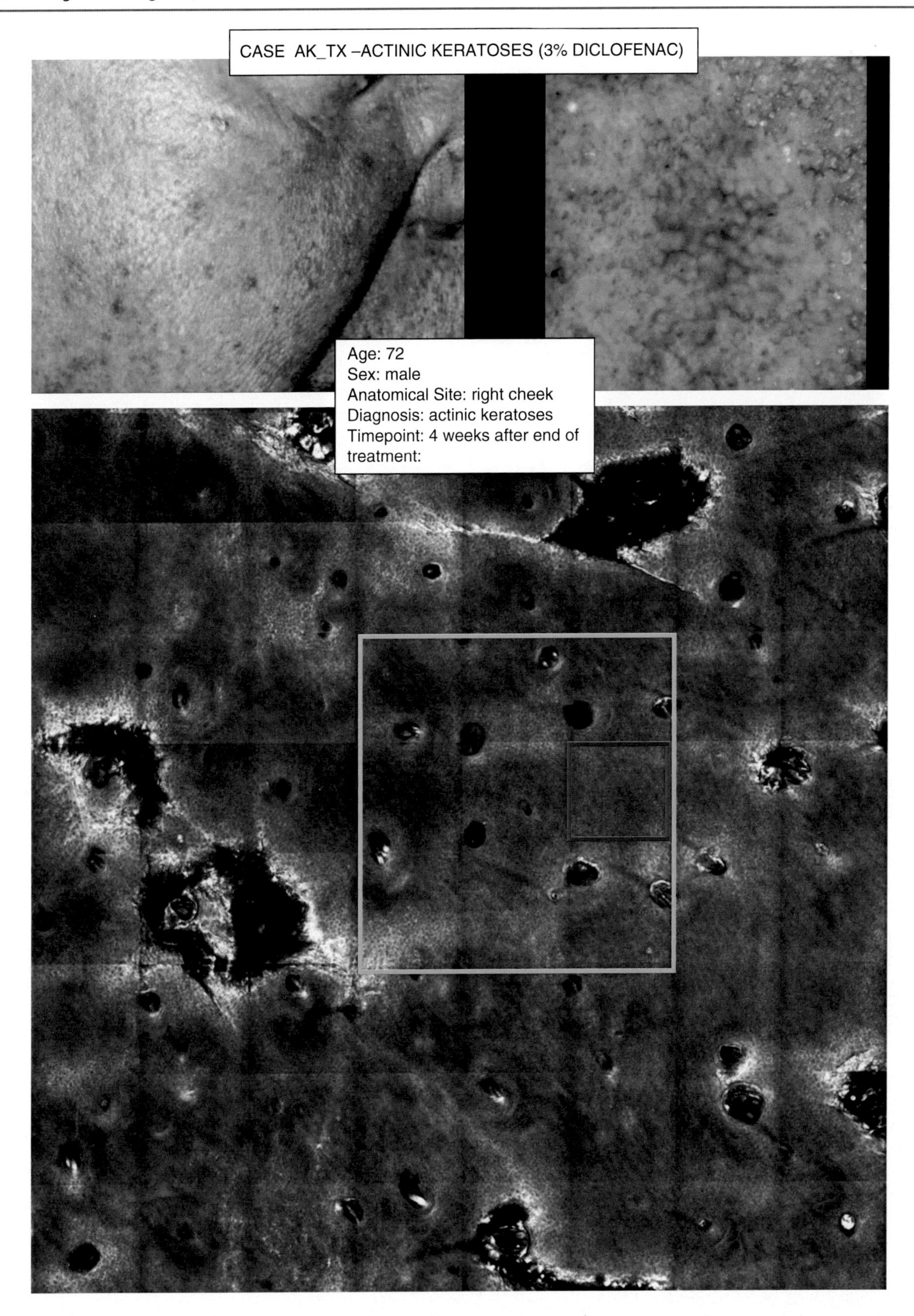

Fig. 32.2.6 RCM mosaic (4 × 4 mm) of the same lesion obtained at the level of the stratum spinosum 4 weeks after end of treatment with 3% Diclofenac in 2.5% hyaluronic acid. Regular appearance of the epidermis can be observed

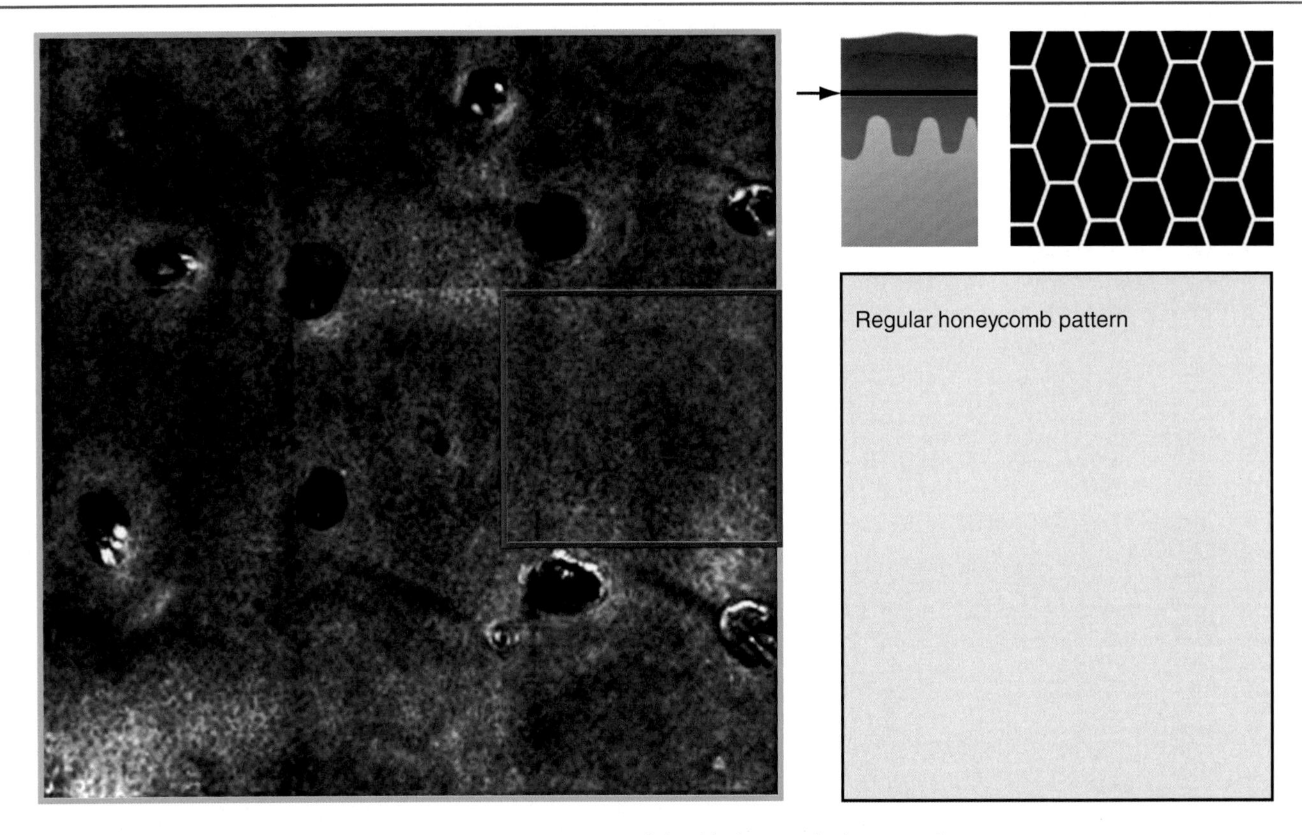

Fig. 32.2.7 RCM mosaic (1.5 × 1.5 mm) illustrating re-arrangement of the skin in a regular honeycomb pattern

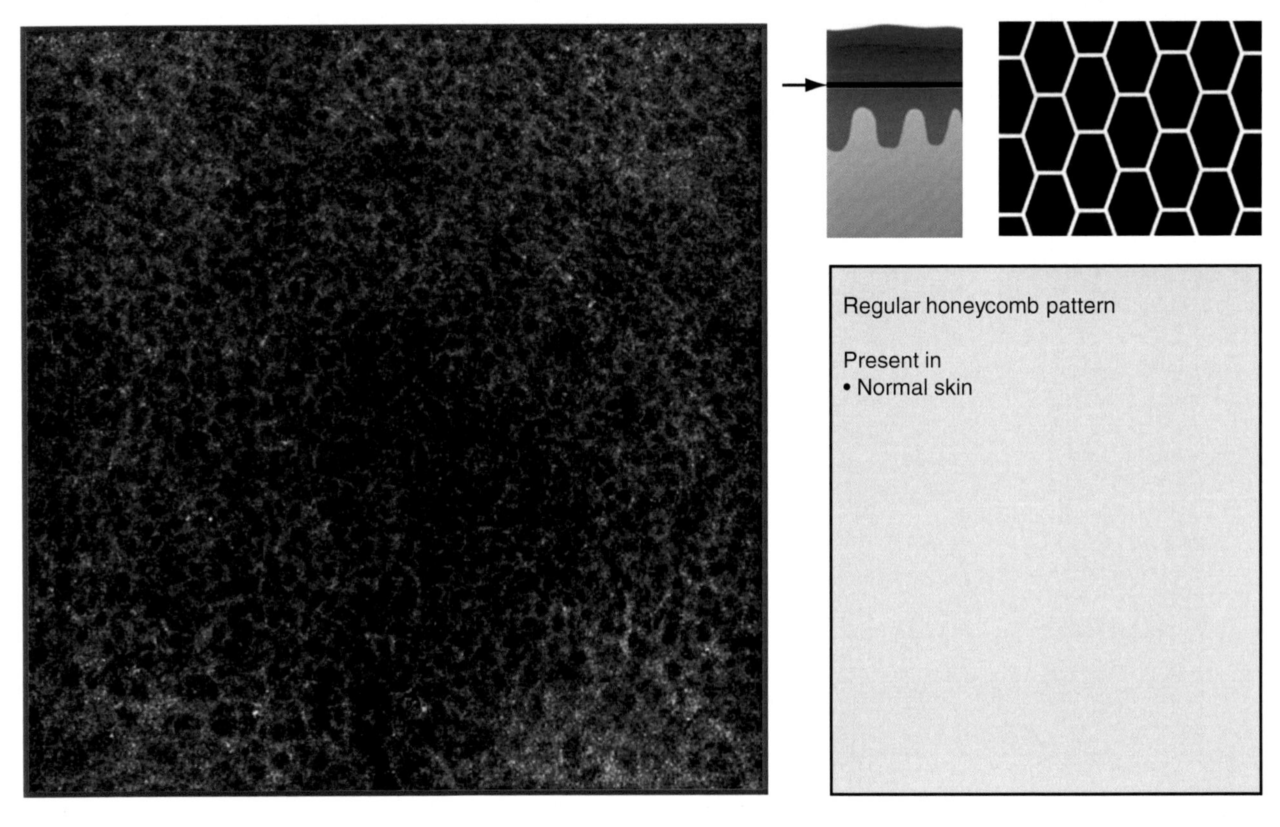

Fig. 32.2.8 Basic image (0.5 × 0.5 mm) illustrating re-arrangement of the epidermis and presence of typical honeycomb pattern

Core Messages

- RCM enables noninvasive diagnosis and margin mapping in clinically challenging skin tumors.
- Treatment effects of nonsurgical antitumor therapies, such as inflammation, apoptosis and necrosis, can be monitored in vivo over a longitudinal period of time.
- Treatment efficacy and necessity of further treatment after cessation of therapy can be noninvasively evaluated by RCM.

References

1. Nori S, Rius-Díaz F, Cuevas J, Goldgeier M, Jaen P, Torres A, González S (2004) Sensitivity and specificity of reflectance-mode confocal microscopy for in vivo diagnosis of basal cell carcinoma: a multicenter study. J Am Acad Dermatol 51(6):923–930
2. Sauermann K, Gambichler T, Wilmert M, Rotterdam S, Stücker M, Altmeyer P, Hoffmann K (2002) Investigation of basal cell carcinoma by confocal laser scanning microscopy *in vivo*. Skin Res Technol 8(3):141–147
3. Torres A, Niemeyer A, Berkes B, Marra D, Schanbacher C, González S, Owens M, Morgan B (2004) 5% imiquimod cream and reflectance-mode confocal microscopy as adjunct modalities to Mohs micrographic surgery for treatment of basal cell carcinoma. Dermatol Surg 30(12 Pt 1):1462–1469
4. Ahlgrimm-Siess V, Horn M, Koller S, Ludwig R, Gerger A, Hofmann-Wellenhof R (2009) Monitoring efficacy of cryotherapy for superficial basal cell carcinomas with in vivo reflectance confocal microscopy: a preliminary study. J Dermatol Sci 53(1):60–64
5. Ulrich M, Maltusch A, Rius-Diaz F, Röwert-Huber J, González S, Sterry W, Stockfleth E, Astner S (2008) Clinical applicability of in vivo reflectance confocal microscopy for the diagnosis of actinic keratoses. Dermatol Surg 34:610–619
6. Horn M, Gerger A, Ahlgrimm-Siess V, Weger W, Koller S, Kerl H, Samonigg H, Smolle J, Hofmann-Wellenhof R (2008) Discrimination of actinic keratoses from normal skin with reflectance mode confocal microscopy. Dermatol Surg 34:620–625
7. Ulrich M, Krueger-Corcoran D, Roewert-Huber J, Sterry W, Stockfleth E, Astner S (2010) Reflectance confocal microscopy for noninvasive monitoring of therapy and detection of subclinical actinic keratoses. Dermatology 220(1):15–24
8. Ahlgrimm-Siess V, Massone C, Scope A, Fink-Puches R, Richtig E, Wolf IH, Koller S, Gerger A, Smolle J, Hofmann-Wellenhof R (2009) Reflectance confocal microscopy of facial lentigo maligna and lentigo maligna melanoma: a preliminary study. Br J Dermatol 161(6):1307–1316
9. Naylor MF, Crowson N, Kuwahara R, Teague K, Garcia C, Mackinnis C, Haque R, Odom C, Jankey C, Cornelison RL (2003) Treatment of lentigo maligna with topical imiquimod. Br J Dermatol 149(Suppl 66):66–70
10. Curiel-Lewandrowski C, Williams CM, Swindells KJ, Tahan SR, Astner S, Frankenthaler RA, González S (2004) Use of in vivo confocal microscopy in malignant melanoma: an aid in diagnosis and assessment of surgical and nonsurgical therapeutic approaches. Arch Dermatol 140(9):1127–1132
11. Nadiminti H, Scope A, Marghoob A, Busam K, Nehal KS (2010) Use of reflectance confocal microscopy to monitor response of Lentigo maligna to nonsurgical treatment. Derm Surg 36(2):177–184
12. Ardigo M, Cameli N, Berardesca E, Gonzalez S (2010) Characterization and evaluation of pigment distribution and response to therapy in melasma using in vivo reflectance confocal microscopy: a preliminary study. J Eur Acad Dermatol Venereol 24(11):1296–1303
13. Ahmed I, Berth-Jones J (2000) Imiquimod: a novel treatment for lentigo maligna. Br J Dermatol 143(4):843–845

33 Confocal Mosaicing Microscopy in Skin Excisions: Feasibility of Cancer Margin Screening at the Bedside to Guide Mohs Surgery

Daniel S. Gareau, Kishwer Nehal, and Milind Rajadhyaksha

33.1 Introduction

Nonmelanoma skin cancers occur most commonly on cosmetically sensitive areas such as on the face and head-and-neck. For the surgical treatment of these cancers, complete resection of diseased tissue is guided by microscopic pathology, with the objective of preserving perilesional healthy tissue. The current method for screening the margins of staged excisions for the presence of residual tumor is frozen histopathology. Histopathology-guided Mohs surgery for basal cell carcinoma (BCC) is effective [1] with 5-year cure rate of about 99% [2]. However, the preparation of histopathology is laborious and time consuming. Up to 20–45 min may be needed for preparation of frozen sections of an excision [3] and a Mohs procedure requires typically from two to several excisions. Thus, the preparation of Mohs histopathology may require up to hours. As an emerging mode of cellular imaging that is being translated for clinical utility, confocal microscopy potentially offers a means for real-time detection of skin cancers at the bedside, either directly on patients in vivo [4] or directly in surgically excised tissue ex vivo [3–5]. Nuclear and cellular morphology is imaged in noninvasive thin optical sections with high resolution. The optical sectioning of 1–5 μm and resolution of 0.1–1.0 μm is comparable to that for physically microtomed sections in histopathology. Thus, confocal imaging may serve as an adjunct to pathology for guiding Mohs surgery in a more efficient manner, while saving labor, time and cost.

Imaging of thin optical sections at high resolution with a confocal microscope requires the use of objective lenses with relatively high numerical apertures of 0.7–1.4 and high magnifications of 20–100×. With such lenses, the field of view is typically 1.0–0.2 mm. For example, we routinely use an objective lens with magnification of 30× that displays a field-of-view of 0.5 mm with resolution of 0.5 μm. However, Mohs surgical excisions are much larger, typically 5–20 mm in size. The Mohs surgeon usually examines the histopathology of the entire excision at low magnification, typically 2×, and with low resolution of 4 μm. To create such a large field-of-view, a two-dimensional sequence of confocal images is captured and stitched together in software into a seamless composite mosaic [6–8]. For example, with the 30× objective lens, up to 35 × 35 images may be stitched into a mosaic that displays a field-of-view of up to 15 × 15 mm. This field-of-view is equivalent to the view with 2× magnification in a standard light microscope and therefore mimics the conventional technique for margin screening.

The acquisition of a contiguous sequence of 35 × 35 images on the entire surface, including the epidermis along the periphery, requires that the tissue be kept stable and flat. A tissue fixture was specially engineered to mount Mohs surgical excisions [7, 8]. The stitching of images into a seamless mosaic requires correction for illumination artifacts, vignetting, field curvature, and lateral and angular registration. An image-stitching algorithm and software was developed to create and display mosaics [6, 7]. The images are stitched together using one of two methods. Either the overlap between adjacent images is cropped and the resultant images merged together, or the overlapping area is averaged following initial feature matching. The cropping-and-merging method is rapid but at the cost of leaving minor seams at the

D.S. Gareau (✉)
Dermatology Service, Memorial Sloan-Kettering Cancer Center, New York, NY, USA

Departments of Dermatology and Biomedical Engineering, Oregon Health & Science University, Portland, OR, USA
e-mail: dan@dangareau.net

K. Nehal • M. Rajadhyaksha
Dermatology Service, Memorial Sloan-Kettering Cancer Center, New York, NY, USA
e-mail: nehalk@mskcc.org; rajadhym@mskcc.org

R. Hofmann-Wellenhof et al. (eds.), *Reflectance Confocal Microscopy for Skin Diseases*,
DOI 10.1007/978-3-642-21997-9_33,

edges, while the averaging-and-feature matching algorithm yields seamless mosaics at the cost of speed. Further details of the tissue fixturing and the crop-and-merge mosaicing algorithm will be found elsewhere [6–8].

A full mosaic at full resolution requires ~325 MB of memory but may be scaled down to ~4 MB with resolution of about 4 μm and pixelation of about 2500 × 2500 that is equivalent to that in a 2× view of histopathology. Viewing the scaled mosaics on a large monitor, with at least 2500 pixels per line, mimics the observation of histopathology at 2× magnification. Furthermore, digital zooming enables closer observation of specific regions with higher magnification at the native 0.5 μm resolution. Examination of mosaics at low (2×) magnification and low resolution, followed by inspection of specific areas in sub-mosaics at higher magnification (4×–30×) and higher resolution, mimics the Mohs surgeons' examination of frozen histopathology sections. The process of confocal mosaic observation provides comparative analytical quality to conventional microscopy on sectioned slides.

33.2 Contrast Agents

As in histopathology, contrast agents may be used in excised tissue. In reflectance, acetic acid was shown to stain and brighten nuclear morphology and enhance tumor-to-dermis contrast [3, 5, 7, 8]. High diagnostic accuracy has been shown for detection of malignant morphologies of BCC [9]. The inter-observer agreement was excellent for identification of peripheral palisading, tumor cell nuclei and tumor nests. In a second study by the same group, on invasive squamous cell carcinoma (SCC), an overall sensitivity of 95% and a specificity of 96.25% were achieved by four observers (positive predictive value 96.25%, negative predictive value 95.23%) [10]. While encouraging, these results were obtained on preselected and single images (i.e., the analysis not blinded and not on large area mosaics). In our experience, large superficial and nodular BCC tumors are easily detected in reflectance mode mosaics but smaller tumors such as micronodular and, especially, tiny strands of infiltrative and sclerosing BCCs are not [7, 8]. Although the acetic acid-stained tumors appear bright, the surrounding strongly-scattering dermis is also relatively bright in reflectance. Thus, large tumors with dense nucleation remain detectable in mosaics. By comparison, small nodules and tiny strands of tumor may contain only 5–10 nuclei. Though these tumors are easily seen in individual confocal images that display small fields of view with high magnification, they are undetectable in mosaics that display large fields of view with low magnification.

Fluorescence provides a better alternative, to specifically stain and brighten nuclear morphology while the dermis appears either dark or, at most, weakly bright due to autofluorescence. Contrast agents such as methylene blue and toluidine blue [11] and acridine orange [6] have been shown to strongly improve tumor-to-dermis contrast. Fluorescence contrast allows the detection of smaller micronodular and infiltrative BCCs [6] that was not possible earlier with reflectance. The shape, size and location of BCC tumors and features such as nuclear atypia, nuclear density (crowding), nuclear/cytoplasm ratio, pleomorphism and peripheral palisading of elongated monomorphic basaloid nuclei are clearly observable. The epidermal margin and normal features such as hair follicles, sebaceous glands and eccrine glands are seen. Inflammatory infiltrates in the dermis are also seen.

Figure 33.1 shows the fluorescence confocal mosaic of a Mohs excision with nodular and micronodular BCC and correlating histopathology. The contrast agent is acridine orange of concentration 1 mM and the treatment (immersion) time was 20 s. The zoomed in single image displays a higher-magnification view of a smaller area, showing nuclear, cellular and morphologic detail with high resolution. With dense nuclear crowding, BCC is easily distinguished within the dermis in both the high-magnification image and the low-magnification mosaics. Mosaics of several BCC tumors of all subtypes can be found in our earlier reports [6–8, 12–14].

33.3 Clinical Accuracy

To determine sensitivity and specificity, a study was performed using 45 mosaics [13, 14]. Two Mohs surgeons were blinded to the cases and to the histopathology and presented mosaics to read. Each mosaic was divided into quarters, where each quarter sub-mosaic displayed tissue with the equivalent of 4× magnification. The reading of mosaics simulated the examination of histopathology sections with varying magnifications. The Mohs surgeons used digital zooming in place of physical switching of objective lenses, to interrogate suspicious regions at higher magnification. They scored each mosaic for the presence or absence of tumor. The scoring was subsequently correlated to the corresponding histopathology. Overall sensitivity of 96.6%, specificity of 89.2%, positive predictive value of 93.0%, and negative predictive value of 94.7% were achieved for detecting BCC with the mosaicing technique [13, 14]. Challenging cases to read were infiltrative BCCs with low tumor burden, small superficial tumors that were difficult to distinguish from the epidermal margin (that was occasionally incomplete), and those with dense inflammatory infiltrates. Such challenges are experienced when examining Mohs histopathology, too. Technical challenges were retention of contrast agent in the dermis (including, in some cases, specific staining of elastin in solar elastosis), resulting in false positive regions that appeared similar in brightness to nodular BCC.

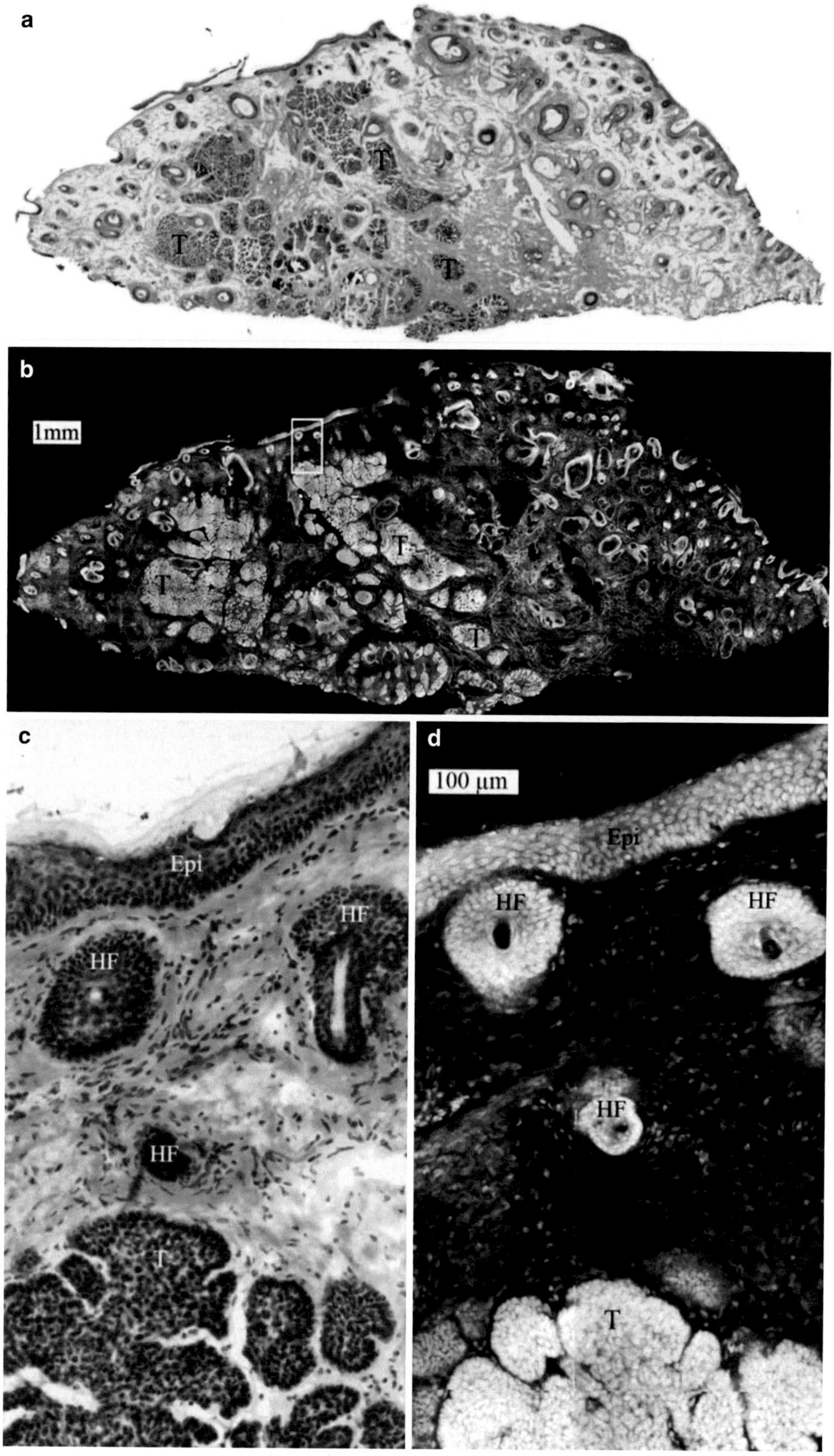

Fig. 33.1 Low and high magnification confocal fluorescence mosaics of skin excisions containing nodular and infiltrative basal cell carcinoma. The conventional histopathology (**a**) at 2× low magnification correlated well with the full confocal mosaic (**b**). At high 30× magnification (**d**), the "zoomed" single image (indicated by the *white box* in **b**) revealed cellular organization of epidermis (*Epi*) and hair follicles (*HF*) and disorganization and nuclear crowding of nodular tumor (*T*) as well as inflammatory infiltrates in surrounding dermis. (**c**) The correlating high-magnification histopathology

33.4 Digital Staining

Ongoing work aims to expand the toolbox of optical modes and contrast agents and apply confocal mosaicing microscopy techniques to squamous cell carcinoma (SCC), which is the other non-melanoma skin cancer. Since the morphological signs of malignancy are more subtle for SCC than for BCC, a more refined approach will likely be required for similarly high sensitivity and specificity. In evaluation of SCC (especially in situ disease), a key diagnostic indication is the absence of the normal differentiation pattern of keratinocytes in their progression from the basal layer through the epidermis to the stratum corneum. Figure 33.2 shows a multimodal confocal mosaic of an SCC in situ from the lip, using the fluorescence and reflectance modes to provide contrast and counter-contrast, respectively, to nuclei. The composite image shows both modes together. The corresponding histopathology shows the correlation. Squamous cell carcinoma in situ is characterized by an intraepidermal proliferation of atypical keratinocytes. Hyperkeratosis, acanthosis, and confluent parakeratosis are seen within the epidermis, and the keratinocytes lie in complete disorder, resulting in the classic "windblown" appearance. Cellular atypia, including pleomorphism, hyperchromatic nuclei, and mitoses, is prominent. Atypical keratinocytes may be found in the basal layer and often extend deeply down hair follicles, but they do not invade the dermis. To reveal these malignant morphologies, similar to the use of two stains in histopathology, a counter-contrast mode is required to represent cytoplasm in the epidermis and collagen in the dermis.

For success in SCC, multiple modes may be required to mimic the labeling in conventional histopathology: acridine orange to label nuclei and reflectance to label dermis and cytoplasm. Fluorescence shows only nuclear detail, similar to hematoxylin-staining in histopathology. Reflectance shows only cellular cytoplasm and collagen, similar to eosin-staining. Though cytoplasmic and collagen components appear bright in reflectance mode, collagen is about fivefold brighter yielding relatively weak contrast of tumor nodules which form dark silhouettes within dermal collagen. A digital staining algorithm is being developed [12] to color the fluorescence mosaic purple and the reflectance mosaic pink, producing composite mosaics with an appearance that resembles that of hematoxylin and eosin in histopathology.

33.5 Alternative Methods

Competing optical technologies for the detection of non-melanoma skin cancers include multiphoton microscopy, wide-field fluorescence spectroscopic imaging, Raman spectroscopy, ultrasound and optical coherence tomography.

The ratio of multiphoton fluorescence (which increases in tumor nodules) to second-harmonic generation (which decreases in tumor nodules) has been shown to be effective in discrimination of nodular BCC tumors from the surrounding dermal stroma [15]. In another study, the multiphoton fluorescence images enabled reproduction of the traditional histopathological diagnostic criteria for BCC and SCC [16]. Fluorescence lifetime imaging has also been used to distinguish BCC from perilesional normal areas [17] as well as fluorescence from tetracycline derivatives with optical polarization [18]. Raman spectroscopy can accurately discriminate nodular- and morphea-type BCC biopsies from perilesional skin samples [19], and spectral analysis on the stratum corneum has shown 100% sensitivity and 100% specificity [20], though it is unclear how much must be present for detection as this technique currently lacks the spatial resolution to detect very sparse tumors. A multimodal approach based on macroscopic mapping of lesions combined aminolaevulinic acid (ALA)-induced protoporphyrin IX fluorescence and autofluorescence followed by Fisher linear discrimination and texture analysis. Good discriminability of BCCs [21] from normal tissue was reported, though ALA-induced fluorescence was inconsistently distributed in some tumor areas.

Similar to confocal microscopy, all these modalities appear promising in feasibility studies and either alone or in multimodal combination may prove useful for clinical applications. Confocal mosaics are currently the only method to achieve nuclear detail on large fields-of view rapidly with high sensitivity and specificity, and are therefore most feasible in the near future for margin screening at the bedside in the surgical theater.

33.6 Future Directions

Preparation and display of confocal mosaics requires, at present, 5–9 min, depending on the size of the Mohs excision [7, 8]. Engineering analysis suggests that, with further improvements in instrumentation, up to 20 × 20 mm may be mosaiced in 2–3 min. Our work in skin serves as a proof-of-feasibility model for applications in other tissues, toward enabling rapid pathology at-the-bedside. For example, breast tissue from needle core biopsies may be rapidly screened with confocal mosaicing microscopy [22, 23]. Other demonstrated applications include screening of head-and-neck, especially for normal versus adenoma parathyroid during surgery, and hepatic tissues [24–26].

Confocal microscopy on whole tissue is a newly developing technique. Confocal mosaicing microscopy may, some day, serve as an adjunct to histopathology or, perhaps, compete as an entirely new alternative. A multicenter clinical trial

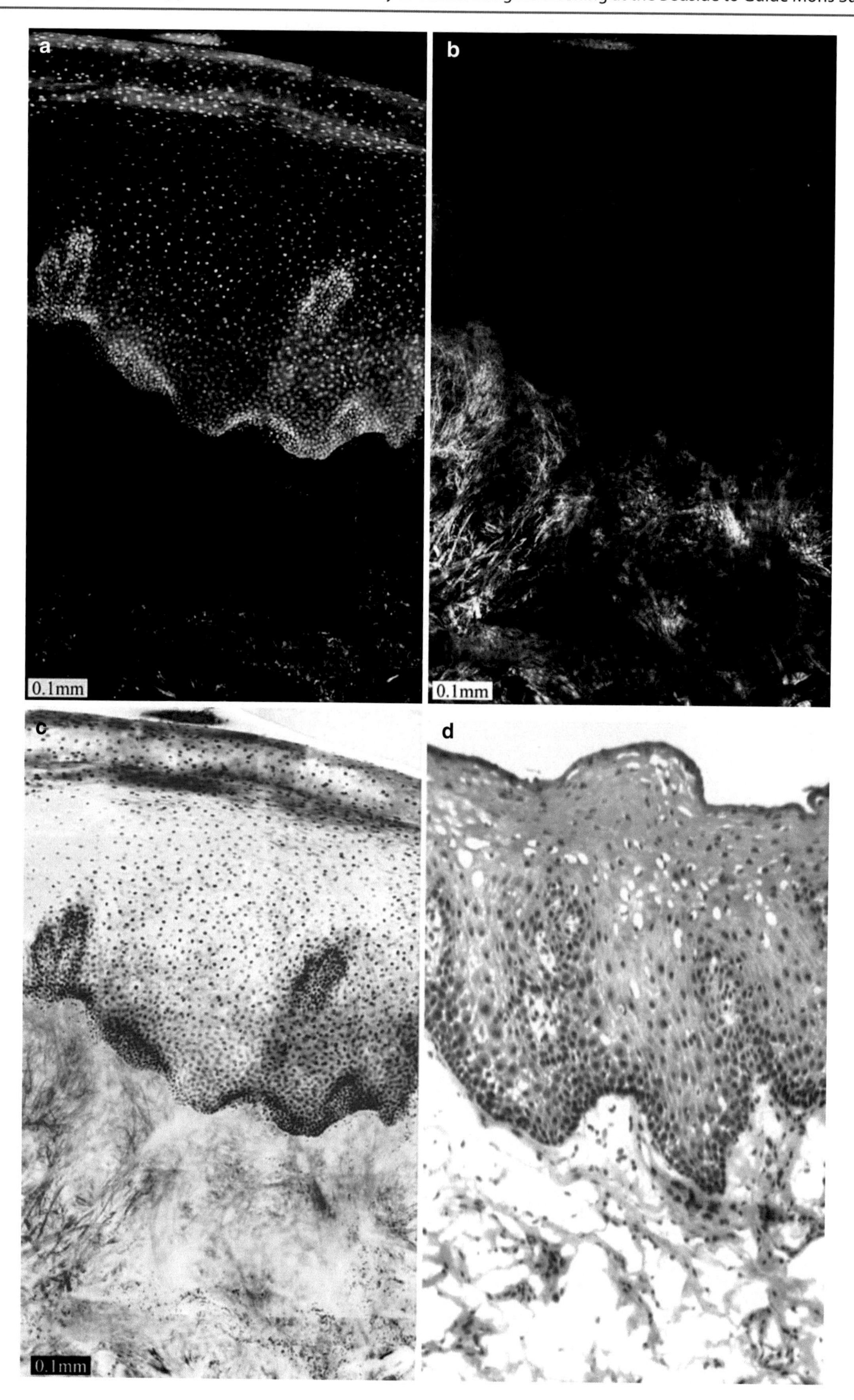

Fig. 33.2 (**a**) fluorescence mode confocal mosaic of SCC in situ with acridine orange staining of nuclei, (**b**) corresponding reflectance mode mosaic where endogenous reflectance labels collagen, (**c**) multimodal digitally stained confocal mosaic (C=A+B), and (**d**) the corresponding histopathology

and acceptance by Mohs surgeons will be required before this technique can be moved out of the laboratory and into routine practice. Beyond detection in excised tissue ex vivo, the next advance will be toward intra-operative imaging directly on patients in situ during surgery. A preliminary study has demonstrated the feasibility of reflectance confocal mosaicing to detect residual BCC tumors in the superficial peripheral epidermal and deeper dermal margins in shave biopsy wounds on patients [27] Shave biopsy wounds are an excellent model for the intraoperative tissue conditions to be expected during Mohs surgery. This study and others [28] on non-Mohs surgery, therefore, are harbingers to an exciting future involving the development of specialized instrumentation, contrast agents and clinical studies toward intraoperative confocal imaging to guide surgery in skin as well as other tissues.

References

1. Tierney EP, Hanke CW (2009) Cost effectiveness of Mohs micrographic surgery: review of the literature. J Drugs Dermatol 8(10):914–922
2. Roenigk RK, Ratz JL, Bailin PL et al (1986) Trends in the presentation and treatment of basal cell carcinomas. J Dermatol Surg Oncol 12(8):860–865
3. Rajadhyaksha M, Menaker G, Flotte T et al (2001) Confocal examination of nonmelanoma cancers in thick skin excisions to potentially guide Mohs micrographic surgery without frozen histopathology. J Invest Dermatol 117:1137–1143
4. Gonzalez S, Halpern AC, Gill M (2008) Reflectance confocal microscopy of cutaneous tumors: an atlas with clinical, dermoscopic and histological correlations. Informa Healthcare, London
5. Chung VQ, Dwyer PJ, Nehal KS et al (2004) Use of *ex vivo* confocal scanning laser microscopy during Mohs surgery for non-melanoma skin cancers. Dermatologi Surg 30:1470–1478
6. Gareau DS, Li Y, Huang B et al (2008) Confocal mosaicing microscopy in Mohs skin excisions: feasibility of rapid surgical pathology. J Biomed Opt 13:054001
7. Gareau DS, Patel YG, Li Y et al (2009) Confocal mosaicing microscopy in skin excisions: a demonstration of rapid surgical pathology. J Microsc 233(1):149–159
8. Patel YG, Nehal KS, Aranda I et al (2007) Confocal reflectance mosaicing of basal cell carcinomas in Mohs surgical skin excisions. J Biomed Opt 12:034027
9. Gerger AG, Horn MD, Koller S et al (2005) Confocal examination of untreated fresh specimens from basal cell carcinoma. Arch Dermatol 141:1269–1274
10. Horn M, Gerger A, Koller S (2007) The use of confocal laser-scanning microscopy in microsurgery for invasive squamous cell carcinoma. Brit J Dermatol 156:81–84
11. Al-Arashi M, Salomatina E, Yaroslavsky AN (2007) Multimodal confocal microscopy for diagnosing nonmelanoma skin cancers. Lasers Surg Med 39(9):696–705
12. Gareau DS (2009) The feasibility of digitally stained multimodal confocal mosaics to simulate histopathology. J Biomed Opt 14:034050
13. Gareau DS, Karen JK, Dusza SW et al (2009) Sensitivity and specificity for detecting basal cell carcinomas in Mohs excisions with confocal fluorescence mosaicing microscopy. J Biomed Opt 14:034012
14. Karen JK, Gareau DS, Dusza SW et al (2009) Detection of basal cell carcinomas in Mohs excisions with fluorescence confocal mosaicing microscopy. Brit J Dermatol 160:1242–1250
15. Lin SJ, Jee SH, Kuo CJ et al (2006) Discrimination of basal cell carcinoma from normal dermal stroma by quantitative multiphoton imaging. Opt Lett 31:2756–2758
16. Paoli J, Smedh M, Wennberg AM et al (2007) Multiphoton laser scanning microscopy on non-melanoma skin cancer: Morphologic features for future non-invasive diagnostics. J Invest Dermatol 128:1248–1255
17. Galletly NP, McGinty J, Dunsby C et al (2008) Fluorescence lifetime imaging distinguished basal cell carcinoma from surrounding uninvolved skin. Brit J Dermatol 159:152–161
18. Yaroslavsky AN, Salomatina EV, Neel V et al (2007) Fluorescence polarization of tetracycline derivatives as a technique for mapping nonmelanoma skin cancers. J Biomed Opt 12:014005
19. Nijssen A, Maquelin K, Santos LF et al (2007) Discriminating basal cell carcinoma from preilisional skin using high wave-number Raman spectroscopy. J Biomed Opt 12:034004
20. Lieber CA, Majumder SK, Billheimer D et al (2008) Raman microscopy for skin cancer detection. J Biomed Opt 13:024013
21. Ericson MB, Uhre J, Strandeberg C et al (2005) Bispectral fluorescence imaging combined texture analysis and linear discrimination correlation with histopathologic extent of basal cell carcinoma. J Biomed Opt 10:034009
22. Schiffhauer LM, Boger JN, Bonfiglio TA et al (2009) Confocal microscopy of unfixed breast needle core biopsies: a comparison to fixed and stained sections. BMC Cancer BMC Cancer 9:265. doi:10.1186/1471-2407-9-265
23. Tilli MT, Cabecabrera MC, Parrish AR et al (2007) Real-time imaging and characterization of human breast tissue by reflectance confocal microscopy. J Biomed Opt 12:051901
24. Campo-Ruiz V, Ochoa ER, Lauwers GY et al (2002) Evaluation of hepatic histology by near-infrared confocal microscopy: a pilot study. Human Pathol 33:975–982
25. White WM, Tearney GJ, Pilch BZ et al (2000) A novel noninvasive imaging technique for intraoperative assessment of parathyroid glands: confocal reflectance microscopy. Surgery 128: 1088–1101
26. White WM, Baldassano M, Rajadhyaksha M et al (2004) Confocal reflectance imaging of head and neck surgical specimens: a comparison with histologic analysis. Arch Otolaryngol Head Neck Surg 130:923–928
27. Scope A, Mahmood U, Gareau DS, Kenkre M, Lieb JA, Nehal K, Rajadhyaksha M. In vivo reflectance confocal microscopy of shave biopsy wounds: feasibility of intra-operative mapping of cancer margins. Pending publication in Brit J Dermatol
28. Nguyen QN, Bainkin AV, Leong WL et al (2009) Real time intraoperative confocal laser microscopy-guided surgery. Ann Surg 249: 735–737

34 Reflectance Confocal Microscopy Applications in Cosmetology

Giovanni Pellacani, Caterina Longo, and Marco Ardigò

Skin is a multi-functional organ that present distinct aspects in physiological and pathological conditions. The two main structural layers of the skin, the epidermis and the dermis, can be either affected by many pathologic processes. An inevitable skin change occurs with the passage of time (skin aging) that can be dramatically accelerated by environmental factors. Since the epidermis is the outer layer of skin, which serves as a physical and chemical barrier to the environment, several damage can affect this compartment, mainly due to irritants or medical treatments such as peelings. Another pathologic phenomenon regards the skin pigmentation that can be located exclusively in the epidermis and at dermo-epidermal junction or deeper into the dermis. The skin comprises also adnexal structures such as hairs that are part of distinct cutaneous entities belonging from the spectrum of inflammatory or degenerative diseases.

To assess the subtle skin changes occurring in different clinical situations, several bioengineering methods have been proposed aiming to evaluate the skin damage and to test cosmetic efficacy of products.

RCM represents an excellent tool to determine whether the pathologic changes are present, adding also cytologic information on what cell population is precisely involved in the process (keratinocytes, melanocytes, inflammatory cells). Additionally, it adds the great opportunity to follow the changes over time while providing the measurement of the efficacy of cosmetics.

Here, we delineate the main confocal findings in distinct skin situations such as skin aging, skin pigmentary disorders, skin barrier function, skin hydration, and hair evaluation.

34.1 Skin Aging

Skin aging is a complex biologic process in which both epidermal and dermal changes play a major role to determine the final skin clinical aspect. The structural changes occurring at epidermal level comprise the progressively transformation of a honeycomb pattern, seen in young subjects, into an irregular honeycomb pattern where the keratinocytes show a more variably size and shape. The skin folds, observable at the top layer of the skin, present a rhomboidal arrangement in the young and a predominantly linear pattern in the elderly. The presence of clinical uneven pigmentation is seen as bright keratinocytes, singly or in cluster, in the context of a honeycomb pattern. This confocal aspect is named mottled pigmentation [1]. Interestingly, RCM is able to detect small foci of mottled pigmentation even when it is not clinically evident (Fig. 34.1). The presence of mottled pigmentation is present in almost all ages with a less predominance in the youngest (>30 years old) and the elderly (>65 years old).

The dermal compartment show distinct collagen type and extent among different age groups. A fine reticulated collagen present in the young subjects become progressively replaced by coarse collagen fibers and, at the end of the degenerative process, a compact collagen occupy the entire dermis. Highly refractive curled fibers corresponding to elastic fibers are observed in severe elastosis.

G. Pellacani (✉)
Department of Dermatology and Venereology, University of Modena and Reggio Emilia, Modena, Italy
e-mail: pellacani.giovanni@unimore.it

C. Longo
Department of Dermatology, Arcispedale S Maria Nuova, Reggio Emilia, Italy

M. Ardigò
San Gallicano Dermatological Institute, Rome, Italy

R. Hofmann-Wellenhof et al. (eds.), *Reflectance Confocal Microscopy for Skin Diseases*,
DOI 10.1007/978-3-642-21997-9_34,

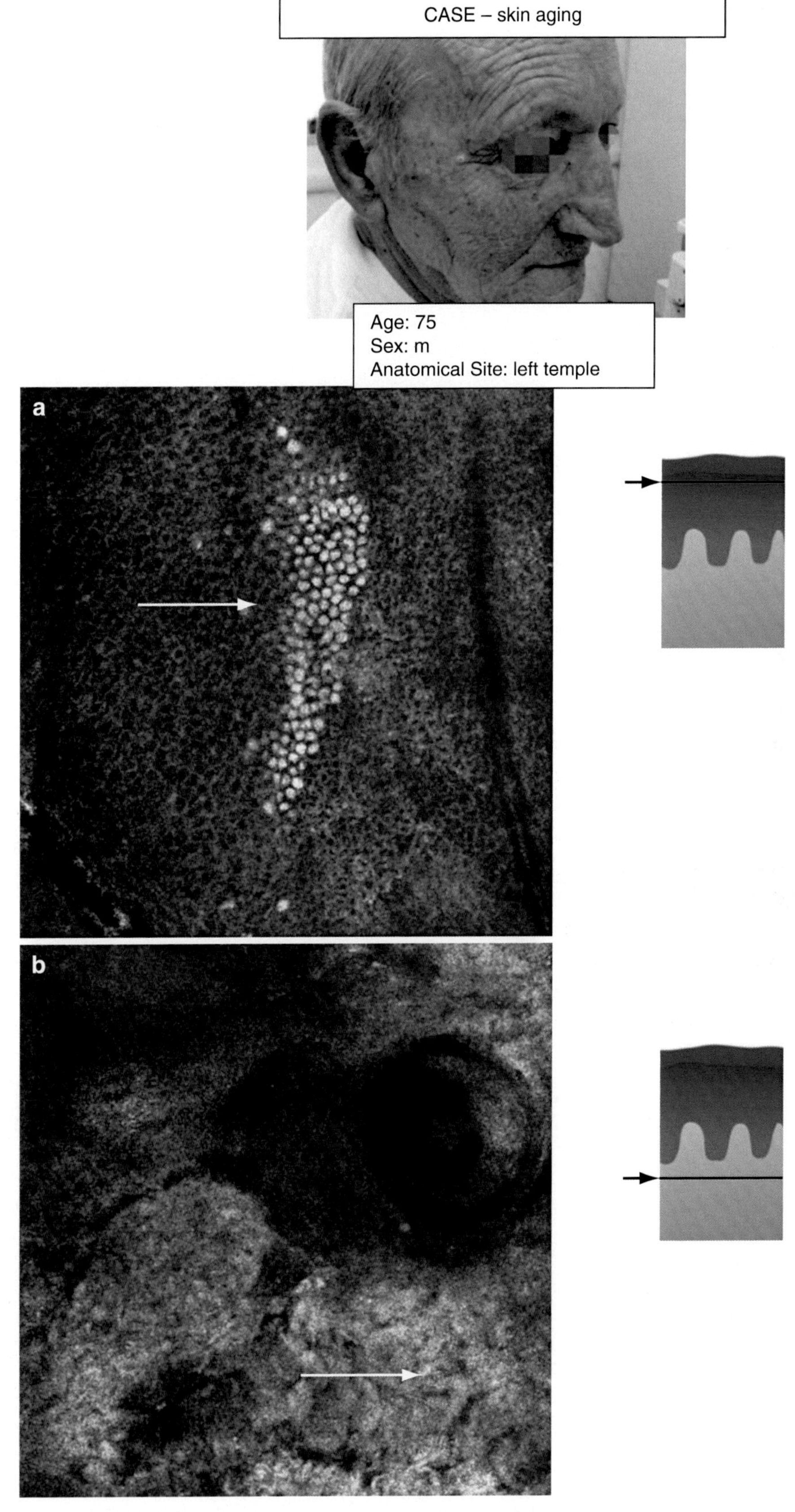

Fig. 34.1 RCM single frames (0.5 × 0.5 mm). At the level of the spinous layer (**a**) there is a mottled pigmentation composed by pigmented keratinocytes (*arrow*) in the context of a honeycombed pattern; (**b**) at the level of the dermis there are huddles of collagen with curled fibers corresponding to elastic fibers (*arrow*)

34.2 Skin Pigmentation in Cosmetology

It is assumed that melanin, that can be found located in melanocytes as well as in keratinocytes or melanophages, represents the main target of RCM examination underling the usefulness of this method for hyper and hypo pigmented skin diseases evaluation [2]. Consequently, a noninvasive microscopical assessment of pigment presence/location in the skin as well as its reduction during treatments represents an unquestionable advantage for cosmetical applications of RCM.

The possibilities of differential diagnosis between pigmented skin tumors with cosmetical implications (i.e. solar lentigo) from others with potential malignancy (i.e. pigmented actinic keratosis or lentigo maligna) let the clinician to select the correct treatment avoiding errors or overtreatment (with unnecessary scar) Guitera [3, 4]. Same, usefulness derives from the application of RCM in hypopigmentary diseases with the possibility of differential diagnosis between vitiligo (Fig. 34.2), characterized by the total absence of pigmentation at the epidermal layer as well as at the level of the DEJ, and other hypopigmentary diseases like pitiriasis alba, in which signs of inflammation like dilated dermal vessels and inflammatory cells infiltration of epidermis (spongiosis) and dermis are generally seen. Furthermore, regarding pigmentary skin disorders, testing the ratio efficacy/side effect of a topical active for pigment elimination in melasma or in post-inflammatory pigmentation represents another goal for a microscopical, high sensitive non invasive technique in cosmetology [5, 6].

34.3 Skin Barrier Function

34.3.1 Mild Damage

The skin is subjected to exposure to irritant agents such as detergents, etc. Usually, the acute exposure to mild irritants is not showing perceivable clinical effects, whereas chronic exposure is responsible for a subtle skin damage due to the loss of lipids and inflammatory phenomena, which lead to a reduced skin barrier function. There are different experimental setting which reproduce a slight irritant damage of the skin. Different concentrations of sodium lauryl solfate (SLS) are able to generate a slight barrier damage and a subclinical skin irritation that can be measured by non invasive biophysical methods, such as trans-epidermal water loss, stratum corneum capacitance and colorimetry. For a more accurate interpretation of the phenomena occurring in the epidermis after irritation, confocal microscopy is able to show modification in the keratinocytes aspect which results correlated with the intensity of the skin damage, as measured by TEWL.

The most striking confocal features correlated with mild irritation are (i) a mild detachment of the superficial corneocytes, which appear brighter than at baseline, with a few cells detectable as discoidal structures separated by a dark halo from the other cells; (ii) decreased brightness of the honeycombed pattern, corresponding to less distinguishable interkeratinocyte borders, which appear blurred and no well outlined (Fig. 34.3). After a mild, subclinical irritation usually inflammatory infiltration, spongiosis and alteration of the vascularization or of the dermal papilla aspects are not observable.

34.3.2 Severe Damage

In addition, the much more severe skin barrier damage induced by chemicals, as peelings application for cosmetical procedures, can be easily evaluated and followed with RCM. In particular, RCM can be used for qualify and quantify the microscopical changes induced by chemical application on stratum corneum, epidermal epithelium and superficial dermis disclosing demonstrated high correlation with TEWL. In specific, the stratum corneum destruction after different type and concentration of the peeling can be estimated in terms of quantification of thickness reduction and qualification of corneocytes destruction (i.e. necrosis, loss of connection, etc.). The consequence is the possibility of an in vivo, real-time assessment of efficacy of the chemical under study, but also the possibility to monitor the clinical effect of the peeling under use directly on the patient and close to the time of application.

So, for example, after salicylic acid application, the disruption of the cohesion proteins between corneocytes became evident immediately after peelings application at RCM as the presence of flotting large corneocytes, but the thickness reduction arise and became evident at RCM only 24 h later. The effects of a peeling on the epidermal epithelium can be seen as keratinocyte necrosis and disruption associated with inflammatory cells infiltration (exocytosis). Also the inflammation induced by an irritant at superficial dermal layer can be seen as presence of dilated vessels generally horizontally oriented to the epidermis and inflammatory cells between collagen bundles.

34.4 Skin Hydration

Skin hydration affects the cosmetic appearance of the skin. A well hydrated skin appears smoother and softer, whereas dry skin is usually scaly and rough. Between different biophysical methods, skin capacitance is the most used method

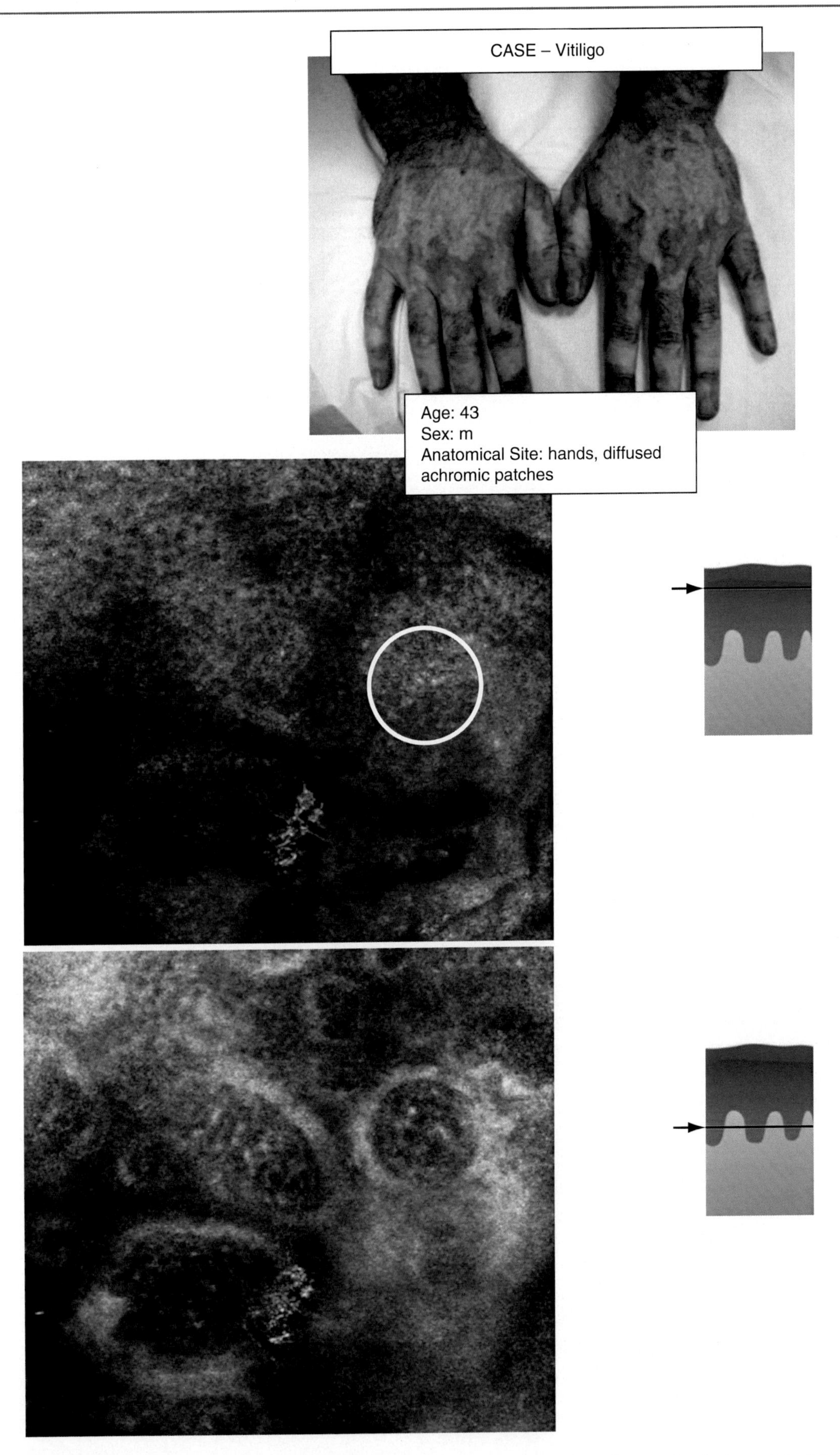

Fig. 34.2.1 and 34.2.2 RCM single frames (0.5 × 0.5 mm) respectively at the level of the spinous layer and at the level of the DEJ showing little remnant of pigmented keratinocytes (*circle*) and absence of pigmentation at the DEJ

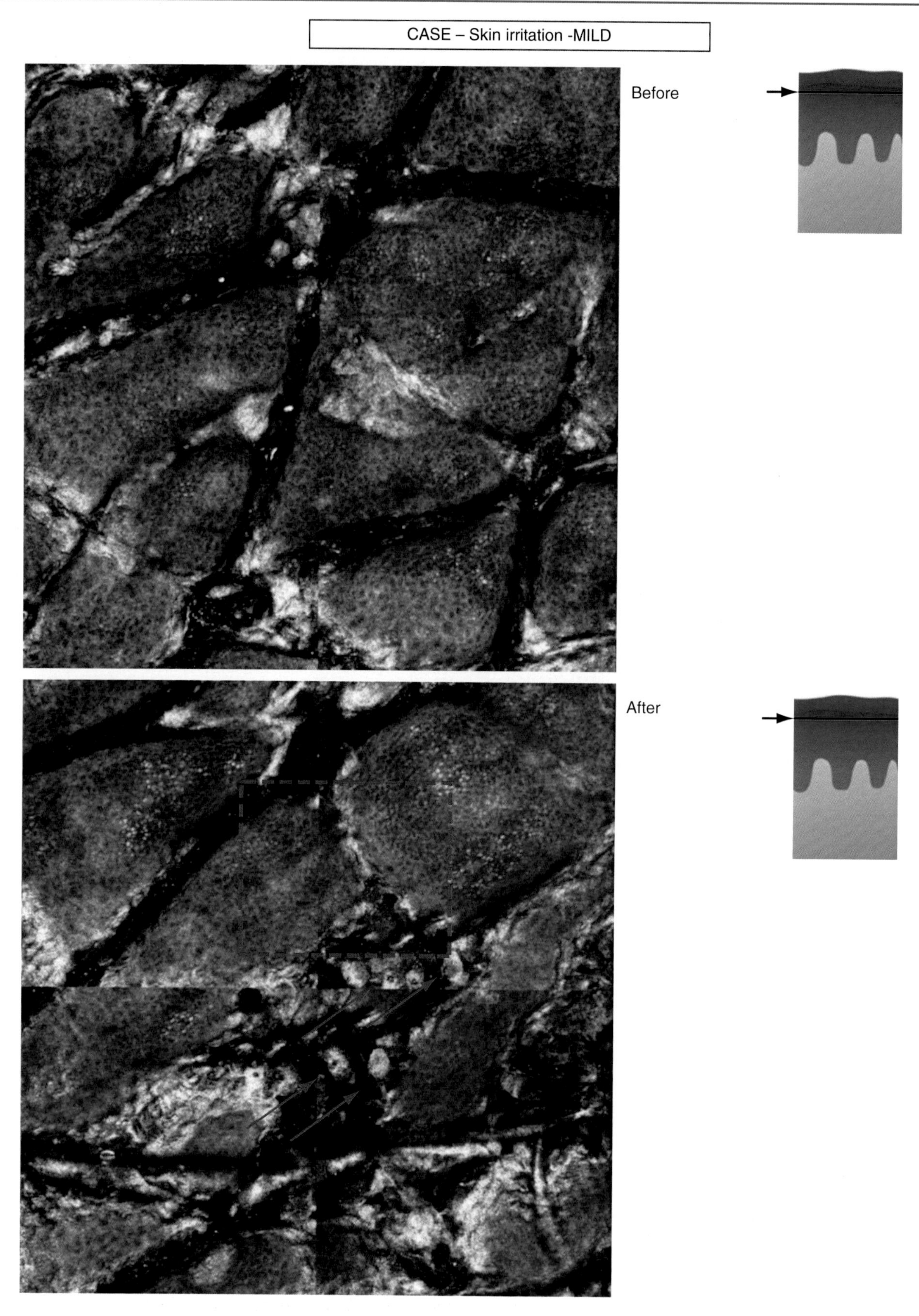

Fig. 34.3.1 RCM (1 × 1 mm) showing the superficial epidermal layers before (1.1) and after (1.2) 30 min exposure to 5% SLS under occlusion. The first image shows a regular epidermis, whereas the second figure shows some detached keratinocytes (→) and more blurred interkeratinocytic contours (*red square*)

CASE – Skin hydration

Fig. 34.4 RCM (1 × 1 mm) showing the superficial epidermal layer changes before (4.1) and after 1 h (4.2) and after 3 h (4.3) from the application of a oil-in-water moisturizer

to evaluate skin hydration. Confocal microscopic changes according with skin hydration can be observed predominantly in the epidermal layers.

After the application of a moisturizer, it is possible to observe by means of confocal microscopy a decrease in brightness in the superficial layers, mostly corresponding to the disappearance of micro-scales. During the time course, it is possible to observe progressive changes in the skin furrow aspect. At short distance from application of a common oil-in-water moisturizer (<1 h), in coincidence with the peak of capacitance, RCM shows the skin fold filled by a bright material, corresponding to remnants, not absorbed, of the moisturizer. After 3 h from the application, in correspondence of the return of the capacitance close to the baseline value, it is possible to observe with RCM a progressive narrowing of the skin furrows which also shows less deep than baseline (Fig. 34.4). It is possible to suppose that moisturizers first increase water content in the superficial layers (corneum), as demonstrated by the increment in capacitance along with the disappearance of the microscales. Subsequently, with the absorption of the product and its distribution between the interkeratinocyte spaces in deeper epidermal layers (granulosum/spinosum), the stratum corneum water content is re-established to its baseline level, as for close to baseline capacitance level, whereas the deep epidermal layers increase their water content, generating a swelling of the whole epidermis which result in narrowed and less deep skin furrows.

34.5 Hairs

Common hair diseases, like alopecia areata, androgenic alopecia or cicatricial alopecias, have high aesthetical impact on the patients. The therapeutical management of alopecias is characterized by a subjective clinical assessments of the response generally focused on the patient impression and on the utilization of tricoscopy that let the clinician use dermoscopical signs (follicular hyperkeratosis and erythema, presence of yellow or white dots, and dilated vessels, etc.) for efficacy of the treatment interpretation, but lack the possibility of a microscopic identification of signs of remnant of diseases activity. That's why RCM, despite its limit in term of "penetration" into the skin, represents a useful device for hair diseases management giving useful microscopic information about inflammatory status of the diseases, the presence of micronized as well as dysmorphic hair, and the presence of dermal scar. Because of the limit in penetration to the superficial dermis, new criteria are needed to be used for RCM in vivo assessment of hair diseases status. So, scientific works devoted to the evaluation of the real utility of RCM on this field have been done and are on work: yellow (alopecia areata) and white (lichen plano pilaris, alopecia androgenetica) dots identification/interpretation, RCM criteria for cicatricial alopecias activity [5].

Using RCM, morphology, quality, dimension, caliber, distribution and density of hair shaft as well as the normotrophysm of the adnexal, distal epithelium can be easily evaluated. The advantage is the possibility of an easy identification of signs of inflammation involving the distal part of the adnexal epithelium, the superficial dermis, and the epidermis in areas of alopecias; also the eventual cicatricial evolution of the alopecia can be assessed with RCM evaluating the superficial dermal changes (Fig. 34.5).

RCM seems to be powerful also in testing hair cosmetical products effects on the hair shaft as well as on the epidermis of the scalp. Moreover, the possibility of a non invasive follow-up of the disease response to treatment represents a big help for patient clinical management and cosmetical result.

34.6 Assessing the Efficacy of Treatments of Skin Diseases

The chance and power of RCM for microscopically modification assessment during the treatment of skin diseases have been already demonstrated and confirmed in literature in both neoplastic as well as inflammatory diseases. In particular, skin inflammation/irritation, pigmentation, aging and dryness evaluation let the clinician to add, noninvasively, and immediately in front to the patient useful microscopical information for skin disease management. If this is a strong advantage for skin tumor non surgical management, regarding inflammatory skin diseases this could represent a real revolution for the therapeutic choice and follow-up in daily practice. That is why several studies have been done and are in course about the application of RCM to drug efficacy evaluation with the advantage of a non invasive, microscopic control of possible local side effects [7, 8]. Regarding this point works on melasma, vitiligo, cicatricial alopecias and psoriasis have been already performed, but the possible application of RCM spread on all the inflammatory and cosmetic skin conditions involving the epidermis, upper dermis and adnex structures. In particular, in relation to pigmentary diseases, starting from the experience with RCM in inflammation estimation, it is possible to follow-up the irritant effects of the actives (hydroquinone) and physical therapies (peelings or laser) in order to reduce the risk of post-inflammatory pigmentation during melasma treatment (Fig. 34.6) or Koebner phenomenon

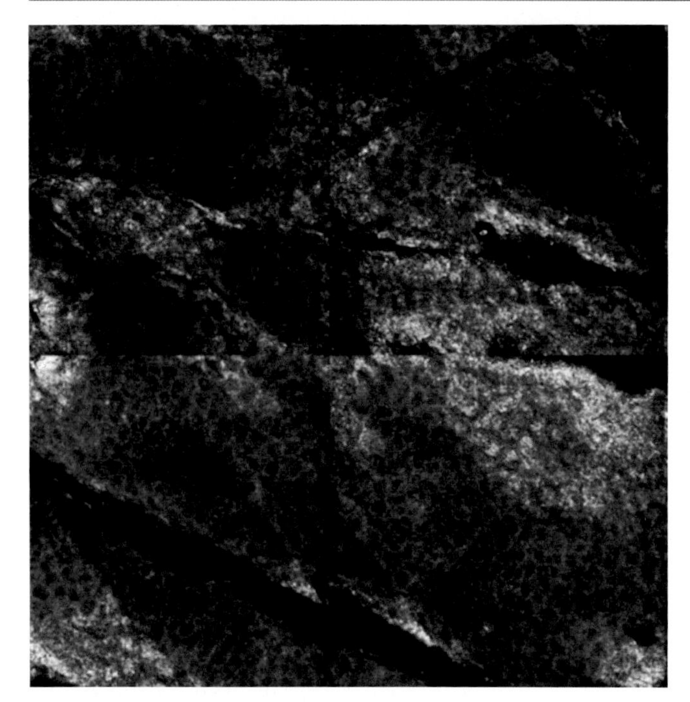

Fig. 34.4.1 Baseline: the epidermis is characterized by microscales (bright areas) (*) and *black lines* corresponding to skin furrows (→)

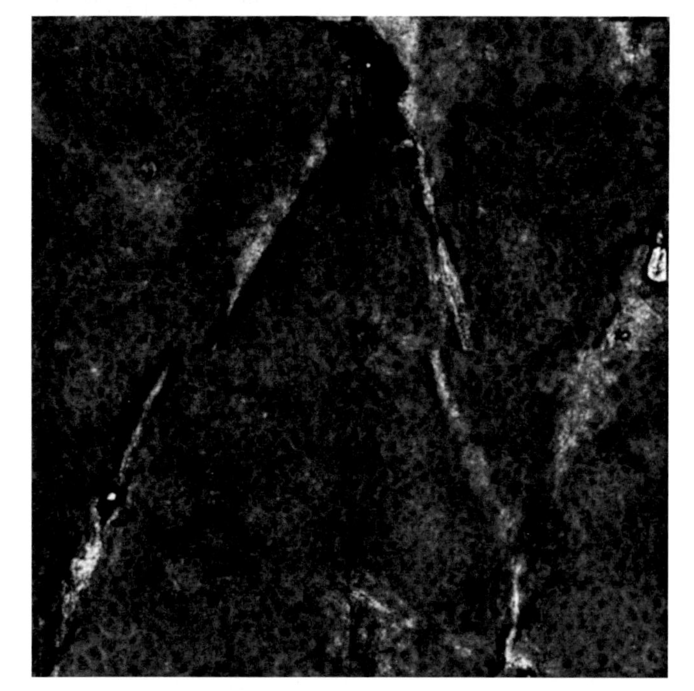

Fig. 34.4.2 After 1 h: disappearance of the scales. Skin furrows appear filled by a bright amorphous material corresponding to remnant of the product

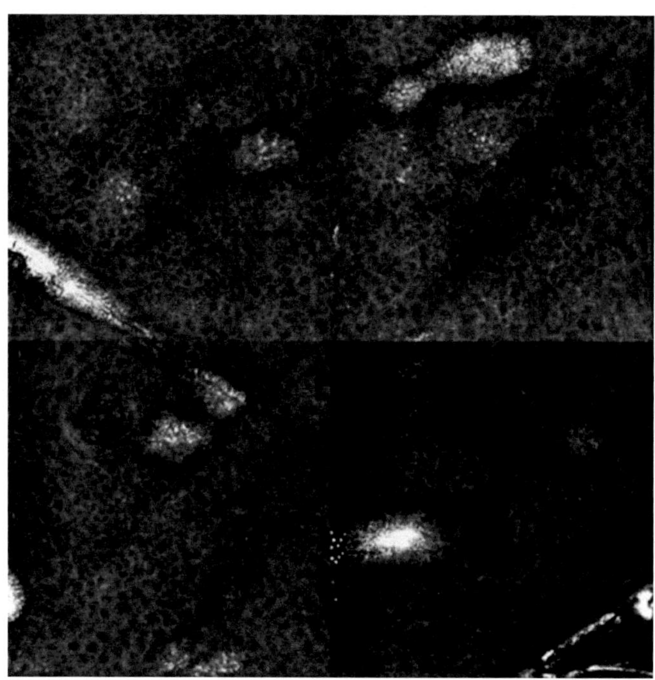

Fig. 34.4.3 After 3 h: narrowing and smoothing of the skin furrows is observable. Some oval roundish structures of amorphous material correspond to artifacts due to the interaction between the water and lipids on the corneum

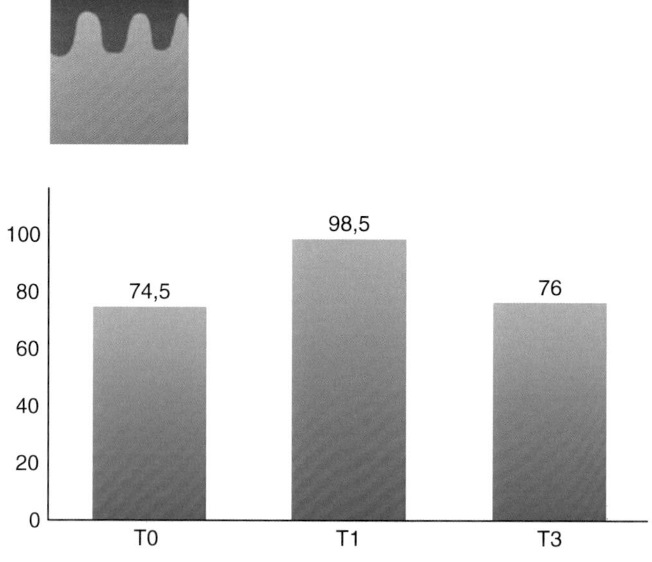

Fig. 34.4.4 Capacitance values recorder at baseline (T0) shows a marked increase after 1 h (T1), and a value close to baseline after 3 h (T3). This can be explained by the fact that capacitance values depends only by the water content in the stratum corneum

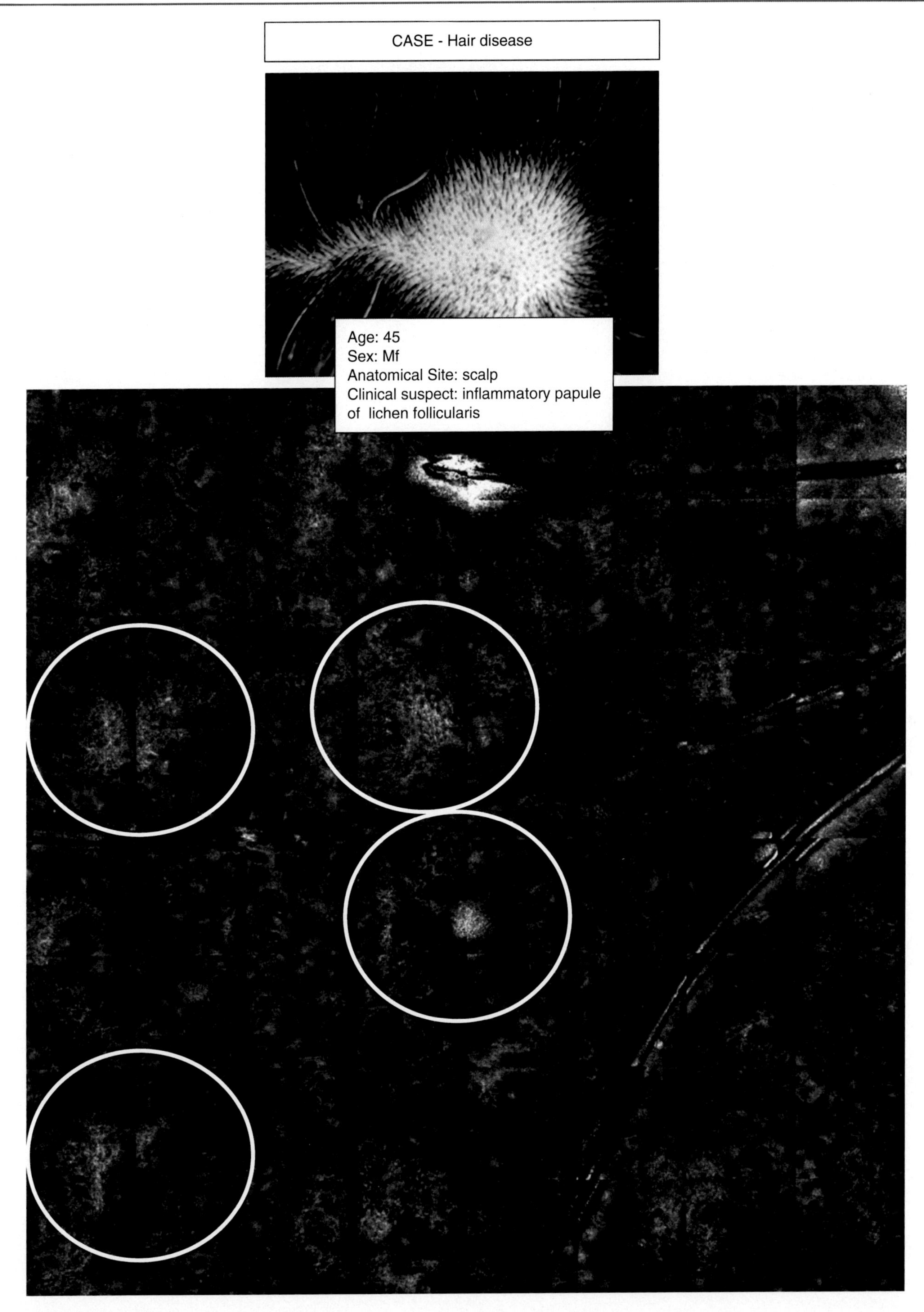

Fig. 34.5 RCM mosaic image (4×4) of a scalp at the level of the DEJ. Follicular openings appear irregularly affected by the inflammatory infiltrate (*circle*) differently from the interfollicular areas that appears normal

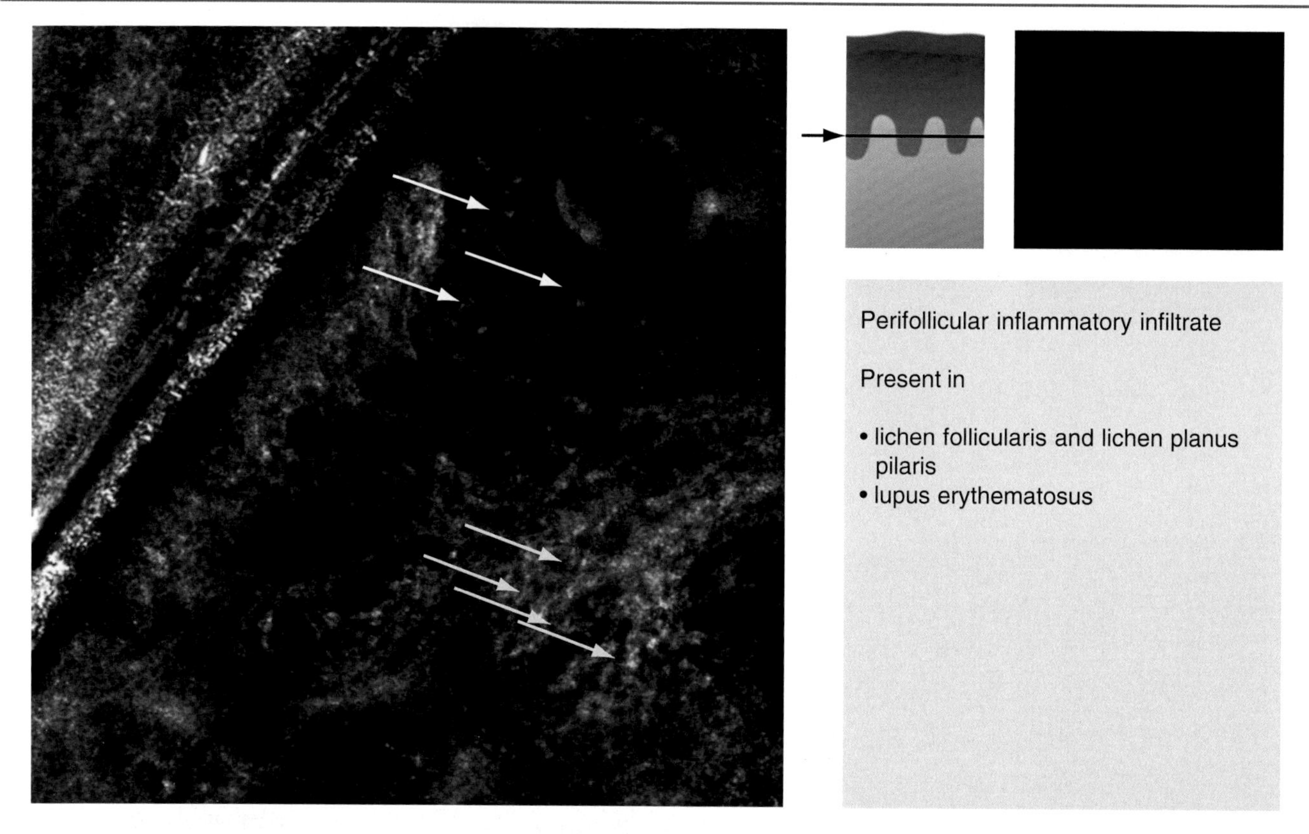

Fig. 34.5.1 RCM single frame (0.5×0.5 mm) at the level of the DEJ showing periadenzal inflammatory cells infiltration (*arrows*) and presence of dermal inflammation (*yellow arrows*). DP are edge but not rimmed

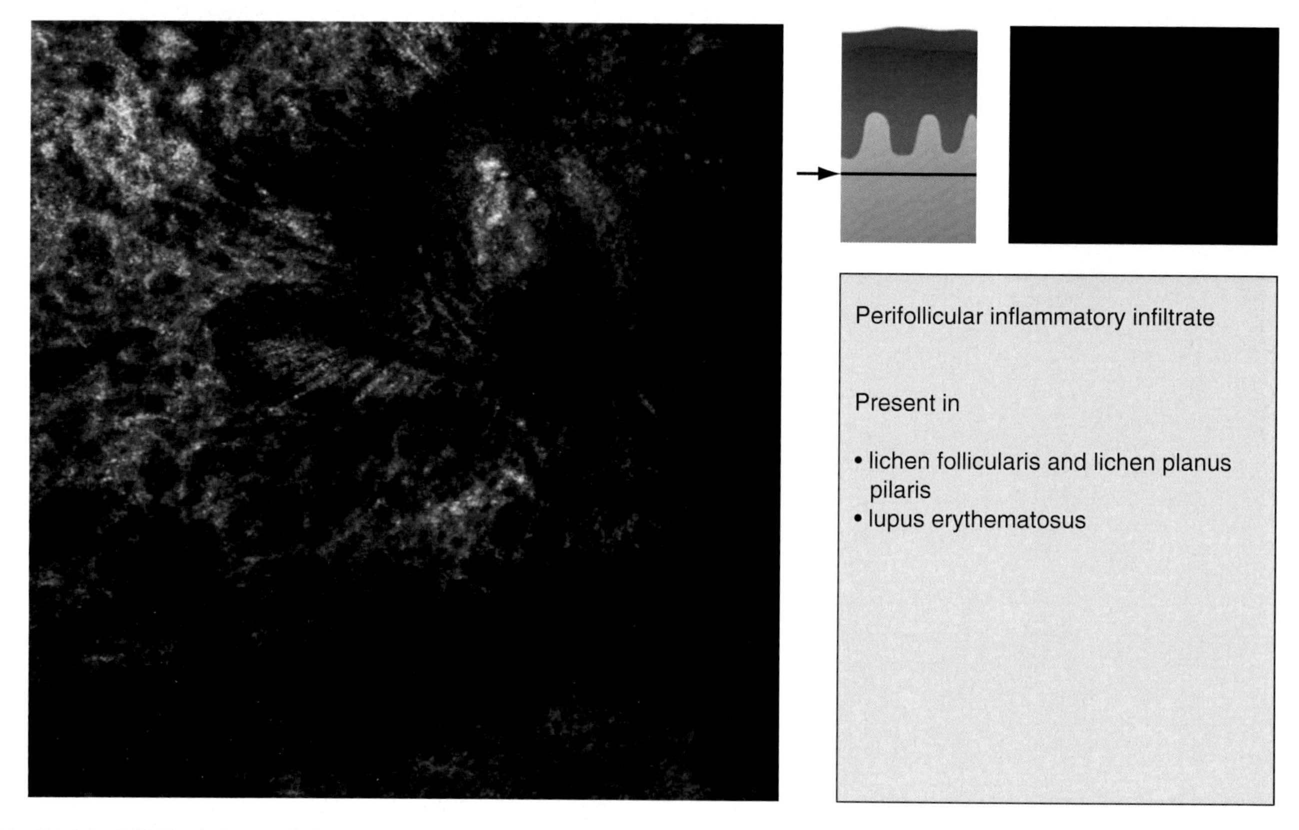

Fig. 34.5.2 RCM basic image (0.5 × 0.5) at the level of upper dermis showing thickening of collagen bundles around adnexal structures

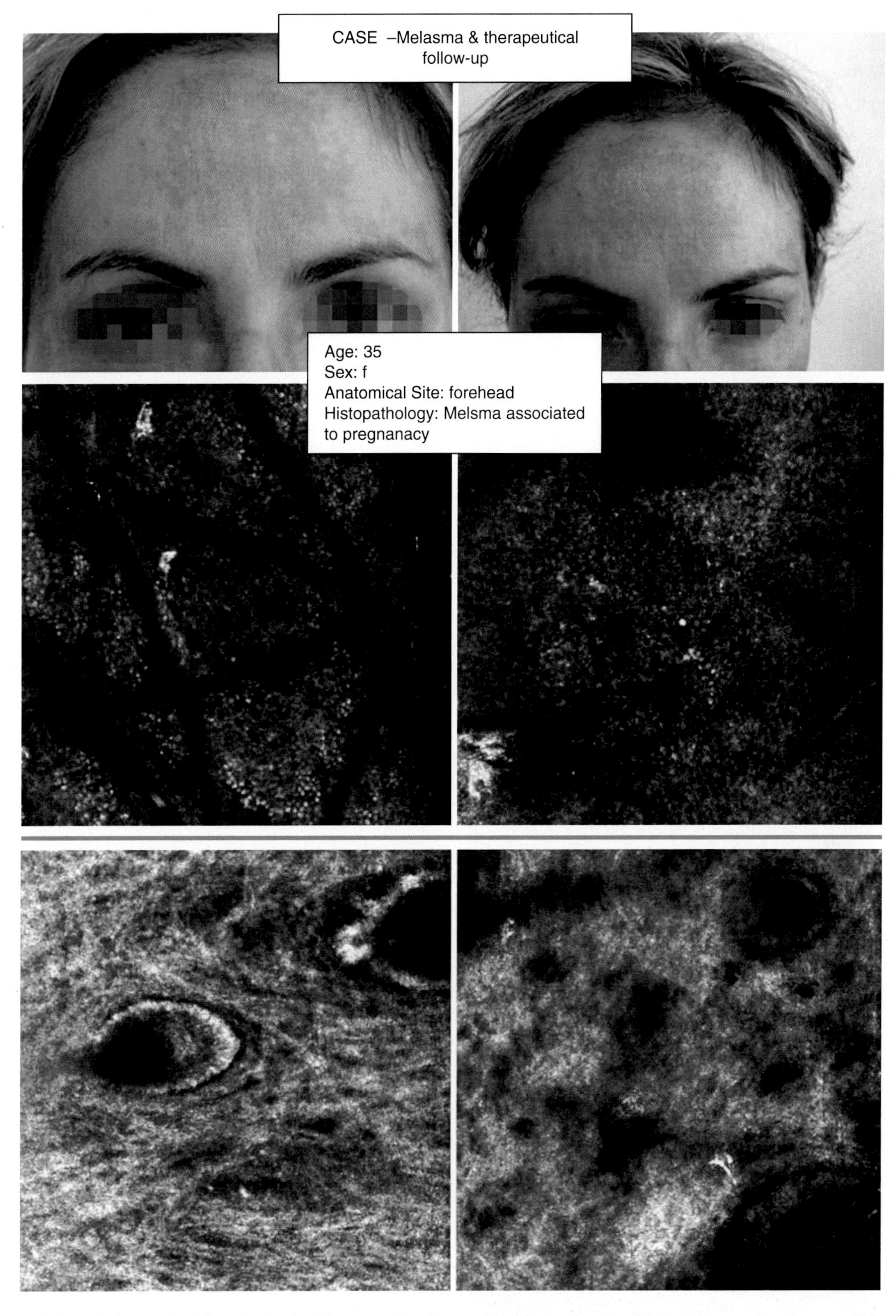

Fig. 34.6 RCM mosaic image (4 × 4) at the level of the upper dermis showing the presence of peri-adnexal epithelium inflammatory infiltrate (*red arrows*), seen as round-to-polygonal, mildly refractile cells around and inside the adnexal epithelium between keratinocytes. Dilated vessels diffused (*red asterisk*) and aggregates of inflammatory cells can be seen associated with thickening of stroma fibers (*white arrows*)

arising in vitiligo patch during UV treatment [7, 8]. So, both aesthetic dermatologists and cosmetic companies could used RCM for manage and testing different actives during the therapeutical follow-up of the patients affected by pigmentary disorders. Not only chemical actives like peeling, hydroquinone or alpha-hydroxy-acyd, but also physical treatment as lasers can be tested with RCM.

Core Messages

- RCM helps in treatment selection for pigment removal.
- Unwanted inflammatory side effect of actives can be monitored with RCM.
- Medium to severe skin damage involving different skin layers be easily assessed with RCM.
- Scalp epidermis and superficial dermis as well as hair shaft and distal adnexal epithelium can be studied with RCM.
- Follow-up of the effects of an active on pathological as well as cosmetological conditions can be easily obtained in real time using RCM.

References

1. Longo C, Casari A, Beretti F, Cesinaro AM, Pellacani G. Skin aging: *In vivo* microscopic assessment of epidermal and dermal changes by means of confocal microscopy. J Am Acad Dermatol 2011 In Press
2. Rajadhyaksha M, Grossman M, Esterowitz D, Webb RH, Anderson RR (1995) *In vivo* confocal scanning laser microscopy of human skin: melanin provides strong contrast. J Invest Dermatol 104(6):946–952
3. Guitera P, Pellacani G, Crotty KA, Scolyer RA, Li LX, Bassoli S, Vinceti M, Rabinovitz H, Longo C, Menzies SW (2010) The impact of in vivo reflectance confocal microscopy on the diagnostic accuracy of lentigo maligna and equivocal pigmented and nonpigmented macules of the face. J Invest Dermatol 130(8):2080–2091
4. Guitera P, Li LX, Scolyer RA, Menzies SW (2010) Morphologic features of melanophages under in vivo reflectance confocal microscopy. Arch Dermatol 146(5):492–498
5. Ardigo M, Tosti A, Cameli N, Vincenzi C, Misciali C, Berardesca E. Reflectance confocal microscopy of the yellow dots pattern in alopecia areata. Arch Dermatol 2011 Jan;147(1):61-4
6. Ardigo M, Cameli N, Berardesca E, Gonzalez S (2010) Characterization and evaluation of pigment distribution and response to therapy in melasma using in vivo reflectance confocal microscopy: a preliminary study. J Eur Acad Dermatol Venereol 24(11):1296–1303
7. Ardigo M, Malizewsky I, Dell'anna ML, Berardesca E, Picardo M (2007) Preliminary evaluation of vitiligo using in vivo reflectance confocal microscopy. J Eur Acad Dermatol Venereol 21(10):1344–1350
8. Ardigò M, Maliszewski I, Cota C, Scope A, Sacerdoti G, Gonzalez S, Berardesca E (2007) Preliminary evaluation of in vivo reflectance confocal microscopy features of Discoid lupus erythematosus. Br J Dermatol 156(6):1196–1203

Part IX

Future Aspects

35 Tele-Reflectance Confocal Microscopy

Elisabeth M.T. Wurm, Caterina Longo, Paul Hemmer, and Giovanni Pellacani

35.1 Introduction

Evaluation of RCM images requires specialized training that is not universally available, despite a growing number of publications in this field and this present work being the second book published in this area. Application of teledermatology in RCM (Tele-RCM) aims to overcome this shortage of distribution of experts and to improve distribution of knowledge by e-learning.

The principle of teledermatology is the use of telecommunication technology to send skin disorder related medical data over distance for the purpose of administration, research, disease prevention, patient management and (continuing) education. It provides access to dermatological specialist knowledge that would be otherwise unavailable at a particular location by transferring the information rather than the patient or professional [1]. Especially for second opinion in dermoscopy, the store-and-forward (SAF) technique is widely used. With SAF teledermatology the referring physician acquires digital still images with accompanying data. This information is subsequently sent to a data storage unit to be assessed by the reviewer at his/her convenience. Computer and internet-based training, better known as e-learning, are becoming increasingly utilized in medical education; saving the required travel and associated attendance of lectures for busy professionals. Herein, we describe current applications and future directions regarding the potential application of RCM for tele-consultation and e-learning.

E.M.T. Wurm (✉)
Dermatology Research Centre, The University of Queensland School of Medicine, Princess Alexandra Hospital, Brisbane, QLD, Australia
e-mail: e.wurm@uq.edu.au; lissy.wurm@gmail.com

C. Longo • G. Pellacani
Department of Dermatology and Venereology,
University of Modena and Reggio Emilia, Modena, Italy
e-mail: caterina.longo@unimore.it

P. Hemmer
Lucid Inc., Rochester, NY, USA
e-mail: phemmer@lucid-tech.com

35.2 E-learning and Tele-consult

35.2.1 Skinconfocalmicroscopy.net

In order to gain expertise in reflectance confocal microscopy a novice has to have viewed and evaluated a high number of lesions which requires a considerable amount of time in a real clinical setting. In order to overcome this, a dedicated web-platform (original web address: http://www.skinconfocalmicroscopy.org) was developed. The Skin Confocal Microscopy Website was initially launched in 2007 with the aim to test the reproducibility of RCM descriptors in terms of inter- and intra-observer agreement [2]. RCM specialists from six centers in three continents were trained by a tutorial on the webpage and then asked to evaluate high resolution basic images (500 × 500 μm) for the presence of specific RCM criteria in a blinded fashion. Remarkably, good reproducibility was generated for most of the evaluated parameters, particularly those previously proposed within diagnostic algorithms [3].

The increasing interest in RCM application in the clinical and research community prompted the need to offer a free on-line tutorial for RCM novices. Therefore, the web-site and the images acquired for the reproducibility study were made available as an open source for users interested in testing their capability of recognizing confocal features and a new interactive web-platform was subsequently developed (new web address: http://www.skinconfocalmicroscopy.net). Features of this e-learning platform comprise a "tutorial" and a "training" section (Figs. 35.1 and 35.2).

In the tutorial section, the major confocal aspects of different skin layers (superficial layer, basal layer, DEJ and

R. Hofmann-Wellenhof et al. (eds.), *Reflectance Confocal Microscopy for Skin Diseases*,
DOI 10.1007/978-3-642-21997-9_35, © Springer-Verlag Berlin Heidelberg 2012

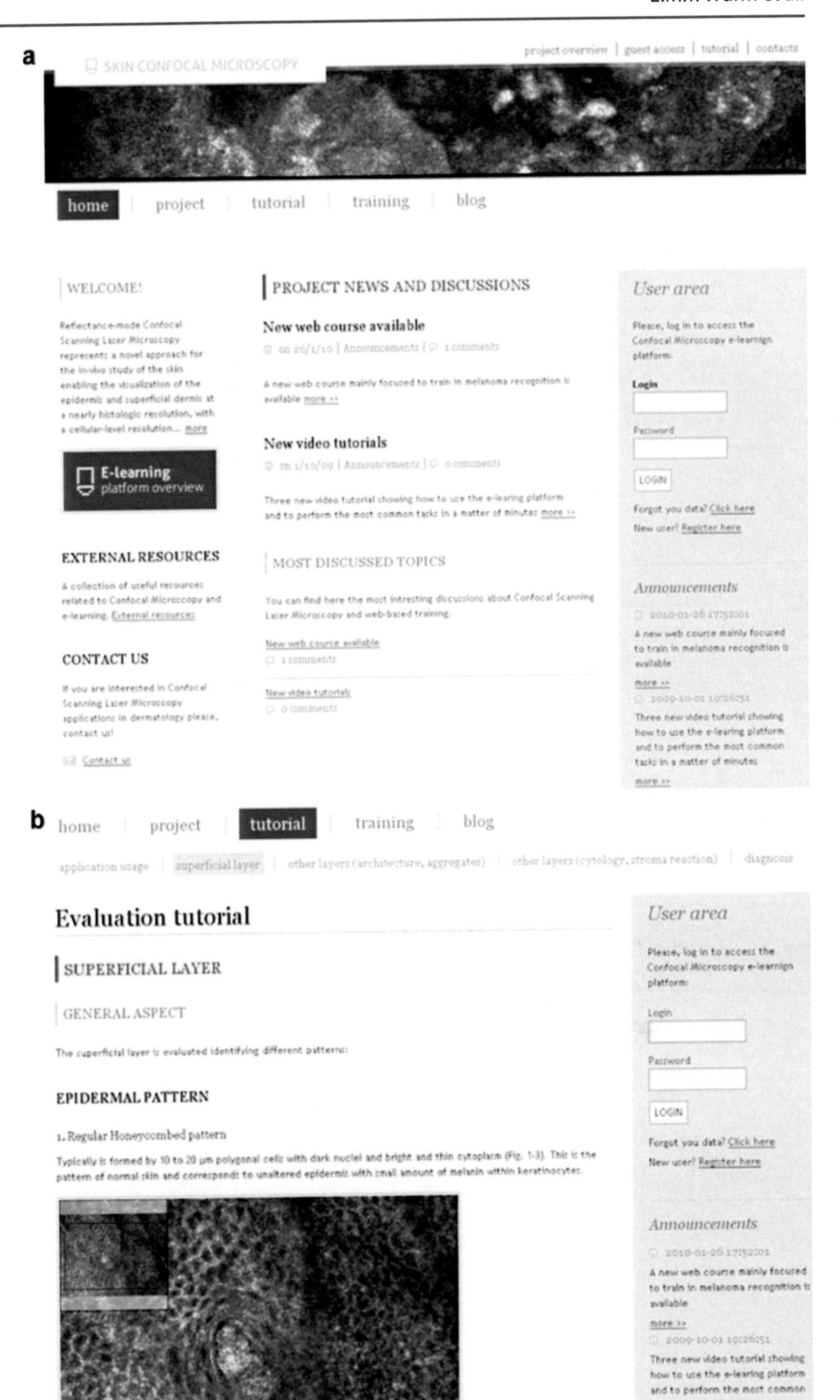

Fig. 35.1 Skinconfocalmicroscopy.net (**a**) offers a free online tutorial for RCM novices. In a tutorial section (**b**), the major confocal aspects of different skin in normal and lesional skin, comprising RCM descriptors, are described by displaying example images with definitions of the single parameters

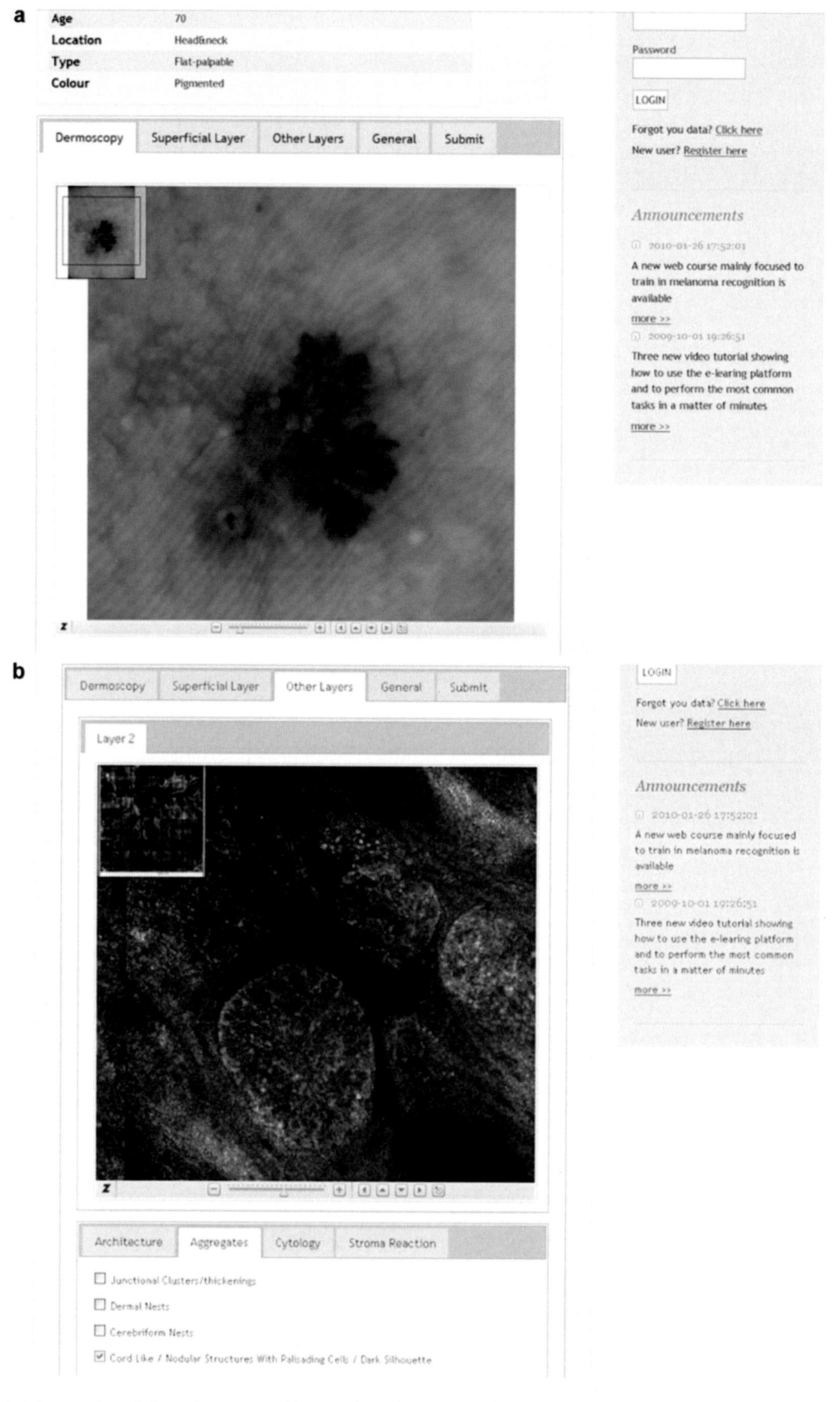

Fig. 35.2 The training section of the web page provides a series of cases in a reproduced clinical setting to be explored and evaluated for pattern identification. A dermoscopic image (**a**) and at least two RCM mosaics (**b**) are displayed. Lists of RCM features to be filled in by the user are displayed below the corresponding RCM mosaics. Following submission of the case evaluation, the user can compare his/her evaluation with that proposed by an expert

upper dermis) in normal skin and in skin lesions, including RCM descriptors, are detailed by displaying example images with definitions of the single parameters.

The training section provides a series of cases in a reproduced clinical setting to be explored and evaluated for pattern identification. A dermoscopic image of a given lesion, along with at least two complete RCM mosaics (blocks) of the lesion (superficial layer, DEJ and, in some cases, a third level corresponding to superficial dermis), rather than high resolution single images, are provided to the users. Basic clinical information is given in order to mimic real-time confocal imaging during an office visit and to test the diagnostic abilities of the user. To accelerate uploading and display of large image files, dedicated software was implemented enabling the rapid navigation and zooming within the RCM mosaics and dermoscopic images. Essential clinical data comprising age and lesion location are included along with clinical characteristics of the lesion. This training section is intended to transfer the know-how of expert centers to distant users that are studying the method. To evaluate diagnostic skills, the user is asked to complete specific forms detailing the identified features and diagnostic suspicion. Separate lists of features for the epidermal layer, DEJ (and dermal layer) are displayed below the corresponding RCM mosaics. The user is first required to submit the evaluation of each case, after which he/she is able to visualize the correct diagnosis and to compare his/her evaluation of every single feature with that proposed by an expert. This expert feedback is designed to assist the participants in learning the criteria for RCM diagnosis and to improve his/her confidence in the decision making process. A recent study, which included six residents as users, has demonstrated the efficacy of the e-learning web platform in melanoma diagnosis for physicians/dermatologists not previously skilled in the use of confocal microscopy (*data not published*). Moreover, it was possible to evaluate the "e-learning curve" that resulted in an improvement of diagnostic accuracy and confidence over the first 50 cases analyzed.

35.3 VivaNet®

Despite the growing body of RCM learning and teaching material, specialist knowledge is not available everywhere and in response to this a net system for RCM image exchange, called VivaNet®, has been developed. As with all teledermatology applications, security of image storage, retrieval and privacy of information is crucial. It is imperative that the quality or content of the acquired images is not altered in any way. Equally important is the protection of patient privacy. VivaNet® is a DICOM (Digital Imaging and Communications in Medicine) and HIPPA (Health Insurance Portability and Accountability Act) compliant server for the storage, retrieval, and transfer of medical images that does not digitize, print, display, process, or irreversibly compress the medical images. From a high-level perspective VivaNet® can be described as a group of high performance computers, all speaking the same language and securely connected to each other over a Virtual Private Network (VPN) in a manner that protects data, prevents intrusion and ensures consistency in presentation while allowing for the seamless sharing of information between medical professionals using the system (Fig. 35.3).

By linking VivaNet® computers to each other over a secure, private and high-speed connection, VivaNet® users are able to share and evaluate these large image sets quickly and effortlessly. Like a tree, VivaNet® has a root server which is responsible for permanently and securely archiving medical records. The branches and leaves of the tree represent the connections to imaging and reading workstations. As is often the case, a primary care physician may have colleagues he or she is accustomed to working with for the examination of excised tissue samples. VivaNet® will allow these collaborations to continue and flourish while opening up a world of additional resources for second opinions and consent-based information sharing to the benefit of all those involved. In some cases, VivaNet® imaging workstations may be directly connected to the expert who will be performing the evaluation. In other cases, where a direct connection between the primary care physician and confocal expert is not possible due to any number of geographic, political or economic limitations, the remote VivaNet® workstations can still communicate with each other by way of the root VivaNet® server. Currently, the VivaNet® implementation is in an experimental phase in Europe and US in order to test its applicability and efficiency.

35.3.1 How Does VivaNet® Work Practically?

Confocal images are acquired in a face-to-face visit as described in Chap. 3 following an imaging protocol (Mosaics at 30, 60 and 90 μm, respectively with two additional stacks, for example). After image acquisition, the confocal imager opens a dedicated web link on the display of the VivaScope. Along with the RCM images and the VivaCam dermoscopic images, patient data can also be transferred. Some required fields (such as patient age and sex have to be completed while additional information can be given in free text or by simple clicking on a box. The information is then sent to the preferred confocal reviewer who can open and assess the cases to his/her convenience.

The confocal reviewer can open and assess the images on a two screen viewing station specifically designed to view RCM cases (Fig. 35.4). On one screen, thumbnail images of the mosaic and dermoscopic images are displayed and a mosaic can be viewed in magnification view with options to navigate

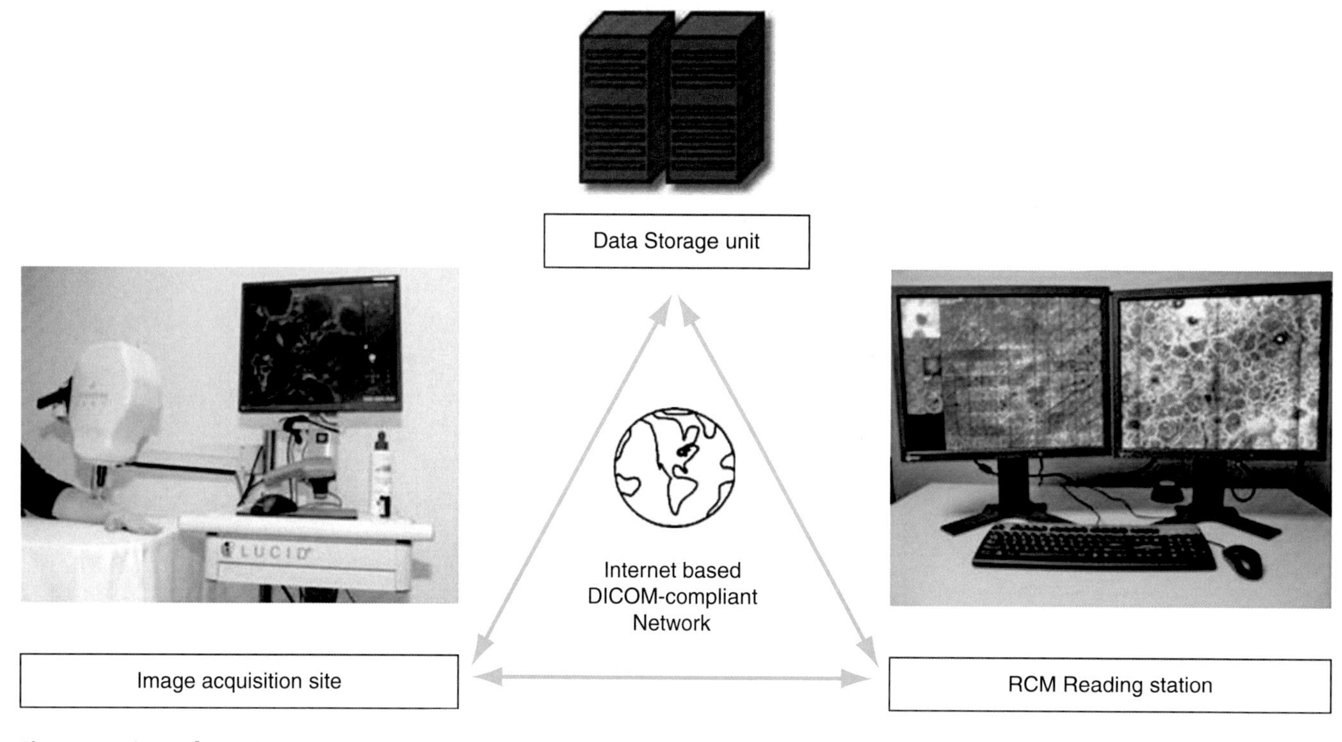

Fig. 35.3 VivaNet® workflow: RCM images are sent from image acquisition site (clinical office where RCM images are acquired in a face-to-face visit) to a reading station where the reviewer can assess the images via an internet-based DICOM-compliant network

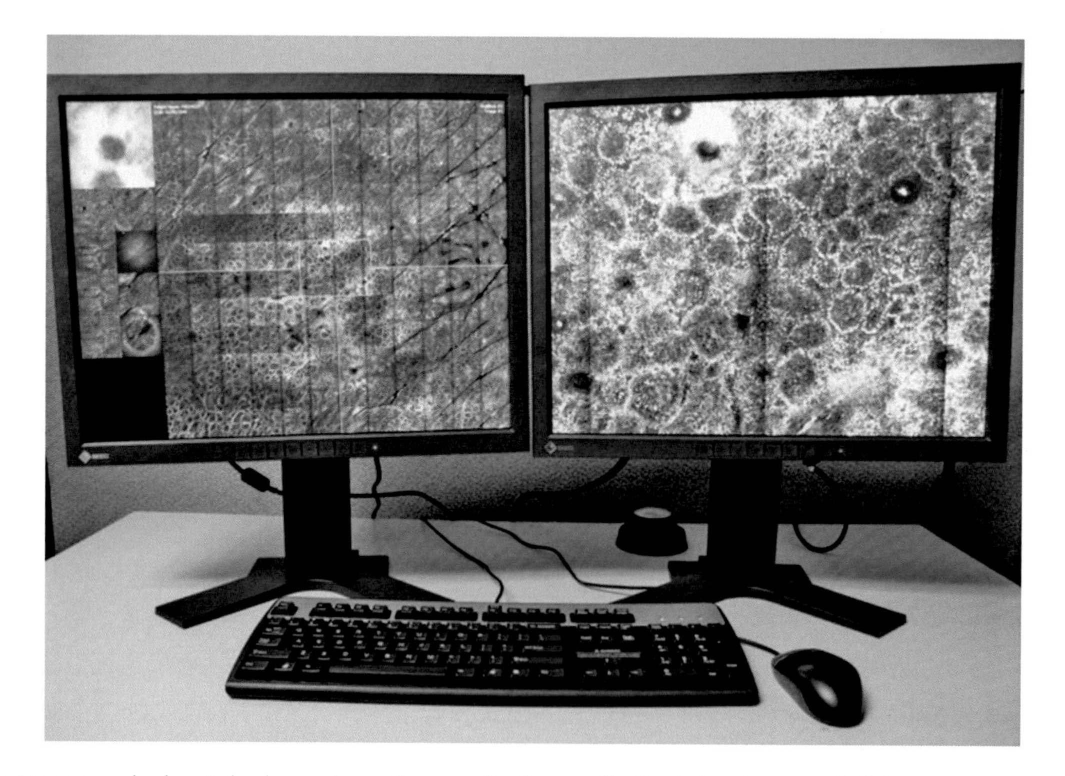

Fig. 35.4 The two screen viewing station is a custom software application specifically designed to assess RCM cases

on the image. On the second screen, the chosen image area is displayed in magnification. This two screen method allows for a quick and easy image assessment and enables the reviewer to have a good correlation between dermoscopic, architectural RCM features and the corresponding cellular features of a lesion. The reviewer then completes a report. Finally, the reviewer's digitally signed evaluation is sent back to the VivaNet® server for archiving as medical record and can be subsequently viewed by the confocal imager.

Core Messages

1. Tele-RCM aims to overcome shortage among the distribution of experts and to improve distribution of knowledge by e-learning.
2. A dedicated e-learning platform (skinconfocalmicroscopy.net) has been created to meet the growing interest in RCM among the scientific community.
3. Features of this website comprise a tutorial displaying and explaining the most common features of benign and malignant skin lesions and a training platform to review single features and diagnose lesions in a reproduced clinical setting.
4. Implementation of a net system for RCM image exchange, called VivaNet®, is in an experimental phase in order to test its applicability and efficiency.
5. With VivaNet® secure storage, retrieval, and transfer of confocal images is made possible. A distant RCM reviewer can assess images sent by a remote physician that acquires the RCM images.

35.4 Conclusion

The requirement of intense training to acquire expertise in evaluation of RCM images could hinder successful application of this novel technique. Tele-RCM is able to link medical institutions specialized in dermatooncology with specialized RCM centers to overcome the current shortage in distribution of RCM experts and enables the fast and accurate transfer of RCM images worldwide. The use of e-learning platforms, such as the Skin Confocal Microscopy webpage described above, might prove crucial in providing continuing medical education and in the sharing of difficult cases. Furthermore, exchange of confocal images for second opinion among the scientific community enhances the diagnostic skills of the participants and is beneficial to all involved.

References

1. Wurm EM, Hofmann-Wellenhof R, Wurm R, Soyer HP (2008) Telemedicine and teledermatology: past, present and future. J Dtsch Dermatol Ges 6:106–112
2. Pellacani G, Vinceti M, Bassoli S, Braun R, Gonzalez S, Guitera P et al (2009) Reflectance confocal microscopy and features of melanocytic lesions: an internet-based study of the reproducibility of terminology. Arch Dermatol 145:1137–1143
3. Pellacani G, Guitera P, Longo C, Avramidis M, Seidenari S, Menzies S (2007) The impact of in vivo reflectance confocal microscopy for the diagnostic accuracy of melanoma and equivocal melanocytic lesions. J Invest Dermatol 127:2759–2765

Automated Diagnosis and Reflectance Confocal Microscopy

36

Marco Wiltgen

36.1 Introduction

In this chapter, we introduce the basic principles of automated diagnosis of CLSM images of skin lesions. Special attention is given to the machine based description and analysis of the tissues in a way that conforms to the diagnostic guidelines of the derma pathologists. Further, the machine learning algorithm for the automated prediction of the pathology and the generated diagnostic rules are discussed and compared with the diagnostic skills of the derma pathologists. The application and performance of the discussed methods are demonstrated by selected studies.

Confocal laser scanning microscopy (CLSM) enables the non-invasive examination of skin lesions in real time [1–4]. In contrast to dermoscopic examinations (with 10× magnification), the CLSM technique allows the viewing of micro-anatomic structures and individual cells. However, training and experience is necessary for a successful and accurate diagnosis in this new and powerful imaging technique. Specialists, trained in CLSM, acquire a considerable improvement in the sensitivity (detection of melanomas) and the specificity (percentage of non-melanomas correctly diagnosed as benign common nevi), compared with dermoscopic methods [5]. To diminish the need for training and to improve diagnostic accuracy, computer aided diagnostic systems are required by the derma pathologists [6, 7].

Automated diagnostic systems provide accurate and reliable detection of skin tumors. Computer aided diagnosis requires no input by the clinician but rather reports a likely diagnosis based on computer algorithms. One of the main tasks in automated image analysis is the selection of appropriate features for a "computer friendly" description of the tissue. The choice and development of such features is determined by the common diagnostic guidelines of the derma pathologists. The experiences of the derma pathologists show that for the diagnosis of CLSM views of skin lesions, architectural structures at different scales play a crucial role. The CLSM images of benign common nevi show pronounced architectural structures, such as arrangements of the small nevi cells around basal structures and tumor cell nests. The images of malignant melanoma show large melanoma cells and connective tissue with few or no architectural structures. Therefore, features enabling an analysis of structures at different scales are suitable for the description of CLSM views of skin lesions. The mathematical background for such an analysis is provided by the so-called wavelet texture analysis. Features based on the wavelet transform enable an adequate description of images at different scales.

A further task in automated analysis is the choice of the machine learning algorithm for classification, which enables it, after training, to predict the class of a lesion (nevi or malignant melanoma). For medical diagnosis, the algorithm should duplicate the automated diagnostic process by making it understandable to the human diagnostician.

36.2 Manual Diagnosis of CLSM Images by the Derma Pathologist

An important step for a successful automated image analysis of histological tissue is the choice of the appropriate texture features. The selection of the features can be made according to the diagnostic guidelines used by the derma pathologist. To gain more insight into the automated diagnostic processes, we will illustrate the diagnostic guidelines in the case of CLSM views of skin lesions.

For the diagnosis of CLSM views [8–12] architectural structures such as: micro-anatomic structures; cell nests etc. play an important role in the diagnosis. The derma pathologist takes melanocytic cytomorphology and architecture and

M. Wiltgen
Institute for Medical Informatics, Statistics and Documentation, Medical University of Graz, Graz, Austria
e-mail: marco.wiltgen@medunigraz.at

R. Hofmann-Wellenhof et al. (eds.), *Reflectance Confocal Microscopy for Skin Diseases*,
DOI 10.1007/978-3-642-21997-9_36, © Springer-Verlag Berlin Heidelberg 2012

keratinocyte cell borders into account for diagnostic decisions. Due to the high refraction of melanin, basal keratinocytes appear very intensive. The images of benign common nevi show, beside the nevi cells, pronounced architectural structures, whereas images of malign melanoma show melanoma cells and connective tissue with little or no architectural structures. Therefore the information at different scales (from coarse structures to detail) plays a crucial role in the diagnosis of CLSM images of skin lesions. This procedure is reflected by the wavelet analysis. Therefore, features based on the properties of the wavelet transform enable an exploration of architectural structures, of different sizes, at different spatial scales. They provide an adequate description of the morphology of CLSM views.

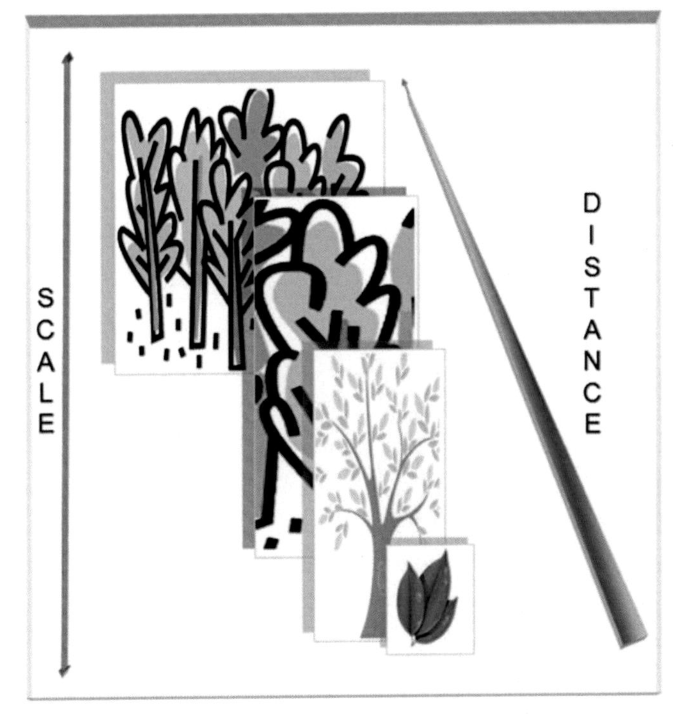

Fig. 36.1 By wavelet analysis, the CLSM views of skin lesions are analyzed at different scales. The principle of this multi-resolution analysis can be illustrated as follows ("see the forest and the trees"): At great distances an observer sees a forest (large scale). When he goes closer to the forest he can see single trees. At a certain distance he can see the branches of the trees (medium scale). When he is close enough, he can distinguish the single leaves and their structures (small scale)

36.3 Computer-Aided Diagnosis of CLSM Images

For an automated, or computer aided, diagnosis of CLSM views of skin lesions, several steps are necessary. First, suitably defined features are calculated from the image matrix. The computer does not see the image in the same way as a human observer. Therefore the tissue properties must be translated by a mathematical procedure into numerical feature values. These values are then processed by the computer. To enable an interpretation by the clinician, the formulation of appropriate features should follow the derma pathologists´ diagnostic guidelines for CLSM views. Secondly, the images must be automatically classified according to their features, enabling a class prediction for every CLSM view of skin lesions. To this purpose, the machine learning algorithm must first be trained on the basis of training images. Then, with the gained knowledge, new samples (test set) are analyzed by the machine learning algorithm resulting in an automated class prediction. For medical purposes, it is important that the knowledge acquired during the training phase of the machine learning algorithm is represented in an understandable and readable form. Thirdly, the automated class prediction performance is evaluated. To this purpose, single classified square elements of the CLSM views are superimposed (relocated) onto the corresponding images using the diagnostic rules generated by the machine learning algorithm. The categorized square elements are highlighted in the images, enabling an identification of diagnostically highly relevant regions and an evaluation of typical diagnostic CLSM features by comparing them with the diagnostic decisions by the human observer.

36.3.1 Wavelet Analysis and Tumor Tissue Description

The terminus "wavelet" is derived from "small waves" which are the basis function of the wavelet transform. (In the early 1980s, the French word "ondelette", meaning "small wave" was used, but soon it was converted to English by translating "onde" into "wave", giving "wavelet".) A wavelet is a fast-decaying wave-like oscillation that starts with amplitude of a non-zero amount and flattens rapidly to zero. It can typically be visualized as a "brief oscillation" similar to the signals recorded by a heart monitor.

The wavelet transform is the representation of a given tissue texture by wavelets. The basis wavelets are scaled and translated copies ("daughter wavelets") of the finite-length waveform ("mother wavelet"). The goal of the transformation is to represent texture data in another way, one which is more suitable for the analysis and interpretation of its global and local structures [13–19]. By use of the wavelet basis functions with increasing spatial extension, the tissue texture can be analyzed at different scales showing detail (local) to coarse (global) properties (Fig. 36.1). This feature gives the wavelet transform a multi resolution property which enables the study of textures properties at varying resolutions.

The wavelet transform shows an analogy to human vision which seems to prefer methods of analysis that run from coarse to fine and, repeating the same process, obtaining new information at the end of each cycle [20]. The principle of the multi resolution can be compared with the impression received by a

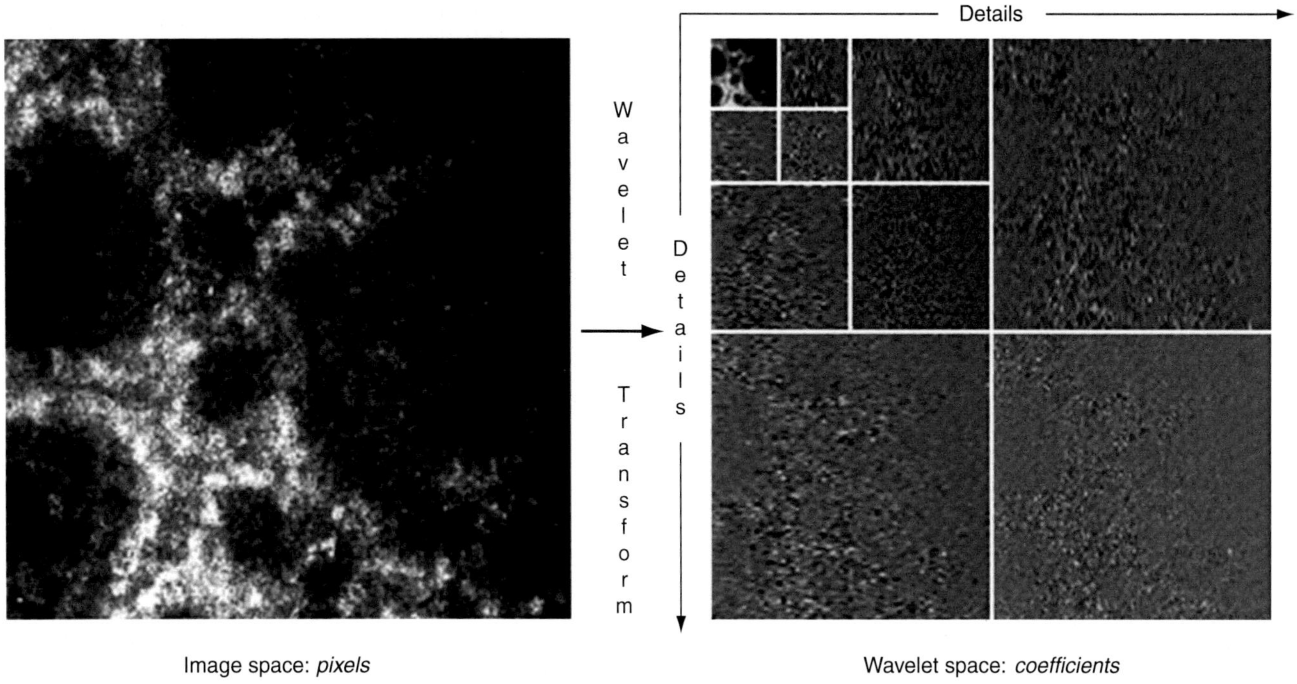

Fig. 36.2 Using the wavelet transform, the CLSM image is dissected into several frequency bands (*right*). Statistical values are calculated inside each frequency band reflecting properties of the CLSM view at different scales. The image in the frequency band on top (*left*) shows large scale structures where details are smoothed out. Outgoing from this low frequency band, the higher frequency bands show successively more and more details (*from top to bottom and from left to right*)

human observer at different distances from an image. When the observer is close enough to the image he can study details (local properties). Then he increases the distance to the image to obtain a general impression (global properties) of the image. The greater the distance between the observer and the image, the better he can study the image as a whole without being overwhelmed by the details, because these are visually smoothed out. In other words, he studies the images at different distances and therefore different scales. The result in wavelet analysis is to "see the forest and the trees" (Fig. 36.1).

By the wavelet transform, the CLSM image is dissected into the so called frequency bands (Fig. 36.2). Each frequency band contains the coefficients of the wavelets, at a given resolution, resulting from the wavelet transform. The frequency bands have different sizes. The detail information is contained in the frequency bands with increasing sizes. The total number of wavelet coefficients equals the number of pixels in the originals image. Large scale information is contained in the low frequency bands, whereas the higher frequency bands contain successively more detail information. The image in the lowest frequency band shows the large scale structures where details are smoothed out. The wavelet coefficients inside the other frequency bands reflect structures at different scales where successively, by increasing frequency bands, more and more details are included. Several statistical values (mean value, deviations and others) are calculated from the wavelet coefficients inside each frequency band, reflecting properties of the CLSM view at different scales. These numerical values are used as features by the computer for the discrimination of skin lesion tissue.

36.3.2 Machine Learning and Skin Lesion Prediction

By means of the classification procedure, the primary inhomogeneous set of CLSM samples, consisting of a mix of malignant melanoma and benign common nevi cases, is split into homogeneous sub-sets, which are assigned to one of the two tumor classes: common benign nevi or malignant melanoma. A homogeneous subset means that it contains only CLSM images with similar feature values, representing one specific kind of tissue.

Classification is done by machine learning algorithms [21–23]. In principle such algorithms work as follows: First, the algorithm learns how to assign the CLSM views to given classes based on a selected training set. Or in other words, it learns to discriminate between the different kinds of tissues. Prior to the training of the machine learning algorithm, the selected CLSM views in the training set are diagnosed by one or more experienced derma pathologists. Then the algorithm determines the feature values of both kinds of tissues and sets threshold values in the range of feature values, separating the tissues into the two classes. After the successful training, the algorithm applies the gained knowledge to predict the class of new and primary unknown samples.

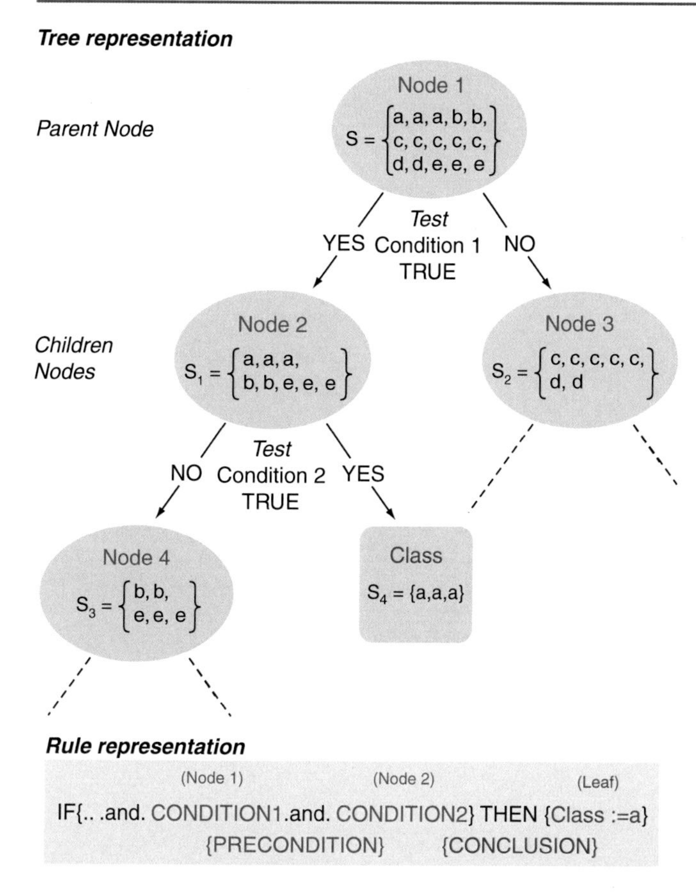

Fig. 36.3 A decision tree consists of a root node (node 1), several inner nodes (node 2, 3, 4) and leaf nodes (Class). Starting from the root node, a set of different samples (a, b, c, d, and e) is routed down the tree until a leaf node is reached. At every node, branching is done according to the feature values so that the children nodes contain sub-sets that are purer than the parent node. This can be done by testing a specific condition, for example; is the selected feature value greater (YES) or smaller (NO) than a threshold value. The inferring rules, containing the test of the conditions down the tree, are automatically generated out of the tree. Knowledge representation by rules, with a syntax that permits their use as diagnostic rules, is suitable for medical diagnosis

In computers, knowledge can be represented in different ways, for example: by numeric values, trees, rules and others. For the discrimination of CLSM views of skin lesions a tree representation (CART: Classification and Regression Trees) that is acquired from the training set is used to represent the knowledge. The tree representation consists of different nodes and branches (Fig. 36.3). There is a root node, several terminal nodes (leafs of the tree) and inner nodes. The first node in the tree is the root node. It contains the inhomogeneous set of samples (or more precisely their feature values). A terminal (leaf) node is a homogeneous node which contains only samples belonging to the same class. The inner nodes contain more or less inhomogeneous sample sets (Fig. 36.3). A branch in the decision tree involves the testing of a particular feature. Then the considered node (parent node) is split into two children nodes. A feature can be tested, for example, by comparing its numerical value with a threshold value that divides its range of values. The threshold value is selected by the algorithm in such a way, that the subsets of samples in the children nodes are purer than the set in the parent node (Fig. 36.3). To this purpose, an information measure is used which indicates the degree of homogeneity; the value in leaf nodes is zero and the higher the value, the higher the corresponding node is inhomogeneous (Fig. 36.4). To classify an unknown sample, it is routed down the tree according to the values of the different features. At every node (except the leaf node), the feature values are tested. When a leaf node is reached, the sample is classified according to the class assigned to the leaf.

For medical diagnosis purposes it is important to duplicate the automated diagnostic process. Therefore, the rules that the algorithm uses to predict the class of an instance should have a syntax that is understandable for the human interpreter. This means that the decision rules (or splitting rules) generated from the tree are sufficiently intelligible to be understood, discussed and explicitly used as diagnostic rules. The generated decision rules have a syntax consisting of an antecedent (precondition) and a consequent (conclusion) part (Fig. 36.3). They are generally expressed as "IF-THEN" rules:

$$\text{IF } \{\text{precondition}\} \text{ THEN } \{\text{conclusion}\}$$

These rules represent knowledge in a form that is easily understandable for the human observer. It enables him to understand why a specific CLSM view is assigned to a benign common nevi or malignant melanoma. The rules can be compared with the diagnostic guidelines of the derma pathologist. According to the guidelines for the diagnosis, the rule can be translated in: if the tissue contains large and medium structures, for example: nevi cells grouped around basal structures, then it is nevus tissue:

$$\text{IF}\left\{\begin{array}{l}\text{The tissue shows}\\ \text{structures of medium size}\\ \text{.and.}\\ \text{The tissue shows}\\ \text{extended structures}\end{array}\right\}\text{THEN}\{\text{tissue} := \text{nevus tissue}\}$$

Some decision trees (like the CART algorithm) have the ability to capture the decision structure explicitly. By using the CART algorithm for classification and class prediction, the decision rules are automatically generated out of the tree, whereby one rule is generated for each terminal node.

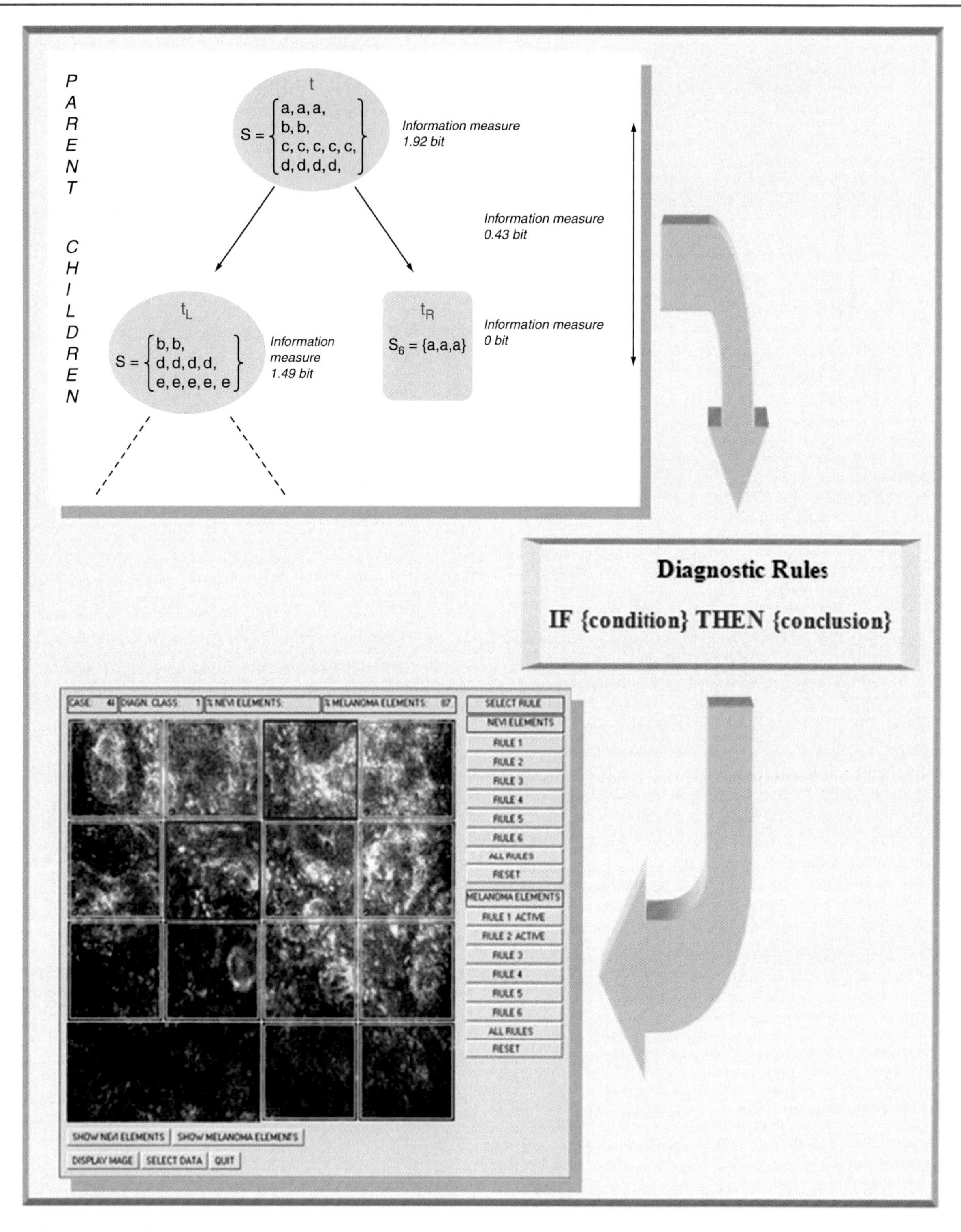

Fig. 36.4 The set of CLSM views is split in such a way that the information difference between the parent node and the children nodes has the greatest value. In other words, they are purer than the parent node. The inferring rules, generated from the decision tree, are implemented as diagnostic rules on a computer. Then, depending on the feature values, the computer generates a class prediction for single square elements of the image. These square elements are superimposed with the image, enabling the derma pathologist to evaluate diagnostic high significant regions in the CLSM image

36.3.3 Evaluation and Visualization of the Automated Diagnostic Process

To verify the performance of computer-aided diagnosis and to interpret the diagnostic process, the automatically generated decision rules are implemented in viewer software (Fig. 36.4). This enables the human interpreter to see an appropriately visualized interpretation of the results of the automated diagnostic. Classified square elements of the images (parts of the images) are indicated in the corresponding CLSM image by the viewer in order to judge the performance of the analysis. For these purposes, square elements of size 128 × 128 pixels are used, because they enable a good localization of the different regions into the images and the texture features still have enough discrimination power. (The CLSM views have a spatial resolution of 512 × 512 pixels). The diagnostic rules are visualized by highlighting the square elements, containing diagnostically highly significant malign melanoma or common benign nevi tissue. The procedure is illustrated in the case of malignant melanoma tissue. Square elements resulting from terminal nodes, with 100% of discrimination power, are taken as highly significant and are drawn with red margins at the graphical user interface of the viewer and labeled with the number 1. Square elements with a discrimination power of 80–99% are drawn with green margins and labeled with the number 2 (Fig. 36.4). The relocated elements mainly show polymorphic tumor cells with structural disarray and are in good accordance with previously published diagnostic CLSM features.

Since the highlighted regions in the CLSM images show tissue structures which comply with the already known diagnostic guidelines, no explicit formulation of the diagnostic rules is necessary for an evaluation. Due to the fact that the tissue features are based on the wavelet transform, reflecting the guidelines of the derma pathologists, the highlighted regions are self-explaining.

36.4 Outlook

Already known, but subjective CLSM criteria are objectively reproduced by the automated diagnosis. The computer aided diagnostic system enables the identification of highly significant parts in CLSM views of malignant melanoma. In a clinical application, the system can be used as a screening tool to improve preventive medical checkups and the early recognition of skin tumors. The automated decisions provided can be used as an expert second opinion and as a training system for inexperienced or student derma pathologists. In another clinical onset, the system may automatically pre-select the cases so that the critical (malignant) cases are first interpreted by the clinician.

Acknowledgment We wish to thank Ms. G. Searle for the critical reading of the text and all the colleagues who enabled this work.

References

1. Rajadhyaksha M, Conzales S, Zavislan JM, Anderson RR, Webb RR (1999) In vivo confocal scanning laser microscopy of human skin: advances in instrumentation and comparison with histology. J Invest Dermatol 113:293–303
2. Busam KJ, Marghoob AA, Halpern AC (2005) Melanoma diagnosis by confocal microscopy: promise and pitfalls. J Invest Dermatol 125:vii
3. Langley RG, Rajadhyaksha M, Dwyer PJ, Sober AJ, Flotte TJ, Anderson RR (2001) Confocal scanning laser microscopy of benign and malignant skin lesions in vivo. J Am Acad Dermatol 45: 365–376
4. Pellacani G, Cesinaro AM, Seidenari S (2005) Reflectance-mode confocal microscopy for the in vivo characterization of pagetoid melanocytosis in melanomas and nevi. J Invest Dermatol 125: 532–537
5. Gerger A, Koller S, Kern T et al (2005) Diagnostic applicability of in vivo confocal laser scanning microscopy in melanocytic skin tumors. J Invest Dermatol 124:493–498
6. Erkol B, Moss RH, Stanley RJ, Stoecker WV, Hvatum E (2005) Automatic lesion boundary detection in dermoscopy images using gradient vector flow snakes. Skin Res Technol 11:17–26
7. She Z, Liu Y, Damatoa A (2007) Combination of features from skin pattern and ABCD analysis for lesion classification. Skin Res Technol 13:25–33
8. Busam KJ, Charles C, Lee G, Halpern AC (2001) Morphologic features of melanocytes, pigmented keratinocytes and melanophages by in vivo confocal scanning laser microscopy. Mod Pathol 14:862–868
9. Pellacani G, Cesinaro AM, Seidenari S (2005) In vivo assessment of melanocytic nests in nevi and melanomas by reflectance confocal microscopy. Mod Pathol 18:469–474
10. Langley RG, Walsh N, Sutherland AE, Propperova I, Delaney L, Morris SF, Gallant C (2007) The diagnostic accuracy of in vivo confocal scanning laser microscopy compared to dermoscopy of benign and malignant melanocytic lesions: a prospective study. Dermatology 215(4):365–372
11. Pellacani G, Cesinaro AM, Longo C, Grana C, Seidenari S (2005) Microscopic in vivo description of cellular architecture of dermoscopic pigment network in nevi and melanomas. Arch Dermatol 141(2):147–154
12. Langley RG, Burton E, Walsh N, Propperova I, Murray SJ (2006) In vivo confocal scanning laser microscopy of benign lentigines: comparison to conventional histology and in vivo characteristics of lentigo maligna. J Am Acad Dermatol 55(1):88–97
13. Wiltgen M, Gerger A, Wagner C, Smolle J (2008) Automatic identification of diagnostic significant regions in confocal laser scanning microscopy of melanocytic skin tumours. Methods Inf Med 47:15–25
14. Press WH, Teukolsky SA, Vetterling WT, Flannery BP (1992) Numerical recipes in C: the art of scientific computing, 2nd edn. Cambridge University Press, New York, pp 591–606
15. Prasad L, Iyengar SS (1997) Wavelet analysis with applications to image processing. CRC Press, Boca Raton

16. Puniena J, Punys V, Punys J (2001) Ultrasound and angio image compression by cosine and wavelet transforms. Int J Med Inform 64:473–481
17. Mello-Thoms C, Dunn SM, Nodine CF, Kundel HL (2001) An analysis of perceptual errors in reading mammograms using quasi-local spatial frequency spectra. J Digital Imaging 14(3):117–123
18. Terae S, Miyasaka K, Kudoh K, Nambu T, Shimizu T, Kaneko K, Yoshikawa H, Kishimoto R, Omatsu T, Fujita N (2000) Wavelet compression on detection of brain lesions with magnetic resonance imaging. J Digital Imaging 13(4):178–190
19. Kerut EK, Given MB, Mc Ilwain E, Allen G, Espinoza C, Giles TD (2000) Echocardio-graphic texture analysis using the wavelet transform: Differentiation of early heart muscle disease. Ultrasound Med Biol 26(9):1445–1453
20. Marr D (1982) Vision. W.H. Freeman, New York
21. Nilsson NJ (1965) Learning machines. McGraw Hill, New York
22. Quinlan JR (1986) Induction of decision trees. Machine Learning 1(1):81–106
23. Quinlan JR (1993) C4.5: Programs for machine learning. Morgan Kaufmann, San Francisco

Experimental Applications and Future Directions

37

Chris Glazowski, Zhao Wang, and James M. Zavislan

37.1 Introduction

As described in detail in the previous chapters, confocal reflectance microscopy has demonstrated the ability to provide images of in vivo or unprocessed ex vivo tissue with sufficient cellular and morphological information to enable the diagnosis of a broad range of dermatological conditions. In many ways, confocal reflectance microscopy provides to clinical dermatology what medical ultrasound did for radiology: a real-time diagnostic imaging modality available in the clinic at the time of care. Although confocal reflectance microscopy and ultrasound operate at different tissue resolutions and imaging depths, there are many analogies between these two modalities. Like ultrasound, a trained observer interprets the image information to make a diagnosis and determine the next steps in care. Tissue information is typically presented as gray scale images. Real-time information can be recorded in cross-sectional image stacks or movies. Examinations can be interpreted in real time or stored and reviewed later or remotely. Like ultrasound, the clinical ergonomics of the reflectance confocal microscope can limit its clinical application and frequency of use. Finally, just as in the case of ultrasound systems, the underlying physics and technology of clinical reflectance confocal microscopes will evolve and improve. In this section we will discuss the progress in development of reflectance confocal microscopy to: (1) enhance clinical ergonomics, (2) improve image fidelity, (3) increase image specificity, and (4) provide for deeper imaging.

C. Glazowski
Memorial Sloan-Kettering Cancer Center, New York, NY, USA
e-mail: glazowsc@mskcc.org; zavislan@optics.rochester.edu

Z. Wang
Department of Biomedical Engineering, University of Rochester, Rochester, NY, USA

Optimedica, Santa Clara, CA, USA
e-mail: jwang@optimedica.com

J.M. Zavislan
Departments of Biomedical Engineering and Ophthalmology, Center for Visual Science, University of Rochester
Rochester, NY, USA
e-mail: zavislan@optics.rochester.edu

37.2 Clinical Ergonomics

Confocal reflectance microscopy for dermatology was introduced in the 1990s. Originally developed as laboratory instruments [1–6], these systems were based on existing scanning microscopes: tandem scanning microscopes (Corcuff and Griem) or scanning laser ophthalmoscopes (Rajadhyaksha). These instruments were the first to produce subcellular resolution images of in vivo skin and they did so over moderately large fields of view of approximately 0.25–0.5 mm. However, they were large stationary instruments that required that the patient be brought to the instrument, not the instrument to the patient. In 1998 Lucid, Inc. introduced the first commercial clinical confocal microscope (VivaScope 1000), based on the system design of Rajadhyaksha and Webb [6], which used a rotating polygon fast scanner and galvanometer slow scanner. While too large to be practical in clinical settings, the VivaScope 1000 was portable, allowing it to be brought to the patient and provided the images in many of the early confocal clinical studies. Lucid further refined the implementation of the polygon/galvanometer scanning into the VivaScope 1500, which dramatically reduced the size of the imaging head. With this system the entire imaging head could be positioned relative to the patient, thus maximizing the locations that could be imaged without requiring the patient to lie down or assume awkward positions.

Clinical reflectance confocal imaging systems require both high numerical objective apertures (NA) and large field of view to provide high resolution images that cover significant areas of a lesion. Because of this there is a limit to how small a polygon/galvanometer optical system can be made and still provide a large field of view, high resolution imaging system. Further reduction in imaging head size requires a different scanning technology to optimize the head volume

R. Hofmann-Wellenhof et al. (eds.), *Reflectance Confocal Microscopy for Skin Diseases*,
DOI 10.1007/978-3-642-21997-9_37, © Springer-Verlag Berlin Heidelberg 2012

for a given resolution and field of view. Two approaches that have been implemented and tested in dermatology clinical trials to further reduce the size of the reflectance confocal imaging head brought to the patient are: resonant galvanometer scanning and slit scanning. Resonant galvanometer systems replace the rotating polygon with a fast-scanning galvanometer driven at its resonant frequency. Replacing the polygon with a single mirror scanner reduces the size of the imaging head (due to the reduced size of the resonant galvanometer relative to the polygon) as well as potentially reducing the number of relay optics within the head. Larger fields of view are possible as well. However, resonant galvanometers, unlike polygon scanners, do not sweep the illumination beam at constant velocity, which then requires variable pixel acquisition and sophisticated electronics to provide an undistorted en face image. This scanning system is now in use in the hand-held Lucid VivaScope 3000.

Slit scanning systems [7–13] project a diffraction-limited illumination line into the tissue and transversely scan the line to illuminate an en-face field of view. The backscattered light is collected and focused onto a one-dimensional array of detectors. This scanning geometry eliminates the need for a fast scanner altogether. This reduces the optical complexity and also allows for each detector element to integrate the optical signal approximately 1000 times longer than in a scanning spot geometry. While this optical geometry is not truly confocal in all directions, the geometry of the illumination and the detection provide comparable axial and lateral resolution to that of point-scan confocal systems. Although the current slit scan systems have image artifacts such as drop-outs, the overall simplicity of the optical system and the reduced detection electrical bandwidth make this attractive for compact imaging systems.

During the time that confocal imaging heads have shrunk to permit straightforward access across the patients skin, advances in electronic imaging and computerized control have also greatly impacted clinical navigation. Digital image sensors have allowed for the integration of a clinical macroscopic image with confocal image locations for systems that use a tissue stabilization ring. This provides for direct navigation of the lesion and greatly assists in correlating areas of cellular abnormality with the clinical lesion. Advanced control software enable automated image stacks and mosaics and when combined with automatic laser power control provide for coordinated image stacks with balanced image brightness.

Looking to the future, high-volume consumer electronics, such as smart phones have introduced inexpensive display components and graphics processors that will likely enable further improvements in system integration and functionality. While fundamental optical principals likely prevent the design of confocal heads that are smaller than 500 mL in volume with the necessary resolution and field of view, continued advances in electronics and display technologies will likely enable integrating image displays with touch screen controls directly on confocal heads as well as providing real-time image enhancement such as tissue highlighting for feature review and quantitative analysis of lesions.

37.3 Image Fidelity

A principal goal of a clinical confocal microscopy image is to accurately report the cellular and tissue morphology. The imaging system collects the backscattered light from a tissue section, and since the backscattering originates from the refractive index distribution within the tissue, the images correlate to cellular and tissue morphology. A fundamental challenge in clinical reflectance confocal imaging is that the illumination light must be focused through the optically thick tissue to the section being imaged. The overlying tissue distorts the incident beam as it focuses into the imaged tissue section. This distortion reduces the amount of irradiance of the illumination and thus, image brightness. Also, the distortion reduces the resolution and contrast of the tissue features imaged within the section. Fortunately, even with this distortion approximately micrometer-level resolution is possible within the epidermis and superficial dermis and increasing the laser power compensates the image brightness. However, light scattered from above and below the imaged tissue section produces background scattering that is also collected by the imaging optics and directed onto the pinhole. That is, a portion of the background scattered light is also collected with the light collected from the imaged tissue section of interest. The amount of light from the imaged section relative to the background decreases with deeper imaging and cannot be compensated by increasing the incident laser power.

The presence of the background signal not only reduces the contrast of the tissue images, it changes the image appearance; the background scatter collected by the pinhole optically interferes with the light from the imaged section and this interference changes the reported image. Mathematically, the light from the tissue and the background scatter collected by the pinhole can be represented by the integrated (within the pinhole aperture) optical powers $\Phi_T(x,y)$ and $\Phi_B(x,y)$, where (x, y) are the coordinates of a pixel in the acquired image. The image collected and displayed by the system is given by

$$I(x,y) = \alpha \left\{ \begin{array}{l} \Phi_T(x,y) + \Phi_B(x,y) \\ +2\sqrt{\Phi_T(x,y)\Phi_B(x,y)}\cos\left[\gamma(x,y)\right] \end{array} \right\},$$

where α is a proportionality constant associated with the detection electronics and $\gamma(x,y)$ is the integrated optical phase difference between the tissue and background scatter at a particular image position (x, y).

The term $\alpha\left\{\Phi_T(x,y)\right\}$ represents the best possible tissue image. It is still affected by the position-varying aberrations accumulated by the light's round trip in the tissue, but contains the desired reflectance information associated with the tissue plane being imaged. The contrast of the tissue image is reduced by the term $\alpha\left\{\Phi_B(x,y)\right\}$, which represents the diffuse and generally uniform "glow" from the scattering within the tissue that actually makes it through the detection pinhole. If the signal only had these two contributions, simple image processing would be largely able to restore the contrast of the tissue image. However, the last term in the equation represents the interference between the tissue signal and the background light that arises from the coherence properties of the small high-brightness illumination source. The interference term modulates the background randomly depending on the particular path the light takes, but the modulation is correlated to image position (x, y) and is essentially repeatable over successive frames. The result of this interference is the production of the image artifact commonly referred to as speckle that results in "grainy" images. Speckle artifacts can produce isolated bright pixels or spots within the image and occur where the tissue and background scatter are in phase, $\cos\left[\gamma(x,y)\right]\approx 1$. Other phase conditions lead to image artifacts of other brightness distributions. This speckle can make a pixel within the displayed image appear brighter or darker than if it only reported the tissue signal $\Phi_T(x,y)$. Also, because speckle artifacts are fixed for a stationary patient, averaging multiple images does not dramatically reduce their appearance. Consequently, speckle distorts the appearance of the images and makes the identification of fine features and overall morphology challenging. When viewing a skin image, one could ask, "Are the bright pixels within the image due to melanin or an image artifact?" and "Is the image *grainy* because the tissue is filled with keratin or because of an image artifact?"

It is possible to directly reduce the effect of the background scatter by altering the optical design of the illumination system, the detection system or both [14–16]. Most often confocal microscopes use a laser illumination beam with a smooth power distribution over its width. However, if this illumination beam is replaced by one with a 180° phase step at its center to produce a bi-lobed distribution, commonly referred as a TEM_{01} beam, the background scattered light from the tissue is split into two components $\Phi_B(x,y)$ anld $\Phi'_B(x,y)$ with one component coming from each lobe of the illumination beam. Because of the phase step in the illumination beam, the two background components are nominally out of phase and partially cancel each other. Unfortunately, the signal strength from the tissue is also reduced when using this illumination beam, but less so than the background is reduced. The result of using this illumination is that the overall signal to background ratio is improved by a factor of 1.8× for the 0.9 NA objectives commonly used in skin imaging. Note the lateral resolution is elongated by approximately √2 in the direction of the phase step placed in the pupil.

Another modified system incorporates a polarizing beam splitter before the objective to produce an illumination focus comprised of two overlapping spots with orthogonal polarizations at the imaged tissue section. Because the tissue is illuminated with two beams the lateral resolution spot becomes slightly elongated, typically by 25% in a 45° direction relative to the scanning direction. This imaging mode is referred to as non-reversible differential interference contrast (NR-DIC) and was included in the VivaScope 1000. The background signal light, $\Phi_B(x,y)$ and $\Phi'_B(x,y)$, originating from these two beams are correlated and again largely optically cancel each other now due to the orthogonal polarization of the incident beams. The tissue signals from the two beams, $\Phi_T(x,y)$ and $\Phi'_T(x,y)$, also partially cancel due to the overlapping illumination spots. However, the background reduction relative to the signal reduction is higher with this imaging mode than with the TEM_{01} illumination beam. With the NR-DIC imaging mode the overall signal to background ratio is improved by a factor of at least 5× when using a 0.9 NA objective.

Figure 37.1 shows epidermal images within the granular and spinous layers of Fitzpatrick type II ex vivo skin from a traditional reflectance confocal microscope operating at 830 nm and 0.9 NA using (a) traditional illumination and detection and (b) orthogonally polarized illumination and detection (NR-DIC mode). Ex vivo tissue was used to allow for the same area to be imaged without motion. The brightness for each image was normalized to be the same. Notice that the image from the standard confocal imaging mode shows a grainy appearance due to speckle. The NR-DIC imaging mode shows clearer outlines of the individual cells and structures within the cells are more clearly evident. Glazowski [17] has developed confocal imaging within skin that suggests various modifications of the illumination and detection systems and allows these to be compared and optimized. Using this work it is likely that further reductions to speckle and overall improvements to image fidelity will be possible.

Another component of image fidelity relates to knowing that the system is imaging within its operation specifications. Clinical confocal imaging is routinely done with tissue windows and immersion liquids and gels that must have the correct optical properties to provide good images. Immersion compounds need to be appropriately cleaned from the objective or otherwise the images degrade. The United States

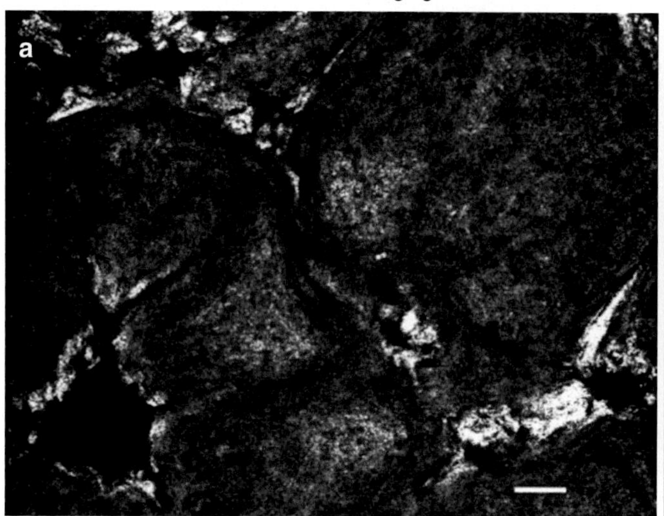

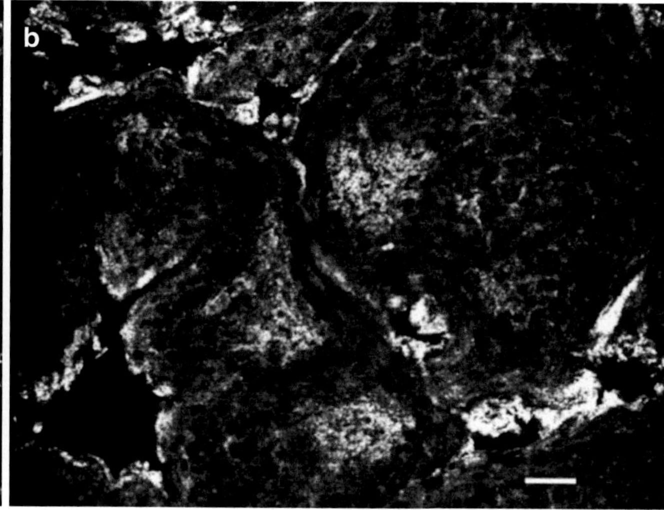

Fig. 37.1 Comparison of confocal imaging modes in the granular and spinous layers of Fitzpatrick type II ex vivo skin within the granular and spinous layers, 830 nm illumination wavelength and 0.9 NA objective operating with water immersion. (**a**) The standard confocal imaging mode, 0.8 μm lateral resolution and 3.3 μm axial resolution. (**b**) The orthogonally polarized NR-DIC imaging mode, 1.0× 0.8 μm lateral resolution and 3.3 μm axial resolution. Both images have been normalized to the same overall brightness. Scale bars are 40 μm.

Clinical Laboratories Improvement Act requires the routine maintenance and calibration of medical instrumentation. Fortunately, the optical quality of reflectance confocal systems, including the immersion compounds and tissue windows can be directly tested using the image of a target formed on the back of a tissue window. Using images from this target and a modified implementation of the ISO-12233 electronic imaging standard, quantitative information on the image quality of scanning confocal systems can be easily measured, recorded and transmitted back to the manufacturer for system verification and tracking [18]. The routine testing of the clinical systems will ensure that image features seen are associated with the tissue and not optical artifact the and will assist in comparing images taken from different instruments.

37.4 Image Specificity

In the absence of background scattered light reflectance confocal images report the light backscattered from the tissue components within the imaged section. Cellular and tissue structures with large refractive index relative to the interstitial components in general appear bright. Homogeneous regions or structures that absorb light appear black. The overall displayed image brightness is dependent on the optical power incident on the imaged section and the overall detection efficiency of the scattered light. In general it is not possible to uniquely know the power within the tissue. Because of this it is difficult to uniquely identify structures by brightness alone, and presently, image interpretation requires strictly morphological interpretation. Image specificity will likely be enhanced by utilizing exogenous contrast labeling agents, applying image-processing algorithms, utilizing polarization information and by imaging at multiple.

37.4.1 Exogenous Contrast Labeling

Exogenous stains are routinely applied to fixed and sectioned tissue to provide the contrast that enables pathological diagnosis. However, most stains used in pathology are not appropriate for in-vivo tissue imaging or even un-processed tissue since they mostly rely on differential absorption, which works well when imaging in transmission but fails in reflection; in reflectance imaging an absorbing region appears similar to a homogenous region without backscatter. For this reason, research and development in reflectance confocal contrast agents have been directed to conjugated gold nanoparticles [19–21]. These particles exhibit enhanced backscatter and can be conjugated to preferentially bind to specific cells or sub-cellular proteins. Current research indicates that these compounds provide in vivo labeling [19] and have the potential to be safely used in humans. However, the specific indications for use in skin have not been developed and clinical use will need to wait for studies to confirm safety and efficacy in specific situations.

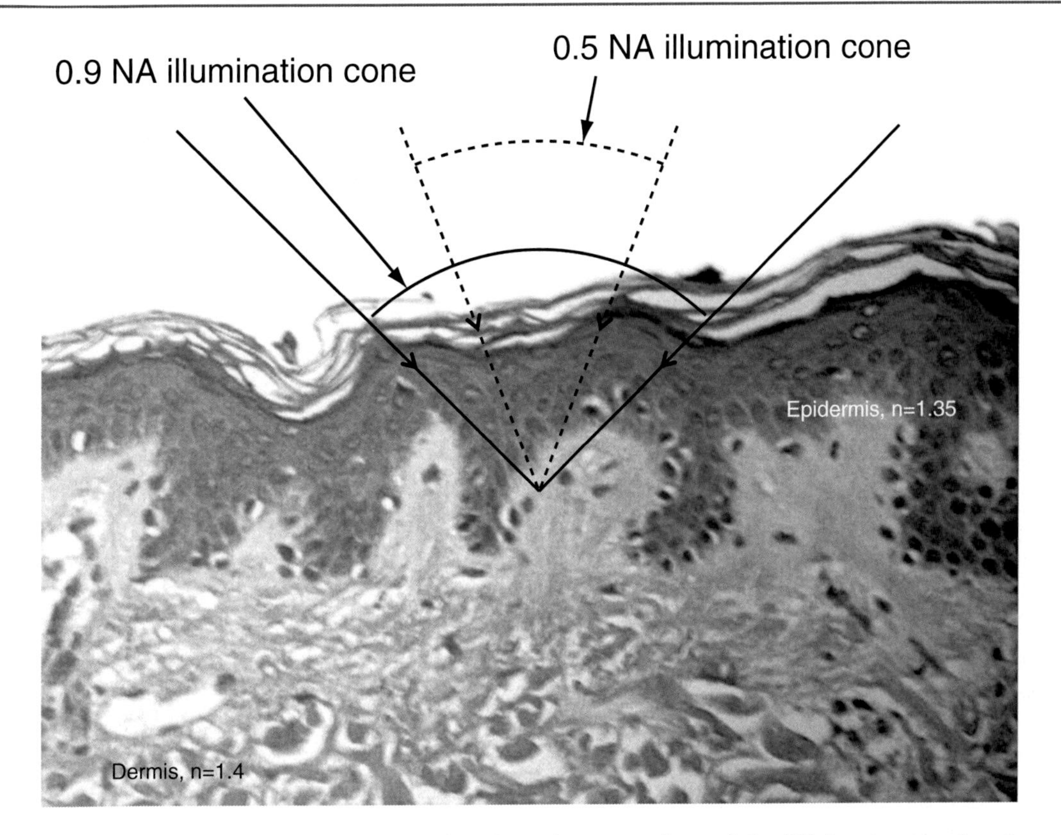

Fig. 37.2 Cross-sectional optical paths of light focusing below the dermal-epidermal (DE) junction for 0.9 and 0.5 NA (water immersed) superimposed on a traditionally stained skin section. The difference in the average refractive index of the dermis and epidermis combined with the corrugations of the DE junction introduce larger optical path differences across the focused beam for the larger NA and limit the ability to produce images significantly below the DE junction at 0.9 NA

37.4.2 Image Processing

When the VivaScope 1000 was initially cleared by the US Food and Drug Administration in the late 1990s, regulators were concerned that the confocal imager would be used as a part of a computer-based diagnostic system and whether the computer could modify or process the confocal images as to change their interpretation when viewed by a human reader. Because the VivaScope 1000 merely presented the cellular images to the user without computer modification or processing, it operated analogously to a pathology microscope but without the need to process and section the tissue. Without any modification of the images there was no need to independently validate any image processing algorithms and the overall imaging system was initially cleared as a Class 1 product exempt from premarket notification. Its initial classification was under CFR 21g§880.6320, AC powered examination light. With this classification, the system could be sold and used in clinical trials without the need to submit investigational device exemptions.

Although the regulators were initially concerned about image processing and automated diagnosis, at the time the VivaScope 1000 was cleared, too few clinical studies were completed in order to even propose trial image processing algorithms using this new imaging modality. Presently, multiple clinical trials have been completed on many of the common neoplastic and inflammatory skin diseases and opportunities and limitations of confocal imaging are better understood. Because reflectance confocal microscopes report endogenous morphology, one of the first applications for image processing is identifying and classifying differential diagnostic criteria. To this end work has begun to automatically identify the dermal-epidermal junction [22], epidermal keratinocytes [23] and melanoma [24,25, 25]. The use of computer algorithms to "over-read" clinical images or to select regions of "interest" is becoming more common in radiology and fixed tissue pathology. These algorithms augment the interpretation and judgment of a clinical observer. Presently, computer systems have sufficient processing power to linearly process video-rate confocal images in real-time. With this processing power and the wisdom gained from the completed and ongoing clinical trials, it is likely that image processing algorithms will be validated that will assist clinicians as they use confocal microscopes in their practices.

37.4.3 Polarization Imaging

The scattering of light from tissues often depends on the polarization and incidence direction of the illumination. Because of this imaging with polarized light has demonstrated enhanced contrast and specificity in macroscopic skin imaging [26–28]. Polarization selective imaging has also been applied to reflectance confocal imaging of ex vivo tissues to highlight and differentiate the epithelium from the collagen [29, 30]. The VivaScope 1000 had an imaging system that could be adjusted between a "bright-field" and "dark-field" polarization mode by rotating the waveplate mounted adjacent to the objective lens. This adjustment changed the polarization state of the illumination to either direct polarization-maintaining scatter or the crossed-polarization scatter back to the detector. Collagen could be detected if the waveplate was rotated during imaging. Collagen fibers, being locally birefringent, would brighten and dim depending on their orientation. Unfortunately, the overall image would brighten and dim as well as the waveplate was rotated, but birefringent structures would evolve differently than non-birefringent or de-polarizing structures.

The present generation of the commercial clinical reflectance confocal imagers do not provide for control of the illumination polarization or the analysis of the detected polarization. However, the same technology that enables flat-panel liquid crystal displays enables rapid modification of the incident polarization and its analysis. It is likely that a polarization-based contrast image will be presented to the user merely by selecting an operation mode where internal liquid crystal polarization switches are actuated as successive frames are scanned and processed to maintain overall image brightness. As a further enhancement, recent work has demonstrated the ability to spatially vary the polarization across the illumination beam and the detection pupil [31]. These so-called "inhomogeneously polarized beams" allow for the light incident at various directions within the focused beam to have a specific polarization state that could be optimized to scatter off particular tissue constituents with a desired return polarization state for enhanced detection. This variable polarization control represents another design tool in optimizing the contrast and specificity of confocal images.

37.4.4 Multiwavelength Imaging

Currently, most clinical reflectance confocal microscopes report tissue images that are grayscale mappings of the collected backscatter at one color, and the pathological identification of various tissue and cellular structures is based on relative brightness and image morphology. A common request from clinicians is to produce "color" images of the tissue that in some way mirror the colors found in traditionally processed sectioned and stained tissue. While this may be possible if exogenous contrast agents and fluorescent detection is used [32] image contrast in reflectance confocal originates in scatter rather than in absorption and simply imaging at multiple wavelengths and displaying the collected image will not likely produce images that directly correlate to histology slides. However, incorporating multiple wavelengths into reflectance confocal microscopy can easily be achieved by combining two or more collimated semiconductor lasers with dichroic beamsplitters into a single illumination beam. Images from each wavelength can be acquired either sequentially onto a single detector in the imaging head or multiple detectors can simultaneously collect images for each wavelength. Images from the various wavelengths encode different scattering signatures that may be used to highlight different cell and tissue types.

The rationale for this imaging mode is as follows. The backscatter of the inter- and intra-cellular structures varies with wavelength and the size, geometry and refractive index of the scattering structure [33, 34]. Thus, the backscatter from inter- and intra-cellular structures of different refractive indices or geometries vary with wavelength. By acquiring reflectance images from multiple wavelengths it is possible to extract "color dependent" information that correlates to tissue properties. Using a three-wavelength reflectance confocal microscope operating at 785, 810 and 850 nm, Wang was able to identify T lymphocytes in whole ex vivo skin specimens [35]. The identified T lymphocytes were correlated to CD3+ cells by fluorescently labeling the cells and imaging with a coincident fluorescent channel. Additionally, Wang showed that the reflectivity of papillary dermis and reticular dermis at each of the three wavelengths could be used as a reflectance standard to estimate the backscattering irradiance of granulocytes and lymphocytes in skin tissue regardless of the imaging depth and illumination power of the optical imaging system.

The Lucid VivaScope 1500 can be configured to operate with up to three wavelengths which will enable clinical researchers to determine if imaging at multiple wavelengths will provide clinical useful tissue information.

37.5 Deeper Imaging

Currently, reflectance confocal systems are able to image to the papillary or reticular dermis in most clinical situations. Although this is sufficient for many clinical needs, deeper imaging would allow for additional applications. A common question is, "Can the confocal imaging systems be configured to image deeper?" The answer to this question is "Yes, but at a penalty." The penalty is resolution. The high-resolution images produced by a reflectance confocal require all the light scattered from a particular structure within the tissue that is collected and focused by the optics onto the detection pinhole have all the optical paths matched to approximately ¼ a wavelength of the illumination light or 0.2 μm for typical near-infrared illumination. This condition must be met over the full numerical aperture cone of the objective. Optical path mismatches from the optical system itself can be minimized by appropriate design and manufacture. However, the tissue above the imaging plane effectively becomes part of the optical system and variations in thickness and average refractive index across the numerical aperture add uncontrollable optical path difference.

Because light must be collected with matched optical paths over the entire numerical aperture, the larger the numerical aperture the more the natural variations of the tissue within this cone influence the optical paths. Figure 37.2 illustrates the optical paths taken by a 0.9 and 0.5 NA cone when imaging inside below the dermal-epidermal (DE) junction. Because the average refractive index of dermis and epidermis is approximately 1.4 and 1.35, respectively, imaging below the DE junction increases the optical path difference for the 0.9 NA beam much more rapidly than at 0.5 or lower NA. Thus, one way to image deeper is to reduce the operating NA of the system. The remarkably deep images obtained by optical coherence tomography systems illustrate this point. Operating with lateral resolutions of 15 μm limited by the NA and axial resolutions of 4 μm limited by the 70 nm spectral width of the illumination, images in skin can be obtained to depths of 1.5 mm [36]. However, with 15 μm lateral resolution no cellular morphology can be determined and clinical interpretations must be made on tissue morphology alone.

Reducing the NA increases the lateral blur proportionally to 1/ NA and increases the axial blur by $1/\text{NA}^2$. Going from 0.9 to 0.5 NA increases the lateral blur from 1 to 2 μm and is usually not objectionable. However, reducing the NA from 0.9 to 0.5 NA increases the axial blur by almost a factor of 4 from 3 μm to approximately 12 μm, which noticeably reduces the overall contrast of the confocal image. Kempe proposed a coherent microscope that combines a multi-wavelength reflectance confocal imaging system with a coherent confocal detector arm similar to that used in time domain OCT [37–39]. By adding a coherent detector and simultaneously illuminating with three semiconductor lasers this imaging system operating at 0.5 NA provides the same axial resolution as a 0.9 NA reflectance confocal system, but because of the lower operating NA it allows for deeper imaging. We have done preliminary ex vivo imaging studies with this system and the results are encouraging. More studies are needed to determine the limitations and applications of this type of confocal system.

37.6 Conclusions

Reflectance confocal systems are the first clinical imaging systems that provide sufficient resolution and information to enable an "optical biopsy" for a wide range of dermatological conditions. This resulted from the diligence of the clinical researchers who helped mold laboratory microscopes into clinical imaging systems compatible with every day workflow. Through the combined work of clinicians and scientists, the applications and the utility of these instruments will continue to develop. It is likely that the confocal imaging systems of the future will be straightforward to use, provide several distinct modes that can highlight particular tissue conditions with diagnostic specificity, and become a routine part of a dermatological exam offering enhanced efficiency and improved patient care.

Acknowledgements We would like to acknowledge the support of the National Institutes of Health, National Cancer Institutes under grant 5R42CA110226 and the New York State Office of Science, Technology and Academic Research and 5T32AR007472, under TTIP Award C020027.

References

1. Corcuff P, Leveque JL (1993) In vivo vision of the human skin with the tandem scanning Microscope. Dermatology 186:50–54
2. Corcuff P, Bertrand C, Leveque JL (1993) Morphometry of human epidermis in vivo by real-time confocal microscopy. Arch Dermatol Res 285:475–481
3. Corcuff P, Gonnord G, Pierard GE, Leveque JL (1996) In vivo confocal microscopy of human skin: a new design for cosmetology and dermatology. Scanning 18:351–355
4. Griem ML, Robotewskyj A, Nagel RH (1994) Potential vascular damage from radiation in the space environment. Adv Space Res 14(10):555–563
5. Rajadhyaksha M, Grossman M, Esterowitz D, Webb RH, Anderson RR (1995) In vivo confocal scanning laser microscopy of human skin: melanin provides strong contrast. J Invest Dermatol 104: 946–952
6. Rajadhyaksha M, Anderson RR, Webb RH (1999) Video-rate confocal scanning laser microscope for imaging human tissues in vivo. Appl Opt 38:2105–2115
7. Maurice DM (1974) A scanning slit optical microscope. Ophthalmologie 13:1033–1037
8. Koester C (1980) Scanning mirror microscope with optical sectioning characteristics: applications in ophthalmology. Appl Opt 19: 1749–1757
9. Wang T, Mandella M, Contag C, Kino G (2003) Dual-axis confocal microscope for high-resolution in vivo imaging. Opt Lett 28: 414–416
10. Dwyer PJ, DiMarzio CA, Zavislan JM, Fox WJ, Rajadhyaksha R (2006) Confocal reflectance theta line scanning microscope for imaging human skin in vivo. Opt Lett 31:942–944
11. Dwyer PJ, DiMarzio CA, Rajadhyaksha M (2007) Confocal theta line-scanning microscope for imaging human tissues. Appl Opt 46: 1843–1851
12. Gareau D, Abeytunge S, Rajadhyaksha M (2009) Line-scanning reflectance confocal microscopy of human skin: comparison of full-pupil and divided-pupil configurations. Opt Lett 34:3235–3237
13. Patel YG, Rajadhyaksha R, DiMarzio CA (2010) Optimal pupil design for confocal microscopy. Proc SPIE 7570:75700P. doi:10.1117/12.842862
14. Zavislan JM (2000) Imaging system using polarization effects to enhance image quality. US Patent 6,134,010, October 17
15. Zavislan JM (2000) Imaging system using polarization effects to enhance image quality. US Patent 6,134,009, October 17

16. Zavislan JM (2001) Imaging system using multi-mode laser illumination to enhance image quality. US Patent 6,304,373, October 16
17. Glazowski C, Zavislan JM (2010) Coherent pupil engineered scanning reflectance confocal microscope (SRCM) for turbid imaging. Proc SPIE 7570:75700O. doi:10.1117/12.842439
18. Wang Z, Glazowski CE, Zavislan JM (2007) Modulation transfer function measurement of scanning reflectance microscopes. J Biomed Opt 12:051802. doi:10.1117/1.2779352
19. Kumar S, Sokolov K, Richards-Kortum R (2006) In vivo optical detection of intranuclear cancer biomarkers using gold nanoparticles. Proc SPIE 6095:609504. doi:10.1117/12.647139
20. Nitin N, Javier DJ, Roblyer DM, Richards-Kortum R (2007) Widefield and high-resolution reflectance imaging of gold and silver nanospheres. J Biomed Opt 12:051505. doi:10.1117/1.2800314
21. Javier DJ, Nitin N, Levy M, Ellington A, Richards-Kortum R (2008) Aptamer-targeted gold nanoparticles as molecular-specific contrast agents for reflectance imaging. Bioconj Chem 19(6):1309–1312
22. Kurugol S, Dy JG, Brooks DH, Rajadhyaksha M (2011) Pilot study of semiautomated localization of the dermal/epidermal junction in reflectance confocal microscopy images of skin. J Biomed Opt 16(3):036005
23. Gareau D (2011) Automated identification of epidermal keratinocytes in reflectance confocal microscopy. J Biomed Opt 16:030502. doi:10.1117/1.3552639
24. Huang B, Gareau D (2009) Toward automated detection of malignant melanoma. Proc SPIE 7169:71690X. doi:10.1117/12.809386
25. Hennessy R, Jacques S, Pellacani G, Gareau D (2010) Clinical feasibility of rapid confocal melanoma feature detection. Proc SPIE 7548:75480Q. doi:10.1117/12.842824
26. Anderson RR (1991) Polarized light examination and photography of the skin. Arch Dermatol 127(7):1000–1005
27. Jacques SL, Lee K (1998) Polarized video imaging of skin. Proc SPIE 3245:356. doi:10.1117/12.312307
28. Jacques SL, Ramella-Roman JC, Lee K (2002) Imaging skin pathology with polarized light. J Biomed Opt 7:329. doi:10.1117/1.1484498
29. Rajadhyaksha M, Menaker G, Gonzalez S (2000) Confocal microscopy of excised human skin using acetic acid and crossed polarization: rapid detection of non-melanoma skin cancers. Proc SPIE 3907:84–88
30. Patel YG, Nehal KS, Aranda I, Li Y, Halpern AC, Rajadhyaksha R (2007) Confocal reflectance mosaicing of basal cell carcinomas in Mohs surgical skin excisions. J Biomed Opt 12:034027. doi:10.1117/1.2750294
31. Spilman A, Brown T (2007) Stress birefringent, space-variant wave plates for vortex illumination. Appl Opt 46:61–66
32. Gareau DS (2009) Feasibility of digitally stained multimodal confocal mosaics to simulate histopathology. J Biomed Opt 14:034050. doi:10.1117/1.3149853
33. Backman V, Gurjar RS, Perelman LT, Gopal V, Kalashnikov M, Badizadegan K, Wax A, Georgakoudi I, Mueller MG, Boone CW, Itzkan I, Dasari RR, Feld MS (2002) Imaging and measurement of cell structure and organization with submicron accuracy using light scattering spectroscopy. Proc SPIE 4613:101. doi:10.1117/12.465234
34. Rajadhyaksha M, Gonzalez S, Zavislan JM (2004) Detectability of contrast agents for confocal reflectance imaging of skin and microcirculation. J Biomed Opt 9:323. doi:10.1117/1.1646175
35. Wang Z (2008) Multiwavelength reflectance confocal microscopy for immune cell identification Thesis (Ph.D.), University of Rochester, Department of Biomedical Engineering
36. Jung W, Kim J, Jeon M, Chaney EJ, Stewart C, Boppart SA (2011) Handheld optical coherence tomography scanner for primary care diagnostics. IEEE Trans Biomed Eng 58(3 part 2):741–744
37. Kempe M (2000) Confocal microscopy. US Patent 6,151,127, November 21
38. Kempe M (2002) Confocal heterodyne interference microscopy. US Patent 6,381,023, April 30
39. Kempe M (2008) Confocal microscopy. US Patent 7,333,213, February 19

Part X

Glossary

Reflectance Confocal Microscopy Imaging: A Glossary of Terminology

38

Joseph Malvehy and Alon Scope

A standardized terminology to describe RCM images is required for successful dissemination of RCM among clinicians and scientists. The glossary of terms in this atlas is another important milestone in achieving a consensus on terminology among experts in the field of RCM [1] (Tables 38.1, 38.2, and 38.3). The present works builds on the terms defined in the "Consensus glossary in confocal reflectance microscopy consensus" and subsequent publications in the scientific literature. In this book many definitions and confocal terms are used. The glossary introduces in this chapter the principal descriptors in normal skin and in neoplasms and hardly to inflammatory skin lesions. These terms and definitions are the result of a previous "Consensus terminology" work published in 2007 and numerous publications in confocal microscopy evolving during last years. Only those criteria that have been considered to be reproducible in the literature or when they were considered of special importance for the consultation by the reader are presented in this chapter organized three different tables: normal skin, [1] melanocytic tumors [2, 3]and nonmelanocytic tumors [4-8]. Other concepts and definitions are included in the book in every single chapter.

J. Malvehy (✉)
Department of Dermatology, Melanoma Unit,
Hospital Clinic of Barcelona,
Barcelona, Spain
e-mail: jmalvehy@clinic.ub.es

A. Scope
Department of Dermatology, Sheba Medical Center, Tel-Aviv, Israel

R. Hofmann-Wellenhof et al. (eds.), *Reflectance Confocal Microscopy for Skin Diseases*,
DOI 10.1007/978-3-642-21997-9_38, © Springer-Verlag Berlin Heidelberg 2012

Table 38.1 RCM terms used to describe normal skin by anatomic level

RCM terms	Definition
Superficial (supra-basal) epidermal layers	
Stratum corneum (skin surface)	Top layer of intact skin with greater brightness compared with other epidermal layers, because of the backscatter of light at the air-stratum corneum interface (skin surface); the keratinocytes appear as 10- to 30-μm, bright polygonal structures with dark outlines
Honeycomb pattern	Normal pattern of the spinous-granular layers formed by bright polygonal outlines of keratinocytes, about 15–25 μm in diameter, with dark central nuclei
Broadened honeycombed pattern	Honeycombed pattern with bright enlarged and broadened intercellular spaces
Cobblestone pattern	Bright round cells without a visible nucleus (pigmented keratinocytes) are closely set, separated by a less refractive polygonal outline. This is the normal pattern of basal keratinocytes at the supra-papillary plates and a variant of the normal pattern of the spinous-granular layers in darkly pigmented skin.
Dermo-epidermal junction	
Basal layer of the epidermis	A single layer of cells arranged as aggregates of refractive cells (forming foci of cobblestone pattern and corresponding to horizontal optical sectioning at the supra-papillary plates) or in a circular pattern around the dermal papillae (forming edged-papillae and corresponding to optical sectioning through the dermal papillae). The basal layer is located 50–100 μm below the stratum corneum, depending on anatomic site
Dermal-epidermal junction (DEJ)	The DEJ is characterized by the presence of dermal papillae - round, oval or polygonal dark areas surrounded by structures of the basal or spinous layers of the epidermis. Observation of blood vessels or collagen in the dermal papillae may facilitate recognition of the DEJ. DEJ that appears flattened on histopathology is less perceptible on RCM than an undulating DEJ
Edged-papillae	Dermal papillae demarcated by a rim of bright cells (pigmented basal keratinocytes and melanocytes)
Superficial dermis	
Coarse collagen structures	Bright fibrillar structures that appear finely reticulated, forming a web-like pattern, or as thicker bundles. Can be described as: – Reticulated – crossing fibers (mostly 1–5 μm in diameter), forming a bright web-like pattern in dermal papillae or superficial dermis – Bundles – parallel fibers creating thick fascicles (5–25 μm in diameter)
Blood vessels	Dark structures in the dermis (i.e., darker than surrounding stroma) in which movement of bright round cells (white blood cells) is seen during real-time imaging or video-mode viewing The outline of the blood vessels can be: – Canalicular (elongated) – the vessel is oriented en-face (parallel to the skin surface) – Round – the vessel is oriented perpendicularly to the plane of RCM imaging

Table 38.2 RCM terms mostly used to describe melanocytic neoplasms by anatomic level

RCM term	Definition
Superficial (supra-basal) epidermal layers	
Pagetoid spread (or pagetoid pattern) of cells	Presence of bright round or dendritic nucleated cells at supra-basal layers of the epidermis. Descriptors of cells in pagetoid spread: – Cell size – "small": diameter > 50 μm; "large": if 50 μm or greater – Cell density – "slight": 1-3 cells per mm²; "medium": 4–6 cells per mm²; "marked": > 6 cells per mm² Low density corresponds to less than 5 cells per square millimeter, moderate to 5 to 10 cells per square millimeter, and high to more than 10 cells per square millimeter – Cell shape – evaluated by appearance, mostly as round or dendritic (or by abnormal shapes, such as triangular) – Pleomorphism – variability of cell shape in the same image (three or more pagetoid cells are needed to evaluate this term)
Roundish pagetoid cells	Large bright cells with well outlined border and dark nucleus within the epidermis
Dendritic pagetoid cells	Large cells with bright cytoplasm and dark nucleus with clearly visible dendrites connected to the cell
Disarranged pattern	Focal or diffuse loss of the normal patterns of the spinous-granular layers (honeycomb or cobblestone) characterized by unevenly distributed bright cells and granular particles

Table 38.2 (continued)

RCM term	Definition
Dermo-epidermal junction	
Ringed pattern	Numerous densely packed bright rings corresponding to papillae surrounded by a rim of small bright cells sharply contrasting with the dark background
Meshwork pattern	Distinctive mesh characterized by small dark holes surrounded by clearly thickened inter-papillary spaces
Clod pattern	Numerous densely packed clods, constituted by clusters of melanocytes usually within dermal papillae
Nonspecific pattern	Nonuniform architecture, noncorresponding to any of the above described patterns
Edged-papillae	Dermal papillae demarcated by a rim of bright cells (pigmented basal keratinocytes and melanocytes). The appearance is that of bright rings
Nonedged papillae	Dermal papillae without a demarcating bright rim at the DEJ, but separated by a series of large reflecting cells
Nonvisible papillae	Papillary architecture obscured by numerous cells or by nonhomogeneously bright and dark areas
Junctional clusters (nests)	Compact, round to oval bright cell aggregates, connected with the basal layer of the epidermis and bulging into the dermal papillae
Junctional thickening	Enlargement of the inter-papillary spaces (i.e. rete ridges) by bright cell aggregates. Outline of individual cells is often indiscernible
Sheet-like distribution (structure) of cells	Round or dendritic nucleated cells (melanocytes) that are not aggregated in nests but closely distributed at the transition of the epidermis and dermis (DEJ) that shows loss of dermal papillae
Superficial dermis	
Clusters (nests)	Compact cell aggregates of variable reflectance located in the dermis without connection with the basal layer of the epidermis. The clusters can be described as: dense, sparse-cell and cerebriform
Dense clusters (nests)	Dense cluster can be described as: – Regular discrete (dense homogenous): round, oval to polygonal compact aggregates with sharp margin in which outline of individual cells is indiscernible or similar in shape, size and refractivity – Irregular-discrete (dense nonhomogenous): round, oval to polygonal compact aggregates with sharp margin, in which outline of individual cells is variable in shape, size and refractivity – Irregular-nondiscrete (dense and sparse): cell aggregates with irregular, discohesive margins showing isolated nucleated cells at the periphery
Sparse clusters (loose sparse nests)	Roundish nonreflecting structures with a well-demarcated border, containing isolated round to oval cells with dark nucleus and reflecting cytoplasm, sometimes presenting in a multilobate configuration
Cerebriform clusters	Confluent aggregates of low reflecting cells in the dermis separated by a darker rim, resulting in a multi-lobate or brain-like appearance; cells often exhibit a granular cytoplasm, without evident nuclei, and ill-defined borders
Nucleated cells	Nonaggregated cells with oval to round shape, hyperrefractyle cytoplasm and visible eccentric dark nuclei
Atypical cells	Large cells showing a bright cytoplasm with clearly outlined borders and sharply contrasted dark nucleus inside, roundish to oval in shapes, sometimes presenting dendritic-like structures, located at the dermal-epidermal junction
Bright stellate spots	Small bright round structures ($\leq$20 μm) without visible nucleus
Small bright particles in papillae	Small cells with very bright hyper-reflecting cytoplasm, sometimes visible nuclei, corresponding to leukocyte infiltration
Plump-bright cells	Large (>20 μm) irregularly shaped bright cells with ill-defined borders and usually no visible nucleus. At times, may be aggregated (>3 cells) within dermal papillae

Table 38.3 RCM terms mostly used to describe nonmelanocytic neoplasms

RCM term	Definition
Basal cell carcinoma	
Tumor islands	Round to oval, cord-like or lobulated structures at the level of DEJ or superficial dermis that can be either darker than the surrounding epidermis or dermis ("dark silhouettes") or bright well-demarcated structures.
Polarization of nuclei (streaming)	Cells within the tumor islands, or overlying basal or spinous keratinocytes, display nuclei that are elongated and distorted into alignment along the same axis
Dark cleft (clefting)	Dark slit-like space observed between tumor island and surrounding dermis
Canalicular blood vessels	Thickened, elongated or tortuous dark structures, oriented parallel to the skin surface, containing moving small, round bright structures (white blood cells)
Actinic keratosis and squamous cell carcinoma	
Parakeratosis	Individual highly-refractile round cells in the stratum corneum
Scale (hyperkeratosis)	Increase of thickness of stratum corneum seen as refractile amorphous material
Irregular (atypical) honeycomb pattern	Abnormal pattern of the spinous-granular layers formed by bright cellular outlines which vary in size and shapes and in the thickness and brightness of the lines.
Round blood vessels	Dilated blood vessels within the dermal papillae that run perpendicular to the horizontal RCM plane of imaging.
Seborrheic keratosis and solar lentigo	
Corneal plugs	Bright laminar onion-like structures on epidermal surface
Corneal cysts	Well-circumscribed large, round, highly refractive intra-epidermal structures
Surface holes and fissures (crypts)	Round to linear structures, darker than the surrounding epidermal surface
Elongated cords	Thickened interwoven or parallel bright tubular structures at the DEJ, containing aggregated bright, monomorphic cells with ill-defined borders
Bulbous Projections	Round to oval structures contiguous with or adjacent to the elongated cords
Vascular neoplasms or hamartomas	
Vascular spaces	Wide dark spaces within the superficial dermis displaying moving small, round bright structures (white blood cells)

References

1. Scope A, Benvenuto-Andrade C, Agero AL, Malvehy J, Puig S, Rajadhyaksha M, Busam KJ, Marra DE, Torres A, Propperova I, Langley RG, Marghoob AA, Pellacani G, Seidenari S, Halpern AC, Gonzalez S. In vivo reflectance confocal microscopy imaging of melanocytic skin lesions: consensus terminology glossary and illustrative images. J Am Acad Dermatol. 2007 Oct;57(4):644-58.
2. Pellacani G, Vinceti M, Bassoli S, Braun R, Gonzalez S, Guitera P, Longo C, Marghoob AA, Menzies SW, Puig S, Scope A, Seidenari S, Malvehy J (2009) Reflectance confocal microscopy and features of melanocytic lesions: an internet-based study of the reproducibility of terminology. Arch Dermatol 145(10):1137–1143
3. Segura S, Puig S, Carrera C, Palou J, Malvehy J (2009) Development of a two-step method for the diagnosis of melanoma by reflectance confocal microscopy. J Am Acad Dermatol 61(2):216–229
4. Braga JC, Scope A, Klaz I, Mecca P, González S, Rabinovitz H, Marghoob AA (2009) The significance of reflectance confocal microscopy in the assessment of solitary pink skin lesions. J Am Acad Dermatol 61(2):230–241
5. Ahlgrimm-Siess V, Horn M, Koller S, Ludwig R, Gerger A, Hofmann-Wellenhof R (2009) Monitoring efficacy of cryotherapy for superficial basal cell carcinomas with in vivo reflectance confocal microscopy: a preliminary study. J Dermatol Sci 53(1):60–64
6. Rishpon A, Kim N, Scope A, Porges L, Oliviero MC, Braun RP, Marghoob AA, Fox CA, Rabinovitz HS (2009) Reflectance confocal microscopy criteria for squamous cell carcinomas and actinic keratoses. Arch Dermatol 145(7):766–772
7. Ulrich M, Stockfleth E, Roewert-Huber J, Astner S (2007) Noninvasive diagnostic tools for nonmelanoma skin cancer. Br J Dermatol 157(Suppl 2):56–58
8. Agero AL, Busam KJ, Benvenuto-Andrade C, Scope A, Gill M, Marghoob AA, González S, Halpern AC (2006) Reflectance confocal microscopy of pigmented basal cell carcinoma. J Am Acad Dermatol 54(4):638–643

Index

R. Hofmann-Wellenhof et al. (eds.), *Reflectance Confocal Microscopy for Skin Diseases*,
DOI 10.1007/978-3-642-21997-9, © Springer-Verlag Berlin Heidelberg 2012